Probiotics, Prebiotics and Synbiotics

Probiotics, Prebiotics and Synbiotics

Technological Advancements Towards Safety and Industrial Applications

Edited by

Parmjit Singh Panesar
Department of Food Engineering & Technology
Sant Longowal Institute of Engineering and Technology
Sangrur, India

Anil Kumar Anal
Food Engineering and Bioprocess Technology
Food Innovation, Nutrition and Health
Department of Food, Agriculture, and Bioresources
School of Environment, Resources, and Development
Asian Institute of Technology
Pathumthani, Thailand

WILEY

This edition first published 2022

Registered Offices
John Wiley & Sons, Inc., 111 River Street, Hoboken, NJ 07030, USA
John Wiley & Sons Ltd, The Atrium, Southern Gate, Chichester, West Sussex, PO19 8SQ, UK

Editorial Office
The Atrium, Southern Gate, Chichester, West Sussex, PO19 8SQ, UK

For details of our global editorial offices, customer services, and more information about Wiley products visit us at www.wiley.com.

Wiley also publishes its books in a variety of electronic formats and by print-on-demand. Some content that appears in standard print versions of this book may not be available in other formats.

Library of Congress Cataloging-in-Publication data applied for

Names: Panesar, P. S. (Parmjit Singh), editor. | Anal, Anil, editor.
Title: Probiotics, prebiotics and synbiotics : technological advancements towards safety and industrial applications / edited by Parmjit Singh Panesar, Department of Food Engineering & Technology, Sant Longowal Institute of Engineering and Technology Sangrur, India, Anil Kumar Anal, Department of Food Agriculture and Bioresources, Asian Institute of Technology Pathumthani, Thailand.
Description: Hoboken, NJ : Wiley, 2022. | Includes bibliographical references and index.
Identifiers: LCCN 2021052437 (print) | LCCN 2021052438 (ebook) | ISBN 9781119701200 (hardback) | ISBN 9781119701224 (adobe pdf) | ISBN 9781119701231 (epub)
Subjects: LCSH: Probiotics–Therapeutic use. | Prebiotics–Therapeutic use. | Functional foods.
Classification: LCC RM666.P835 P7894 2022 (print) | LCC RM666.P835 (ebook) | DDC 613.2/6–dc23/eng/20211202
LC record available at https://lccn.loc.gov/2021052437
LC ebook record available at https://lccn.loc.gov/2021052438

Cover Design: Wiley
Cover Images: Rasi/Adobe Stock Photo, Lotus_studio/Shutterstock, Radoslav Zilinsky/Getty Images

Set in 9.5/12.5pt STIXTwoText by Straive, Pondicherry, India

Printed and bound by CPI Group (UK) Ltd, Croydon, CR0 4YY

C9781119701200_040122

Contents

List of Contributors

Cristóbal N. Aguilar
Bioprocesses & Bioproducts Research Group
Food Research Department
School of Chemistry
Universidad Autónoma de Coahuila
Saltillo
Coahuila
Mexico

Ali Akbar
Department of Microbiology
Faculty of Life Sciences
University of Balochistan
Quetta
Balochistan
Pakistan

Anil Kumar Anal
Food Engineering and Bioprocess Technology
Food Innovation, Nutrition and Health
Department of Food, Agriculture, and Bioresources
School of Environment, Resources, and Development
Asian Institute of Technology
Pathumthani, Thailand

Juan A. Ascacio-Valdés
Bioprocesses & Bioproducts Research Group
Food Research Department
School of Chemistry
Universidad Autónoma de Coahuila
Saltillo
Coahuila
Mexico

Nuntarat Boonlao
Food Engineering and Bioprocess Technology
Department of Food Agriculture and Bioresources
School of Environment and Resources
Asian Institute of Technology
Pathumthani
Thailand

Chaichawin Chavapradit
Food Engineering and Bioprocess Technology
Department of Food Agriculture and Bioresources
School of Environment and Resources
Asian Institute of Technology
Pathumthani
Thailand

Son Chu-Ky
Laboratory of Applied Microbiology
School of Biotechnology and Food Technology
Hanoi University of Science and Technology
Hai Ba Trung
Hanoi
Vietnam

Hang-Thuy Dam
Laboratory of Applied Microbiology
School of Biotechnology and Food Technology
Hanoi University of Science and Technology
Hai Ba Trung
Hanoi
Vietnam

Orlando de la Rosa
Bioprocesses & Bioproducts Research Group
Food Research Department
School of Chemistry
Universidad Autónoma de Coahuila
Saltillo
Coahuila
Mexico

Raj Kumar Duary
Department of Food Engineering and Technology
Tezpur University
Napaam
Sonitpur
Assam
India
Department of Dairy Science and Food Technology
Institute of Agricultural Sciences
Banaras Hindu University
Varanasi
Uttar Pradesh
India

Elizabethe Adriana Esteves
Faculty of Biological Sciences and Health
Federal University of Jequitinhonha and Mucuri Valeys
Diamantina
MG
Brazil

Adriana C. Flores-Gallegos
Bioprocesses & Bioproducts Research Group
Food Research Department
School of Chemistry
Universidad Autónoma de Coahuila
Saltillo
Coahuila
Mexico

Phu-Ha Ho
Laboratory of Applied Microbiology
School of Biotechnology and Food Technology
Hanoi University of Science and Technology
Hai Ba Trung
Hanoi
Vietnam

Rupinder Kaur
Food Biotechnology Research Laboratory
Department of Food Engineering & Technology
Sant Longowal Institute of Engineering and Technology
Longowal
Punjab
India

Ghulam Ishaq Khan
Department of Microbiology
Faculty of Life Sciences
University of Balochistan
Quetta
Balochistan
Pakistan

Muhammad Iftikhar Khan
Department of Zoology
Abdul Wali Khan University
Khyber Pakhtunkhwa
Pakistan

Sushil Koirala
Department of Food, Agriculture and Bioresources
School of Environment, Resources, and Development, Asian Institute of Technology
Pathumthani
Thailand

Simmi Ranjan Kumar
Food Engineering and Bioprocess Technology, Department of Food Agriculture and Bioresources
School of Environment and Resources
Asian Institute of Technology
Pathumthani
Thailand

Shweta Kumari
Department of Biochemical Engineering & Biotechnology
Indian Institute of Technology
Hauz Khas
New Delhi
India

Julio C. Montáñez
Bioprocesses & Bioproducts Research Group
Food Research Department
School of Chemistry, Universidad Autónoma de Coahuila
Saltillo
Coahuila
Mexico

Lauane Gomes Moreno
Faculty of Biological Sciences and Health
Federal University of Jequitinhonha and Mucuri Valeys
Diamantina
MG
Brazil

Chinh-Nghia Nguyen
Laboratory of Applied Microbiology
School of Biotechnology and Food Technology
Hanoi University of Science and Technology
Hai Ba Trung
Hanoi
Vietnam

Ha-Anh Nguyen
Laboratory of Applied Microbiology
School of Biotechnology and Food Technology
Hanoi University of Science and Technology
Hai Ba Trung
Hanoi
Vietnam

Hoang Anh Nguyen
Faculty of Food Science and Technology
Vietnam National University of Agriculture
Trau Quy
Gia Lam
Hanoi
Vietnam

Lan-Huong Nguyen
Laboratory of Applied Microbiology
School of Biotechnology and Food Technology
Hanoi University of Science and Technology
Hai Ba Trung
Hanoi
Vietnam

Tien-Thanh Nguyen
Laboratory of Applied Microbiology
School of Biotechnology and Food Technology
Hanoi University of Science and Technology
Hai Ba Trung
Hanoi
Vietnam

Parmjit Singh Panesar
Food Biotechnology Research Laboratory
Department of Food Engineering & Technology
Sant Longowal Institute of Engineering and Technology
Longowal
Punjab
India

Suwan Panjanapongchai
Food Engineering and Bioprocess Technology
Department of Food Agriculture and Bioresources
School of Environment and Resources
Asian Institute of Technology
Pathumthani
Thailand

Krisha Pant
Food Engineering and Bioprocess Technology
Department of Food Agriculture and Bioresources
School of Environment and Resources
Asian Institute of Technology
Pathumthani
Thailand

Divyani Panwar
Food Biotechnology Research Laboratory
Department of Food Engineering & Technology
Sant Longowal Institute of Engineering and Technology
Longowal
Punjab
India

Falguni Patra
Mansinhbhai Institute of Dairy & Food Technology
Dudhsagar Dairy campus
Mehsana
Gujarat
India

Giorgia Perpetuini
Faculty of Bioscience and Technology for Food
Agriculture and Environment
University of Teramo
Teramo
Italy

Tuan-Anh Pham
Laboratory of Applied Microbiology
School of Biotechnology and Food Technology
Hanoi University of Science and Technology
Hai Ba Trung
Hanoi
Vietnam

Quyet-Tien Phi
Institute of Biotechnology
Vietnam Academy of Science and Technology
Cau Giay
Hanoi
Vietnam

Yudi Pranoto
Department of Food and Agricultural Product Technology
Faculty of Agricultural Technology
Universitas Gadjah Mada
Yogyakarta
Indonesia

Cíntia Lacerda Ramos
Faculty of Biological Sciences and Health
Federal University of Jequitinhonha and Mucuri Valeys
Diamantina
MG, Brazil

Sujitta Raungrusmee
Program in Food, Nutrition and Dietetics
Department of Home Economics
Faculty of Agriculture, Kasetsart University
Bangkok
Thailand

Muhammad Bilal Sadiq
School of Life Sciences
Forman Christian College (A Chartered University)
Lahore
Pakistan

Anuradha Saini
Food Biotechnology Research Laboratory
Department of Food Engineering & Technology
Sant Longowal Institute of Engineering and Technology
Longowal
Punjab
India

Rosane Freitas Schwan
Biology Department
Federal University of Lavras
Lavras
MG, Brazil

Leonardo Sepúlveda
Bioprocesses & Bioproducts Research Group
Food Research Department
School of Chemistry
Universidad Autónoma de Coahuila, Saltillo
Coahuila
Mexico

Gisha Singla
Food Biotechnology Research Laboratory
Department of Food Engineering & Technology
Sant Longowal Institute of Engineering and Technology
Longowal
Punjab
India

Waraporn Sorndech
Expert Centre of Innovative Health Food (InnoFood)
Thailand Institute of Scientific and Technological Research (TISTR)
Khlong Ha
Khlong Luang
Pathumthani
Thailand

Sarina Pradhan Thapa
Department of Food, Agriculture and Bioresources
School of Environment, Resources and Development
Asian Institute of Technology
Pathumthani
Thailand

Rosanna Tofalo
Faculty of Bioscience and Technology for Food
Agriculture and Environment
University of Teramo
Teramo
Italy

Quoc-Phong Truong
Laboratory of Applied Microbiology
School of Biotechnology and Food Technology
Hanoi University of Science and Technology
Hai Ba Trung
Hanoi
Vietnam

Yves Waché
Tropical Fermentation Network, France,
International Joint Laboratory, Tropical Bioresources & Biotechnology
Université Bourgogne Franche-Comté
AgroSup Dijon
France
School of Biotechnology and Food Technology
Hanoi University of Science and Technology
Hanoi
Vietnam
School of Food Science and Technology
Faculty of Science and Technology
Thammasat University
Thailand

Nayara Martins Zille de Miranda
Faculty of Biological Sciences and Health
Federal University of Jequitinhonha and Mucuri Valeys
Diamantina, MG, Brazil

Preface

This book is launched at the height of the COVID-19 pandemic that has given rise to increased food and nutrition insecurity for individuals, families and communities. The COVID-19 crisis threatens the food security and nutrition of millions of people. In the longer term, the world will face other possible disruptions to the functioning of food systems, with severe consequences for health and nutrition. With concerted action, it can not only avoid some of the worst impacts but do so in a way that supports a transition to more sustainable food systems that are in better balance with nature and that support healthy diets – and thus better health prospects – for all. There is an urgency to develop nutritionally enhanced foods to boost immune systems including probiotics and prebiotics-based food systems. Commensal organisms that constitute the gut microbiome compete with each other for the ability to grow in the intestine, and ultimately secrete protective or disease-causing mediators. As ever-increasing levels and types of antibiotics are used, not only are pathogens affected but beneficial gut flora are also likely to be mutated and killed.

This book focuses on the various aspects of functional foods (probiotics, prebiotics and synbiotics) and provides information about the various facets of the production of these health-beneficial compounds, recent technological developments and the present as well as future market scenario. Moreover, their mechanism of action and their significant applications in the different sectors are also discussed. This book contains detailed information about the different probiotics and prebiotics, their production strategies, and new developments in production techniques in a concise manner including the safety regulations and policies as well as future perspectives.

This book is divided into five sections. The first section provides general information about the pro-, pre- and synbiotics, and their relationship with the gut microflora. The second part of the book covers probiotics, in which their properties, types, production, health benefits, and mode of action are discussed. In addition, the commercially available probiotics and their prospects are elaborated in this section. Part three provides comprehensive information about the different prebiotics and their functionalities. Each prebiotic component is discussed in detail in terms of its properties, production strategies and the recent technological developments in the production. The fourth section discusses synbiotics, their health applications, and prospects. In the last part, information about the various regulatory claims of the use of these functional components and their potential applications is provided.

This book can be used by students, researchers, industry personnel and policy developers. It is a sort of encyclopedia, which contains all the necessary information about the pro-, pre- and synbiotics and will provide a basic understanding of the basic concepts as well as the production strategies, health benefits, mechanism of action, ongoing developments in this area and the future of these products in the market.

It is the ambient relationship that exists between probiotics and other pathogens that will influence the health and wellness of people at a time when we are faced with a pandemic.

The editors:
Professor Parmjit Singh Panesar
Professor Anil Kumar Anal

1

Probiotics, Prebiotics and Synbiotics: Opportunities, Health Benefits and Industrial Challenges

Parmjit Singh Panesar[1]*, Anil Kumar Anal*[2] *and Rupinder Kaur*[1]

[1] *Food Biotechnology Research Laboratory, Department of Food Engineering & Technology, Sant Longowal Institute of Engineering and Technology, Longowal-, 148 106, Punjab, India*
[2] *Department of Food Agriculture and Bioresources, School of Environment, Resources and Development, Asian Institute of Technology, Pathumthani, Thailand*

1.1 Introduction

Ever since the "Theory of Longevity" was proposed by Elie Metchnikoff and was correlated with prolonged youth and healthy old age, the search for food components as well as nutrients that not only enhance health but also help prevent disease has expanded, as has understanding of their role. Over the past few decades a plethora of novel foods have indicated specific health benefits, and those foods have been termed "functional foods" (Anal 2019; Noomhorm *et al.* 2014). The functional foods concept applies to those food products that exhibit various health beneficial properties to the host, apart from nutrition; hence this has become a recent area of research worldwide (Rastall 2010). Since its introduction, the global market demand for these foods has enlarged and market size is predicted to increase from USD 150 billion in 2018 to USD 250 billion in the next few years. The major leaders in this market are the United States, Europe and Japan, whereas China, India, Latin America and some of the other Asian countries are emerging as the fastest growing market (Patel and Goyal, 2012). In recent years, the functional food concept has moved progressively towards the development of dietary supplements that may have a profound effect on the gut microbial composition and activities.

The human microbiota comprises approximately 10^{14} microbial cells, which are 10 times greater in number than the cells of the human body (Savage 1970). Among all the parts or surface of the human body, the gastrointestinal tract is one of the most heavily colonized organs, accommodating about 70% of all the microbes in the human body (Figure 1.1) and playing a crucial role in health and disease (Ley *et al.* 2006). Changes in the gastrointestinal ecosystem or an imbalanced gut microflora have been associated with the occurrence of several diseases, including inflammatory bowel disease, diarrhea, colon cancer and many others.

Probiotics, Prebiotics and Synbiotics: Technological Advancements Towards Safety and Industrial Applications, First Edition. Edited by Parmjit Singh Panesar and Anil Kumar Anal.

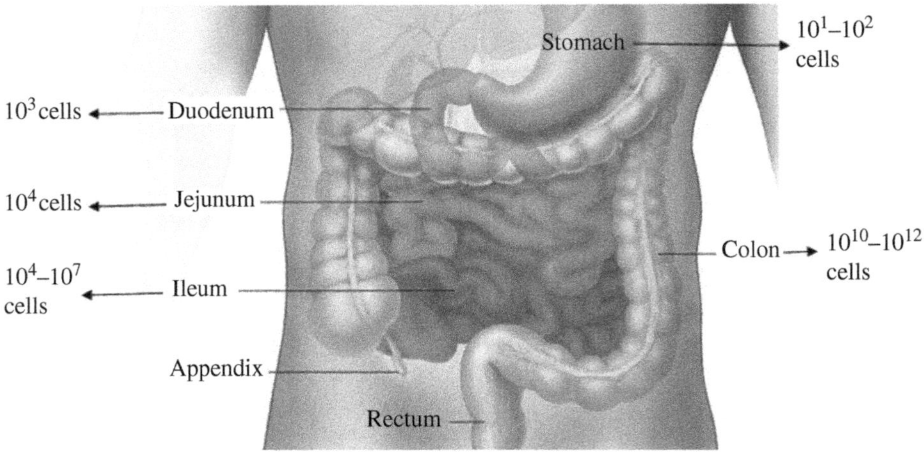

Figure 1.1 Human intestine and the number of microflora in the gut. *Source:* Modified from Vyas, U. and Ranganathan, N. (2012). Probiotics, prebiotics, and synbiotics: gut and beyond. *Gastroenterology Research and Practice*, 2012: 872716.

Studies have revealed that several dietary supplements, such as probiotics and prebiotics, have a positive impact on the gut microbiota and can be used to combat various diseases. In addition, the synergistic combination of probiotics and prebiotics, known as synbiotics, is known to impart greater efficiency than probiotic or prebiotic supplements used in isolation. Further, combinations of synbiotics have shown therapeutic effects against various diseases, such as those of the gastrointestinal and respiratory tracts, allergy, diabetes and cancer (Dinleyici *et al.* 2013; Rayes *et al.* 2002). Various examples of probiotics, prebiotics and synbiotics are described in Table 1.1. In United States, several foods incorporating probiotics and prebiotics have been introduced to the market and novel techniques are being developed to enhance shelf life and consumer acceptability (Koirala and Anal 2021).

In this context, this chapter provides a comprehensive overview of probiotics and prebiotics as well as synbiotics. Their mechanism of action in the body and significant health beneficial applications are also discussed in detail.

1.2 Probiotics

The term "probiotic" originates from the Greek word meaning "for life". The term was first invented by Ferdinand Vergin in 1954 as "probiotika", denoting something observed to be favorable to the gut microflora (Vergin 1954).This term was further refined by Lilly and Stillwell in 1965 as "a product produced by one microorganism stimulating the growth of another microorganism" (Lilly and Stillwell 1965). Subsequently, the term was redefined by Fuller in 1989 as "non-pathogenic microorganisms which when ingested exert a positive influence on host's health or physiology" (Fuller 1989). The latest definition was formulated in 2002 by the Food and Agriculture Organization (FAO) and World Health Organization (WHO), and states "live strains of strictly selected microorganisms, which when administered in adequate amounts, confer a health benefit on the host" (FAO 2002).

Table 1.1 Examples of probiotics, prebiotics and synbiotics.

Functional foods	Examples
Probiotics	*Lactobacillus acidophilus, L. rhamnosus, L. reuteri, L. bulgaricus, L. plantarum, L. casei, L. lactis, L. johnsonii, L. delbrueckii, L. fermentum, L. gasseri, L. helveticus, L. pentosus, Bacillus coagulans, Bifidobacterium bifidum, B. longum, B. breve, B. infantis, B. lactis, B. adolescentis, B. animalis, B. thermophilum, Streptococcus thermophilus, S. diactylactis, Saccharomyces cerevisiae, S. boulardii, Lactococcus lactis, Enterococcus*
Prebiotics	Galactooligosaccharides (GOS), fructooligosaccharides (FOS), inulin, xylooligosaccharides (XOS), isomaltooligosaccharides (IMO), lactulose, tagatose, lactosucrose, resistant starch, lactitol
Synbiotics	*Saccharomyces boulardii* + *Lactobacillus sporogenes* + FOS *Lactobacillus* + *Bifidobacterium* + inulin *Lactobacillus* + *Bifidobacterium* + *Enterococcus* + FOS *Lactobacillus* + *Bifidobacterium* + *Streptococcus* + FOS *L. rhamnosus* + inulin

Sources: Based on Tadesse, S. (2012). Probiotics, prebiotics and synbiotics as functional food ingredients: production, health benefits and safety. *Journal of Biologically Active Products from Nature*, 2(3): 124–134; Pandey, K.R., Naik, S.R. and Vakil, B.V. (2015). Probiotics, prebiotics and synbiotics-a review. *Journal of Food Science and Technology*, 52(12): 7577–7587; Markowiak, P. and Śliżewska, K. (2018). The role of probiotics, prebiotics and synbiotics in animal nutrition. *Gut Pathogens*, 10(1): 21; Mofid, V., Izadi, A., Mojtahedi, S.Y. and Khedmat, L. (2020). Therapeutic and nutritional effects of synbiotic yogurts in children and adults: a clinical review. *Probiotics and Antimicrobial Proteins* 12(3): 851–859.

The most common microbial strains are *Lactobacillus rhamnosus, L. reuteri, L. casei, L. acidophilus, Bacillus coagulans, Bifidobacterium,* etc. Probiotic products may comprise either a single strain or a combination of two or more strains (Chapman *et al.* 2011). As per the guidelines of the FAO, WHO and European Food Safety Authority (EFSA) on the selection of probiotic strains, the strains must satisfy safety as well as functionality criteria and technological usability. The safety of the strain is characterized by its origin and absence of association with pathogens and antibiotic resistance, whereas functional aspects include its survival in the gastrointestinal tract and its immunomodulatory properties. On the other hand, technological usability is related to its production and is correlated with its survival and maintenance of properties throughout the storage and distribution period (Lee 2009). In addition, in the USA, the microorganisms used for consumption must have a Generally Recognized As Safe (GRAS) status regulated by the FDA; in Europe the EFSA has introduced Qualified Presumption of Safety (QPS), which involves additional criteria for the safety of bacterial supplements (Anadón *et al.* 2006; Gaggìa *et al.* 2010).

1.2.1 Mechanism of Action

Probiotics play a significant role in the host, especially in the development of the microbiota, ensuring a balance between the pathogens and bacteria necessary for the normal function of the host (Schachtsiek *et al.* 2004). A few microorganisms, such as *L. plantarum,*

L. reuteri, *Bifidobacterium adolescentis* and *B. pseudocatenulatum*, have been reported as natural producers of B-group vitamins (Li and Gu 2016), immunomodulators, increase the absorption of vitamins as well as minerals and allow the production of amino acids and organic acids (Nova *et al.* 2007). Apart from this, some probiotic microorganisms are known to generate enzymes such as esterase and lipase, and coenzymes (A, Q, NAD, NADP), and the products of bacterial metabolism have anticancerogenic, immunosuppressive and antibiotic properties (Ishikawa *et al.* 2005).

On the basis of molecular and genetic studies, the health beneficial properties of probiotic microorganisms involve four basic mechanisms: (i) antagonism through secretion of antimicrobial substances; (ii) competition with pathogens for adhesion to the epithelium and for nutrients; (iii) immunomodulation of the host; and (iv) inhibition of toxin production (Guillot 2003; Isolauri *et al.* 2001).

Probiotic microorganisms prevent colonization by pathogens of the epithelial cells by adhesion, which further activates the signalling cascade or releases some of the components that lead to the activation of immunological cells and helps in the prevention of contagious disease (Collado *et al.* 2007). Further, immunomodulation can also be due to the enhanced production of immunoglobulins, increase in the production of macrophages and lymphocytes and production of γ-interferon (Oelschlaeger 2010).

1.3 Prebiotics

Prebiotics are defined as "non-digestible food ingredients that beneficially affect the host by selectively stimulating the growth and/or activity of one or a limited number of bacteria in the colon, which can improve host health" (Gibson and Roberfroid 1995). Any food can be considered a prebiotic if it meets some specific criteria, such as: (i) it must pass into the colon in the intact form and must not be hydrolyzed in the upper gastrointestinal tract by digestive enzymes; (ii) it must be fermented in the colon by the colonic microflora; and (iii) it must enhance the activity and/or growth of beneficial microflora, particularly *Lactobacillus* and *Bifidobacterium* (Gibson *et al.* 2004).

There are several types of prebiotics available, for example galactooligosaccharides, lactulose, fructooligosaccharides, tagatose, maltooligosaccharides, inulin, resistant starch, and lactitol that are composed of 2–10 sugar moieties linked together by glycosidic bonds, which makes them resistant to digestion in the upper gastrointestinal tract (Grajek *et al.* 2005; Panesar *et al.* 2018). Thus, these functional components reach the colon in the intact form where they are fermented, leading to the production of short chain fatty acids (SCFAs) such as acetate, propionate and butyrate as well as other metabolites that exhibit various health benefits on the host (Panesar *et al.* 2013a; Sarbini and Rastall 2011). These health benefits include modulation of the immune system, absorption of minerals, prevention of cancer, prevention of irritable bowel syndrome and reduction in gastrointestinal as well as other inflammatory conditions (Kaur and Panesar 2020; Lomax and Calder 2008).

Prebiotics are naturally present in Jerusalem artichoke, chicory, rye, milk, honey, asparagus, onion, leek, banana, garlic, wheat bran, flour, barley and other sources; however the concentration is less and varies with the source. Thus, in order to meet demand from consumers, there is a need for the production of prebiotics. Generally, prebiotics can be extracted from plants. Enzymatic synthesis is achieved either by the hydrolysis of plant polysaccharides or transgalactosylation of carbohydrates (Panesar *et al.* 2013b; Torres *et al.* 2010).

1.3.1 Mechanism of Action

Prebiotics act as substrates of fermentation by the colonic microflora, resulting in the production of SCFAs with a decrease in colonic pH. The reduction in pH creates a colonic environment less favorable for the survival of pathogens. In addition, SCFAs act as a fuel for epithelial cells, helping to maintain the integrity of the colon wall and allowing the absorption of water and electrolytes, thereby diminishing the risk of diarrhea (Panesar *et al.* 2009).

1.4 Applications of Synbiotics

The combined effect of probiotics and prebiotics is known to impart various health beneficial properties, such as antimicrobial, anticarcinogenic, immunomodulatory, antidiarrheal, antiallergenic, hypolipidemic and hypoglycemic activities. Besides this, synbiotics also enhance the absorption of minerals, thus possessing anti-osteoporotic activity (Holzapfel and Schillinger 2002; Zubillaga *et al.* 2001). Prebiotics help to nourish probiotic microorganisms, further imparting a positive impact on the health of the host (Figure 1.2). The various applications of synbiotics are described in detail in the following sections.

1.4.1 Diarrhea

According to the WHO, diarrhea is defined as three or more watery stools during a period of 24 hours. It is often caused by infectious agents, especially pathogens that cause changes in the gut microflora, hence outnumbering the beneficial microflora of the gut (Narayan *et al.* 2010). Studies have indicated that probiotic bacteria interfere with the colonisation and proliferation of pathogens through the release of antibacterial and inhibitory substances, thereby preventing the manifestations of infection (Dinleyici *et al.* 2013).

A combination of fructooligosaccharides (FOS) along with a consortium of probiotic microorganisms (*L. paracasei, L. rhamnosus, L. acidophilus* and *B. lactis*) were tested for their efficacy in the treatment of diarrhea, which revealed that there was a significant reduction in diarrhea among the patients (da Silveira *et al.* 2017).

1.4.2 Lactose Intolerance

Lactose intolerance is of the most prevalent problems, affecting approximately 70% worldwide. It is associated with inability to digest lactose because of lower levels of the enzyme β-galactosidase (Lactose Intolerance – Scientific status report 2011). The most common symptoms include diarrhea, bloating, abdominal pain and flatulence. To alleviate this problem, two possible interventions have been proposed: treatment either with lactase or with probiotics. The combination of *L. casei* Shirota and *B. breve* Yakult has been reported to have better effects and to eliminate the problem of lactose intolerance significantly (Vonk *et al.* 2012).

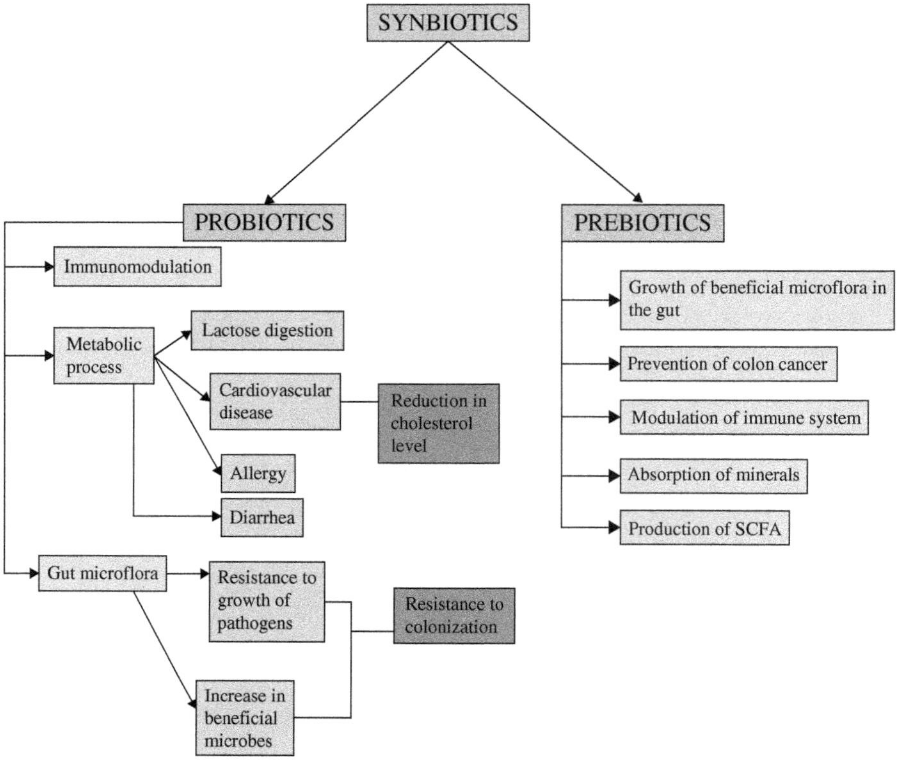

Figure 1.2 Health applications of probiotics, prebiotics and synbiotics. SCFA, short chain fatty acids. *Source:* Based on Markowiak, P. and Śliżewska, K. (2018). The role of probiotics, prebiotics and synbiotics in animal nutrition. *Gut Pathogens*, 10(1): 21.

1.4.3 Modulation of the Immune System

Probiotics have immunomodulatory properties as well as anti-inflammatory activity that have a profound effect on cell mediated immunity. Probiotics are known to secrete factors that help in immune enhancement, for example secreted factor from *L. reuteri* minimizes NF-κB dependent gene expression, an important process for inducing apoptosis (Delcenserie *et al.* 2008). The mechanism of the effect of prebiotics on the immune system has not yet been well established, however a few mechanisms have been proposed, such as: (i) mucin production; (ii) the SCFAs produced help in the down regulation of hepatic lipogenic enzymes; (iii) increased IgA secretion; (iv) butyrate acts as a modulator of histone tail acetylation (Schley and Field 2002). Synbiotics also seem to be an attractive candidate for modulation of the immune system. A combination of inulin and *B. coagulans* in the diet resulted in enhancement of glutathione levels and decrease in C-reactive protein levels (Panda *et al.* 2006).

1.4.4 Prevention of Colon Cancer

Colon cancer is one of the most common cancers worldwide. The major factors responsible are genetic, environmental (radiation, chemical carcinogens) and diet (Willet 2000). Treatments involve a high complication rate and lower success rate. Studies on pre-, pro- and synbiotics in rodents have implied that these foods may have therapeutic properties. Study of the synbiotic combination of resistant starch and *B. lactis* on colorectal carcinogenesis revealed that such a combination had significant impact on the gut microflora as compared to probiotic or prebiotic treatments alone (Worthley *et al.* 2009). Moreover, studies in in vitro systems provide evidence that probiotics, prebiotics and synbiotics have antineoplastic effects (Fotiadis *et al.* 2008).

1.4.5 Cardiovascular Disease

Probiotics are reported to reduce the risk of cardiovascular disease by lowering blood cholesterol levels, which may be achieved either by decreasing hydroxyl-methyl-glutaryl-coenzyme A reductase in the liver, or by conversion of cholesterol to bile salts. Another possible mechanism may be removal of cholesterol by the probiotics during growth (Teitelbaum and Walker 2002). Synbiotic formulations comprising *L. acidophilus* ATCC 4962, FOS, mannitol and inulin fed to hypercholesterolemic pigs for 8 weeks revealed positive results with a decrease in the total plasma triacylglycerol, total cholesterol and low density lipoprotein (LDL) levels (Liong *et al.* 2007).

1.4.6 Gut–brain Axis: Role of Probiotics

The main site of action of probiotics is the gut. While studies have shown that probiotic administration has positive effects of on sound gut health, it may also enhance brain health (Mörkl *et al.* 2020; Skonieczna-Żydecka *et al.* 2018). Gut and brain are connected, a partnership known as the gut–brain axis, linked through biochemical and neuro-electrical signalling between the central nervous system and digestive tract (Figure 1.3). The gut is also termed "the second brain" because it produces 90% of the total serotonin and other neurotransmitters such as dopamine and γ-aminobutyric acid, which help to regulate the human mood (Carabotti *et al.* 2015). This axis can be defined in many ways. The gut receives warning signals when our brain senses trouble, resulting in an upset stomach, whereas gastrointestinal issues such as irritable bowel syndrome (IBS), Crohn's disease or chronic constipation trigger anxiety or depression in the brain. The regulation of appetite is also modulated through the gut–brain axis (Sinagra *et al.* 2020). Various biochemical

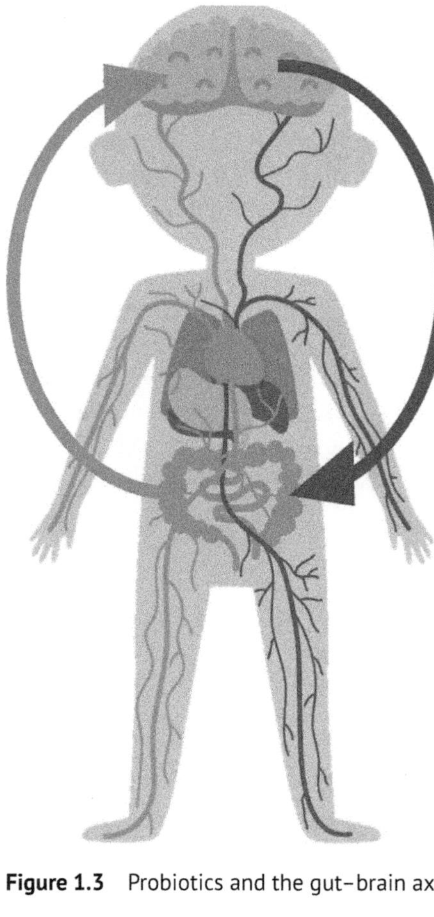

Figure 1.3 Probiotics and the gut–brain axis.

signals coordinate to inform the brain when it is time to eat and when to stop eating. Different proteins and other molecules are produced by gut microbes, helping to suppress the appetite when people start to begin to feel full (Galland 2014).

Now, how might probiotics fit in the gut–brain axis? Rigorous scientific research and animal studies are showing that probiotics help to boost mood and cognitive function, and lower stress and anxiety (Sarkar *et al.* 2016). Akbari *et al.* (2016) studied the effect of probiotic supplementation on cognitive function and metabolic status in patients with Alzheimer's disease in a randomized, double-blind and controlled trial. The authors found that patients who took milk made with four probiotic bacteria species (*Lactobacillus acidophilus, L. casei, Bifidobacterium bifidum* and *Lactobacillus fermentum* [2×10^9 colony forming units/g for each]) for 12 weeks scored better on a test to measure cognitive impairment compared with those who drank regular milk.

It is too early to determine the exact role of probiotics in the gut–brain axis as this research is still ongoing. Probiotics may not only support a healthier gut, but a healthier brain too.

1.5 Current Outlook and Industrial Challenges

The global market for probiotics and prebiotics in 2018 was more than USD 40 billion and USD 5 billion, respectively (Belorkar and Gupta 2016; Buriti *et al.* 2016). Despite the increasing consumer demand and growing market opportunities, scientific and industrial barriers exist along with the lack of clinical evidence (Van den Nieuwboer *et al.* 2016). The evidence to support health claims varies from country to country, for example both the EFSA and FDA have not approved health claims for any probiotic or synbiotic combinations (Van Loveren *et al.* 2012). Apart from this, another hindrance is the discrimination of these components either as pharmaceutical or food products (Govender *et al.* 2014).

Synbiotics are incorporated into various food products including cultured dairy as well as non-dairy products and delivered to consumers. Although prebiotics can be used in an array of food products, the environmental sensitivity of probiotics and synbiotics limits their usage in non-refrigerated products (Saulnier 2008). However, innovative processing techniques such as microencapsulation and bioencapsulation that protect the bacteria against the harsh processing conditions have led to the development of novel food products such as desserts, juices, cheese and chocolate incorporated with synbiotic formulations (Anal and Singh 2007; Kumaree *et al.* 2015; Praepanitchai *et al.* 2019; Xu *et al.* 2020).

1.6 Conclusion

The gut microbiota contributes to every aspect of human growth and development, thus an array of diseases and dysfunctions are associated with imbalance either in its composition or numbers. Probiotics, prebiotics and synbiotics have systemic effects on metabolism and the immune system and have been clinically proven to be effective against various gut related disorders. Although several studies have helped our understanding of the basic functions of these functional components, establishing the underlying mechanisms of probiotics, prebiotics and synbiotics and clinical evidence of effective synbiotic combinations is the challenging issue of today's era. Further, the ability to target a specific organism in the colon for a defined health beneficial activity is the need of the hour, as the carbohydrate utilization pattern varies with the bacterial species and strain, and this would be beneficial for the development of new synbiotic formulations. With innovations in molecular as well as microbiological techniques, there is a possibility in the future for the development of detailed profiles of target bacteria that would be useful to test the efficiency of candidate synbiotic compounds and tailor them to achieve the desired health outcome. The use of synbiotics in food is a promising area; however, they should be administered cautiously by determining the minimum effective doses, and this is possible only on the basis of strong scientific evidence.

References

Akbari, E., Asemi, Z., Daneshvar Kakhaki, R., Bahmani, F., Kouchaki, E., Tamtaji, O.R., Hamidi, G.A. and Salami, M. (2016). Effect of probiotic supplementation on cognitive function and metabolic status in Alzheimer's disease: a randomized, double-blind and controlled trial. *Frontiers in Aging Neuroscience*, 8: 256.

Anadón, A., Martínez-Larrañaga, M.R. and Martínez, M.A. (2006). Probiotics for animal nutrition in the European Union. Regulation and safety assessment. *Regulatory Toxicology and Pharmacology*, 45(1): 91–95.

Anal, A.K. (2019). Quality ingredients and safety concerns for traditional fermented foods and beverages from Asia: A review. *Fermentation*, 5(1): 8.

Anal, A.K. and Singh, H. (2007). Recent advances in microencapsulation of probiotics for industrial applications and targeted delivery. *Trends in Food Science & Technology*, 18(5): 240–251.

Belorkar, S.A. and Gupta, A.K. (2016). Oligosaccharides: a boon from nature's desk. *AMB Express*, 6(1): 82.

Buriti, F.C., Bedani, R. and Saad, S.M. (2016). Probiotic and prebiotic dairy desserts. In: *Probiotics, Prebiotics and Synbiotics* (ed. R.R. Watson and V.R. Preedy), 345–360. Elsevier.

Carabotti, M., Scirocco, A., Maselli, M.A. and Severi, C. (2015). The gut-brain axis: interactions between enteric microbiota, central and enteric nervous systems. *Annals of Gastroenterology: Quarterly Publication of the Hellenic Society of Gastroenterology*, 28(2): 203.

Chapman, C.M.C., Gibson, G.R. and Rowland, I. (2011). Health benefits of probiotics: are mixtures more effective than single strains? *European Journal of Nutrition*, 50(1): 1–17.

Collado, M.C., Meriluoto, J. and Salminen, S. (2008). Adhesion and aggregation properties of probiotic and pathogen strains. *European Journal of Food Research and Technology*, 226(5): 1065–1073.

da Silveira, E.A., Falco, M.O., Nery, M.W. and Turchi, M.D. (2017). Effectiveness of nutritional treatment and synbiotic use on gastrointestinal symptoms reduction in HIV-infected patients: Randomized clinical trial. *Clinical Nutrition*, 36(3): 680–685.

Delcenserie, V., Martel, D., Lamoureux, M., Amiot, J., Boutin, Y. and Roy, D. (2008). Immunomodulatory effects of probiotics in the intestinal tract. *Current Issues in Molecular Biology*, 10(1/2): 37.

Dinleyici, E.C., Dalgic, N., Guven, S., Ozen, M., Kara, A., Arica, V., Metin-Timur, O., Sancar, M., Kurugol, Z., Tanir, G. and Ozturk, D. (2013). The effect of a multispecies synbiotic mixture on the duration of diarrhea and length of hospital stay in children with acute diarrhea in Turkey: single blinded randomized study. *European Journal of Pediatrics*, 172(4): .459–464.

Food and Agriculture Organization (FAO). (2002). *Guidelines for the Evaluation of Probiotics in Food*. Joint FAO/WHO Working Group on Drafting Guidelines for the Evaluation of Probiotics in Food, 30 April–1 May 2002. London, ON, Canada: FAO.

Fotiadis, C.I., Stoidis, C.N., Spyropoulos, B.G. and Zografos, E.D. (2008). Role of probiotics, prebiotics and synbiotics in chemoprevention for colorectal cancer. *World Journal of Gastroenterology: WJG*, 14(42): 6453.

Fuller, R. (1989). Probiotics in man and animals. *Journal of Applied Microbiology*, 66: 365–378.

Gaggìa, F., Mattarelli, P. and Biavati, B. (2010). Probiotics and prebiotics in animal feeding for safe food production. *International Journal of Food Microbiology*, 141: S15–S28.

Galland, L. (2014). The gut microbiome and the brain. *Journal of Medicinal Food*, 17(12): 1261–1272.

Gibson, G.R. and Roberfroid, M.B. (1995). Dietary modulation of the human colonic microbiota: introducing the concept of prebiotics. *The Journal of Nutrition*, 125(6): 1401–1412.

Gibson, G.R., Probert, H.M., Van Loo, J., Rastall, R.A. and Roberfroid, M.B. (2004). Dietary modulation of the human colonic microbiota: updating the concept of prebiotics. *Nutrition Research Reviews*, 17(2): 259–275.

Govender, M., Choonara, Y.E., Kumar, P., du Toit, L.C., van Vuuren, S. and Pillay, V. (2014). A review of the advancements in probiotic delivery: Conventional vs. non-conventional formulations for intestinal flora supplementation. *AAPS PharmSciTech*, 15(1): 29–43.

Grajek, W., Olejnik, A. and Sip, A. (2005). Probiotics, prebiotics and antioxidants as functional foods. *Acta Biochimica Polonica*, 52(3): 665–671.

Guillot, J.F. (2003). Probiotic feed additives. *Journal of Veterinary and Pharmacology and Therapeutics*, 26: 52–55.

Holzapfel, W.H. and Schillinger, U. (2002). Introduction to pre-and probiotics. *Food Research International*, 35(2-3): 109–116.

Ishikawa, H., Akedo, I., Otani, T., Suzuki, T., Nakamura, T., Takeyama, I., Ishiguro, S., Miyaoka, E., Sobue, T. and Kakizoe, T. (2005). Randomized trial of dietary fiber and Lactobacillus casei administration for prevention of colorectal tumors. *International Journal of Cancer*, 116(5): 762–767.

Isolauri, E., Sütas, Y., Kankaanpää, P., Arvilommi, H. and Salminen, S. (2001). Probiotics: effects on immunity. *The American Journal of Clinical Nutrition*, 73(2): 444s–450s.

Kaur, R. and Panesar, P.S. (2020). Enzyme systems for high-value biomolecule production. In: *Biomass, Biofuels, Biochemicals*, 273–308. Elsevier.

Koirala, S. and Anal, A.K. (2021). Probiotics-based foods and beverages as future foods and their overall safety and regulatory claims. *Future Foods*, 3: 100013.

Kumaree, K.K., Akbar, A. and Anal, A.K. (2015). Bioencapsulation and application of Lactobacillus plantarum isolated from catfish gut as an antimicrobial agent and additive in fish feed pellets. *Annals of Microbiology*, 65(3): 1439–1445.

Lactose Intolerance – Scientific Status Report (2011). http://www.nationaldairycouncil.org/SiteCollectionDocuments/research/research-summaries/ScientificStatusReportLactoseIntolerance.pdf (accessed February 21, 2021).

Lee, Y.K. (2009). Selection and maintenance of probiotic microorganisms. *Handbook of Probiotics and Prebiotics*, 177–187. Weinheim: Wiley-VCH.

Ley, R.E., Peterson, D.A. and Gordon, J.I. (2006). Ecological and evolutionary forces shaping microbial diversity in the human intestine. *Cell*, 124(4): 837–848.

Li, P. and Gu, Q. (2016). Complete genome sequence of *Lactobacillus plantarum* LZ95, a potential probiotic strain producing bacteriocins and B-group vitamin riboflavin. *Journal of Biotechnology*, 229: 1–2.

Lilly, D.M. and Stillwell, R.H. (1965). Probiotics: growth-promoting factors produced by microorganisms. *Science*, 147(3659): 747–748.

Liong, M.T., Dunshea, F.R. and Shah, N.P. (2007). Effects of a synbiotic containing Lactobacillus acidophilus ATCC 4962 on plasma lipid profiles and morphology of erythrocytes in hypercholesterolaemic pigs on high-and low-fat diets. *British Journal of Nutrition*, 98(4): 736–744.

Lomax, A.R. and Calder, P.C. (2008). Prebiotics, immune function, infection and inflammation: a review of the evidence. *British Journal of Nutrition*, 101(5): 633–658.

Markowiak, P. and Śliżewska, K. (2018). The role of probiotics, prebiotics and synbiotics in animal nutrition. *Gut Pathogens*, 10(1): 21.

Mofid, V., Izadi, A., Mojtahedi, S.Y. and Khedmat, L. (2020). Therapeutic and nutritional effects of synbiotic yogurts in children and adults: a clinical review. *Probiotics and Antimicrobial Proteins*, 12(3): 851–859.

Mörkl, S., Butler, M.I., Holl, A., Cryan, J. F. and Dinan, T.G. (2020). Probiotics and the microbiota-gut-brain axis: focus on psychiatry. *Current Nutrition Reports*, 9(3): 171–182.

Narayan, S.S., Jalgaonkar, S., Shahani, S. and Kulkarni, V.N. (2010). Probiotics: current trends in the treatment of diarrhoea. *Hong Kong Medical Journal*, 16(3): 213–218.

Noomhorm, A., Ahmad, I. and Anal, A. K. (2014). *Functional Foods and Dietary Supplements: Processing Effects and Health Benefits*. John Wiley & Sons.

Nova, E., Warnberg, J., Gomez-Martinez, S., Diaz, L.E., Romeo, J. and Marcos, A. (2007). Immunomodulatory effects of probiotics in different stages of life. *Brazilian Journal of Nutrition*, 98: S90–S95.

Oelschlaeger, T.A. (2010). Mechanisms of probiotic actions–a review. *International Journal of Medical Microbiology*, 300(1): 57–62.

Panda, A.K., Rao, S.V.R., Raju, M.V. and Sharma, S.R. (2006). Dietary supplementation of Lactobacillus sporogenes on performance and serum biochemico-lipid profile of broiler chickens. *The Journal of Poultry Science*, 43(3): 235–240.

Pandey, K.R., Naik, S.R. and Vakil, B.V. (2015). Probiotics, prebiotics and synbiotics-a review. *Journal of Food Science and Technology*, 52(12): 7577–7587.

Panesar, P.S., Bali, V., Kumari, S., Babbar, N. and Oberoi H.S. (2013b). Prebiotics. In: *Biotransformation of Waste Biomass into High Value Biochemicals* (ed. S.K. Brar et al.). New York: Springer.

Panesar, P.S., Kaur, G., Panesar, R. and Bera, M.B. (2009). Synbiotics: potential dietary supplements in functional foods. *FST Bulletin*. UK: Food Science Central, IFIS Publishing.

Panesar, P.S., Kaur, R., Singh, R.S. and Kennedy, J.F. (2018). Biocatalytic strategies in the production of galacto-oligosaccharides and its global status. *International Journal of Biological Macromolecules*, 111: 667–679.

Panesar, P.S., Kumari, S. and Panesar, R. (2013a). Biotechnological approaches for the production of prebiotics and their potential applications. *Critical Reviews in Biotechnology*, 33(4): 345–364.

Patel, S. and Goyal, A. (2012). The current trends and future perspectives of prebiotics research: a review. *3 Biotech*, 2(2): 115–125.

Praepanitchai, O.-A., Noomhorm, A. and Anal, A. K. (2019). Survival and behavior of encapsulated probiotics (Lactobacillus plantarum) in calcium-alginate-soy protein isolate-based hydrogel beads in different processing conditions (pH and temperature) and in pasteurized mango juice. *BioMed Research International*, 2019: 9768152.

Rastall, R.A. (2010). Functional oligosaccharides: application and manufacture. *Annual Review of Food Science and Technology*, 1: 305–339.

Rayes, N., Seehofer, D., Hansen, S., Boucsein, K., Müller, A.R., Serke, S., Bengmark, S. and Neuhaus, P. (2002). Early enteral supply of *Lactobacillus* and fiber versus selective bowel decontamination: a controlled trial in liver transplant recipients. *Transplantation*, 74(1): 123–128.

Sarbini, S.R. and Rastall, R.A. (2011). Prebiotics: metabolism, structure, and function. *Functional Food Reviews*, 3(3): 93–106.

Sarkar, A., Lehto, S. M., Harty, S., Dinan, T. G., Cryan, J. F., and Burnet, P. W. (2016). Psychobiotics and the manipulation of bacteria–gut–brain signals. *Trends in Neurosciences*, 39(11): 763–781.

Saulnier, D.M. (2008). Synbiotics: making the most of probiotics and prebiotics by their combinations. *Food Science and Technology Bulletin: Functional Foods*, 4: 9–19.

Savage, D.C. (1970). Associations of indigenous microorganisms with gastrointestinal mucosal epithelia. *The American Journal of Clinical Nutrition*, 23(11): 1495–1501.

Schachtsiek, M., Hammes, W.P. and Hertel, C. (2004). Characterization of *Lactobacillus coryniformis* DSM 20001T surface protein Cpf mediating coaggregation with and aggregation among pathogens. *Applied and Environmental Microbiology*, 70(12): 7078–7085.

Schley, P.D. and Field, C.J. (2002). The immune-enhancing effects of dietary fibres and prebiotics. *British Journal of Nutrition*, 87(S2): S221–S230.

Sinagra, E., Utzeri, E., Morreale, G. C., Fabbri, C., Pace, F. and Anderloni, A. (2020). Microbiota-gut-brain axis and its affect in flammatory bowel disease: Pathophysiological concepts and insights for clinicians. *World Journal of Clinical Cases*, 8(6): 1013.

Skonieczna-Żydecka, K., Marlicz, W., Misera, A., Koulaouzidis, A. and Łoniewski, I. (2018). Microbiome—the missing link in the gut-brain axis: focus on its role in gastrointestinal and mental health. *Journal of Clinical Medicine*, 7(12): 521.

Tadesse, S. (2012). Probiotics, prebiotics and synbiotics as functional food ingredients: production, health benefits and safety. *Journal of Biologically Active Products from Nature*, 2(3): 124–134.

Teitelbaum, J.E. and Walker, W.A. (2002). Nutritional impact of pre-and probiotics as protective gastrointestinal organisms. *Annual Review of Nutrition*, 22(1): 107–138.

Torres, D.P.M., Goncalves, M.P.F., Teixeira, J.A. and Rodrigues, L.R. (2010). Galacto-oligosaccharides: production, properties, applications, and significance as prebiotics. *Comprehensive Reviews in Food Science and Food Safety*, 9: 438–454.

Van den Nieuwboer, M., Van De Burgwal, L.H.M. and Claassen, E. (2016). A quantitative key-opinion-leader analysis of innovation barriers in probiotic research and development: valorisation and improving the tech transfer cycle. *PharmaNutrition*, 4(1): 9–18.

van Loveren, H., Sanz, Y. and Salminen, S. (2012). Health claims in Europe: probiotics and prebiotics as case examples. *Annual Review of Food Science and Technology*, 3: 247–261.

Vergin, F. 1954. Anti-und Probiotica. *Hipokrates*, 25: 116–119.

Vonk, R.J., Reckman, G.A., Harmsen, H.J. and Priebe, M.G. (2012). Probiotics and lactose intolerance. *Intech*, 7: 149–160.

Vyas, U. and Ranganathan, N. (2012). Probiotics, prebiotics, and synbiotics: gut and beyond. *Gastroenterology Research and Practice*, 2012: 872716.

Willett, W.C. (2000). Diet and cancer. *The Oncologist*, 5(5): 393–404.

Worthley, D.L., Le Leu, R.K., Whitehall, V.L., Conlon, M., Christophersen, C., Belobrajdic, D., Mallitt, K.A., Hu, Y., Irahara, N., Ogino, S. and Leggett, B.A. (2009). A human, double-blind, placebo-controlled, crossover trial of prebiotic, probiotic, and synbiotic supplementation: effects on luminal, inflammatory, epigenetic, and epithelial biomarkers of colorectal cancer. *The American Journal of Clinical Nutrition*, 90(3): 578–586.

Xu, K., Cai, H., Shen, Y., Ni, Q., Chen, Y., Hu, S., Li, J., Wang, H., Yu, L. and Huang, H. (2020). [Management of corona virus disease-19 (COVID-19): the Zhejiang experience.] *Zhejiang Da Xue Xue Bao Yi Xue Ban*, 49(1): 147–157.

Zubillaga, M., Weill, R., Postaire, E., Goldman, C., Caro, R. and Boccio, J. (2001). Effect of probiotics and functional foods and their use in different diseases. *Nutrition Research*, 21(3): 569–579.

2

Isolation, Identification and Characterization of Beneficial Microorganisms from Traditional Fermented Foods

Phu-Ha Ho[1], Tuan-Anh Pham[1], Quoc-Phong Truong[1], Lan-Huong Nguyen[1], Tien-Thanh Nguyen[1], Hang-Thuy Dam[1], Chinh-Nghia Nguyen[1], Ha-Anh Nguyen[1], Quyet-Tien Phi[2], Hoang Anh Nguyen[3] and Son Chu-Ky[1]

[1] *Laboratory of Applied Microbiology, School of Biotechnology and Food Technology, Hanoi University of Science and Technology, 1, Dai Co Viet, Hai Ba Trung, Hanoi 100000, Vietnam*
[2] *Institute of Biotechnology, Vietnam Academy of Science and Technology, 18 Hoang Quoc Viet, Cau Giay, Hanoi, 100000, Vietnam*
[3] *Faculty of Food Science and Technology, Vietnam National University of Agriculture, Trau Quy, Gia Lam, Hanoi, 100000, Vietnam*

2.1 Introduction

Traditional fermented foods, either of plant or animal origin, play a key role in the diet of people around the world. Traditional fermented foods not only provide important sources of nutrients but also offer important potential in order to maintain health and prevent diseases. Probiotics are the major group of microorganisms associated with traditional fermented foods. In tropical countries, traditional fermented foods are usually homemade products obtained through spontaneous fermentation or backslopping. Nowadays, they are demanding to respond to quality, safety and mass production issues. This requires the acquisition of knowledge on the microbial biodiversity, raw materials and production processes.

2.2 Fermented Food as a Source of Probiotic Microorganisms

2.2.1 Fermented Food and Health Benefits

Fermented food has existed for thousands of years. Fermentation is initially known as a method of food preservation. The shelf life of the substrate food is extended, and digestibility and organoleptic properties of food are also improved. Based on substrates of

Probiotics, Prebiotics and Synbiotics: Technological Advancements Towards Safety and Industrial Applications, First Edition. Edited by Parmjit Singh Panesar and Anil Kumar Anal.

fermentation, fermented foods can be characterized as dairy, meat, fish, vegetables and fruits, cereals and legumes products, such as yoghurt, cheese, fermented sausage, kimchi, natto, etc. Raw materials that contain high concentrations of carbohydrate such as sugars, and in few cases starch, are normally fermented by yeast and lactic acid bacteria. High enzyme producers such as fungi and bacilli are usually applied in proteolysis and saccharification of materials. Fermented foods can also be described based on the metabolites of the microorganisms involved, for instance alcoholic products fermented by yeast (e.g. *Saccharomyces*), acetic acid by *Acetobacter*, or lactic acid by lactic acid bacteria (LAB) such as *Lactobacillus, Leuconostoc, Streptococcus*, etc. Due to the metabolisms of fermenting microorganisms (producing enzymes, organic acids, alcohols), substrates can be transformed into nutritive, bioactive and bioavailable end products.

Health beneficial effects of fermented foods are described as whole products and recently have been reviewed in Xiang *et al.* (2019).

Fermented dairy products such as yoghurt, Bulgarian butter milk, acidophilus milk, kefir, koumiss, dahi and cheese are common around the world. They are well known as sources of fatty acids, vitamins, free amino acids and other useful compounds. Reported health benefits include improved lactose maldigestion, anti-inflammatory and anti-stress effects, memory-improving, neuroprotective and cognition enhancing effects, enhanced absorption of nutrients (including minerals) and gut-associated immune response, decreased cholesterol levels, shortening of the duration of diarrheal bouts, and improvements in the incidence of arrhythmias, ischemia and cancer.

The claimed health benefits of fermented cereals and legumes arise from the combination of probiotics and prebiotics present in these products, for example the probiotic microorganisms lactobacilli and bifidobacteria and raw materials containing prebiotic carbohydrates (e.g. beta-glucan, arabinoxylan, galacto-/fructooligosaccharides and resistant starch). Chinese red rice has been reviewed in Kalaivani *et al.* (2010) as an exceptional source of bioactive compounds. Rice fermented with *Monascus purpureus* became red in color and was found to contain elevated sterols, unsaturated fatty acids and phytochemicals (e.g. vitamins and phenolics). Animal and clinical studies showed that red rice consumption could improve type 2 diabetes, cardiovascular disease, Alzheimer's disease, cancer and human B lymphomas. A range of functionalities such as antioxidant, lipid metabolism-regulating, osteoporosis-fighting, appetite-improving, fatigue-reducing, as well as antibacterial, anti-infection and blood glucose-lowering effects are exhibited in vinegars and fermented products from sugar and alcohol. Other products, such as amazake (Japan), ogi (Nigeria), pozol (Pre-Columbian Mexico), and kvass (Ukraine, Russia and Belarus), also are well known to have antioxidant, blood glucose-lowering and appetite-improving functionality (Ampe *et al.* 1999). Various fermented soy products are consumed all over the world. Soybean is fermented with mold, bacteria, yeast or their combination to obtain products such as soy sauce, miso, tempeh and natto. The health-promoting properties of fermented soy products with high nutritional value have been evidenced in in vitro and in vivo experiments to improve cardiovascular health (Steinkraus 2004).

Fermented vegetables provide dietary fiber, minerals, antioxidants and vitamins that can positively influence human health. Products such as kimchi, sauerkraut, fermented carrots, cauliflowers, tomatoes, olives, green peas and peppers are traditional foods made at home or produced industrially. Their claimed health benefits include anti-aging, anti-inflammatory, antibacterial, anti-obesity and anticancer effects due to the probiotic micro-organisms and antioxidants contained in the final products (Park *et al.* 2014).

Fermented fish is normally produced using Gram-positive bacteria including LAB such as lactobacilli, pediococci and streptococci (Kuda *et al.* 2010). Fermented fish contains minerals and is rich in protein-based compounds such as amino acid and soluble nitrogen. It also possesses antioxidative, angiotensin-1 converting enzyme (ACE)-inhibitory, γ-aminobutyric acid (GABA)-producing, cholesterol-reducing and antitumor effects.

A large number of other fermented products can be found worldwide. Fermented tea is traditionally served in many Asian countries. Kombucha (fermented by a mixture of yeast and LAB) is becoming common outside its original country, Indonesia, because the tea has properties against undesirable microorganisms and contributes to the prevention and treatment of cardiovascular diseases and cancer. Improvement of gastrointestinal infection and diabetes has also been demonstrated (Fu *et al.* 2011; Martínez Leal *et al.* 2018).

2.2.2 Occurrence of Probiotics in Fermented Foods

There are thousands of types of fermented foods all over the world. Substrates undergo a fermentation process with fermenting microorganisms either by purposefully adding starter cultures, backslopping or spontaneous fermentation. Yoghurt is the most common fermented dairy product. Fermenting microorganisms commonly found in different countries are the same starter culture of *Streptococcus thermophilus* and *Lactobacillus delbrueckii* spp. *bulgaricus*. Alcoholic drinks (wine, beer) and breads are also fermented by starter culture (*Saccharomyces*). Popular fermented soy products such as natto and tempeh are produced on a large scale with a starter culture of *Bacillus subtilis* var. *natto* and *Rhizopus*, respectively. Vegetables are found to be fermented in different areas and countries by very similar fermenting microorganisms: *Leuconostoc mesenteroides, L. plantarum* and *L. brevis* (Marco *et al.* 2017). Spontaneous or backslopping fermentation is normally used for home-made, local, ethnic foods. Microorganisms can originate from the air, environment, soil, irrigation water, raw materials or equipment (Lortal *et al.* 2014).

Probiotics are defined as "live microorganisms that, when administered in adequate amounts, confer a health benefit on the host" (FAO/WHO 2001). Spontaneously fermented foods might contain probiotic microorganisms; however, they are not necessarily regarded as probiotic foods. Examples include kefir made with undefined kefir grain (microbiota), sauerkraut and kombucha made with spontaneous microbiota. These are not probiotic foods, although they can have health benefits. Nowadays, probiotic fermented foods are produced by supplementing probiotic microorganisms in adequate amounts, such as yoghurt supplemented with probiotic *L. acidophilus* and bifidobacteria. They can also be produced using probiotics as the starter culture (e.g. Yakult).

Lactic acid bacteria (LAB) are most commonly used in the production of fermented foods. A number of LAB have been isolated from foods and tested for their probiotic properties. It is worthy of note that commercial probiotics have mostly been isolated from the human compartment, such as *L. rhamnosus* GG (ATCC 53103), isolated from human feces (ATCC 2007); *L. reuteri Protectis* (ATCC 55730) (BioGaia 2007) and *L. casei* strain Shirota isolated from the human intestine (Yakult 2007). There have been numerous reviews about probiotics isolated from fermented foods. The diversity of probiotic strains depends on diversity of foods, localities and fermentation conditions. With industrialization, in order to standardize the final products, many fermented foods are produced by starter cultures, which narrows the diversity of the fermenting microorganisms isolated. Sources of newly isolated probiotics are mostly ethnic, spontaneously fermented products. Zhao *et al.* (2019) have established a database to document probiotic microorganisms isolated from different fermented foods. Although the health benefits of fermented foods in many cases are anecdotal, and clinical databases on the health benefits of probiotics from fermented food are still limited, there is a vast diversity of probiotic sources. Representative potential probiotic microorganisms isolated from fermented foods are presented in Table 2.1.

Many of the species found in fermented foods are either identical to or share physiological traits with species relevant to promoting gastrointestinal tract health (Marco *et al.* 2017). Fermented foods were found to contain high cell counts of strains of the species recognized as probiotics. *Lactobacillus acidophilus, L. casei* and *L. paracasei* were discovered in non-starter LAB long-ripening cheese; *L. johnsonii* was found in kefir grain; bushera and other African cereal porridge and beverages contained *L. fermentum; L. fermentum* was found in salami, sauerkraut, kimchi, and olives.

Live LAB are consumed as fermented foods are digested. However, it is still inconclusive whether they thrive in the human intestine and become part of the gut's microbiome. Several reports have tried to explain LAB diffusion and phylogenetic diversity. As reviewed in De Filippis *et al.* (2020), LAB are widely distributed in nutrient-rich habitats associated with food, plants, soil, animals and human hosts (Duar *et al.* 2017). In recent years, comparative and evolutionary studies have been reported. Lactic acid bacteria are allocated in three clusters: (i) free living: those bacteria that do not rely on a eukaryotic host and live on plant materials in the environment; (ii) host adapted: bacteria that live in association with a eukaryotic host with the ability to adapt to the host and persistence; (iii) nomadic: non-specific bacteria that thrive in both environments and host niches (Martino *et al.* 2016; Sun *et al.* 2015; Zheng *et al.* 2015). *L. buchneri* and *L. collinoides* groups, and all the species *L. brevis, L. composti* and *L. perolens* are free-living bacteria. Free-living species are consistently capable of growing at lower temperatures, whereas host-adapted species grow optimally at temperatures close to the body temperature of their corresponding hosts (Duar *et al.* 2017). *L. casei/paracasei, L. plantarum* and *L. rhamnosus, L. amylovorus, L. iners, L. johnsonii, L. reuteri, L. ruminis* and *L. salivarius* were found to be adapted to vertebrate hosts, although some of them are also relevant in food fermentation (De Filippis *et al.* 2020).

By analyzing 9445 metagenomes from human samples, Pasolli *et al.* (2020) demonstrated that the prevalence and abundance of LAB species in stool samples is generally low. The chance of occurrence is linked to age, lifestyle and geography, with *Streptococcus thermophilus* and *Lactococcus lactis* being most prevalent. Six hundred and sixty-six metagenome-assembled genomes (MAGs) newly reconstructed from fermented food microbiomes along with 154 723 human MAGs and 193 078 reference genomes were considered. Closely related LAB strains could be found in both food and gut environments. This evidenced that fermented foods can be regarded as a possible source of LAB for the gut microbiome (Pasolli *et al.* 2020).

Table 2.1 Representative potential probiotic microorganisms isolated from fermented foods in different continents.

Substrate products	Africa	Asia	EU	America
Dairy	Zimbabwe, amasi or mukaka, wakora or zifa. Potential probiotics are *Lactococcus lactis* subsp. *lactis*, *Lactococcus lactis* subsp. *lactis* biovar *diacetylactis*,*Lactobacillus paracasei* subsp.*paracasei*, *Lactobacillus plantarum*, *Lactobacillus acidophilus*, *Leuconostoc mesenteroides* subsp.*mesenteroides*, *Enterococcus faecium*, *Enterococcus faecalis* (Shah and Swami 2017) Ayib, ergo, Ethiopia. Cow milk, Potential probiotics are *Lactobacillus* sp.*Streptococcus* sp.; Susa (camel milk), Kenya. Potential probiotics are *Lactobacillus acidophilus*,*Kluyveromyces fragilis*,*Saccharomyces cerevisiae* (Tamime and Marshall 1997)	Dahi (Indian yoghurt), India. Cow milk or buffalo milk. Potential probiotics are *Lactococcus lactis* subsp. *cremoris*, *Lactococcus lactis* subsp. *lactis*, *Streptococcus thermophilus*, *Lactobacillus delbrueckii* subsp. *bulgaricus*,*Lactobacillus acidophilus*,*Lactobacillus helveticus*, *Lactobacillus fermentum*, *Lactobacillus casei*, *Lactobacillus plantarum* (Steinkraus 1983)	Nordic or Scandinaviansour milk (various local names). Norway, Sweden. Lactic acid bacteria,*Lactococcus lactis* subsp.*lactis*, *Lactococcus lactis* subsp. *cremoris*, *Lactococcus lactis* subsp.*lactis* biovar *diacetylactis*,*Leuconostoc mesenteroides* subsp. *cremoris* (Tamime and Marshall 1997) Žinčica (in Slovakia), Žinčice(in the Czech Republic), Żentyca (in Poland). Potential probiotics are *Lactobacillus casei*,*Lactobacillus plantarum*,*Lactococcus lactis* and*Leuconostocmesenteroides* (Oyewole 1997)	
Meat		Nahm, Thailand. Pork, rice. Potential probiotics are *Pediococcus* sp., *P. cerevisiae*, providing vitamins (Noonpakdee *et al.* 2003) Nem-chua, Vietnam. Pork, rice. *Pediococcus* sp, *Lactobacillus* sp. preventing constipation and lowering cholesterol (Lee 1997)	Sausage	
Fish	Bonome (stink fish), Ghana. Fish with significantly increased lactic acid content (Franz *et al.* 2014)	Burong dalag, Philippines. Fish (dalag), rice. *Ln. mesenteroides*,*P. cerevisiae*, *Lactobacillus plantarum*, *S. faecalis*, *Micrococcus* sp. inhibiting the proliferation of harmful bacteria (Steinkraus 1983)	Anchovy, Mediterraneancountries. Lactic acid bacteria, yeasts improve liver function and immunity (Aubert 1985)	Anchovy, Argentina. Anchovy. Lactic acid bacteria, yeastsimprove liver function and immunity (Aubert 1985)

		Kungchao, Thailand. Shrimp, rice. *P. cerevisiae* provides vitamins (Oyewole 1997)
Vegetables	Kawal, North Africa. Vegetables. *L. plantarum* enhancing food quality and safety (Oyewole 1997)	Duamuoi, Vietnam. Cabbage,various vegetables. Potential probiotics are *Ln. mesenteroides,Lactobacillus. plantarum;* removal of antinutrient compounds (Lee 1997)
		Kimchi, Korea. Korean cabbage, radish, various vegetables. Contains *Ln. mesenteroides,Lactobacillus brevis, Lactobacillus plantarum* providing antimicrobial properties, antitumor activity, preventing constipation (Lee 1997)
Cereals, legumes	Dawadawa, Nigeria. Locust beans (*Parkia biglobosa*) seeds. Contains *Bacillus* sp. (Mensah 1997; Steinkraus 1997)	Doenjang, Korea. Soybeans. *Aeromonas oryzae* (Surh *et al.* 2008)
	Soumbara, Ivory Coast. Locust beans,*Parkia biglobosa* seed. *Bacillus* sp., antinutrient reduction (Steinkraus 1997)	Hama-natto, Japan. Soybeans, *Aeromonas oryzae, Streptococcus* sp., *Pediococcus* sp. Strong cytotoxic activity against cancer cells (Steinkraus 1997)
		Miso, Japan. Soybeans, *Aeromonas oryzae, Torulopsis etchellsii,Lactobacillus* sp. enhances the lingering after taste (Blandino *et al.* 2003)
		Tempeh, Indonesia. Soybeans, Rhizopus mold. Prevention of atherosclerosis, cancer, osteoporosis and menopausal disorders (Steinkraus 1983)

2.2.3 Probiotic Viability in Fermented Food

Traditional fermented foods contain different numbers and species of live microorganisms which transform the raw material into new products with high nutritional value. The diversity and viability of probiotics, especially LAB, in fermented foods depend on food properties, geographical areas and fermentation conditions. Probiotics should be maintained in fermented foods at levels above 10^7 viable cells per gram or milliliter until consumption.

Fermented dairy products are extensively consumed worldwide. Humans around the world have been consuming these products for millennia by exploiting the microorganisms naturally present in raw milk. The production of dairy products is commonly carried out through the coagulation of milk, with or without the elimination of serum, by bacterial cultures, where the transformation of lactose into lactic acid plays an important role. There are three categories of milk fermentation: thermophilic fermentation at 40–45 °C with lactic acid production (i.e. matzoon, yoghurt, cheese); mesophilic fermentation at 20–30 °C with lactic acid production (i.e. cultured buttermilk, ymer, skyr); and acid and alcoholic fermentation at 15-25 °C with the production of some alcohol in addition to lactic acid and carbon dioxide (i.e. kefir) (Macori and Cotter 2018). The cultures of microorganisms will be viable, active and abundant in the fermented milk. The most common LAB used for fermentation of milk are strains of bifidobacteria (i.e. *Bifidobacterium breve* C50, *Bifidobacterium lactis*, *Bifidobacterium longum* and *Bifidobacterium animalis*) and lactobacilli (i.e., *Lactobacillus acidophilus*, *Lactobacillus rhamnosus*, *Lactobacillus johnsonii* and *Lactobacillus casei*), usually together with *Streptococcus thermophilus* (Granier *et al.* 2013).

Besides milk, cereal grains represent a major source of dietary nutrients throughout the world. Compared to unfermented cereals, fermented cereal foods tend to be more palatable and have lower antinutritional effects and higher bioavailability of minerals (Katina *et al.* 2005). In an earlier study, Blandino *et al.* (2003) established a database on the most common indigenous cereal and cereal–legume-based fermented foods and beverages. It is reported that most of those products are produced in Asia and Africa. Indigenous rice-based fermented foods are used in several traditional foods in Asian countries (i.e. idli and dosa originated in India, me originated in Vietnam and takju from Korea). Rice is usually mixed with other ingredients (i.e. black gram, wheat or soybean), steamed or non-steamed, followed by natural fermentation at room temperature for varying duration (La Anh 2015; Nagaraju and Manohar 2000; Nout 2003). The LAB have been found to be responsible for the fermentation process in those foods. In soy sauce, production consists of a two-step fermentation process called koji (solid-state fermentation) and moromi (brine fermentation) (Devanthi and Gkatzionis 2019). While fungi play an important role in the koji fermentation (25–35 °C for 3 days) by producing proteolytic and amylase enzymes, moromi fermentation (3–6 months) is mainly driven by the indigenous halotolerant LAB and yeast that create the soy sauce flavor. LAB proliferate quickly at the beginning of the moromi fermentation and result in a gradual decrease in pH due to lactic acid fermentation and other metabolic products. However, while fermentation by LAB can significantly improve the structure and taste of starch-based foods (Falade *et al.* 2014; Wan *et al.* 2011), most LAB are unable to degrade starch due to their lack of amylolytic activity (Aguilar *et al.* 2000). Furthermore, it is noted that malted cereal substrates promote LAB growth and aroma compound generation better than non-malted cereals (Charalampopoulos *et al.* 2003; Coda *et al.* 2011; Gebremariam *et al.* 2015; Salmerón *et al.* 2015).

Fermented vegetable products, such as kimchi, sauerkraut, carrots, cauliflowers, tomatoes, olives, green peas and peppers, and duamuoi, can positively influence human health thanks to their abundance of dietary fiber, minerals, antioxidants and vitamins. Sauerkraut, a popular fermented vegetable in Europe and China, is made via lactic acid fermentation of salted white cabbage (*Brassica oleracea* var. *capitata*) (Yang *et al.* 2020). Korean kimchi is mainly made by LAB fermentation of baechu cabbage, radish, green onion, red pepper powder, garlic, ginger and fermented seafoods (jeotgal). The LAB profile during kimchi fermentation varies with pH and acidity. *Leu. mesenteroides* is observed during early fermentation (pH 5.6–4.3 and acidity 0.5–0.9%); *L. plantarum* and *L. sakei* dominate later in the fermentation (pH 4.2 and acidity 1.0%) (Lee *et al.* 2008). Normally, fermented kimchi contains high levels of LAB (about 10^8–10^9 CFU/g) (Park and Jeong 2016).

The lactic acid fermentation of seafoods is usually produced with Gram-positive cocci including LAB such as lactobacilli, pediococci and streptococci (Xiang *et al.* 2019). The most common products of seafood fermentation are fish sauce and seasoning, made by lengthy fermentation. Nare-zushi is a Japanese fermented sushi made from raw fish (e.g. mackerel, salmon, crucian carp or sandfish) along with rice or other carbohydrate-based materials (Kuda *et al.* 2010). Vietnamese fish sauce, nuoc mam, mostly made from anchovy, is produced over 12–18 months via the following steps. Fish and salt are mixed at a ratio of 25–33% (w/w) in vessels made of different materials depending on the local custom (e.g. wood, ceramic or cement). After maturation, the extract is drained from the ripened fish mass, pomaced several times, and filtered to obtain a transparent liquid (the fish sauce) (Nguyen *et al.* 2011).

In addition, there are a wide range of fermented meat products globally. It is suggested that fermented meat sausages in Europe have been produced since Roman times in Mediterranean countries (Hammes *et al.* 1990). The fermentation of meat products is produced by utilizing naturally occurring microflora, or by using one or more species of commercial preparations of bacteria, yeasts and molds (such as LAB, micrococci and staphylococci). In Europe, Mediterranean sausage production can be carried out at high temperature fermentation (18–24 °C) for 1–2 days or at a low temperature (10–12 °C) for 1 week (Comi *et al.* 2005; Lebert *et al.* 2007). Similarly, temperatures for drying/ripening range mainly between 10 and 14 °C from 4 to 12 weeks for French, Italian or Greek sausages (Oliveira *et al.* 2018). In some South East Asia tropical countries, the fermented sausages (i.e. nem chua in Vietnam) are fermented by LAB at ambient temperature (from 20 to 37 °C), ripened for only 1–2 days, and must be consumed in a short time (La Anh 2015). Along with sausage elaboration, the microorganisms present (mainly LAB) transform the raw materials, providing different physicochemical, sensory and microbiological properties. Furthermore, some LAB are able to produce bacteriocins that inhibit pathogenic microorganisms and increase the shelf life and microbial diversity of the sausage, thus providing unique sensory properties (Benito *et al.* 2007; Lücke, 2000).

2.3 Probiotic Isolation

2.3.1 Traditional Culture-dependent Approach

Microorganisms with probiotic properties are phylogenetically and metabolically diverse. They can be isolated from a variety of habitats including traditional fermented food sources as mentioned in the previous section. Therefore, there is no single method to isolate probiotic microorganisms.

Samples containing potential probiotic microorganisms are processed according to their physical characteristics. Sample homogenization can be achieved using conventional pestles and mortars. High-speed blenders and stomacher blenders are alternative methods to efficiently and uniformly transfer microorganisms from the food matrix into dilution buffers.

Tenfold dilutions are prepared serially in sterile water or in an appropriate buffer such as saline solution (0.85% NaCl), phosphate saline buffer (137 mM NaCl, 10 mM phosphate, 2.7 mM KCl, pH 7.4), peptone water (10 g/L peptone, 5 g/L NaCl, pH 7.2). In the case of isolating anaerobic probiotic groups such as *Lactobacillus* and *Bifidobacterium*, L-cysteine hydrochloride is added at a nominal concentration of 0.25% as the reducing agent to the dilution buffer to maintain low oxygen levels. The dilution should be performed over no more than 15 min to keep exposure of the bacteria to oxygen at a minimal level. Dilutions of samples are inoculated onto Petri dishes containing culture media suitable for the microorganisms of interest. Lactic acid bacteria such as *Lactobacillus, Lactococcus, Leuconostoc* and *Bifidobacterium* are anaerobic microorganisms that can tolerate a small quantity of oxygen. They are grown under anaerobic conditions in anaerobic jars (e.g. GasPak™) or in anaerobic cabinets supplied with a mixture of anaerobic gas (for example, 82% N_2, 10% CO_2 and 5% H_2). Alternatively, the dilution containing the seed microbes can be mixed with liquefied agar and poured onto the plates, or a layer of sterile agar medium can be overlaid on the spread plate to minimize exposure of the inoculum to oxygen. The plates can then be incubated in an ambient atmosphere. Many LAB can tolerate small amounts of oxygen diffused through the agar and therefore can be isolated using this simple method.

de Man, Rogosa and Sharpe (MRS) medium is most commonly used to isolate LAB. MRS medium was developed based on the tomato juice medium of Briggs and All Purpose Tween (APT) medium of Evans and Niven (1951) in which tomato juice was omitted and replaced by defined growth factors of *Lactobacillus* including ions (Mg^{2+} and Mn^{2+}) and Tween 80 (De Man *et al.* 1960; Evans and Niven 1951). The latter component provides lactobacilli with essential fatty acids and thus shortens the lag phase of LAB cultures.

MRS supports the growth of a wide range of LAB including bacteria belonging to the genera *Lactobacillus, Leuconostoc, Streptococcus, Enterococcus* and *Bifidobacterium*, which share the same types of habitat. MRS medium can be modified to be more selective to isolate a particular group of lactobacilli. Decreasing the pH of MRS medium to about 5.5–6 effectively inhibits streptococci and enterococci. In attempts to isolate LAB from high-salt habitats such as fermented fish, sodium chloride is added at a higher concentration (e.g. 2%). MRS is the basal medium subjected to modification to enhance the selectivity of particular groups of LAB. Two research groups simultaneously developed modified MRS media (i.e. LcS Select medium and maltose–MRS–vancomycin [MMV] medium) to select

Table 2.2 Composition of MRS medium, LcS select medium and MMV medium.

		Composition		
No.	**Ingredients**	**MRS medium**	**LcS select medium**	**MMV medium**
1	Tryptic digest of casein	10 g	10 g	10 g
2	Beef extract	8 g	8 g	–
3	Yeast extract	4 g	4 g	4 g
4	Glucose	20 g	20 g	–
5	Maltose	–	–	10 g
6	Sorbitan monooleate (Tween 80)	1 g	1 g	1 g
7	Dipotassium hydrogen phosphate	2 g	2 g	2 g
8	$MgSO_4.7H_2O$	0.2 g	0.2 g	0.2 g
9	$MnSO_4.4H_2O$	0.05 g	0.05 g	0.05 g
10	Ammonium citrate	2 g	2 g	2 g
11	Sodium acetate.$3H_2O$	5 g	5 g	5 g
12	Agar	15 g	15 g	15 g
13	L-cysteine hydrochloride	–	0.05%	0.05%
14	Bromophenol Blue	–	0.002%	–
15	Bromocresol purple 1.6% (w/v)	–	–	3 mL
16	Vancomycin	–	1%	1 %
17	Distilled water	1000 mL	1000 mL	1000 mL
18	pH	6.2	6.2	6.9–7.0

Sources: Based on Di Lena, M., Quero, G.M., Santovito, E., Verran, J., De Angelis, M. and Fusco, V. (2015). A selective medium for isolation and accurate enumeration of Lactobacillus casei-group members in probiotic milks and dairy products. *International Dairy Journal*, 47: 27–36 and Sutula, J., Coulthwaite, L. and Verran, J. (2012). Culture media for differential isolation of Lactobacillus casei Shirota from oral samples. *Journal of Microbiological Methods*, 90(1): 65–71.

for *Lactobacillus casei* group (Table 2.2) (Di Lena *et al.* 2015; Sutula *et al.* 2012). Vancomycin is the selective agent that inhibits the growth of co-inhabitants of *Lactobacillus casei* group, including *Enterococcus, Streptococcus*, and *Bifidobacterium,* and allows for the growth of the vancomycin-resistant *Lactobacillus casei* group. L-cysteine hydrochloride not only promotes the growth of anaerobic *Lactobacillus* but also provides them with a source of nitrogen. Bromophenol Blue is a pH indicator allows for recognition of carbohydrate fermentation and production of acid as the fermentation products. In MMV medium, maltose is supplied as the sole carbon source to promote the growth of LAB capable of fermenting maltose and acidifying the medium. *Lactobacillus casei* groups are easily recognized on these media by their typical colonies (round, domed, off-white colonies with yellowish halos around the colonies indicating a pH 3.0 and lower resulting from carbohydrate fermentation).

Table 2.3 Composition of *Leuconostoc* selective medium (LUSM).

No.	Ingredient	Composition
1	Glucose	10 g
2	Bacto Peptone	10 g
3	Yeast extract	5 g
4	Meat extract	5 g
5	Gelatin	2. g
6	Calcium lactate	5 g
7	Sorbic acid	0.5 g
8	Sodium acetate	2.5 g
9	Tween 80	1 mL
10	Sodium azide	75 ppm
11	Tomato juice	15%
12	Vancomycin	30 μg/mL
13	Tetracycline	20 μg/mL
14	L-cysteine hydrochloride	0.5 mg/mL
15	pH	5.3–5.8

Vancomycin is prepared in water at a concentration of 10 μg/mL, filter sterilized before adding into the cooling autoclaved medium. Bromophenol Blue is prepared in 1 M NaOH solution at a concentration of 0.02 g/L. Maltose and vancomycin are added from filter sterilized solution into the autoclaved medium when it cools.

Leuconostoc are commonly found in a variety of fermented vegetables. They also co-inhabit with other LAB in dairy products, including naturally fermented milk. Several media have been developed to selectively isolate *Leuconostoc* from these samples (Benkerroum *et al.* 1993). Selective factors include sodium azide, sorbic acid and a combination of several antibiotics to which *Leuconostoc* are resistant, including vancomycin and tetracycline (Table 2.3). Tomato juice is prepared by blending fresh tomatoes in water (1 : 1 volume ratio), then centrifuging at 8000 G for 15 min, and is used without filtration. Vancomycin, tetracycline and L-cysteine hydrochloride are added after the rest of the medium is autoclaved and cooled.

Bifidobacterium are anaerobic, non-spore-forming lactic bacteria belonging to the phylum Actinobacteria. They are common inhabitants in human and animal intestinal tracts and are then subsequently discharged into sewage systems. Therefore, a vast majority of *Bifidobacterium* strains have been isolated from feces of humans and animals, and from sewage systems. *Bifidobacterium* is also found in naturally fermented milk (e.g. *Bifidobacterium lactis*, *Bifidobacterium mongoliense*). In addition to using MRS as an isolation non-selective medium, several selective media have been formulated to isolate *Bifidobacterium* from a variety of habitats and thus can be used to isolate them from traditional fermented food. Those media include TOS propionate medium, LP and BFM (*Bifidobacterium* medium) (Table 2.4) (Lapierre *et al.* 1992; Nebra and Blanch 1999).

Table 2.4 Composition of TOS propionate agar, BFM agar and LP agar.

		Composition		
No.	**Ingredients**	**TOS propionate agar**	**BFM agar**	**LP agar**
1	Trypticase peptone	10 g	–	–
2	Liver infusion	–	–	35 g
3	Yeast extract	1 g	7 g	–
4	Meat extract	–	2 g	–
5	Peptone	–	5 g	–
6	Bacto Peptone	–	–	10 g
7	Tryptone	–	2 g	–
8	Galactooligosaccharide	10 g	–	–
9	Starch	–	2 g	–
10	Lactose	–	–	10 g
11	Sodium chloride	–	5 g	2 g
12	Lithium chloride	–	2 g	2 g
13	KH_2PO_4	3 g	–	–
14	K_2HPO_4	4.8 g	–	–
15	$(NH_4)_2SO_4$	3 g	–	–
16	$MgSO_4.7H_2O$	0.2 g	–	–
17	L-cysteine hydrochloride	0.5 mg/mL	0.5 g	–
18	Lactulose	–	5 g	–
19	Riboflavin	–	1 mg	–
20	Thiamine chloride	–	1 mg	–
21	Methylene Blue	–	16 mg	–
22	Propionic acid	–	5 mL	–
23	Sodium propionate	15 g	–	3 g
24	Agar	15 g	15 g	20 g
25	Water	1000 mL	1000 mL	1000 mL
26	pH	6.3–6.7	5.5	6.7

Sources: Based on Lapierre, L., Undeland, P. and Cox, L.J. (1992). Lithium chloride-sodium propionate agar for the enumeration of bifidobacteria in fermented dairy products. *Journal of Dairy Science*, 75(5): 1192–1196 and Nebra, Y. and Blanch, A.R. (1999). A new selective medium for Bifidobacterium spp. *Applied and Environmental Microbiology*, 65(11): 5173–5176.

The selectivity of media used in isolation and enumeration of *Bifidobacterium* is determined by the presence of some substances (e.g. propionic acid, lithium chloride) that inhibit the growth of unwanted *Enterobacteriaceae* or LAB that may be present in the same habitats with *Bifidobacterium*. Lactulose and galactooligosaccharide are a non-digestible oligo- and di-saccharide, respectively, which are not readily digestible by a wide variety of microorganisms. They are supplemented into isolation medium to selectively enhance the growth of *Bifidobacterium*.

Bacillus is a remarkably diverse bacterial genus inhabiting essentially every habitat. *Bacillus* is present in many traditional legume and grain-based fermented foods. It acts as the natural starter of the fermentation process and confers probiotic benefits to human health when the fermented food is consumed. Probiotic *Bacillus* strains can be successfully isolated from legume and grain-based fermented food by plating an appropriately diluted sample on a nutrient-rich medium. A protein-rich medium such as casein agar may be used to isolate *Bacillus* strains with alkaline proteolytic activity. For the isolation of probiotic *Bacillus* which are present at a relatively lower abundance in naturally fermented grains, vegetative cells of co-inhabitants can be removed by treating the diluted sample at 75–95 °C for 20 min (Chantawannakul *et al.* 2002). *Bacillus* spores remain and germinate when on isolation media. *Bacillus*-like colonies are then selected and transferred into fresh medium to make pure cultures.

Bacteria are predominantly present in commercialized probiotic products worldwide. So far, microorganisms of eukaryotic origin harboring probiotic properties are limited to the genus *Saccharomyces* (e.g. *Saccharomyces boulardii*). Having similar growth characteristics and 99% genomic similarity to *Saccharomyces cerevisiae*, isolation of *Saccharomyces boulardii* is fairly similar to that of *Saccharomyces cerevisiae*. The common isolation media are potato dextrose agar (PDA), Sabouraud dextrose agar, malt extract agar, etc. The final pH of *Saccharomyces* isolating medium of 5.6 is a selective factor against bacteria present in the same food matrix with the targeted *Saccharomyces* strains. Bacteriocides such as chloramphenicol or kanamycin can also be added to enhance the selectivity of the isolation medium. Incubating the isolation plate at 37 °C also selects for potential probiotic activities of *Saccharomyces* since many non-probiotic *Saccharomyces* strains are sensitive to temperature as high as 37 °C.

2.3.2 Culturomics Approach

As mentioned previously, many strains of microorganisms with probiotic activity are isolated using traditional culture methods through sequential steps including: sample treatment (grinding, homogenization, heating), sample dilution, plating on culture media suitable for the targeted organisms such as MRS, PDA, etc., and incubating under defined conditions. When the targeted probiotic microorganisms are present at low abundance in the sample or vulnerable to homogenization effects during sample processing, enrichment is an option to increase their viable cell numbers prior to isolation. The isolated strains are then subjected to identification and testing for probiotic activities (Figure 2.1).

Several nutrient media such as Luria–Bertani (LB) and PDA have been used for isolating probiotic microorganisms; some selective media were employed to facilitate the isolation of the targeted microorganisms. However, the above-mentioned sequential process can only be used to grow culturable microorganisms, and thus does not reflect the complete microbial composition of natural environments (Stackebrandt and Embley 2000). The growth and activity of a microorganism is greatly influenced by the microorganisms sharing the same niche, and our knowledge about microbial communities is therefore limited (Fleet 1999).

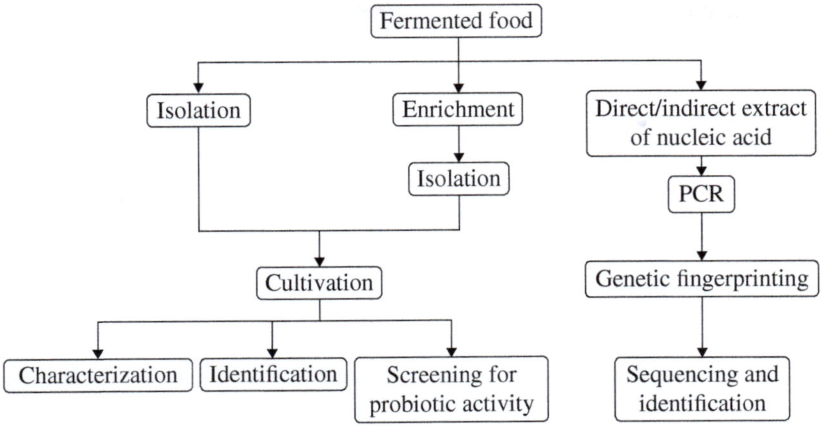

Figure 2.1 Schema of probiotic isolation. PCR, polymerase chain reaction. *Source:* Adapted from Rizo, J., Guillén, D., Farrés, A., Díaz-Ruiz, G., Sánchez, S., Wacher, C. and Rodríguez-Sanoja, R. (2020). Omics in traditional vegetable fermented foods and beverages. *Critical Reviews in Food Science and Nutrition*, 60(5): 791–809.

Fei *et al.* (2018) used media including MRS medium, Elliker's medium, LB medium and PDA medium for the isolation of 13 microbial species in naturally fermented tofu whey. Compared to metagenomics analysis, the authors noticed that only four species were similar for both methods. Moreover, no streptococci were isolated from Mexican pozol, a fermented maize dough beverage, using a culture-dependent method while the genus *Streptococcus* represents 25–50% of the microbiota as revealed by denaturing gradient gel electrophoresis (DGGE) fingerprinting and rRNA quantification (Ampe *et al.* 1999). These observations show the limitations of culture-dependent methods. Therefore, to characterize microbial diversity and composition, a combination of both culture-dependent and molecular biology methods is required (Rizo *et al.* 2020)

However, culture-independent methods do not result in pure microbial cultures. Thus, "culturomics" was employed to study the complex microbial ecosystems. This new approach has many advantages: (i) culturomics has the capability to detect minority populations; (ii) the application of this method is not restricted to eubacteria; and (iii) the method results in novel species and allows for studying the interactions between different bacterial strains (Greub 2012).

Culturomics may be defined as an approach involving extensive assessment of the microbial composition and using high-throughput culture to provide rich nutrients and suitable culture conditions for fastidious bacteria, allowing microorganisms that were previously uncultured to be cultured (Bilen *et al.* 2018). Thus, it is a new and powerful methodology to study microbiology.

In 2015, more than 604 prokaryotic species isolated from the human body as pathogens or commensals were reported, of which 400 species were found using the culturomic approach, accounting for 66.2% (Bilen *et al.* 2018). Through culturomics, several anticancer and anti-Listeria microorganisms have been isolated and identified (Lagier *et al.* 2019). Recently, Xu *et al.* (2020) used a culturomics approach for bacterial isolation from pit muds of Baijiu. Twenty-seven culture conditions were applied in order to investigate bacterial diversity. Two hundred and fifteen prokaryotic strains were isolated and identified, which were assigned to four phyla, 41 genera and 66 species, including 19 potentially new species. The culturable bacteria in pit muds were increased by 273.33% at the genus level, and gas conditions were key factors in this isolation attempt (Xu *et al.* 2020).

2.4 Identification of Probiotic Microorganisms

2.4.1 Phenotypic Identification

For preliminary description of taxa up to family, phenotypic features including colony appearance, cell morphology and growth conditions (temperatures, pH and salt tolerance) are a particularly useful data source. For many years, these morphological and physiological tests were the most important, if not the only, identification methods of probiotic microorganisms. This approach, however, is insufficient when differentiating closely related species, genus or families, in which case other biochemical, molecular, proteomic or metabolomics methods are required.

2.4.2 Biochemical Identification

The principle of biochemical identification of microorganisms is based on their metabolic activities such as metabolism of carbon and nitrogen sources, sugar fermentation, secondary metabolite generation and enzyme production. Biochemical tests were used to identify LAB and yeasts from fermented buttermilk (Gebreselassie, Abay and Beyene 2016) and the Beninese fermented food degue (Angelov *et al.* 2017). There have been several identification kits developed for commercial use such as: API 50CH (bioMerieux, France) a carbohydrate fermentation test; the Biolog Microbial Identification System for identification of more than 2200 species of bacteria, yeast and fungi (RIGEL, Italy); and the KB001 HiIMViC biochemical test kit (HiMedia, India) for differentiation of *Enterobacteriaceae* species.

2.4.3 Molecular Identification

Molecular identification has become a suitable and effective tool for identification of microorganisms from traditional fermented foods. This approach is widely applied in identification of both cultured and uncultured microorganisms. In identifying probiotic microorganisms, some of the most popular techniques include PCR, qPCR, RAPD, rep-PCR, mCOLD-PCR, AFLP, mtDNA-RFLP, ARDRA, DGGE, TGGE, MLSA and MLST.

2.4.3.1 Specific Gene Analysis

The polymerase chain reaction (PCR) technique allows the specific amplification of a target nucleotide sequence. PCR with gene-specific primers is commonly used to identify a particular species, specifically LAB isolated from fermented foods, such as native LAB strains from Vietnamese nem chua (Doan *et al.* 2012), Thai fermented meat (Phoottosavako *et al.* 2015; Tanasupawat *et al.* 2015) and Thai pickled vegetable phak-dong (Meidong *et al.* 2017). Thirty-seven species-specific primer pairs have been designed to detect

Lactobacillus species, which are commonly used in probiotics and fermented food, by PCR method in a single 96 well plate (Kim *et al.* 2020).

Specific real-time quantitative PCR (qPCR) primers can be used to identify and quantify microbial species in fermented foods (Park *et al.* 2009; Wang *et al.* 2016; Yu *et al.* 2015), particularly LAB in traditional dairy foods of Russia (Yu *et al.* 2015) and Baotou and Bayannur of Midwestern Inner Mongolia (Wang *et al.* 2016). This method was applied to enumerate total bacterial, archaeal and yeast strains in kimchi (Park *et al.* 2009). The microbial community in Chinese traditional fermented vegetable food – Chinese homemade paocai – was characterized by real-time PCR (Liang *et al.* 2016). In recent years, qPCR has been used to identify lactic acid cocci from dairy products (Damnjanovic, *et al.* 2019) as well as yeasts and acid acetic bacteria from fermented cocoa beans (Visintin *et al.* 2016).

The random amplification of polymorphic DNA (RAPD) technique was generally applied to assess the diversity of LAB strains from fermented foods (Chao *et al.* 2008; Schillinger *et al.* 2003), and to analyze different *Leuconostoc mesenteroides* strains from vegetables and food products from Korea (Kaur *et al.* 2017).

At a subspecies level, the repetitive element palindromic sequence-based PCR (rep-PCR) technique can unveil significant differences in genotypes of various bacterial strains of the same species from fermented foods (Tamang *et al.* 2008) and differentiate various yeasts in clinical microbiology laboratories (Zhao *et al.* 2018).

A modified co-amplification at lower denaturation temperature PCR (mCOLD-PCR) method has been developed by using a double-strand RNA probe to inhibit the amplification of the sequence of a major microorganism. This method is suitable to detect low-abundant microorganisms, such as detection of *Schizosaccharomyces pombe* from a sample containing 10 000 times more *Saccharomyces cerevisiae* (Takahashi *et al.* 2014).

Based on the selective amplification and separation of genomic restriction fragments, the amplified fragment length polymorphism (AFLP) technique is commonly applied in identification of various LAB strains in fermented foods (Tanigawa and Watanabe 2011), different species/strains of wine yeast (Baselga *et al.* 2017), and *Lactobacillus brevis* from sourdough (Fusco *et al.* 2016).

The mtDNA-RFLP technique, along with microsatellite typing and interdelta analysis, is a widely used genetic marker for distinction of *Saccharomyces cerevisiae* (Schuller *et al.* 2007), specifically strains in amylolytic starters used for the production of rice-based fermented beverage in North East India (Jeyaram *et al.* 2010) and fermented grapes (de Ponzzes-Gomes *et al.* 2014).

Amplified ribosomal DNA restriction analysis (ARDRA) has been utilized in identification of uncultivable microorganisms in fermented bamboo shoot production in India (Jeyaram *et al.* 2010) and characterization of LAB and yeast of Protected Designation of Origin (PDO) Tuscan bread sourdough (Palla *et al.* 2017).

Based on sequence-specific distinctions of PCR-produced 16S rDNA or 26S rDNA amplicons, cultural-independent methods such as DGGE and temperature gradient gel electrophoresis (TGGE) have been developed for assessing microbial populations in fermented food (Alegría *et al.* 2011) and identifying specific groups of bacteria, for example histamine-producing bacteria (Diaz *et al.* 2016).

Multilocus sequence analysis (MLSA) and multilocus sequence typing (MLST) techniques have been used for identification and classification of LAB species found in fermented foods (Bao *et al.* 2016; De Bruyne *et al.* 2010).

2.4.3.2 Metagenomic Analysis

Pyrosequencing has been the most common metagenomics approach in identifying microorganisms. This technique is high-throughput in screening and identification of microorganisms (Cummings *et al.* 2013; Petrosino *et al.* 2009).

Pyrosequencing of 16S rRNA has been utilized to study microbial populations in a variety of traditional fermented foods (Oki *et al.* 2014). Using this method, researchers reported microbial diversity and predominant species present in different fermented foods. Metagenomic analysis of cocoa bean fermentation revealed dominance by *Hanseniaspora uvarum*, *Hanseniaspora opuntiae*, *Saccharomyces cerevisiae*, *Lactobacillus fermentum* and *Acetobacter pasteurianus*. Other genera such as *Erwinia*, *Lactobacillus*, *Lactococcus*, *Leuconostoc* and *Oenococcus* were also revealed (Illeghems *et al.* 2012). In Brazilian kefir grains, the microbial ecology is dominated by *Lactobacillus* (96%), while *Leuconostoc*, *Lactococcus*, *Acetobacter* and *Streptococcus* were at low levels (Leite *et al.*, 2012). LAB were found mainly in gajami-sikhae by pyrosequencing analysis (Kim *et al.* 2014).

2.4.3.3 Proteomics

Mass spectrometry is a crucial technique of proteomics in identification of proteins, in which matrix-assisted laser desorption ionization–time of flight mass spectrometry (MALDI-TOF MS) has been widely used to identify microorganisms based on identification of their protein profile (Singhal *et al.* 2015). Researchers reported multiple uses of MALDI-TOF MS in identification of probiotic microorganisms such as lactobacilli isolates from food (Dušková *et al.* 2012), LAB from French cheese (Nacef *et al.* 2017), bacteria from probiotics and yoghurts (Angelakis *et al.* 2011) and LAB in fruit pulp processing byproducts (Garcia *et al.* 2016). MALDI-TOF MS was also used to validate rapid classification and identification of lactic acid isolates (Doan *et al.* 2012).

2.4.3.4 Metabolomics

Metabolomics is the comprehensive and quantitative analysis of wide ranges of metabolites in biological samples (Kim and Heyman 2018). Techniques in metabolomics such as mass spectrometry could be used to study the metabolite profiles of fermented foods (Mozzi *et al.* 2013).

2.5 Characterization of Probiotic Microorganisms

The first and foremost important characteristic required from probiotic bacteria is the ability to well withstand the stress of the gastrointestinal tract (GIT). Besides traditional in vivo research using only treatment with low pH and high concentration of bile salt (Kavitha *et al.* 2018; Manhar *et al.* 2015; Uma Maheshwari *et al.* 2019), counting of the survival rate after treatment with simulated gastric conditions and simulated intestinal fluids containing pepsin and pancreatin respectively has recently been applied (Jeon *et al.* 2018; Lee *et al.* 2017). Second, in order for them to be widely accepted and used, the safety of these strains needs to be reviewed, for example their properties of autoaggregation, co-aggregation (Trunk *et al.* 2018) and undesirable hemolytic activity, which was analyzed by streaking fresh cultures on blood agar plate – all used strains were γ-hemolytic (Jeon *et al.* 2018; Kavitha *et al.* 2018; Lee *et al.* 2017). The ability to adhere to mucus and epithelial cells is proposed as an important selection criterion for potential probiotic strains (Xu *et al.* 2009). The adhesion of probiotic bacteria varies among strains. Hence, in order to evaluate the physicochemical properties and adhesion ability of probiotic strains available for human use, some examined hydrophobicity (Kavitha *et al.* 2018), while others studied exopolysaccharides (EPS) –extracellular macromolecules excreted – or biofilm formation using assay by the Congo red agar (CRA) method (Uma Maheshwari *et al.* 2019). The antimicrobial or antagonistic activity of probiotics is a vital property that includes the production of antimicrobial compounds, competitive exclusion of pathogens, enhancement of intestinal barrier function and others (Fijan 2016). in vivo methods include various modifications of the spot-on lawn assay, agar well diffusion assay (Borah *et al.* 2019; Manhar *et al.* 2015; Uma Maheshwari *et al.* 2019) and others. Furthermore, since antibiotic gene transfer has become a concern, antibiotic resistance of these probiotic strains must be investigated via microbiological cut-off values, quantitative methods of the minimum inhibitory concentration (MIC) or genetic basis of resistance following the method as per the guidelines of the Clinical and Laboratory Standards Institute (CLSI) and European Food Safety Authority (EFSA). Lastly, in the interest of using supplements not only for nutrition but also for health improvement, the antioxidant and anticancer activities of these strains are gaining more attention. Tests to measure phenolic compounds, which contribute to antioxidant potential, are largely used (Jeon *et al.* 2018). Meanwhile, anticancer ability was tested in an MTT cytotoxicity assay against lung cancer cell line A549 (Uma Maheshwari *et al.* 2019).

Bacillus, a genus of spore-forming bacteria, is increasingly being used as probiotics, as their spores are more stable during processing and storage of food and pharmaceutical preparations, making them more suitable candidates for health promoting formulations (Elshaghabee *et al.* 2017). The characterization of potential probiotic *Bacillus* species isolated from traditional fermented foods is shown in Table 2.5.

A number of studies have focused on the tolerance of probiotic bacteria to gastric acid and bile salts. In the study of Jeon *et al.* (2018), the resistance of *B. subtilis* P229 (isolated from Cheonggukjang-fermented soybean food) to artificial gastric juice and bile salts was investigated to evaluate its survival in the gastrointestinal (GI) tract in vitro. In artificial gastric acid (0.3% pepsin pH 2.5, 3 h), the number of *B. subtilis* P229 vegetative and spore cells decreased from 6.79 and 4.88 to 4.58 and 4.87 log CFU/mL, whereas following exposure to bile salts (0.3% oxgall, 24 h), the number of vegetative cells and spores increased from 6.79 and 4.88 to 7.48 and 7.01 log CFU/mL, respectively. The relative survival ratios (RSR) of *B. subtilis* MKSK-E1, J1 (isolated from Korean traditional soy sauces) after exposure to 0.1% pepsin solution (pH 2.0) for 3 h were 93.14%, 91.85%; MKSK-E1 had high tolerance against 3% bile salt solution (92.50%) followed by MKSK-J1 (90.31%) (Lee *et al.* 2017). These probiotic *B. subtilis* strains showed strong tolerance against gastric juice compared to other reported values for probiotic *Bacillus* species. *B. amyloliquefaciens* AMS1 (isolated from churpi – traditional fermented soybean) only survived 70.07% after 3 h at pH 2.0 but had a survival rate of 94.69% (pH 6.8) and 84.75% (pH 8.0) in 0.3% oxgall after 4 h (Manhar *et al.* 2015). Also, *B. safensis* M5S2B8 and *B. velezensis* M4S1B1 (isolated from panchamirtham – fermented fruit mix) showed high bile salt tolerance (Uma Maheshwari *et al.* 2019). In a recent study, Borah *et al.* (2019) evaluated *B. velezensis* strain DU14 (isolated from apong – traditionally fermented rice beer of Assam, India) for its resistance to acid and bile salt. It can tolerate pH 2.0–3.0 and can survive significantly at up to pH 9.0 ($p < 0.05$), at least for 5 h, which is sufficient for a probiotic microbe to reach the colon, and could withstand 0.2–1.0% (w/v) bile salt for 18 h. *B. velezensis* DU14 also shows a substantial level of growth even in the presence of lysozyme (400 μg/mL), as compared to its absence, which may help the isolate against digestion if administered orally, since the first biological barrier swallowed probiotic bacteria encounter is lysozyme in saliva. Additionally, other *Bacillus* sp. possess the primary requirement of gastrointestinal stress and small intestinal fluid tolerance. Kavitha *et al.*'s 2018 study of *Bacillus* strains isolated from Indian carp *L. calbasu* in the Stanley River, India, shows that FS1 (*B. subtilis* KX756706), FC3 (*B. cereus* KX756707) and FC6 (*B. amyloliquefaciens* KX775224) only survive 43.96%, 56.87% and 68.51%, respectively, in gastric juice after 3 h. Of all the above-mentioned isolated strains (Table 2.5), MKSK-M1 (63.8%, similar to *B. megaterium*) has the highest tolerance of 95.98% to 0.1% pepsin solution (pH 2.0) after 3 h and 99.31% RSR against 3% bile salt solution (Lee *et al.* 2017).

Of all the tested strains mentioned in Table 2.5, *B. subtilis* P229 (Jeon *et al.* 2018), MKSK-E1, J1 and M1 (Lee *et al.* 2017) are revealed to produce esterase, esterase lipase and naphthol-AS-BI-phosphohydrolase. Moreover, P229 has trypsin activity while three strains in Lee *et al.*'s study also possess alkaline phosphatase and acid phosphatase activity. In addition, MKSK-E1 has enzymatic characteristics of α-galactosidase, MKSK-J1 has α-chymotrypsin activity, and MKSK-M1 has both α-chymotrypsin and N-acetyl-β-glucosaminidase activity. β-Glucosidase is an enzyme important in flavor enhancement. It hydrolyzes glucosides to release aglycones aroma precursors that are bound to a sugar molecule thereby making them available to contribute to the flavor of foods and beverages (Stradwick *et al.* 2017). β-Glucosidase activity is an important characteristic of *Lactobacillus* and *Bacillus* species. In a recent study, *B. subtilis* MKSK-J1, *B. velezensis* M4S1B1 and *B. safensis* M5S2B8 were reported to exhibit this characteristic (Uma Maheshwari *et al.* 2019).

The safety of these isolates was evaluated by autoaggregation, co-aggregation and hemolytic activity. One possible application of autoaggregation may be the neutralization of pathogenic strains by co-aggregation with probiotic bacteria (Bujnakova and Kmet 2002). In the aggregated state, pathogens, especially of the gastrointestinal and urinary tracts, would not be able to reach the mucosal surface to colonize the host. This may actually be one of the mechanisms by which some probiotic strains exert their beneficial effects, though it has not been widely released (Reid *et al.* 1988). Jeon *et al.* (2018) demonstrated that *B. subtilis* P229 has co-aggregation ability with *Staphylococcus aureus* ATCC 6538, *Salmonella enteritidis* ATCC 13076, *Listeria monocytogenes* ATCC 15313 and *Escherichia coli* ATCC 93 25922 (64.20% after 24 h), while AMS1 showed co-aggregation with *S. enterica typhimurium* MTCC 1252, *L. monocytogenes* KF894986 and *B. cereus* MTCC 430 (highest, 56.6–60.3%) (Manhar *et al.* 2015). The autoaggregation of *B. subtilis* P229 after 4 h was 49.18%, which is much lower than that of MKSK-E1, J1 (89.6%) and MKSK-M1 (90.4% after 3 h) (Lee *et al.* 2017), and 78.83% after 24 h, which is higher than that of AMS1 (65–75%).

Table 2.5 Characterization of potential probiotic *Bacillus* species isolated from traditional fermented foods.

		Characterization						
SPECIES	SOURCE	Survival under GIT conditions	Safety for the use in human nutrition	Colonization ability	Antimicrobial	Antibiotic sensitivity	Others	Reference
B. licheniformis								
B. subtilis	Cheonggukjang (fermented soybean food)	• 0.3% pepsin pH 2.5 for 3 h, viable cell number : 4.58 (log CFU/mL) • 0.3% oxgall for 24 h, viable cell number : 7.48 (log CFU/mL)	• 49.18% autoaggregation after 4 h 78.83% autoaggregation after 24 h • Co-aggregation ability with *Staphylococcus aureus* ATCC 6538, *Salmonella enteritidis* ATCC 13076, *Listeria monocytogenes* ATCC 15313, and *Escherichia coli* ATCC 93 25922 • Esterase, esterase lipase, trypsin, naphthol-AS286 BI-phosphohydrolase • γ -hemolysis	-	-	• Susceptible to ampicillin, gentamicin, tetracycline, chloramphenicol, cephalexin, erythromycin, penicillin and vancomycin	• Antioxidant activity	Jeon *et al.*, (2018)
	Korean traditional soy sauces	• Survival rate (%) after 3 h in pepsin (0.1%, pH 2.0): 91.85% • Survival rate (%) after 3 h in bile salt (3%): 90.31%	• Autoaggregation (%): 1 h: 91.5%; 2 h: 89.4%; 3 h: 89.6% • Amylase; protease; alkaline phosphatase; esterase; esterase lipase; α-chymotrypsin; acid phosphatase; naphtol-AS-BI-phosphohydrolase; β-glucosidase • γ -hemolysis	• Hydrophobicity(%): xylene (28.1%); chloroform (88.2%); ethyl acetate (21.5%)	• *Staphylococcus aureus* • *B. cereus* • *E. coli* • *Shigella sonnei* • *S. flexneri* • *Pseudomonas fluorescens* • *Klebsiella pneumoniae*	• Susceptible to ampicillin, cephalexin, penicillin G, vancomycin, chloramphenicol, erythromycin, gentamicin and tetracycline.	–	Lee *et al.* (2017)

(*Continued*)

Table 2.5 (Continued)

SPECIES	SOURCE	Characterization: Survival under GIT conditions	Safety for the use in human nutrition	Colonization ability	Antimicrobial	Antibiotic sensitivity	Others	Reference
		• Survival rate (%) after 3 h in pepsin (0.1%, pH 2.0): 93.14% • Survival rate (%) after 3 h in bile salt (3%): 92.5%	• Autoaggregation (%): 1 h: 90.3%; 2 h: 88.9%; 3 h: 89.6% • Amylase; protease; alkaline phosphatase; esterase; esterase lipase; acid phosphatase; naphtol-AS-BI-phosphohydrolase; α-galactosidase • γ -hemolysis	• Hydrophobicity(%): xylene (25.7%); chloroform (80%); ethyl acetate (26.1%)	• *Staph. aureus* • *B. cereus* • *E. coli* • *S. sonnei* • *S. flexneri* • *Pseudo. fluorescens* • *K. pneumoniae*	• Susceptible to ampicillin, cephalexin, penicillin G, vancomycin, chloramphenicol, erythromycin, gentamicin and tetracycline.	Non-biogenic amine formation	
B. amyloliquefaciens	Fermented soybean	• pH 2–8, Survival rate (%) after 3 h at pH 2.0 = 70.07% • Survival rate (%) after 4 h in bile salt (0.3% oxgall), pH 6.8 = 94.69% • Survival rate (%) after 4 h in bile salt (0.3% oxgall), pH 8.0 = 84.75%	• Autoaggregation (%): 65.5–75.5% after 24 h • Co-aggregation with *Salmonella enterica typhimurium* MTCC 1252, *Listeria monocytogenes* KF894986 and *B. cereus* MTCC 430 (56.6–60.3%) • Cellulase • γ -hemolysis	• Hydrophobicity(%): n-hexadecane (68.5–77.9%), chloroform 63.5–74.3%	• *Listeria monocytogenes* • *K. pneumoniae*	• Susceptible to chloramphenicol, streptomycin, sulphatriad , tetracycline	–	Manhar *et al.* (2015)
	Indian carp *L. calbasu* in Stanley River, Mettur Dam, Salem District, Tamil Nadu, India	• pH 1–10 for 24 h • Bile salt 1%, 2,5%; 5,0%; 7.5% for 6 h	• γ-hemolysis	• Hydrophobicity (%): xylene (86.65%), ethyl acetate (69.14%), chloroform (65.71%), toluene (57.07%) • Biofilm formation	• *Aeromonas hydrophila* • *Acinetobacter tandoii* • *Acinetobacter* sp.	• Susceptible to ampicillin, amoxicillin, penicillin, vancomycin, gentamicin, erythromycin, chloramphenicol and ciprofloxacin	–	Kavitha *et al.* (2018)

B. safensis	Panchamirtham (fermented fruit mix)	• pH 3–8 for 48 h • Bile salt 0.3% for 8 h: high tolerance	• β-glucosidase • γ -hemolysis	• Exopolysaccharide 0.55 μg EPS/mL/min	• *E. coli MTCC 2622*	Less susceptible to 30 μg novobiocin, 30 μg kanamycin, 30 μg vancomycin, 5 μg trimethoprim, 100 μg carbenicillin , 30 μg tetracy-cline, 100 μg spectinomycin 10 μg, streptomycin, 300 μg polymyxin--B, 30 μg cefotaxime, 5 μg rifampicin, 15 μg erythromycin, 30 μg chloramphenicol, 10 μg colistin, 10 μg ampicillin, 30 μg doxycycline hydrochloride, 8 μg bacitracin, 30 μg nalidixic acid, 5 μg ciprofloxacin except 10 μg colistin / methane sulfonate and 100 μg polymyxin	–	Uma Maheshwari *et al.* (2019)

(Continued)

Table 2.5 (Continued)

		Characterization						
SPECIES	**SOURCE**	**Survival under GIT conditions**	**Safety for the use in human nutrition**	**Colonization ability**	**Antimicrobial**	**Antibiotic sensitivity**	**Others**	**Reference**
B. velezensis	Apong (traditionally fermented rice beer of Assam)	• pH 2–10 for 5 h (survive significantly) • Bile salt: 0,2%, 0,4%, 0,6%, 0,8%, 1% for 18 h; • 400 μg/mLlysozyme for 7 h	• 51.66% autoaggregation • γ -hemolysis	• Hydrophobicity (%) = 39.2%	• *B. cereus ATCC-11778* • *E. coli ATCC-25922*	• Susceptibility against ampicillin (10 μg/disc), amikacin (30 μg/disc), ceftriaxone (30 μg/ disc), ciprofloxacin (5 μg/disc), chloramphenicol (30 μg/disc), clindamycin (30 μg/disc), erythromycin (15 μg/disc), gentamicin (10 μg/disc), imipenem (10 μg/disc), ofloxacin (5 μg/disc), penicillin (10 μg/disc), and vancomycin (g/disc) • Resist ceftazidime (30 μg/disc), metronidazole (5 μg/disc) and rifampicin (5 μg/disc)	–	Borah *et al.* (2019)

	Panchamirtham (fermented fruit mix)	• pH 3–8 for 48 h • Bile salt 0.3% for 8 h	• β-glucosidase • γ -hemolysis	• Exopolysaccharide 1.00 μg EPS/mL/min	• *Listeria monocytogenes MTCC 1143*	–	• Potential activity against lung cancer cell line A549 with low IC50 values (402 μg/mL)	Uma Maheshwari *et al.* (2019)
Bacillus spp.	Korean traditional soy sauces	• Survival rate (%) after 3 h in pepsin (0.1%, pH 2.0): 95.98% • Survival rate (%) after 3 h in bile salt (3%): 99.31%	• Autoaggregation (%): 1 h: 92%; 2 h: 88.3%; 3 h: 90.4% • Amylase; protease; alkaline phosphatase; esterase; esterase lipase;leucine arylamidase; crystine arylamidase; α-chymotrypsin; acid phosphatase; naphtol-AS-BI-phosphohydrolase; N-Acetyl-β glucose	• Hydrophobicity (%):xylene (89.8%); chloroform (93.8%); ethyl acetate (34.3%)	• *Staph. aureus* • *B. cereus* • *E. coli* • *S. sonnei* • *S. flexneri* • *Pseudo. fluorescens* • *K. pneumoniae*	• Susceptible to ampicillin, cephalexin, penicillin G, vancomycin, chloramphenicol, erythromycin, gentamicin and tetracycline.	-	Lee *et al.* (2017)

GIT, gastrointestinal tract.

Many types of bacteria exhibit hemolytic activity (Adimpong *et al.* 2012). In the above-mentioned studies, hemolytic activity was analyzed by streaking fresh cultures on blood agar plate and all used strains were γ-hemolytic (i.e. no hemolysis).

The ability to adhere to mucus and epithelial cells is proposed to be an important selection criterion for potential probiotic strains (Xu *et al.* 2009). In order to evaluate the physicochemical properties and adhesion ability of probiotic strains available for human use, some examined hydrophobicity by the adhesive characteristics of probiotic strains and foodborne pathogens to xylene, chloroform and ethyl acetate. Among the strains mentioned in Table 2.5, the adhesion capacity to xylene of *Bacillus* MKSK-M1 (89.8%) was the highest, followed by that of *B. amyloliquefaciens* FC6 (86.65%). Furthermore, the percentages of recorded hydrophobicity of MKSK-M1, J1 and E1 in chloroform were 93.8%, 88.2% and 80.0%, respectively, significantly higher than those of other strains. However, FC6 has the highest ability to adhere to ethyl acetate (69.14%). Kavitha *et al.* (2018) also studied toluene adhesion of FC6, which is 57.07%.

Exopolysaccharides (EPS) play the most prominent role in protection of the secreted microorganisms against unfavorable conditions such as desiccation, phagocytosis, cell recognition, phage attack, antibiotics or toxic compounds and osmotic stress (Angelin and Kavitha 2020). Given this well-established role and the health-promoting potential regarding the application of EPS in the regulation of different pathophysiological conditions, many studies have investigated the ability of exopolysaccharide to inhibit pathogens or to abrogate the cytotoxic effect of bacterial toxins (Ruas-Madiedo *et al.* 2010). EPS production of *B. velezensis* M4S1B1 and *B. safensis* M5S2B8 was 1.00 μg EPS/mL/min and 0.55 μg EPS/mL/min, respectively (Uma Maheshwari *et al.* 2019).

Biofilm formation by probiotic microorganisms could promote colonization and enable them to become the dominant microflora in host intestinal mucosa (Salas-Jara *et al.* 2016). In a study of biofilm formation assay by the Congo red agar (CRA) method, FC6 displayed black colonies with dry crystalline morphology, suggesting that FC6 has the ability to form biofilm (Kavitha *et al.* 2018).

The antimicrobial or antagonistic activity of probiotics is an important property that enhances intestinal barrier function, among others (Fijan 2016). The antimicrobial/antagonistic effect of the isolate was tested against both Gram-positive and -negative pathogens by using either well diffusion (Borah *et al.* 2019; Manhar *et al.* 2015; Uma Maheshwari *et al.* 2019) or spot-on assay (Lee *et al.* 2017). In both methods, microbial activity is evaluated by measuring the clear zone excluding colonies. There is one paper that presented results from using two different methods at the same time (Kavitha *et al.* 2018), the cross streak method (Lertcanawanichakul and Sawangnop 2008) and the agar well diffusion method (Schillinger and Lücke 1989).

Among all the articles that have been reviewed in this section, S. Lee *et al.* (2017) successfully tested antimicrobial ability against the widest range of pathogenic bacteria, which included *Staph. aureus, B. cereus, E. coli, Shigella sonnei, S. flexneri, Pseudomonas fluorescens,* and *Klebsiella pneumoniae.* All three *Bacillus* strains tested in this research showed resistance to these seven pathogens, however the best activity was exhibited against *B. cereus* and *E. coli.* When examined against the same pathogen but using the diffusion method with a cell-free solution, *B. velezensis* isolated from apong (traditionally fermented rice beer of Assam) also showed an antimicrobial effect with zone of inhibition of 16 ± 2 and 11 ± 1.5 mm respectively against *B. cereus* ATCC 11778 and *E. coli* ATCC 25922. Two other potential probiotics of the *Bacillus* species, *B. velezensis* M4S1B1 and *B. safensis* M5S2B8, also exhibited antagonistic capability against *Listeria monocytogenes* MTCC 1143 and *E. coli* MTCC 2622, respectively. In Kavitha's research (2018), pathogens that were used to examine antimicrobial activity are quite different from the others, as they are target fish pathogens. The six Gram-negative bacteria included *Aeromonas hydrophila*, *Aeromonas veronii*, *Acinetobacter junii*, *Acinetobacter* spp., *Acinetobacter tandoii* and *Pseudomonas stutzeri*. Nevertheless, *Bacillus* spp. were isolated from *Labeo calbasu* inhibitory activity of probiotics. Among the three bacterial strains, only one showed potential antagonistic activity against three Gram-negative fish pathogenic bacteria (*A. hydrophila, A. tandoii* and *Acinetobacter* sp.) (Kavitha *et al.* 2018).

Antibiotic susceptibility is considered to be the best probiotic characteristic (Patel *et al.* 2009), because it is believed to be the substantial solution for traditional antibiotics that have been used. It should be tested for safety purposes, as 293 antibiotic resistance can be transferred to other bacterial species by transposons and plasmids 294 and as a result of gene mutations (Khochamit *et al.* 2015). All of the *B. subtilis* strains in the above-mentioned articles (Jeon *et al.* 2018; Lee *et al.* 2017) showed high vulnerability to different panels of ampicillin, gentamicin, tetracycline, chloramphenicol, cephalexin, erythromycin and vancomycin. Whereas a *B. subtilis* strain from cheongukjang (Jeon *et al.* 2018) was tested on penicillin, two strains isolated from Korean traditional soy sauces (Lee *et al.* 2017) were tested with penicillin G. However, all showed susceptibility. *B. amyloliquefaciens* is also a popular species to be examined for their probiotic potential, however they are less susceptible to certain antibiotics. Chloramphenicol is the only antibiotic against which all three *B. amyloliquefaciens* strains show no resistance. Meanwhile, antibiotics against which *B. subtilis* showed high vulnerability (ampicillin, gentamicin, tetracycline, chloramphenicol, cephalexin, erythromycin, vancomycin) can only be resisted by two-thirds of the *B. amyloliquefaciens* strains. Some other antibiotics have also been tested with this species, for example penicillin, amoxicillin, ciprofloxacin, sulphatriad, but only one strain showed susceptibility (Kavitha *et al.* 2018; Lee *et al.* 2017; Manhar *et al.* 2015). The other two species have been tested for antibiotic susceptibility in this review are *B. velezensis* (Borah *et al.* 2019) and *B. safensis* (Uma Maheshwari *et al.* 2019). The strain in the Borah study was found sensitive against many antibiotics belonging to two groups categorized by their mechanisms.. The two groups were cell wall inhibitors, including ampicillin, cephalexin, penicillin G and vancomycin, and protein synthesis inhibitors including chloramphenicol, erythromycin, gentamicin and tetracycline (Argyri *et al.* 2013). The other strain from Uma Maheshwari's research was also evaluated against a wide range of different antibiotic agents. It was vulnerable to ampicillin (10 μg/disc), ciprofloxacin (5 μg/disc), chloramphenicol (30 μg/disc), clindamycin (30 μg/disc), erythromycin (15 μg/disc), penicillin (10 μg/ disc) and vancomycin (30 μg/disc), and even some others such as amikacin (30 μg/ disc), ceftriaxone (30 μg/ disc), imipenem (10 μg/disc) and ofloxacin (5 μg/disc) (Uma Maheshwari *et al.* 2019).

Other properties of probiotic bacteria worth mentioning are their antioxidant and anticancer activity. Jeon *et al.* (2018) performed tests of total polyphenolic content as a measure of antioxidant potential. Total phenolic content and antioxidant activity are known to be strongly correlated (Lee and Teo 2005). Lee and Teo (2005) have explained that the increase

Table 2.6 Characterization of potential probiotic *Lactobacillus* species isolated from traditional fermented foods.

Species	Sources	Characterization							Reference
		Survival under gastrointestinal tract conditions	Safety for use in human nutrition	Colonization ability	Antimicrobial	Antibiotic sensitivity	in vitro anticancer models	Anonymous	
Lactobacillus fermentum	Iranian koozeh traditional cheese	• Able to grow in bile salt up to 3% in agar medium • Survived at pH 2.2 after 1.5 h	NA	• Cell surface hydrophobic index 47–58% (with hexadecane)	• *S. aureus* (+); • *P. aeruginosa* (+) • *S. enterica* (+) • *E. coli* (+) • *E. hirae* (+)	Vancomycin (30 μg)^R, gentamicin (10 μg)^R, tetracycline (30 μg)^R, streptomycin (10 μg)^R ceftriaxone (30 μg)^R, chloramphenicol (30 μg)^R, amoxicillin (25 μg)^R, erythromycin (15 μg)^R, streptomycin (10 μg)^R	NA	β-Galactosidase activity (+) H_2O_2 production (6-7%)	Gebreselassie *et al.* (2016)
	Indian traditional fermented food	• ~100 % survived for 6 h in 0.5% pancreatin • 95% survived for 6 h in 0.3% bile salt • 95% survived for 3 h at pH 2.5	• Negative hemolytic activity	• Autoaggregation 60% after 4 h	NA	• Susceptible to chloramphenicol, erythromycin, gentamicin and penicillin • Intermediate sensitivity to nalidixic acid and streptomycin	NA		Angelov *et al.* (2017)
	Vietnamese fermented eggplant	• No loss of viability at pH 3.0, slightly reduced viability to approximately 90% when grown at pH 2.5	NA	• Adhered to the surface of human Caco-2 cells	• Strong and broad inhibitory spectrum activity against 7 out of 11 indicator mold and yeast strains *(Aspergillus terreus, A. fumigatus, A. niger, Absidia corymbifera, Paecilomyces lilacinus, Geotrichum candidum, Fusarium* sp., *Scopulariopsis brevicaulis, Curvularia lunata, Penicillium* sp, *and Candida albicans)*	NA	Inhibited the proliferation of human cancer cell lines in vitro: 90% (melanoma cell line MM200), 60% (breast cancer cell line MCF7); 40% (colon cancer cell line HT29)	PepX activity (+)	Doan *et al.* (2012)
Lactobacillus plantarum	Iranian koozeh traditional cheese	• Survived at pH 2.2 after 1.5 h • Able to grow in agar medium with 1% bile salt	NA	• Cell surface hydrophobic index 22–63% with hexadecan	• *S. aureus* (+) • *P. aeruginosa* (+) • *S. enterica* (+) • *E. coli* (+) • *E. hirae* (+)	Vancomycin (30 μg)^R, gentamicin (10 μg)^R, tetracycline (30 μg)^R; streptomycin (10 μg)^R ceftriaxone (30 μg)^S; chloramphenicol (30 μg)^S; amoxicillin (25 μg)^S; erythromycin (15 μg)^S; streptomycin (10 μg)^R	NA	β-Galactosidase activity (+) H_2O_2 production (0–7%)	Gebreselassie et al. (2016)

Traditional fermenting green olives	• Survival rate of 56.51–83.19% at pH 3, 0.3% bile salt for 5 h in MRS medium	• Negative mucinolytic activity • No hemolytic, DNase or gelatinase activities • Negative α-chymotrypsin, β-glucuronidase and N-acetyl-β-glucosaminidase	• Autoaggregation 10.29–41.34% • Hydrophobic 16.66–33.23% (with xylene)	Inhibition zone cause by cell free crude extract • *C. pelliculosa* (18.20–24.5 mm) • *L. innocua* (10.15-13.8 mm) • *M. luteus* (11.4-13.9 mm) • *S. aureus* (10.10–12.25 mm) • *E. coli* (11.75 -13.8 mm • *P. aeruginosa* (10.25–12.5 mm)	Oxacillin (1 μg)^{R,S}, cephalothin (30 μg)^{S}, vancomycin (30 μg)^{R,S}, amoxicillin (25 μg)^{R,S}, erythromycin (15 μg)^{R,S}, ampicillin (10 μg^{R,S}, 25 μg^{R,S}), chloramphenicol (30 μg)^{R,S}, penicillin G (10 μg)^{R,S}	NA	β-Galactosidase activity (+) EPS production (+) Antioxidant 49.81–52.00%	Phoottosavako *et al.* (2015)
Fermented ragi millet (*Eleusine coracana*), India	• Showed significant (*P* <0.05) survival rate at pH 3, 0.3% bile salt for 3 h	NA	NA	NA	Ampicillin^{S}, gentamicin^{R}, kanamycin^{R}, streptomycin^{R}, erythromycin$^{(R,S)}$	NA	Antioxidant activity (+) Cholesterol assimilation rate: the degradation rates of cholesterol were 56.2–61.9%	Tanasupawat *et al.* (2015)
Bhatoroo (indigenous bread)	• Mild growth at pH 2.5 • Good growth with 4% NaCl • Survival at 2% bile salt	• Negative hemolytic activity	• Autoaggregation 8.23% after 3 h and 54.09% after 24 h • Co-aggregation with *L. monocytogenes* 15.43% (3 h) and 56.21% (24 h) • Hydrophobic index (%) to hexadecane (<5%), xylene (20%), octane and toluene (<10%)	Inhibition zone • *S. aureus* (17.5 mm) • *B.subtilis* (15.5 mm) • *P. aeruginosa* (-) • *S. dysenteriae* (12.4 mm) • *E. coli* (12.2 mm)	Penicillin G (10 Units)^{R}; clindamycin (2 μg)^{R}; co-trimoxazole (25 μg)^{R}; erythromycin (15 μg)^{R}; vancomycin (30 μg)^{R}; ampicillin (10 μg)^{S}; carbenicillin (100 μg)^{S}; cefotaxime (30 μg)^{S}; chloramphenicol (30 μg)^{S}; co-trimazine (25 μg)^{R}; gentamicin (10 μg)^{S}; norfloxacin (10 μg)^{S}; oxacillin (5 μg)]^{R}	NA	Heterofermentation	Meidong *et al.* (2017)
Indian traditional fermented food	• ~100% survived for 6 h in 0.5% pancreatin • 98% survived for 6 h in 0.3% bile salt • 95% survived for 3 h at pH 2.5	• Negative hemolytic activity	• Autoaggregation 80% after 4 h	NA	Susceptible to chloramphenicol, erythromycin, gentamicin and penicillin • Intermediate sensitivity to nalidixic acid and streptomycin	NA		Angelov *et al.* (2017)

(Continued)

Table 2.6 (Continued)

		Characterization							Reference
Species	Sources	Survival under gastrointestinal tract conditions	Safety for use in human nutrition	Colonization ability	Antimicrobial	Antibiotic sensitivity	in vitro anticancer models	Anonymous	
	Chinese fermented cereal foods	• Maintained optical density of cell suspension in medium with 0.6% bile salt of 0.16–0.18 after 48 h • Good growth at pH 3	NA	• Autoaggregation after 24 h of 45–80% • Co-aggregation with 5 indicator strains including *E. coli, S. typhimurium, S. aureus, S. enteritidis, L. monocytogenes* of 20–35% after 24 h	• *E. coli* ATCC 25922 (+) • *S. enteritidis* ATCC 13076 (+) • *S. typhimurium* ATCC 14028 (+) • *S. aureus* ATCC 29213 (+) • *L. monocytogenes* EGD-e (+)	Ciprofloxacin (5 μg)^R, amikacin (30 μg$)^R$, gentamicin (10 μg)^R, trimethoprim-sulfamethoxazole (25 μg)^S, ampicillin–sulbactam (20 μg)^S, ceftriaxone (30 μg)^S, chloramphenicol (30 μg)^S, aztreonam (30 μg)^R, tetracycline (30 μg)^S, cefoxitin (30 μg)^R, ampicillin (30 μg)^S	NA	Amylase activity (+)	Kim *et al.* (2020)
Lactobacillus casei	Churpe (dried cheese), seera (cereal-based fermented product), chilra (barley pancake)	Good survival at pH 2.0 and bile salt of 2%	• Negative hemolytic activity	• Autoaggregation 10.75% after 3 h and 47.42% after 24 h • Co-aggregation with *L. monocytogenes* 16.45% (3 h) and 42.76% (24 h) • Hydrophobic index (%) to hexadecane (11%), xylene (31%), octane (15%) and toluene (10%)	Inhibition zone • *Staphylococcus aureus* (16.1 mm) • *Bacillus subtilis* (18.3 mm) • *Pseudomonas aeruginosa* (-) • *Shigella dysenteriae* (7.2 mm) • *Escherichia coli* (9.02 mm)	Penicillin G (10 Units)^R; clindamycin (2 μg)^R; co-trimoxazole (25 μg)^R; erythromycin (15 μg)^R; vancomycin (30 μg)^R; ampicillin (10 μg)^R; carbenicillin (100 μg)^S; cefotaxime (30 μg)^R; chloramphenicol (30 μg)^R; co-trimazine (25 μg)^R; gentamicin (10 μg)^S; norfloxacin (10 μg)^S oxacillin (5 μg)^R	NA	Heterofermentative	Meidong *et al.* (2017)
	Iranian koozeh traditional cheese	• Survived at pH 2.2 after 1.5 h • Able to grow in agar medium with 1% bile salt	NA	• Cell surface hydrophobic index 14.56% (with hexadecane)	• *S. aureus* (+); • *P. aeruginosa* (+) • *S. enterica* (-) • *E. coli* (+) • *E. hirae* (+)	Vancomycin (30 μg)^R, gentamicin (10 μg)^S; tetracycline (30 μg)^S; streptomycin (10 μg)^S ceftriaxone (30 μg)^S; chloramphenicol (30 μg)^S; amoxicillin (25 μg)^S; erythromycin (15 μg)^S; streptomycin (10 μg)^R	NA	β-Galactosidase activity (+) H_2O_2 production (7.12%)	Gebreselassie *et al.* (2016)
Lactobacillus pentosus	Iranian koozeh traditional cheese	• Survived at pH 2.2 after 1.5 h • Able to grow in agar medium with 0.5% bile salt	NA	• Cell surface hydrophobic index 41.61% with hexadecan	• *St. aureus* (+); • *P. aeruginosa* (+) • *S. enterica* (-) • *E. coli* (-) • *E. hirae* (-)	Vancomycin (30 μg)^R, gentamicin (10 μg)^R; tetracycline (30 μg)^R; streptomycin (10 μg)^R ceftriaxone (30 μg)^S; chloramphenicol (30 μg)^S; amoxicillin(25 μg)^S; erythromycin (15 μg)^R; streptomycin (10 μg)^R	NA	β-Galactosidase (-) H_2O_2 production (6.26%)	Gebreselassie *et al.* (2016)

	Traditional fermenting green olives	• Survival rate of 67.33–81.04% at pH 3, 0.3% bile salt for 5 h in MRS medium	• Negative mucinolytic activity • No hemolytic, DNase or gelatinase activities • Negative α-chymotrypsin, β-glucuronidase, and N-acetyl-β-glucosaminidase	• Autoaggregation 13.15–33.63% • Hydrophobic index: 19.86–23.05% (with xylene)	Inhibition zone caused by cell free crude extract • *C. pelliculosa* (18.8–20.15 mm) • *L. innocua* (11.45–13.45 mm) • *M. luteus* (11.5–13.5 mm) • *S. aureus* (10.5–12.1 mm) • *E. coli* (11.75–14.1 mm • *P. aeruginosa* (10.8–12.3 mm)	Oxacillin (1 μg)$^{(R,S)}$, cephalothin (30 μg)^{R,S}, vancomycin (30 μg)$^{(R)}$, amoxicillin (25 μg)$^{(R,S)}$, erythromycin (15 μg) $^{(R,S)}$, ampicillin (10 μg^{R,S}, 25 μg^{R,S}), chloramphenicol (30 μg)$^{(R,S)}$, penicillin G (10 μg)$^{(R,S)}$	NA	β-Galactosidase activity (+) EPS production (+) Antioxidant 51–52%	Phoottosavako *et al.* (2015)
Lactobacillus brevis	Traditional fermenting green olives	• Survival rate of 68.12–82.06% at pH 3, 0.3% bile salt for 5 h in MRS medium	• Negative mucinolytic activity • No hemolytic, DNase or gelatinase activities • Negative α-chymotrypsin, β-glucuronidase, and N-acetyl-β-glucosaminidase	• Autoaggregation 12.11–30.46% • Hydrophobic 15.06–34.67% (with xylene)	Inhibition zone caused by cell free crude extract • *C. pelliculosa* (20.30–24.48 mm) • *L. innocua* (11.40–12.8 mm) • *M. luteus* (12.15–13.4 mm) • *S. aureus* (10.25–11.8 mm) • *E. coli* (11.7–13.4 mm • *P. aeruginosa* (10.2–12.4 mm)	Oxacillin (1 μg)$^{(R,S)}$, cephalothin (30 μg)^{R,S}, vancomycin (30 μg)$^{(R)}$, amoxicillin (25 μg)$^{(R,S)}$, erythromycin (15 μg) $^{(R,S)}$, ampicillin (10 μg^{S}, 25 μg^{S}), chloramphenicol (30 μg)$^{(R,S)}$, penicillin G (10 μg)$^{(R,S)}$	NA	β-Galactosidase activity (+) EPS production (+) Antioxidant 43.11 –52.54%	Phoottosavako *et al.* (2015)
	Channg, phab, dheli, kronto, pole, babroo	• Mild growth at pH 2.5, • Survived well at 2% bile salt	• Negative hemolytic activity	• Autoaggregation 12.19–16.10 % after 3 h and 59.35– 68.22% after 24 h • Co-aggregation with *L. monocytogenes* 5.84– 23.43% (3 h) and 50.19– 72.11% (24 h) • Hydrophobic index (%) to hexadecane (15–20 %), xylene (5–20%), octane (10–20%) and toluene (10–12%) • Adherence to HT29 cells 15.26%	Inhibition zone • *Staphylococcus aureus* (13.1–18.0 mm) • *Bacillus subtilis* (13.0–20.5 mm) • *Pseudomonas aeruginosa* (8.4–10.3 mm) • *Shigella dysenteriae* (12.4 –17.2 mm) • *Escherichia coli* (8.5–10.1 mm)	Penicillin G (10 Units)^{S,R}; clindamycin (2 μg)^{S}; co-trimoxazole (25 μg)^{R,S}; erythromycin (15 μg)^{S}; vancomycin (30 μg)^{R}; ampicillin (10 μg)^{S}; carbenicillin (100 μg)^{S}; cefotaxime (30 μg)^{S}; chloramphenicol (30 μg)^{S,R}; co-trimazine (25 μg)^{R}; gentamicin (10 μg)^{S}; norfloxacin (10 μg)^{S,R} oxacillin (5 μg)^{S}	NA	Heterofermentation	Meidong *et al.* (2017)

(Continued)

Table 2.6 (Continued)

Species	Sources	Characterization: Survival under gastrointestinal tract conditions	Safety for use in human nutrition	Colonization ability	Antimicrobial	Antibiotic sensitivity	in vitro anticancer models	Anonymous	Reference
Lactobacillus paracasei	Chilra (barley pancake), pole (fermented fried bread)	• Mild growth at pH 2.5 • Good survival at pH 2 and bile salt 2%	• Negative hemolytic activity	• Autoaggregation 9.15% after 3 h and 50.86 % after 24 h • Co-aggregation with *Listeria monocytogenes* (3 h) and 42.21% (24 h) • Hydrophobic index HI (%) to hexadecane (25%), xylene (12%), octane (18%) and toluene (9%) • Adherence to HT29 cells 21.21%	Inhibition zone • *Staphylococcus aureus* (16.3 mm) • *Bacillus subtilis* (17.2 mm) • *Pseudomonas aeruginosa* (9.2 mm) • *Shigella dysenteriae* (10.1 mm) • *Escherichia coli* (14.0 mm)	Penicillin G (10 Units)^{S},^{R}; clindamycin (2 μg)^{S}; co-trimoxazole (25 μg)^{S}; erythromycin (15 μg)^{S}; vancomycin (30 μg$^{)R}$; ampicillin (10 μg)^{S}; carbenicillin (100 μg)^{S}; cefotaxime (30 μg)^{S}; chloramphenicol (30 μg)^{R}; co-trimazine (25 μg)^{R}; gentamicin (10 μg)^{S}; norfloxacin (10 μg)^{R} oxacillin (5 μg)^{R}	NA	Homofermentative	Meidong *et al.* (2017)
Lactobacillus curvatus	Traditional fermented meat product (Greece)	• Reduction of <2.5 log after 4 h exposed to bile salts 0.5%	• Negative hemolytic activity	NA	• *Listeria monocytogenes* (-) • *Salmonella enterica subsp. enterica serovar* Enteritidis (-), • *Staphylococcus epidermidis* (-) • *E. coli* (-)	NA	NA		Park *et al.* (2009)
Lactobacillus sakei	Traditional fermented meat product (Greece)	• Survival rate at pH 2.5 after 3 h of 71.65–79.86% • Survival rate in 0.5% bile salt of 87.11–94.14% after 4 h	• Negative hemolytic activity	NA	• *Listeria monocytogenes* (-) • *Salmonella enterica* subsp. *enterica serovar* Enteritidis (-) • *Staphylococcus epidermidis* -) • *E. coli* (-)	MIC concentration (μg/mL) of different antibiotics: vancomycin (256–512), gentamicin (8–16), kanamycin (32), streptomycin (64), erythromycin (<1), tetracycline (2–4), chloramphenicol (0.5–1)	NA		Park *et al.* (2009)
Lactobacillus helveticus	Nakham (fermented fish), Meghalaya, India	• At pH 2.0, after 4 h, reduction of 4.5 logs • In 0.5% bile salt, after 4 h, log reduction from 7.33 to 4.27	• Negative hemolytic activity	• Co-aggregation with 5 test strains (*Salmonella typhi Staphylococcus aureus, Bacillus cereus, Listeria monocytogenes, Escherichia coli*) of 28.83–39.16% after 24 h • Cell surface hydrophobicity of 55% (hexadecane) • Cell autoaggregation of 62%	Inhibition zone: • *Bacillus cereus* ATCC 14459 (13 mm) • *Enterococcus faecalis* NCDC 115 (15 mm) • *Shigella dysenteriae* NCDC 107 (25 mm) • *Escherichia coli* ATCC 25922 (22 mm) • *Salmonella typhi* NCTC 5017(17 mm)	Azithromycin (15 μg)^{R}, ampicillin (10 μg)^{S}, vancomycin (30 μg)^{R}, methicillin (15 μg)^{S}, oxacillin (1 μg)^{S}; norfloxacin (10 μg)^{S}; kanamycin (30 μg)^{S}, streptomycin (10 μg)^{R}, erythromycin (15 μg)^{S}, tetracycline (30 μg)^{S}	NA	Cholesterol assimilation of 25% Inhibition of free radical of 60% (after 6 h). EPS production (500 mg/L) β-Glucosidase (+) α-Galactosidase (+)	Yu *et al.* (2015)

EPS, exopolysaccharide; MIC, minimum inhibitory concentration; NA, not applicable.*Source:* Based on Doan *et al.* (2012). Validation of MALDI-TOF MS for [illegible]id classification and in total phenolic content, including levels of gentisic acid, caffeic acid and ferulic acid, caused by fermentation has strong antioxidant effects. Application of *B. subtilis* P229 in soybean fermentation resulted in a fermented soybean extract with high total phenolic content of 74.56 GAE mg/g, which elevated antioxidant activity. In Uma Maheshwari *et al.*'s study (2019), anticancer activity of selected bacteria against lung cancer cell line A549 was tested in an MTT cytotoxicity assay. The results revealed that *B. velezensis* M4S1B1 showed potential activity against lung cancer cell line A549 with low IC50 values (402 μg/mL). Further, its toxic effect was analyzed based on morphological changes of cancer cell lines. Treatment with *B. velezensis* M4S1B1 cells showed greater morphological changes, including cellular shrinkage and membrane damage, than control cells on 48 h incubation, which confirmed the toxic effect of selected bacteria against lung cancer cell line A549.

Lactic acid bacteria strains isolated from traditional fermented products were characterized by several criteria relevant to their probiotic properties. In general, the criteria include tolerance to gastrointestinal conditions, colonization ability, antimicrobial activity, susceptibility to antibiotics, cancer cell interaction and other beneficial properties. Characteristics of some potential probiotic *Lactobacillus* species isolated from traditional fermented foods are described in Table 2.6 (studies since 2015).

Since 2015, most of characterized *Lactobacillus* species have been isolated from traditional fermented food from Asian countries such as Vietnam, India, Iran and China where there is a huge diversity of food products. These fermented foods, in fact, are valuable sources for a lot of beneficial microorganisms, not only for human health (probiotics) but also for many other biotechnology fields (e.g. lactic acid production, bacteriocin, peptide) and food processing. Among them, *L. plantarum* is the most abundant species in food products, because most products are of plant-related origin such as pickled vegetables and fermented cereals. Other species such as *L. fermentum*, *L. sakei*, *L. brevis* are less common but can be isolated from food sources. Depending on species, strains and isolation source, the characteristics of some LAB are different from others. The wide variety of characteristics of LAB from fermented foods is shown in Table 2.6.

For probiotic application, the first characteristic of LAB considered is resistance against gastrointestinal tract conditions such as low pH and presence of digestive enzymes and bile salts. To assess this feature, strains were incubated under low pH (2–5) and bile salt concentration of 0.1–0.6%. The bacteria cell number (log) or the culture turbidity was monitored during incubation. It can be seen that several strains grow well at pH 3 or higher, and some are resistant at pH 2.2–2.5 for a period of 1.5 2 h, equivalent to the retention time of food in the human stomach. However, at pH 2.0, very few strains can survive and grow. Regarding bile salt concentration, the strains of *Lactobacillus* are tolerant up to 0.5–0.6% after 6 h of incubation with a survival rate of over 90%. Some strains are able to survive at 1–2% bile salt concentration.

Colonization ability, especially adhesion of bacteria to mucus and epithelial cells, is an important indicator of the probiotic cells' ability to interact with the host. This ability is defined by the cell surface properties of *Lactobacillus* strains. The cell surface characteristics were assessed through the hydrophobicity index (interaction with hydrocarbons such as hexadecane, toluene, octane and xylene), self-autoaggregation or co-aggregation with other bacteria (especially pathogens). In addition, the ability to interact with intestinal cells is considered. The hydrophobicity of *Lactobacillus* strains assessed with hydrocarbons, mainly hexadecane and xylene, showed that for strains from different species, from the same food source, this value varied from a few to over 50%. These *Lactobacillus* strains also exhibited relatively good autoaggregation: 10–20% after 3 h and 50–80% after 24 h. Among them, autoaggregation can reach 80% in 4 h with some strains. Moreover, some authors have shown that *Lactobacillus* can adhere to HT29 cells, for example at the rate of 20% (Meidong *et al.* 2017). Similarly, some strains have shown the ability to adhere to human intestinal Caco-2 cells (Doan *et al.* 2012).

Lactic acid bacteria, including *Lactobacillus*, often produce acids and bacteriocin during growth, so they can inhibit other pathogenic bacteria, molds and yeasts. In general, *Lactobacillus* species obtained from fermented food sources mostly inhibit or kill food-borne pathogens such as *Staphylococcus aureus*, *Bacillus subtilis*, *Pseudomonas aeruginosa*, *Shigella dysenteriae*, *Escherichia coli*, *Salmonella typhi* and *L. monocytogenes*. Growth of *Lactobacillus* strains can result in an inhibition zone on agar medium or inhibit the growth of pathogens in liquid media. The inhibitory effect is due to the formation of organic acids (lactic acid, acetic acid) (mainly for Gram-negative bacteria) and bacteriocins such as plantaricin and sakacin (for Gram-positive bacteria). The inhibition zone on agar media produced was therefore larger with Gram-positive bacteria than for Gram-negative bacteria. Of course, this antimicrobial effect varies widely between species and between strains within species from different sources. For example, with *P. aeruginosa* (Gram negative), many strains do not have an inhibitory effect. Surprisingly, *L. curvatus* and *L. sakei* (isolated from Greek fermented meat) were shown not to have antibacterial properties against *L. monocytogenes*, *Salmonella enterica* subsp. *enterica* serovar Enteritidis, *Staphylococcus epidermidis* or *E. coli* (Park *et al.* 2009). *Lactobacillus* strains also showed co-aggregation with pathogens. When being incubated with a pathogen such as *Salmonella typhi*, *Staphylococcus aureus*, *Bacillus cereus*, *L. monocytogenes* or *E. coli*, after 24 h, the co-aggregation rates were 20–35% depending on the strain. Especially with *L. monocytogenes*, some *Lactobacillus* strains showed a co-aggregation rate of up to 50% after 24 h. This characteristic is supportive for antimicrobial properties of probiotics against foodborne pathogens, thus preventing the negative effect of "free" pathogens to the host.

Antibiotic susceptibility/resistance of *Lactobacillus* strains isolated from fermented food was also assessed. Various common antibiotics were used including penicillin, clindamycin, co-trimoxazole, erythromycin, vancomycin, ampicillin, carbenicillin, cefotaxime, chloramphenicol, co-trimazine, gentamicin, norfloxacin, oxacillin, streptomycin, tetracycline, kanamycin, etc. The resistance to antibiotics depends on *Lactobacillus* strain and antibiotic concentration. There is no strain that is resistant to all the antibiotics mentioned. Vancomycin is shown to be the weakest of the antibiotics. At a concentration of 30 μg/mL, it did not inhibit the growth of any *Lactobacillus*. In contrast, ampicillin exhibited the strongest effect. At a concentration of 10 μg/mL, this antibiotic inhibited most tested strains of *Lactobacillus*.

The ability to inhibit cancer cells was less investigated in the reviewed studies, except for *L. fermentum* HA6, which has been shown to inhibit (in vitro) the proliferation of some types of cancer cells (Doan *et al.* 2012) (see Table 2.6). It is possible that the formation of short-chain organic acids contributes to this effect, as some studies have shown previously.

In addition to such properties, other beneficial properties of *Lactobacillus* derived from traditional fermented foods have been considered, such as the ability to produce the enzyme lactase or β-galactosidase, which is an important enzyme in the dairy industry, as well as the ability to assimilate cholesterol, exopolysaccharide production and antioxidant activity (see Table 2.6). These properties enhance the value of *Lactobacillus* strains.

Last, but not least, for human application the safety properties of *Lactobacillus* strains are also important. Most *Lactobacillus* strains were demonstrated to have negative hemolytic activity (see Table 2.6).

2.6 Conclusion

Traditional fermented foods in tropical countries with a source of diverse microorganisms, including probiotic ones which confer positive health effects on humans and animals, have been explored. Isolation of probiotic microorganisms can be done using the most used medium (i.e. MRS), although modifications have been made to selectively isolate the targeted probiotic microorganisms. Recently developed high-throughput isolation and identification strategies result in massive information on beneficial organisms present on fermented foods and substantially increase the number of hard-to-culture organisms in axenic cultures which may have potential probiotic capabilities. Resistance to gastrointestinal stress, ability to adhere to the epithelial cells and antimicrobial and antagonistic activities are among the important characteristics of probiotic microorganisms. Such activities need to be determined via well-established methodologies before an isolated strain can be considered as a probiotic to be used on humans and animals.

Acknowledgements

This work was supported by grants from The Ministry of Education and Training (MOET), Vietnam, through the project entitled "Genetic preservation of lactic acid bacteria capable of producing PepX and *Bacillus subtilis* capable of producing Nattokinase and excreting low PGA", The Ministry of Science and Technology (MOST) Vietnam, through the project entitled "Study on biological characteristics and activity of *Bacillus* strains to produce safe probiotic preparations for animal husbandry" (grant number ĐTĐL.CN-17/19), and Vietnam Academy of Scienceand Technology (VAST) through the grant number CN40SH.01/18-21.

References

Adimpong, D.B., Nielsen, D.S., Sørensen, K.I., Derkx, P.M.F. and Jespersen, L. (2012). Genotypic characterization and safety assessment of lactic acid bacteria from indigenous African fermented food products. *BMC Microbiology*, 12(1): 75.

Aguilar, G., Morlon-Guyot, J., Trejo-Aguilar, B. and Guyot, J.P. (2000). Purification and characterization of an extracellular α-amylase produced by Lactobacillus manihotivorans LMG 18010T, an amylolytic lactic acid bacterium. *Enzyme and Microbial Technology*, 27(6): 406–413.

Alegría, A., González, R., Díaz, M. and Mayo, B. (2011). Assessment of microbial populations dynamics in a blue cheese by culturing and denaturing gradient gel electrophoresis. *Current Microbiology*, 62(3): 888–893.

Ampe, F., Omar, N. ben and Guyot, J.-P. (1999). Culture-independent quantification of physiologically-active microbial groups in fermented foods using rRNA-targeted oligonucleotide probes: application to pozol, a Mexican lactic acid fermented maize dough. *Journal of Applied Microbiology*, 87(1): 131–140.

Angelakis, E., Million, M., Henry, M. and Raoult, D. (2011). Rapid and accurate bacterial identification in probiotics and yoghurts by MALDI-TOF mass spectrometry. *Journal of Food Science*, 76(8): M568–572.

Angelin, J. and Kavitha, M. (2020). Exopolysaccharides from probiotic bacteria and their health potential. *International Journal of Biological Macromolecules*, 162: 853–865.

Angelov, A.I., Petrova, G., Angelov, A.D., Stefanova, P., Bokossa, I.Y., Tchekessi, C.K.C., Marco, M.L. and Gotcheva, V. (2017). Molecular identification of yeasts and lactic acid bacteria involved in the production of Beninese fermented food degue. *The Open Biotechnology Journal*, 11(1): 94–104.

Argyri, A.A., Zoumpopoulou, G., Karatzas, K.-A.G., Tsakalidou, E., Nychas, G.-J.E., Panagou, E.Z. and Tassou, C.C. (2013). Selection of potential probiotic lactic acid bacteria from fermented olives by in vitro tests. *Food Microbiology*, 33(2): 282–291.

Aubert, C. (1985). *Les aliments fermentés traditionnels. Une richesse méconnue*. Terre Vivante.

Bao, Q., Song, Y., Xu, H., Yu, J., Zhang, W., Menghe, B., Zhang, H. and Sun, Z. (2016). Multilocus sequence typing of Lactobacillus casei isolates from naturally fermented foods in China and Mongolia. *Journal of Dairy Science*, 99(7): 5202–5213.

Baselga, I., Zafra, O., Pérez Lago, E., Francisco-Álvarez, R., Rodriguez-Tarduchy, G. and Santos, C. (2017). An AFLP based method for the detection and identification of indigenous yeast in complex must samples without a microbiological culture. *International Journal of Food Microbiology*, 241: 89–97.

Benito, M.J., Martín, A., Aranda, E., Pérez-Nevado, F., Ruiz-Moyano, S. and Córdoba, M.G. (2007). Characterization and selection of autochthonous lactic acid bacteria isolated from traditional Iberian dry-fermented Salchichón and Chorizo sausages. *Journal of Food Science*, 72(6): M193–201.

Benkerroum, N., Misbah, M., Sandine, W.E. and Elaraki, A.T. (1993). Development and use of a selective medium for isolation of Leuconostoc spp. from vegetables and dairy products. *Applied and Environmental Microbiology*, 59(2): 607–609.

Bilen, M., Dufour, J.-C., Lagier, J.-C., Cadoret, F., Daoud, Z., Dubourg, G. and Raoult, D. (2018). The contribution of culturomics to the repertoire of isolated human bacterial and archaeal species. *Microbiome*, 6(1): 94.

Blandino, A., Al-Aseeri, M.E., Pandiella, S.S., Cantero, D. and Webb, C. (2003). Cereal-based fermented foods and beverages. *Food Research International*, 36(6): 527–543.

Borah, T., Gogoi, B., Khataniar, A., Gogoi, M., Das, A. and Borah, D. (2019). Probiotic characterization of indigenous Bacillus velezensis strain DU14 isolated from Apong, a traditionally fermented rice beer of Assam. *Biocatalysis and Agricultural Biotechnology*, 18: 101008.

Bujnakova, D. and Kmet, V. (2002). Aggregation of animal Lactobacilli with O157 enterohemorrhagic Escherichia coli. *Journal of Veterinary Medicine, Series B*, 49(3): 152–154.

Chantawannakul, P., Oncharoen, A., Klanbut, K., Chukeatirote, E. and Lumyong, S. (2002). Characterization of proteases of Bacillus subtilis strain 38 isolated from traditionally fermented soybean in Northern Thailand. *ScienceAsia*, 28(3): 241.

Chao, S.-H., Tomii, Y., Watanabe, K. and Tsai, Y.-C. (2008). Diversity of lactic acid bacteria in fermented brines used to make stinky tofu. *International Journal of Food Microbiology*, 123(1–2): 134–141.

Charalampopoulos, D., Pandiella, S.S. and Webb, C. (2003). Evaluation of the effect of malt, wheat and barley extracts on the viability of potentially probiotic lactic acid bacteria under acidic conditions. *International Journal of Food Microbiology*, 82(2): 133–141.

Coda, R., Rizzello, C.G., Trani, A. and Gobbetti, M. (2011). Manufacture and characterization of functional emmer beverages fermented by selected lactic acid bacteria. *Food Microbiology*, 28(3): 526–536.

Comi, G., Urso, R., Iacumin, L., Rantsiou, K., Cattaneo, P., Cantoni, C. and Cocolin, L. (2005). Characterisation of naturally fermented sausages produced in the North East of Italy. *Meat Science*, 69(3): 381–392.

Cummings, P.J., Ahmed, R., Durocher, J.A., Jessen, A., Vardi, T. and Obom, K.M. (2013). Pyrosequencing for microbial identification and characterization. *Journal of Visualized Experiments : JoVE*, (78): e50405.

Damnjanovic, D., Harvey, M. and Bridge, W.J. (2019). Application of colony BOXA2R-PCR for the differentiation and identification of lactic acid COCCI. *Food Microbiology*, 82: 277–286.

De Bruyne, K., Camu, N., De Vuyst, L. and Vandamme, P. (2010). Weissella fabaria sp. nov., from a Ghanaian cocoa fermentation. *International Journal of Systematic and Evolutionary Microbiology*, 60(Pt 9): 1999–2005.

De Filippis, F., Pasolli, E. and Ercolini, D. (2020). The food-gut axis: lactic acid bacteria and their link to food, the gut microbiome and human health. *FEMS Microbiology Reviews*, 44(4): 454–489.

De Man, J.C., Rogosa, M. and Sharpe, M.E. (1960). A medium for the cultivation of Lactobacilli. *Journal of Applied Bacteriology*, 23(1): 130–135.

de Ponzzes-Gomes, C.M.P.B.S., de Mélo, D.L.F.M., Santana, C.A., Pereira, G.E., Mendonça, M.O.C., Gomes, F.C.O., Oliveira, E.S., Barbosa, A.M.J., Trindade, R.C. and Rosa, C.A. (2014). Saccharomyces cerevisiae and non-Saccharomyces yeasts in grape varieties of the São Francisco Valley. *Brazilian Journal of Microbiology : [Publication of the Brazilian Society for Microbiology]*, 45(2): 411–416.

Devanthi, P.V.P. and Gkatzionis, K. (2019). Soy sauce fermentation: Microorganisms, aroma formation, and process modification. *Food Research International*, 120: 364–374.

Di Lena, M., Quero, G.M., Santovito, E., Verran, J., De Angelis, M. and Fusco, V. (2015). A selective medium for isolation and accurate enumeration of Lactobacillus casei-group members in probiotic milks and dairy products. *International Dairy Journal*, 47: 27–36.

Diaz, M., Ladero, V., Redruello, B., Sanchez-Llana, E., del Rio, B., Fernandez, M., Martin, M.C. and Alvarez, M.A. (2016). A PCR-DGGE method for the identification of histamine-producing bacteria in cheese. *Food Control*, 63: 216–223.

Doan, N.T.L., Van Hoorde, K., Cnockaert, M., De Brandt, E., Aerts, M., Le Thanh, B. and Vandamme, P. (2012). Validation of MALDI-TOF MS for rapid classification and identification of lactic acid bacteria, with a focus on isolates from traditional fermented foods in Northern Vietnam. *Letters in Applied Microbiology*, 55(4): 265–273.

Duar, R.M., Lin, X.B., Zheng, J., Martino, M.E., Grenier, T., Pérez-Muñoz, M.E., Leulier, F., Gänzle, M. and Walter, J. (2017). Lifestyles in transition: evolution and natural history of the genus Lactobacillus. *FEMS Microbiology Reviews*, 41(Supp_1): S27–48.

Dušková, M., Šedo, O., Kšicová, K., Zdráhal, Z. and Karpíšková, R. (2012). Identification of lactobacilli isolated from food by genotypic methods and MALDI-TOF MS. *International Journal of Food Microbiology*, 159(2): 107–114.

Elshaghabee, F.M.F., Rokana, N., Gulhane, R.D., Sharma, C. and Panwar, H. (2017). Bacillus As Potential Probiotics: Status, Concerns, and Future Perspectives. *Frontiers in Microbiology*, 8: 1490.

Evans, J.B. and Niven, C.F.J. (1951). Nutrition of the heterofermentative Lactobacilli that cause greening of cured meat products. *Journal of Bacteriology*, 62(5): 599–603.

Falade, A.T., Emmambux, M.N., Buys, E.M. and Taylor, J.R.N. (2014). Improvement of maize bread quality through modification of dough rheological properties by lactic acid bacteria fermentation. *Journal of Cereal Science*, 60(3): 471–476.

FAO/WHO (2001). Health and nutritional properties of probiotics in food including powder milk with live lactic acid bacteria. Amerian Córdoba Park Hotel, Córdoba, Argentina, 1–4 October 2001.

Fei, Y., Li, L., Chen, L., Zheng, Y. and Yu, B. (2018). High-throughput sequencing and culture-based approaches to analyze microbial diversity associated with chemical changes in naturally fermented tofu whey, a traditional Chinese tofu-coagulant. *Food Microbiology*, 76: 69–77.

Fijan, S. (2016). Antimicrobial effect of probiotics against common pathogens. In: *Probiotics and Prebiotics in Human Nutrition and Health* (ed. V. Rao and L. Rao), 191–221. doi: DOI: 10.5772/63141

Fleet, G.H. (1999). Microorganisms in food ecosystems. *International Journal of Food Microbiology*, 50(1–2): 101–117.

Franz, C.M.A.P., Huch, M., Mathara, J.M., Abriouel, H., Benomar, N., Reid, G., Galvez, A., and Holzapfel, W.H. (2014). African fermented foods and probiotics. *International Journal of Food Microbiology*, 190: 84–96.

Fu, D., Ryan, E.P., Huang, J., Liu, Z., Weir, T.L., Snook, R.L. and Ryan, T.P. (2011). Fermented Camellia sinensis, Fu Zhuan Tea, regulates hyperlipidemia and transcription factors involved in lipid catabolism. *Food Research International*, 44(9): 2999–3005.

Fusco, V., Quero, G.M., Chieffi, D. and Franz, C.M.A.P. (2016). Identification of Lactobacillus brevis using a species-specific AFLP-derived marker. *International Journal of Food Microbiology*, 232: 90–94.

Garcia, E.F., Luciano, W.A., Xavier, D.E., da Costa, W.C.A., de Sousa Oliveira, K., Franco, O.L., de Morais Júnior, M.A., Lucena, B.T.L., Picão, R.C., Magnani, M., Saarela, M. and de Souza, E.L. (2016). Identification of lactic acid bacteria in fruit pulp processing byproducts and potential probiotic properties of selected Lactobacillus strains. *Frontiers in Microbiology*, 7: 1371.

Gebremariam, M.M., Hassani, A., Zarnkow, M. and Becker, T. (2015). Investigation of fermentation conditions for teff (Eragrostis tef) malt-wort by Lactobacillus amylolyticus. *LWT - Food Science and Technology*, 61(1): 164–171.

Gebreselassie, N., Abay, F. and Beyene, F. (2016). Biochemical and molecular identification and characterization of lactic acid bacteria and yeasts isolated from Ethiopian naturally fermented buttermilk. *Journal of Food Science and Technology* 53(1): 184–196.

Granier, A., Goulet, O. and Hoarau, C. (2013). Fermentation products: Immunological effects on human and animal models. *Pediatric Research*, 74(2): 238–244.

Greub, G. (2012). Culturomics: a new approach to study the human microbiome. *Clinical Microbiology and Infection: The Official Publication of the European Society of Clinical Microbiology and Infectious Diseases*, 18(12): 1157–1159.

Hammes, W.P., Bantleon, A. and Min, S. (1990). Lactic acid bacteria in meat fermentation. *FEMS Microbiology Letters*, 87(1): 165–173.

Illeghems, K., De Vuyst, L., Papalexandratou, Z. and Weckx, S. (2012). Phylogenetic analysis of a spontaneous cocoa bean fermentation metagenome reveals new insights into its bacterial and fungal community diversity. *PLOS ONE*, 7(5): e38040.

Jeon, H.-L., Yang, S.-J., Son, S.-H., Kim, W.-S., Lee, N.-K. and Paik, H.-D. (2018). Evaluation of probiotic Bacillus subtilis P229 isolated from cheonggukjang and its application in soybean fermentation. *LWT*, 97: 94–99.

Jeyaram, K., Romi, W., Singh, T.A., Devi, A.R. and Devi, S.S. (2010). Bacterial species associated with traditional starter cultures used for fermented bamboo shoot production in Manipur state of India. *International Journal of Food Microbiology*, 143(1–2): 1–8.

Kalaivani, M., Sabitha, R., Kalaiselvan, V. and Rajasekaran, A. (2010). Health benefits and clinical impact of major nutrient, red yeast rice: a review. *Food and Bioprocess Technology*, 3(3): 333–339.

Katina, K., Arendt, E., Liukkonen, K.-H., Autio, K., Flander, L. and Poutanen, K. (2005). Potential of sourdough for healthier cereal products. *Trends in Food Science & Technology*, 16(1): 104–112.

Kaur, J., Lee, S., Park, Y.-S. and Sharma, A. (2017). RAPD analysis of Leuconostoc mesenteroides strains associated with vegetables and food products from Korea. *LWT*, 77: 383–388.

Kavitha, M., Raja, M. and Perumal, P. (2018). Evaluation of probiotic potential of Bacillus spp. isolated from the digestive tract of freshwater fish Labeo calbasu (Hamilton, 1822). *Aquaculture Reports*, 11: 59–69.

Khochamit, N., Siripornadulsil, S., Sukon, P. and Siripornadulsil, W. (2015). Antibacterial activity and genotypic-phenotypic characteristics of bacteriocin-producing Bacillus subtilis KKU213: potential as a probiotic strain. *Microbiological Research*, 170: 36–50.

Kim, E., Yang, S.-M., Lim, B., Park, S.H., Rackerby, B. and Kim, H.-Y. (2020). Design of PCR assays to specifically detect and identify 37 Lactobacillus species in a single 96 well plate. *BMC Microbiology*, 20(1): 96.

Kim, H.J., Kim, M.J., Turner, T.L., Kim, B.S., Song, K.M., Yi, S.H. and Lee, M.K. (2014). Pyrosequencing analysis of microbiota reveals that lactic acid bacteria are dominant in Korean flat fish fermented food, gajami-sikhae. *Bioscience, Biotechnology and Biochemistry*, 78(9): 1611–1618.

Kim, Y.-M. and Heyman, H.M. (2018). Mass spectrometry-based metabolomics. *Methods in Molecular Biology (Clifton, N.J.)*, 1775: 107–118.

Kuda, T., Kaneko, N., Yano, T. and Mori, M. (2010). Induction of superoxide anion radical scavenging capacity in Japanese white radish juice and milk by Lactobacillus plantarum isolated from aji-narezushi and kaburazushi. *Food Chemistry*, 120(2): 517–522.

La Anh, N. (2015). Health-promoting microbes in traditional Vietnamese fermented foods: A review. *Food Science and Human Wellness*, 4(4): 147–161.

Lagier, J.-C., Million, M., Togo, A.H., Khelaifia, S. and Raoult, D. (2019). Culturomics provides critical prokaryote strains for anti-Listeria and anti-cancer probiotics. *International Journal of Antimicrobial Agents*, 54(4): 407–409.

Lapierre, L., Undeland, P. and Cox, L.J. (1992). Lithium chloride-sodium propionate agar for the enumeration of bifidobacteria in fermented dairy products. *Journal of Dairy Science*, 75(5): 1192–1196.

Lebert, I., Leroy, S., Giammarinaro, P., Lebert, A., Chacornac, J.P., Bover-Cid, S., Vidal-carou, M.C. and Talon, R. (2007). Diversity of microorganisms in the environment and dry fermented sausages of small traditional French processing units. *Meat Science*, 76(1): 112–122.

Lee, C.-H. (1997). Lactic acid fermented foods and their benefits in Asia. *Food Control*, 8(5): 259–269.

Lee, D., Kim, S., Cho, J., and Kim, J. (2008). Microbial population dynamics and temperature changes during fermentation of kimjang kimchi. *The Journal of Microbiology*, 46(5):590–93.

Lee, K.K. and Teo, E.C. (2005). Material sensitivity study on lumbar motion segment (L2-L3) under sagittal plane loadings using probabilistic method. *Journal of Spinal Disorders & Techniques*, 18(2): 163–170.

Lee, S., Lee, J., Jin, Y.-I., Jeong, J.-C., Chang, Y.H., Lee, Y., Jeong, Y. and Kim, M. (2017). Probiotic characteristics of Bacillus strains isolated from Korean traditional soy sauce. *LWT - Food Science and Technology*, 79: 518–524.

Leite, A.M.O., Mayo, B., Rachid, C.T.C.C., Peixoto, R.S., Silva, J.T., Paschoalin, V.M.F. and Delgado, S. (2012). Assessment of the microbial diversity of Brazilian kefir grains by PCR-DGGE and pyrosequencing analysis. *Food Microbiology*, 31(2): 215–221.

Lertcanawanichakul, M. and Sawangnop, S. (2008). A comparison of two methods used for measuring the antagonistic activity of Bacillus species. *Walailak Journal of Science and Technology (WJST)*, 5(2): 161–171.

Liang, H., Zhang, A., Wu, Z., Liu, C. and Zhang, W. (2016). Characterization of microbial community during the fermentation of Chinese homemade paocai, a traditional fermented vegetable food. *Food Science and Technology Research*, 22(4): 467–475.

Lortal, S., Licitra, G. and Valence, F. (2014). Wooden tools: reservoirs of microbial biodiversity in traditional cheesemaking. *Microbiology Spectrum*, 2(1): CM-0008–2012.

Lücke, F.-K. (2000). Utilization of microbes to process and preserve meat. *Meat Science*, 56(2): 105–115.

Macori, G. and Cotter, P.D. (2018). Novel insights into the microbiology of fermented dairy foods. *Current Opinion in Biotechnology*, 49: 172–178.

Manhar, A.K., Saikia, D., Bashir, Y., Mech, R.K., Nath, D., Konwar, B.K. and Mandal, M. (2015). in vitro evaluation of celluloytic Bacillus amyloliquefaciens AMS1 isolated from traditional fermented soybean (Churpi) as an animal probiotic. *Research in Veterinary Science*, 99: 149–156.

Marco, M.L., Heeney, D., Binda, S., Cifelli, C.J., Cotter, P.D., Foligné, B., Gänzle, M., Kort, R., Pasin, G., Pihlanto, A., Smid, E.J. and Hutkins, R. (2017). Health benefits of fermented foods: microbiota and beyond. *Current Opinion in Biotechnology*, 44: 94–102.

Martínez Leal, J., Valenzuela Suárez, L., Jayabalan, R., Huerta Oros, J. and Escalante-Aburto, A. (2018). A review on health benefits of kombucha nutritional compounds and metabolites. *CyTA - Journal of Food*, 16(1): 390–399.

Martino, M.E., Bayjanov, J.R., Caffrey, B.E., Wels, M., Joncour, P., Hughes, S., Gillet, B., Kleerebezem, M., van Hijum, S.A.F.T. and Leulier, F. (2016). Nomadic lifestyle of Lactobacillus plantarum revealed by comparative genomics of 54 strains isolated from different habitats. *Environmental Microbiology*, 18(12): 4974–4989.

Meidong, R., Doolgindachbaporn, S., Jamjan, W., Sakai, K., Tashiro, Y., Okugawa, Y. and Tongpim, S. (2017). A novel probiotic Bacillus siamensis B44v isolated from Thai pickled vegetables (Phak-dong) for potential use as a feed supplement in aquaculture. *The Journal of General and Applied Microbiology*, 63(4): 246–253.

Mensah, P. (1997). Fermentation — the key to food safety assurance in Africa? *Food Control*, 8(5): 271–278.

Mozzi, F., Ortiz, M.E., Bleckwedel, J., De Vuyst, L. and Pescuma, M. (2013). Metabolomics as a tool for the comprehensive understanding of fermented and functional foods with lactic acid bacteria. *Food Research International*, 54(1): 1152–1161.

Nacef, M., Chevalier, M., Chollet, S., Drider, D. and Flahaut, C. (2017). MALDI-TOF mass spectrometry for the identification of lactic acid bacteria isolated from a French cheese: The Maroilles. *International Journal of Food Microbiology*, 247: 2–8.

Nagaraju, V.D. and Manohar, B. (2000). Rheology and particle size changes during Idli fermentation. *Journal of Food Engineering*, 43(3): 167–171.

Nebra, Y. and Blanch, A.R. (1999). A new selective medium for Bifidobacterium spp. *Applied and Environmental Microbiology*, 65(11): 5173–5176.

Nguyen, T.X., Bui, H.T.T. and Pham, D.T. (2011). Study on quality of fish sauce at production facilities in Vietnam. *Vietnam Journal of Science and Technology*, 49(6A): 120–126.

Noonpakdee, W., Santivarangkna, C., Jumriangrit, P., Sonomoto, K. and Panyim, S. (2003). Isolation of nisin-producing Lactococcus lactis WNC 20 strain from nham, a traditional Thai fermented sausage. *International Journal of Food Microbiology*, 81(2): 137–145.

Nout, M.J.R. (2003). Traditional fermented products from Africa, Latin America and Asia. In: *Yeasts in Food, Woodhead Publishing Series in Food Science, Technology and Nutrition* (ed. T. Boekhout and V. Robert), 451–473. Woodhead Publishing. doi: https://doi.org/10.1533/9781845698485.451

Oki, K., Dugersuren, J., Demberel, S. and Watanabe, K. (2014). Pyrosequencing analysis of the microbial diversity of airag, khoormog and tarag, traditional fermented dairy products of Mongolia. *Bioscience of Microbiota, Food and Health*, 33(2): 53–64.

Oliveira, M., Ferreira, V., Magalhães, R. and Teixeira, P. (2018). Biocontrol strategies for Mediterranean-style fermented sausages. *Food Research International*, 103: 438–449.

Oyewole, O.B. (1997). Lactic fermented foods in Africa and their benefits. *Food Control*, 8(5):289–97.

Palla, M., Cristani, C., Giovannetti, M. and Agnolucci, M. (2017). Identification and characterization of lactic acid bacteria and yeasts of PDO Tuscan bread sourdough by culture dependent and independent methods. *International Journal of Food Microbiology*, 250: 19–26.

Park, E.-J., Chang, H.-W., Kim, K.-H., Nam, Y.-D., Roh, S.W. and Bae, J.-W. (2009) .Application of quantitative real-time PCR for enumeration of total bacterial, archaeal, and yeast populations in kimchi. *Journal of Microbiology (Seoul, Korea)*, 47(6): 682–685.

Park, K.Y., Jeong, J.K., Lee, Y.-E. and Daily, J.W. (2014). Health benefits of kimchi (Korean fermented vegetables) as a probiotic food. *Journal of Medicinal Food*, 17(1): 6–20.

Park, K.Y. and Jeong, J.K. (2016). *Kimchi (Korean fermented vegetables) as a Probiotic Food*. Elsevier. doi: 10.1016/B978-0-12-802189-7.00026-5

Pasolli, E., De Filippis, F., Mauriello, I.E., Cumbo, F., Walsh, A.M., Leech, J., Cotter, P.D., Segata, N. and Ercolini, D. (2020). Large-scale genome-wide analysis links lactic acid bacteria from food with the gut microbiome. *Nature Communications*, 11(1): 2610.

Patel, A.K., Ahire, J.J., Pawar, S.P., Chaudhari, B.L. and Chincholkar, S.B. (2009). Comparative accounts of probiotic characteristics of Bacillus spp. isolated from food wastes. *Food Research International*, 42(4): 505–510.

Petrosino, J.F., Highlander, S., Luna, R.A., Gibbs, R.A. and Versalovic, J. (2009). Metagenomic pyrosequencing and microbial identification. *Clinical Chemistry*, 55(5): 856–866.

Phoottosavako, M., Keeratipibul, S., Techo, S. and Tanasupawat, S. (2015). Identification and characterization of lipolytic bacteria from Thai fermented foods. *Malaysian Journal of Microbiology*, 11(3): 231–239.

Reid, G., McGroarty, J.A., Angotti, R. and Cook, R.L. (1988). Lactobacillus inhibitor production against Escherichia coli and coaggregation ability with uropathogens. *Canadian Journal of Microbiology*, 34(3): 344–351.

Rizo, J., Guillén, D., Farrés, A., Díaz-Ruiz, G., Sánchez, S., Wacher, C. and Rodríguez-Sanoja, R. (2020). Omics in traditional vegetable fermented foods and beverages. *Critical Reviews in Food Science and Nutrition*, 60(5): 791–809.

Ruas-Madiedo, P., Medrano, M., Salazar, N., De Los Reyes-Gavilán, C.G., Pérez, P.F. and Abraham, A.G. (2010). Exopolysaccharides produced by Lactobacillus and Bifidobacterium strains abrogate in vitro the cytotoxic effect of bacterial toxins on eukaryotic cells. *Journal of Applied Microbiology*, 109(6): 2079–2086.

Salas-Jara, M.J., Sanhueza, E.A., Retamal-Díaz, A., González, C., Urrutia, H. and García, A. (2016). Probiotic Lactobacillus fermentum UCO-979C biofilm formation on AGS and Caco-2 cells and Helicobacter pylori inhibition. *Biofouling*, 32(10): 1245–1257.

Salmerón, I., Thomas, K. and Pandiella, S.S. (2015). Effect of potentially probiotic lactic acid bacteria on the physicochemical composition and acceptance of fermented cereal beverages. *Journal of Functional Foods*, 15: 106–115.

Schillinger, U. and Lücke, F.K. (1989). Antibacterial activity of Lactobacillus sake isolated from meat. *Applied and Environmental Microbiology*, 55(8): 1901–1906.

Schillinger, U., Yousif, N.M.K., Sesar, L. and Franz, C.M.A.P. (2003). Use of group-specific and RAPD-PCR analyses for rapid differentiation of Lactobacillus strains from probiotic yogurts. *Current Microbiology*, 47(6): 453–456.

Schuller, D., Pereira, L., Alves, H., Cambon, B., Dequin, S. and Casal, M. (2007). Genetic characterization of commercial Saccharomyces cerevisiae isolates recovered from vineyard environments. *Yeast (Chichester, England)*, 24(8): 625– 636.

Shah, N.J. and Swami, O.C. (2017). Role of probiotics in diabetes: A review of their rationale and efficacy. *EMJ Diabetes*, 5(1): 104–110.

Singhal, N., Kumar, M., Kanaujia, P.K. and Virdi, J.S. (2015). MALDI-TOF mass spectrometry: an emerging technology for microbial identification and diagnosis. *Frontiers in Microbiology*, 6: 791.

Stackebrandt, E. and Embley, T.M. (2000). Diversity of uncultured microorganisms in the environment. In: *Nonculturable microorganisms in the Environment* (ed. R.R. Colwell and D.J. Grimes),. 57–75. Boston, MA: Springer US. doi: 10.1007/978-1-4757-0271-2_5

Steinkraus, K.H. (1983). Indigenous fermented foods involving an acid fermentation/Acid fermented cereal gruel. In: *Handbook of Indigenous Fermented Foods,* 189–218. New York: Mariel Dekkes.

Steinkraus, K.H. (1997). Classification of fermented foods: worldwide review of household fermentation techniques. *Food Control*, 8(5): 311–317.

Steinkraus, K.H. (2004). Origin and history of food fermentations. In: *Handbook of Food and Beverage Fermentation Technology* (ed. Y. H. Hui, L. Meunier-Goddik, J. Josephsen, W.-K. Nip and P. S. Stanfield), 1–9. CRC Press.

Stradwick, L., Inglis, D., Kelly, J. and Pickering, G. (2017). Development and application of assay for determining β-glucosidase activity in human saliva. *Flavour*, 6(1): 1.

Sun, Z., Harris, H.M.B., McCann, A., Guo, C., Argimón, S., Zhang, W., Yang, X., Jeffery, I.B., Cooney, J.C., Kagawa, T.F., Liu, W., Song, Y., Salvetti, E., Wrobel, A., Rasinkangas, P., Parkhill, J., Rea, M.C., O'Sullivan, O., Ritari, J., Douillard, F.P., Paul Ross, R., Yang, R., Briner, A.E., Felis, G.E., de Vos, W.M., Barrangou, R., Klaenhammer, T.R., Caufield, P.W., Cui, Y., Zhang, H. and O'Toole, P.W. (2015). Expanding the biotechnology potential of lactobacilli through comparative genomics of 213 strains and associated genera. *Nature Communications*, 6(1): 8322.

Surh, J., Kim, Y.-K.L. and Kwon, H. (2008). Korean fermented foods: Kimchi and Doenjang. In: *Handbook of Fermented Functional Foods* (ed E.R. Farnsworth). CRC Press.

Sutula, J., Coulthwaite, L. and Verran, J. (2012). Culture media for differential isolation of Lactobacillus casei Shirota from oral samples. *Journal of Microbiological Methods*, 90(1): 65–71.

Takahashi, M., Masaki, K., Mizuno, A. and Goto-Yamamoto, N. (2014). Modified COLD-PCR for detection of minor microorganisms in wine samples during the fermentation. *Food Microbiology*, 39: 74–80.

Tamang, B., Tamang, J.P., Schillinger, U., Franz, C.M.A.P., Gores, M. and Holzapfel, W.H. (2008). Phenotypic and genotypic identification of lactic acid bacteria isolated from ethnic fermented bamboo tender shoots of North East India. *International Journal of Food Microbiology*, 121(1): 35–40.

Tamime, A.Y. and Marshall, V.M.E. (1997). Microbiology and technology of fermented milks. In: *Microbiology and Biochemistry of Cheese and Fermented Milk*, (ed. B.A. Law), 57–152. Boston, MA: Springer US. doi: 10.1007/978-1-4613-1121-8_3

Tanasupawat, S., Phoottosavako, M. and Keeratipibul, S. (2015). Characterization and lipolytic activity of lactic acid bacteria isolated from Thai fermented meat. *Journal of Applied Pharmaceutical Science*, 5(3): 6–12.

Tanigawa, K. and Watanabe, K. (2011). Multilocus sequence typing reveals a novel subspeciation of Lactobacillus delbrueckii. *Microbiology (Reading, England)*, 157(Pt 3): 727–738.

Trunk, T., Khalil, H.S. and Leo, J.C. (2018). Bacterial autoaggregation. *AIMS Microbiology*, 4(1): 140–164.

Uma Maheshwari, S., Amutha, S., Anandham, R., Hemalatha, G., Senthil, N., Kwon, S.W. and Sivakumar, N. (2019). Characterization of potential probiotic bacteria from "panchamirtham"; A Southern Indian ethinic fermented fruit mix. *LWT*, 116: 108540.

Visintin, S., Alessandria, V., Valente, A., Dolci, P. and Cocolin, L. (2016). Molecular identification and physiological characterization of yeasts, lactic acid bacteria and acetic acid bacteria isolated from heap and box cocoa bean fermentations in West Africa. *International Journal of Food Microbiology*, 216: 69–78.

Wan, J., Huang, W., Zhong, J., Huang, L., Rayas-Duarte, P. and Liu, B. (2011). Effects of LAB fermentation on physical properties of oat flour and its suitability for noodle making. *Cereal Chemistry*, 88(2): 153–158.

Wang, D., Liu, W., Ren, Y., De, L., Zhang, D., Yang, Y., Bao, Q., Zhang, H. and Menghe, B. (2016). Isolation and identification of lactic acid bacteria from traditional dairy products in Baotou and Bayannur of Midwestern Inner Mongolia and q-PCR analysis of predominant species. *Korean Journal for Food Science of Animal Resources*, 36(4): 499–507.

Xiang, H., Sun-Waterhouse, D., Waterhouse, G.I.N., Cui, C. and Ruan, Z. (2019). Fermentation-enabled wellness foods: A fresh perspective. *Food Science and Human Wellness*, 8(3): 203–243.

Xu, H., Jeong, H.S., Lee, H.Y. and Ahn, J. (2009). Assessment of cell surface properties and adhesion potential of selected probiotic strains. *Letters in Applied Microbiology*, 49(4): 434–442.

Xu, J., Sun, L., Xing, X., Sun, Z., Gu, H., Lu, X., Li, Z. and Ren, Q. (2020). Culturing bacteria from fermentation Pit Muds of Baijiu with culturomics and amplicon-based metagenomic approaches. *Frontiers in Microbiology*, 11: 1223.

Yakult. (2007). Www.yakult.co.jp. Retrieved 24 July 2021.

Yang, Xiaozhe, Hu, W., Xiu, Z., Jiang, A., Yang, Xiangyan, Sarengaowa, Ji, Y., Guan, Y. and Feng, K. (2020). Comparison of northeast sauerkraut fermentation between single lactic acid bacteria strains and traditional fermentation. *Food Research International*, 137: 109553.

Yu, J., Wang, H.M., Zha, M.S., Qing, Y.T., Bai, N., Ren, Y., Xi, X.X., Liu, W.J., Menghe, B.L.G. and Zhang, H.P. (2015). Molecular identification and quantification of lactic acid bacteria in traditional fermented dairy foods of Russia. *Journal of Dairy Science*, 98(8): 5143–5154.

Zhao, W., Liu, Y., Latta, M., Ma, W., Wu, Z. and Chen, P. (2019). Probiotics database: a potential source of fermented foods. *International Journal of Food Properties*, 22(1): 197–216.

Zhao, Y., Tsang, C.-C., Xiao, M., Chan, J.F.W., Lau, S.K.P., Kong, F., Xu, Y. and Woo, P.C.Y. (2018). Yeast identification by sequencing, biochemical kits, MALDI-TOF MS and rep-PCR DNA fingerprinting. *Medical Mycology*, 56(7): 816–827.

Zheng, J., Ruan, L., Sun, M. and Gänzle, M. (2015). A genomic view of Lactobacilli and Pediococci demonstrates that phylogeny matches ecology and physiology. *Applied and Environmental Microbiology*, 81(20): 7233–7243.

3

Lactic Acid Bacteria as Potential Probiotics

Muhammad Bilal Sadiq

School of Life Sciences, Forman Christian College (A Chartered University) Lahore, 54600, Pakistan

3.1 Introduction

Lactic acid bacteria (LAB) are group Gram-positive, catalase-negative and oxygen-resistant bacteria (Domingos-Lopes *et al.* 2017). The most used probiotic LAB genera are *Lactobacillus*, *Lactococcus*, *Carnobacterium*, *Enterococcus*, *Streptococcus*, *Pediococcus*, *Propionibacterium* and *Leuconostoc*. Lactic acid is the main product of LAB and is produced by the fermentation of carbohydrates. LAB are generally recognized as safe (GRAS) by the United States Food and Drug Administration (Ma *et al.* 2019). Many LAB exhibit probiotic characteristics and are therefore considered as a leading source of potential probiotics. Probiotic LAB are non-pathogenic and maintain the microbial gut balance (Pringsulaka *et al.* 2015). The major probiotic attributes of LAB include tolerance to gastrointestinal tract (GIT) conditions, survival in low pH and health benefits associated with their consumption (Evivie *et al.* 2017). LAB were reported to exhibit antibacterial, anticancer, anti-inflammatory, anti-obesity and antidiabetic effects (Evivie *et al.* 2017; Tsai *et al.* 2014; Wang *et al.* 2019). LAB have been used for the formulation of fermented food products and play an important role in organoleptic value and preservation of food (Sáez *et al.* 2018). Probiotic LAB have been isolated and characterized from various sources such as dairy products, fermented foods, fruits and vegetables (Abushelaibi *et al.* 2017; Fessard and Remize 2019; Tamang *et al.* 2016). In the food industry LAB are used as a starter culture for acidification of food by lactic acid and not as a starter culture to produce aromatic flavoring agents (Motta and Gomes 2015). LAB serve as a functional food ingredient due to their probiotic attributes, fermentation and preservation potential (Fessard and Remize 2019). Probiotic LAB-based feed has been recommended as an alternative to antibiotics for farm animals (Vieco-Saiz *et al.* 2019). For commercial applications of LAB as probiotics, safety evaluation and probiotic characterization should be evaluated by in vitro and in vivo screening tests (Koirala and Anal 2021). LAB, being the most prominent source of probiotics, can be used in the formulation of various fermented food products (Anal 2019).

Probiotics, Prebiotics and Synbiotics: Technological Advancements Towards Safety and Industrial Applications, First Edition. Edited by Parmjit Singh Panesar and Anil Kumar Anal.

3.2 Isolation and Identification of Lactic Acid Bacteria

LAB are isolated from various sources by using de Man, Rogosa and Sharpe (MRS) agar. Samples are serially diluted and plated on MRS agar plates followed by incubation (24–48 h) at 37 °C. After incubation, LAB are primarily identified by the criteria of being Gram positive and catalase negative, and gas and acid production (Figure 3.1). After phenotypic characterization, LAB strains are identified by 16S r-RNA sequence analysis (Pringsulaka *et al.* 2015; Taroub *et al.* 2019).

3.3 Characterization of Lactic Acid Bacteria

Numerous strains and species of microorganisms have been classified as probiotics but LAB are being used most often in foods and their probiotic potential has been well reported (Rama *et al.* 2019). LAB are Gram-positive, catalase-negative, anaerobe or facultative aerobe, non-pathogenic inhabitants of the GIT of most animals (Byakika *et al.* 2019). Among LAB, *Lactobacillus*, *Lactococcus*, *Carnobacterium*, *Enterococcus*, *Streptococcus*, *Pediococcus*, *Propionibacterium* and *Leuconostoc* are the most common genera used as probiotics and their ingestion as probiotics has been associated with various host health benefits (Pinto *et al.* 2020). To declare LAB or any other microorganism as a probiotic various factors are

(a) (b) (c)

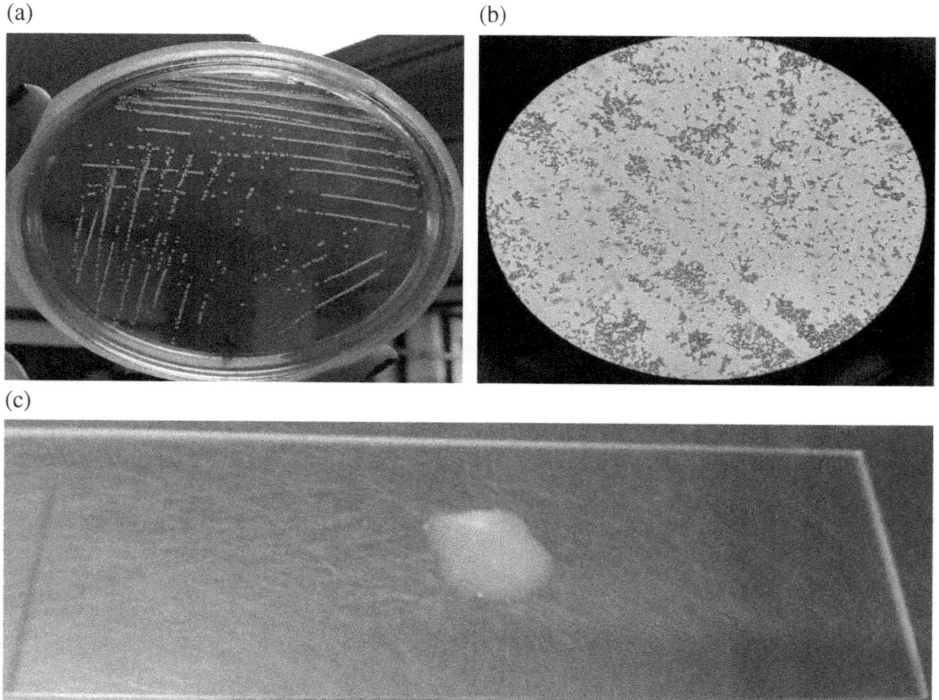

Figure 3.1 Isolation of lactic acid bacteria from raw goat milk on MRS agar plate (a), preliminary identification as Gram positive (b) and catalase negative (c). (Data not published.)

generally considered such as safety, a suitable source of isolation, evaluation of pathogenicity (phenotypic and genotypic), identification (biochemical and molecular), antibiotic susceptibility, resistance to low pH, tolerance to heat and bile salts, antagonistic effect against pathogens, genetic stability, host immune modulation and anticancer potential (FAO/WHO 2002; Saadat *et al.* 2019).

3.4 Criteria for Selection of Lactic Acid Bacteria as Potential Probiotic Candidates

The established and widely accepted criteria to declare LAB or any other microbe as a probiotic were fully published by a joint group of the FAO/WHO (FAO/WHO 2002). The criteria to evaluate the probiotic potential of LAB were aimed at ensuring the safety and claimed health benefits of putative probiotics (Byakika *et al.* 2019). However, the health benefits of LAB and other probiotics are strain dependent (Ramos *et al.* 2013). LAB characterization involves both in vitro and in vivo tests; however, in vitro tests may not depict the real functionality of a putative probiotic in a human or animal system. Therefore, complete characterization of LAB to be declared as a probiotic should be a blend of in vitro and in vivo trials. There are various tests for characterization of LAB such as resistance to gastric acid, bile tolerance, adherence to epithelial cells, safety profile analysis, antimicrobial potential against pathogens, etc. (FAO/WHO 2002) (Figure 3.2).

3.4.1 Evaluation of Gastric Survival

For LAB to be candidate probiotics, survival in the GIT is essential, as the putative probiotic has to pass through the acidic environment of the stomach and bile secretion. Therefore, tolerance to low pH and bile salts is considered as a prerequisite for an LAB to be a probiotic. LAB tolerance to low pH and bile salts is evaluated mostly by in vitro tests, as in vivo tests are expensive and laborious and involve expertise and ethical considerations. in vitro screening tests are rapid and result oriented, but, in some cases, in vivo tests become essential for commercial recognition of putative probiotics. For example, during in vitro assay of tolerance to low pH, only LAB with survivability in very low pH (2–3) are selected by neglecting the strains with survival in pH 4 or above; however, in practical cases ingestion of probiotics with food may raise the pH of the stomach to 4–5 (Papadimitriou *et al.* 2015). Moreover, tolerance to low pH can be achieved by encapsulation of LAB, if the putative probiotic exhibits other technological, probiotic and functional attributes (Kavitake *et al.* 2018). For evaluation of bile salt tolerance of LAB, 0.15–0.3% concentration of bile salts is recommended as it is the normal physiological range found in the GIT (Akbar *et al.* 2019).

The most widely used in vitro method for evaluation of LAB resistance to low pH is based on adjustment of broth or phosphate buffer saline (PBS) pH (1.5–3) with HCl. LAB as a putative probiotic candidate is inoculated in acidified broth or PBS for 2–4 h to imitate gastric conditions, followed by viable cell count by plating or measuring optical density at various time intervals (Abushelaibi *et al.* 2017; Pringsulaka *et al.* 2015). Furthermore, LAB tolerance to gastric juice can be evaluated by inoculation of LAB in PBS or broth by

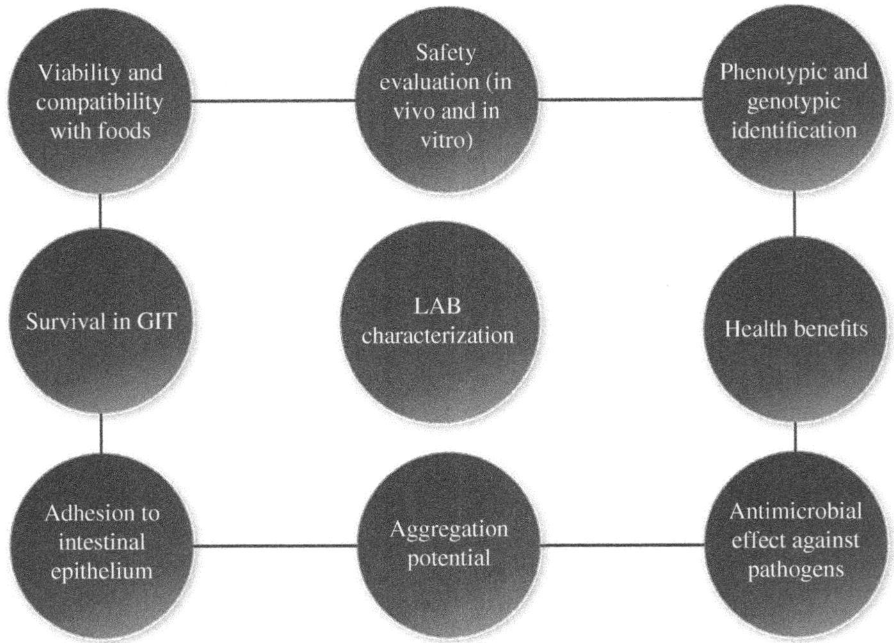

Figure 3.2 Criteria for the characterization of lactic acid bacteria as probiotic. GIT, gastrointestinal tract; LAB, lactic acid bacteria. *Source:* Based on Food and Agriculture Organization/World Health Organization. "Guidelines for the Evaluation of Probiotics in Foods", Report of a Joint FAO/WHO Working Group on Drafting Guidelines for the Evaluation of Probiotics in Food; World Health Organization: Geneva, Switzerland, 2002.

adjusting pH to 2 and addition of pepsin. For bile tolerance, LAB are inoculated in PBS or broth containing bile salts (0.3%) followed by incubation for 0–4 h, cells are counted by plating, and bile tolerance is determined with respect to change in viable cell count after exposure to bile salts (Adesulu-Dahunsi *et al.* 2018).

3.4.2 Bile Salt Hydrolysis Activity

Deconjugated bile salts have a strong antimicrobial effect and are produced by hydrolysis of bile salts (Bermudez-Brito *et al.* 2012). Deconjugated bile salts produced by LAB or putative probiotics can reduce cholesterol and contribute towards the management of hypercholesteremia (Yadav *et al.* 2016). Bile salt hydrolysis (BSH) ability ensures the survival of LAB in the intestine and add to the health benefits of the LAB strain. BSH ability can be evaluated by inoculating the freshly grown LAB on agar plates containing bile salts. The plates are incubated under specific conditions depending on the type of LAB. BSH ability is assessed by precipitation of deconjugated salts around the LAB colonies and can be classified based on zone of precipitation as low (less than or equal to 10 mm), medium (11–15 mm) or high BSH (16 mm or above). Abushelaibi *et al.* (2017) reported that LAB strains isolated from camel milk were able to hydrolyze bile salts and produce free cholic acid; furthermore, LAB were able to remove cholesterol from media.

3.4.3 Adhesion to Epithelium

Attachment to the epithelial cell lining is an important criterion for selection of LAB as a potential probiotic. The health benefits of probiotics are associated with their attachment to intestinal epithelium, as failure to do so may remove them from the GIT due to peristaltic movements. The adhesion and colonization of probiotics at the intestinal epithelium inhibits the growth of pathogens by competing for attachment site and nutrients (Collado *et al.* 2007). The probiotics should be consumed on a regular basis as they are short-term colonizers or inhabitants of intestine. The adhesion capacity of LAB can be evaluated by using human cell lines, i.e. colon cell lines, cancer coli-2 (Caco-2) lines, Hep-2 and HeLa cell lines. When these cell lines are cultured under specific conditions, their morphology and functionality imitate the enterocytes of the ileum (Haeri *et al.* 2012; Tropcheva *et al.* 2011). The adhesion capacity of LAB can also be evaluated by using animal ileum or by using genomic analysis for the presence of adhesion proteins (Azcarate-Peril *et al.* 2008; Kos *et al.* 2003).

3.4.4 Hydrophobicity

The probiotic bacteria attach to host epithelial cells through non-polar interactions between bacterial and host cells. Hydrophobicity is the measure of LAB or potential probiotic ability to interact with host cells by minimizing the GIT aqueous interactions. High hydrophobicity indicates that LAB have high potential for adhesion to the epithelial cell lining of host and can resist peristaltic movements (Shobharani and Agrawal 2011). Hydrophobicity is evaluated by estimating the adhesion capacity of LAB to a hydrocarbon such as xylene. The culture of LAB grown overnight is suspended in PBS and later hydrocarbon is added to develop a two-phase system. After vortexing, the aqueous layer is removed and the hydrophobicity of LAB is determined by measuring relative abundance (absorbance at 600 nm) of LAB in the hydrocarbon phase and the initial aqueous phase (Ding *et al.* 2017).

3.4.5 Aggregation Ability

The aggregation ability of LAB is evaluated in terms of autoaggregation and co-aggregation. Autoaggregation indicates the ability of identical bacteria to aggregate with each other, whereas co-aggregation indicates the ability of bacteria to aggregate with other types of bacterial cells (Tomáška *et al.* 2015). Autoaggregation is the measure of LAB ability to colonize and adhere to intestinal epithelium, and co-aggregation represents their ability to aggregate with pathogenic bacteria and prevent their colonization and attachment to intestinal epithelium. High autoaggregation and co-aggregation ability indicate that LAB are capable of colonizing in intestine and can prevent the adherence of pathogens to intestine (Kos *et al.* 2003).

3.4.6 Antimicrobial Potential

One of the important characteristics of LAB and other probiotics is the inhibition of growth of pathogens in GIT or even within a food system (Fessard and Remize 2019). The antimicrobial effects of LAB are associated with various mechanisms, such as production of various metabolites (i.e. organic acids, bacteriocins, hydrogen peroxide) and competition with pathogens for nutrition or attachment sites in host epithelium (Angmo *et al.* 2016; Collado *et al.* 2007). The antimicrobial potential of LAB is mostly evaluated by agar well diffusion method and spot-on lawn assay. Agar well diffusion assay is based on the evaluation of LAB for production of antimicrobial metabolites. Cell free supernatant (CFS) of LAB is obtained by centrifugation and introduced in agar plate wells to evaluate the antimicrobial potential against pathogens. The spot-on lawn assay evaluates the potential of viable LAB bacteria to inhibit the growth of pathogens in agar medium. LAB are spot inoculated on agar plate followed by overlaying with another layer of molten agar containing the pathogens (Figure 3.3). After incubation, clear zones around the LAB spot indicate the antimicrobial potential of the LAB (Tejero-Sariñena *et al.* 2012). Xu *et al.* (2020) reported that LAB isolated from fermented cereal-based products showed antimicrobial potential against various indicator strains including *Escherichia coli*, *Staphylococcus aureus* and *Listeria monocytogenes*. LAB have also been reported for their antifungal potential. Ma *et al.* (2019) isolated LAB from citrus sources and reported their antifungal activity against *Penicillium digitatum*. Taroub *et al.* (2019) isolated LAB from grapes and reported their antifungal and ochratoxin degradation activity.

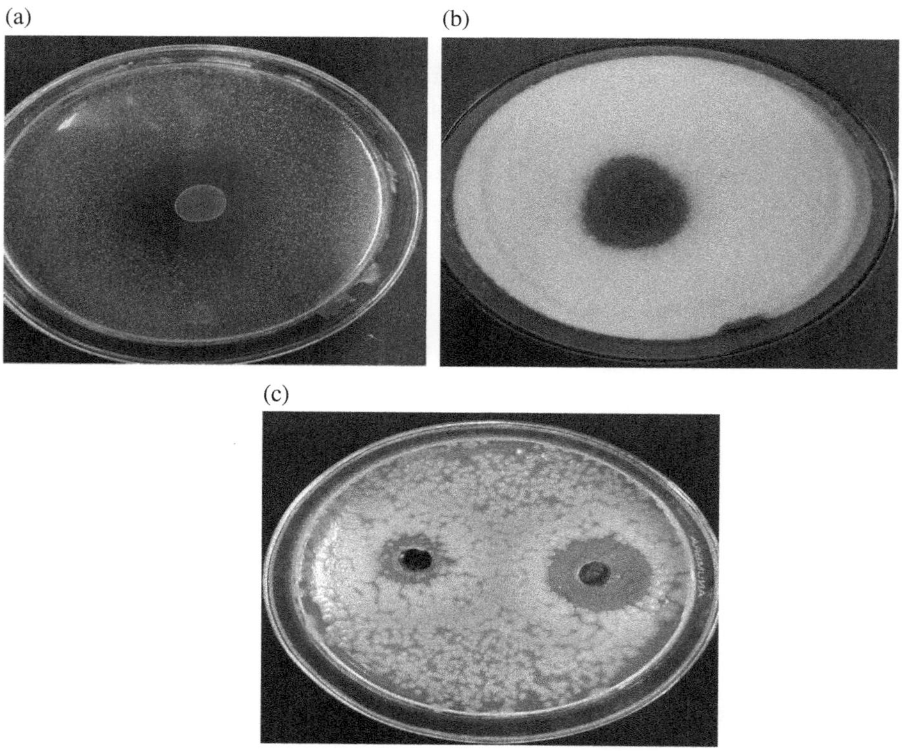

Figure 3.3 Antimicrobial effect of lactic acid bacteria isolated from raw goat milk against *Salmonella typhimurium* (a) and *Penicillium* spp. (b) by spot-on lawn assay (c) cell free supernatant of LAB against *S. typhimurium* by agar well diffusion assay. (Data not published.)

3.4.7 Amylolytic Property

Fermentation by LAB can improve the taste and texture of starch-containing foods (Falade *et al.* 2014). Starch degradation by LAB is associated with the ability of LAB to produce amylase. Due to lack of amylolytic activity, most LAB cannot hydrolyze starch. Several starch-degrading LAB have been previously isolated such as *L. lactis* from pickle and *L. plantarum* from fermented cereal (Bhanwar and Ganguli 2014; Xu *et al.* 2020). Amylolytic activity of LAB is determined by inoculating freshly grown culture of LAB on modified MRS agar plates prepared by replacing glucose with starch. After the incubation period, the results are interpreted by observing halo zones around colonies of LAB after the addition of a few drops of Gram's iodine (Adesulu-Dahunsi *et al.* 2018). The amylase activity can also be determined by measuring the reducing sugars released during starch hydrolysis (Bozic *et al.* 2014).

3.4.8 Safety Evaluation

Lactic acid bacteria or other putative probiotics should be evaluated for the production of harmful secondary metabolites such as biogenic amines. Various tests are performed to evaluate the safety potential of probiotic candidates, including antibiotic susceptibility and evaluation of hemolysis, toxin production, etc. Antibiotic susceptibility of LAB is usually evaluated by agar disc diffusion assay (Thapa *et al.* 2020). The antibiotic resistance of probiotics may ensure their survival during antibiotic treatment, however at the same time the transfer of antibiotic resistance genes from probiotics to other gut microflora may raise serious concerns (Gueimonde *et al.* 2013). Biogenic amines produce various health hazards, therefore production of biogenic amines from LAB is not desirable (Gardini *et al.* 2016). Hemolysis is an important criterion to declare a potential probiotic candidate safe for commercialization, as LAB or probiotic candidates should not produce lysis of red blood cells. The hemolysis of LAB is evaluated by inoculating on Columbia agar plates supplemented with sterile sheep blood, and results are interpreted as β-hemolysis (clear zones around colonies), α-hemolysis (green zones around colonies) or γ-hemolysis (no zones) (Tejero-Sariñena *et al.* 2012).

3.5 Lactic Acid Bacteria as Sources of Probiotics

Lactic acid bacteria are one of the most well-known sources of probiotics due to their ability to tolerate the extreme environment of the GIT (low pH, enzymes, bile salts, etc.) and confer health benefits to the host (Xu *et al.* 2020). Probiotic LAB have been isolated from various sources including fruits, vegetables, fermented food products, dairy products and animal or human gut.

3.5.1 Fruits and Vegetables

Raw fruits and vegetables contain various microbes including bacteria, yeast and molds. The microbial diversity in fruits and vegetables is dependent on agriculture practices, cultivation season, irrigation water and environmental conditions (Leff and Fierer 2013). The potential of LAB to ferment and confer health benefits and biopreservation incited scientists to find various new sources of LAB. Fruit- and vegetable-based foods with moderately acidic and anaerobic conditions are the preferred environment for probiotic LAB. Therefore, LAB have been isolated and characterized from various fermented vegetables and fruits (Tamang *et al.* 2016).

Fessard and Remize (2019) isolated LAB from white cabbage, papaya and tomatoes. They characterized the probiotic potential of LAB and after genetic characterization found that putative probiotics belonged to *Lactobacillus*, *Lactococcus*, *Leuconostoc*, *Weissella* and *Fructobacillus* genera of LAB.

LAB have gained interest in the food industrial sector due to their fermentation ability. Xu *et al.* (2020) isolated amylolytic LAB from fermented cereal-based products in China and amylolytic LAB with probiotic characteristics (antimicrobial effect, pH, salt and bile tolerance, aggregation potential) were identified as *L. plantarum*.

Taroub *et al.* (2019) isolated LAB from grapes with probiotic potential and antifungal effect against *Aspergillus* spp. LAB with probiotic attributes, antifungal activity and ochratoxin detoxification potential were identified as *Pediococcus pentosaceus* and *L. plantarum*. LAB produce various antifungal compounds such as organic acids and peptides.

3.5.2 Animal Sources

Pringsulaka *et al.* (2015) studied the probiotic attributes of LAB isolated from animal fecal samples (cow, pig, duck and hen). Fecal isolates of LAB showed antimicrobial potential against pathogens and demonstrated various probiotic attributes. Based on probiotic characterization, the selected LAB were identified by 16S rRNA as *L. plantarum*, *L. paraplantarum* and *L. reuteri*. Pringsulaka *et al.* (2015) suggested that these isolated LAB can be used as probiotics in animal feed.

Alonso *et al.* (2019) isolated putative probiotic LAB from fresh marine fish gut and identified them as *L. lactis*, *Enterococcus* spp., *L. plantarum* and *Leuconostoc mesenteroides*. They also reported that putative LAB from fish gut exhibited antimicrobial potential against aquaculture pathogens and could be used as potential probiotics in aquaculture feed.

Probiotic LAB have been isolated from poultry gut and genetically characterized under *Enterococcus*, *Lactobacillus* and *Pediococcus* genera. Poultry gut-based LAB isolates showed antibacterial activity against both Gram-positive and Gram-negative bacteria and were proposed to be used as potential probiotics in poultry feed (Reuben *et al.* 2019). LAB with probiotic potential have been isolated from human infant fecal samples and identified as *Enterococcus* spp. and *Lactobacillus* spp. (Rubio *et al.* 2014).

3.5.3 Dairy Products

Probiotic LAB can provide health benefits to the host and are categorized as generally recognized as safe (FAO/WHO 2002). Probiotic LAB have been isolated and characterized from cow milk, goat milk, camel milk and even human milk (Abushelaibi *et al.* 2017; da Silva Ferrari *et al.* 2016; Rajoka *et al.* 2017). Probiotic LAB have been isolated and characterized from various ethnic fermented dairy products such as shubat, a Kazakh camel milk fermented product, raabadi, and Indian fermented milk drink, and kefir from Eastern Europe (Fiorda *et al.* 2017; Manaer *et al.* 2015; Yadav *et al.* 2016).

Domingos-Lopes *et al.* (2017) isolated LAB from raw cow milk cheese. After genetic and technological characterization they found that most of the LAB belonged to *Lactobacillus* and *Enterococcus* genera. Further safety screening of LAB resulted in the selection of *L. paracasei* as a starter culture for cheese.

3.6 Health Benefits and Probiotic Mechanisms of Lactic Acid Bacteria

3.6.1 Host Immunity

The intestinal mucosa of the host serves as a barrier to protect against pathogens. Intestinal mucosa plays an important role in host immunity, which is regulated by diverse gut microbiota. The variation in the composition of the gut microbiota directly influences the host's immunity. LAB are predominant bacteria in gut microbiota and their adhesion to intestinal epithelium regulates the immune response by activating lymphoid tissues. The interaction between the host mucosal membrane and LAB improves the intestinal barrier, activates phagocytes and immune cells to regulate the inflammatory response, and enhances the activity of natural killer cells and antibody production (Wang *et al.* 2019). *L. plantarum* isolated from traditional Greek dairy products showed a tendency to modulate the anti-inflammatory response and increase the production of interleukins (Zoumpopoulou *et al.* 2018).

Lactic acid bacteria exert their influence on the immune system not only when they are viable: LAB metabolites such as exopolysaccharides (EPS) play an important role in immunomodulation by suppressing pathogens, preventing GIT cancers and regulating the production of various cytokines (Saadat *et al.* 2019).

3.6.2 Beneficial Metabolites

Lactic acid bacteria fermentation of sugars and amino acids produces secondary metabolites which increase the growth of beneficial intestinal bacteria. Lactic acid and EPS produced by LAB help to balance the host gut microbial community and serve as an energy source for microbial symbiosis, respectively. LAB induced regulation of gut microbial flora helps to prevent cancer, inflammation, allergy and various intestinal infections (Ren *et al.* 2021). Administration of *L. rhamnosus* for 1 week can regulate gut immunity and prevent *Salmonella* translocation into liver (Zhang *et al.* 2018). Lactic acid and short chain fatty acids (SCFAs) produced by LAB inhibit the growth of intestinal pathogens. Lactic acid exhibits a direct antibacterial effect by the lysis of the outer membrane of pathogenic bacteria (*E. coli, Salmonella, L. monocytogenes*, etc.) (Wang *et al.* 2015). SCFAs produced by LAB alleviate cancer by promoting apoptosis of cancer cells (dos Reis *et al.* 2017). LAB also produce various other antibacterial metabolites such as bacteriocins and hydrogen peroxide (Ren *et al.* 2021).

3.6.3 Lactose Intolerance

Inability to digest lactose is called lactose intolerance (LI) and is characterized by the symptoms of flatulence, bloating, abdominal cramps and diarrhea. The consumption of LAB lowers LI, as lactose in yoghurt is better tolerated than the lactose in milk. This can be explained by the fact that either yoghurt contains the lactase enzyme, or LAB such as *Lactobacillus* spp. produce lactase, helping to manage LI. Therefore, consumption of fermented dairy products is recommended in the management of LI (Evivie *et al.* 2017; Masood *et al.* 2011).

3.6.4 Gastric Ulcer

Lactic acid bacteria have been reported to alleviate the symptoms of gastric ulcer. LAB administration improved gastric ulcer recovery when combined with anti-ulcer treatment. The anti-ulcer effect of LAB was proposed due to their potential to inhibit the growth of *Helicobacter pylori* (Masood *et al.* 2011). Lam *et al.* (2007) reported that *L. rhamnosus* has been recommended in ulcer treatment as an adjuvant, due to its ability to eradicate *H. pylori* and reduce mucosal lesions.

3.6.5 Obesity and Diabetes Management

Obesity is a complex disease defined by the accumulation of excessive body fat; it is recognized as one of the major health problems across the globe. Obesity is a triggering factor for various other diseases such as cardiovascular problems, cancer and diabetes (Wang *et al.* 2015). LAB have been reported previously in the management of obesity. Supernatant of soy milk fermented by *L. paracasei* was reported to have anti-obesity effects in high fat diet (HFD) administered mice; the anti-obesity effects were marked with a decrease in accumulation of body fat (Lee *et al.* 2013). LAB play a role in the management of obesity by modulating the GIT enzymes involved in energy metabolism and dietary fiber metabolism (Tsai *et al.* 2014). The metabolic syndrome, caused by various factors including obesity, was treated in mice by modulation of GIT microbiota after the administration of *L. rhamnosus*, *Bifidobacterium lactis* and *L. paracasei* (Wang *et al.* 2015). Probiotic LAB can be an effective treatment in the management of obesity (Mekkes *et al.* 2014).

Obesity has been reported to be the major factor contributing to the increase in the number of type 2 diabetic patients across the globe. Type 2 diabetes is defined by the combination of various factors such as insulin resistance, low-level inflammation and exhausted β cells (Xu *et al.* 2015). LAB (*L. rhamnosus*) were reported to have antidiabetic effects in rats by delaying glucose intolerance and hyperglycemia (Tabuchi *et al.* 2003). *L. acidophilus* and *L. casei* were reported to delay diabetes progression in HFD administered animals (Yadav *et al.* 2007). *L. rhamnosus* GG viable cells were reported to decrease glucose absorption and thus reduce the postprandial glucose level in rats (Honda *et al.* 2012). The antidiabetic effects of LAB are strain dependent, and previous clinical studies also reported that breastfeeding was found to be related to a decrease in the incidence of diabetes as maternal milk is a source of various LAB strains (Evivie *et al.* 2017).

3.6.6 Role of Lactic Acid Bacteria Probiotics in Cancer

Lactic acid bacteria have been reported to have anticancer potential such as prevention of colon cancer (Shukla *et al.* 2014). Disturbances in the gut environment such as changes in the normal microbiota or mucosal immunity may potentiate various ailments including cancer. The natural microbiota of the gut exhibit a negative effect on cancer development (Zitvogel *et al.* 2017). Probiotic LAB produce an anticancer effect by the inhibition of microbes involved in carcinogen production, immunomodulation, altering cancer gene expression, modulation of gut microbiota, apoptosis and cell cycle control (Raman *et al.* 2013). LAB fermented dairy products such as kefir were reported to regulate gene expression for apoptosis in cancer cells (Khoury *et al.* 2014). *L. rhamnosus* GG was reported to express p50 and p75 proteins which inhibit cancer cell proliferation (Liévin-Le Moal and Servin 2014). *L. plantarum* and *L. lactis* subsp. *Lactis* were reported to have anticancer activity against various types of cancer cell lines. *L. plantarum* and *L. casei* were reported to have anticancer and antimutagenic effects (Abbas Ahmadi *et al.* 2014). Metabolites of LAB such as EPS have also been reported to have anticancer effects by modulating host immunity (Saadat *et al.* 2019).

3.7 Industrial Applications of Probiotic Lactic Acid Bacteria

Lactic acid bacteria have gained importance for food industries owing to their fermentative potential. LAB are used for the development of fermented products at the industrial scale such as yoghurt, sourdough, cheese and pickles (Corona *et al.* 2016; Evivie *et al.* 2017). Probiotic LAB are also used in the preservation of food products. The combination of probiotic LAB such as *L. delbrueckii* with *S. thermophilus* in the development of yoghurt was reported to have synergistic effects against pathogens (Aslim *et al.* 2011). LAB metabolites such lactic acid and bacteriocins exhibit food preservation potential. Among bacteriocins, nisin has been used commercially in the preservation of various food products such as canned foods, milk, cheese and baby formulas (Quinto *et al.* 2014). The LAB metabolite lactic acid is of great interest for industries as it serves a precursor for polylactic acid, which in turn is used as biodegradable plastic (Singhvi *et al.* 2018).

3.8 Challenges for Lactic Acid Bacteria as Probiotics

Lactic acid bacteria are the main source of probiotics, however certain limitations or challenges are associated with them for probiotic applications. LAB probiotic candidates should maintain high viability in the GIT and tolerate low pH in the GIT and fermented foods (Evivie *et al.* 2017). The viability and survival of probiotics are crucial for their applications. The viability and survival of probiotics can be ensured in the GIT and food formulations by using microencapsulation. Encapsulation of probiotic LAB can also mask the tastes of probiotic foods (Kavitake *et al.* 2018). The other challenges for probiotic LAB are to ensure the viability and enumeration of cells when mixed LAB cultures are used, to study the interaction of probiotic LAB with host microbiota and, most importantly, safety evaluation and GRAS status of probiotic LAB for commercial applications (Evivie *et al.* 2017).

3.9 Conclusion and Future Perspectives

Most of the commercially used probiotics belong to LAB, due to their potential for fermentation, food preservation and host health benefits. For better understanding of the potential of LAB as probiotics and functional food ingredients, detailed genetic characterization such as whole genome sequencing should be taken into consideration. After characterization of LAB as probiotics, detailed safety and characterization should be carried out by combining in vitro and in vivo tests. Due to their health benefits, probiotic LAB-based food products are gaining the consumer's interest and leading the food market. LAB provide not only health benefits but also flavor, taste and preservation potential for food products. LAB metabolites such as lactic acid, bacteriocins and EPS have potential for industrial applications and should be incorporated in various foods and feed products.

References

Abbas Ahmadi, M., Tajabadi Ebrahimi, M., Mehrabian, S., Tafvizi, F., Bahrami, H. and Dameshghian, M. (2014). Antimutagenic and anticancer effects of lactic acid bacteria isolated from Tarhana through Ames test and phylogenetic analysis by 16S rDNA. *Nutrition and Cancer*, 66(8): 1406–1413.

Abushelaibi, A., Al-Mahadin, S., El-Tarabily, K., Shah, N.P. and Ayyash, M. (2017). Characterization of potential probiotic lactic acid bacteria isolated from camel milk. *LWT-Food Science and Technology*, 79: 316–325.

Adesulu-Dahunsi, A.T., Jeyaram, K. and Sanni, A.I. (2018). Probiotic and technological properties of exopolysaccharide producing lactic acid bacteria isolated from cereal-based Nigerian fermented food products. *Food Control*, 92: 225–231.

Akbar, A., Sadiq, M.B., Ali, I., Anwar, M., Muhammad, N., Muhammad, J. and Ahmad, S. (2019). Lactococcus lactis subsp. lactis isolated from fermented milk products and its antimicrobial potential. *CyTA-Journal of Food*, 17(1): 214–220.

Alonso, S., Castro, M.C., Berdasco, M., de la Banda, I.G., Moreno-Ventas, X. and de Rojas, A.H. (2019). Isolation and partial characterization of lactic acid bacteria from the gut microbiota of marine fishes for potential application as probiotics in aquaculture. *Probiotics and Antimicrobial Proteins*, 11(2): 569–579.

Anal, A.K. (2019). Quality ingredients and safety concerns for traditional fermented foods and beverages from Asia: A review. *Fermentation*, 5(1): 8.

Angmo, K., Kumari, A. and Bhalla, T.C. (2016). Probiotic characterization of lactic acid bacteria isolated from fermented foods and beverage of Ladakh. *LWT-Food Science and Technology*, 66: 428–435.

Aslim, B., Onbasili, D. and Yuksekdag, Z.N. (2011). Determination of lactic acid production and antagonistic activity against Helicobacter pylori of L. delbrueckii subsp. bulgaricus and S. thermophilus strains. *Kafkas Univ Vet Fak Derg*, 17(4): 609–614.

Azcarate-Peril, M.A., Altermann, E., Goh, Y.J., Tallon, R., Sanozky-Dawes, R.B., Pfeiler, E. A., et al. (2008). Analysis of the genome sequence of Lactobacillus gasseri ATCC 33323 reveals the molecular basis of an autochthonous intestinal organism. *Applied and Environmental Microbiology*, 74(15): 4610–4625.

Bermudez-Brito, M., Plaza-Díaz, J., Muñoz-Quezada, S., Gómez-Llorente, C. and Gil, A. (2012). Probiotic mechanisms of action. *Annals of Nutrition and Metabolism*, 61(2): 160–174.

Bhanwar, S. and Ganguli A. (2014). Amylase and galactosidase production on potato starch waste by *Lactococcus lactis* subsp. lactic isolated from pickled yam. *Journal of Scientific and Industrial Research*, 73: 324–330.

Bozic N., Slavic M.S. and Gavrilovic A. (2014). Production of raw-starch-digesting α-amylase isoform from *Bacillus sp.* under solid-state fermentation and biochemical characterization. *Bioprocess and Biosystems Engineering*, 37: 1353–1360.

Byakika, S., Mukisa, I.M., Byaruhanga, Y.B. and Muyanja, C. (2019). A review of criteria and methods for evaluating the probiotic potential of microorganisms. *Food Reviews International*, 35(5): 427–466.

Collado, M.C., Meriluoto, J., and Salminen, S. (2007). Role of commercial probiotic strains against human pathogen adhesion to intestinal mucus. *Letters in Applied Microbiology*, 45(4): 454–460.

Corona, O., Alfonzo, A., Ventimiglia, G., Nasca, A., Francesca, N., Martorana, A. et al. (2016). Industrial application of selected lactic acid bacteria isolated from local semolinas for typical sourdough bread production. *Food Microbiology*, 59: 43–56.

da Silva Ferrari, I., de Souza, J.V., Ramos, C.L., da Costa, M.M., Schwan, R.F. and Dias, F.S. (2016). Selection of autochthonous lactic acid bacteria from goat dairies and their addition to evaluate the inhibition of Salmonella typhi in artisanal cheese. *Food Microbiology*, 60: 29–38.

Ding, W., Shi, C., Chen, M., Zhou, J., Long, R. and Guo, X. (2017). Screening for lactic acid bacteria in traditional fermented Tibetan yak milk and evaluating their probiotic and cholesterol-lowering potentials in rats fed a high-cholesterol diet. *Journal of Functional Foods*, 32: 324–332.

Domingos-Lopes, M.F.P., Stanton, C., Ross, P.R., Dapkevicius, M.L.E. and Silva, C.C.G. (2017). Genetic diversity, safety and technological characterization of lactic acid bacteria isolated from artisanal Pico cheese. *Food Microbiology*, 63: 178–190.

dos Reis, S.A., da Conceição, L.L., Siqueira, N.P., Rosa, D.D., da Silva, L.L., and Maria do Carmo, G.P. (2017). Review of the mechanisms of probiotic actions in the prevention of colorectal cancer. *Nutrition Research*, 37: 1–19.

Evivie, S.E., Huo, G.C., Igene, J.O., and Bian, X. (2017). Some current applications, limitations and future perspectives of lactic acid bacteria as probiotics. *Food and Nutrition Research*, 61(1): 1318034.

Falade A.T., Emmambux M.N., Buys E.M. and Taylor J.R.N. (2014). Improvement of maize bread quality through modification of dough rheological properties by lactic acid bacteria fermentation. *Journal of Cereal Science*, 60: 471–476.

Fessard, A. and Remize, F. (2019). Genetic and technological characterization of lactic acid bacteria isolated from tropically grown fruits and vegetables. *International Journal of Food Microbiology*, 301: 61–72.

Fiorda, F.A., de Melo Pereira, G.V., Thomaz-Soccol, V., Rakshit, S.K., Pagnoncelli, M.G.B., de Souza Vandenberghe, L.P. and Soccol, C.R. (2017). Microbiological, biochemical, and functional aspects of sugary kefir fermentation-A review. *Food Microbiology*, 66: 86–95.

Food and Agriculture Organization/World Health Organization. (2002). *Guidelines for the Evaluation of Probiotics in Foods*. Report of a Joint FAO/WHO Working Group on Drafting Guidelines for the Evaluation of Probiotics in Food; World Health Organization: Geneva, Switzerland. http://www.who.int/foodsafety/fs_management/en/probiotic_guidelines.pdf.

Gardini, F., Özogul, Y., Suzzi, G., Tabanelli, G. and Özogul, F. (2016). Technological factors affecting biogenic amine content in foods: a review. *Frontiers in Microbiology*, 7: 1218.

Gueimonde, M., Sánchez, B., de los Reyes-Gavilán, C.G., and Margolles, A. (2013). Antibiotic resistance in probiotic bacteria. *Frontiers in Microbiology*, 4: 202.

Haeri, A., Khodaii, Z., Ghaderian, S.M.H., Panah, A.S.T., and Najar, R.A. (2012). Comparison of adherence patterns of a selection of probiotic bacteria to Caco-2, HEp-2, and T84 cell lines. *Annals of Microbiology*, 62(1): 339–344.

Honda, K., Moto, M., Uchida, N., He, F. and Hashizume, N. (2012). Anti-diabetic effects of lactic acid bacteria in normal and type 2 diabetic mice. *Journal of Clinical Biochemistry and Nutrition*, 51(2): 96–101.

Kavitake, D., Kandasamy, S., Devi, P.B. and Shetty, P.H. (2018). Recent developments on encapsulation of lactic acid bacteria as potential starter culture in fermented foods–A review. *Food Bioscience*, 21: 34–44.

Khoury, N., El-Hayek, S., Tarras, O., El-Sabban, M., El-Sibai, M. and Rizk, S. (2014). Kefir exhibits anti-proliferative and pro-apoptotic effects on colon adenocarcinoma cells with no significant effects on cell migration and invasion. *International Journal of Oncology*, 45(5): 2117–2127.

Koirala, S., and Anal, A.K. (2021). Probiotics-based foods and beverages as future foods and their overall safety and regulatory claims. *Future Foods*: 100013.

Kos, B.V.Z.E., Šušković, J., Vuković, S., Šimpraga, M., Frece, J. and Matošić, S. (2003). Adhesion and aggregation ability of probiotic strain Lactobacillus acidophilus M92. *Journal of Applied Microbiology*, 94(6): 981–987.

Lam, E.K., Tai, E.K., Koo, M.W., Wong, H.P., Wu, W.K., Yu, L., et al. (2007). Enhancement of gastric mucosal integrity by Lactobacillus rhamnosus GG. *Life Sciences*, 80(23): 2128–2136.

Lee, B.H., Lo, Y.H. and Pan, T.M. (2013). Anti-obesity activity of Lactobacillus fermented soy milk products. *Journal of Functional Foods*, 5(2): 905–913.

Leff, J.W., and Fierer, N. (2013). Bacterial communities associated with the surfaces of fresh fruits and vegetables. *PloS One*, 8(3): e59310.

Liévin-Le Moal, V. and Servin, A.L. (2014). Anti-infective activities of lactobacillus strains in the human intestinal microbiota: from probiotics to gastrointestinal anti-infectious biotherapeutic agents. *Clinical Microbiology Reviews*, 27(2): 167–199.

Ma, J., Hong, Y., Deng, L., Yi, L., and Zeng, K. (2019). Screening and characterization of lactic acid bacteria with antifungal activity against Penicillium digitatum on citrus. *Biological Control*, 138: 104044.

Manaer, T., Yu, L., Zhang, Y., Xiao, X.J., and Nabi, X.H. (2015). Anti-diabetic effects of shubat in type 2 diabetic rats induced by combination of high-glucose-fat diet and low-dose streptozotocin. *Journal of Ethnopharmacology*, 169: 269–274.

Masood, M.I., Qadir, M.I., Shirazi, J.H., and Khan, I.U. (2011). Beneficial effects of lactic acid bacteria on human beings. *Critical Reviews in Microbiology*, 37(1): 91–98.

Mekkes, M.C., Weenen, T.C., Brummer, R.J., and Claassen, E. (2014). The development of probiotic treatment in obesity: a review. *Beneficial Microbes*, 5(1): 19–28.

Motta, A.D.S., and Gomes, M.D.S.M. (2015). Technological and functional properties of lactic acid bacteria: the importance of these microorganisms for food. *Revista do Instituto de Laticínios Cândido Tostes*, 70(3): 172–184.

Papadimitriou, K., Zoumpopoulou, G., Foligné, B., Alexandraki, V., Kazou, M., Pot, B. and Tsakalidou, E. (2015). Discovering probiotic microorganisms: in vitro, in vivo, genetic and omics approaches. *Frontiers in Microbiology*, 6: 58.

Pinto, A., Barbosa, J., Albano, H., Isidro, J. and Teixeira, P. (2020). Screening of bacteriocinogenic lactic acid bacteria and their characterization as potential probiotics. *Microorganisms*, 8(3): 393.

Pringsulaka, O., Rueangyotchanthana, K., Suwannasai, N., Watanapokasin, R., Amnueysit, P., Sunthornthummas, S., et al. (2015). in vitro screening of lactic acid bacteria for multi-strain probiotics. *Livestock Science*, 174: 66–73.

Quinto, E.J., Jiménez, P., Caro, I., Tejero, J., Mateo, J. and Girbés, T. (2014). Probiotic lactic acid bacteria: a review. *Food and Nutrition Sciences*, 5(18): 1765.

Rajoka, M.S.R., Mehwish, H.M., Siddiq, M., Haobin, Z., Zhu, J., Yan, L., et al. (2017). Identification, characterization, and probiotic potential of Lactobacillus rhamnosus isolated from human milk. *LWT*, 84: 271–280.

Rama, G.R., Kuhn, D., Beux, S., Maciel, M.J. and de Souza, C.F.V. (2019). Potential applications of dairy whey for the production of lactic acid bacteria cultures. *International Dairy Journal*, 98: 25–37.

Raman, M., Ambalam, P., Kondepudi, K.K., Pithva, S., Kothari, C., Patel, A.T., et al. (2013). Potential of probiotics, prebiotics and synbiotics for management of colorectal cancer. *Gut Microbes*, 4(3): 181–192.

Ramos, C.L., Thorsen, L., Schwan, R.F. and Jespersen, L. (2013). Strain-specific probiotics properties of Lactobacillus fermentum, Lactobacillus plantarum and Lactobacillus brevis isolates from Brazilian food products. *Food Microbiologyogy* 36(1): 22–29.

Ren, C., Faas, M.M. and de Vos, P. (2021). Disease managing capacities and mechanisms of host effects of lactic acid bacteria. *Critical Reviews in Food Science and Nutrition*, 61(8): 1365–1393.

Reuben, R.C., Roy, P.C., Sarkar, S.L., Alam, R.U. and Jahid, I.K. (2019). Isolation, characterization, and assessment of lactic acid bacteria toward their selection as poultry probiotics. *BMC Microbiology*, 19(1): 253.

Rubio, R., Jofré, A., Martin, B., Aymerich, T. and Garriga, M. (2014). Characterization of lactic acid bacteria isolated from infant faeces as potential probiotic starter cultures for fermented sausages. *Food Microbiology*, 38: 303–311.

Saadat, Y.R., Khosroushahi, A.Y. and Gargari, B.P. (2019). A comprehensive review of anticancer, immunomodulatory and health beneficial effects of the lactic acid bacteria exopolysaccharides. *Carbohydrate Polymers*, 217: 79–89.

Sáez, G.D., Saavedra, L., Hebert, E.M. and Zárate, G. (2018). Identification and biotechnological characterization of lactic acid bacteria isolated from chickpea sourdough in northwestern Argentina. *LWT*, 93: 249–256.

Shobharani, P. and Agrawal, R. (2011). A potent probiotic strain from cheddar cheese. *Indian Journal of Microbiology*, 51(3): 251–258.

Shukla, R., Iliev, I. and Goyal, A. (2014). Leuconostoc mesenteroides NRRL B-1149 as probiotic and its dextran with anticancer properties. *Journal of BioScience and Biotechnology*, 3(1): 79–87.

Singhvi, M., Zendo, T. and Sonomoto, K. (2018). Free lactic acid production under acidic conditions by lactic acid bacteria strains: challenges and future prospects. *Applied Microbiology and Biotechnology*, 102(14): 5911–5924.

Tabuchi, M., Ozaki, M., Tamura, A., Yamada, N., Ishida, T., Hosoda, M. and Hosono, A. (2003). Antidiabetic effect of Lactobacillus GG in streptozotocin-induced diabetic rats. *Bioscience, Biotechnology, and Biochemistry*, 67(6): 1421–1424.

Tamang, J.P., Watanabe, K., and Holzapfel, W.H. (2016). Diversity of microorganisms in global fermented foods and beverages. *Frontiers in Microbiology*, 7: 377.

Taroub, B., Salma, L., Manel, Z., Ouzari, H.I., Hamdi, Z. and Moktar, H. (2019). Isolation of lactic acid bacteria from grape fruit: Antifungal activities, probiotic properties, and in vitro detoxification of ochratoxin A. *Annals of Microbiology*, 69(1): 17–27.

Tejero-Sariñena, S., Barlow, J., Costabile, A., Gibson, G.R. and Rowland, I. (2012). in vitro evaluation of the antimicrobial activity of a range of probiotics against pathogens: evidence for the effects of organic acids. *Anaerobe*, 18(5): 530–538.

Thapa, S.P., Shrestha, S., and Anal, A.K. (2020). Addressing the antibiotic resistance and improving the food safety in food supply chain (farm-to-fork) in Southeast Asia. *Food Control*, 108: 106809.

Tomáška, M., Drončovský, M., Klapáčová, L., Slottová, A. and Kološta, M. (2015). Potential probiotic properties of Lactobacilli isolated from goat's milk. *Potravinarstvo Slovak Journal of Food Sciences*, 9(1): 66–71.

Tropcheva, R., Georgieva, R. and Danova, S. (2011). Adhesion ability of Lactobacillus plantarum AC131. *Biotechnology and Biotechnological Equipment*, 25(suppl): 121–124.

Tsai, Y.T., Cheng, P.C. and Pan, T.M. (2014). Anti-obesity effects of gut microbiota are associated with lactic acid bacteria. *Applied Microbiology and Biotechnology*, 98(1): 1–10.

Vieco-Saiz, N., Belguesmia, Y., Raspoet, R., Auclair, E., Gancel, F., Kempf, I. and Drider, D. (2019). Benefits and inputs from lactic acid bacteria and their bacteriocins as alternatives to antibiotic growth promoters during food-animal production. *Frontiers in Microbiology*, 10: 57.

Wang, J., Tang, H., Zhang, C., Zhao, Y., Derrien, M., Rocher, E. et al. (2015). Modulation of gut microbiota during probiotic-mediated attenuation of metabolic syndrome in high fat diet-fed mice. *The ISME Journal*, 9(1): 1–15.

Wang, L., He, Z., Tian, P. and Wang, G. (2019). Lactic acid bacteria and host immunity. In: *Lactic Acid Bacteria*, (261–296). Singapore: Springer.

Xu, J., Lian, F., Zhao, L., Zhao, Y., Chen, X., Zhang, X., et al. (2015). Structural modulation of gut microbiota during alleviation of type 2 diabetes with a Chinese herbal formula. *The ISME Journal*, 9(3): 552–562.

Xu, Y., Zhou, T., Tang, H., Li, X., Chen, Y., Zhang, L. and Zhang, J. (2020). Probiotic potential and amylolytic properties of lactic acid bacteria isolated from Chinese fermented cereal foods. *Food Control*, 111: 107057.

Yadav, H., Jain, S. and Sinha, P.R. (2007). Antidiabetic effect of probiotic dahi containing Lactobacillus acidophilus and Lactobacillus casei in high fructose fed rats. *Nutrition*, 23(1): 62–68.

Yadav, R., Puniya, A.K. and Shukla, P. (2016). Probiotic properties of Lactobacillus plantarum RYPR1 from an indigenous fermented beverage Raabadi. *Frontiers in Microbiology*, 7: 1683.

Zhang, W., Zhu, Y.H., Yang, G.Y., Liu, X., Xia, B., Hu, X., et al. (2018). Lactobacillus rhamnosus GG affects microbiota and suppresses autophagy in the intestines of pigs challenged with Salmonella infantis. *Frontiers in Microbiology*, 8: 2705.

Zitvogel, L., Daillère, R., Roberti, M.P., Routy, B. and Kroemer, G. (2017). Anticancer effects of the microbiome and its products. *Nature Reviews Microbiology*, 15(8): 465.

Zoumpopoulou, G., Tzouvanou, A., Mavrogonatou, E., Alexandraki, V., Georgalaki, M., Anastasiou, R., et al. (2018). Probiotic features of lactic acid bacteria isolated from a diverse pool of traditional Greek dairy products regarding specific strain-host interactions. *Probiotics and Antimicrobial Proteins*, 10(2): 313–322.

4

Non-Lactic Acid Bacteria as Probiotics and their Functional Roles

Cíntia Lacerda Ramos[1], *Elizabethe Adriana Esteves*[1], *Nayara Martins Zille de Miranda*[1], *Lauane Gomes Moreno*[1] and *Rosane Freitas Schwan*[2]

[1] *Faculty of Biological Sciences and Health, Federal University of Jequitinhonha and Mucuri Valeys, CEP, 39100-000, Diamantina, MG, Brazil*
[2] *Biology Department, Federal University of Lavras, CEP, 37200-000, Lavras, MG, Brazil*

4.1 Spore-forming Bacteria

Spore-forming bacteria are Gram-positive bacteria belonging to the phylum Firmicutes, especially the aerobic Bacillaceae and the anaerobic Clostridia. This group of bacteria shares the common characteristic of spore (also called endospore) production, a bacterial survival strategy in response to adverse environmental conditions such as starvation of nutrients, extreme temperatures, low water activity, exposure to toxic substances and radiation. According to some reports, the bacteria may remain dormant in sporulating form for as long as 40 million years, as observed for *Bacillus sphaericus* detected in the gut of bees preserved in Dominican amber, or 250 million years as reported for *Virgibacillus* spp. in salt crystals from the Salado Formation in New Mexico (Nicholson *et al.* 2000; Nicholson 2004). In general, when favorable conditions return, the bacterial spores germinate, reestablishing the vegetative state. Each vegetative bacteria cell originates a spore, which may germinate in a vegetative cell again. Thus, the bacterial spore is a resistant structure and not related to reproduction.

The principal genera of spore-forming bacteria from the health and biotechnological point of view are *Bacillus* and *Clostridium*. Because of their resistance characteristic, spore-forming bacteria have been the subject of increased interest in human and animal use as probiotics. *Lactobacillus* spp. and *Bifidobacterium* spp. are the most studied and employed genera as probiotics since they are part of the natural gut microbiota (Hardy *et al.* 2013). However, these microorganisms may show the disadvantage of a prolonged storage period at environmental temperature (Corona-Hernandez *et al.* 2013; Succi *et al.* 2017). Strategies such as microencapsulation and refrigeration may be employed to overcome this problem (Andrade *et al.* 2019). However, this increases the cost of production and, consequently, the final product for the consumers. In this sense, spore-forming bacteria may display some

Probiotics, Prebiotics and Synbiotics: Technological Advancements Towards Safety and Industrial Applications, First Edition. Edited by Parmjit Singh Panesar and Anil Kumar Anal.

advantages which enable them to reach the desired viable number of cells in the product and after gastrointestinal transit to cause probiotic benefit to the host. These microorganisms are generally resistant to high temperature, industrial processing production and gut conditions, and are viable after a prolonged storage period at environmental temperature (Elshaghabee *et al.* 2017; Majeed *et al.* 2019).

Several spore-forming *Bacillus* species have been studied and applied as probiotics for both animals and humans, such as *B. coagulans, B. subtilis, B. licheniformis, B. pumilus, B. amyloliquefaciens, B. clausii*, and *B. polyfermentans* (Elshaghabee *et al.* 2017). An exciting characteristic demonstrated by some *Bacillus* species is the antagonistic effect on several pathogenic microorganisms (Al-Ajlani and Hasnain 2010; Amin *et al.* 2015).

The *Clostridium* genus is widely distributed in the environment and is found in the intestinal tract of animals and humans. They are involved in a wide range of infectious diseases depending on the species, e.g. *C. difficile, C septicum, C. perfringens, C. botulinum,* and *C. tetani*, which are generally related to toxin production (Guo *et al.* 2020). However, non-pathogenic *Clostridium* species, mainly *C. butyricum*, commonly found in human and animal gut, has been employed as a probiotic by the Asian population, especially in Japan, Korea and China (Cassir *et al.* 2016; Guo *et al.* 2020). This species was first isolated from pig intestines 140 years ago and can produce high amounts of butyric acid (Vos *et al.* 2009). The beneficial effect demonstrated by *Clostridium* strains is generally related to enhancing the capacity of the intestinal barrier and immunomodulation. These improved properties are probably due to some metabolites such as butyrate, secondary bile acids and indole propionic acid.

4.1.1 Types, Structure and Formation of Spores

Sporulation of *Bacillus* and some *Clostridium* species has been extensively studied and described at morphological, metabolic and physiological levels (Galperin *et al.* 2012; Gauvry *et al.* 2017). *B. subtilis* is one of the most thoroughly studied bacteria, serving as a model to study sporulation and the regulatory networks controlling this differentiation system. On the other hand, studies on *Clostridium* spp.'s sporulation to understand the complete regulatory cycle are still scarce. According to Talukdar et al. (2015), the early stage of *Clostridium* sporulation differs from *Bacillus* due to the absence of a phosphorelay system. This system is the principal regulator for sporulation, Spo0A, and the downstream signaling systems are mostly conserved. Studies employing industrial and pathogenic *Clostridium* species revealed intragenic differences in sporulation regulation (Talukdar *et al.* 2015).

Knowledge of spore structure and formation is of great interest to the health and industry fields. The spores' high resistance, their adhesion properties and their capacity to form biofilms make these anaerobic clostridia and facultative anaerobic bacilli challenging to eliminate, having a direct economic impact upon the food industry and human health (Carlin 2011). In contrast, this characteristic may be advantageous for probiotic use because it makes these bacteria easier to store and manipulate. To better manage and control these bacteria, it is crucial to know what initiates and modulates sporulation and identify their structure and composition.

The spore is located in different portions of the bacterial cell, classified as central, terminal or subterminal (Figure 4.1a). Central spores are formed in the middle of the bacterial

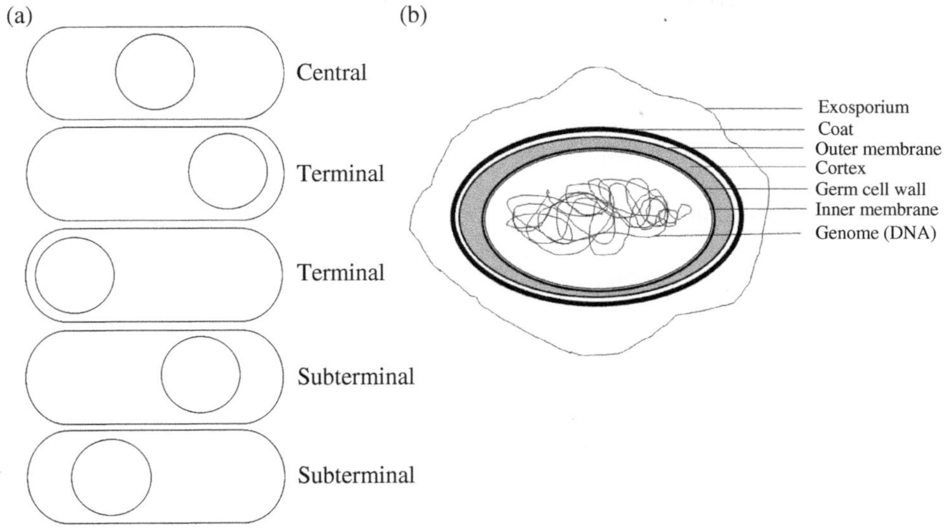

Figure 4.1 Scheme of spore types according to localization in the cell (central, terminal, and subterminal) (a); and spore structure (b). Exosporium presence and coat layers vary according to species. (b) *Sources:* Based on Driks A, Eichenberger P. (2016) The Spore Coat. *Microbiol spectr.* 4(2); Henriques AO, Charles PMJ. (2007) Structure, assembly, and function of the spore surface layers. *Annu Rev Microbiol.* 61: 555–588 and McKenney PT, Driks A, Eichenberger P. (2013) The Bacillus subtilis endospore: assembly and functions of the multilayered coat. *Nat Rev Microbiol.* 11(1): 33–44.

cell, while the terminal spore is located at the cells' poles. The subterminal type of spore is present between the middle and the end of the cell (Cavalcante *et al.* 2019). Terminal spores are observed in *C. tetani*, while *B. cereus* shows central spores.

4.1.1.1 Structure

The structure of bacterial spores shares a general and typical architecture. The genome DNA is located in the partially dehydrated central core surrounded by the inner spore membrane, followed by a germ cell wall (a thin peptidoglycan layer which will become the cell wall of the bacterium after spore germination), cortex, outer spore membrane, and coat, consecutively (Figure 4.1b). Additional outer layers vary in number and structure according to species. Furthermore, some species may show an exosporium as the outermost layer (Driks and Eichenberger 2016). For instance, *B. subtilis* has the coat as the outermost spore layer, while *B. anthracis* and *B. megaterium* have two additional layers and an exosporium (Bozue *et al.* 2016; McKenney *et al.* 2013). In studies of coat genes in *Clostridium* spp. the genome has shown some differences regarding *B. subtilis* (Galperin *et al.* 2012; Henriques and Charles 2007). However, there are significant similarities among closely related species, as demonstrated for *B. subtilis* and closely related species. These bacteria have similar coat structures, and the exosporium is absent. All *B. cereus* groups (including *B. anthracis*) have similar exosporium structures (Cavalcante *et al.* 2019). The outer spore layers, including exosporium, may influence spores' adherence to surfaces, which plays a crucial role in their survival and spread in different environments (Huang *et al.* 2020; Malyshev and Baillie 2020; McKenney *et al.* 2013).

During spore germination, the coat is removed, and cell wall hydrolases degrade the cortex. The germ cell originates the vegetative cell wall, whereas the inner spore membrane becomes the cytoplasmic membrane. The outer spore membrane may be lost during spore maturation, although for *Acetonema longum* it persists after germination, thus generating a double membrane vegetative cell (Tocheva *et al.* 2011).

4.1.1.2 Spore Formation

The sporulation process in bacterial cells happens by asymmetric cell division, and the genome copies are partitioned into each of the two cells (Errington 2003). The smaller cell (prespore) develops until it forms the mature endospore, while the larger cell (mother cell) contributes to spore formation by providing essential conditions and substances for the process. Following cell division, the prespore is engulfed by the mother cell in a process similar to phagocytosis. Thus, a prespore structure with a double membrane isolated from the external medium is generated (Narula *et al.* 2016). Following the process, two peptidoglycan layers are assembled between the inner and outer membranes surrounding the prespore. The primordial germ cell wall is a thin layer of peptidoglycan assembled from the inner spore membrane's surface. This layer is similar in composition to the vegetative cell wall and originates when the spore germinates. The spore cortex is a thicker and chemically distinct layer of peptidoglycan assembled from the outer prespore membrane. This structure is directly related to the spore core's dehydrated state and crucial for spore mineralization and dormancy, providing thermal resistance of spores (Driks and Eichenberger 2016; McKenney *et al.* 2013).

Simultaneously with cortex development, the protein coat is deposited around the outer membrane's outer surface. Assembly of the glycoprotein exosporium layer also becomes visible at this stage. Synthesis of the cortex, coat and exosporium is performed by the mother cell. The germ cell wall, cortex and coat layers are close to one another. In contrast, the exosporium assumes an irregular form (see Figure 4.1b) (Driks and Eichenberger 2016; Henriques and Charles 2007; McKenney *et al.* 2013).

Many factors are involved in modulating sporulation, including nutrient starvation and cell density. Nutrient starvation and cell density are related factors that lead to activation of the molecular master regulator of sporulation, Spo0A, by phosphorylation. The cell's communication via quorum-sensing signals transmits the information among cells, "there is sufficient/insufficient nutrient per cell", which allows reservation of energy for the sporulation process (Bischofs *et al.* 2009). Although nutrient starvation induces sporulation, this process requires energy and only starts when enough nutrients are available. Nutrient starvation concerns either amino acids or carbon sources and even minerals (Gauvry *et al.* 2017). Other environmental factors, such as temperature, pH, water activity, aeration and others, may also affect the sporulation process (Gauvry *et al.* 2017). There is still no evidence that bacterial sporulation occurs outside the growth range of temperature, pH and water activity. Studies about spore structure and sporulation conditions are crucial to understanding the impact on the gastric survival of spores administered as probiotics and their interactions with the gut microbiota and mucosa (Bressuire-Isoard *et al.* 2018). Although the life cycle, including the sporulating process, of pathogenic *Bacillus* in the human gastrointestinal tract is well known (Hutchison *et al.* 2014; Narula *et al.* 2016), literature on the life cycle of beneficial spore formers is still scarce. According to Bernardeau *et al.* (2017), spore properties such as proteinaceous coat, high resilience in macrophages and dipicolinic acid improve the absorption, competitiveness for adhesion and immune response modulation, and survival of spore-forming bacteria in the gastrointestinal tract.

4.1.2 Sources and Probiotic Potential of Spore-forming Strains

Spore-forming bacteria have exceptional diversity and adaptability, which makes them ubiquitous microorganisms. The richness of the mechanisms, in addition to their resistance characteristics, mainly associated with sporulation capacity, allows this microbial group to occupy many ecological niches. They are found in soil, water, air and the gastrointestinal tract of various animals (Atarashi *et al.* 2013; Fakhry *et al.* 2008; Gu *et al.* 2015; Hong *et al.* 2005; Kuebutornye *et al.* 2020; Zhou *et al.* 2019).

Studies regarding potential probiotic spore-forming bacteria isolated from different sources have been performed, and some examples are shown in Table 4.1. For a probiotic to benefit human or animal health, it must survive passage through the gastrointestinal tract and function in the gut environment (Giraffa *et al.* 2010). Thus, it is common to search for novel probiotic strains in animal and human gut or feces since they are probably resistant to these harsh conditions. On the other hand, researchers have demonstrated potential probiotic strains in different environments, particularly in fermented foods (Ramos *et al.* 2013; Sui *et al.* 2020). In aquaculture, *Bacillus* species have been used as probiotics. They have been isolated from a variety of sources, including soil, water, decaying matter, commercial sources and the gastrointestinal tract of fish and other vertebrates (Gu *et al.* 2015; Kuebutornye *et al.* 2020; Pereira *et al.* 2019; Zhou *et al.* 2019). However, some authors have commented that commercial probiotics are often relatively ineffective because they are isolated from non-fish sources, making their colonization process difficult in the fish gut (Kavitha *et al.* 2018; Nandi *et al.* 2017).

The spore-producing species most used as probiotics are those of the *Bacillus* genus. Most of these genus strains do not demonstrate high toxicity and fulfill the typical probiotic strain characterization (Cutting 2011; Nithya and Halami 2013). They are microorganisms that can survive under gastrointestinal conditions by the sporulating process (Miller and Ouwehand 2013).

The main probiotic *Bacillus* strains are: *B. cereus*, *B. subtilis* natto, *B. licheniformis* Me1, *B. flexus* Hk1, *B. subtilis* Bn1, *B. subtilis* PY79, *B. clausii*, *B. indicus* HU36, *B. mojavensis* KJS-3, *B. coagulans*, *B. subtilis* KD1, *B. polyfermenticus* SDC, *B. pumilus*, *B. laterosporus* and *B. polymyxa* (Cutting 2011; Hong *et al.* 2008; Kim *et al.* 2011; Nithya and Halami 2013).

The form of intervention of the strains is varied, often promoting benefits to specific targets. For instance, *B. subtilis* natto is related to modulation of the immune system (Hosoi and Kiuchi 2004), while *B. coagulans* BC_{30} can be used to aid in the treatment of rheumatoid arthritis (Mandel *et al.* 2010). The strains of *B. clausii* are usually used for clinical occurrences of childhood diarrhea and *Helicobacter pylori* treatment (Cutting 2011). Finally, strains of *B. cereus* and *B. licheniformis* are commonly associated with therapies for animals.

To a lesser extent, another spore-forming genus, *Clostridium*, has been applied for potential probiotic use. In 1968, in Japan, although known as a virulent species to the human organism, the *C. butyricum* MIYAIRI 588 (CBM588) strain was validated to be used

Table 4.1 Examples of spore-forming bacteria strains and their source, use indication, and potential as probiotics.

Strains	Source	Indication	Probiotic potential	Reference
B. velezensis TPS3N, *B. subtilis* TPS4, *B. amyloliquefaciens* TPS17	Gut of Nile tilapia	Potential probiotics in tilapia aquaculture	High survivability after heat treatment, non-hemolytic nature, broad antimicrobial activities, and safety	Kuebutornye *et al.* (2020)
B. subtilis	Gastrointestinal tract of Hulong grouper	Potential probiotic in aquatic culture	Antimicrobial compound production towards pathogens improved performance in the non-specific immune response of grouper and increased the expression of immune-related genes under virus infection	Zhou *et al.* (2019)
B. coagulans CGMCC 9551	Healthy piglet feces	Animal probiotic	Antibacterial activity against pathogens, bile and low pH tolerance, mucus adherence, safety assessment, and extracellular hydrolase activity improving animal digestibility	Gu *et al.* (2015)
Bacillus spp.	Feces and ileal biopsies of healthy human volunteers	Potential probiotic for human use and as oral vaccine vehicles	Resistance of cells and spores to simulated gastric conditions, the ability to grow and sporulate in anaerobic conditions, and the presence of toxin-encoding genes in their genome	Fakhry *et al.* (2008)
B. velezensis FTC01	Probiotic feed supplement for farm and domestic animals (Biotop®)	Animal probiotic	Presence of gene clusters involved in the synthesis of antimicrobial peptides and hydrolases (peptidases, phytases and glycosidases), improving animal digestion and preventing intestinal disorders. Presence of a peptidylprolyl isomerase (prsA) gene, suggesting effects on bacterial adhesion and biofilm formation, protecting intestinal cells against toxicogenic microorganisms and their products	Pereira *et al.* (2019)

B. subtilis HU58	Human	Spores as probiotic supplements in wholemeal biscuits and a range of novel food products due to their survival after the baking process	Resistance to gastric fluids, rapid sporulation, and biofilms formation	Permpoonpattana *et al*. (2012)
B. coagulans T242	Fermentation samples of a spice factory in Dalian	Potential probiotic for human use	Viability at gastrointestinal condition, adhesion to HT-29 cells, inhibiting growth and adhesion of *E. coli* to intestinal epithelial cells, safety, cholesterol assimilation, and antioxidant capacity	Sui *et al*. (2020)
Clostridium spp.	Human fecal samples	Potential probiotic for human use	Counterbalance dysbiosis, induce Treg cells, and aid in the management of allergic and inflammatory conditions	Atarashi *et al*. (2013)
C. butyricum MIYAIRI 588 (CBM588)	Commercial probiotic in Japan isolated from human	Probiotic for human use	Inhibition of *C. difficile* toxicity, probably by the inhibition of toxin protein production. The low pH due to organic acid production may also have inhibitory effects on *C. difficile* growth, metabolism, and toxicity	Woo *et al*. (2011)

clinically for diarrhea prevention and treatment caused by the use of antimicrobials (Ito *et al.* 1997; Kamiya *et al.* 1997). *C. butyricum* MIYAIRI 588 (CBM588) is a Japanese probiotic strain isolated from a patient in 1933 and is currently commercially available. When these probiotic strains are orally consumed, the spores of *C. butyricum* can germinate and develop in the gastrointestinal tract (Waligora-Dupriet *et al.* 2009). They produce high amounts of short-chain fatty acids, such as acetate and butyrate, through the fermentation of undigested carbohydrates (Waligora-Dupriet *et al.* 2009). These short-chain fatty acids stimulate the proliferation of desired enterocytes (Hamer *et al.* 2008).

Among the observed therapeutic effects, it is possible to report that the probiotic *C. butyricum* strain may act on inflammatory bowel disease (Okamoto *et al.* 2000), *C. difficile* infections (Woo *et al.* 2011), gastric ulcers (Wang *et al.* 2015) and diarrhea and have immunomodulatory effects on colon inflammation (Hamer *et al.* 2008). Although the presented benefits are innovative, most *Clostridium* strains may show implications for human health. Probiotic and pathogenic properties are strain-specific, highlighting the need to evaluate the strain used as a probiotic.

Sporulated inoculum-based probiotics in foods are still restricted due to consumer safety (Jafari *et al.* 2017). The virulence genes and toxicity capacity of some spore-forming bacteria associated with food spoilage and foodborne diseases are factors of concern because they are often related to outbreaks of foodborne infections. Germination of these microorganisms in the food matrix is therefore contraindicated to avoid microbial proliferation and food deterioration (Ranadheera *et al.* 2010).

The spore-forming bacteria as probiotics for human consumption are generally available in medical form, usually lyophilized and sold in microcapsules to protect the product from the oxidation process and minimize undesirable odors and flavors (Pande *et al.* 2012). It is possible to find some spore-forming probiotics as food supplements that are useful for maintaining gastrointestinal tract integrity and stimulating human well-being.

4.1.3 Spore Formers as Gut Microbiota

The term "gut microbiota" covers all microorganisms that colonize the enteric portion of humans and animals. Microbial colonization is found throughout the gastrointestinal tract. In the small intestine, the conditions are limited for microbial colonization since food transit is accelerated in this region, thus preventing adequate microbial adhesion to the mucosa. Furthermore, there is the presence of pancreatic secretions, bile acids and remarkable peristalsis. On the other hand, there is an excellent nutritional supply and absence of intestinal fluids in the large intestine, which allows a quantitative and diverse prevalence of microbial populations (Walter and Ley 2011).

Colonization by microbes is associated with their ability to adhere to the receptors of gut cells. Gut microbiota can be classified as autochthonous (permanent) or allochthonous (transient). Autochthonous microbiota are regularly found in the gastrointestinal tract, and, in conditions of dysbiosis, they can quickly reestablish. On the other hand, allochthonous microorganisms reach the gastrointestinal tract and remain in this region temporarily. They are eliminated through the feces in a short period (Brandt *et al.* 2006). The principal genera considered permanent in the gastrointestinal tract are *Bacteroides, Bifidobacterium, Eubacterium, Clostridium, Lactobacillus, Escherichia, Enterobacter,*

Enterococcus, Klebsiella, Methanobrevibacter, Peptococcus, Peptostreptococcus, Proteus, Ruminococcus, Staphylococcus and *Streptococcus* (Brandt *et al.* 2006; Guarner and Malagelada 2003).

It is known that during the gestational period, the fetus is mostly free of microorganisms. At birth, even during childbirth, microbial colonization starts. Maternal vaginal contact and exposure to the hospital environment promote the microbial population's first insertion (Nuriel-Ohayon *et al.* 2016). The lactation process is another fundamental mechanism that affects microbial colonization in the first months of life due to bifidobacterial factors and is a source of bacteria to the infant gut (Funkhouser and Bordenstein 2013; Rodríguez 2014). Bacteria were detected in human milk (Funkhouser and Bordenstein 2013; Rodríguez 2014); however, their origin and impact on neonatal gut microbiota establishment are still unknown.

Studies indicate that neonates fed with milk formulas in the first months of life have a higher incidence of the spore-forming bacteria *Clostridium* in the initial microbiota than neonates who are exclusively breastfed (Stürmer *et al.* 2012). The type of childbirth also demonstrates an influence on gut microbiota colonization: babies born through surgical procedures, such as cesarean sections, have also shown a high incidence of *Clostridium* spp. and other potential pathogens (Nuriel-Ohayon *et al.* 2016).

C. difficile species is a common spore-forming bacterium found in the healthy adult population. It is an autochthonous bacterial species, which does not expose the individual to relevant pathological risks when present in low concentrations. However, a high population of this bacterium in the intestine can cause clinical disorders that manifest from diarrhea to infectious conditions, and in some cases, cause death (Kotowska *et al.* 2005). *C. difficile* may increase their adhesion area in the intestinal mucosa in conditions of dysbiosis, causing damage to the host. This bacterium acts as an opportunistic pathogen by secreting toxins A and B. These toxins affect the actin fiber structure of the cytoskeleton of epithelial cells of the intestine. This process may generate inflammatory conditions and intestinal lesions (Berkes *et al.* 2003). The leading cause of dysbiosis and damage caused by *C. difficile* is administration of antibiotics, especially those with a broad spectrum of action (Carlet 2012). The antimicrobial substances can eliminate the target microorganisms. However, they also destroy beneficial bacteria (Langdon *et al,* 2016).

Another species of *Clostridium* resident in the gut microbiota of healthy individuals is *C. perfringens*, which, in the same way, in conditions of dysbiosis can cause gastrointestinal infections to the host and diarrhea related to the ingestion of antimicrobials. This bacterium releases an enterotoxin that causes damage to the intestinal mucosa and elimination of electrolytic fluids (Berkes *et al.* 2003).

Regarding the spore-forming bacteria belonging to the *Bacillus* genus, they are considered transient microorganisms ingested in spoiled foods or as probiotic consumption in the case of beneficial strains. In this last case, when the bacteria are consumed in the spore form, they undergo physical–chemical processes throughout the gastrointestinal region through enzymatic activity, and can then exert their protective effect (Hong *et al.* 2005).

Bacillus spp. have been found in daily human and animal feces for a limited time after their initial ingestion, which confirms that they remain in the intestinal tract for a specific period (Hong *et al.* 2005; Vesa *et al.* 2000). The same pattern is observed with pathogenic strains such as *B. cereus*. The microorganism is eliminated within 24–48 h after ingestion of the strain when the infectious process caused to the host is temporary (Granum 2002; Kotiranta *et al.* 2000). However, it has been reported that the transit time of some *Bacillus* spp. in the intestinal microbiota can last approximately 10 days, which corresponds to a period longer than the generally reported microbial intestinal transit. Thus, it suggests that *Bacillus* spp. in contact with the intestinal colon may establish a symbiotic relationship with the host, developing the ability to multiply and re-sporulate (Graff *et al.* 2001; Hong *et al.* 2005).

Bacillus spp. have also been isolated from the gastrointestinal tract of animals and applied as a feed supplement for animals. Researchers have shown positive effects on chickens, pigs and aquaculture growth and inhibiting pathogens in the treated animals' intestine (Abriouel *et al.* 2011; Cavazzoni *et al.* 1998; Hendricks and Guo 2006; Murillo and Villamil 2011; Permpoonpattana *et al.* 2012; Thirabunyanon and Thongwittaya 2012). Probiotic *Bacillus* spp. administration for animals has also been used as an alternative to antimicrobial substances (Gu *et al.* 2015; Thirabunyanon and Thongwittaya 2012).

4.1.4 Interaction with the Intestinal Cells

Bacterial spore formers, mostly of the genus *Bacillus* as mentioned previously, are among a large number of probiotic products on the market today, mostly in their spore form. They have been shown to prevent several gastrointestinal conditions and diseases, and the diversity of species and their applications are remarkable. The interest in these species for humans is their tolerance and ability to survive in gastric acid and the hostile intestinal environment (Hong *et al.* 2005). Presently, *Bacillus* spp. are some of the most studied and well-characterized probiotics; their use as probiotics is expanding rapidly because of their inherent ability to form endospores (Elisashvili *et al.* 2019).

Several *Bacillus* strains have human and animal health benefit potential, directly associated with their ability to interact with the host's gastrointestinal tract because of their adhesion and attachment features. In general, it has been shown that different *Bacillus* strains have antimicrobial (Khochamit *et al.* 2015), antioxidant (Gobi *et al.* 2016) and immune modulatory (Foligné *et al.* 2012; Lefevre *et al.* 2015) activity in the host. Also, they may modulate the composition of gut microbiota (Nyangale *et al.* 2014).

Among the elements behind the beneficial effects of *Bacillus* spp. probiotics stand out for their ability to interact with intestinal cells, especially immune cells (Elshaghabee *et al.* 2017; Gobi *et al.* 2016). This interaction may also be between their spores or their vegetative forms and the intestinal immune cells.

Although several in vitro and in vivo animal models (Choi *et al.* 2016; Dudonné *et al.* 2015) have shown the efficacy as probiotics of the vegetative forms of *Bacillus* spp., few reports describe the health benefits of their spore form (Foligné *et al.* 2012; Mazzoli *et al.* 2019). Some of these studies provide evidence that oral administration of spores stimulates the intestinal immune system and could be beyond their probiotic effect (Elshaghabee *et al.* 2017). It seems that spores can interact with the gut-associated lymphoid tissue (GALT). The oral administration of *B. subtilis* spores led to their dissemination into the Peyer's patches and mesenteric lymph nodes (MLN), which points out they are immunogenic (Duc *et al.* 2003). Also, in vitro studies have shown that phagocytosed spores can germinate and express vegetative genes, even though they cannot replicate (Duc *et al.* 2004b).

The evidence about the immune stimulation of *Bacillus* spores is extensive. Kosaka *et al.* (1998) have shown that orally administered *B. subtilis* led to the rapid induction of interferon production by mononuclear cells in the peripheral blood, which stimulated the activity of both macrophages and natural killer (NK) cells. Furthermore, two other studies showed that *Bacillus* strains led to an increase in Th1 responses of GALT in mice (Duc *et al.* 2004a, 2004b). Th1 responses drive IgG synthesis, but, more importantly, cytotoxic T-cell recruitment, which is essential for the destruction of intracellular microorganisms (e.g. viruses, bacteria such as *Salmonella* spp.). The authors showed that *B. subtilis* or *B. pumilus* orally administered to mice induced an increase of interferon-γ (IFN-γ) and tumor necrosis factor-α (TNF-α) synthesis in the GALT and the secondary lymphoid organs (Duc *et al.*, 2004a, 2004b). IFN-γ is an effector of cellular responses and can be produced by an innate immune response, probably including NK cells, so these findings reinforced a Th1 response after intake of those bacilli. Recently, Mazzoli *et al.* (2019) showed that orally administered spores of strain SF185, a human isolate of *B. megaterium*, to mice with dextran sulfate sodium (DSS)-induced colitis reduced lipid peroxidation, TNF-α levels and IL-12/IL-10 cytokine ratio in the colonocytes, indicating antioxidant and anti-inflammatory effects. Because of that, they speculated that spores prevented cell damage, maintaining colon integrity, as seen in the histological analysis. They also recommended further studies to elucidate mechanisms beyond these effects.

In humans, one of the first studies showing that spore-forming bacteria can interact with the intestinal immune system and produce systemic immune responses was the randomized trial conducted by Fiorini *et al.* (1985). In this trial, 30 elderly patients received *B. subtilis* spores of Enterogermina® orally. In peripheral blood mononuclear cells, the authors observed a significant increase of IgA-producing B cells but not an unrestricted proliferation of all B cells. These results indicated that orally ingested spores could be interacting with the GALT, priming B cells for IgA synthesis.

The effects of a spore-based probiotic formulation in patients with irritable bowel syndrome (IBS) were investigated recently by Catinean *et al.* (2019). IBS is an intestinal functional disorder, and as yet its pathophysiology remains unclear and controversial. Several mechanisms have been investigated, ranging from inflammation and immunological involvement to dysbiosis, genetic, brain–gut interaction or dietary factors (Holtmann *et al.* 2016; Kennedy *et al.* 2014). In the Catinean *et al.* (2019) study, the authors compared the effects of treatment with a spore-based probiotic formulation (five *Bacillus* spp. strains: MegaSporeBiotic, Microbiome Labs, St. Augustine, FL, USA) with two standard treatments: rifaximin followed by a nutraceutical agent (*Lactobacillus* strain, prebiotics and vitamins) or rifaximin followed by a low-fermentable oligosaccharide, disaccharides, monosaccharides and polyols diet (Low-FODMAP diet). The spore-based probiotic formulation led to the same outcomes as the two standard treatments regarding the impact on severity score and all the rectal volume sensation test parameters, and a significantly better effect on the quality of life (Catinean *et al.* 2019). Although not mechanistic, this study also showed *Bacillus* spores' potential as probiotics interacting with intestinal cells in humans and contributing to disease treatment.

In addition to the *Bacillus* genus, another group of spore-forming bacteria that have received attention as potential probiotics is the genus *Clostridium*. *Clostridium* spp., as commensal bacteria in our gut, exert beneficial effects on our intestinal homeostasis.

Clostridium spp. have been reported to attenuate inflammation and allergic diseases effectively due to some of their specific biological activities. Like butyrate, secondary bile acids and indole propionic acid, their cellular components and metabolites play a probiotic role by providing energy to intestinal epithelial cells, strengthening the intestinal barrier and interacting with the immune system. Because of their health effects, *Clostridium* species have considerable potential as probiotics, *Faecalibacterium prausnitzii* being a representative of *Clostridium* species in recent studies.

In this context, *F. prausnitzii* and its culture supernatant exhibited anti-inflammatory effects under recovery from chronic colitis and colitis reactivation in animal models (Kiely *et al.* 2018, Richard *et al.* 2018). Umesaki *et al.* (1999) found that a defined mixture of 46 strains of *Clostridium* species modified the intraepithelial lymphocyte profile in the large intestine of gnotobiotic mice (Umesaki *et al.* 1999). *Clostridium* strains also promoted mucosal Treg cell accumulation in the colon, and a cocktail of 46 *Clostridium* strains increased transforming growth factor-β in the colon of mice (Atarashi *et al.* 2011). Similarly, oral administration of 17 strains of clostridia induced the expansion and differentiation of Treg cells in the intestine, attenuating colitis and allergic diarrhea of mice (Atarashi *et al.* 2013).

A recent study discovered a new gut-derived Treg cell subpopulation in humans, named DP8α, which could express CD4 and CD8α. Among DP8α T cells, *F. prauspecific* T cells were co-expressing CCR6 and CXCR6, decreasing inflammatory bowel disease (IBD) in patients (Godefroy *et al.* 2018). These authors suggested that *Clostridium* spp. could powerfully improve gut immune tolerance.

It is relevant to point out that, despite the fact that *Bacillus* and *Clostridium* strains can interact with intestinal immune cells and promote health benefits, their application in specific immune-deficient populations, especially the critically ill, neonates and the elderly, should be carefully evaluated and regulated. Some reports have described bacteremia in immune-compromised patients treated with spore-forming and other probiotics (Doron and Snydman 2015). Therefore, it is also essential to detect and eliminate any link between probiotics and strains isolated from immune-compromised hosts. Clinical trials of these formulations should cover a sufficient ratio of the target population, including people with low immunity.

The data presented showed that several *Bacillus* and *Clostridium* strains possess potent probiotic characteristics for intestinal homeostasis, primarily because of their interaction with the GALT, so promising a great future as probiotics. Further research will accelerate the development and achievement of species as probiotics in the future.

4.2 Propionibacteria

4.2.1 Phenotypic and Genotypic Characterization

Propionibacteria are mesophilic, Gram-positive, catalase-positive, non-motile pleomorphic rods, belonging to the Actinobacteria class. These bacteria are anaerobic or aerotolerant, and they do not form spores. The growth temperature ranges from 15 to 40 °C (optimal at 30 °C), at a pH range of 5.1 to 8.5.

In general, the species of *Propionibacterium* genus are divided into two groups: (i) "dairy" or "classical", primarily isolated from milk and dairy environments, and composed of *P. acidipropionici, P. cyclohexanicum, P. freudenreichii, P. jensenii, P. microaerophilum* and *P. thoenii*; and (ii) "cutaneous", primarily isolated from skin and occasionally associated with infections, and composed of *P. acidifaciens, P. acnes, P. australiense, P. avidum, P. granulosum, P. humerusii* and *P. propionicus* (Cummins and Johnson 1986). Although these species are grouped as "dairy" and "cutaneous", they have also been isolated from other environments: "dairy" *Propionibacterium* spp. have been isolated from silages, vegetables, and rumen, intestine and feces of animals (Argañaraz-Martínez *et al.* 2013; Mantere-Alhonen and Ryhaenen 1994), and "cutaneous" *Propionibacterium* spp. have been isolated from the intestine of humans and animals (Argañaraz-Martínez *et al.* 2013; Macfarlane *et al.* 1988; Mantere-Alhonen and Ryhaenen 1994).

Among "dairy" species, *P. freudenreichii* is associated with developing the typical holes due to carbon dioxide production and contributing to the flavor of Swiss cheese (Falentin *et al.* 2010; Langsrud and Reinbold 1973). *Propionibacterium* spp. can convert different carbohydrates (e.g. glucose, galactose, lactose, fructose), alcohols (e.g. glycerol and erythritol) and organic acids (lactic and gluconic acids) into propionic and acetic acids and carbon dioxide. Moreover, *Propionibacterium* spp. can produce a wide variety of biological and bioactive compounds such as folic acid, proline, conjugated linoleic acid (CLA), vitamin B_{12}, bacteriocins and antifungals (Ho *et al.* 2009). Some strains have shown to remain viable throughout the gastrointestinal tract and be beneficial to the host, suggesting a potential probiotic use (Freitas *et al.* 2015). They may enhance immune system activity, prevent infections and allergies, and reduce cancer risk because they remove and metabolize carcinogenic compounds like mycotoxins, plant lectins and heavy metals.

Genetic characterization of *Propionibacterium* spp. has been performed using different approaches, such as random amplified polymorphic DNA (RAPD), pulsed-field gel electrophoresis (PFGE), multilocus sequence analysis (MLSA), for differentiation of bacteria species and strains (Freitas *et al.* 2015; Kaufmann 1998; Lomholt and Kilian 2010; Maiden *et al.* 1998; Perry *et al.* 2003; Rossetti and Giraffa 2005). Molecular typing of "dairy" and "cutaneous" propionibacteria is essential to relate the isolates taxonomically and phylogenetically to characterize strains with interesting industrial characteristics or those responsible for infections, even belonging to the same species. Freitas *et al.* (2015) evaluated the biodiversity of *Propionibacterium* in Brazilian dairy farms that produce Swiss-type cheeses. Using the PFGE technique, these authors found heterogeneity among the same species' strains when isolated from different geographical regions, suggesting that each location represents a specific niche. Gautier *et al.* (1996) described that *P. freudenreichii* strains isolated from milk or cheese from different geographical origins also displayed different PFGE restriction patterns. Lomholt and Kilian (2010) described similar finds, evaluating subpopulations of *P. acnes*, which may be responsible for infections and non-pathogenic strains. Strains of *P. acnes* showed phenotypic and genotypic variability (Lomholt and Kilian 2010). The strains have been classified into three groups according to their serological differentiation of cell wall carbohydrates, phage typing, and analysis of recA, tly and CAMP gene sequences (Johnson and Cummins 1972; McDowell *et al.* 2005; Valanne *et al.* 2005). Furthermore, fermentation and PFGE profiles have also suggested heterogeneity among the *P. acnes* strains (Kishishita *et al.* 1979; Oprica *et al.* 2004). Regarding their pathogenic potential, it seems that the strains may vary in their ability to induce human β-defensin 2. Moreover, they may differently affect the growth, differentiation and viability of keratinocytes and sebocytes (Nagy *et al.* 2005, 2006).

Strain phenotypic and genotypic characterization of *Propionibacterium* spp. is crucial to search for novel probiotic isolates once it is shown that probiotic potential is strain specific (Ramos *et al.* 2013). In general, the environment of dairy farms and milk production has proved to be a reservoir of a great diversity of *Propionibacterium* spp. with the potential to be used as starter cultures and probiotics (Freitas *et al.* 2015).

4.2.2 Probiotic Properties and Potential Mechanisms of Action

An increasing number of reports on propionibacteria's potential probiotic properties have been published in the past decades. Among the significant number of strains, some dairy propionibacteria have shown probiotic effects, alone or in combination with lactic acid bacteria and bifidobacteria (Rabah *et al.* 2017).

Several dairy propionibacteria strains tolerate upper gastrointestinal tract conditions and easily adhere to intestinal epithelial cells (Campaniello *et al.* 2015; Zárate *et al.* 2016) and human and animal intestinal mucus (Ganan *et al.* 2013; Ouwehand *et al.* 2000). It seems their tolerance to digestive stresses and epithelial cell adhesion are due to several metabolites produced by them, allowing close contact of the probiotic and the target cells (Guan *et al.* 2014).

Dairy propionibacteria produce nutraceuticals and beneficial metabolites responsible for their versatile probiotic attributes, including surface proteins, short-chain fatty acids (SCFAs), conjugated fatty acids and 1,4-dihydroxy-2-naphthoic acid (DHNA). These metabolites possess beneficial properties, and their production depends on the strain and the growth medium. Therefore, in general, the reported probiotic effects of dairy propionibacteria are described according to their ability to modulate the microbiota and the immune system and show cancer modulation (Rabah *et al.* 2017).

4.2.2.1 Immunomodulation

Probiotic consumption has been indicated, as supplements, to treat or ameliorate acute episodes of inflammatory diseases such as inflammatory bowel disease (IBD). Ulcerative colitis (UC) and Crohn's disease (CD) are the two main IBD. It seems they result from an imbalance of the intestinal immune response, probably because some specific microbiota components occur in genetically predisposed individuals (Sánchez *et al.* 2017).

It has been shown that dairy propionibacteria, specifically *P. freudenreichii*, can modulate the intestinal immune system and improve inflammation in the context of IBD. For example, intake of *P. freudenreichii* was able to prevent trinitrobenzene sulfonic acid (TNBS)-induced colitis in mice in a strain-dependent manner (Foligné *et al.* 2013). A probiotic mixture of *Lactobacillus rhamnosus* and *P. freudenreichii* was given to mice fed a high-fat diet. The intestinal and systemic pro-inflammatory markers induced by high-fat feeding were down-regulated (Oksaharju *et al.* 2013). In human peripheral blood mononuclear cells (PBMCs), some strains caused high levels of interleukin 10 (IL-10), a regulatory interleukin that is thought to be the most effective in improving TNBS-induced colitis (Cousin *et al.* 2012a). Selected strains of *P. freudenreichii* also decreased plasma haptoglobulin, gut mucosa IL8 and TNF-α (pro-inflammatory cytokines), after lipopolysaccharide (LPS) stimulation ex vivo (Cousin *et al.* 2012a). In humans, patients with active UC receiving cell-free culture supernatant of *P. freudenreichii* (BGS) experienced improvement in clinical activity index score (Suzuki *et al.* 2006). In IBS patients, a probiotic mixture of *Lactobacillus rhamnosus* and *P. freudenreichii* alleviated symptoms and balanced the gut microbiota (Kajander *et al.* 2008).

Different characteristics of dairy propionibacteria that trigger several molecular mechanisms seem to be underlying their anti-inflammatory effects, such as:

1) *Short-chain fatty acid production.* Short-chain fatty acids (SCFAs) are known for their ability to modulate the immune system. They are produced in the colon through fiber or complex carbohydrate fermentation by colonic bacteria. Butyrate, propionate and acetate are the main SCFAs produced. They are used primarily as an energy source by colonocytes and hepatocytes. There is an excellent scope of scientific data on the crucial role of SCFAs in intestinal immune regulation (Kim *et al.* 2014; Ratajczak *et al.* 2019; Tan *et al.* 2014). Dairy propionibacteria produce acetate and propionate in a 2 : 1 ratio by anaerobic fermentation of carbohydrates or organic acids. Transcriptomic analysis of HT29 cells (a human cell line of colorectal adenocarcinoma) showed a modulation by treatments with *P. freudenreichii* or SCFAs of nucleotide-binding and oligomerization domain (NOD)-like receptors and cytokine–cytokine receptor interaction gene expression, both being known to play a critical role in immune response (Cousin *et al.* 2016). Dairy propionibacteria could also exert a histone deacetylase (HDAC) inhibitory activity, modulating gut inflammation through SCFAs (Zimmerman *et al.* 2012). SCFAs may activate G protein-coupled receptors, inducing HDAC inhibition. This event could modulate intestinal inflammation by regulating activation, proliferation and differentiation of immune and epithelial cells (Kim *et al.* 2014; Tan *et al.* 2014; Zimmerman *et al.* 2012).
2) *Conjugated fatty acid production.* Many probiotics also can convert linoleic (LA), α-linolenic (LNA), γ-linolenic (GLA) and stearidonic acids (SA, C18:4) into their respective conjugated fatty acid (CLA, CLNA, CGLA and CSA, respectively) (Hennessy *et al.* 2012; McIntosh *et al.* 2009). Conjugated fatty acids (CFA) produced by propionibacteria could inhibit bacterial growth (Rainio *et al.* 2001). *P. freudenreichii* produces the *cis*-9, *trans*-11 octadecadienoic isomer in culture, and fermented dairy products from LA. Furthermore, it isomerizes the c12-double bond of LNA and GLA. Although there have been just a few studies reporting CFA production by propionibacteria (Gorissen *et al.* 2015; Rainio *et al.* 2001), their biological effects have not been investigated. It seems the anti-inflammatory effects of CFA, including those produced by propionibacteria, occur at different levels of modulation and isomer type. CLA and CLNA act as peroxisome proliferator-activated receptor γ (PPAR-γ) agonists. PPAR-γ is a nuclear receptor and, when activated, can regulate the expression of its target genes involved in lipid metabolism, inflammation, adipogenesis and maintenance of metabolic homeostasis (Kim *et al.* 2016; Yuan *et al.* 2015). PPAR-γ also impacts other proteins and transcription factor function mechanisms (Yuan *et al.* 2015). Regarding dairy propionibacteria, *P. freudenreichii*, alone or in combination with lactic acid bacteria in the cheese's matrix, increased PPAR-γ mRNA levels in the colon of TNBS-induced colitis

mice. The authors attributed this effect to the presence of CFAs in fermented cheeses. However, they alert that further investigation is needed to clarify the link between the increase of PPAR-γ gene expression and CFA production by dairy propionibacteria (Plé *et al.* 2015, 2016).

3) *Presence of surface layer proteins.* Surface layer proteins (Slps) form a surface-exposed proteinaceous network present in many Gram-positive bacteria other than propionibacteria and archaebacteria (Lortal *et al.* 1993). A wide variety of gene sequences encode Slps among species and within the same species. Therefore, they show tremendous functional diversity: molecule transport, adhesion, disguising receptors to phages, virulence factors and protection against environmental stresses (Fagan and Fairweather 2014). For example, in other species in *Lactobacillus acidophilus*, the S-layer protein A interacts with immune cells, such as dendritic cells, via specific receptors (Konstantinov *et al.* 2008; Lightfoot *et al.* 2015), inducing tolerance response and ameliorating colonic inflammation. Slps from propionibacteria also have been reported for their anti-inflammatory effects. In *P. freudenreichii*, three Slps proteins were identified by proteomic analysis (SlpA, SlpB and SlpE) (Le Maréchal *et al.* 2015). In an ex vivo study, the treatment of PBMCs with this protein mixture induced IL-10 (an anti-inflammatory cytokine) release in a dose-dependent manner, with little or no secretion of IL-12, TNF-α and IL-6 (pro-inflammatory cytokines) (Le Maréchal *et al.* 2015). Later, when this protein mixture was used with a pro-inflammatory strain (*Lactococcus lactis* MG1363) in PBMCs, it reduced the production of IL-12, IFN-γ and TNF-α (Deutsch *et al.* 2017). These studies have confirmed that surface proteins of these bacteria modulate the release of immunomodulatory factors. The *P. freudenreichii* CIRM-BIA 129 strain, which has a very marked anti-inflammatory profile, has been mutated for the SlpB and SlpE genes suppression of the anti-inflammatory effect of this strain on human PBMCs (Deutsch *et al.* 2017). It seems that this strain's anti-inflammatory effect depends on the combination of several surface proteins. Another compelling piece of evidence is that strains of *P. freudenreichii* that fail to modulate the immune response have an extracellular capsule of exopolysaccharides. When this capsule is removed, the strain shows immunomodulatory effects (Deutsch *et al.* 2010, 2012). Therefore, it seems that surface proteins from dairy propionibacteria have a crucial role in their anti-inflammatory potential.

4) *DHNA production.* In several murine colitis models, DHNA from propionibacteria, especially *P. freudenreichii*, has been able to reduce the expression of adhesion molecules such as MAdCAM-1 or VCAM-1, showing anti-inflammatory properties. In humans affected by IBD, these molecules increase immune cell infiltration into the tissue and worsen the inflammation (Okada *et al.* 2006, 2013). Indeed, in colitis mice intestine and a human intestinal epithelial cell line (Caco2 cells), DHNA from *P. freudenreichii* ET-3 isolated from Swiss-type cheese reduced lymphocyte infiltration and pro-inflammatory cytokine expression within macrophage cells after endotoxin stimulation. This study showed that DHNA activated the aryl hydrocarbon receptor (AhR), a transcriptional factor involved in inflammation. AhR activation is involved in the inhibition of the secretion of pro-inflammatory cytokines. Indeed, the inhibition of pro-inflammatory cytokine IL-6 in LPS-stimulated macrophages was related to AhR activation by DHNA (Fukumoto *et al.* 2014).

4.2.2.2 Microbiota Modulation

The consumption of *P. freudenreichii* and *P. acidipropionici* has been reported as modulating the gut microbiota in animals and human beings, in the context of UC (Fukumoto *et al.* 2014; Plé *et al.* 2015) and healthy subjects (Hojo *et al.* 2002; Seki *et al.* 2004). An increase in the genus of *Bifidobacterium* in feces has been observed (Miller and Ouwehand 2013; Nithya and Halami 2013), and these bacteria are well known for their positive health benefits to the host via several metabolic activities (O'Callaghan and Sinderen 2016). Dairy propionibacteria also showed *Bacteroides* genus-lowering properties. This genus produces an enterotoxin associated with inflammatory bowel disease occurrence (Wexler 2007). They also have reduced the *Clostridium* genus, several strains of which are associated with severe intestinal infections (Hudson *et al.* 2017).

The mechanisms underlying microbiota modulation by dairy propionic bacteria favoring symbiotic bacteria such as *Bifidobacterium* at the expense of opportunistic pathogens are not fully understood. However, they seem to be linked to their ability to produce and release two small molecules: DHNA and 2-amino-3-carboxy-1,4-naphthoquinone (ACNQ) (Isawa *et al.* 2002).

DHNA is an intermediate molecule from the menaquinone (vitamin K_2) biosynthetic pathway (Furuichi *et al.* 2006). It has been shown to induce the expression of the C-type lectin Reg III protein family, which has antimicrobial properties and affects microbiota (Fukumoto *et al.* 2014). Indeed, in mice with DSS-induced colitis, DHNA treatment restored *Lactobacillus* and *Enterobacteriaceae* populations (Okada *et al.* 2006).

ACNQ is an electron acceptor of NAD(P)H diaphorase and an electron donor of NAD(P)H peroxidase (Kaneko 1999; Yamazaki *et al.* 1999). It has been shown that ACNQ raises the activity of NADH peroxidase and NADH oxidase cofactors in *Bifidobacterium,* and the regeneration of them stimulates their growth (Kaneko 1999; Yamazaki *et al.* 1999). Indeed, the intake of dried cultures of *P. freudenreichii* ET-3 led to an increase in the *Bifidobacterium* population in the gut microbiota of healthy male and female volunteers (Hojo *et al.* 2002).

Likewise, cell-free culture supernatant of *P. freudenreichii*, named bifidogenic growth stimulator (BGS), showed similar modulation (Kaneko *et al.* 1994; 1999; Seki *et al.* 2004). Moreover, Uchida *et al.* (2011) showed no adverse effects of BGS in humans at high doses, up to 45 tablets daily. Therefore, BGS showed the potential and safety of using those components as prebiotics (Uchida *et al.* 2011).

4.2.2.3 Cancer Modulation

In this field, although many studies connect probiotic intake and beneficial effects in different types of cancer, most reports relate to colorectal cancer (CRC). CRC is one of the most common cancers and incurs substantial morbidity and mortality (Bultman 2017). Among the factors associated with CRC, unhealthy diet and gut inflammation stand out, the latter being governed by the microbiota, especially its metabolites (Bultman 2017; O'Keefe 2016). Therefore, probiotic propionibacteria strains could help to modulate gut microbiota metabolism to prevent CRC. Their short and conjugated fatty acid production and their ability to bind heavy metals or toxins are, possibly, factors underlying their anti-CRC effects.

Several dairy propionibacteria strains have shown the ability to induce apoptosis in CRC and gastric cancer cells in vitro (Caco2, HGT-1 and HT29, and cancerous cell lines). This ability was observed for *P. acidipropionici*, *P. freudenreichii* subsp. *freudenreichii,* and

P. freudenreichii subsp. *shermanii* (Cousin *et al.* 2016; Jan *et al.* 2002) in human microbiota-associated rats (Lan *et al.* 2008). Propionate and acetate, produced by them, were identified as the main factors in this effect (Cousin *et al.* 2012b, 2016; Jan *et al.* 2002; Lan *et al.* 2008). It seems these SCFAs act on the mitochondrial adenine nucleotide translator (ANT) pore, causing mitochondrial depolarization and permeabilization, leakage of cytochrome C, and caspase activation (Cousin *et al.* 2016; Jan *et al.* 2002). Furthermore, the TNF-related apoptosis-inducing ligand (TRAIL) has been increased by these SCFAs from dairy propionibacteria. TRAIL is a death receptor, which mediates apoptosis by activating the extrinsic apoptotic death pathway (Plé *et al.* 2015). In the Cousin *et al.* (2016) study, these SCFAs increased TRAIL expression in HT29 cells. The authors also showed that the HDAC inhibition in HT29 cells by SCFAs led to growth inhibition and cell cycle arrest. Also, regarding other mechanisms, a probiotic mixture containing both lactic acid bacteria and propionibacteria led to a reduction in fecal α-glucosidase, which is also associated with carcinogenesis (Hatakka *et al.* 2008; Kekkonen *et al.* 2011).

Conjugated fatty acids, including those produced by dairy propionibacteria (Gorissen *et al.* 2015; Hennessy *et al.* 2012; Rainio *et al.* 2001), have shown antiproliferative properties in various cancerous cells (Kim *et al.* 2016). The antiproliferative effect seems to be time and dose dependent. Also, for some CFA isomers, the antiproliferative mechanisms on cancerous cells were characterized at a molecular level, and they involve cycle cell arrest, lipid peroxidation and activation of apoptotic pathways (Hennessy *et al.* 2016).

Many probiotic bacteria, including dairy propionibacteria, can bind heavy metals or toxins associated with a high risk of cancers, reducing risk. *P. acidipropionici* removed two plant lectins, concanavalin A and jacalin, in colonic cells, reducing lectin toxicity in those cells (Zárate and Chaia 2009). The intestinal absorption of aflatoxin B1 was prevented, and cadmium and lead were removed from the intestine by selected strains of dairy propionibacteria (El-Nezami *et al.* 2000; Gratz *et al.* 2004, 2005; Lee *et al.* 2003). A clinical trial with Chinese people exposed to aflatoxin contamination showed the detoxification effect on aflatoxin B1 of dairy propionibacteria (El-Nezami *et al.* 2006). Still, regarding CRC, clinical evidence of bioremediation against carcinogenic components for propionibacteria is weak.

4.3 Conclusion and Future Trends

Nowadays, substantially increased interest has driven probiotic studies and evaluations. Among probiotic strains, *Lactobacillus* and *Bifidobacterium* are the most mentioned in the literature and commercially available. However, these bacteria have the disadvantage of long storage periods at environmental temperatures. As a consequence, there has been increased interest in spore-forming bacteria in human and animal use as probiotics due to the resistance characteristic offered by spore production. Among spore-forming bacteria, *Bacillus* spp. are some of the most studied and well-characterized probiotics, and their use as probiotics is expanding rapidly. They have shown potential human and animal health benefits associated with their ability to interact with the host's gastrointestinal tract because of their adhesion and attachment properties. It has been reported that spore administration may prevent cell damage, maintaining colonic integrity, and stimulate the immune system of the host. However, further studies to elucidate mechanisms beyond these effects are needed. Most of the studies are related to the use of vegetative cells. Few reports describe the health benefits of the spore form. Other non-LAB reported as probiotic are the species of *Propionibacterium*, especially those isolated from dairy environments. Dairy propionibacteria strains can tolerate gastrointestinal tract conditions and adhere to intestinal epithelial cells and human and animal intestinal mucus. These bacteria produce nutraceuticals and beneficial metabolites such as surface proteins, short-chain fatty acids (SCFAs), conjugated fatty acids and 1,4-dihydroxy-2-naphthoic acid (DHNA), conferring on them probiotic potential. In general, the reported probiotic effects of dairy propionibacteria are described according to their ability to modulate the microbiota and the immune system and show cancer modulation. Although several studies have demonstrated the potential probiotic effect of *Propionibacterium* spp., clinical evidence is still necessary, mainly regarding the anticarcinogenic effect.

Non-LAB bacteria have shown important probiotic features, and some strains are successfully employed for animals and humans. However, probiotic properties are strain specific, and the search for and evaluation of novel strains from different sources are essential issues to be exploited. Furthermore, some mechanisms of action are still unknown, and their elucidation is necessary to improve the use of non-LAB probiotic strains.

References

Abriouel, H., Franz, C.M., Omar, N.B. and Gálvez, A. (2011). Diversity and applications of *Bacillus* bacteriocins. *FEMS Microbiol Rev*, 35(1): 201–232.

Al-Ajlani, M.M. and Hasnain, S. (2010). Bacteria exhibiting antimicrobial activities; screening for antibiotics and the associated genetic studies. *Open Conf Proc J*, 1: 230–238.

Amin, M., Rakhisi, Z. and Ahmady, Z.A. (2015). Isolation and identification of *Bacillus* species from soil and evaluation of their antibacterial properties. *Avicenna J Clin Microbiol Infect*, 2(1): 23233.

Andrade, D.P., Ramos, C.L., Botrel, D.A., Borges, S.V., Schwan, R.F. and Dias, D.R. (2019). Stability of microencapsulated lactic acid bacteria under acidic and bile juice conditions. *International Food Science and Technology*, 54(7): 2355–2362.

Argañaraz-Martínez, E., Babot, J.D., Apella, M.C. and Chaia, A.P. (2013). Physiological and functional characteristics of *Propionibacterium* strains of the poultry microbiota and relevance for the development of probiotic products. *Anaerobe*, 23: 27–37.

Atarashi, K., Tanoue, T., Oshima, T., Imaoka, A., Kuwahara, T., Momose, Y., et al. (2011). Induction of colonic regulatory T cells by indigenous *Clostridium* species. *Science*, 331(6015): 337–341.

Atarashi, K., Tanoue, T., Oshima, K., Suda, W., Nagano, Y., Nishikawa, H., et al. (2013). Treg induction by a rationally selected mixture of *Clostridia* strains from the human microbiota. *Nature*, 500(7461): 232–236.

Berkes, J., Viswanathan, V., Savkovic, S. and Hecht, G. (2003) Intestinal epithelial responses to enteric pathogens: effects on the tight junction barrier, ion transport, and inflammation. *Gut*, 52(3): 439–451.

Bernardeau, M., Lehtinen, M.J., Forssten, S.D. and Nurminen, P. (2017). Importance of the gastrointestinal life cycle of *Bacillus* for probiotic functionality. *J Food Sci Technol*, 54(8): 2570–2584.

Bischofs, I.B., Hug, J.A., Liu, A.W., Wolf, D.M. and Arkin, A.P. (2009). Complexity in bacterial cell–cell communication: Quorum signal integration and subpopulation signaling in the *Bacillus subtilis* phosphorelay. *PNAS*, 106(16): 6459–6464.

Bozue, J.A., Welkos, S. and Cote, C.K. (2016). The *Bacillus anthracis* exosporium: what's the big "hairy" deal? *Microbiol Spectr*, 3(5): TBS0021.

Brandt, K.G., Sampaio, M., Carneiro, M. and Miuki, C.J. (2006). Importância da microflora intestinal. *Pediatria*, 28(2):117–127.

Bressuire-Isoard, C., Broussolle, V. and Carlin, F. (2018). Sporulation environment influences spore properties in *Bacillus*: evidence and insights on underlying molecular and physiological mechanisms. *FEMS Microbiol Rev*, 42(5): 614–626.

Bultman, S.J. (2017). Interplay between diet, gut microbiota, epigenetic events, and colorectal cancer. *Mol Nutr Food Res*, 61(1): 10.1002/mnfr.201500902.

Campaniello, D., Bevilacqua, A., Sinigaglia, M. and Altieri, C. (2015). Screening of *Propionibacterium* spp. for potential probiotic properties. *Anaerobe*, 34: 169–173.

Carlet J. (2012). The gut is the epicentre of antibiotic resistance. *Antimicrob Resist Infect Control*, 1(1): 39.

Carlin F. (2011). Origin of bacterial spores contaminating foods. *Food Microbiol*, 28(2): 177–182.

Cassir, N., Benamar, S. and La Scola, B. (2016). *Clostridium butyricum*: from beneficial to a new emerging pathogen. *Clin Microbiol Infect*, 22(1): 37–45.

Catinean, A., Neag, A.M., Nita, A., Buzea, M. and Buzoianu, A.D. (2019). *Bacillus* spp. spores—A promising treatment option for patients with irritable bowel syndrome. *Nutrients*, 11(9): 1968.

Cavalcante, D.A., De-Souza, M.T., de Orem, J.C., de Magalhães, M.I.A., Martins, P.H., Boone, T.J., et al. (2019). Ultrastructural analysis of spores from diverse Bacillales species isolated from Brazilian soil. *SfAM*, 11(2): 155–164.

Cavazzoni, V., Adami, A. and Castrovilli, C. (1998). Performance of broiler chickens supplemented with *Bacillus coagulans* as probiotic. *Br Poult Sci*, 39(4): 526–529.

Choi, J.-H., Pichiah, P.B.T., Kim, M.-J. and Cha, Y.-S. (2016). Cheonggukjang, a soybean paste fermented with *B. licheniformis*-67 prevents weight gain and improves glycemic control in high fat diet induced obese mice. *J Clin Biochem Nutr*, 59(1): 31–38.

Corona-Hernandez, R.I., Álvarez-Parrilla, E., Lizardi-Mendoza, J., Islas-Rubio, A.R., de la Rosa, L.A., Wall-Medrano, A., et al. (2013). Structural stability and viability of microencapsulated probiotic bacteria: a review. *Compr Rev Food Sci F*, 12(6): 614–628.

Cousin, F.J., Foligné, B., Deutsch, S.M., Massart, S., Parayre, S., Le Loir, Y., et al. (2012a). Assessment of the probiotic potential of a dairy product fermented by *Propionibacterium freudenreichii* in piglets. *J Agric Food Chem*, 60(32): 7917–7927.

Cousin, F.J., Jouan-Lanhouet, S., Dimanche-Boitrel, M.-T., Corcos, L. and Jan, G. (2012b). Milk fermented by *Propionibacterium freudenreichii* induces apoptosis of HGT-1 human gastric cancer cells. *PLOS ONE* 7(3): e31892.

Cousin, F.J., Jouan-Lanhouet, S., Théret, N., Brenner, C., Jouan, E., Le Moigne-Muller, G., et al. (2016). The probiotic *Propionibacterium freudenreichii* as a new adjuvant for TRAIL-based therapy in colorectal cancer. *Oncotarget* 7(6): 7161–7178.

Cummins, C.S. and Johnson, J.L. (1986). Genus 1. *Propionibacterium* Orla-Jensen 1909. In: *Bergey's Manual of Systematic Bacteriology* (ed. P.H.A. Sneath, N.S. Mair, M.E. Sharpe, and J.G. Holt), 2 1346–1353. Baltimore MD: Williams & Wilkins.

Cutting, S.M. (2011). *Bacillus* probiotics. *Food Microbiol.* 28(2): 214–220.

Deutsch, S.M., Le Bivic, P., Hervé, C., Madec, M.N., LaPointe, G., Jan, G., et al. (2010). Correlation of the capsular phenotype in *Propionibacterium freudenreichii* with the level of expression of gtf, a unique polysaccharide synthase-encoding gene. *Appl Environ Microbiol*, 76(9): 2740–2746.

Deutsch, S.M., Mariadassou, M., Nicolas, P., Parayre, S., Le Guellec, R., Chuat, V., et al. (2017). Identification of proteins involved in the anti-inflammatory properties of *Propionibacterium freudenreichii* by means of a multi-strain study. *Sci Rep.* 7: 46409.

Deutsch, S.M., Parayre, S., Bouchoux, A., Guyomarc'h, F., Dewulf, J., Dols-Lafargue, M., et al. (2012). Contribution of surface β-glucan polysaccharide to physicochemical and immunomodulatory properties of *Propionibacterium freudenreichii*. *Appl Environ Microbiol*, 78(6): 1765–1775.

Doron, S. and Snydman, D.R. (2015). Risk and safety of probiotics. *Clin Infect Dis*, 60(Suppl 2): S129–S34.

Driks, A. and Eichenberger, P. (2016). The spore coat. *Microbiol Spectr*, 4(2).

Duc, L.H., Hong, H.A., Barbosa, T.M., Henriques, A.O. and Cutting, S.M. (2004a). Characterization of *Bacillus* probiotics available for human use. *Appl Environ Microbiol*, 70(4): 2161–2171.

Duc, L.H., Hong, H.A., Fairweather, N., Ricca, E. and Cutting, S.M. (2003). Bacterial spores as vaccine vehicles. *Infect Immun*, 71(5): 2810–2818.

Duc, L.H., Hong, H.A., Uyen, N.Q. and Cutting, S.M. (2004b). Intracellular fate and immunogenicity of *B. subtilis* spores. *Vaccine*, 22(15-16): 1873–1885.

Dudonné, S., Varin, T.V., Anhê, F.F., Dubé, P., Roy, D., Pilon, G., et al. (2015). Modulatory effects of a cranberry extract co-supplementation with *Bacillus subtilis* CU1 probiotic on phenolic compounds bioavailability and gut microbiota composition in high-fat diet-fed mice. *Pharma Nutrition*, 3(3): 89–100.

Elisashvili, V., Kachlishvili, E. and Chikindas, M.L. (2019). Recent advances in the physiology of spore formation for *Bacillus* probiotic production. *Probiotics Antimicrob Proteins*, 11(3): 731–747.

El-Nezami, H., Mykkänen, H., Kankaanpää, P., Salminen, S. and Ahokas, J. (2000). Ability of *Lactobacillus* and *Propionibacterium* strains to remove aflatoxin B_1 from the chicken duodenum. *J. Food Prot*, 63(4): 549–552.

El-Nezami, H.S., Polychronaki, N.N., Ma, J., Zhu, H., Ling, W., Salminen, E.K., et al. (2006). Probiotic supplementation reduces a biomarker for increased risk of liver cancer in young men from Southern China. *Am J Clin Nutr*, 83(5): 1199–1203.

Elshaghabee, F.M., Rokana, N., Gulhane, R.D., Sharma, C. and Panwar, H. (2017). *Bacillus* as potential probiotics: status, concerns, and future perspectives. *Front Microbiol*, 8: 1490.

Errington, J. (2003). Regulation of endospore formation in *Bacillus subtilis*. *Nature Rev Microbiol*, 1(2): 117–126.

Fagan, R.P. and Fairweather, N.F. (2014). Biogenesis and functions of bacterial S-layers. *Nat Rev Microbiol*, 12(3): 211–222.

Fakhry, S., Sorrentini, I., Ricca, E., De Felice, M. and Baccigalupi, L. (2008). Characterization of spore forming Bacilli isolated from the human gastrointestinal tract. *Journal of Applied Microbiology*, 105(6): 2178–2186.

Falentin, H., Deutsch, S.-M., Jan, G., Loux, V., Thierry, A., Parayre, S., et al. (2010). The complete genome of *Propionibacterium freudenreichii* CIRM-BIA1 T, a hardy Actinobacterium with food and probiotic applications. *Plos One*, 5(7): e11748.

Fiorini, G., Cimminiello, C., Chianese, R., Visconti, G., Cova, D., Uberti, T., et al. (1985). *Bacillus subtilis* selectively stimulates the synthesis of membrane bound and secreted IgA. *Chemioterapia*, 4(4): 310.

Foligné, B., Breton, J., Mater, D. and Jan, G. (2013). Tracking the microbiome functionality: focus on *Propionibacterium* species. *Gut*, 62(8): 1227–1228.

Foligné, B., Peys, E., Vandenkerckhove, J., Dewulf, J., Breton, J. and Pot, B. (2012). Spores from two distinct colony types of the strain *Bacillus subtilis* PB6 substantiate anti-inflammatory probiotic effects in mice. *Clin Nutr*, 31(6): 987–994.

Freitas, R., Chuat, V., Madec, M.-N., Nero, L.A., Thierry, A., Valence, F., et al. (2015). Biodiversity of dairy *Propionibacterium* isolated from dairy farms in Minas Gerais, Brazil. *Int J Food Microbiol*, 203: 70–77.

Fukumoto, S., Toshimitsu, T., Matsuoka, S., Maruyama, A., Oh-Oka, K., Takamura, T., et al. (2014). Identification of a probiotic bacteria-derived activator of the aryl hydrocarbon receptor that inhibits colitis. *Immunol Cell Biol*, 92(5): 460–465.

Funkhouser, L.J. and Bordenstein, S.R. (2013). Mom knows best: the universality of maternal microbial transmission. *Plos Biol*, 11(8): e1001631.

Furuichi, K., Hojo, K., Katakura, Y., Ninomiya, K. and Shioya, S. (2006). Aerobic culture of *Propionibacterium freudenreichii* ET-3 can increase production ratio of 1,4-dihydroxy-2-naphthoic acid to menaquinone. *J Biosci Bioeng*, 101(6): 464–470.

Galperin, M.Y., Mekhedov, S.L., Puigbo, P., Smirnov, S., Wolf. Y.I., Rigden, D.J. (2012). Genomic determinants of sporulation in Bacilli and Clostridia: towards the minimal set of sporulation-specific genes. *Environ Microbiol*, 14(11): 2870–2890.

Ganan, M., Martinez-Rodriguez, A.J., Carrascosa, A.V., Vesterlund, S., Salminen, S. and Satokari, R. (2013). Interaction of *Campylobacter* spp. and human probiotics in chicken intestinal mucus. *Zoonoses and Public Health*, 60(2): 141–148.

Gautier, M., de Carvalho, A. and Rouault, A. (1996). DNA fingerprinting of dairy *Propionibacteria* strains by pulsed-field gel electrophoresis. *Curr Microbiol*, 32(1): 17–24.

Gauvry, E., Mathot, A.-G., Leguérinel, I., Couvert, O., Postollec, F., Broussolle, V., et al. (2017). Knowledge of the physiology of spore-forming bacteria can explain the origin of spores in the food environment. *Res Microbiol*, 168(4): 369–378.

Giraffa, G., Chanishvili, N. and Widyastuti, Y. (2010). Importance of lactobacilli in food and feed biotechnology. *Res Microbiol*, 161(6): 480–487.

Gobi, N., Malaikozhundan, B., Sekar, V., Shanthi, S., Vaseeharan, B., Jayakumar, R., et al. (2016). GFP tagged *Vibrio parahaemolyticus* Dahv2 infection and the protective effects of the probiotic *Bacillus licheniformis* Dahb1 on the growth, immune and antioxidant responses in *Pangasius hypophthalmus*. *Fish Shellfish Immunol*, 52: 230–238.

Godefroy, E., Alameddine, J., Montassier, E., Mathé, J., Desfrançois-Noël, J., Marec, N., et al. (2018). Expression of CCR6 and CXCR6 by gut-derived CD4(+)/CD8α(+) T-regulatory cells, which are decreased in blood samples from patients with inflammatory bowel diseases. *Gastroenterology*, 155(4): 1205–1217.

Gorissen, L., Leroy, F., De Vuyst, L., De Smet, S. and Raes, K. (2015). Bacterial production of conjugated linoleic and linolenic acid in foods: a technological challenge. *Crit Rev Food Sci Nutr*, 55(11): 1561–1574.

Graff, J., Brinch, K. and Madsen, J.L.J.C.P. (2001). Gastrointestinal mean transit times in young and middle-aged healthy subjects. *Clin Physiol*, 21(2): 253–259.

Granum, P. (2002). *Bacillus cereus* and food poisoning. In: *Applications and Systematics of Bacillus and Relatives* (ed. R. Berkeley, M. Heyndrickx, N.A. Logan amd P. De Vos). Oxford: Blackwell Science.

Gratz, S., Mykkänen, H. and El-Nezami, H. (2005). Aflatoxin B1 binding by a mixture of *Lactobacillus* and *Propionibacterium*: *in vitro* versus *ex vivo*. *J Food Prot*, 68(11): 2470–2474.

Gratz, S., Mykkänen, H., Ouwehand, A.C., Juvonen, R., Salminen, S. and El-Nezami, H. (2004). Intestinal mucus alters the ability of probiotic bacteria to bind aflatoxin B1 in vitro. *Appl Environ Microbiol*, 70(10): 6306–6308.

Gu, S.B., Zhao, LN., Wu, Y., Li, S.C., Sun, J.R., Huang, J.F., et al. (2015). Potential probiotic attributes of a new strain of *Bacillus coagulans* CGMCC 9951 isolated from healthy piglet feces. *World J Microbiol Biotechnol*, 31(6): 851–863.

Guan, N., Shin, H.-d., Chen, R.R., Li, J., Liu, L., Du, G., et al. (2014). Understanding of how *Propionibacterium acidipropionici* respond to propionic acid stress at the level of proteomics. *Sci Rep*, 4(1): 6951.

Guarner, F. and Malagelada, J.-R. (2003). Gut flora in health and disease. *Lancet*, 361(9356): 512–519.

Guo, P., Zhang, K., Ma, X. and He, P. (2020). *Clostridium* species as probiotics: potentials and challenges. *J Anim Sci Biotechnol*, 11: 24.

Hamer, H.M., Jonkers, D., Venema, K., Vanhoutvin, S., Troost, F.J., Brummer, R.J. (2008). Review article: the role of butyrate on colonic function. *Aliment Pharmacol Ther*, 27(2): 104–119.

Hardy, H., Harris, J., Lyon, E., Beal, J. and Foey, A.D. (2013). Probiotics, prebiotics and immunomodulation of gut mucosal defences: homeostasis and immunopathology. *Nutrients*, 5(6): 1869–1912.

Hatakka, K., Holma, R., El-Nezami, H., Suomalainen, T., Kuisma, M., Saxelin, M., et al. (2008). The influence of *Lactobacillus rhamnosus* LC705 together with *Propionibacterium freudenreichii* ssp. *shermanii* JS on potentially carcinogenic bacterial activity in human colon. *Int J Food Microbiol*, 128(2): 406–410.

Hendricks, G. and Guo, M. (2006). Significance of milk fat in infant formulae. In: *Advanced Dairy Chemistry, Volume 2 Lipids* (ed. P.F. Fox and P.L.H. McSweeney). Boston: Springer.

Hennessy, A.A., Barrett, E., Paul Ross, R., Fitzgerald, G.F., Devery, R. and Stanton, C. (2012). The production of conjugated α-linolenic, γ-linolenic and stearidonic acids by strains of bifidobacteria and propionibacteria. *Lipids*, 47(3): 313–327.

Hennessy, A.A., Ross, P.R., Fitzgerald, G.F. and Stanton C. (2016). Sources and bioactive properties of conjugated dietary fatty acids. *Lipids*, 51(4): 377–397.

Henriques, A.O. and Charles, P.M.J. (2007). Structure, assembly, and function of the spore surface layers. *Annu Rev Microbiol*, 61: 555–588.

Ho, P.-H., Luo, J. and Adams, M.C. (2009). Lactobacilli and dairy propionibacterium with potential as biopreservatives against food fungi and yeast contamination. *Biochem Microbiol*, 45(4): 414–418.

Hojo, K., Yoda, N., Tsuchita, H., Ohtsu, T., Seki, K., Taketomo, N., et al. (2002). Effect of ingested culture of *Propionibacterium freudenreichii* ET-3 on fecal microflora and stool frequency in healthy females. *Biosci Microflora*, 21: 115–120.

Holtmann, G.J., Ford, A.C. and Talley, N.J. (2016). Pathophysiology of irritable bowel syndrome. *Lancet Gastroenterol*, 1(2): 133–146.

Hong, H.A., Duc, L.H. and Cutting, S.M. (2005). The use of bacterial spore formers as probiotics. *FEMS Microbiol Rev*, 29(4): 813–835.

Hong, H.A., Huang, J.-M., Khaneja, R., Hiep, L.V., Urdaci, M.C. and Cutting, S.M. (2008). The safety of *Bacillus subtilis* and *Bacillus indicus* as food probiotics. *J Appl Microbiol*, 105(2): 510–520.

Hosoi, T. and Kiuchi, K. (2004). Production and probiotic effects of natto. In: *Bacterial Spore Formers: Probiotics and Emerging Applications* (ed. E. Ricca, A.O. Henriques and S. Cutting). Horizon Bioscience.

Huang, Y., Flint, S.H. and Palmer, J.S. (2020). *Bacillus cereus* spores and toxins – The potential role of biofilms. *Food Microbiol*, 90: 103493.

Hudson, L.E., Anderson, S.E., Corbett, A.H. and Lamb, T.J. (2017). Gleaning insights from fecal microbiota transplantation and probiotic studies for the rational design of combination microbial therapies. *Clin Microbiol Rev*, 30(1): 191–231.

Hutchison, E.A., Miller, D.A. and Angert, E.R. (2014). Sporulation in bacteria: beyond the standard model. *Microbiol Spectr*, 2(5).

Isawa, K., Hojo, K., Yoda, N., Kamiyama, T., Makino, S., Saito, M., et al. (2002). Isolation and identification of a new bifidogenic growth stimulator produced by *Propionibacterium freudenreichii* ET-3. *Biosci Biotechnol Biochem*, 66(3): 679–681.

Ito, I., Hayashi, T., Iguchi, A., Endo, H., Nakao, M., Kato, S., et al. (1997). Effects of administration of *Clostridium butyricum* to patients receiving long-term tube feeding. *Nihon Ronen Igakkai zasshi Japanese journal of geriatrics*, 34(4): 298–304.

Jafari, M., Mortazavian, A.M., Hosseini, H., Safaei, F., Khaneghah, A.M. and Sant'Ana, A.S. (2017). Probiotic *Bacillus*: Fate during sausage processing and storage and influence of different culturing conditions on recovery of their spores. *Food Res Int*, 95: 46–51.

Jan, G., Belzacq, A.S., Haouzi, D., Rouault, A., Métivier, D., Kroemer, G., et al. (2002). Propionibacteria induce apoptosis of colorectal carcinoma cells via short-chain fatty acids acting on mitochondria. *Cell Death Differ*, 9(2): 179–188.

Johnson, J. and Cummins, C.S. (1972). Cell wall composition and deoxyribonucleic acid similarities among the anaerobic coryneforms, classical propionibacteria, and strains of *Arachnia propionica*. *J Bacteriol*, 109(3): 1047–1066.

Kajander, K., Myllyluoma, E., Rajilić-Stojanović, M., Kyrönpalo, S., Rasmussen, M., Järvenpää, S., et al. (2008). Clinical trial: multispecies probiotic supplementation alleviates the symptoms of irritable bowel syndrome and stabilizes intestinal microbiota. *Aliment Pharmacol Ther*, 27(1): 48–57.

Kamiya, S., Taguchi, H., Yamaguchi, H., Osaki, T., Takahashi, M. and Nakamura, S. (1997). Bacterioprophylaxis using *Clostridium butyricum* for lethal caecitis by *Clostridium difficile* in gnotobiotic mice. *Rev Med Microbiol*, 8: S60.

Kaneko, T. (1999). A novel bifidogenic growth stimulator produced by *Propionibacterium freudenreichii*. *Biosci Microflora*, 18(2): 73–80.

Kaneko, T., Mori, H., Iwata, M. and Meguro, S. (1994). Growth stimulator for bifidobacteria produced by *Propionibacterium freudenreichii* and several intestinal bacteria. *J Dairy Sci*, 77(2): 393–404.

Kaufmann, M.E. (1998). Pulsed-field gel electrophoresis. In: *Methods in Molecular Medicine. Molecular Bacteriology 15.* (ed. N.W. Woodford and A. Johnson), 33–50. Totowa, New Jersey: Humana Press.

Kavitha, M., Raja, M. and Perumal, P. (2018). Evaluation of probiotic potential of *Bacillus* spp. isolated from the digestive tract of freshwater fish *Labeo calbasu* (Hamilton, 1822). *Aquacult Rep*, 11: 59–69.

Kekkonen, R.A., Holma, R., Hatakka, K., Suomalainen, T., Poussa, T., Adlercreutz, H., et al. (2011). A probiotic mixture including galactooligosaccharides decreases fecal β-glucosidase activity but does not affect serum enterolactone concentration in men during a two-week intervention. *J Nutr*, 141(5): 870–876.

Kennedy, P.J., Cryan, J.F., Dinan, T.G. and Clarke, G. (2014). Irritable bowel syndrome: a microbiome-gut-brain axis disorder? *World J Gastroenterol*, 20(39): 14105–14125.

Khochamit, N., Siripornadulsil, S., Sukon, P. and Siripornadulsil, W. (2015). Antibacterial activity and genotypic–phenotypic characteristics of bacteriocin-producing *Bacillus subtilis* KKU213: Potential as a probiotic strain. *Microbiol Res*, 170: 36–50.

Kiely, C.J., Pavli, P. and O'Brien, C.L. (2018). The role of inflammation in temporal shifts in the inflammatory bowel disease mucosal microbiome. *Gut Microbes*, 9(6): 477–485.

Kim, C.H., Park, J. and Kim, M. (2014). Gut microbiota-derived short-chain fatty acids, T cells, and inflammation. *Immune Netw*, 14(6): 277–288.

Kim, J.H., Kim, Y., Kim, Y.J. and Park, Y. (2016). Conjugated linoleic acid: potential health benefits as a functional food ingredient. *Annu Rev Food Sci Technol*, 7(1): 221–244.

Kim, K.M., Jung, T.S., Ok, S., Ko, C.Y. and Kang, J.S. (2011). in vitro characterization study of *Bacillus mojavensis* KJS-3 for a potential probiotic. *Food Sci Biotechnol*, 20(4): 1155.

Kishishita, M., Ushijima, T., Ozaki, Y. and Ito, Y. (1979). Biotyping of *Propionibacterium acnes* isolated from normal human facial skin. *Applied Environment Microbiol*, 38(4): 585–589.

Konstantinov, S.R., Smidt, H., de Vos, W.M., Bruijns, S.C.M., Singh, S.K., Valence, F., et al. (2008). S layer protein A of *Lactobacillus acidophilus* NCFM regulates immature dendritic cell and T cell functions. *Proc Natl Acad Sci U S A*, 105(49): 19474–19479.

Kosaka, T., Maeda, T., Nakada, Y., Yukawa, M. and Tanaka, S. (1998). Effect of *Bacillus subtilis* spore administration on activation of macrophages and natural killer cells in mice. *Vet Microbiol*, 60(2-4): 215–225.

Kotiranta, A., Lounatmaa, K. and Haapasalo, M. (2000). Epidemiology and pathogenesis of *Bacillus cereus* infections. *Microbes and Infect*, 2(2): 189–198.

Kotowska, M., Albrecht, P. and Szajewska, H. (2005). Therapeutics *Saccharomyces boulardii* in the prevention of antibiotic-associated diarrhoea in children: a randomized double-blind placebo-controlled trial. *Aliment Pharmacol Ther*, 21(5): 583–590.

Kuebutornye, F.K.A., Lu, Y., Abarike, E.D., Wang, Z., Li, Y. and Sakyi, M.E. (2020). *in vitro* assessment of the probiotic characteristics of three *Bacillus* species from the gut of Nile Tilapia, *Oreochromis niloticus*. *Probiotics Antimicro*, 12(2): 412–424.

Lan, A., Bruneau, A., Bensaada, M., Philippe, C., Bellaud, P., Rabot, S., et al. (2008). Increased induction of apoptosis by *Propionibacterium freudenreichii* TL133 in colonic mucosal crypts of human microbiota-associated rats treated with 1,2-dimethylhydrazine. *Br J Nutr*, 100(6): 1251–1259.

Langdon, A., Crook, N. and Dantas, G. (2016). The effects of antibiotics on the microbiome throughout development and alternative approaches for therapeutic modulation. *Genome Med*, 8(1): 39.

Langsrud, T. and Reinbold, G.W. (1973). Flavor development and microbiology of Swiss cheese-A review: III. Ripening and flavor production. *J. Milk Food Technol*, 36(12): 593–609.

Le Maréchal, C., Peton, V., Plé, C., Vroland, C., Jardin, J., Briard-Bion, V., et al. (2015). Surface proteins of *Propionibacterium freudenreichii* are involved in its anti-inflammatory properties. *J Proteomics*, 113: 447–461.

Lee, Y.K., El-Nezami, H., Haskard, C.A., Gratz, S., Puong, K.Y., Salminen, S., et al. (2003). Kinetics of adsorption and desorption of aflatoxin B1 by viable and nonviable bacteria. *J. Food Prot*, 66(3): 426–430.

Lefevre, M., Racedo, S.M., Ripert, G., Housez, B., Cazaubiel, M, Maudet, C., et al. (2015). Probiotic strain *Bacillus subtilis* CU1 stimulates immune system of elderly during common infectious disease period: a randomized, double-blind placebo-controlled study. *Immun Ageing*, 12(1): 1–11.

Lightfoot, Y.L., Selle, K., Yang, T., Goh, Y.J., Sahay, B., Zadeh, M., et al. (2015). SIGNR3-dependent immune regulation by *Lactobacillus acidophilus* surface layer protein A in colitis. *EMBO J*, 34(7): 881–895.

Lomholt, H.B. and Kilian, M. (2010). Population genetic analysis of *Propionibacterium acnes* identifies a subpopulation and epidemic clones associated with acne. *PLoS ONE*, 5(8): e12277.

Lortal, S., Rouault, A., Cesselin, B. and Sleytr, U.B. (1993). Paracrystalline surface layers of dairy propionibacteria. *Appl Environ Microbiol*, 59(8): 2369–2374.

Macfarlane, G., Allison, C., Gibson, S. and Cummings, J.H. (1988). Contribution of the microflora to proteolysis in the human large intestine. *J Appl Bacteriol*, 64(1): 37–46.

Maiden, M.C., Bygraves, J.A., Feil, E., Morelli, G., Russell, J.E., Urwin, R., et al. (1998). Multilocus sequence typing: a portable approach to the identification of clones within populations of pathogenic microorganisms. *Proc Natl Acad Sci U S A*, 95(6): 3140–3145.

Majeed, M., Majeed, S., Nagabhushanam, K., Arumugam, S., Beede, K. and Ali, F. (2019). Evaluation of probiotic *Bacillus coagulans* MTCC 5856 viability after tea and coffee brewing and its growth in GIT hostile environment. *Food Res Int*, 121: 497–505.

Malyshev, D. and Baillie, L. (2020). Surface morphology differences in *Clostridium difficile* spores, based on different strains and methods of purification. *Anaerobe*, 61:102078.

Mandel, D.R., Eichas, K. and Holmes, J. (2010). *Bacillus coagulans*: a viable adjunct therapy for relieving symptoms of rheumatoid arthritis according to a randomized, controlled trial. *BMC Complem Altern M*, 10: 1.

Mantere-Alhonen, S. and Ryhaenen, E.-L. (1994). Lactobacilli and propionibacteria in living food. *Aliments Nutr*, 12(4): 399–405.

Mazzoli, A., Donadio, G., Lanzilli, M., Saggese, A., Guarino, A.M., Rivetti, M., et al. (2019). *Bacillus megaterium* SF185 spores exert protective effects against oxidative stress in vivo and in vitro. *Sci Rep*, 9(1): 1–10.

McDowell, A., Valanne, S., Ramage, G., Tunney, M.M., Glenn, J.V., McLorinan, G.C., et al. (2005). *Propionibacterium acnes* types I and II represent phylogenetically distinct groups. *J Clin Microbiol*, 43(1): 326–334.

McIntosh, F.M., Shingfield, K.J., Devillard, E., Russell, W.R. and Wallace, R.J. (2009). Mechanism of conjugated linoleic acid and vaccenic acid formation in human faecal suspensions and pure cultures of intestinal bacteria. *Microbiology*, 155: 285–294.

McKenney, P.T., Driks, A. and Eichenberger, P. (2013). The *Bacillus subtilis* endospore: assembly and functions of the multilayered coat. *Nat Rev Microbiol*, 11(1): 33–44.

Miller, L.E. and Ouwehand, A.C. (2013). Probiotic supplementation decreases intestinal transit time: meta-analysis of randomized controlled trials. *World J Gastroenterol*, 19(29): 4718–4725.

Murillo, I. and Villamil, L. (2011). *Bacillus cereus* and *Bacillus subtilis* used as probiotics in rotifer (*Brachionus plicatilis*) cultures. *J Aquac Res Dev*, S1: 007.

Nagy, I., Pivarcsi, A., Kis, K., Koreck, A., Bodai, L., McDowell, A., et al. (2006). *Propionibacterium acnes* and lipopolysaccharide induce the expression of antimicrobial peptides and proinflammatory cytokines/chemokines in human sebocytes. *Microbes Infect*, 8(8): 2195–2205.

Nagy, I., Pivarcsi, A., Koreck, A., Széll, M., Urbán, E. and Kemény, L. (2005). Distinct strains of *Propionibacterium acnes* induce selective human β-defensin-2 and interleukin-8 expression in human keratinocytes through toll-like receptors. *J Invest Dermatol*, 124(5): 931–938.

Nandi, A., Dan, S.K., Banerjee, G., Ghosh, P., Ghosh, K., Ringø, E., et al. (2017). Probiotic potential of autochthonous bacteria isolated from the gastrointestinal tract of four freshwater teleosts. *Probiotics Antimicrob Proteins*, 9(1): 12–21.

Narula, J., Fujita, M. and Igoshin, O.A. (2016). Functional requirements of cellular differentiation: lessons from *Bacillus subtilis*. *Curr Opin Microbiol*, 34: 38–46.

Nicholson, W.L. (2004). Ubiquity, longevity, and ecological roles of *Bacillus* spores. In: *Bacterial Spore Formers: Probiotics And Emerging Applications* (ed. E. Ricca, A.O. Henriques and S.M. Cutting), 1–15. Norfolk: Horison Bioscience.

Nicholson, W.L., Munakata, N., Horneck, G., Melosh, H.J. and Setlow, P. (2000). Resistance of *Bacillus* endospores to extreme terrestrial and extraterrestrial environments. *Microbiol Mol Biol Rev*, 64(3): 548–572.

Nithya, V. and Halami, P.M. (2013). Evaluation of the probiotic characteristics of *Bacillus* species isolated from different food sources. *Ann Microbiol*, 63(1): 129–137.

Nuriel-Ohayon, M., Neuman, H. and Koren, O. (2016). Microbial changes during pregnancy, birth, and infancy. *Front Microbiol*, 7:1031.

Nyangale, E.P., Farmer, S., Keller, D., Chernoff, D. and Gibson, G.R. (2014). Effect of prebiotics on the fecal microbiota of elderly volunteers after dietary supplementation of *Bacillus coagulans* GBI-30, 6086. *Anaerobe*, 30: 75–81.

O'Callaghan, A. and van Sinderen, D. (2016). Bifidobacteria and their role as members of the human gut microbiota. *Front Microbiol*, 7: 925.

Okada, Y., Tsuzuki, Y., Miyazaki, J., Matsuzaki, K., Hokari, R., Komoto, S., et al. (2006). *Propionibacterium freudenreichii* component 1.4-dihydroxy-2-naphthoic acid (DHNA) attenuates dextran sodium sulphate induced colitis by modulation of bacterial flora and lymphocyte homing. *Gut*, 55(5):681–688.

Okada, Y., Tsuzuki, Y, Narimatsu, K., Sato, H., Ueda, T., Hozumi, H., et al. (2013). 1,4-Dihydroxy-2-naphthoic acid from *Propionibacterium freudenreichii* reduces inflammation in interleukin-10-deficient mice with colitis by suppressing macrophage-derived proinflammatory cytokines. *J. Leukoc Biol*, 94(3): 473–480.

Okamoto, T., Sasaki, M., Tsujikawa, T., Fujiyama, Y., Bamba, T. and Kusunoki, M. (2000). Preventive efficacy of butyrate enemas and oral administration of *Clostridium butyricum* M588 in dextran sodium sulfate-induced colitis in rats. *J Gastroenterol*, 35(5): 341–346.

O'Keefe, S.J. (2016). Diet, microorganisms and their metabolites, and colon cancer. *Nat Rev Gastroenterol Hepatol*, 13(12): 691–706.

Oksaharju, A., Kooistra, T., Kleemann, R., van Duyvenvoorde, W., Miettinen, M., Lappalainen, J., et al. (2013). Effects of probiotic *Lactobacillus rhamnosus* GG and *Propionibacterium freudenreichii* ssp. *shermanii* JS supplementation on intestinal and systemic markers of inflammation in ApoE*3Leiden mice consuming a high-fat diet. *Br J Nutr*, 110(1): 77–85.

Oprica, C., Emtestam, L., Lapins, J., Borglund, E., Nyberg, F., Stenlund, K., et al. (2004). Antibiotic-resistant *Propionibacterium acnes* on the skin of patients with moderate to severe acne in Stockholm. *Anaerobe*, 10(3): 155–164.

Ouwehand, A.C., Tölkkö, S., Kulmala, J., Salminen, S. and Salminen, E. (2000). Adhesion of inactivated probiotic strains to intestinal mucus. *Lett Appl Microbiol*, 31(1): 82–86.

Pande, R., Bagad, M., Dubey, V. and Ghosh, A.R. (2012). Prospectus of probiotics in modern age diseases. *Asian Pac J Trop Biomed*, 2(3): S1963–S74.

Pereira, J.Q., Ritter, A.C., Cibulski, S. and Brandelli, A. (2019). Functional genome annotation depicts probiotic properties of *Bacillus velezensis* FTC01. *Gene*, 713: 143971.

Permpoonpattana, P., Hong, H., Khaneja, R. and Cutting, S.M. (2012). Evaluation of *Bacillus subtilis* strains as probiotics and their potential as a food ingredient. *Benef Microbes*, 3(2): 127–135.

Perry, A.L., Worthington, T., Hilton, A.C., Lambert, P.A., Stirling, A.J. and Elliott, T.S.J. (2003). Analysis of clinical isolates of *Propionibacterium acnes* by optimised RAPD. *FEMS Microbiol*, 228(1): 51–55.

Plé, C., Breton, J., Richoux, R., Nurdin, M., Deutsch, S.M., Falentin, H., et al. (2016). Combining selected immunomodulatory *Propionibacterium freudenreichii* and *Lactobacillus delbrueckii* strains: Reverse engineering development of an anti-inflammatory cheese. *Mol Nutr Food Res*, 60(4): 935–948.

Plé, C., Richoux, R., Jardin, J., Nurdin, M., Briard-Bion, V., Parayre, S., et al. (2015). Single-strain starter experimental cheese reveals anti-inflammatory effect of *Propionibacterium freudenreichii* CIRM BIA 129 in TNBS-colitis model. *J Funct Foods*, 18: 575–585.

Rabah, H., Rosa do Carmo, F.L. and Jan, G. (2017). Dairy Propionibacteria: Versatile Probiotics. *Microorganisms*, 5(2): 24.

Rainio, A., Vahvaselkä, M., Suomalainen, T. and Laakso, S. (2001). Reduction of linoleic acid inhibition in production of conjugated linoleic acid by *Propionibacterium freudenreichii* ssp. *shermanii*. *Can J Microbiol*, 47(8): 735–740.

Ramos, C.L., Thorsen, L., Schwan, R.F. and Jespersen, L. (2013). Strain-specific probiotics properties of *Lactobacillus fermentum, Lactobacillus plantarum* and *Lactobacillus brevis* isolates from Brazilian food products. *Food Microbiol*, 36(1): 22–29.

Ranadheera, R., Baines, S. and Adams, M.C. (2010). Importance of food in probiotic efficacy. *Food Res Int*, 43(1): 1–7.

Ratajczak, W., Rył, A., Mizerski, A., Walczakiewicz, K., Sipak, O. and Laszczyńska, M. (2019). Immunomodulatory potential of gut microbiome-derived short-chain fatty acids (SCFAs). *Acta Biochim Pol*, 66(1): 1–12.

Richard, M.L., Liguori, G., Lamas, B., Brandi, G., da Costa, G., Hoffmann, T.W., et al. (2018). Mucosa-associated microbiota dysbiosis in colitis associated cancer. *Gut Microbes*, 9(2): 131–142.

Rodríguez, J.M. (2014). The origin of human milk bacteria: is there a bacterial entero-mammary pathway during late pregnancy and lactation? *Adv Nutr*, 5(6): 779–784.

Rossetti, L. and Giraffa, G. (2005). Rapid identification of dairy lactic acid bacteria by M13-generated, RAPD-PCR fingerprint databases. *J Microbiol Methods*, 63(2): 135–144.

Sánchez, B., Delgado, S., Blanco-Míguez, A., Lourenço, A., Gueimonde, M. and Margolles, A. (2017). Probiotics, gut microbiota, and their influence on host health and disease. *Mol Nutr Food Res*, 61(1).

Seki, K., Nakao, H., Umino, H., Isshiki, H., Yoda, N., Tachihara, R., et al. (2004). Effects of fermented milk whey containing novel bifidogenic growth stimulator produced by *Propionibacterium* on fecal bacteria, putrefactive metabolite, defecation frequency and fecal properties in senile volunteers needed serious nursing-care taking enteral nutrition by tube feeding. *J Intest Microbiol*, 18(2): 107–115.

Stürmer, E.S., Casasola, S., Gall, M.C. and Gall, M.C. (2012). A importância dos probióticos na microbiota intestinal humana. *Rev Bras Nutr Clin*, 27(4): 264–272.

Succi, M., Tremonte, P., Pannella, G., Tipaldi, L., Cozzolino, A., Coppola, R. and Sorrentino, E. (2017). Survival of commercial probiotic strains in dark chocolate with high cocoa and phenols content during the storage and in a static in vitro digestion model. *J Funct Foods* 35: 60–67.

Sui, L., Zhu, X., Wu, D., Ma, T., Tuo, Y., Jiang, S., et al. (2020). *in vitro* assessment of probiotic and functional properties of *Bacillus coagulans* T242. *Food Biosci*, 36:100675.

Suzuki, A., Mitsuyama, K., Koga, H., Tomiyasu, N., Masuda, J., Takaki, K., et al. (2006). Bifidogenic growth stimulator for the treatment of active ulcerative colitis: a pilot study. *Nutrition*, 22(1): 76–81.

Talukdar, P.K., Olguín-Araneda, V., Alnoman, M., Paredes-Sabja, D. and Sarker, M.R. (2015). Updates on the sporulation process in *Clostridium* species. *Res Microbiol*, 166(4): 225–235.

Tan, J., McKenzie, C., Potamitis, M., Thorburn, A.N., Mackay, C.R. and Macia, L. (2014). The role of short-chain fatty acids in health and disease. *Adv Immunol*, 121: 91–119.

Thirabunyanon, M. and Thongwittaya, N. (2012). Protection activity of a novel probiotic strain of *Bacillus subtilis* against *Salmonella Enteritidis* infection. *Res Vet Sci*, 93(1): 74–81.

Tocheva, E.I., Matson, E.G., Morris, D.M., Moussavi, F., Leadbetter, J.R. and Jensen, G.J. (2011). Peptidoglycan remodeling and conversion of an inner membrane into an outer membrane during sporulation. *Cell*, 146(5): 799–812.

Uchida, M., Tsuboi, H., Takahashi Arita, M., Nemoto, A., Seki, K., Tsunoo, H., et al. (2011). Safety of high doses of *Propionibacterium freudenreichii* ET-3 culture in healthy adult subjects. *Regul Toxicol Pharmacol*, 60(2): 262–267.

Umesaki, Y., Setoyama, H., Matsumoto, S., Imaoka, A. and Itoh, K. (1999). Differential roles of segmented filamentous bacteria and clostridia in development of the intestinal immune system. *Infect Immun*, 67(7): 3504–3511.

Valanne, S., McDowell, A., Ramage, G., Tunney, M.M., Einarsson, G.G., O'Hagan, S., et al. (2005). CAMP factor homologues in *Propionibacterium acnes*: a new protein family differentially expressed by types I and II. *Microbiology*, 151(5): 1369–1379.

Vesa, T., Pochart, P. and Marteau, P. (2000). Pharmacokinetics of *Lactobacillus plantarum* NCIMB 8826, *Lactobacillus fermentum* KLD, and *Lactococcus lactis* MG 1363 in the human gastrointestinal tract. *Aliment Pharmacol Ther*, 14(6): 823–828.

Vos, P., Garrity, G., Jones, D., Krieg, N.R., Ludwig, W., Rainey, F.A., et al. (2009). Genus I. *Clostridium* Prazmowski. In: *Bergey's Manual of Systematic Bacteriology: The Firmicutes*, 9th ed., vol. 3, 739–740. New York: Springer.

Waligora-Dupriet, A.J., Dugay, A., Auzeil, N., Nicolis, I., Rabot, S., Huerre, M.R., et al. (2009). Short-chain fatty acids and polyamines in the pathogenesis of necrotizing enterocolitis: Kinetics aspects in gnotobiotic quails. *Anaerobe*, 15(4): 138–144.

Walter, J. and Ley, R. (2011). The human gut microbiome: ecology and recent evolutionary changes. *Annu Rev Microbiol*, 65: 411–429.

Wang, F.-Y., Liu, J.-M., Luo, H.-H., Liu, A.-H. and Jiang, Y. (2015). Potential protective effects of *Clostridium butyricum* on experimental gastric ulcers in mice. *World J Gastroenterol*, 21(27): 8340–8351.

Wexler, H.M. (2007). Bacteroides: the good, the bad, and the nitty-gritty. *Clin Microbiol Rev*, 20(4): 593–621.

Woo, T.D.H., Oka, K., Takahashi, M., Hojo, F., Osaki, T., Hanawa, T., et al. (2011). Inhibition of the cytotoxic effect of *Clostridium difficile in vitro* by *Clostridium butyricum* MIYAIRI 588 strain. *J Med Microbiol*, 60: 1617–1625.

Yamazaki, S., Kano, K., Ikeda, T., Isawa, K. and Kaneko, T. (1999). Role of 2-amino-3-carboxy-1,4-naphthoquinone, a strong growth stimulator for bifidobacteria, as an electron transfer mediator for NAD(P)(+) regeneration in *Bifidobacterium longum*. *Biochim Biophys Acta*, 1428(2-3): 241–250.

Yuan, G., Chen, X. and Li, D. (2015). Modulation of peroxisome proliferator-activated receptor gamma (PPAR γ) by conjugated fatty acid in obesity and inflammatory bowel disease. *J Agric Food Chem*, 63(7): 1883–1895.

Zárate, G., Chaia, A.P. (2009). Dairy bacteria remove in vitro dietary lectins with toxic effects on colonic cells. *J. Appl. Microbiol.* 106(3): 1050–1057.

Zárate, G., Palacios, J.M., Villena, J. and Zúñiga-Hansen, M.E. (2016). Inhibition of enteropathogens adhesion to human enterocyte-like HT-29 cells by a dairy strain of *Propionibacterium acidipropionici*. *Benef Microbes*, 7(3): 431–441.

Zhou, S., Song, D., Zhou, X., Mao, X., Zhou, X., Wang, S., et al. (2019). Characterization of *Bacillus subtilis* from gastrointestinal tract of hybrid Hulong grouper (*Epinephelus fuscoguttatus* × *E. lanceolatus*) and its effects as probiotic additives. *Fish Shellfish Immunol*, 84: 1115–1124.

Zimmerman, M.A., Singh, N., Martin, P.M., Thangaraju, M., Ganapathy, V., Waller, J.L., et al. (2012). Butyrate suppresses colonic inflammation through HDAC1-dependent Fas upregulation and Fas-mediated apoptosis of T cells. *Am J Physiol Gastrointest Liver Physiol*, 302(12): G1405–1415.

5

Yeasts as Probiotics and their Functional Roles

Giorgia Perpetuini[1], *Yves Waché*[2,3,4] *and Rosanna Tofalo*[1]

[1] *Faculty of Bioscience and Technology for Food, Agriculture and Environment, University of Teramo, Teramo, Italy*
[2] *Tropical Fermentation Network, France, International Joint Laboratory, Tropical Bioresources & Biotechnology, Université Bourgogne Franche-Comté, AgroSup Dijon, PAM UMR A 02, .102, France*
[3] *School of Biotechnology and Food Technology, Hanoi University of Science and Technology, Hanoi, Vietnam*
[4] *School of Food Science and Technology, Faculty of Science and Technology, Thammasat University, 12120, Thailand*

5.1 Yeasts: General Considerations and Taxonomy

Yeasts are involved in food and beverage fermentations. They positively influence safety and sensory qualities of the final product. In addition, they can exert beneficial health effects including probiotic, antigenotoxic and antioxidant activities (Tofalo and Suzzi 2016).

The name yeast originates from the German word *gift*, which refers to the foam typical of beer fermentation, and the French word "levure" (role in bread dough leavening).

Yeasts are eukaryotic microorganisms with vegetative growth through budding or fission and do not form their sexual states within or upon a fruiting body (Kurtzman *et al.* 2011; Tofalo and Suzzi 2016). Yeast taxonomy is evolving on the basis of the latest discoveries in biochemistry and molecular biology. According to Kurtzman *et al.* (2011), spore and cell morphology, type of conidiogenesis, life cycles, biochemical features, type of coenzyme Q, and G+C content are used to differentiate yeast genera, while DNA hybridization or reassociation is applied to establish relationships among yeast species.

The molecular methods mainly used for yeast identification rely on ribosomal genes (e.g. 5.8S, 18S and 26S rRNA) variability since they show a low intraspecific polymorphism and a high interspecific variability. The first marker used for this purpose was the 18S rRNA gene. Actually, the D1/D2 domain of the 26S rRNA gene (600 bp) is used to differentiate basidiomycetes, hemiascomycetes and filamentous euascomycetes. Whole-genome sequence analysis of yeasts is revolutionizing the taxonomy resulting in new description of yeast phylogeny (Kurtzman *et al.* 2011; Tofalo and Suzzi 2016).

Yeasts are heterotroph and require several elements for their growth including carbon (glucose, fructose, galactose, mannose, maltose or sucrose) and nitrogen sources, phosphate, sulfate, potassium, magnesium, calcium, iron, zinc and vitamins (e.g. biotin, thiamine or

Probiotics, Prebiotics and Synbiotics: Technological Advancements Towards Safety and Industrial Applications, First Edition. Edited by Parmjit Singh Panesar and Anil Kumar Anal.

Table 5.1 Main effects of yeasts in food production and in human health.

Yeast species	Activity	Effect
Candida humilis, Debaryomyces hansenii, Galactomyces candidum, Hanseniaspora uvarum, Kluyveromyces marxianus, K. lactis, Schizosaccharomyces pombe, S. cerevisiae, Kazachstania exigua, Torulaspora delbrueckii, Zygosaccharomyces rouxii, Yarrowia lipolytica	Fermentation of foods and beverages	Fermentation, determination of flavor and color
Cyberlindnera jadinii, K. marxianus, S. cerevisiae, Y. lipolytica, Rhodotorula glutinis, Sporidiobolus salmonicolor	Food additive production	Release of vitamins of group B, proteins, peptides, amino acids, minerals, antioxidants, aromas, colorants, glutamic acids, nucleotides, vanillin, citronellol, linalool, geraniol, β-glucans
Saccharomyces boulardii	Probiotic effect	Maintenance of epithelial barrier integrity and permeability, restoration of the tight-junction structure, reduction of inflammation, immunomodulation
Saccharomyces spp.; *Metschnikowia lochheadii, Priceomyces melissophilus, Schwanniomyces vanrijiae* var. *vanrijiae, Debaryomyces hansenii, Yamadazyma philogaea, Kodamaea anthophila, Kurtzmaniella cleridarum, Candida drosophilae, Candida humilis, T. delbrueckii, Kazachstania exigua, Pichia fermentans, Whycheramomyces anomalus, Candida glabrata, Kluyveromyces marxianus, Pichia kudriavzevii*	Folate production	Prevention of neural tube defects in the fetus, and reduction of the risk for cardiovascular disease, cancer and Alzheimer's disease

Source: Modified from Tofalo, R. and Suzzi, G. (2016). Yeasts. In Caballero, B., Finglas, P., Toldrá, F. (eds.) *The Encyclopedia of Food and Health*, 5, 593–599. Oxford: Academic Press.

pantothenic acid) (Hatoum *et al.* 2012; Rodrigues *et al.* 2006; Tofalo and Suzzi 2016). However, they can also employ other molecules such as alcohols and organic acids under aerobic conditions (Deak 2006).

Yeasts are probably the main microbial group exploited for fermentation of foods (Table 5.1). During the fermentation process mixed cultures of yeasts, bacteria and fungi are involved in parallel or in a sequential manner to transform raw materials into safer final products with an added value. Some yeast species – mainly belonging to *Saccharomyces* genus – are used as starter cultures for the production of fermented beverages such as wine, cider and beer and foods like cheese, bread, sourdoughs, fermented meats and fermented vegetable products (Hatoum *et al.* 2012; Tofalo and Suzzi 2016).

Many species of yeasts are recognized as food-grade and are used as sources of high-nutritional-value proteins, enzymes and vitamins or nutritional supplements, or food additives, conditioners and flavoring agents. Last but not least the antifungal activity of yeasts is exploited to control food spoilage (Hatoum *et al.* 2012).

Yeasts are also used for their probiotic properties (Tofalo and Suzzi 2016). The word "probiotic" derives from the Greek words *pro* and *bios* (promoter of life) (McFarland 2017). The World Health Organization (WHO) defines probiotics as "viable microorganisms that can provide benefits to human (and animals) health when administered in adequate amounts" (Hill *et al.* 2014).

The most common probiotics are bacteria (Plaza-Diaz *et al.* 2019). However, some eukaryotic probiotics are available. *Saccharomyces* spp. and *Kluyveromyces* spp. are the only commercially available. However, other species such as *D. hansenii*, *T. delbrueckii* (Perpetuini *et al.* 2020; Psani and Kotzekidou 2006), *K. lactis*, *K. marxianus* and *K. lodderae* (Kumura *et al.* 2004) have shown antagonistic activity against pathogenic bacteria and tolerance of passage through the gastrointestinal tract.

5.2 *Saccharomyces boulardii*

Saccharomyces boulardii was first isolated from litchi fruit in Indochina by Henri Boulard in the 1920s and is the only species used in the pharmaceutical industry as a yeast preparation with proven probiotic efficiency in double-blind studies (Khatri *et al.* 2017; Pais *et al.* 2020). Its taxonomic position as a distinct species from *S. cerevisiae* is still controversial (Khatri *et al.* 2017). Molecular typing studies revealed that *S. boulardii* strains from distinct origins clustered separately from *S. cerevisiae* species (Fietto *et al.* 2004; Mitterdorfer *et al.* 2002; Pais *et al.* 2020). On the contrary, a DNA/RNA hybridization spotted microarray study revealed that *S. boulardii* is not different from *S. cerevisiae*; it only lacks the intact Ty1/2 elements (Edwards-Ingram *et al.* 2004).

Several studies have been performed to highlight the genetic differences between *S. boulardii* and *S. cerevisiae* genomes. Edwards-Ingram *et al.* (2007) showed some differences in the copy number of genes in three chromosomes (chromosomes I, VII and XII). Other differences include those in flocculation genes responsible for a different adhesion profile of *S. boulardii* when compared to *S. cerevisiae* (Edwards-Ingram *et al.* 2007). All flocculins except FLO5 protein and adhesins were present in *S. boulardii*. This yeast showed a higher number of repeats in the *FLO1* gene than *S. cerevisiae*. This additional number of repeats could influence its adhesion and flocculation ability, as well as environmental stress response.

Recently, Khatri *et al.* (2017) compared the genome of a commercial strain of *S. boulardii* with 145 strains of *S. cerevisiae* to highlight genetic differences. The data obtained revealed that Ty1/3/4 were absent elements in *S. boulardii*, but not Ty2/5. Moreover, *S. boulardii* strains presented both MAT alleles and the *HO* gene which confer on them homothallic and diploid characteristics. Even if they are diploid, they cannot sporulate. This feature depends on the deficiency in mating genes and not simply on the absence/divergence of sporulation genes or respiration efficiency. An introgression of five genes from *Zygosaccharomyces bailii* into chromosome IV of *S. boulardii* and wine strains of *S. cerevisiae* was found. In fact, *S. boulardii* clustered closely to *S. cerevisiae* wine strains (Khatri *et al.* 2017).

Physiological and biochemical aspects are more useful to differentiate *S. cerevisiae* and *S. boulardii*. Fietto *et al.* (2004) compared physiological characteristics in these two species. *S. boulardii* was more resistant to high temperatures, growing up to 55 °C, and showed fast

Table 5.2 Some characteristics of *S. boulardii* strains.

Nitrogen utilization	Nitrate	–
	Peptone	+
	Ammonium sulfate	+
Carbon utilization	Glucose	+
	Fructose	+
	Sucrose	+
	Lactose	–
	Starch	+
Urea hydrolysis		–
Gelatin liquefaction test		–
Optimal growth temperature		37 °C
Ploidy		Always diploid
Homo- or heterothallic		Both
Sporulation		Asporogenous
Retrotransposon (Ty elements)		No intact Ty1, 3 or 4 elements

Source: Modified from Pais, P., Almeida, V., Yilmaz, M., Teixeira, M.C. (2020). *Saccharomyces boulardii*: What makes it tick as successful probiotic? *J Fungi*, 6: 78 and Hossain, M.N., Afrin, S., Humayun, S., Ahmed, M.M., Saha, B.K. (2020). Identification and growth characterization of a novel strain of *Saccharomyces boulardii* isolated from soya paste. *Front Nutr*, 7: 27.

growth at 30 °C and 37 °C. Other studies showed other different metabolic traits in these species. As stated earlier, *S. boulardii* does not form ascospores, and does not use galactose as a carbon source (Hossain *et al.* 2020; Khatri *et al.* 2017; Mitterdorfer *et al.* 2001). It is more resistant to temperature and acidic stresses, but less resistant to bile salts (Pais *et al.* 2020) (Table 5.2).

S. boulardii exhibits benefits to human health and shows several probiotic characteristics such as the ability to survive in the gastrointestinal tract and face different stressing conditions (Rajkowska and Kunicka-Styczynska 2012; Romanin *et al.* 2010). This last trait is linked to its ability to tolerate a wide range of temperatures and pH levels (Romero-Luna *et al.* 2019). Once in the gastrointestinal tract it exerts several positive effects including inhibition of bacterial toxins and reduction of toxin-induced inflammation (Anoop *et al.* 2015). Moreover, it is able to modulate the host immune system and intestinal enzymes that enhance nutrient digestion and absorption (Ansari *et al.* 2019).

Moreover, *S. boulardii* decreased the incidence of antibiotic-associated diarrhea (Gut *et al.* 2018) and diminished the risk of recurrence of *Clostridium difficile* infection and Crohn's disease (Chen *et al.* 2006; Stier and Bischoff 2016). This yeast is also employed for restoration of intestinal homeostasis, lactose intolerance, urinary tract infections, vaginal yeast infections, treatment of high cholesterol levels, fever blisters and teenage acne (Palma *et al.* 2015; van der Aa Kühle *et al.* 2005; Zanello *et al.* 2009).

S. boulardii is also used as a cell factory for the production of molecules with industrial and biotherapeutics potential and as a drug delivery agent targeted to the gastrointestinal tract (Lin 2003).

5.3 Mechanism of Action of Yeast Probiotics

The mechanisms involved in the probiotic action of yeasts are not completely understood. They mainly include: improvement of gut epithelia physical barriers, regulation of cytokine secretion, modulation of the immune system and trophic effect on intestinal mucosa (O'Toole and Cooney 2008) (Figure 5.1).

Concerning the enhancement of the epithelial barrier it is important to note that intestinal barrier defects are associated with inflammation and immune system alteration (Terciolo *et al.* 2017). These alterations negatively influence the intestinal epithelial barrier, which represents the starting point for diseases affecting the gut, such as infectious enterocolitis, small intestinal bacterial overgrowth, inflammatory bowel disease (IBD) and irritable bowel syndrome (IBS) (Lee 2015). Intestinal permeability is mainly regulated by tight junctions which seal the intercellular space between adjacent epithelial intestinal cells. Previous reports suggested that probiotics can improve intestinal permeability by improving tight junctions and excluding some pathogens by adhering to the intestinal mucosa (Sen and Mansell 2020).

Previous studies highlighted that *S. boulardii* conferred beneficial effects against various enteric pathogens through the following mechanisms:

1) *Inhibition of bacterial adherence and translocation in the intestinal epithelium. S. boulardii* CNCM I-745 probiotic strain is able to interact with pathogens and the intestinal mucosa (Canonici *et al.* 2012; Moré and Swidsinski 2015). It seems that yeast cells, as well as cell wall particles, can alter surface receptors involved in *C. difficile* adhesion (Tasteyre *et al.* 2002). This *S. boulardii* strain is also able to protect the intestinal barrier in colitis caused by *Escherichia coli* (Czerucka *et al.* 2007). The administration of *S. boulardii* reduced the *E. coli* adherence to mesenteric lymph node in pig's intestine (Lessard

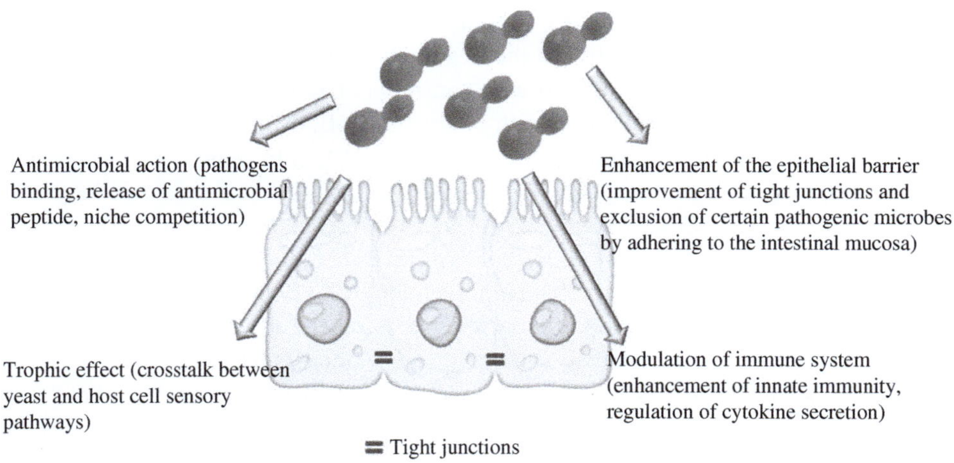

Figure 5.1 Overview of the main modes of action of yeast probiotics in the intestinal epithelium. The majority of studies are focused on *S. boulardii*. However, the genetic basis is not completely understood. *Source:* Based on O'Toole, P.W. and Cooney, J.C. (2008). Probiotic bacteria influence the composition and function of the intestinal microbiota. *Interdiscip Perspect Infect Dis*, 175285.

et al. 2009). This activity has also been described in *S. cerevisiae* UFMG A-905, which is able to adhere to some enteropathogenic bacteria, such as *E. coli*, *Salmonella typhi* and *S. typhimurium* (Tiago *et al.* 2012).

2) *Antimicrobial activity*. This effect can be achieved through different mechanisms. First of all, probiotics compete with pathogens by consuming nutrients and causing a nutrient limitation for pathogenic organisms (Bermudez-Brito *et al.* 2012). On the other hand, probiotics release specific molecules able to reduce gut pH, creating a hostile environment for pathogens (Bermudez-Brito *et al.* 2012). Moreover, they produce factors that neutralize bacterial toxins: it has been demonstrated that the pathogenic effects of *C. difficile* mainly rely on the release of toxin A and toxin B. *S. boulardii* releases a 54 kDa serine protease able to hydrolyze these toxins as well as to inhibit toxin binding to intestinal glycoprotein receptor (Psani and Kotzekidou 2006). Another mechanism used by *S. boulardii* against *C. difficile* is the release of factors able to inhibit pathogen growth and its toxins' production and stimulation of host mucosal disaccharidase activity (Buts *et al.* 1990). Other studies demonstrated the ability of *S. boulardii* to inhibit *E. coli* surface endotoxins by dephosphorylation (Buts *et al.* 2006), the production of a protein which reduces the chloride secretions stimulated by cholera toxin by reducing cAMP levels (Czerucka *et al.* 1994) and its ability to bind the cholera toxin, blocking its toxic effect (Brandão *et al.* 1998).
3) *Modulation of inflammation*. Moslehi-Jenabian *et al.* (2010) performed *in vitro* studies revealing that *S. boulardii* can influence pathways involved in the pro-inflammatory response by inhibiting nuclear factor-kappa B (NF-κB) and mitogen activated protein kinase (MAPK) causing a decrease of inflammation-associated cytokines such as interleukin 8 (IL-8), tumor necrosis factor alpha (TNF-α) and interferon gamma (IFN-γ).

S. boulardii affects the host's pathways at various positions. For instance, the decrease of pro-inflammatory response and/or regulation of epithelial barrier integrity represent the main protective strategies exerted by *S. boulardii* against diarrheal pathogens. In fact, *S. boulardii* CNCM I-745 is effective in the treatment of IBD and IBS (Abbas *et al.* 2014). Moreover, it releases a 10 kDa protein with anti-inflammatory effects in the presence of *C. difficile* toxin A. This protein causes both a reduction of IL-8 secretion in human colonocytes and the activation of protein kinases 1 and 2 (ERK1/2) in human colonocytes and murine ileal loops (Chen *et al.* 2006). Another study showed that *S. boulardii* released a protein preventing NF-κB activation and IL-8 gene expression in intestinal epithelial cells and monocytes (Sougioultzis *et al.* 2006). Pontier-bres *et al.* (2014) showed that *S. boulardii* activates the release of IFN-γ, inhibits the production of IL-10 in the small intestine and enhances IFN-γ and IL-10 release in the cecum, indicating the ability of *S. boulardii* to differentially modulate immune activity through the gastrointestinal tract.

A similar behavior was observed for *S. cerevisiae* UFMG A-905 in mouse typhoid fever models. In fact, a reduction of inflammation and IL-6, TNF-α, IFN-γ and IL-10 levels was observed (Martins *et al.* 2011).

The modulation of the immune system by probiotic yeasts can be explained in different ways including the release of molecules preventing the secretion of pro-inflammatory cytokines and the modulation of ERK1/2 and p38 proteins (for a review see Pothoulakis 2009).

In particular, *S. boulardii* is able to promote peroxisome proliferator-activated receptor γ (PPAR-γ) expression. PPAR-γ plays positive roles in host health including protection from gut inflammation and IBD and inhibition of bacterial overgrowth and adhesion to host cells (Pothoulakis 2009). Sougioultzis *et al.* (2006) studied the effect of *S. boulardii* in murine models of colitis and showed that it released a *Saccharomyces* anti-inflammatory factor (SAIF) able to inhibit pro-inflammatory cytokine gene expression. Finally, *S. boulardii* stimulates short chain fatty acids (SCFAs) release with immunomodulatory properties. In patients requiring total enteral nutrition the administration of *S. boulardii* enhanced the amount of butyrate in the gut (Schneider *et al.* 2005). This type of action is also involved in the inhibition of *C. difficile* growth and in the reduction of diarrhea incidence in patients needing enteral nutrition (Schneider *et al.* 2005).

Similarly, *S. cerevisiae* 982 – isolated from feta cheese – showed immunomodulatory activity in the small intestine of mice, favoring the release of immunoglobulin A (IgA), TNF-α, IFN-γ, IL-5, IL-6, IL-10 and IL-12 (Kourelis *et al.* 2010).

Another important mechanism is the trophic effect on intestinal mucosa (Pais *et al.* 2020). Probiotic yeasts stimulate brush border membrane, digestive enzymes and nutrient transporter activity. They modulate SCFAs and branched-chain fatty acids (BCFAs) synthesis (Pais *et al.* 2020). In particular, *S. boulardii* play a central role in the reestablishment of SCFA levels after diseases (Girard-Pipau *et al.* 2002; Schneider *et al.* 2005). Several studies demonstrated the ability of *S. boulardii* to release polyamines regulating digestive enzymes and nutrient transporters (for a review see Moré and Vandenplas 2018).

5.4 Health Benefits of Yeast Probiotics

The majority of studies concerning the health benefits resulting from the oral administration of probiotic yeasts have been performed on *S. boulardii* and include probiotic and nutritional effects (Figure 5.2).

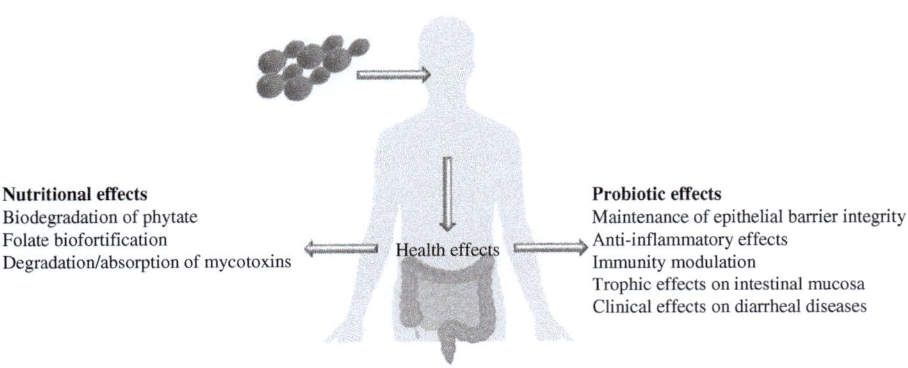

Figure 5.2 Health effects exerted by yeast probiotics.

5.4.1 Probiotic Effects

Saccharomyces boulardii is often used as model organism to describe the probiotic effects of yeasts. As stated in the previous paragraph, probiotic effects are exerted through different mechanisms: a general immune stimulation, an anti-inflammatory and antisecretory action, influencing the signaling pathways NF-κB and MAP in the host intestinal cells, elimination of bacterial toxins and pathogen binding and physical barrier and colonization resistance (Arevalo-Villena *et al.* 2017). The main reported probiotic effects of probiotic yeasts are as follows.

Antibiotic-associated Diarrhea This condition is associated with an intestinal inflammation caused by antibiotics. In fact, even if antibiotic treatment is essential to eliminate pathogens, it also alter gut microbiota, causing diarrhea and the promotion of intestinal permeability, which can lead to bacterial and viral translocation. The most common opportunistic pathogens related to this condition are *C. difficile, C. perfringens, Staphylococcus aureus, Klebsiella oxytoca, Candida* spp. and *Salmonella* spp. Szajewska and Kołodziej (2015) and Terciolo *et al.* (2019) showed that *S. boulardii* administration reduced the risk of *C. difficile*-associated diarrhea in children and not in adults.

Traveler's Diarrhea This represents a common health problem in developing countries and is caused by *E. coli, Shigella* and *Salmonella*. McFarland (2007) in a meta-analysis study revealed that this condition can be prevented through the administration of a mixture made up of *S. boulardii, L. acidophilus* and *Bifidobacterium bifidum.*

Acute Diarrhea in Children *S. boulardii* is also used for the treatment of gastroenteritis in children. A clinical trial performed on 200 children revealed that the administration of this yeast reduced the defecation frequency as well as the duration of this condition (Sharif *et al.* 2016). This effect could be associated with ability of this yeast to restore the healthy gut microbiota.

Diarrhea Associated with Tube-feeding and AIDS Several studies demonstrated the effectiveness of the addition of *S. boulardii* to nutrient supplements in the treatment of diarrhea in patients with enteral nutrition or with AIDS (Bleichner *et al.* 1997; Czerucka *et al.* 2007; Sougioultzis *et al.* 2006).

Irritable Bowel Diseases and Irritable Bowel Syndrome IBDs are multifactorial diseases with two main subtypes: Crohn's disease (CD) and ulcerative colitis (UC). IBS is a functional gastrointestinal disorder characterized by intermittent abdominal pain and transit disorders such as diarrhea, constipation or alternating diarrhea/constipation. The effect of *S. boulardii* administration to IBD patients is controversial. Bourreille *et al.* (2013) performed a clinical study with 159 patients and showed that *S. boulardii* did not have a significant effect on IBD. On the other hand, another study indicated that *S. boulardii* could have beneficial effects in the treatment and prevention of intestinal permeability in patients with IBD (Canonici *et al.* 2011, 2012).

Administration of *S. boulardii* has shown positive effects also in the case of steatosis when administered in obese and diabetes 2 mice (Everard *et al.* 2014), and it enhances the viability of probiotic bacteria, probably related to the co-aggregation of yeast/probiotic due to yeast cell wall and glucans (Moslehi-Jenabian *et al.* 2010). Finally, the administration of *S. boulardii* in cases of vaginal candidiasis enhanced the clearance of *C. albicans*, probably through its co-aggregation ability and capability to suppress the adherence of *Candida* to the epithelium (Pericolini *et al.* 2017).

5.4.2 Nutritional Effects

Biodegradation of Phytate Phytic acid or phytate (*myo*-inositol hexaphosphate, IP6) is a molecule made up of six phosphate groups linked to inositol. Because of its negative charge, it forms insoluble complexes with multivalent cations (Mg^{2+}, Ca^{2+}, Zn^{2+} and Fe^{3+}), reducing their bioavailability (Reddy and Pierson 1994; Vohra and Satyanarayana 2003). The presence of phytase (*myo*-inositol-hexakisphosphate 6-phosphohydrolases) – able to dephosphorylate IP6 in inorganic phosphate (Pi) and inositol phosphate esters – has been reported in several yeast species including *C. krusei, D. castellii, Arxula adeninivorans, W. anomalus, Pichia rhodanensis, P. spartinae, Cryptococcus laurentii, Rhodotorula gracilis, S. cerevisiae, S. kluyveri, T. delbrueckii, Candida* spp. and *K. lactis* (Moslehi-Jenabian *et al.* 2010). However, this activity is relatively low and is influenced by pH. In fact, it is weak in a medium with pH 6 and in presence of phosphate (Andlid *et al.* 2004). Yeasts or yeast phytases could be exploited to decrease the concentration of IP6 in fermented foods or used as a food supplement to favor IP6 hydrolysis after digestion.

Folate Biofortification Folate or vitamin B_9 is part of a family of compounds containing a pteridine moiety associated with para-aminobenzoic acid and with one or more glutamyl residues (Saubade *et al.* 2017). There are different forms of vitamin B_9, called vitamers. Folate contains only a glutamate residue and fully oxidized pteridine ring, while vitamers are characterized by the presence of a polyglutamate chain and partially or fully reduced pteridine rings. Thanks to their chemical structure, vitamers are more stable and resistant to oxidation, acid pH and heat treatments (Saubade *et al.* 2017). Several studies highlighted a positive role of folate on human health since it is involved in several physiological functions including amino acid metabolism and DNA replication and repair. Unfortunately, humans have to obtain folate from the diet because they are not able to synthesize folate de novo (Saubade *et al.* 2017). The FAO/WHO established that the recommended dietary intake (RDI) of folate is 200–300 μg/day for males and 170–300 μg/day for females (FAO/WHO 2005). Folate deficiency is a problem worldwide and is related to several health problems, such as megaloblastic anemia, cardiovascular risks and neural tube defects (Saubade *et al.* 2017). Some yeast species are able to produce folate, suggesting their possible use as a biofortificant in fermented foods.

Folate production has been reported in *Issatchenkia orientalis, W. anomalus, S. cerevisiae, K. marxianus, Candida milleri, C. glabrata* and *T. delbrueckii*. Among them *S. cerevisiae* is considered a high producer with 3 mg of folate per 100 g dry weight (Moslehi-Jenabian *et al.* 2010).

Several studies have been performed to test the effect of yeasts on folate biofortification of food. Unfortunately, the final content of folate is often low because it is partially lost during food processing. For instance, Jägerstad *et al.* (2005) observed that, in beer, the amount of folate enhanced during the first steps of fermentation because of yeast production but, because yeast folate is intracellular, after cropping its content was strongly reduced. Patring *et al.* (2006) isolated folate vitamers-producing yeasts from kefir offering new insights concerning folate stability during fermentation and storage, useful to enhance its concentration in kefir products. Cereals represent the main folate source in the diet. The sourdough used and the baking process applied influence folate content. In particular, folate concentration is higher in sourdough fermentation, while it is degraded during baking (Kariluoto *et al.* 2004).

Further studies are necessary to select high folate vitamers-producing strains and to optimize food processes. It is essential to evaluate the effect of technological parameters in situ in order to limit folate losses. Finally, the direct use of probiotic yeasts could be an advantage, because folate could be produced in the gut.

Degradation/Absorption of Mycotoxins Mycotoxins are toxic compounds produced by fungi which can contaminate food and animal feeds. The main mycotoxins are the aflatoxins, ochratoxins (OTA), fumonisins, deoxynivalenol (DON), zearalenone (ZEA) and trichothecenes (Pfliegler *et al.* 2015). They are associated with various diseases in humans and animals, ranging from gastrointestinal and kidney disorders to immune deficiency and cancer (Pfliegler *et al.* 2015). Different approaches have been proposed to control contamination by mycotoxins, and the exploitation of yeasts is the most promising (Pfliegler *et al.* 2015; Russo *et al.* 2016). Yeasts can eliminate mycotoxins through two different mechanisms: biodegradation and absorption of mycotoxins to cell-wall components. The majority of studies have focused on the decontamination of animal feeds by yeast, while only a few data are available concerning decontamination of foods and beverages. For instance, Moss and Long (2002) showed that *S. cerevisiae* can degrade patulin releasing E-ascladiol and Z-ascladiol as major metabolites. This yeast is also able to reduce the content of OTA and fumonisins B1 and B2 in foods (Scott *et al.* 1995).

Shetty *et al.* (2007) tested some wine *S. cerevisiae* strains for their ability to absorb OTA in synthetic and natural grape juice. Heat-treated cells showed higher absorption than viable cells. In the same study they also investigated the abilities of *S. cerevisiae* to bind aflatoxin B1. This ability was strain specific, with heat- and acid-treated cells showing higher binding capacity. *Phaffia rhodozyma* and *Xanthophyllomyces dendrorhous* convert ochratoxin A to ochratoxin α (Péteri *et al.* 2007).

Other examples of yeast effects on mycotoxins are reported in Table 5.3.

5.5 Other Yeast Strains with Probiotic Potential

Studies concerning eukaryotic probiotics have increased in the last years, especially because they offer several advantages compared to prokaryotic probiotics. In particular, eukaryotic probiotics showed resistance to antibiotics and inability for horizontal gene transfer. However, only *S. boulardii* and *K. marxianus* (formerly *K. fragilis*) B0399 are approved for human and animal application and are commercially available (Quarella *et al.* 2016). The last species is commonly isolated from kefir, cheese, whey and curds of cow milk. It is able to face the stressing conditions of the gastrointestinal tract and colonize the intestinal

Table 5.3 Some examples of exploitation of yeasts to reduce/eliminate the content of mycotoxins in food.

Yeast species	Target	Type of action
S. cerevisiae	OTA	Absorption
S. cerevisiae	ZEN	Biodegradation
Rhodosporidium paludigenum	Patulin	Biodegradation
D. hansenii	OTA	Inhibition of toxinogenic strains of *Penicillium nordicum*
W. anomalus and *S. cerevisiae*	OTA	Inhibition of OTA production by *Penicillium verrucosum*

OTA, ochratoxins.
Source: Modified from Arevalo-Villena, M., Briones-Perez, A., Corbo, M. R., Sinigaglia, M., Bevilacqua, A. (2017). Biotechnological application of yeasts in food science: Starter cultures, probiotics and enzyme production. *J Appl Microbiol*, 123: 1360–1372.

epithelium (Maccaferri *et al.* 2012a, 2012b). Therefore, it seems to be able to modulate intestinal activity when antibiotics are administered (Maccaferri *et al.* 2012a, 2012b) and to degrade lactose, reducing its adverse effects in susceptible individuals (Fonseca *et al.* 2008). Moreover, it decreases pro-inflammatory cytokine concentration, favors the growth of bifidobacteria, shows an antimycotic action (e.g. against *Candida albicans*) and competes against pathogens through different mechanisms including: adhesion to the epithelium, competition for nutrients, enhancement of epithelial cell growth and reinforcement of the gut barrier (Lisotti *et al.* 2011; Nigro *et al.* 2014).

Some studies revealed the probiotic potential of some fungi such as *Aspergillus awamori*. When administered to broiler chickens it increased body weight (Saleh *et al.* 2014). Sugiharto *et al.* (2018) evaluated the probiotic effects of *Chrysonilia crassa* administration to broiler chickens. The group administered with *C. crassa* showed better growth and immune responses. Gil de Los Santos *et al.* (2018) demonstrated that administration of *Pichia pastoris* along with *S. boulardii* to broiler chickens improved feed efficiency.

Several studies highlighted the ability of *D. hansenii*, *T. delbrueckii* (Psani and Kotzekidou 2006), *K. lactis, Y. lipolytica* (Chen *et al.* 2010), *K. marxianus* and *K. lodderae* to inhibit development of pathogens and to tolerate passage through the gastrointestinal tract (Kumura *et al.* 2004).

5.6 Encapsulation

Although probiotic yeast cells are rather resistant to conditions encountered during human or animal digestion, it is possible to improve the efficacy of the yeast by means of encapsulation. Encapsulation consists in coating yeast cells with materials that can protect them, target them to their compartment of action and release them at this place. There is not one type of encapsulation; many materials and techniques can be used to reach these objectives. Indeed, many types of protection may be required (against acid environment, oxidation, heat, dryness, etc.), many strategies of release may be of interest (the coating material can be solubilized in the presence of water, it can be hydrolyzed by enzymes or bile acids, or destructured when pH changes, etc) and, finally, many targets can be identified for yeast. In addition to these functionalities, the capsules can also play a sensorial role to decrease the impact of yeast cells on the flavor or color of the product. They can also be used to mimic a natural environment of a biofilm, thereby enhancing the resistance of the cells or modifying their physiological state to increase their colonization properties.

Although there are many techniques and materials that can be used for encapsulation, when living cells and contact with human are concerned, the number of techniques drops, as detailed in several review papers on the subject (Anal and Singh 2007; Krasaekoopt and Bhandari 2012; Rathore *et al.* 2013). One popular way consists in mixing cells in a monomer solution and adding a polymerizing agent. Cells are often mixed in alginate solution, and polymerization occurs in presence of a divalent salt (e.g. $CaCl_2$). To obtain particles, droplets of the solution are usually extruded into a solution containing the polymerizing agent. Although very simple, this technique faces several challenges to diminish the size of the capsules to less than the threshold of perception (for instance, the mouth perception threshold can be around 100 μm for structured foods) and to increase production (several techniques are available to produce small capsules but the price increases rapidly when the size drops). Among these techniques are air atomization (concentric air jet technique), electrostatic atomization, the jet break-up method or spinning-disc atomization, or all techniques making emulsions (Chan *et al.* 2009; Krasaekoopt and Bhandari 2012).

Other popular encapsulation techniques like spray-drying or freeze-drying can be used. Rapidity of drying with a coating material is important to retain the activity of the probiotic cell (Krasaekoopt and Bhandari 2012). This coating process can be added on alginate droplets to achieve protection or to use a coating that will be degraded in the target compartment.

Besides alginate, several materials can be used, usually of natural origin such as chitosan, gellan gum, γ-carrageenan, xanthan, starch, etc. Proteins are also increasingly used with development in more developed countries, whereas development in developing countries was primarily based on low-cost by-product materials (Waché *et al.* 2014).

The physicochemical or chemical properties of the outside layer are very important for protection, targeting and release. It is possible to add such a layer on alginate particles by several of the techniques cited previously. It is also possible to use a layer-by-layer technique (Nguyen *et al.* 2015). In this technique, polyelectrolytes will organize at the surface of yeast cells based on electrostatic properties. Usually, one cationic compound will adsorb to the negatively-charged surface of the cells, resulting in a global positive charge that will be used to attract an anionic compound for the next layer. Special attention has to be paid to the choice of cationic compounds as many of them exhibit antimicrobial properties.

5.7 Conclusion and Future Challenges

Increasing scientific reports are confirming the therapeutic potential of eukaryotic probiotics. In fact, only *S. boulardii* and *K. marxianus* (formerly *K. fragilis*) B0399 are commercially available. Several studies are ongoing to characterize new eukaryotic probiotics, especially for their advantages compared to prokaryotic ones in terms of antibiotic resistance, rich enzymatic reservoir, better action on the immune system, improved defense against pathogens and toxic compounds, promotion of bacterial probiotics development, and their employment as vectors for bioactive molecules.

Several studies are focusing on the characterization of new eukaryotic probiotics, but they are extremely laborious, costly and time consuming. Beneficial traits are often strain specific, and because of the complexity of the possible interactions with host microbiota and various mechanisms of action it is essential to characterize strains thoroughly and understand their metabolic and physiological traits. Concerning *S. boulardii*, its probiotic potential is still underestimated and genome engineering is limited. In this sense several researchers are exploiting molecular tools (e.g. the CRISPR-Cas9 system) developed for *S. cerevisiae* with good results because of the great similarity between these two species. These studies are offering new insights concerning *S. boulardii* probiotic attributes.

References

Abbas, Z., Yakoob, J., Jafri, W., Ahmad, Z., Azam, Z., Usman, M.W., Shamim, S. and Islam, M. (2014). Cytokine and clinical response to *Saccharomyces boulardii* therapy in diarrhoea-dominant irritable bowel syndrome: a randomized trial. *Eur J Gastroenterol Hepatol*, 26: 630–639.

Anal, A.K. and Singh H. (2007). Recent advances in microencapsulation of probiotics for industrial applications and targeted delivery. *Tds Food Sci Technol*, 18: 240–251.

Andlid, T.A., Veide, J. and Sandberg, A.S. (2004). Metabolism of extracellular inositol hexaphosphate (phytate) by *Saccharomyces cerevisiae. Int J Food Microbiol*, 97: 157–169.

Anoop, V., Rotaru, S., Shwed, P.S., Tayabali, A.F. and Arvanitakis G. (2015). Review of current methods for characterizing virulence and pathogenicity potential of industrial *Saccharomyces cerevisiae* strains towards humans. *FEMS Yeast Res*, 15: 57.

Ansari, J.M., Colasacco, C., Emmanouil, E., Kohlhepp, S. and Harriott, O. (2019). Strain level diversity of commercial probiotic isolates of *Bacillus, Lactobacillus*, and *Saccharomyces* species illustrated by molecular identification and phenotypic profiling. *PLoS ONE*, 14: e0213841.

Arevalo-Villena, M., Briones-Perez, A., Corbo, M. R., Sinigaglia, M. and Bevilacqua, A. (2017). Biotechnological application of yeasts in food science: Starter cultures, probiotics and enzyme production. *J Appl Microbiol*, 123: 1360–1372.

Bermudez-Brito, M., Plaza-Díaz, J., Muñoz-Quezada, S., Gómez-Llorente, C. and Gil, A. (2012). Probiotic mechanisms of action. *Ann Nutr Metab*, 61: 160–174.

Bleichner, G., Blehaut, H., Mentec, H. and Moyse, D. (1997). *Saccharomyces boulardii* prevents diarrhoea in critically ill tube-fed patients – A multicenter, randomized, double-blind placebo-controlled trial. *Intensive Care Med*, 23: 517–523.

Bourreille, A., Cadiot, G., Le Dreau, G., Laharie, D., Beaugerie, L., Dupas, J. L., Marteau, P., Rampal, P., Moyse, D., Saleh, A., Le Guern, M. E., Galmiche, J. P., FLORABEST Study Group (2013). *Saccharomyces boulardii* does not prevent relapse of Crohn's disease. *Clin Gastroenterol Hepatol*, 11: 982–987.

Brandão, R.L., Castro, I.M., Bambirra, E.A., Amaral, S.C., Fietto, L.G., Tropia, M.J.M., Neves, M.J., Dos Santos, R.G., Gomes, N.C.M. and Nicoli, J.R. (1998). Intracellular signal triggered by cholera toxin in *Saccharomyces boulardii* and *Saccharomyces cerevisiae. Appl Environ Microbiol*, 64, 564–568.

Buts, J.P., Bernasconi, P., Vaerman, J.P. and Dive, C. (1990). Stimulation of secretory IgA and secretory component of immunoglobulins in small intestine of rats treated with *Saccharomyces boulardii*. *Dig Dis Sci*, 35: 251–256.

Buts, J.P., Dekeyser, N., Stilmant, C., Delem, E., Smets, F. and Sokal, E. (2006). *Saccharomyces boulardii* produces in rat small intestine a novel protein phosphatase that inhibits *Escherichia coli* endotoxin by dephosphorylation. *Pediatr Res*, 60: 24–29.

Canonici, A., Pellegrino, E., Siret, C., Terciolo, C., Czerucka, D., Bastonero, S., Marvaldi, J., Lombardo, D., Rigot, V. and André, F. (2012). *Saccharomyces boulardii* improves intestinal epithelial cell restitution by inhibiting $\alpha v\beta 5$ integrin activation state. *PLoS ONE*, 7: e45047.

Canonici, A., Siret, C., Pellegrino, E., Pontier-Bres, R., Pouyet, L., Montero, M. P., Colin, C., Czerucka, D., Rigot, V. and André, F. (2011). *Saccharomyces boulardii* improves intestinal cell restitution through activation of the $\alpha 2\beta 1$ integrin collagen receptor. *PLoS ONE*, 6: e18427.

Chan, E.S., Lee, B.B., Ravindra, P. and Poncelet, D. (2009). Prediction models for shape and size of ca-alginate macrobeads produced through extrusion–dripping method. *J Colloid Interf Sci*, 338: 63–72.

Chen, X., Kokkotou, E.G., Mustafa, N., Bhaskar, K.R., Sougioultzis, S., O'Brien, M., Pothoulakis, C. and Kelly, C.P. (2006). *Saccharomyces boulardii* inhibits ERK1/2 mitogen-activated protein kinase activation both *in vitro* and *in vivo* and protects against *Clostridium difficile* toxin A induced enteritis. *J Biol Chem*, 281: 24449–24454.

Czerucka, D., Piche, T. and Rampal, P. (2007). Review article: yeast as probiotics – *Saccharomyces boulardii*. *Aliment Pharmacol Ther*, 26: 767–778.

Czerucka, D., Roux, I. and Rampal, P. (1994). *Saccharomyces boulardii* inhibits secretagogue-mediated adenosine 30, 50-cyclic monophosphate induction in intestinal cells. *Gastroenterol*, 106: 65–72.

Deak, T. (2006). Environmental factors influencing yeasts. In: *Biodiversity and Ecophysiology of Yeasts* (The Yeast Handbook series), (ed. G. Péter and C. Rosa), 155–174. Berlin: Springer.

Edwards-Ingram, L.C., Gent, M.E., Hoyle, D.C., Hayes, A., Stateva, L.I. and Oliver, S.G. (2004). Comparative genomic hybridization provides new insights into the molecular taxonomy of the *Saccharomyces Sensu Stricto* complex. *Genome Res*, 14: 1043–1051.

Edwards-Ingram, L., Gitsham, P., Burton, N., Warhurst, G., Clarke, I., Hoyle, D., Oliver, S.G. and Stateva, L. (2007). Genotypic and physiological characterization of *Saccharomyces boulardii*, the probiotic strain of *Saccharomyces cerevisiae*. *Appl Environ Microbiol*, 73: 2458–2467.

Everard, A., Matamoros, S., Geurts, L., Delzenne, N.M. and Cani, P.D. (2014). *Saccharomyces boulardii* administration changes gut microbiota and reduces hepatic steatosis, low-grade inflammation, and fat mass in obese and type 2 diabetic db/db mice. *mBio*, 5: e01011–e01014.

FAO/WHO (2005). Vitamin and mineral requirements in human nutrition, Second edition. Available from http://apps.who.int/iris/bitstream/handle/10665/42716/9241546123.pdf;jsessionid=E546F6BC9471B3E3789DDCB2BBA37390?sequence=1.

Fietto, J.L., Araújo, R.S., Valadão, F.N., Fietto, L.G., Brandão, R.L., Neves, M.J., Gomes, F.C., Nicoli, J.R. and Castro, I.M. (2004). Molecular and physiological comparisons between *Saccharomyces cerevisiae* and *Saccharomyces boulardii*. *Can J Microbiol*, 50: 615–621.

Fonseca, G.G., Heinzle, E., Wittmann, C. and Gombert. A.K. (2008). The yeast *Kluyveromyces marxianus* and its biotechnological potential. *Appl Microbiol Biotechnol*, 79: 339–354.

Gil de Los Santos, D., Gil de Los Santos, J.R., Gil-Turnes, C., Gaboardi, G., Fernandes Silva, L., França, R., Gevehr Fernandes, C. and Rochedo Conceição, F. (2018). Probiotic effect of *Pichia pastoris* X-33 produced in parboiled rice effluent and YPD medium on broiler chickens. *PLoS ONE*, 13, e0192904.

Girard-Pipau, F., Pompei, A., Schneider, S., Nano, J.L., Hebuterne, X., Boquet, P. and Rampal, P. (2002). Intestinal microflora, short chain and cellular fatty acids, influence of a probiotic *Saccharomyces boulardii*. *Microb Ecol Health Dis*, 14: 221–228.

Gut, A.M., Vasiljevic, T., Yeager, T. and Donkor, O. (2018). *Salmonella* infection – prevention and treatment by antibiotics and probiotic yeasts: a review. *Microbiol*, 164: 1327–1344.

Hatoum, R., Labrie, S. and Fliss, I. (2012). Antimicrobial and probiotic properties of yeasts: from fundamental to novel applications. *Front Microbiol*, 3: 421.

Hill, C., Guarner, F., Reid, G., Gibson, G.R., Merenstein, D.J., Pot B., Morelli, L., Canani, R.B., Flint, H.J., Salminen, S., Calder, P.C. and Sanders, M.E. (2014). Expert consensus document. The International Scientific Association for Probiotics and Prebiotics consensus statement on the scope and appropriate use of the term probiotic. *Nat Rev Gastroenterol Hepatol*, 11: 506–514.

Hossain, M.N., Afrin, S., Humayun, S., Ahmed, M.M. and Saha, B.K. (2020). Identification and growth characterization of a novel strain of *Saccharomyces boulardii* isolated from soya paste. *Front Nutr*, 7: 27.

Jägerstad, M., Piironen, V., Walker, C., Ros, G., Carnovale, E., Holasova, M. and Nau, H. (2005). Increasing natural-food folates through bioprocessing and biotechnology. *Trends Food Sci Technol*, 16: 298–306.

Kariluoto, S., Vahteristo, L., Salovaara, H., Katina, K., Liukkonen, K.H. and Piironen, V. (2004). Effect of baking method and fermentation on folate content of rye and wheat breads. *Cereal Chem*, 81: 134–139.

Khatri, I., Tomar, R., Ganesan, K., Prasad, G.S. and Subramanian, S. (2017). Complete genome sequence and comparative genomics of the probiotic yeast *Saccharomyces boulardii*. *Sci Rep*, 7: 1–13.

Kourelis, A., Kotzamanidis, C., Litopoulou-Tzanetaki, E., Papaconstantinou, J., Tzanetakis, N. and Yiangou M. (2010). Immunostimulatory activity of potential probiotic yeast strains in the dorsal air pouch system and the gut mucosa. *J Appl Microbiol*, 109: 260–271.

Krasaekoopt, W. and Bhandari, B. (2012). Properties and applications of different probiotic delivery systems. In: *Encapsulation Technologies and Delivery Systems for Food Ingredients and Nutraceuticals* (ed. N. Garti and D.J. McClements), 541–594. Woodhead Publishing.

Kumura, H., Tanoue, Y., Tsukahara, M., Tanaka, T. and Shimazaki, K. (2004). Screening of dairy yeast strains for probiotic applications. *J Dairy Sci*, 87: 4050–4056.

Kurtzman, C.P., Fell, J.W. and Boekhout, T. (2011). *The Yeasts: A Taxonomic Study*. Elsevier.

Lee, S.H. (2015). Intestinal permeability regulation by tight junction: implication on inflammatory bowel diseases. *Intest Res*, 13: 11–18.

Lessard, M., Dupuis, M., Gagnon, N., Nadeau, E., Matte, J.J., Goulet, J. and Fairbrother, J.M. (2009). Administration of *Pediococcus acidilactici* or *Saccharomyces cerevisiae boulardii* modulates development of porcine mucosal immunity and reduces intestinal bacterial translocation after *Escherichia coli* challenge. *J Anim Sci*, 87: 922–934.

Lin, D.C. (2003). Probiotics as functional foods. *Nutr Clin Pract*, 18: 497–506.

Lisotti, A., Cornia, G.L., Morselli-Labate, A.M., Sartini, A., Turco, L., Grasso, V., Cavina, P., Mazzella, G. and Roda, E. (2011). Effects of a fermented milk containing *Kluyveromyces marxianus* B0399 and *Bifidobacterium lactis* BB12 in patients with irritable bowel syndrome. *Minerva Gastroenterol Dietol*, 57: 1–12.

Maccaferri, S., Candela, M., Turroni. S., Centanni, M., Severgnini, M., Consolandi, C., Cavina, P. and Brigidi, P. (2012b). IBS-associated phylogenetic unbalances of the intestinal microbiota are not reverted by probiotic supplementation. *Gut Microbes*, 3: 406–413.

Maccaferri, S., Klinder, A., Brigidi, P., Cavina, P. and Costabile, A. (2012a). Potential probiotic *Kluyveromyces marxianus* B0399 modulates the immune response in Caco-2 cells and peripheral blood mononuclear cells and impacts the human gut microbiota in an in vitro colonic model system. *Appl Environ Microbiol*, 78: 956–964.

Martins, F.S., Elian, S.D.A., Vieira, A.T., Tiago, F.C.P., Martins, A.K.S., Silva, F.C.P., Souza, E.L.S., Sousa, L.P., Araújo, H.R.C., Pimenta, P.F., Bonjardim, C.A., Arantes, R.M.E., Teixeira, M.M. and Nicoli, J.R. (2011). Oral treatment with *Saccharomyces cerevisiae* strain UFMG 905 modulates immune responses and interferes with signal pathways involved in the activation of inflammation in a murine model of typhoid fever. *Int J Med Microbiol*, 301: 359–364.

McFarland, L.V. (2007). Meta-analysis of probiotics for the prevention of traveler's diarrhoea. *Travel Med Infect Dis*, 5: 97–105.

McFarland, L.V. (2017). Common organisms and probiotics: *Saccharomyces boulardii*. In: *The Microbiota in Gastrointestinal Pathophysiology*, 145–164. Cambridge, MA: Academic Press.

Mitterdorfer, G., Kneifel, W. and Viernstein H. (2001). Utilization of prebiotic carbohydrates by yeasts of therapeutic relevance. *Lett Appl Microbiol*, 34: 251–255.

Mitterdorfer, G., Mayer, H.K., Kneifel, W. and Viernstein, H. (2002). Clustering of *Saccharomyces boulardii* strains within the species *S. cerevisiae* using molecular typing techniques. *J Appl Microbiol*, 93: 521–530.

Moré, M.I. and Swidsinski, A. (2015). *Saccharomyces boulardii* CNCM I-745 supports regeneration of the intestinal microbiota after diarrheic dysbiosis – a review. *Clin Exp Gastroenterol*, 8: 237–255.

Moré, M.I. and Vandenplas, Y. (2018). *Saccharomyces boulardii* CNCM I-745 improves intestinal enzyme function: a trophic effects review. *Clin Med Insights Gastroenterol*, 11: 1179552217752679.

Moslehi-Jenabian, S., Pedersen, L.L. and Jespersen, L. (2010). Beneficial effects of probiotic and food borne yeasts on human health. *Nutrients*, 2: 449–473.

Moss, M.O. and Long, M.T. (2002). Fate of patulin in the presence of the yeast *Saccharomyces cerevisiae*. *Food Addit Contam*, 19: 387–399.

Nguyen, T.D., Guyot, S., Lherminier, J., Waché, Y., Saurel, R. and Husson, F. (2015). Protection of living yeast cells by micro-organized shells of natural polyelectrolytes. *Process Biochem*, 50: 1528–1536.

Nigro, A., Nicastro, A. and Trodella, R. (2014). Retrospective observational study to investigate Sinerga, a multifactorial nutritional product, and bacterial extracts in the prevention of recurrent respiratory infections in children. *Int J Immunopathol Pharmacol*, 27: 455–460.

O'Toole, P.W. and Cooney, J.C. (2008). Probiotic bacteria influence the composition and function of the intestinal microbiota. *Interdiscip Perspect Infect Dis*, 175285.

Pais, P., Almeida, V., Yilmaz, M. and Teixeira, M.C. (2020). *Saccharomyces boulardii*: What makes it tick as successful probiotic? *J Fungi*, 6: 78.

Palma, M.L., Zamith-Miranda, D., Martins, F.S., Bozza, F.A., Nimrichter, L., Montero-Lomeli, M., Marques, E.T. Jr. and Douradinha, B. (2015). Probiotic *Saccharomyces cerevisiae* strains as biotherapeutic tools: is there room for improvement? *Appl Microbiol Biotechnol*, 99: 6563–6570.

Patring, J.D.M., Hjortmo, S.B., Jastrebova, J.A., Svensson, U.K., Andlid, T.A. and Jägerstad, I.M. (2006). Characterization and quantification of folates produced by yeast strains isolated from kefir granules. *Eur Food Res Technol*, 223: 633–637.

Pericolini, E., Gabrielli, E., Ballet, N., Sabbatini, S., Roselletti, E., Cayzeele Decherf, A., Pélerin, F., Luciano, E., Perito, S., Jüsten, P. and Vecchiarelli, A. (2017). Therapeutic activity of a *Saccharomyces cerevisiae*-based probiotic and inactivated whole yeast on vaginal candidiasis. *Virulence*, 8: 74–90.

Perpetuini, G., Prete, R., Garcia-Gonzalez, N., Khairul Alam, M. and Corsetti, A. (2020). Table olives more than a fermented food. *Foods*, 9: 178.

Péteri, Z., Teren, J., Vagvolgyi, C. and Varga, J. (2007). Ochratoxin degradation and adsorption caused by astaxanthin-producing yeasts. *Food Microbiol*, 24: 205–210.

Pfliegler, W.P., Pusztahelyi, T. and Pocsi, I. (2015). Mycotoxins – prevention and decontamination by yeasts. *J Bas Microbiol*, 55: 805–818.

Plaza-Diaz, J., Ruiz-Ojeda, F.J., Gil-Campos, M. and Gil, A. (2019). Mechanisms of action of probiotics. *Adv Nutr*, 10: S49–S66.

Pontier-bres, R., Munro, P., Boyer, L., Anty, R., Rampal, P. and Lemichez, E. (2014). *Saccharomyces boulardii* modifies *Salmonella typhimurium* traffic and host immune responses along the intestinal tract. *PLoS ONE*, 9: e103069.

Pothoulakis, C. (2009). Review article: anti-inflammatory mechanisms of action of *Saccharomyces boulardii*. *Aliment Pharmacol Ther*, 30: 826–833.

Psani, M. and Kotzekidou, P. (2006). Technological characteristics of yeast strains and their potential as starter adjuncts in Greek-style black olive fermentation. *World J Microbiol Biotechnol*, 22: 1329–1336.

Quarella, S., Lovrovich, P., Scalabrin, S., Campedelli, I., Backovic, A., Gatto, V., Cattonaro, F., Turello, A., Torriani, S., Felis, G.E. (2016). Draft genome sequence of the probiotic yeast *Kluyveromyces marxianus fragilis* B0399. *Genome Announc*, 4: e00923–16.

Rajkowska, K. and Kunicka-Styczynska, A. (2012). Probiotic activity of *Saccharomyces cerevisiae* var. *boulardii* against human pathogens. *Food Technol Biotechnol*, 50: 230–236.

Rathore, S., Desai, P.M., Liew, C.V., Chan, L.W. and Heng, P.W.S. (2013). Microencapsulation of microbial cells. *J Food Engin*, 116: 369–381.

Reddy, N.R. and Pierson, M.D. (1994). Reduction in antinutritional and toxic components in plant foods by fermentation. *Food Res Int*, 27: 281–290.

Rodrigues, F., Ludovico, P. and Leão, C. (2006). Sugar metabolism in yeasts: an overview of aerobic and anaerobic glucose catabolism. In: *The Yeast Handbook* (ed. G. Péter and C. Rosa), 101–121. Berlin: Springer.

Romanin, D., Serradell, M., Maciel, D.G., Lausada, N., Garrote, G.L. and Rumbo, M. (2010). Down-regulation of intestinal epithelial innate response by probiotic yeasts isolated from kefir. *Int J Food Microbiol*, 140: 102–108.

Romero-Luna, H.E., Hernández-Sánchez, H., Ribas-Aparicio, R.M., CauichSánchez, P.I. and Dávila-Ortiz, G. (2019). Evaluation of the probiotic potential of *Saccharomyces cerevisiae* strain (C41) isolated from Tibicos by *in vitro* studies. *Probiot Antimicrob Prot*, 11: 794–800.

Russo, P., Capozzi, V., Spano, G., Corbo, M.R., Sinigaglia, M. and Bevilacqua, A. (2016). Metabolites of microbial origin with an impact on health: ochratoxin A and biogenic amines. *Front Microbiol*, 7: 482.

Saleh, A., Hayashi, K., Ijiri, D. and Ohtsuka, A. (2014). Beneficial effects of *Aspergillus awamori* in broiler nutrition. *World's Poultry Science Journal*, 70: 857–864.

Saubade, F., Hemery, Y.M., Guyot, J.P. and Humblot, C. (2017). Lactic acid fermentation as a tool for increasing the folate content of foods. *Crit Rev Food Sci Nutr*, 57: 3894–3910.

Schneider, S.M., Girard-Pipau, F., Filippi, J., Hebuterne, X., Moyse, D., Hinojosa, G.C., Pompei, A. and Rampal, P. (2005). Effects of *Saccharomyces boulardii* on fecal short-chain fatty acids and microflora in patients on long-term total enteral nutrition. *World J Gastroenterol*, 11: 6165–6169.

Scott, P.M., Kanhere, S.R., Lawrence, G.A., Daley, E.F. and Farber, J.M. (1995). Fermentation of wort containing added ochratoxin A and fumonisins B1 and B2. *Food Addit Contam*, 12: 31–40.

Sen, S. and Mansell, T.J. (2020). Yeasts as probiotics: mechanisms, outcomes, and future potential. *Fungal Genet Biol*, 137: 103333.

Sharif, M.R., Kashani, H.H., Ardakani, A.T., Kheirkhah, D., Tabatabaei, F. and Sharif, A. (2016). The effect of a yeast probiotic on acute diarrhoea in children. *Probiotics Antimicrob Proteins*, 8: 211–214.

Shetty, P.H., Hald, B. and Jespersen, L. (2007). Surface binding of aflatoxin B1 by *Saccharomyces cerevisiae* strains with potential decontaminating abilities in indigenous fermented foods. *Int J Food Microbiol*, 113:41–46.

Sougioultzis, S., Simeonidis, S., Bhaskar, K.R., Chen, X., Anton, P.M., Keates, S., Pothoulakis, C. and Kelly, C.P. (2006). *Saccharomyces boulardii* produces a soluble anti-inflammatory factor that inhibits NF-κB-mediated IL-8 gene expression. *Biochem Biophys Res Commun*, 343: 69–76.

Stier, H. and Bischoff, SC. (2016). Influence of *Saccharomyces boulardii* CNCM I745 on the gut-associated immune system. *Clin Exp Gastroenterol*, 9: 269.

Sugiharto, S., Yudiarti, T., Isroli, I., Widiastuti, E., Wahyuni, H. and Sartono, T. (2018). The effect of fungi-origin probiotic *Chrysonilia crassa* in comparison to selected commercially used feed additives on broiler chicken performance, intestinal microbiology, and blood indices. *J Adv Vet Anim Res*, 5: 332.

Szajewska, H. and Kołodziej, M. (2015). Systematic review with meta-analysis: *Saccharomyces boulardii* in the prevention of antibiotic-associated diarrhoea. *Aliment Pharmacol Ther*, 42: 793–801.

Tasteyre, A., Barc, M.C., Karjalainen, T., Bourlioux, P. and Collignon, A. (2002). Inhibition of *in vitro* cell adherence of *Clostridium difficile* by *Saccharomyces boulardii*. *Microb Pathog*, 32: 219–225.

Terciolo, C., Dapoigny, M. and Andre, F. (2019). Beneficial effects of *Saccharomyces boulardii* CNCM I-745 on clinical disorders associated with intestinal barrier disruption. *Clin Exp Gastroenterol*, 12: 67–82.

Terciolo, C., Dobric, A., Ouaissi, M., Siret, C., Breuzard, G., Silvy, F., Marchiori, B., Germain, S., Bonier, R., Hama, A., Owens, R., Lombardo, D., Rigot, V. and André, F. (2017). *Saccharomyces boulardii* CNCM I-745 restores intestinal barrier integrity by regulation of E-cadherin recycling. *J Crohns Colitis*, 11: 999–1010.

Tiago, F.C.P., Martins, F.S., Souza, E.L.S., Pimenta, P.F.P., Araujo, H.R.C., Castro, I.M., Brandão, R.L. and Nicoli, J.R. (2012). Adhesion to the yeast cell surface as a mechanism for trapping pathogenic bacteria by *Saccharomyces* probiotics. *J Med Microbiol*, 61: 1194–1207.

Tofalo, R. and Suzzi, G. (2016). Yeasts. In: *The Encyclopedia of Food and Health* (ed. B. Caballero, P. Finglas and F. Toldrá), 5, 593–599. Oxford: Academic Press.

van der Aa Kühle, A., Skovgaard, K. and Jespersen, L. (2005). *in vitro* screening of probiotic properties of *Saccharomyces cerevisiae* var. *boulardii* and foodborne *Saccharomyces cerevisiae* strains. *Int J Food Microbiol*, 101: 29–39.

Vohra, A. and Satyanarayana, T. (2003). Phytases: Microbial sources, production, purification, and potential biotechnological applications. *Crit Rev Biotechnol*, 23: 29–60.

Waché, Y., Anal, A.K., Chan, E.S., Heng, P.W.S. and Ngo, D.N., In, S., Poncelet, D., Phan-Thi, H. (2014). Meeting report: The 1st BRG-training school in Asia, a first step in the building of an ASEAN encapsulation network. *Biotechnol J*, 9: 1473–1475.

Zanello, G., Meurens, F., Berri, M. and Salmon, H.Y. (2009). *Saccharomyces boulardii* effects on gastrointestinal diseases. *Curr Issues Mol Biol*, 11: 47.

6

Determination and Safety Aspects of Probiotic Cultures

Falguni Patra[1] *and Raj Kumar Duary*[2,3]

[1] *Mansinhbhai Institute of Dairy & Food Technology, Dudhsagar Dairy campus, Mehsana, Gujarat-, 384002, India*
[2] *Department of Food Engineering and Technology, Tezpur University, Napaam, Sonitpur, Assam-, 784028, India*
[3] *Department of Dairy Science and Food Technology, Institute of Agricultural Sciences, Banaras Hindu University, Varanasi, Uttar Pradesh-, 221005, India*

6.1 Introduction

The market and demand for probiotic products are increasing tremendously. Analysis of reports and data showed that the global probiotics market was USD 47.1 billion in 2018 and is projected to increase at a compound annual growth rate of 6.8% from 2019 to 2026 (https://www.globenewswire.com/news-release/2020/02/06/1981205/0/en/Probiotics-Market-To-Reach-USD-78-3-Billion-By-2026-Reports-And-Data.html). Currently available products containing probiotics on the market can be found in different sections such as food matrix, dietary supplements or additives, drugs or neutraceutical components and cosmetics. A probiotic has been defined as a microorganism that in its live state shows health-promoting functionalities when given in adequate doses (FAO/WHO 2002). There are numerous functional or health benefits associated with probiotic activities such as: lactose metabolism and food digestion, improved immunity, cholesterol normalization, reduction of blood pressure, improvement of oral health, and treatment of urogenital and upper respiratory tract infection, inflammatory bowel disease (IBD), irritable bowel syndrome (IBS), Crohn's disease, antibiotic associated diarrhea, *Clostridium difficile* infection, diabetes, obesity, etc. Recently, strains of lactobacilli and *Bifidobacterium* have been the most often used probiotics on the market, although other organisms such as lactococci, enterococci, *Streptococcus thermophilus*, spore-forming probiotics belonging to genus *Bacillus* and yeasts such as *Saccharomyces boulardii* are also used (Anal 2019; Koirala and Anal 2021).

Generally, lactic acid bacilli (LAB) are food-grade organisms regarded as safe as they have a long and safe association with humans through consumption of fermented foods. However, certain reports regarding their pathogenicity question their infinite safety for human consumption. Strains of both lactobacilli and bifidobacteria have been associated

Probiotics, Prebiotics and Synbiotics: Technological Advancements Towards Safety and Industrial Applications, First Edition. Edited by Parmjit Singh Panesar and Anil Kumar Anal.

with bacteremia, sepsis, endocarditis, meningitis and abscesses in specifically immune-compromised individuals (Castro-Gonzalez *et al.* 2019; Pradhan *et al.* 2020). Further, several metabolic activities (e.g. bile salt deconjugation, D-lactate production, biogenic amine production, the presence of glycosidase and β-glucuronidase activities, mucin degradation, platelet aggregation, etc.) may raise safety issues with these probiotic organisms in humans upon administration. Additionally, the presence of virulence determinants, toxin genes, antibiotic resistance potential and transferability of probiotic strains are other safety concerns which also should be taken into consideration. Thus, safety assessment is the top priority before a probiotic can be launched into the market. Countries have developed their own guidelines for safety assessment of probiotics. The European Food Safety Authority (EFSA) has introduced Qualified Presumption of Safety (QPS) status for microorganisms intended to be added to foods for human consumption. The United States Food and Drug Administration (FDA) have the designation Generally Recognized As Safe (GRAS) and quote "a chemical or substance added to food is considered safe by experts, and so is exempted from the usual Federal Food, Drug, and Cosmetic Act (FFDCA) food additive tolerance requirements". The FAO/WHO (2002) jointly put forward guidelines for assessment of safety of a probiotic candidate, which begins with proper identification of the specific strain, determination of antibiotic resistance and transferability, harmful metabolites, virulence factor, toxins, safety study in an in vivo animal model, human clinical trial and post-marketing surveillance.

6.2 Assessments of Probiotics in the Gut

Probiotics can be used or explored either prophylactically or as a biotherapeutic alternative to pharmaceutical or drug interventions to target specific groups. Probiotics are found to be safer and can overcome the physiological barriers of human anatomy. Still, various claims related to efficacy or functional attributes for the host's health are unsubstantiated and yet to be properly established. Morbidity, mortality and adverse effects related to probiotics intervention have also been reported, as in immune-compromised subjects (Bafeta *et al.* 2018; Vogel 2008).

For safety assessments, the suitable and accurate identification of probiotic strains at species and strain level plays an important role. To establish the commercial value and credibility of a particular probiotic culture, its identification at strain level is very important. The estimation and assessment of the probiotic in the gut environment can be done by both direct and indirect methods with respect to labeling safety and integrity of the strain used. Various molecular biological tools such as gene sequencing, specific primer based polymerase chain reaction (PCR) techniques, genetic fingerprinting, etc., are being explored for assessment of probiotics. Even various functional attributes can be assessed by various direct and indirect techniques.

6.2.1 Direct Method

Culture-based methods alone cannot provide accurate information in identification of a particular probiotic strain. Generally, biochemical-based approaches along with genetic-based approaches are employed for identification or assessment of probiotic strains. Earlier, molecular-based techniques such as genus and species specific PCR, random amplified polymorphic DNA (RAPD), fluorescent in situ hybridization (FISH), pulsed-field gel electrophoresis (PFGE), temperature gradient gel electrophoresis (TGGE)/denaturing gradient gel electrophoresis (DGGE) and probe-based PCR, etc., were explored to differentiate between closely related species of a particular probiotic strain (Kaushik *et al.* 2009; McCartney 2002).

Analyses of whole genomes or some conserved genes such as 16S and 18S rRNA/rDNA (ribosomal RNA/DNA) for prokaryotes and eukaryotes are included in nucleic acid approaches. The 16S rRNA gene is considered the gold standard for phylogenetic studies of different microbes and is generally targeted as the marker gene of choice for bacterial and archaeal communities, even uncultured ones. Recently, Zmora *et al.* (2018) urged researchers to look beyond using 16S rDNA analysis for assessment of probiotic strains in relation to their strain-specific effects. Recently, with the availability of different high-throughput molecular methods (sequencing), it has become relatively easier to study the human gut flora accurately. The genetic sequence of bacteria can be effectively detected by metagenomics approaches. Quantitative PCR (qPCR) or metagenomics sequencing like high-throughput sequencing (Solexa or 454 pyrosequencing or SOLID system targeting 16S DNA) can be effective methods.

Still, there is a debate that microbiome analysis through stool samples for probiotic numbers or effects can be an effective tool to establish functionality in the host. Zmora *et al.* (2018) reported that the mucosal microbiome and stool microbiome correlate partially, suggesting personalized probiotics based approaches. They employed endoscopy and colonoscopy methods in healthy human subjects during feeding of 11 probiotic strains (Supherb Bio-25, a cocktail of probiotics). They also reported that the tested probiotic organisms in feces get enriched during the feeding schedule.

Other techniques such as propidium monoazide (PMA; an intercalating dye for nucleic acid) coupled with qPCR can be effective in quantification of viable bacteria in food matrices based on integrity of the cell membrane. Scariot *et al.* (2018) used PMA-qPCR to detect and quantify *Lactobacillus paracasei* in probiotic yoghurt targeting the *tuf* (related with elongation factor) gene. *Bifidobacterium animalis* subsp. *lactis* BB-12 was rapidly and effectively enumerated in a probiotic-based passion fruit juice formulation stored at 4 °C for 30 days (Dias *et al.* 2020). Flow cytometry has also been explored as a powerful tool for assessing the viability of probiotic strains using viable staining dye and a flow cytometer (Chiron *et al.* 2018; Raymond and Champagne 2015).

The genes involved in acid and bile stress tolerance in *Lactobacillus* spp. have been identified using advanced genomic and proteomic analysis tools (Altermann *et al.* 2005; Sánchez *et al.* 2006). The acid and bile salt tolerance of probiotic strain/s is because of expression of ATP synthase (*atp*), bile salt hydrolase (*Bsh*) and some transporter proteins under gut conditions (Duary *et al.* 2010, 2012; Kim and Lee 2008). Wall *et al.* (2003), working on the probiotic bacterium *L. reuteri*, reported the role of 52 novel genes encoding for various transmembrane and extracellular proteins in adherence to the epithelial cell lines of the gut. The role and importance of *Mub* and *Map*A (mucus adhesion genes) along with EF-Tu (adhesion-like factor) have been established in *L. plantarum* in relation to adhesion in the gut (Duary *et al.* 2012; Ramiah *et al.* 2007). Ramiah *et al.* (2009) also stated that the expressions of these surface proteins are very strain specific. The quantification of probiotic attributes and study of the exact mechanism of their strategies to overcome the physiological barriers of host gut are important parameters for both in vivo function and fermentation stability. Exploring the gene expression profile using microarray and reverse transcription quantitative PCR (RT-qPCR) on selected strains to overcome host physiological conditions (like high acid and bile containing simulated medium), adhesion mechanisms (involvement of surface proteins like elongation factor Tu [EF-Tu], mucus-binding protein [*mub*], mucus adhesion promoting protein [*mapA*], fibronectin-binding protein [*Fbp*], collagen-binding protein [*CnBP*]), synthesis of nutrients (pathways for folate, vitamin B_1, vitamin B_{12}, vitamin K, pyridoxine, biotin, riboflavin, pantothenate), essential amino acids (threonine, phenylalanine, leucine, tryptophan, lysine, valine, methionine and isoleucine) and production of lactic acid, butyrate, short chain fatty acids, antimicrobial compounds (bacteriocin), etc., will establish the efficiency. Hence, the expression of various genes in probiotics during the transit period under gut conditions can be reliably used as one of the important biomarkers for assessing the functional efficacy of probiotic strains.

6.2.2 Indirect Method

The indirect method involves an in vitro gut or colon model simulating the gut physiology of humans and in vivo tests in various animal models to assess the safety of a probiotic strain. Programmed computer-controlled sophisticated and reliable in vitro systems mimicking gastrointestinal environment based digesters can be utilized to assess the efficiency and safety of a probiotic culture. Duysburgh *et al.* (2018) proposed an in vitro technology platform called Simulator of the Human Intestinal Microbial Ecosystem (SHIME®), which mimics the gut conditions of an adult human. The SHIME® model consists of five reactors mimicking the gastric tract, intestinal tract and ascending, transverse and descending colon respectively. This model is effective in correlating the mechanism, antipathogenic activity and mucosal colonization, etc., of a probiotic strain. The developed model can be extended with various cell culturing models such as human epithelial colorectal adenocarcinoma cells (Caco-2) or human colorectal adenocarcinoma (HT29) cells, peripheral blood mononuclear cells (PBMCs), monocyte-like cell line (THP1 macrophages), etc.

Duary *et al.* (2010, 2011, 2012) have reported the probiotic potential of two promising indigenous *L. plantarum* isolates, namely Lp9 and Lp91, against colitis mice models. The animal models are usually designed to mimic disease conditions to assess the acute (single dose, 14 days), subacute (repeated dose, 28 days) and chronic toxicity (repeated dose, 90 days) of ingestion of probiotics (Organization for Economic Cooperation and Development [OECD] 2001). Also, the production of any toxic metabolites by the targeted probiotic strain should be also assessed in animal models. Immune-compromised mouse models should be explored for assessing safety, i.e. causing no infectivity (Ganguly *et al.* 2011). The translocation, if any, of probiotics to the bloodstream and mucosal tissues from the host' gut after consumption along with probabilities of infection should be assessed in diseased in vivo models (Pradhan *et al.* 2020). The final safety aspects of the probiotic strain should be assessed in healthy human subjects (over the short or long term) as well as in the group of targeted patients.

6.3 Dosage for Probiotic Effect

Effective probiotic influence on human health is correlated with sufficient doses of probiotic strain/s. The legal guidelines/definition laid down by various agencies such as the FAO/WHO, European Union (EU) and Indian Council of Medical Research (ICMR) emphasize the importance of adequate amounts/dose to exert health-promoting effects in humans. As per the legislation of the EU, there are no specific dose-based regulations on safety of probiotics (guidelines of the Scientific Committee on Animal Nutrition [SCAN] and Council Directive 70/254/EEC) (Von Wright 2005). Also, there is no mentioning of clear dosing of probiotics in the FAO/WHO (2002) and ICMR-DBT guidelines (Ganguly *et al.* 2011). They have only quoted "The suggested serving size must deliver the effective dose of probiotics related to the health claim" (FAO/WHO 2002).

A minimum dose of 10^6 CFU/mL has been recommended for probiotic-based formulations during the time of consumption (Tripathi and Giri 2014). Karimi *et al.* (2011) earlier stated that approximately 10^9 viable cells can effectively reach the intestinal environment with consumption of 100 g of probiotic products daily. However, the effective probiotic doses in relation to specific functional health benefits should be established through clinical trials on specific strains in humans. In general, assessments of doses are performed by taking a 10-fold overdose of the final product/formulation of the particular probiotic in the target animal model. Meta-analysis (mostly published reports of clinical trials on humans) can be effective in evaluating the dose-response of the probiotic organism. Through meta-analysis, Zhang *et al.* (2016) reported that a low dose of single probiotics in a short treatment duration improved responses in patients with irritable bowel syndrome (IBS). Ouwehand (2017) reported meta-analysis data of probiotic strains in relation to necrotizing enterocolitis (NEC) and antibiotic-associated diarrhea (AAD). In AAD a positive dose-dependent effect was clearly observed, while no dose-dependent responses were noted for NEC (because of lack of studies). The author suggested meta-analysis of a particular probiotic strain before commercializing its use with dose-dependent labeling on the product. In general, industries prefer to use overages of probiotic organisms in products to maintain the target dose during shelf-life. Thus, it is mandatory to define minimal/maximal doses along with the frequency of probiotic administration to be in accordance with the specific health claims made by the producer on their product.

6.4 Pathogenicity and Inefficiency of Probiotic Culture

6.4.1 Pathogenicity of Probiotics

Probiotic organisms, particularly lactobacilli, have been reported to be responsible for meningitis, endometritis, peritonitis, pneumonia, bacteremia and endocarditis, mainly in immune-compromised individuals, those with a dysfunctional gut barrier, and patients with underlying diseases (Table 6.1). Translocation of probiotic bacteria from the gastrointestinal tract (GIT) to extraintestinal sites (i.e. the bloodstream) occurs due to gut immaturity, impaired intestinal barrier function and immune suppression.

Table 6.1 Incidence of infections linked to probiotic organisms.

Infection	Patient reports	Probiotic organism	References
Bacteremia	17-year-old boy with ulcerative colitis	*Lb. rhamnosus* GG	Vahabnezhad *et al.* (2013)
Bacteremia	6-day-old newborn with intrauterine growth restriction (IUGR) symptoms	*Lb. rhamnosus* GG ATCC 53103	Sadowska-Krawczenko *et al.* (2014)
Bacteremia associated with candidemia	Adult patient with severe active ulcerative colitis	*Lb. rhamnosus* GG	Meini *et al.* (2015)
Bacteremia	75-year-old patient with end-stage renal disease and type 2 diabetes mellitus	*Lb. rhamnosus*	Sendil *et al.* (2020)
Bacteremia	Two premature babies (26 2/7 weeks and 28 6/7 weeks)	*Bifidobacterium longum* subspecies *infantis*	Bertelli *et al.* (2015)
Bacteremia	Three preterm babies (23–24 weeks)	*B. longum* ssp. *infantis*	Esaiassen *et al.* (2016)
Liver abscess and bacteremia	82-year-old woman with a history of diabetes mellitus, hypertension and end-stage renal disease	Lactobacilli	Sherid *et al.* (2016)
Pneumonia	11-month-old female	*Lb. rhamnosus* GG	Doern *et al.* (2014)
Endocarditis	77-year-old man with prostate cancer	*Lb. paracasei*	Franko *et al.* (2013)
Endocarditis	80-year-old man	*Lb. rhamnosus*	Aaron *et al.* (2017)
Endocarditis	80-year-old male	*Lb. rhamnosus*	Pararajasingam and Uwagwu (2017)
Endocarditis	36-year-old woman with a history of complicated cirrhosis and prior *Clostridium difficile* colitis	*Lb. rhamnosus*	Naqvi *et al.* (2018)
Endocarditis	>65-year-old patient with hereditary hemorrhagic telangiectasia, aortic bioprosthesis, and a history of repeated serious infections with hospitalizations	*Lb. rhamnosus*	Boumis *et al.* (2018)
Sepsis	24-year-old female patient after an aortic valve replacement	*Lb. rhamnosus*	Kochan *et al.* (2011)
Sepsis	54-year-old male patient with acute promyelocytic leukemia	*Lb. rhamnosus* GG (ATCC 53103)	Koyama *et al.* (2019)

Bacteremia was identified in a 17-year-old boy with ulcerative colitis after 1 week of probiotic *Lb. rhamnosus* GG administration. The blood culture method detected a strain of *Lb. rhamnosus* by 16S rRNA gene sequencing that was 99.78% identical with the probiotic strain present in the tablet (Vahabnezhad *et al.* 2013). In a 6-day-old newborn with symptoms of intrauterine growth restriction (IUGR), *Lb. rhamnosus* GG (ATCC 53103) infection was reported (Sadowska-Krawczenko *et al.* 2014). The baby was administered with antibiotics, and a probiotic was given to prevent antibiotic-associated gastrointestinal disorder. The blood sample was positive for lactobacilli on day 6; the strain identified was *Lb. rhamnosus* GG (confirmed by PCR and 16S rRNA sequencing) and showed 100% similarity with the probiotic product as confirmed by rep-PCR and amplified fragment length polymorphism (AFLP). Meini *et al.* (2015) reported a case of *Lb. rhamnosus* GG bacteremia in an adult patient with severe active ulcerative colitis. The patient was taking a probiotic formulation and the bacteremia was associated with candidemia. PFGE typing confirmed that the bacteremia strain was identical with the probiotic formulation. Yelin *et al.* (2019) reported that the rate of *Lactobacillus* bacteremia was higher for intensive care unit (ICU) patients treated with probiotics as compared to those without probiotics, and whole genome sequencing revealed that blood isolate and probiotic strains were phylogenetically similar. A total of 22 174 cases (ICU patients at Boston Children's Hospital, Massachusetts, USA, over the period of 5.5 years) were analyzed: 522 patients were given *Lb. rhamnosus* strain GG, and the rate of bacteremia was 1.1 and 0.009% with and without probiotic administration, respectively. Most recently, Sendil *et al.* (2020) reported bacteremia caused by *Lb. rhamnosus* identified by 16S rRNA sequencing in a 75-year–old patient with type 2 diabetes mellitus and end-stage renal disease. The patient had a history of consumption of a probiotic supplement containing *Lb. acidophilus, Lb. bulgaricus* and *Bifidobacterium longum* ssp. *infantis*. Bacteremia was reported in two premature babies (female infants of 26 2/7 weeks and 28 6/7 weeks respectively) upon administration of probiotic, and genome analysis revealed that the strain from blood culture was similar to that of the commercial probiotic preparation (Bertelli *et al.* 2015). Esaiassen *et al.* (2016) also reported bacteremia cases in three preterm babies (23–24 weeks) due to *B. longum* ssp. *infantis*, and whole genome analysis along with matrix-assisted laser desorption ionization time-of-flight (MALDI-TOF) mass spectrometry data revealed the strain to be similar to the probiotics administered.

Lb. paracasei endocarditis was reported in a 77-year-old man with prostate cancer (Franko *et al.* 2013). The patient consumed a probiotic yoghurt containing *Lb. paracasei* on a daily basis. Aaron *et al.* (2017) reported *Lb. rhamnosus* endocarditis following upper endoscopy in an 80-year-old man whose blood sample and mitral valve culture were positive for *Lb. rhamnosus*. The patient frequently consumed yoghurt containing the organism, although the authors could not conclusively state that his diet was responsible for the causative organism. *Lactobacillus paracasei* bacteremia with a complex liver abscess was reported in a 65-year-old female with a medical history of hypertension, type 2 diabetes mellitus (T2DM) and hypercholesterolemia (Pararajasingam and Uwagwu 2017). Naqvi *et al.* (2018) reported fatal *Lb. rhamnosus* endocarditis in a 36-year-old woman who had prior *Clostridium difficile* colitis and a history of complicated cirrhosis. The patient was self-medicating with two commercially available probiotic capsules daily (*Lb. acidophilus* 32×10^9 CFU organisms, *Lb. rhamnosus* 4×10^9 CFU organisms and *S. cerevisiae* 4×10^9

CFU) as per the manufacturer's information. Her blood culture and operative aortic valve tissue culture were positive for *Lb. rhamnosus.*

An 82-year-old woman with a history of hypertension, diabetes mellitus and end-stage renal disease during treatment of *Cl. difficile* colitis showed symptoms of liver abscess and bacteremia due to intake of probiotic-containing lactobacilli (Sherid *et al.* 2016). A purulent fluid sample from the liver lesion was positive for lactobacilli but the strain was not identified.

Pre-operative probiotic administration was found to cause sepsis due to *Lb. rhamnosus* in a 24-year-old female patient after an aortic valve replacement (Kochan *et al.* 2011). The patient's blood sample was positive for *Lb. rhamnosus* and PFGE analysis confirmed the strain to be similar with the probiotic strain in the drug. Doern *et al.* (2014) reported a case of pneumonia in an 11-month-old female baby associated with probiotic *Lb. rhamnosus* GG consumption (the patient was taking *Lb. rhamnosus* LGG) for 3 months before her illness.

6.4.2 Inefficiency of Probiotics

Of the strains confirmed to have probiotic properties in vitro, not all will actually show health-promoting effects on the host. There are reports that show that a probiotic strain did not show any effect or any favorable effects, and additionally may be associated with undesirable effects.

Soh *et al.* (2009) reported that early probiotic supplementation feeding of infants between birth and 6 months of age (253 infants with a family history of allergic disease in Singapore) was not effective in reducing the risk of allergic sensitization and eczema at the age of 1 year. The infants were given ≥60 mL/day of commercially available cow's milk-based formula and a probiotics formulation (*B. longum,* 10^7 CFU/g, and *Lb. rhamnosus,* 2×10^8 CFU/g) from birth to the age of 6 months. The authors reported that there was no difference in the rate of sensitization and incidence of eczema between the placebo and probiotic groups. This group also carried out a follow-up study up to 5 years to monitor the effect of early probiotic supplementation on long-term outcome but concluded that probiotic administration (from birth to 6 months of age) had not had any preventive effect on allergic diseases (Loo *et al.* 2014). Cohen *et al.* (2013) reported a study in which administration of probiotics (*S. thermophilus* NCC 2496, *S. salivarius* DSM 13084, *Lb. rhamnosus* LPR CGMCC 1.3724) and prebiotics (Raftilose/Raftiline) in the follow-on formula were not effective in reduction of risk of acute otitis media (AOM), recurrent AOM, antibiotic use or lower respiratory tract infections in 7- to 13-month- old children. The trial (randomized, double-blind and placebo-controlled) was conducted with 224 children enrolled by 37 pediatricians in France for 12 months. Stevenson *et al.* (2014) reported that *Lb. plantarum* 299 v administration at 5×10^9 CFU per capsule (2 capsules/day) daily for 8 weeks was not effective in relieving symptoms like bloating, abdominal pain and quality of life in IBS patients. Schwenger *et al.* (2015) collected data and analyzed them to record the effect of probiotic strains on prevention of urinary tract infections (UTIs) in children and adults. The analysis was done in four groups of nine studies with 735 participants: seven studies in girls or women with recurrent UTIs; one in healthy women with UTI; and one in children with abnormal urinary tracts. The authors concluded that probiotics did not significantly reduce the recurrence of symptomatic bacterial UTIs as compared to placebo and groups with antibiotic treatment, although the studies included in the analysis used different strains of probiotics, different dosages, different forms of administration) (vaginal, oral), and the period of probiotic administration was also variable. A meta-analysis was done to evaluate the effect of a probiotic as an adjunct in AAD in adults (18–64 years old) and elderly persons (≥65 years old) and reported that probiotic as an adjunct reduced the risk of AAD in adults but showed no positive effect on elderly patients (Jafarnejad *et al.* 2016). Lu *et al.* (2016) conducted a meta-analysis to determine the effect of probiotic supplementation on *Helicobacter pylori* eradication rates. In the study, 21 randomized control trials with or without placebo were included, and effect of probiotics was co-related with standard therapy. The authors concluded that probiotics with triple therapy and a 14-day course of treatment did not improve *H. pylori* eradication rates as compared to placebo, although administration of probiotics improved the adverse effects of diarrhea and nausea. Probiotic administration as an adjunct to standard care for 5 days did not have any beneficial effect on children with acute watery diarrhea. Chau *et al.* (2018) conducted a randomized double-blind, placebo-controlled study in Vietnam with *Lb. acidophilus* culture fed twice daily (4×10^8/day) for 5 days in a study group of 150 children. No significant difference was observed between the probiotic group and placebo group in the duration of diarrhea, duration of hospitalization, stool frequency (in the first 3 days) and daily rotavirus and norovirus fecal loads. A study (randomized, double-blind, placebo-controlled) was conducted with 46 chronic kidney disease patients undergoing maintenance hemodialysis (HD) to evaluate the effect of probiotics administration for 3 months; it was found that probiotic supplementation did not reduce uremic toxins and inflammatory markers (e.g. C-reactive protein and interleukin-6) (Borges *et al.* 2018).

6.5 Safety Assessment of Probiotic Cultures

Currently "probiotics" are available on the market as live biotherapeutics for use in humans as medical therapeutics, probiotic foods (e.g. fermented, non-fermented foods), food for special medical purposes, food ingredients, dietary supplements and directly fed microorganisms for use in animals, respectively. Probiotic microorganisms have been reported to cause four types of side/negative effects (FAO/WHO 2002):

1) *Systemic infections such as bacteremia, endocarditis, meningitis, endometritis, peritonitis and pneumonia, mainly in immune-compromised individuals.* Probiotic organisms belonging to the genera *Lactobacillus* (particularly a very popular strain, *Lb. rhamnosus* GG) (Sendil *et al.* 2020), *Bifidobacterium* (Esaiassen *et al.* 2016), and spore-forming *Bacillus* were demonstrated to cause infections.
2) *Deleterious metabolic activities.* Bile salt hydrolysis (BSH) by bacteria is referred to as a risk factor in the development of colon cancer as deconjugated bile salts can be altered into harmful secondary bile acids (Jarocki *et al.* 2014). As commonly used probiotic organisms, lactobacilli and bifidobacteria have BSH activity. Bile salt deconjugation by probiotics is included as a side effect in determining the safety of probiotics.

Species of lactobacilli produce L+, D− and DL− lactic acid. The D- form has been linked to D-lactic acidosis in excess of 3 mmol/L D-lactate levels in plasma in subjects with short bowel syndrome (also known as D-lactate encephalopathy with severe neurological impairment). D-lactic acidosis rarely occurs in healthy humans (Vitetta *et al.* 2017). Patients with short bowel syndrome who had previously administered probiotics were reported with D-lactic acidosis (Łukasik *et al.* 2018). Łukasik *et al.* (2018) stated that infants are more susceptible to D-lactic acidosis due to weak barrier function of the GIT and reduced renal excretion. Thus it is advisable to take precautions in vulnerable consumers such as newborns and patients who have previously undergone bowel surgery before administering probiotics (Sanders *et al.* 2010).

Other metabolic activities such as mucin degradation, biogenic amine production and production of harmful enzymes also contribute to the side effects of probiotics consumption.

3) *Excessive immune stimulation in susceptible subjects.* In theory, probiotics may cause excessive immune stimulation due to elicited cytokine production in immune-compromised people, which may lead to autoimmune disease or certain inflammations. However there has not as yet been any report of occurrence of this risk in humans (Kothari *et al.* 2019).
4) *Gene transfer.* Strains of lactobacilli and bifidobacteria are intrinsically resistant to antibiotics such as vancomycin, aminoglycosides, ciprofloxacin, nalidixic acid, mupirocin, streptomycin, etc.; however, the presence of transferable antibiotic resistance genes has also been reported (Gueimonde *et al.* 2013; Wei *et al.* 2012). In vitro studies (filter mating assay) and an in vivo model proved transfer of antibiotic resistance genes between probiotics (Vieira de Souza *et al.* 2012) and from probiotics to other organisms including pathogens (Thumu and Halami 2019); thus the nature of antibiotic resistance genes present in a probiotic organism is a criterion for probiotic organisms to get approval for qualified presumption of safety (QPS) status (European Food Safety Authority, EFSA, 2008).

It is evident that probiotic organisms may cause certain infections, particularly in vulnerable groups of consumers such as those who are immune-suppressed or pregnant, patients with structural heart diseases, etc., so safety evaluation of probiotics should be done before their application in humans.

6.5.1 Current Proposal on Probiotic Safety

Countries all over the world have developed their own legislative systems to ensure the safety of probiotic foods or probiotic products. The United States, European Union, Japan and Canada have different guidelines (Narayanan 2013). The US FDA, European Food Safety Authority (EFSA) and Canadian Natural Health Product Directorate are leading authorities to give the most inclusive principles and guidelines regarding safety of probiotics. The Ministry of Health and Welfare (Japan), Norwegian Scientific Committee for Food Safety (VKM), Indian Council of Medical Research/Department of Biotechnology (ICMR/DBT, India) and other countries also have laid down their guidelines for assessing probiotic safety (Halvorsen *et al.* 2009; Pradhan *et al.* 2020; Sanders *et al.* 2010; Yazdankhah *et al.* 2014).

The European Union (EFSA) has introduced QPS criteria for microorganisms which are safe for human consumption. Thus, no microorganism having QPS status will need to undergo a full safety assessment. To be granted QPS status, the tested microorganism must fulfill the following criteria (https://www.efsa.europa.eu/en/topics/topic/qualified-presumption-safety-qps):

- Well-defined taxonomic identification.
- Safety aspects have been established.
- Evidence on its pathogenic properties has been established.
- Clear indication on its use.

The criteria for QPS status of microorganisms are presented in Figure 6.1. QPS-approved microorganisms, especially *Lactobacillus* and *Bifidobacterium* species, are listed in Table 6.2. In 2007, EFSA recommended that the QPS-based approach must be used/implemented for assessing the safety of microorganisms for application in the food chain.

The Norwegian Scientific Committee for Food Safety (VKM) from 2009 also provided guidelines for assessment of safety aspects of probiotic (food) products (Halvorsen *et al.* 2009). The regulation states that probiotic food products should only contain probiotic bacteria granted QPS4 and/or GRAS status; they cannot be prescribed to critically ill patients, or to those having *Clostridium difficile* infection or AAD (Norwegian Scientific Committee for Food Safety 2009).

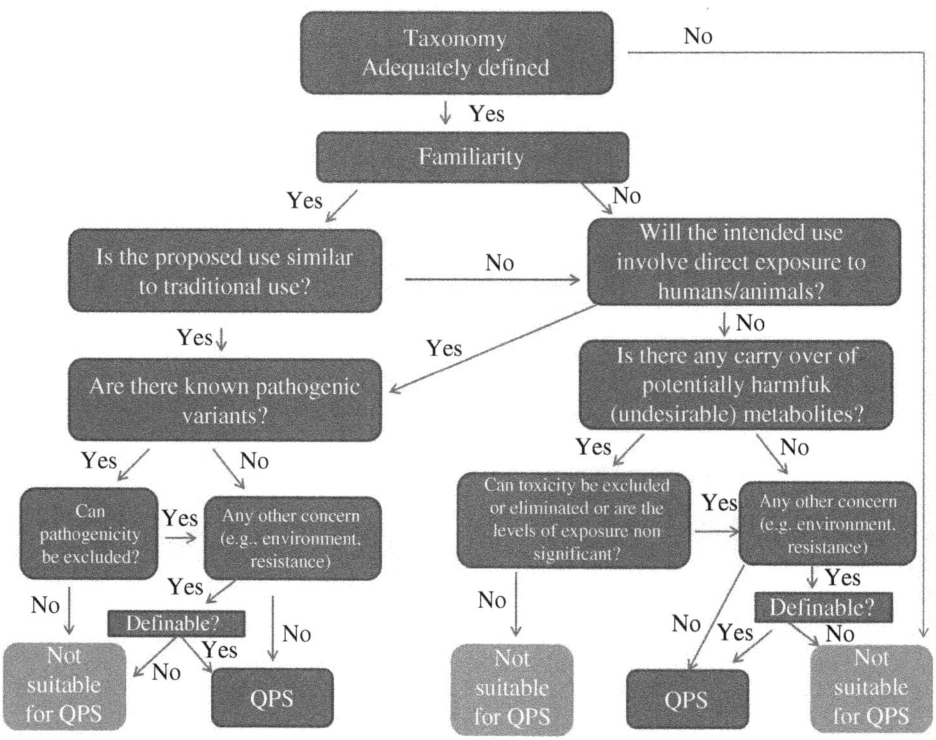

Figure 6.1 General scheme for the assessment of suitability for qualified presumption of safety (QPS) status of microorganisms.

Table 6.2 List of QPS-granted lactobacilli and bifidobacteria.

"Classical" denomination	"Updated" denomination*
Lactobacillus acidophilus	*Lactobacillus acidophilus*
Lactobacillus alimentarius	*Companilactobacillus alimentarius*
Lactobacillus amylolyticus	*Lactobacillus amylolyticus*
Lactobacillus amylovorus	*Lactobacillus amylovorous*
Lactobacillus animalis	*Ligilactobacillus animalis*
Lactobacillus aviarius	*Ligilactobacillus aviarius*
Lactobacillus brevis	*Levilactobacillus brevis*
Lactobacillus buchneri	*Lentilactobacillus buchneri*
Lactobacillus casei	*Lacticaseibacillus casei*
Lactobacillus collinoides	*Secundilactobacillus collinoides*
Lactobacillus coryniformis	*Loigolactobacillus coryniformis*
Lactobacillus crispatus	*Lactobacillus crispatus*
Lactobacillus curvatus	*Latilactobacillus curvatus*
Lactobacillus delbrueckii	*Lactobacillus delbrueckii*
Lactobacillus dextrinicus	*Lapidilactobacillus dextrinicus*
Lactobacillus diolivorans	*Lentilactobacillus dioliovorans*
Lactobacillus farciminis	*Companilactobacillus farciminis*
Lactobacillus fermentum	*Limosilactobacillus fermentum*
Lactobacillus gallinarum	*Lactobacillus gallinarum*
Lactobacillus gasseri	*Lactobacillus gasseri*
Lactobacillus helveticus	*Lactobacillus helveticus*
Lactobacillus hilgardii	*Lentilactobacillus hilgardii*
Lactobacillus johnsonii	*Lactobacillus johnsonii*
Lactobacillus kefiranofaciens	*Lactobacillus kefiranofaciens*
Lactobacillus kefiri	*Lentilactobacillus kefiri*
Lactobacillus mucosae	*Limosilactobacillus mucosae*
Lactobacillus panis	*Limosilactobacillus panis*
Lactobacillus paracasei	*Lacticaseibacillus paracasei*
Lactobacillus paraplantarum	*Lactiplantibacillus paraplantarum*
Lactobacillus pentosus	*Lactiplantibacillus pentosus*
Lactobacillus plantarum	*Lactiplantibacillus plantarum*
Lactobacillus pontis	*Limosilactobacillus pontis*
Lactobacillus reuteri	*Limosilactobacillus reuteri*
Lactobacillus rhamnosus	*Lacticaseibacillus rhamnosus*
Lactobacillus sakei	*Latilactobacillus sakei*
Lactobacillus salivarius	*Ligilactobacillus salivarius*
Lactobacillus sanfranciscensis	*Fructilactobacillus sanfranciscensis*
Bifidobacterium: *B. adolescentis, B. animalis, B. bifidum, B. breve, B. longum*	

* The genus *Lactobacillus* has been recently divided into 25 new genera. The 37 species that are considered as QPS became classified into 13 genera. *Source:* EFSA Panel on Biological Hazards (BIOHAZ), Koutsoumanis, K., Allende, A., Alvarez-Ordóñez, A., Bolton, D., Bover-Cid, S., Chemaly, M., Davies, R., De Cesare, A., Hilbert, F. and Lindqvist, R., 2020. Update of the list of QPS-recommended biological agents intentionally added to food or feed as notified to EFSA 12: suitability of taxonomic units notified to EFSA until March 2020. *EFSA Journal*, 18(7), p.e06174. Licensed under CC BY-ND 4.0.

As per US law, the FDA does not have much regulatory authority over probiotic food products, and food products do not need approval from the FDA prior to marketing. Live probiotic organisms were recognized as drugs by the FDA in 2010 in the field of treatment. The probiotic product should be classified as an Investigational New Drug (IND) based on the definition "an article that is intended for use in the diagnosis, cure, mitigation, treatment, or prevention of disease in humans or in other animals". The FDA recognizes microorganisms that are used for manufacturing fermented foods and have long and safe history of association with humans as GRAS microorganisms. In Canada, use of probiotics is regulated by the project "Health Canada" (a division that regulates natural health products). It is a part of the Canadian Food and Drugs Act, following the joint FAO/WHO recommendation for evaluation of probiotics intended to be applied in food products. In the Canadian Food and Drugs Act, food probiotics are classified in a different category called "natural health products" (Zielińska *et al.* 2018b).

In India, the statutory body called the Food Safety and Standards Authority of India (FSSAI) has drafted regulations for probiotic marketing from January 2018 and listed around 28 probiotic microorganisms, which can be used either singly or in combination, to be marketed (Pradhan *et al.* 2020).

The WHO/FAO recommended that various sets of tests related to antibiotic resistance, determining harmful metabolic activities like D-lactate production, toxin production, bile salt deconjugation activities and hemolytic potentiality should be carried out, ideally in immune-compromised animals, to study infectivity in the immune-compromised host, and conducting human clinical trials to evaluate adverse side effects followed by post-marketing surveillance of commercial consumers for the new probiotic strains in relation with their safety (FAO/WHO 2002). A systematic approach for the safety evaluation of probiotics in food/s (FAO/WHO 2002) is depicted in Figure 6.2.

6.5.2 Identification of Individual Strains

Safety assessment of a probiotic candidate begins with proper identification of the strain. As the probiotic properties of an organism are strain specific, it is absolutely necessary that the strain be identified at strain level so that specific health effects can be linked to it and also that appropriate surveillance and epidemiological studies can be conducted. The FAO/WHO has recommended that the most current and valid methods should be used for proper and complete identification of the strain: a combination of both phenotypic and genetic tests should be applied. Nomenclature of the probiotic strain should conform to the International Code of Nomenclature, as recognized by the International Union of Microbiological Societies (IUMS), and the strain should also be deposited in an international culture collection center (for quality control and scientific purposes).

Preliminary identification of LAB, including probiotic lactobacilli and bifidobacteria, is traditionally based on morphology, physiological and biochemical tests such as sugar fermentation profile, fermentation products and enzymatic activities, which are important to identify family, genus and species taxa. Phenotypic tests are not sufficient for identification of probiotics; they have poor reproducibility (Donelli *et al.* 2013). API 50 CH (Biomerieux) is the most commonly used strip-based carbohydrate fermentation (49 carbohydrates) analysis carried out by most researchers for identification of *Lactobacillus* species within 48 h.

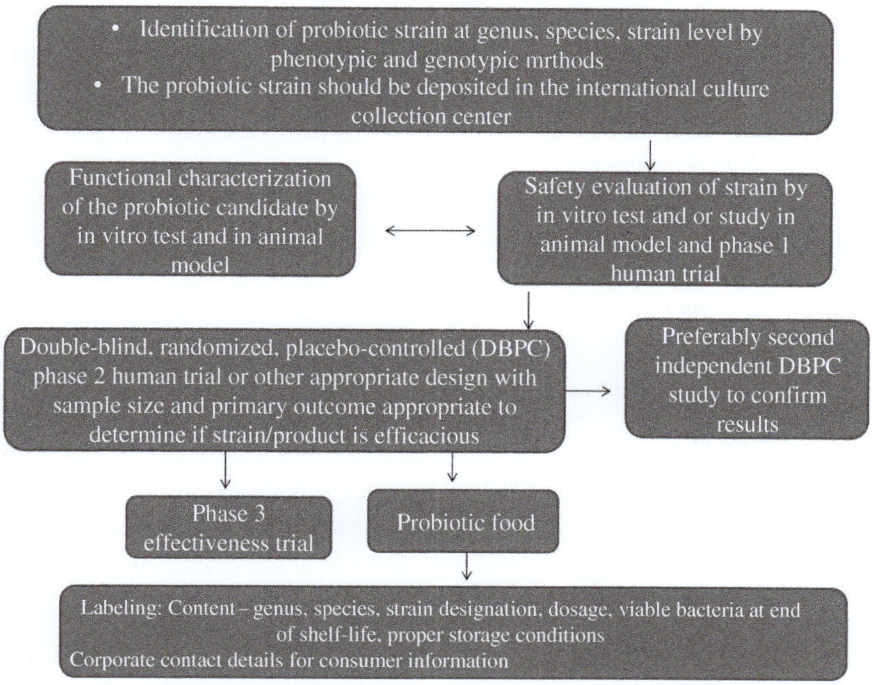

Figure 6.2 Guidelines for the evaluation of probiotic safety (FAO/WHO 2002). *Source:* Modified from FAO/WHO (2002). Working group report on drafting guidelines for the Evaluation of probiotics in food. London, Ontario, Canada.

There was a report that the API 50 CH test was not accurate for identification of *Lactobacillus* species (Boyd *et al.* 2005).

For species level identification, DNA–DNA hybridization technique, amplified ribosomal DNA restriction analysis (ARDRA) (Srutkova *et al.* 2011), 16S and 23S rDNA sequencing (Dimitonova *et al.* 2008) are commonly done (Donelli *et al.* 2013). For identification of probiotic microorganisms at strain level, various techniques such as pulse field gel electrophoresis (PFGE) (Xu *et al.* 2018), random amplified polymorphic DNA-PCR (RAPD-PCR) (Galanis *et al.* 2015), amplified fragment length polymorphism (AFLP) (Makino *et al.* 2011) and ribotyping can be explored (Coudeyras *et al.* 2008). PFGE and RAPD-PCR are considered gold standard for strain typing of probiotics (Zielińska *et al.* 2018a). Further, for identification and strain typing of probiotic organisms, whole genome sequencing is one of the most reliable methods (Kothari *et al.* 2019; Li *et al.* 2017). At present, integration of phenotypic and genotypic methods, i.e. a "polyphasic taxonomy" based approach is suggested to appropriately identify probiotic strains.

6.5.3 In vitro studies

The FAO has recommended the carrying out of various in vitro tests (e.g. hemolytic activity, metabolic activity, analysis of antibiotic resistance, toxin production) for determining safety of probiotic microorganisms. The advantage of in vitro safety tests is that one can easily exclude a pathogenic strain when evaluating a new probiotic candidate based on toxin production, hemolytic activity and other properties rather than moving into more tedious in vivo animal and human trials. However, if a virulence factor related gene is not expressed or is down regulated, which may remain undetectable in in vitro safety assessment, alternative strategies should be adopted.

In vitro safety assessment includes different intrinsic properties of strains such as:

- Antibiotic resistance.
- Hemolytic activity.
- Adhesion to mammalian cells.
- Production of toxin.
- Production of enzymes.
- Production of ammonia.
- Production of biogenic amines.
- Mucin degradation activity.
- Platelet aggregation ability.

The FAO/WHO has recommended that if a probiotic strain belongs to species having hemolytic potentiality, then its respective activity has to be determined. Strains with hemolytic potential are of concern due to the risk of occurrence of edema and anemia in the host. Hemolytic activity is determined by growing the organism in a medium supplemented with animal or human blood (Kim *et al.* 2018). Production of ammonia by intestinal microorganisms due to proteolysis in the large intestine is known to affect the liver and is linked with chronic liver damage. Production of intestinal harmful enzymes such as β-glucuronidase and β-glucosidase, and other enzymes (e.g. glycosidases, proteases and gelatinases) by probiotic microorganisms is also used as potential pathogenicity marker. Biogenic amines (e.g. tyramine, cadaverine, putrescine and histamine) are necessary for normal physiological functions (acting as hormones, neurotransmitters) in humans at lower concentrations. However, high concentrations of these biogenic amines are associated with digestive problems, hypo- or hypertension, headache, migraine, nausea and skin allergy. They also act as the precursors of nitrosamines which have carcinogenic and mutagenic activity. Biogenic amines are produced by microbial action, by endogenous enzymatic activity or by decarboxylation of amino acids or amination of ketones and aldehydes. Thus, it is of uttermost importance to determine whether the pools of biogenic amines are contributed by probiotic organisms or not in the host. Mucus layers in the intestine are the first line of defense of the host against microbes, particularly pathogens. However, there are several reports regarding translocation of probiotic microorganisms in infants and in immune-compromised patients causing bacteremia and endocarditis. Some microorganisms have been reported to degrade mucin or harbor genes to induce mucin degradation. Thus, to ensure safety, mucin degradation ability is determined to evaluate translocation ability of the probiotic organisms. Pathogens such as *Salmonella*, *Shigella*, *Helicobacter pylori* and *Vibrio cholerae* degrade mucin and this is considered a potential virulence trait. Intestinal bacteria including probiotics can enter the bloodstream and subsequently may cause platelet aggregation or may be involved in platelet–fibrin clot formation leading to sepsis and infective endocarditis. Production of human toxins such as cytolysin is also evaluated by in vitro testing.

Safety parameters such as biogenic amine production, antibiotic resistance and presence of virulence determinants such as *agg, cpd, esp, efaAfm, cylA, clyM, gelE, cylB, ccf, ace, cob* and *hyl* were determined for the strain *Enterococcus faecium* KH 24. This strain showed no resistance towards any tested antibiotics, biogenic amines were not produced and only virulence factor *efaAfm* was detected in the strain (Bhardwaj *et al.* 2010). Singh *et al.* (2014) reported that seven probiotic strains of *Lb. reuteri* were safe based on in vitro tests such as biogenic amine production, antibiotic resistance, DNase activity, gelatinase activity and hemolysis. Bujnakova *et al.* (2014) also evaluated safety of lactobacilli strains by determining their antibiotic resistance profile, production of harmful β-glucuronidase and β-glucosidase and identifying genes of amino acid decarboxylase such as tyrosine decarboxylase (*tyrdc*), histidine decarboxylase (*hdc*), agmatine deiminase (*agdi*) and ornithine decarboxylase (*odc*). The safety of the probiotic strain, *Lb. helveticus* (MTCC 5463) was assessed based on genome mining for presence of virulence genes, antibiotic resistance genes and genes producing harmful metabolites (Senan *et al.* 2015). Different strains of *Lb. fermentum, Lb. casei* and *Lb. delbrueckii* subsp. *bulgaricus* were evaluated for their safety using various in vitro tests for mucin degradation, antibiotic resistance, hemolytic activity and the presence of virulence genes (Casarotti *et al.* 2017). The probiotic strains were negative for hemolytic and mucin degradation ability, showed presence of limited virulence genes and were intrinsically resistant to several antibiotics. Whole genome sequencing of the probiotic strain *Lb. helveticus* KLDS1.8701 revealed absence of genes encoding β-glucuronidase, β-glucosidase, azoreductase and arylsulfatase. Genes for D-lactate dehydrogenase and nitroreductase were detected, however in vitro testing did not detect nitroreductase, and D-lactic acid was produced in negligible amounts to cause a health hazard in humans (Li *et al.* 2017). Also, the *Lb. helveticus* KLDS1.8701 strain did not produce biogenic amines, and genes encoding histamine, tyramine, phenylethylamine and cadaverine were not detected in the genome. Genes encoding invasiveness or toxicity and other potential virulence determinants were not detected. Two commercially exploited probiotic strains, *B. longum* BORI and *B. bifidum* BGN4, were subjected to in vitro tests such as hemolysis, ammonia production, biogenic amine production, mucin degradation and antibiotic resistance and transferability to determine their safety (Kim *et al.* 2018). The strains were negative for ammonia production, hemolysis, mucin degradation and production of cadaverine, histamine or tyramine; however, a small amount of putrescine was produced by both strains. Rastogi *et al.* (2019) evaluated safety of probiotic strains of *Lb. mucosae* SRV5 and *Lb. mucosae* SRV10 (isolated from donkey milk) by in vitro tests such as antibiotic resistance, hemolytic ability, DNase, gelatinase and mucin degradation ability and reported that both the strains were safe. Probiotic potential and safety of the bacteriocinogenic strain *E. lactis* PMD74 were evaluated by various in vitro tests such as antibiotic resistance, hemolysis, gelatinase activity, biogenic amine production and presence of virulence genes for enterococcal surface protein, collagen-binding protein, serine protease and gelatinase (Uymaz Tezel 2019). Recently, Pradhan *et al.* (2019b) reported that the probiotic strains *Lb. plantarum* (MTCC 5690) and *Lb. fermentum* (MTCC 5689) showed negative results when tested in vitro for properties such as hemolytic activity, mucin degradation, biogenic amine (histamine, tyramine, cadavarine and putrescine) production and platelet aggregation.

6.5.4 Animal Studies

There are no clear-cut guidelines for safety regulation of functional and novel foods in relation to probiotic preparations, thus for initial safety evaluation of new candidate probiotics traditional toxicological testing as proposed by the OECD is done (Pradhan *et al.* 2020). It includes 14 days of single-dose acute oral toxicity testing, 28 days of repeated dose subacute oral toxicity testing and 90 days of repeated dose sub-chronic oral toxicity testing (Pradhan *et al.* 2020). According to the OECD guidelines, acute oral toxicity testing alone is not enough for safety evaluation, a repeated dose subacute oral toxicity study should be done based on the initial acute oral toxicity test (OECD/OCDE guideline 2008). In animal models, various parameters such as changes in body weight, mortality, feed consumption, relative organ weights (e.g. heart, liver, kidney, brain, lung, spleen, epididymis, adrenal, thymus, uterus, ovary, etc.), histopathological examination (showing loss of normal architecture, fibrosis, necrosis, inflammation or atrophy in various organs), hematological parameters (hemoglobin count, red blood cell count, white blood cell count, thrombocyte count, packed cell volume, mean corpuscular hemoglobin concentration and mean corpuscular volume), biochemical characterization of serum (total cholesterol triglycerides level, LDL cholesterol level, HDL cholesterol level, alanine aminotransferase, albumin content, total bilirubin content, alkaline phosphatase, aspartate aminotransferase, glucose level, urea level, total protein amount, creatinine, calcium, inorganic phosphorus and electrolytes – mostly potassium, sodium and chloride contents) are measured for safety evaluation of probiotics. Alteration in body weight and feed consumption in animal studies are considered good indicators of negative effects of the feed; there should not be more than a 10% reduction in the animals' body weight (Raza *et al.* 2002). Abotsi *et al.* (2011) stated that changes in organ weights are an alternate sign of toxicity in a short-term toxicity study. Reports regarding safety studies of probiotics carried out in in vivo animal models are presented in Table 6.3.

Bhardwaj *et al.* (2010) evaluated the safety of the probiotic strain *E. faecium* KH 24 in a mouse model and reported that the strain was safe, showing weight gain in the probiotic group. The probiotic strain *B. licheniformis* Me1 was tested for acute toxicity and subchronic oral toxicity in male albino Wistar rats. There was no mortality or treatment-related illness in the 14-day acute oral toxicity test with a single dose of 1.1×10^{11} CFU/kg body weight (BW). In a 13-week repeated-dose toxicity test in rats (for no-observed-adverse-effect level, NOAEL), there was no mortality, toxicity or allergy in the treated group. The probiotic dose did not have any genotoxicity in mice as revealed by micronucleus assay (Nithya *et al.* 2012). A probiotic strain of *Saccharomyces cerevisiae* RC 016 was subjected to genotoxicity testing caused by dietary aflatoxin and cytotoxicity (with the bone marrow micronuclei assay, the comet assay) in Wistar rats for 60 days at 10^8 viable *S. cerevisiae* cells; no genotoxicity or cytotoxicity was detected (Gonzalez Pereyra *et al.* 2014). A 90-day subchronic oral toxicity study in rat models at 300 and 1000 mg/kg BW/day (5.55×10^{10} and 1.85×10^{11} CFU/kg BW/day) of the probiotic product AB-LIFE® (consisting of three strains of *Lb. plantarum* CECT 7527, 7528 and 7529) showed no BW gain, mortality or change in BW or food consumption, without any clinical signs of toxicity (Mukerji *et al.* 2016). A translocation study revealed AB-LIFE® colonies in low numbers during culturing from the mesenteric lymph nodes (MLN) or liver samples of treated animals; however, the researchers concluded that it did not pose any safety concern. AB-LIFE® was concluded to be safe with NOAEL in rats

Table 6.3 Safety studies of probiotics in in vivo animal models.

Probiotic strain	Study	References
Enterococcus faecium KH 24	Mice model	Bhardwaj *et al.* (2010)
Bacillus licheniformis Me1	Acute toxicity 14 days and subchronic oral toxicity 13 weeks in male albino Wistar rats, single dose of 1.1×10^{11} CFU/kg body weight and genotoxicity in mice	Nithya *et al.* (2012)
Saccharomyces cerevisiae RC 016	Genotoxicity and cytotoxicity (with the bone marrow micronuclei assay, the comet assay) in Wistar rats for 60 days at 10^8 viable *S. cerevisiae* cells	Gonzalez Pereyra *et al.* (2014)
AB-LIFE® (composed of three strains of *Lactobacillus plantarum* CECT 7527, 7528 and 7529)	90-day subchronic oral toxicity study in rats at 300 and 1000 mg/kg BW/day (5.55×10^{10} and 1.85×10^{11} CFU/kg BW/day)	Mukerji *et al.* (2016)
Lb. fermentum HM3 and *Lb. buchneri* DF2	Acute oral toxicity 14 day and subacute oral toxicity tests 28 day in rat model, dosage 10^{10} CFU/kg BW/day	Shokryazdan *et al.* (2016)
B. clausii UBBC07	Acute oral toxicity at 5000 mg/kg for 15 days and 28 days subacute toxicity at 1000 mg/kg BW in rats	Lakshmi *et al.* (2017)
Lb. mali APS1	Genotoxicity in mice at doses up to 2000 mg/kg BW/day Developmental toxicity in rats at 500–1670 mg/kg BW/day	Lin *et al.* (2018)
Lb. plantarum MTCC 5690 and *Lb. fermentum* MTCC 5689	Dextran sodium sulfate (DSS)-induced colitis mouse model	Pradhan *et al.* (2019a)
Lb. plantarum MTCC 5690 and *Lb. fermentum* MTCC 5689	Acute oral toxicity test, subacute oral toxicity, subchronic oral toxicity, single dose intravenous toxicity, single dose intraperitoneal toxicity and genotoxicity (in vivo chromosomal aberration assay and micronucleus assay in bone marrow cells) in murine model	Pradhan *et al.* (2019b)
Lb. fermentum NCMR 2826 and FIX	Acute oral toxicity study for 14 days (daily dose of probiotics 10^{16} CFU/mL) and subchronic oral toxicity study for 13 weeks at 10^7, 10^8 and 10^{10} CFU/mL probiotics daily in Wistar rats	Thumu and Halami (2020)

BW, body weight.

at 1000 mg/kg BW/day, i.e. 1.85×10^{11} CFU of AB-LIFE®/kg BW/day. Shokryazdan *et al.* (2016) evaluated safety of *Lb. fermentum* HM3 and *Lb. buchneri* DF2 in a rat model using subacute oral toxicity and acute oral toxicity tests and concluded that both strains were safe at 10^{10} CFU/kg BW/day. Acute oral toxicity evaluation revealed no mortality in the probiotic-treated rats. In the treated animal group no reduction of BW, no sign of toxicity and no change in the animals' behavior was noted. In the repeated-dose subacute oral toxicity test, in the probiotic-treated group there was no sign of toxicity and no adverse effect on feed consumption; also, in male rats improvement in BW was evident. These researchers also found that probiotic-treated rats showed significantly lower amounts of harmful intestinal enzyme β-glucuronidase in comparison to control rats. *B. clausii* UBBC07, a spore-forming probiotic, was evaluated for acute oral toxicity at 5000 mg/kg for 15 days and subacute toxicity at 1000 mg/kg BW for 28 days in rats, and no sign of abnormality or toxicity was identified (Lakshmi *et al.* 2017). Administration of the probiotic strain did not significantly affect hematological or clinical chemistry profile, BW, general health and diet of the treated animals. NOAEL for 1000 mg/kg BW as evidenced by the subacute toxicity test was noted. Lin *et al.* (2018) found that the probiotic strain *Lb. mali* APS1 showed no genotoxicity in mice at doses up to 2000 mg/kg BW/day. The strain was also tested for developmental toxicity in rats; when administered at 500–1670 mg/kg BW/day no toxicity was identified as there were no developmental changes or external, visceral and skeletal malformations in fetuses in the treatment group. Therapeutic effect and safety of the probiotic strains *Lb. plantarum* MTCC 5690 and *Lb. fermentum* MTCC 5689 were evaluated in a dextran sodium sulfate (DSS)-induced colitis mouse model. No adverse effect (no inflammation, normal colon, cecum length, blood biochemistry, hematology) was found in colitic mice fed with both probiotics; however, the researchers observed that the probiotic strains were translocated into extraintestinal organs (Pradhan *et al.* 2019a). The same group of researchers also studied acute oral, subacute oral, and subchronic oral toxicity tests along with single-dose intravenous toxicity, single-dose intraperitoneal toxicity and genotoxicity (in vivo micronucleus assay and chromosomal aberration assay in bone marrow cells) in a murine model. The authors concluded that both the probiotic strain MTCC 5690 and MTCC 5689 are safe as there was no cytogenic damage and no mortality or treatment-related clinical aberrations were noted (Pradhan *et al.* 2019b). Thumu and Halami (2020) assessed the safety of two *Lb. fermentum* strains, NCMR 2826 and FIX, in vivo in Wistar rats in an acute oral toxicity study for 14 days (daily dose of probiotics 10^{16} CFU/mL) and a subchronic oral toxicity study for 13 weeks at 10^{7}, 10^{8} and 10^{10} CFU/mL probiotics daily. Administration of probiotics was safe as there were no toxic effects on survival, BW or feed consumption; hematological and serum biochemical parameters measured along with organ weight were similar in both probiotic group and control group.

6.5.5 Human Clinical Studies

Standard human clinical studies consist of a phase 1 trial related to safety, a phase 2 trial related to efficacy, a phase 3 trial related to a effectiveness and phase 4 trial related to surveillance. Probiotics have been studied for various clinical conditions; generally these studies are double-blind, randomized and placebo-controlled, where safety and efficacy are measured by comparing a probiotic group with a placebo group (Table 6.4). Safety of probiotics is measured based on no adverse effects being observed. Probiotic foods are not generally evaluated by a phase 3 trial; the FAO/WHO has recommended that human clinical trials should be undertaken by more than one center for result confirmation.

Xu *et al.* (2015) reported a meta-analysis regarding the safety and efficacy of *Lb. reuteri* DSM 17938 in the treatment of infantile colic. A total of 423 infants were included (in six

Table 6.4 Safety studies of probiotics in human clinical trials.

Study	Population	Study design	Outcome	Reference
Randomized, double-blind, placebo-controlled	Infants 1–6 months of age	Infant formula supplemented with *Lb. fermentum* CECT5716, administered for 5 months	Well tolerated and safe	Gil-Campos *et al.* (2012)
Systematic review and meta- analysis	423 infants (6 randomized trials): 213 probiotics, 210 placebo	Safety and efficacy of *Lb. reuteri* DSM 17938 on the treatment of infantile colic	No severe adverse effect was noted	Xu *et al.* (2015)
Randomized, double-blind placebo-controlled	45 participants (18–70 years of age) with celiac disease	Commercial multistrain probiotic VSL#3 (VSL Pharma, USA) containing 450 billion viable lyophilized bacteria: *S. thermophilus*, *B. breve*, *B. longum*, *B. infantis*, *Lb. acidophilus*, *Lb. plantarum*, *Lb. paracasei*, and *Lb. delbrueckii* subsp. *bulgaricus* one sachet twice daily for 12 weeks	Well tolerated, although two participants each from probiotic and placebo group reported mild bloating	Harnett *et al.* (2016)
Randomized, double-blind, placebo-controlled	96 healthy male workers aged 30–49 years	Efficacy of *Lb. casei* strain *Shirota*-fermented milk (LcS-FM) for preventing upper respiratory tract infections, 1.0×10^{11} viable LcS cells once daily for 12 weeks	There were no adverse effects associated with consumption of the test drinks during the test period	Shida *et al.* (2017)
Systematic review and meta- analysis	31 randomized controlled trials including 8672 patients	Effect of probiotics on prevention of *Clostridium difficile*-associated diarrhea in adults and children	The short-term use of probiotics appears to be safe and effective when used along with antibiotics in patients who are not immunocompromised or severely debilitated. Common side effects reported are abdominal cramping, nausea, fever, soft stools, flatulence, and taste disturbance	Goldenberg *et al.* (2017)

(*Continued*)

Table 6.4 (Continued)

Study	Population	Study design	Outcome	Reference
Randomized, double-blind, placebo-controlled	100 elderly subjects 60–74 years of age	*B. subtilis* CU1. One capsule containing 2×10^9 spores was administered daily for 16 weeks, comprised of four consumption periods of 10 days each separated by 18-day washout periods	Safe, well-tolerated without adverse effects compared to placebo group	Lefevre *et al.* (2017)
Phase 1 clinical trial, partially randomized, controlled	68 infants, Day 7 postnatal, Infant Microbiota Probiotic Intake (IMPRINT) trial	*B. infantis* EVC001 $1.8–2.8 \times 10^{10}$ CFU daily in breast milk	*B. infantis* EVC001 was safe and well tolerated. No difference in adverse events between probiotic and control groups. The events were not serious, normal for infants of that age and not related to probiotics	Smilowitz *et al.* (2017)
Randomized, double-blind, placebo-controlled	32 ICU patients, mean age 59.9 and 57.5 years	*Lb. casei* drink. Danactive® drink was given twice daily for prevention of antibiotic-associated diarrhea (AAD) and *C. difficile* infections (CDI)	Two patients developed AAD, one patient developed CDI. Three cases of emesis in probiotic group	Alberda *et al.* (2018)
Randomized, double-blind, placebo-controlled	53 breastfed infants: 27 in probiotic group	Effectiveness and safety of multistrain probiotic mixture Vivomixx®, Visbiome®, DeSimone Formulation® (Danisco-DuPont) on infantile colic, 21-day trial	Safe as there were no adverse side effects	Baldassarre *et al.* (2018)
Systematic review and meta- analysis	6 randomized controlled trials: 1298 patients	*Bacillus clausii* in treating acute childhood diarrhea	Effective with a good safety profile	Ianiro *et al.* (2018)
Randomized, double-blind placebo-controlled	Celiac disease patients (age 18 and above) with irritable bowel syndrome (IBS)-type symptoms	One sachet daily of multistrain probiotic composed of *Lb. casei, Lb. plantarum*, *B. animalis* subsp. *lactis, B. breve*, *B. breve* Bl10 LMG, 6-week probiotic treatment period preceded by a 2-week run-in and followed by a 6-week follow-up	Probiotic preparation was safe without any incidence of adverse effects	Francavilla *et al.* (2019)

Systematic review and meta- analysis	10 randomized, placebo-controlled studies with 2321 participants with bacterial vaginosis	Efficacy and safety of probiotic use on bacterial vaginosis, 1-month follow-up, probiotic intervention	Beneficial effect without extra adverse events on gastrointestinal tract and genitourinary system including superinfection, such as vulvovaginal candidiasis	Wang *et al.* (2019)
Randomized, double-blind placebo-controlled	100 individuals with mild cognitive impairment (MCI)	Efficacy and safety of *Lb. plantarum* C29-fermented soybean (DW2009) as a nutritional supplement for cognitive enhancement for 12 weeks	Safely administered to enhance cognitive function in individuals with MCI	Hwang *et al.* (2019)
Randomized, double-blind placebo-controlled	50 Vietnamese patients with unconstipated IBS	Mixture of lactobacilli probiotics, 4 weeks	No adverse events in either group during the study period	Oh *et al.* (2019)
Systematic review and meta- analysis	IBS patients, 59 studies, including 6761 patients	To study efficacy and safety of probiotics; 40 studies evaluated safety of probiotic administration	No adverse effects in 14 trials; in 4 trials adverse events were noted. Safe and effective in the treatment of IBS with a single dose of probiotics 10^{10} CFU/day for short duration <8 weeks	Li *et al.* (2020)

randomized trials): 213 were given probiotics, 210 were in the placebo group. No severe adverse effect was noted. A commercial multistrain probiotic, VSL#3 (contains viable lyophilized bacteria *Lb. plantarum*, *S. thermophilus*, *Lb. acidophilus*, *Lb. paracasei*, *B. breve*, *B. infantis*, *B. longum*, and *Lb. delbrueckii* subsp. *bulgaricus* around 450 billion; VSL Pharma, USA) was tested on celiac disease (CoeD) patients to alter their intestinal microbiota as a new therapy. The probiotic preparation was given to 45 participants (18–70 years of age) with CoeD one sachet twice daily for 12 weeks. Safety of the probiotic preparation was evaluated based on monitoring blood and adverse events. The researchers found that CoeD patients tolerated VSL#3 well, although two participants each from the probiotic and placebo groups reporting mild bloating (Harnett *et al.* 2016). Another trial was done on CoeD patients (aged 18 and above) with irritable bowel syndrome (IBS) type symptoms. The participants were given one sachet daily of a multistrain probiotic composed of *Lb. plantarum* CECT 4528 (5×10^9 CFU/sachet), *Lb. casei* LMG 101/37 P-17504 (5×10^9 CFU/sachet), *B. breve* Bbr8 LMG P-17501 (10×10^9 CFU/sachet), *B. animalis* subsp. *lactis* Bi1 LMG P-17502 (10×10^9 CFU/sachet) and *B. breve* Bl10 LMG P-17500 (10×10^9 CFU/sachet) (Francavilla *et al.* 2019). The authors concluded that the probiotic preparation was safe without any incidence of adverse effects in the probiotic group. The study was randomized, double-blind, placebo-controlled with 6 weeks of probiotic treatment period preceded by a 2-week run-in and followed by a 6-week follow-up phase. *B. subtilis* CU1 was evaluated for safety in a randomized, double-blind, placebo-controlled human clinical study, where a total of 100 elderly subjects aged between 60 and 74 years old were divided into control and probiotic-administered groups and the probiotic group- were given daily one capsule containing 2×10^9 spores of *B. subtilis* CU1 (Lefevre *et al.* 2017). The study was conducted for a total of 16 weeks, divided into 10-day consumption periods separated by 18-day washout periods, with monitoring of hematological changes and safety parameters such as adverse events, clinical chemistry and hemodynamic parameters. The authors concluded that daily consumption of 2×10^9 spores of *B. subtilis* CU1 for the test period was safe and well tolerated without adverse effects compared to the placebo group. The Infant Microbiota Probiotic Intake (IMPRINT) trial (phase 1 clinical trial) was conducted in infants Day 7 postnatal for 21 days. The infants were administered *B. infantis* EVC001 1.8–2.8×10^{10} CFU daily in breast milk, and adverse events in terms of illnesses, number of visits to doctor with sickness, presence of colic, eczema diagnoses and use of antibiotics or gas-relieving medications were noted (Smilowitz *et al.* 2017). The study revealed that no difference in adverse events was noted between the probiotic-supplemented and non-supplemented groups, further the events were not serious and were normal for infants of that age and not related to feeding of *B. infantis*. The researchers concluded that *B. infantis* EVC001 supplement was safe and well tolerated. Alberda *et al.* (2018) evaluated the effect of Danactive® drink containing 10 billion CFU *Lb. casei* sp. *paracasei* CNCM I-1518 (Danone, Boucherville, QC, Canada) in the intensive care unit for prevention of *Clostridium difficile* infections (CDI) and antibiotic-associated diarrhea (AAD). The study was conducted in 32 patients (mean age of 59.9 and 57.5 years in the probiotic and control groups, respectively) fed with the probiotic drink twice daily; only two patients (12.5%) developed AAD in the probiotic group compared to five (31.3%) in the control group; one patient developed CDI at Day 5 (6%) in the probiotic group compared to three in the control group (18.75%). Three adverse events were noted in the control group whereas three cases of emesis occurred in the probiotic group. Baldassarre *et al.* (2018) studied the effectiveness and safety of the multistrain probiotic mixtures Vivomixx®, DeSimone Formulation®; Visbiome® (Danisco-DuPont) containing *Lb. acidophilus* DSM 24735, *Lb. paracasei* DSM 24733, *Lb. delbrueckii* subsp. *bulgaricus* DSM 24734 and *Lb. plantarum* DSM 24730), one strain of *S. thermophilus* DSM 24731, and three strains of bifidobacteria (*B. breve* DSM 24732, *B. longum* DSM 24736 and *B. infantis* DSM 24737) on infantile colic in breastfed infants. The randomized, double-blind, placebo-controlled study was conducted with 53 infants: 27 were administered 10 drops of probiotic mixture (5 billion CFU) for 21 days and the authors stated that the probiotic was safe as there were no adverse side effects. A meta-analysis was done to determine efficacy and safety of probiotic use in bacterial vaginosis (Wang *et al.* 2019). The analysis included 10 randomized placebo-controlled studies with 2321 participants with at least 1 month follow-up. Probiotic intervention was found beneficial with no extra adverse events (on genitourinary system, including superinfection such as vulvovaginal candidiasis, and gastrointestinal tract). To study the safety and efficacy of probiotics in IBS patients, a meta-analysis was done which included 59 studies, including 6761 patients. Out of these, only 40 studies evaluated safety of probiotic administration based on adverse events (Li *et al.* 2020). There were no adverse effects observed in 14 trials, while in four trials adverse events were reported, although there was low heterogeneity in the difference between probiotics and placebo groups. The authors concluded that probiotics administration was effective and safe in the treatment of IBS with a single dose of probiotics 10^{10} CFU/day for a short duration of less than 8 weeks.

6.5.6 Antibiotic Resistance – the Probability of Transfer of Resistance

Probiotic organisms have been reported to be intrinsically resistant to an array of antibiotics; however, major safety concerns arise when the organisms carry resistant genes in the plasmid or transposon with the possibility of antibiotic resistance transfer to other intestinal bacteria, particularly pathogenic bacteria. The EFSA recommended that probiotic organisms carrying transferable antibiotic resistance genes should not be used in probiotic and fermented food for human and animal feeds use. The authority agency has also specified antibiotic minimum inhibitory concentration (MIC) breakpoints of selected LAB in order to distinguish between antibiotic-resistant strains and antibiotic-susceptible ones, as shown in Table 6.5. Several studies have reported that strains of *Bifidobacterium* have intrinsic resistance against antibiotics such as nalidixic acid, ciprofloxacin, streptomycin, mupirocin and aminoglycosides (Varankovich *et al.* 2015; Wei *et al.* 2012) while macrolides, lincosamides, tetracycline and streptogramin B resistance genes were transposons mediated antibiotic resistance genes (Gueimonde *et al.* 2013). *Lactobacillus* spp. are also well known for their intrinsic resistance to vancomycin.

Probiotic organisms such as *B. lactis* DSM 10140 and *Lb. reuteri* SD 2112 showed presence of the tetracycline resistance gene *tet*(W), while *Lb. reuteri* SD 2112 showed the lincosamide resistance gene *lnu*(A) (Kastner *et al.* 2006). Probiotic bifidobacteria strains (a total of 23 in Japan) isolated from foods, supplements, pharmaceuticals and reference strains were tested for antibiotic resistance. All the *B. animalis* subsp. *lactis* strains were resistant to tetracycline, and genetic analysis revealed presence of *tet*(W) genes (Xiao *et al.* 2010). The authors also found that bifidobacteria strains were intrinsically resistant to

Table 6.5 Microbiological cut-off (mg/L) values for lactic acid bacteria and others for antibiotics.

Organism	Amp	Van	Gen	Kan	Str	Ery	Clin	Tet	Chlo	Ty	Ci	Co	Fo
Lactobacillus obligate homofermentative[a]	2	2	16	16	16	1	4	4	4	n.r.	n.r.	n.r.	n.r.
Lactobacillus acidophilus group	1	2	16	64	16	1	4	4	4	n.r.	n.r.	n.r.	n.r.
Lactobacillus obligate heterofermentative[b]	2	n.r.	16	64	64	1	4	8[c]	4	n.r.	n.r.	n.r.	n.r.
Lactobacillus reuteri	2	n.r.	8	64	64	1	4	32	4	n.r.	n.r.	n.r.	n.r.
Lactobacillus facultative heterofermentative[d]	4	n.r.	16	64	64	1	4	8	4	n.r.	n.r.	n.r.	n.r.
Lactobacillus plantarum /pentosus	2	n.r.	16	64	n.r.	1	4	32	8	n.r.	n.r.	n.r.	n.r.
Lactobacillus rhamnosus	4	n.r.	16	64	32	1	4	8	4	n.r.	n.r.	n.r.	n.r.
Lactobacillus casei/paracasei	4	n.r.	32	64	64	1	4	4	4	n.r.	n.r.	n.r.	n.r.
Bifidobacterium	2	2	64	n.r.	128	1	1	8	4	n.r.	n.r.	n.r.	n.r.
Pediococcus	4	n.r.	16	64	64	1	1	8	4	n.r.	n.r.	n.r.	n.r.
Leuconostoc	2	n.r.	16	16	64	1	1	8	4	n.r.	n.r.	n.r.	n.r.
Lactococcus lactis	2	4	32	64	32	1	1	4	8	n.r.	n.r.	n.r.	n.r.
Streptococcus thermophilus	2	4	32	n.r.	64	2	2	4	4	n.r.	n.r.	n.r.	n.r.
Bacillus	n.r.	4	4	8	8	4	4	8	8	n.r.	n.r.	n.r.	n.r.
Propionibacterium	2	4	64	64	64	0.5	0.25	2	2	n.r.	n.r.	n.r.	n.r.
Enterococcus faecium	2	4	32	1024	128	4	4	4	16	4	n.r.	n.r.	n.r.
Corynebacterium and other Gram positive	1	4	4	16	8	1	4	2	4	n.r.	n.r.	n.r.	n.r.
Enterobacteriaceae	8	n.r.	2	8	16	n.r.	n.r.	8	n.r.	n.r.	0.06	2	8

Amp, ampicillin; Chlo, chloramphenicol; Ci, ciprofloxacin; Clin, clindamycin; Co, colistin; Gen, gentamicin; Ery, erythromycin; Fo, fosfomycin; n.r., not required; Str, streptomycin; Tet, tetracycline; Ty, tylosin; Van, vancomycin.

[a] Including *Lb. delbrueckii, Lb. helveticus.*

[b] Including *Lb. fermentum.*

[c] For *Lb. buchneri* the cut-off for tetracycline is 128.

[d] Including the homofermentative species *Lb. salivarius.*

Source: EFSA Panel on Additives and Products or Substances used in Animal Feed (FEEDAP), Rychen, G., Aquilina, G., Azimonti, G., Bampidis, V., Bastos, M.L., et al. 2018. Guidance on the characterisation of microorganisms used as feed additives or as production organisms. *EFSA Journal*, 16(3), pe05206.

aminoglycosides. Lactobacilli strains such as *Lb. plantarum, Lb. helveticus, Lb. casei/paracasei, Lb. fermentum* and *Lb. rhamnosus* were isolated from the gastrointestinal microbiome and tested for antibiotic resistance against penicillins, aminoglycosides, macrolides, lincosamides, tetracyclines, chloramphenicol and rifampicin, and *Lb. plantarum* strains showed a broad spectrum of antibiotic resistance (Botina *et al.* 2011). Strains were resistant against antibiotics like tetracycline, aminoglycosides, clindamycin, lincomycin and benzylpenicillin. Cross resistance to two to five different aminoglycosides was detected in strains of *Lb. helveticus, Lb. rhamnosus, Lb. casei/paracasei,* and *Lb. fermentum*. The researchers also identified *tetM* gene of conjugative transposon in the strains *Lb. casei/paracasei* and *Lb. helveticus*. Wei *et al.* (2012) reported the presence of the transferable tetracycline resistance gene in *B. longum* JDM301 after complete genome sequencing, although experimental validation is required. Wong *et al.* (2015) screened five commercially available probiotic dietary supplements (from Malaysia, the USA and Austria) for antibiotic resistance and found that probiotics in all the supplements were resistant to vancomycin; resistance to gentamicin, aztreonam, streptomycin and/or ciprofloxacin was also detected in different probiotics. The probiotic product AB-LIFE® (consisting of three strains of *Lb. plantarum* CECT 7527, 7528 and 7529) was studied for antibiotic resistance and transferability by whole genome sequencing and genome mining. For the strains CECT 7527 and 7528, kanamycin and clindamycin resistance exceeded EFSA microbiological cut-off values. A chloramphenicol resistance gene was identified which is not encoded in the plasmid or in the insertion element and therefore poses no threat of resistance transferability (Mukerji *et al.* 2016). Antibiotic resistance of 33 *Lactobacillus* strains isolated from fermented milk belonging to the species *Lb. plantarum, Lb. casei* and *Lb. helveticus* was evaluated and all the strains were found to be resistant to vancomycin. Genetic analysis determined the presence of *van*(E), *van*(X), *tet*(M) and *gyr*(A) genes, and filter mating assay showed no transfer of antibiotic resistance from the culture (Guo *et al.* 2017). Sharma *et al.* (2016) isolated 30 probiotic lactobacilli from commercial probiotic products belonging to the species *Lb. casei, Lb. rhamnosus, Lb. reuteri, Lb. acidophilus, Lb. fermentum* and *Lb. plantarum* and evaluated their antibiotic resistance profile against 45 antibiotics. The isolates showed higher resistance against antibiotics such as kanamycin, nalidixic acid, co-trimoxazole, vancomycin, teicoplanin, streptomycin, amikacin, nitrofurantoin, norfloxacin and cefepime, but lower resistance against methicillin, ampicillin, tobramycin, penicillin, gentamicin, cefaclor, tetracycline, chloramphenicol, cloxacillin, levofloxacin, ofloxacin, azithromycin, amoxiclav, oxacillin, sulbactam, novobiocin and ciprofloxacin. The spore-forming probiotic *B. clausii* UBBC07 exhibited resistance towards antibiotics like clindamycin, erythromycin and chloramphenicol, however the resistance was non-transferable as the antibiotic-resistant gene was detected in chromosomal DNA as determined by whole genome sequencing (Lakshmi *et al.* 2017). Morovic *et al.* (2017) evaluated the probiotic strains *Lb. paracasei* Lpc-37®, *Lb. acidophilus* NCFM®, *B. animalis* subsp. *lactis* strains Bl-04®, and Bi-07®, and their combination (HOWARU® Restore) for antibiotic resistance and reported that only *B. lactis* Bl-04 was resistant towards tetracycline due to a *tet*W gene which was previously found to be non-transferable one. In a study with two commercial probiotic strains used globally, *B. longum* BORI and *B. bifidum* BGN4, the *B. bifidum* BGN4 strain showed gentamicin resistance at a higher concentration even than that of the cut-off value given by EFSA. Although the strain was resistant to gentamicin, there was no plasmid for resistance transfer and in a conjugation study gentamicin resistance was not transferred to *Lb. acidophilus* ATCC 4356 (susceptible to gentamicin). Similarly, *B. longum* BORI was intrinsically resistant to tetracycline due to the chromosomal presence of a *tet*(W) gene and a conjugation study revealed no tetracycline resistance transfer to *Lb. fermentum* AGBG1, which is susceptible to tetracycline (Kim *et al.* 2018). Kang *et al.* (2019) evaluated antibiotic resistance of oral care probiotic strains available in Korea – *Weissella cibaria* CMU and CMSI, *Lb. reuteri, Lb. salivarius, Lb. rhamnosus* (commercial probiotic isolates) and *E. faecalis* ATCC 29,212 – and reported that strains were particularly resistant to vancomycin and kanamycin. To evaluate antibiotic resistance transferability, *E. faecalis* ATCC 29212 and *Lb. rhamnosus* GG were conjugally mated with *W. cibaria* by filter mating and the authors concluded that the resistance was non-transferable. The authors also mentioned that *E. faecalis* ATCC 29212 harbored the *tet*(M) gene and a conjugative element "Tn916/Tn1545" which is a carrier of the tetracycline resistance gene. Antibiotic resistance of 182 *Lactobacillus* type strains was determined and was compared to their genotypes (with genome-wide annotations of antibiotic resistance genes) (Campedelli *et al.* 2019). The majority of the strains were resistant to trimethoprim, vancomycin and kanamycin. *Lb. ingluviei, Lb. amylophilus* and *Lb. amylotrophicus* harbored tetracycline and erythromycin resistance genes with the possibility of resistance transfer as these genes were flanked in the genome by mobile genetic elements.

Antibiotic resistance gene transfer has been reported previously between probiotic LAB and other microorganisms including pathogens. in vitro and in vivo (in the gut of mice) high-frequency vancomycin resistance gene (*van*A cluster) transfer from enterococci to a *Lb. acidophilus* commercial probiotic strain was reported (Mater *et al.* 2008). Feld *et al.* (2008) also found erythromycin resistance gene *erm*(B) transfer from *Lb. plantarum* which harbors a plasmid pLFE1 carrying the *erm*(B) gene to *E. faecalis* in an in vitro filter mating assay and an in vivo gnotobiotic rat model. *Lb. paracasei* have been reported to transfer the tetracycline resistance gene (*tet* M) present in the conjugative transposon Tn*916* to an opportunistic pathogen, *E. faecalis,* in a filter mating assay (Devirgiliis *et al.* 2009). Vieira de Souza *et al.* (2012) demonstrated that antibiotic resistance transfer occurs between lactobacilli species such as *Lb. acidophilus* strains, *Lb. vaginalis, Lb. salivarius* and *Lb. reuteri* in the gut of chicken. Transfer of erythromycin and tetracycline resistance (due to the presence of *erm*B, *tet*M, *tet*L and *tet*W on single plasmids) was reported from strains of *Lb. salivarius* (CHS-1E and CH7-1E) and *Lb. reuteri* (CH2-2) to *E. faecalis* in vitro and in vivo in albino Wistar rats (Thumu and Halami 2019). The researchers also showed that antibiotic resistance was transferable during food fermentation (e.g., fermented milk, chicken sausage and idli batter) from the lactobacilli to pathogens such as *Listeria monocytogenes* and *Yersinia enterocolitica.*

6.5.7 Post-marketing Surveillance – Genotoxic Studies, Toxin and Virulence Factors

It is the utmost responsibility of probiotic product manufacturers to ensure the safety of consumers. Thus, after the probiotics are released into the market, post-markeing surveillance should be done to detect any cases of pathogenicity, virulence or diseases and these should be reported. One of the safety parameters of probiotics is genotoxicity study. The most commonly used methods to detect genotoxicity are DNA strand break measurements in cells, bacterial Ames test, and cytogenetic assays (including chromosomal and micronucleus aberration assays) in addition to the use of chromosome painting and fluorescence in situ hybridization assays. The majority of researchers use the Ames test, micronucleus assay and chromosomal aberration assay to detect genotoxicity in probiotics.

Endres *et al.* (2009) evaluated the safety of a commercial preparation of *B. coagulans* known as GanedenBC^{30TM} (Ganeden Biotech) by acute oral toxicity test for 14 days and subchronic oral toxicity test for 13 weeks' duration in rats and concluded that GanedenBC^{30TM} was safe for chronic human consumption. GanedenBC^{30TM} tested negative for mutagenicity (by in vitro bacterial reverse mutation assay), genotoxicity and cytogenicity (by in vitro chromosomal aberration assay and micronucleus assay) in mice. Further, GanedenBC^{30TM} was subjected to a 1-year chronic oral toxicity and one-generation reproduction toxicity study in rats. Chronic consumption of GanedenBC30™ at 9.38×10^{10} CFU/day was concluded to be safe as there was no sign of toxicity; toxicity in the parental generation and in offspring was also not evidenced (Endres *et al.* 2011). Whole genome sequencing was done to evaluate the safety of *B. longum* JDM301 (a commercial probiotic strain marketed in China); a total of 162 virulence genes mainly coding for adhesion, transcriptional regulation, amino acid and sugar transport and five enzymes linked to harmful metabolites were detected (Wei *et al.* 2012). However, the authors concluded that in vivo studies should be conducted to validate the safety of the strain effectively. Zhang *et al.* (2012) evaluated a commercially popular probiotic strain in China, *Lb. plantarum* JDM1, for presence of virulence genes, genes associated with toxins, hemolysin, antibiotic resistance and biogenic amine production based on whole genome sequencing. They reported the presence of 126 virulence associated genes, 23 genes associated with adverse metabolism and 51 antibiotic resistance genes. The researchers also reported that genes associated with toxins and hemolysins were not detected and the transferability of virulence genes was rare. Vigiis 101 powder (containing probiotic bacteria *Lb. paracasei* subsp. *paracasei* NTU 101) when studied showed no genotoxicity as assessed using the Ames test, micronucleus assay and mammalian chromosomal aberration test. Further, a 28-day oral toxicity test in Wistar rats identified NOAEL of Vigiis 101 5000 mg/kg/day without any mortality, change in BW or toxicopathological lesions (Tseng *et al.* 2015). *Clostridium butyricum* MIYAIRI 588®, a probiotic strain, has a long history of safe use in humans in Asia, particularly in Japan (where it is classed as pharmaceutical drugs, "quasi drugs" and over-the-counter probiotics) (Isa *et al.* 2016). It was found to be negative for genes encoding for α, β or ε toxins along with botulin neurotoxins types A, B, E or F; when tested in an animal model it did not show any harmful effect on developmental toxicity and reproductive testing in mice. Individual strains of *Lb. acidophilus* NCFM, *Lb. paracasei* Lpc-37, *B. lactis* Bl-04 and *B. lactis* Bi-07 and their commercial preparation HOWARU® Restore (Danisco, Dupoint) was evaluated for acute toxicity in rats for 14 days individually and a dose of $1.7–4.1 \times 10^{12}$ CFU/kg BW proved to be safe as there was no mortality or treatment-related abnormality. Whole genome sequencing and genome mining revealed absence of bacterial toxin genes harmful for the mammalian host in all the probiotic strains (Morovic *et al.* 2017). *B. longum* BORI and *B. bifidum* BGN4 (two well-known probiotics available in the market globally, e.g. in Korea, New Zealand, China, Singapore, Germany, Thailand, Jordan, Lithuania, Poland, Vietnam and Turkey) were studied for genetic stability using whole genome sequencing by comparing the first and 25th generations (Kim *et al.* 2018). The researchers concluded that the genetic information remained stable between first and 25th generations and little genetic mutation was observed. Genes for virulence determinants such as *S. aureus* exoenzyme genes and *E. coli* Shiga toxin gene, host immune alteration or evasion genes and toxin genes were also evaluated by comparing the whole genome of probiotic strains with the pathogens *Enterococcus, E. coli, Staphylococcus aureus* and *Listeria*; none of these virulence factors was detected in either of the probiotic strains.

6.6 Conclusion

Most of the probiotic organisms currently on the market have been consumed by humans regularly for decades through fermented/probiotic foods. Thus, these strains are considered as safe as they do not pose adverse side effects or any threat in healthy individuals. It has been accepted that the risk of causing infections by LAB (except enterococci) is very rare. However, elderly people, premature babies, persons with a previous history of diabetes, hypertension, ulcerative colitis, cardiac valve disease or other conditions such as cancer, cirrhosis, hereditary hemorrhagic telangiectasia, etc., are in the potential risk category. For susceptible individuals who belong to the risk category, administration of probiotics should be made under a doctor's supervision or the manufacturer should issue a warning on the product's labeling. With the increasing market for probiotics, people make the assumption that probiotics are always beneficial, thus it is the responsibility of both regulatory bodies and manufacturers to ensure the safety of probiotics. For a new probiotic candidate, an inclusive and systematic safety assessment should be conducted starting with proper strain identification, determination of antibiotic resistance and transferability, adverse metabolite, virulence and toxin in vivo trials in animal models and human clinical trials. Stringent regulation should be made before releasing probiotics in the market, whether as supplements or biotherapeutic agents.

References

Aaron, J.G., Sobieszczyk, M.E., Weiner, S.D., Whittier, S. and Lowy, F.D. (2017). *Lactobacillus rhamnosus* endocarditis after upper endoscopy. In: *Open Forum Infectious Diseases*, Vol. 4, No. 2, ofx085. US: Oxford University Press.

Abotsi, W.K.M., Ainooson, G.K. and Gyasi, E.B. (2011). Acute and sub-acute toxicity studies of the ethanolic extract of the aerial parts of *Hilleria Latifolia* (Lam.) H. Walt. (Phytolaccaceae) in rodents. *West African Journal of Pharmacy*, 22(1): 27–35.

Alberda, C., Marcushamer, S., Hewer, T., Journault, N. and Kutsogiannis, D. (2018). Feasibility of a *Lactobacillus casei* drink in the intensive care unit for prevention of antibiotic associated diarrhea and *Clostridium difficile*. *Nutrients*, 10(5): 539.

Altermann, E., Russell, W.M., Azcarate-Peril, M.A., Barrangou, R., Buck, B.L., McAuliffe, O., Souther, N., Dobson, A., Duong, T., Callanan, M. and Lick, S. (2005). Complete genome sequence of the probiotic lactic acid bacterium Lactobacillus acidophilus NCFM. *Proceedings of the National Academy of Sciences*, 102(11): 3906–3912.

Anal, A.K. (2019). Quality ingredients and safety concerns for traditional fermented foods and beverages from Asia: a review. *Fermentation*, 5(1): 8.

Bafeta, A., Koh, M., Riveros, C. and Ravaud, P. (2018). Harms reporting in randomized controlled trials of interventions aimed at modifying microbiota: a systematic review. *Annals of Internal Medicine*, 169(4): 240–247.

Baldassarre, M.E., Di Mauro, A., Tafuri, S., Rizzo, V., Gallone, M.S., Mastromarino, P., Capobianco, D., Laghi, L., Zhu, C., Capozza, M. and Laforgia, N. (2018). Effectiveness and safety of a probiotic-mixture for the treatment of infantile colic: a double-blind, randomized, placebo-controlled clinical trial with fecal real-time PCR and NMR-based metabolomics analysis. *Nutrients*, 10(2): 195.

Bertelli, C., Pillonel, T., Torregrossa, A., Prod'hom, G., Fischer, C.J., Greub, G. and Giannoni, E. (2015). *Bifidobacterium longum* bacteremia in preterm infants receiving probiotics. *Clinical Infectious Diseases*, 60(6): 924–927.

Bhardwaj, A., Gupta, H., Kapila, S., Kaur, G., Vij, S. and Malik, R.K. (2010). Safety assessment and evaluation of probiotic potential of bacteriocinogenic *Enterococcus faecium* KH 24 strain under *in vitro* and *in vivo* conditions. *International Journal of Food Microbiology*, 141(3): 156–164.

Borges, N.A., Carmo, F.L., Stockler-Pinto, M.B., de Brito, J.S., Dolenga, C.J., Ferreira, D.C., Nakao, L.S., Rosado, A., Fouque, D. and Mafra, D. (2018). Probiotic supplementation in chronic kidney disease: a double-blind, randomized, placebo-controlled trial. *Journal of Renal Nutrition*, 28(1): 28–36.

Botina, S.G., Poluektova, E.U., Glazova, A.A., Zakharevich, N.V., Koroban, N.V., Zinchenko, V.V., Babykin, M.M., Zhilenkova, O.G., Amerkhanova, A.M. and Danilenko, V.N. (2011). Antibiotic resistance of potential probiotic bacteria of the genus Lactobacillus from human gastrointestinal microbiome. *Microbiology*, 80(2): 164.

Boumis, E., Capone, A., Galati, V., Venditti, C. and Petrosillo, N. (2018). Probiotics and infective endocarditis in patients with hereditary hemorrhagic telangiectasia: a clinical case and a review of the literature. *BMC Infectious Diseases*, 18(1): 65.

Boyd, M.A., Antonio, M.A. and Hillier, S.L. (2005). Comparison of API 50 CH strips to whole-chromosomal DNA probes for identification of Lactobacillus species. *Journal of Clinical Microbiology*, 43(10): 5309–5311.

Bujnakova, D., Strakova, E. and Kmet, V. (2014). *in vitro* evaluation of the safety and probiotic properties of Lactobacilli isolated from chicken and calves. *Anaerobe*, 29: 118–127.

Campedelli, I., Mathur, H., Salvetti, E., Clarke, S., Rea, M.C., Torriani, S., Ross, R.P., Hill, C. and O'Toole, P.W. (2019). Genus-wide assessment of antibiotic resistance in Lactobacillus spp. *Applied and Environmental Microbiology*, 85(1).

Casarotti, S.N., Carneiro, B.M., Todorov, S.D., Nero, L.A., Rahal, P. and Penna, A.L.B. (2017). in vitro assessment of safety and probiotic potential characteristics of Lactobacillus strains isolated from water buffalo mozzarella cheese. *Annals of Microbiology*, 67(4): 289–301.

Castro-González, J.M., Castro, P., Sandoval, H. and Castro-Sandoval, D. (2019). Probiotic lactobacilli precautions. *Frontiers in Microbiology*, 10: 375.

Chau, T.T.H., Chau, N.N.M., Le, N.T.H., The, H.C., Vinh, P.V., To, N.T.N., Ngoc, N.M., Tuan, H.M., Ngoc, T.L.C., Kolader, M.E. and Farrar, J.J. (2018). A double blind, randomized, placebo-controlled trial of *Lactobacillus acidophilus* for the treatment of acute watery diarrhea in Vietnamese children. *The Pediatric Infectious Disease Journal*, 37(1), 35.

Chiron, C., Tompkins, T. A. and Burguiere, P. (2018). Flow cytometry: a versatile technology for specific quantification and viability assessment of micro-organisms in multistrain probiotic products. *Journal of Applied Microbiology*, 124(2): 572–584.

Cohen, R., Martin, E., de La Rocque, F., Thollot, F., Pecquet, S., Werner, A., Boucherat, M., Varon, E., Bingen, E. and Levy, C. (2013). Probiotics and prebiotics in preventing episodes of acute otitis media in high-risk children: a randomized, double-blind, placebo-controlled study. *The Pediatric Infectious Disease Journal*, 32(8): 810–814.

Coudeyras, S., Marchandin, H., Fajon, C. and Forestier, C. (2008). Taxonomic and strain-specific identification of the probiotic strain *Lactobacillus rhamnosus* 35 within the *Lactobacillus casei* group. *Applied and Environmental Microbiology*, 74(9): 2679–2689.

Devirgiliis, C., Coppola, D., Barile, S., Colonna, B. and Perozzi, G. (2009). Characterization of the Tn916 conjugative transposon in a food-borne strain of *Lactobacillus paracasei*. *Applied and Environmental Microbiology*, 75(12): 3866–3871.

Dias, C.O., Scariot, M.C., Amboni, R.D.D.M.C. and Arisi, A.C.M. (2020). Application of propidium monoazide coupled with quantitative PCR to evaluate cell viability of *Bifidobacterium animalis* subsp. *lactis* in a non-dairy probiotic beverage. *Annals of Microbiology*, 70(1): 1–7.

Dimitonova, S.P., Bakalov, B.V., Aleksandrova-Georgieva, R.N. and Danova, S.T. (2008). Phenotypic and molecular identification of lactobacilli isolated from vaginal secretions. *Journal of Microbiology, Immunology and Infection*, 41(6): 469–477.

Doern, C.D., Nguyen, S.T., Afolabi, F. and Burnham, C.A.D. (2014). Probiotic-associated aspiration pneumonia due to *Lactobacillus rhamnosus*. *Journal of Clinical Microbiology*, 52(8): 3124–3126.

Donelli, G., Vuotto, C. and Mastromarino, P. (2013). Phenotyping and genotyping are both essential to identify and classify a probiotic microorganism. *Microbial Ecology in Health and Disease*, 24(1): 20105.

Duary, R.K., Batish, V.K. and Grover, S. (2010). Expression of atpD gene in putative indigenous probiotic *L. plantarum* strains under in vitro acidic conditions by RT-qPCR. *Research in Microbiology*, 161: 399–405.

Duary, R.K., Batish, V.K. and Grover, S. (2012). Relative gene expression of bile salt hydrolase and surface proteins in two putative indigenous *Lactobacillus plantarum* strains under in vitro gut conditions. *Molecular Biology Reports*, 39(3): 2541–2552.

Duary, R.K., Rajput, Y.S., Batish, V.K. and Grover, S. (2011). Assessing the adhesion of putative indigenous probiotic lactobacilli to human colonic epithelial cells. *The Indian Journal of Medical Research*, 134(5): 664.

Duysburgh, C., Van den Abbeele, P. and Marzorati, M. (2018). SHIME®: an advanced *in vitro* technology platform for studying the mode-of-action of probiotics in the gastrointestinal tract. *Nutrafoods*, 17: 213–217.

EFSA. (2008). Update of the criteria used in the assessment of bacterial resistance to antibiotics of human or veterinary importance. *EFSA Journal*, 732: 1–15.

EFSA Panel on Additives and Products or Substances used in Animal Feed (FEEDAP), Rychen, G., Aquilina, G., Azimonti, G., Bampidis, V., Bastos, M. L., et al. (2018). Guidance on the characterisation of microorganisms used as feed additives or as production organisms. *EFSA Journal*, 16(3): e05206.

EFSA Panel on Biological Hazards (BIOHAZ), Koutsoumanis, K., Allende, A., Alvarez-Ordóñez, A., Bolton, D., Bover-Cid, S., Chemaly, M., Davies, R., De Cesare, A., Hilbert, F. and Lindqvist, R. (2020). Update of the list of QPS-recommended biological agents intentionally added to food or feed as notified to EFSA 12: suitability of taxonomic units notified to EFSA until March 2020. *EFSA Journal*, 18(7): e06174.

Endres, J.R., Clewell, A., Jade, K.A., Farber, T., Hauswirth, J. and Schauss, A.G. (2009). Safety assessment of a proprietary preparation of a novel probiotic, *Bacillus coagulans*, as a food ingredient. *Food and Chemical Toxicology*, 47(6): 1231–1238.

Endres, J.R., Qureshi, I., Farber, T., Hauswirth, J., Hirka, G., Pasics, I. and Schauss, A.G. (2011). One-year chronic oral toxicity with combined reproduction toxicity study of a novel probiotic, *Bacillus coagulans*, as a food ingredient. *Food and Chemical Toxicology*, 49(5): 1174–1182.

Esaiassen, E., Cavanagh, P., Hjerde, E., Simonsen, G.S., Stoen, R. and Klingenberg, C. (2016). *Bifidobacterium longum* subspecies *infantis* bacteremia in 3 extremely preterm infants receiving probiotics. *Emerging Infectious Diseases*, 22(9): 1664.

FAO/WHO (2002). Working group report on drafting guidelines for the Evaluation of probiotics in food. London, ON, Canada.

Feld, L., Schjørring, S., Hammer, K., Licht, T.R., Danielsen, M., Krogfelt, K. and Wilcks, A. (2008). Selective pressure affects transfer and establishment of a *Lactobacillus plantarum* resistance plasmid in the gastrointestinal environment. *Journal of Antimicrobial Chemotherapy*, 61(4): 845–852.

Francavilla, R., Piccolo, M., Francavilla, A., Polimeno, L., Semeraro, F., Cristofori, F., Castellaneta, S., Barone, M., Indrio, F., Gobbetti, M. and De Angelis, M. (2019). Clinical and microbiological effect of a multispecies probiotic supplementation in celiac patients with persistent IBS-type symptoms: a randomized, double-blind, placebo-controlled, multicenter trial. *Journal of Clinical Gastroenterology*, 53(3): e117.

Franko, B., Vaillant, M., Recule, C., Vautrin, E., Brion, J.P. and Pavese, P. (2013). Lactobacillus paracasei endocarditis in a consumer of probiotics. *Médecine et Maladies Infectieuses*, 43(4): 171–173.

Galanis, A., Kourkoutas, Y., Tassou, C.C. and Chorianopoulos, N. (2015). Detection and identification of probiotic *Lactobacillus plantarum* strains by multiplex PCR using RAPD-derived primers. *International Journal of Molecular Sciences*, 16(10): 25141–25153.

Ganguly, N.K., Bhattacharya, S.K., Sesikeran, B., Nair, G.B., Ramakrishna, B.S., Sachdev, H.P.S., Batish, V.K., Kanagasabapathy, A.S., Muthuswamy, V., Kathuria, S.C. and Katoch, V.M. (2011). ICMR-DBT guidelines for evaluation of probiotics in food. *The Indian Journal of Medical Research*, 134(1): 22.

Gil-Campos, M., Lopez, M.A., Rodriguez-Benítez, M.V., Romero, J., Roncero, I., Linares, M.D., Maldonado, J., Lopez-Huertas, E., Berwind, R., Ritzenthaler, K.L. and Navas, V. (2012). *Lactobacillus fermentum* CECT 5716 is safe and well tolerated in infants of 1–6 months of age: a randomized controlled trial. *Pharmacological Research*, 65(2): 231–238.

Goldenberg, J.Z., Yap, C., Lytvyn, L., Lo, C.K.F., Beardsley, J., Mertz, D. and Johnston, B.C. (2017). Probiotics for the prevention of *Clostridium difficile*-associated diarrhea in adults and children. *Cochrane Database of Systematic Reviews*, (12): CD006095.

Gonzalez Pereyra, M.L., Dogi, C., Torres Lisa, A., Wittouck, P., Ortíz, M., Escobar, F., Bagnis, G., Yaciuk, R., Poloni, L., Torres, A. and Dalcero, A.M. (2014). Genotoxicity and cytotoxicity evaluation of probiotic *Saccharomyces cerevisiae* RC 016: a 60-day subchronic oral toxicity study in rats. *Journal of Applied Microbiology*, 117(3): 824–833.

Gueimonde, M., Sanchez, B., De Los Reyes-Gavilan, C. G., Margolles A. (2013). Antibiotic resistance in probiotic bacteria. *Frontiers in Microbiology*, 4: 202.

Guo, H., Pan, L., Li, L., Lu, J., Kwok, L., Menghe, B., Zhang, H. and Zhang, W. (2017). Characterization of antibiotic resistance genes from Lactobacillus isolated from traditional dairy products. *Journal of Food Science*, 82(3): 724–730.

Halvorsen, R., Berstad, A., Lassen, J., Midtvedt, T., Narvhus, J. (2009). The use of probiotics forpatients in hospitals: A benefit and risk assessment. Opinion of the Steering Committee of the Norwegian Scientific Committee for Food Safety. *VKM Rep*, Norway.

Harnett, J., Myers, S.P. and Rolfe, M. (2016). Probiotics and the microbiome in celiac disease: a randomised controlled trial. *Evidence-Based Complementary and Alternative Medicine*, 2016.

Hwang, Y.H., Park, S., Paik, J.W., Chae, S.W., Kim, D.H., Jeong, D.G., Ha, E., Kim, M., Hong, G., Park, S.H. and Jung, S.J. (2019). Efficacy and safety of *Lactobacillus plantarum* C29-fermented soybean (DW2009) in individuals with mild cognitive impairment: a 12-week, multi-center, randomized, double-blind, placebo-controlled clinical trial. *Nutrients*, 11(2): 305.

Ianiro, G., Rizzatti, G., Plomer, M., Lopetuso, L., Scaldaferri, F., Franceschi, F., Cammarota, G. and Gasbarrini, A. (2018). *Bacillus clausii* for the treatment of acute diarrhea in children: a systematic review and meta-analysis of randomized controlled trials. *Nutrients*, 10(8): 1074.

Isa, K., Oka, K., Beauchamp, N., Sato, M., Wada, K., Ohtani, K., Nakanishi, S., McCartney, E., Tanaka, M., Shimizu, T. and Kamiya, S. (2016). Safety assessment of the *Clostridium butyricum* MIYAIRI 588® probiotic strain including evaluation of antimicrobial sensitivity and presence of Clostridium toxin genes *in vitro* and teratogenicity *in vivo*. *Human & Experimental Toxicology*, 35(8): 818–832.

Jafarnejad, S., Shab-Bidar, S., Speakman, J.R., Parastui, K., Daneshi-Maskooni, M. and Djafarian, K. (2016). Probiotics reduce the risk of antibiotic-associated diarrhea in adults (18–64 years) but not the elderly (> 65 years) a meta-analysis. *Nutrition in Clinical Practice*, 31(4): 502–513.

Jarocki, P., Podleśny, M., Glibowski, P. and Targoński, Z. (2014). A new insight into the physiological role of bile salt hydrolase among intestinal bacteria from the genus Bifidobacterium. *PLoS One*, 9(12): e114379.

Kang, M.S., Yeu, J.E. and Hong, S.P. (2019). Safety evaluation of oral care probiotics *Weissella cibaria* CMU and CMS1 by phenotypic and genotypic analysis. *International Journal of Molecular Sciences*, 20(11): 2693.

Karimi, R., Mortazavian, A.M. and Da Cruz, A.G. (2011). Viability of probiotic microorganisms in cheese during production and storage: a review. *Dairy Science and Technology*, 91(3): 283–308.

Kastner, S., Perreten, V., Bleuler, H., Hugenschmidt, G., Lacroix, C. and Meile, L. (2006). Antibiotic susceptibility patterns and resistance genes of starter cultures and probiotic bacteria used in food. *Systematic and Applied Microbiology*, 29(2): 145–155.

Kaushik, J.K., Kumar, A., Duary, R.K., Mohanty, A.K., Grover, S. and Batish, V.K. (2009). Functional and probiotic attributes of an indigenous isolate of *Lactobacillus plantarum*. *PloS ONE*, 4(12): e8099.

Kim, G.B. and Lee, B.H. (2008). Genetic analysis of a bile salt hydrolase in *Bifidobacterium animalis* subsp. *lactis* KL612. *Journal of Applied Microbiology*, 105(3): 778–790.

Kim, M.J., Ku, S., Kim, S.Y., Lee, H.H., Jin, H., Kang, S., Li, R., Johnston, T.V., Park, M.S. and Ji, G.E. (2018). Safety evaluations of *Bifidobacterium bifidum* BGN4 and *Bifidobacterium longum* BORI. *International Journal of Molecular Sciences*, 19(5): 1422.

Kochan, P., Chmielarczyk, A., Szymaniak, L., Brykczynski, M., Galant, K., Zych, A., Pakosz, K., Giedrys-Kalemba, S., Lenouvel, E. and Heczko, P.B. (2011). *Lactobacillus rhamnosus* administration causes sepsis in a cardiosurgical patient—is the time right to revise probiotic safety guidelines? *Clinical Microbiology and Infection*, 17(10): 1589–1592.

Koirala, S. and Anal, A.K. (2021). Probiotics-based foods and beverages as future foods and their overall safety and regulatory claims. *Future Foods*, 100013.

Kothari, D., Patel, S. and Kim, S.K. (2019). Probiotic supplements might not be universally-effective and safe: A review. *Biomedicine & Pharmacotherapy*, 111: 537–547.

Koyama, S., Fujita, H., Shimosato, T., Kamijo, A., Ishiyama, Y., Yamamoto, E., Ishii, Y., Hattori, Y., Hagihara, M., Yamazaki, E. and Tomita, N. (2019). Septicemia from *Lactobacillus rhamnosus* GG, from a probiotic enriched yogurt, in a patient with autologous stem cell transplantation. *Probiotics and Antimicrobial Proteins*, 11(1): 295–298.

Lakshmi, S.G., Jayanthi, N., Saravanan, M. and Ratna, M.S. (2017). Safety assessment of *Bacillus clausii* UBBC07, a spore forming probiotic. *Toxicology Reports*, 4: 62–71.

Lefevre, M., Racedo, S.M., Denayrolles, M., Ripert, G., Desfougères, T., Lobach, A.R., Simon, R., Pelerin, F., Justen, P. and Urdaci, M.C. (2017). Safety assessment of *Bacillus subtilis* CU1 for use as a probiotic in humans. *Regulatory Toxicology and Pharmacology*, 83: 54–65.

Li, B., Jin, D., Etareri Evivie, S., Li, N., Yan, F., Zhao, L., Liu, F. and Huo, G. (2017). Safety assessment of *Lactobacillus helveticus* KLDS1. 8701 based on whole genome sequencing and oral toxicity studies. *Toxins*, 9(10): 301.

Li, B., Liang, L., Deng, H., Guo, J., Shu, H. and Zhang, L. (2020). Efficacy and safety of probiotics in irritable bowel syndrome: a systematic review and meta-analysis. *Frontiers in Pharmacology*, 11: 332.

Lin, Y.C., Chen, Y.T. and Chen, M.J. (2018). Lack of mutagenicity, genotoxicity and developmental toxicity in safety assessment tests of *Lactobacillus mali* APS1. *PLoS One*, 13(12): e0208881

Loo, E.X., Llanora, G.V., Lu, Q., Aw, M.M., Lee, B.W. and Shek, L.P. (2014). Supplementation with probiotics in the first 6 months of life did not protect against eczema and allergy in at-risk Asian infants: a 5-year follow-up. *International Archives of Allergy and Immunology*, 163(1): 25–28.

Lu, C., Sang, J., He, H., Wan, X., Lin, Y., Li, L., Li, Y. and Yu, C. (2016). Probiotic supplementation does not improve eradication rate of *Helicobacter pylori* infection compared to placebo based on standard therapy: a meta-analysis. *Scientific Reports*, 6: 23522.

Łukasik, J., Salminen, S. and Szajewska, H. (2018). Rapid review shows that probiotics and fermented infant formulas do not cause d-lactic acidosis in healthy children. *Acta Paediatrica*, 107(8): 1322–1326.

Makino, H., Kushiro, A., Ishikawa, E., Muylaert, D., Kubota, H., Sakai, T., Oishi, K., Martin, R., Amor, K.B., Oozeer, R. and Knol, J. (2011). Transmission of intestinal *Bifidobacterium longum* subsp. *longum* strains from mother to infant, determined by multilocus sequencing typing and amplified fragment length polymorphism. *Applied and Environmental Microbiology*, 77(19): 6788–6793.

Mater, D.D., Langella, P., Corthier, G. and Flores, M.J. (2008). A probiotic Lactobacillus strain can acquire vancomycin resistance during digestive transit in mice. *Journal of Molecular Microbiology and Biotechnology*, 14(1-3): 123–127.

McCartney, A.L. (2002). Application of molecular biological methods for studying probiotics and the gut flora. *British Journal of Nutrition*, 88(S1): s29–s37.

Meini, S., Laureano, R., Fani, L., Tascini, C., Galano, A., Antonelli, A. and Rossolini, G.M. (2015). Breakthrough *Lactobacillus rhamnosus* GG bacteremia associated with probiotic use in an adult patient with severe active ulcerative colitis: case report and review of the literature. *Infection*, 43(6): 777–781.

Morovic, W., Roper, J.M., Smith, A.B., Mukerji, P., Stahl, B., Rae, J.C. and Ouwehand, A.C. (2017). Safety evaluation of HOWARU® Restore (*Lactobacillus acidophilus* NCFM, *Lactobacillus paracasei* Lpc-37, *Bifidobacterium animalis* subsp. *lactis* Bl-04 and *B. lactis* Bi-07) for antibiotic resistance, genomic risk factors, and acute toxicity. *Food and Chemical Toxicology*, 110: 316–324.

Mukerji, P., Roper, J.M., Stahl, B., Smith, A.B., Burns, F., Rae, J.C., Yeung, N., Lyra, A., Svärd, L., Saarinen, M.T. and Alhoniemi, E. (2016). Safety evaluation of AB-LIFE® (*Lactobacillus plantarum* CECT 7527, 7528 and 7529): Antibiotic resistance and 90-day repeated-dose study in rats. *Food and Chemical Toxicology*, 92: 117–128.

Naqvi, S.S.B., Nagendra, V. and Hofmeyr, A. (2018). Probiotic related *Lactobacillus rhamnosus* endocarditis in a patient with liver cirrhosis. *IDCases*, 13: e00439.

Narayanan, R. (2013). Current legislations on probiotic products. *Journal of Agriculture Sciences*, 1(2): 18–24.

Nithya, V., Muthukumar, S.P. and Halami, P.M. (2012). Safety assessment of *Bacillus licheniformis* Me1 isolated from milk for probiotic application. *International Journal of Toxicology*, 31(3): 228–237.

OECD (2001). Test No. 423: Acute oral toxicity – acute toxic class method. Paris: OECD Publishing.

OECD/OCDE (2008). OECD Guideline for the Testing of Chemicals No. 407, Repeated Dose 28-Day Oral Toxicity Study in Rodents. Organisation for Economic Co-operation and Development/Organisation de Coopération et de Développement Economiques. 2008: 13.

Oh, J.H., Jang, Y.S., Kang, D., Chang, D.K. and Min, Y.W. (2019). Efficacy and safety of new lactobacilli probiotics for unconstipated irritable bowel syndrome: a randomized, double-blind, placebo-controlled trial. *Nutrients*, 11(12): 2887.

Ouwehand, A.C. (2017). A review of dose-responses of probiotics in human studies. *Beneficial Microbes*, 8(2), p.143–151.

Pararajasingam, A. and Uwagwu, J. (2017). *Lactobacillus*: the not so friendly bacteria. *Case Reports*, 2017: bcr-2016.

Pradhan, D., Mallappa, R.H. and Grover, S. (2020). Comprehensive approaches for assessing the safety of probiotic bacteria. *Food Control*, 108: 106872.

Pradhan, D., Singh, R., Tyagi, A., Rashmi, H.M., Batish, V.K. and Grover, S. (2019a). Assessing the safety and efficacy of *Lactobacillus plantarum* MTCC 5690 and *Lactobacillus fermentum* MTCC 5689 in colitis mouse model. *Probiotics and Antimicrobial Proteins*, 11(3): 910–920.

Pradhan, D., Singh, R., Tyagi, A., Rashmi, H.M., Batish, V.K. and Grover, S. (2019b). Assessing safety of *Lactobacillus plantarum* MTCC 5690 and *Lactobacillus fermentum* MTCC 5689 using *in vitro* approaches and an *in vivo* murine model. *Regulatory Toxicology and Pharmacology*, 101: 1–11.

Ramiah, K., Van Reenen, C.A. and Dicks, L.M.T. (2007). Expression of the mucus adhesion genes Mub and MapA, adhesion-like factor EF-Tu and bacteriocin gene plaA of *Lactobacillus plantarum* 423, monitored with real-time PCR. *International Journal of Food Microbiology*, 116(3): 405–409.

Ramiah, K., van Reenen, C.A. and Dicks, L.M.T. (2009). Expression of the mucus adhesion gene mub, surface layer protein slp and adhesion-like factor EF-TU of *Lactobacillus acidophilus* ATCC 4356 under digestive stress conditions, as monitored with real-time PCR. *Probiotics and Antimicrobial Proteins*, 1(1): 91.

Rastogi, S., Mittal, V. and Singh, A. (2019). *In vitro* evaluation of probiotic potential and safety assessment of *Lactobacillus mucosae* strains isolated from donkey's lactation. *Probiotics and Antimicrobial Proteins*, 1–12.

Raymond, Y. and Champagne, C.P. (2015). The use of flow cytometry to accurately ascertain total and viable counts of *Lactobacillus rhamnosus* in chocolate. *Food Microbiology*, 46: 176–183.

Raza, M., Al-Shabanah, O.A., El-Hadiyah, T.M. and Al-Majed, A.A. (2002). Effect of prolonged vigabatrin treatment on hematological and biochemical parameters in plasma, liver and kidney of Swiss albino mice. *Scientia Pharmaceutica*, 70(2): 135–145.

Sadowska-Krawczenko, I., Paprzycka, M., Korbal, P., Wiatrzyk, A., Krysztopa-Grzybowska, K., Polak, M., Czajka, U. and Lutyńska, A. (2014). *Lactobacillus rhamnosus* GG suspected infection in a newborn with intrauterine growth restriction. *Beneficial Microbes*, 5(4): 397–402.

Sánchez, B., De Los Reyes-Gavilán, C.G. and Margolles, A. (2006). The F1F0-ATPase of *Bifidobacterium animalis* is involved in bile tolerance. *Environmental Microbiology*, 8(10): 1825–1833.

Sanders, M.E., Akkermans, L.M., Haller, D., Hammerman, C., Heimbach, J.T., Hörmannsperger, G. and Huys, G. (2010). Safety assessment of probiotics for human use. *Gut Microbes*, 1(3): 164–185.

Scariot, M.C., Venturelli, G.L., Prudêncio, E.S. and Arisi, A.C.M. (2018). Quantification of *Lactobacillus paracasei* viable cells in probiotic yoghurt by propidium monoazide combined with quantitative PCR. *International Journal of Food Microbiology*, 264: 1–7.

Schwenger, E.M., Tejani, A.M. and Loewen, P.S. (2015). Probiotics for preventing urinary tract infections in adults and children. *Cochrane Database of Systematic Reviews*, (12):CD008772.

Senan, S., Prajapati, J.B. and Joshi, C.G. (2015). Feasibility of genome-wide screening for biosafety assessment of probiotics: a case study of *Lactobacillus helveticus* MTCC 5463. *Probiotics and Antimicrobial Proteins*, 7(4): 249–258.

Sendil, S., Shrimanker, I., Mansoora, Q., Goldman, J. and Nookala, V.K. (2020). *Lactobacillus rhamnosus* bacteremia in an immunocompromised renal transplant patient. *Cureus*, 12(2): e6887.

Sharma, P., Tomar, S.K., Sangwan, V., Goswami, P. and Singh, R. (2016). Antibiotic resistance of *Lactobacillus* sp. isolated from commercial probiotic preparations. *Journal of Food Safety*, 36(1): 38–51.

Sherid, M., Samo, S., Sulaiman, S., Husein, H., Sifuentes, H. and Sridhar, S. (2016). Liver abscess and bacteremia caused by *lactobacillus*: role of probiotics? Case report and review of the literature. *BMC Gastroenterology*, 16(1): 138.

Shida, K., Sato, T., Iizuka, R., Hoshi, R., Watanabe, O., Igarashi, T., Miyazaki, K., Nanno, M. and Ishikawa, F. (2017). Daily intake of fermented milk with *Lactobacillus casei* strain Shirota reduces the incidence and duration of upper respiratory tract infections in healthy middle-aged office workers. *European Journal of Nutrition*, 56(1): 45–53.

Shokryazdan, P., Faseleh Jahromi, M., Liang, J.B., Kalavathy, R., Sieo, C.C. and Ho, Y.W. (2016). Safety assessment of two new *Lactobacillus* strains as probiotic for human using a rat model. *PLoS One*, 11(7): e0159851.

Singh, T.P., Malik, R.K. and Gurpreet, K. (2014). Safety assessment and evaluation of probiotic potential of *Lactobacillus reuteri* strains under *in vitro* conditions. *International Journal of Current Microbiology and Applied Sciences*, 3(2): 335–348.

Smilowitz, J.T., Moya, J., Breck, M.A., Cook, C., Fineberg, A., Angkustsiri, K. and Underwood, M.A. (2017). Safety and tolerability of *Bifidobacterium longum* subspecies *infantis* EVC001 supplementation in healthy term breastfed infants: a phase I clinical trial. *BMC Pediatrics*, 17(1): 133.

Soh, S.E., Aw, M., Gerez, I., Chong, Y.S., Rauff, M., Ng, Y.P.M., Wong, H.B., Pai, N., Lee, B.W. and Shek, L.C. (2009). Probiotic supplementation in the first 6 months of life in at risk Asian infants–effects on eczema and atopic sensitization at the age of 1 year. *Clinical & Experimental Allergy*, 39(4): 571–578.

Srutkova, D., Spanova, A., Spano, M., Drab, V., Schwarzer, M., Kozakova, H. and Rittich, B. (2011). Efficiency of PCR-based methods in discriminating *Bifidobacterium longum* ssp. *longum* and *Bifidobacterium longum* ssp. *infantis* strains of human origin. *Journal of Microbiological Methods*, 87(1): 10–16.

Stevenson, C., Blaauw, R., Fredericks, E., Visser, J. and Roux, S. (2014). Randomized clinical trial: effect of *Lactobacillus plantarum* 299 v on symptoms of irritable bowel syndrome. *Nutrition*, 30(10): 1151–1157.

Thumu, S.C.R. and Halami, P.M. (2019). Conjugal transfer of erm (B) and multiple tet genes from *Lactobacillus* spp. to bacterial pathogens in animal gut, *in vitro* and during food fermentation. *Food Research International*, 116: 1066–1075.

Thumu, S.C.R. and Halami, P.M. (2020). *In vivo* safety assessment of *Lactobacillus fermentum* strains, evaluation of their cholesterol-lowering ability and intestinal microbial modulation. *Journal of the Science of Food and Agriculture*, 100(2): 705–713.

Tripathi, M.K. and Giri, S.K. (2014). Probiotic functional foods: Survival of probiotics during processing and storage. *Journal of Functional Foods*, 9: 225–241.

Tseng, W.T., Shih, T.W., Liu, S.H. and Pan, T.M. (2015). Safety and mutagenicity evaluation of Vigiis 101 powder made from *Lactobacillus paracasei* subsp. *paracasei* NTU 101. *Regulatory Toxicology and Pharmacology*, 71(2): 148–157.

Uymaz Tezel, B. (2019). Preliminary *in vitro* evaluation of the probiotic potential of the bacteriocinogenic strain *Enterococcus lactis* PMD74 isolated from ezine cheese. *Journal of Food Quality*, 2019.

Vahabnezhad, E., Mochon, A.B., Wozniak, L.J. and Ziring, D.A. (2013). *Lactobacillus* bacteremia associated with probiotic use in a pediatric patient with ulcerative colitis. *Journal of Clinical Gastroenterology*, 47(5): 437–439.

Varankovich, N.V., Nickerson, M.T. and Korber, D.R. (2015). Probiotic-based strategies for therapeutic and prophylactic use against multiple gastrointestinal diseases. *Frontiers in Microbiology*, 6: 685.

Vieira de Souza, F., Roque, R., Silva Moreira, J.L., Resende de Souza, M., Nicoli, J.R., Neumann, E. and Cantini Nunes, A. (2012). Transfer of antibiotic resistance determinants between lactobacilli isolates from the gastrointestinal tract of chicken. *Beneficial Microbes*, 3(2): 137–144.

Vitetta, L., Coulson, S., Thomsen, M., Nguyen, T. and Hall, S. (2017). Probiotics, D-Lactic acidosis, oxidative stress and strain specificity. *Gut Microbes*, 8(4): 311–322.

Vogel, G. (2008). Deaths prompt a review of experimental probiotic therapy. *Science*, 319(5863): 557.

Von Wright, A. (2005). Regulating the safety of probiotics – The European approach. *Current Pharmaceutical Design*, 11: 17–23.

Wall, T., Roos, S., Jacobsson, K., Rosander, A. and Jonsson, H. (2003). Phage display reveals 52 novel extracellular and transmembrane proteins from *Lactobacillus reuteri* DSM 20016T. *Microbiology*, 149: 3493–3505.

Wang, Z., He, Y. and Zheng, Y. (2019). Probiotics for the treatment of bacterial vaginosis: A meta-analysis. *International Journal of Environmental Research and Public Health*, 16(20): 3859.

Wei, Y.X., Zhang, Z.Y., Liu, C., Malakar, P.K. and Guo, X.K. (2012). Safety assessment of *Bifidobacterium longum* JDM301 based on complete genome sequences. *World Journal of Gastroenterology: WJG*, 18(5): 479.

Wong, A., Saint Ngu, D.Y., Dan, L.A., Ooi, A. and Lim, R.L.H. (2015). Detection of antibiotic resistance in probiotics of dietary supplements. *Nutrition Journal*, 14(1): 1–6.

Xiao, J.Z., Takahashi, S., Odamaki, T., Yaeshima, T. and Iwatsuki, K. (2010). Antibiotic susceptibility of bifidobacterial strains distributed in the Japanese market. *Bioscience, Biotechnology, and Biochemistry*, 74(2): 336–342.

Xu, F., Wang, J., Guo, Y., Fu, P., Zeng, H., Li, Z., Pei, X., Liu, X. and Wang, S. (2018). Antibiotic resistance, biochemical typing, and PFGE typing of *Bifidobacterium* strains commonly used in probiotic health foods. *Food Science and Biotechnology*, 27(2): 467–477.

Xu, M., Wang, J., Wang, N., Sun, F., Wang, L. and Liu, X.H. (2015). The efficacy and safety of the probiotic bacterium *Lactobacillus reuteri* DSM 17938 for infantile colic: a meta-analysis of randomized controlled trials. *PloS ONE*, 10(10).

Yazdankhah, S.P., Eckner, K.F., Halvorsen, R., Kapperud, G., Lassen, J.F., Narvhus, J., Nesbakken, T., Robertson, L., Rosnes, J.T., Skjerdal, T. and Skjerve, E. (2014). Guidelines for assessment of safety aspects of probiotic (food) products. Opinion of the Panel on Biological Hazards of the Norwegian Scientific Committee for Food Safety. *VKM Report*.

Yelin, I., Flett, K.B., Merakou, C., Mehrotra, P., Stam, J., Snesrud, E., Hinkle, M., Lesho, E., McGann, P., McAdam, A.J. and Sandora, T.J. (2019). Genomic and epidemiological evidence of bacterial transmission from probiotic capsule to blood in ICU patients. *Nature Medicine*, 25(11): 1728–1732.

Zhang, Y., Li, L., Guo, C., Mu, D., Feng, B., Zuo, X. and Li, Y. (2016). Effects of probiotic type, dose and treatment duration on irritable bowel syndrome diagnosed by Rome III criteria: a meta-analysis. *BMC Gastroenterology*, 16(1): 62.

Zhang, Z.Y., Liu, C., Zhu, Y.Z., Wei, Y.X., Tian, F., Zhao, G.P. and Guo, X.K. (2012). Safety assessment of *Lactobacillus plantarum* JDM1 based on the complete genome. *International Journal of Food Microbiology*, 153(1-2): 166–170.

Zielińska, D., Ołdak, A., Rzepkowska, A. and Zieliński, K. (2018a). Enumeration and identification of probiotic bacteria in food matrices. In: *Advances in Biotechnology for Food Industry*, 167–196. Academic Press.

Zielińska, D., Sionek, B. and Kołożyn-Krajewska, D. (2018b). Safety of probiotics. In: *Diet, Microbiome and Health*, 131–161. Academic Press.

Zmora, N., Zilberman-Schapira, G., Suez, J., Mor, U., Dori-Bachash, M., Bashiardes, S. and Federici, S. (2018). Personalized gut mucosal colonization resistance to empiric probiotics is associated with unique host and microbiome features. *Cell*, 174(6): 1388–1405.

7

Probiotics in Biodegradation of Microbial Toxins: Principles and Mechanisms

Ali Akbar[1], *Muhammad Iftikhar Khan*[2] *and Ghulam Ishaq Khan*[1]

[1] *Department of Microbiology, Faculty of Life Sciences, University of Balochistan, Quetta, 87300, Balochistan, Pakistan*
[2] *Department of Zoology, Abdul Wali Khan University, Khyber Pakhtunkhwa, Pakistan*

7.1 Microbial Toxins

The word "toxin" is derived from Greek and means something that causes harm to living cells or life. Microbial toxins as a poison are inconvenient to human health and well-being. Historical records show various events of death and suffering brought about by pathogens and their toxins, such as *Yersinia pestis* (bubonic plague or Black Death), *Corynebacterium diphtheria* and *Vibrio cholerae*, the causative agents of diphtheria and cholera, respectively, *Bordetella pertussis* (the causative agent of whooping cough) and *Salmonella enterica* subsp. *enterica* serotype Typhi, which causes typhoid (Early and Tamime 2017).

Toxins are usually proteins and associated to both prokaryotic and eukaryotic organisms. A toxin can cause abnormalities in living things after its ingestion, which can be deadly. Toxins are powerful particles produced by a huge variety of pathogens that target the cells and play a key part in the host–pathogen discourse. They are major harmful components that may result in the contamination of several commodities. For the host, production of a toxin serves diverse capacities in the environment, such as paralyzing prey and eluding predators. Prokaryotic and eukaryotic microbes and parasites utilize it for the expulsion of other communities competing for food supplements and occupying the same ecological niche (de Wit 2013).

Verifying its significance in pathogenesis, the infusion of a very small amount of poison can cause serious illness. Bacterial toxins can be separated into a few groups with respect to their nature and mode of activity (do Vale *et al.* 2016).

Microbes produce toxins that can be classified as either exotoxins or endotoxins. Exotoxins are produced by pathogenic bacteria and then secreted to the surroundings, whereas endotoxins stay as an integral part of the microbes. Usually, an endotoxin is incorporated in the bacterial external layer and is not discharged until the bacterium dies and the cell breaks apart (Bordoloi and Ganguly 2014).

Probiotics, Prebiotics and Synbiotics: Technological Advancements Towards Safety and Industrial Applications, First Edition. Edited by Parmjit Singh Panesar and Anil Kumar Anal.

Numerous microorganisms may possibly work as probiotics, of which *Lactobacillus* and *Bifidobacterium* species are the most commonly utilized. Probiotics are live microorganisms thought to be advantageous to living beings. According to the recent definition by the FAO/WHO, probiotics are live microorganisms that can be used for the welfare of human beings. Probiotics influence the host advantageously, which may be coordinate or circuitous, including upgrading the ability to obstruct pathogens by balancing the mucosal resistant framework, production of antimicrobial substances, upgrading assimilation of nutrients, and changing the intestinal microflora (Hemaiswarya *et al.* 2013).

Probiotic strains appear to be very useful against infections such as *H. pylori* contamination, irritable bowel disorder, and inflammatory bowel disease (ulcerative colitis and Crohn's disease) as well as boosting the defenses of healthy people (Lam *et al.* 2016).

The following species have been screened for their use in enhancing well-being: *Lactobacillus casei, L. acidophilus, L. paracasei, L. rhamnosus, L. gasseri, L. plantarum, L. reuteri, L. crispatus, L. johnsonii, L. fermentum, Bifidobacterium bifidum, B. infantis, B. adolescentis, B. lactis, B. breve, B. longum, Saccharomyces boulardii* and *S. cerevisiae*, among others. *Enterococcus faecium* strains have also been assessed; concerns have been raised about their utilization as probiotics, as their role in producing illness and the chance of antibiotic resistance transfer are as yet a matter of discussion regarding their use in humans (Vinderola and Ritieni 2014). Figure 7.1 shows the antibacterial activities of probiotic bacteria against common foodborne and toxin-producing bacteria.

7.1.1 Health Benefits

The most important benefits of these probiotics in the field of health are in pharmaceutics, production of different dairy products, enhancing gut immunity, increasing bowel regulation, inhibition of stomach infection, prevention of enterococcal infections such as diarrhea, and reducing the rate of lactose intolerance. They may also decrease the risk of mutation, carcinogenicity and other genetic disorders in the human body (Kechagia *et al.* 2013). Oral administration is the most efficient route for optimal intake of probiotics as the vital properties of the organisms, such as cell viability, are not as greatly affected (Kataria *et al.* 2009). The reported mechanisms of action of probiotics are competition with other pathogenic microorganisms for survival, conversion of glucose to organic acids which lower the pH of the intestine, production of some important bioactive compounds and displacement of pathogenic bacteria from their adhesion site (Oelschlaeger 2010). Among all the mechanisms of action of probiotics, the most important is the activation of the gut immune system of the host (Koirala and Anal 2021). Dose of microorganism, route of administration and time period of interaction can significantly affect the function of probiotics (Hardy *et al.* 2013).

7.1.2 Mycotoxins and Probiotics

The filamentous fungi produce toxins, called mycotoxins, as secondary metabolites at a late stationary phase of growth. Mycotoxins are considered the most toxic compounds for both humans and animals when they contaminate food and feeds. These toxins are commonly present in almonds, rice, wheat and other cereals. The food and feed products are

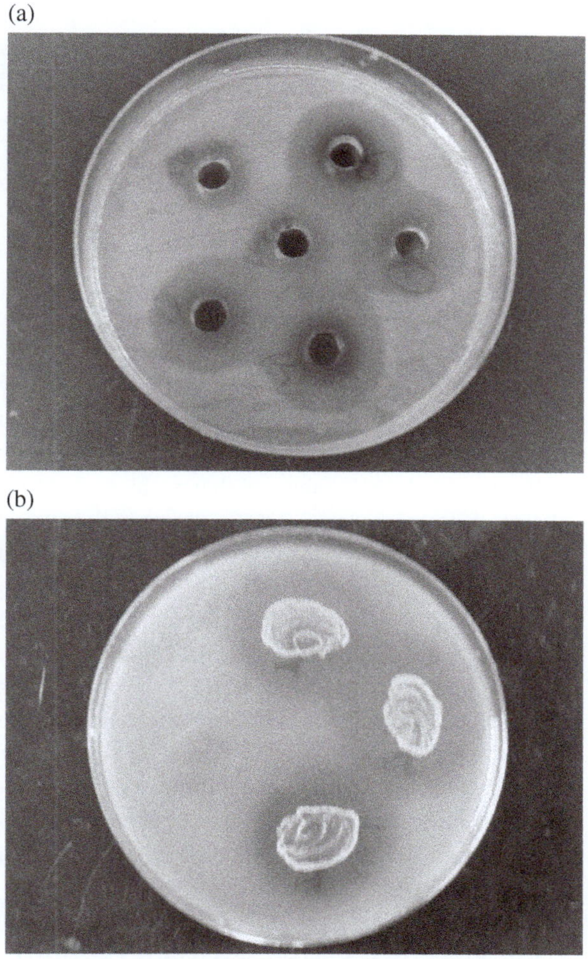

Figure 7.1 Antibacterial activity of probiotic bacteria. (a) Agar well method. (b) Spot-on lawn method.

contaminated in the field during harvesting and cutting and during storage. Mycotoxins causes serious health problems in humans and animals such as nephrotoxicity, hepatotoxicity, immunosuppression and carcinogenic effects (Bezerra *et al.* 2016). As with other toxicological diseases, mycotoxicity can be acute or chronic. Acute toxicity typically has a fast onset of symptoms and a direct toxic reaction, whereas chronic toxic effects are characterized by a long exposure that causes DNA damage and cancer. The three most common fungal genera, Penicillium, Fusarium and Aspergillus, are responsible for the production of mycotoxins in food and feed products Groopman *et al.* (2014). More than 200 different types of mycotoxins have been identified, while the most prominent mycotoxins found in food and feed products are aflatoxin, fumonisin, ochratoxin, zearalenone and trichothecenes (Zain 2011) According to current information obtained by in vitro (liquid medium and cell culture) and in vivo studies (animal and human studies) investigating the function or harmful impact of probiotic bacteria against mycotoxins, probiotics can have a role in prevention or restoration of chronic damage caused by mycotoxins.

It is concluded from different experiments performed on the interaction of probiotics with mycotoxins that the presence of a third factor can significantly affect the efficiency of this interaction such as the presence of epithelial cells in the lamina propria which separates the luminal fluid from internal tissue. Probiotics (*L. rhamnosus* GG, LGG) can reduce the transportation, metabolism and other harmful effects of aflatoxin in the cell. During cell line culture, it was observed that aflatoxin was reduced by about half when it moved from the apical to the basolateral chamber. During this experiment it was clearly observed that aflatoxin reduced the function of epithelial cells (Gratz *et al.* 2007). The same experiment was repeated by (Groopman *et al.* 2014). According to these researchers, with the addition of probiotics a reduction was found in the toxicity of aflatoxin against the epithelial cell. There were some DNA fragments found in the cells which interacted with the aflatoxin only used as a negative control, while these were absent in the cell that interacted with aflatoxin with addition of probiotics, thus it is observed that aflatoxin can affect the structure of DNA while probiotics can inhibit this harmful effect of mycotoxins. The results of Bezerra *et al.* (2016) showed that probiotic bacteria also have an impact on the harmful effects of deoxynivalenol (DON). These collective results demonstrated the key effect of LGG on preserving alkaline phosphatase activity, and therefore the segregation of Caco-2 cells was due to the specific binding of DON and the potentially minor role of unspecified bacterial interference. To elucidate the effect of mycotoxins on immune cells, Mechoud *et al.* (2012) used a specific probiotic, *L. reuteri*, in combination with ochratoxin, which has an effect on the immune system. As in the previous two experiments, when the researchers incubated the ochratoxin with immune cells, they found a clear reduction in the production of interferon and other interleukins. When they used the specific probiotic with the combination of ochratoxin and immune cells, after incubation they found that the effect of ochratoxin was significantly lessened by the probiotic. This experiment also showed that these toxins also have effects on the production of immune cell secretion such as chemotaxis.

7.2 Dual Interaction between Probiotics and Microbial Toxins

One criterion in the selection of a new probiotic strain for medical use is its protective impact and competitive exclusion during its activities in the gastrointestinal tract. It is widely unclear how probiotics impact the host in an advantageous way. The proposed mechanisms include reduction of the pH of the luminal contents, competition for niche and nutrients, antimicrobial release, inactivation of toxins and immune stimulation (Akbar *et al.* 2016; Kumaree *et al.* 2015; Salminen *et al.* 2010).

Host cell and bacterial communication elements include physical interaction between bacteria and epithelial cells of the host (Ohland and MacNaughton 2010). Each probiotic bacterium has its own target on every host cell where it can attach to the cell. Bacteria of the same group may have different impacts on the host cell, due to the attachment site on the cell. Single bacteria can behave differently as they attach to different attachment sites on the same cell. Variation occurring in the genome of any bacterium can change its function and lifestyle in a specific environment. Due to this variation, probiotics adapt to any environment and start responding accordingly to that environment (Timmerman *et al.* 2004).

Probiotic bacteria have the ability to adjust to tough conditions. These environmental changes cause stress and affect the activity of probiotics, but they can adapt to the environmental conditions and resume their normal activity. As discussed earlier, all the probiotics have important positive impacts on human health. These impacts are due to their mechanism of action. They enhance the immunity of the host cell by the production of some valuable compounds. They also change the pH of the gastrointestinal tract by converting available sugar compounds to a variety of organic acids, which alters the environment for other pathogenic bacteria. Probiotic bacteria engage with all the possible adhesion sites on the cell. When the receptor sites of the cell are blocked by probiotics, the chance of attachment of other bacteria is reduced. Other than these mechanisms, these bacteria also produce antibiotics called bacteriocins, which inhibit the growth of other bacteria (Salminen *et al.* 2010)

7.2.1 Clinical Trials

Human ethical research concerns do not allow the injection of toxins into humans for experiments to check the interaction of mycotoxins with probiotics. Humans and animals are however exposed to toxins, particularly mycotoxins, due to their presence in food commodities which are consumed on a daily basis. In a research study conducted in Egypt, El-Nezami *et al.* (2000) confirmed a reduction in levels of mycotoxins in humans by checking the feces of trial volunteers. A similar study conducted in rats by Gratz *et al.* (2004) also confirmed the reducing impact of probiotics on mycotoxins. In another animal study, *L. casei* L1 and *L. reuteri* L2 showed promising results in protection against oxidative stress when an aflatoxin B1 contaminated feed was given to 4-week-old rats (Hathout *et al.* 2011).

7.2.2 Types of Microbial Adsorbents for Mycotoxin Adsorption

7.2.2.1 Lactic Acid Bacteria

Lactic acid bacteria are considered the safest bacteria for humans as they have been used in dairy products and other foods for many years. They also contribute to the normal flora of human intestine, producing some important compounds that not only affect the growth of other bacteria but also boost the immune system in humans (Akbar *et al.* 2016; Settanni and Corsetti 2008). Different species of lactic acid bacteria have the ability to produce antagonistic compounds that control unwanted spoilage during the fermentation of food and bacterial growth (Akbar and Anal 2014). It is also reported that these bacteria produce antibacterial as well as antifungal compounds. The biodegradation properties of these bacteria are high as compared to other bacterial species. *Lactobacillus* species, *Bifidobacterium*, *Streptococcus* and *Lactococcus* are frequently used bacteria for the biocontrol of mycotoxins. They have been used for the biodegradation of mycotoxins in food and feed products. These bacteria not only degrade mycotoxins but also add some valuable products to the food and feed products that increase the value of those particular products (Akbar *et al.* 2016; Zendo 2013).

Other than biodegradation of mycotoxins, lactic acid bacteria have the ability to adsorb aflatoxin, as the cell wall facilitates the adsorption process of aflatoxin. *Streptococcus thermophiles*, usually present in milk, are widely used for adsorption (Settanni and Corsetti 2008). The ochratoxin adsorption ability of lactic acid bacteria has been reported, whereas biodegradation studies of ochratoxin with lactic acid bacteria are limited. More than 50 different species of lactic acid bacteria are used for adsorption. In in vitro experiments adsorption works best in a liquid medium, compared to a solid medium (Del Prete *et al.* 2007). Three different strains of lactic acid bacteria, *L. plantarum*, *L. brevis* and *L. sanfranciscensis*, were used in two different forms (living and inactive) and it was observed that the inactive forms had high activity (59.8%) as compared to living cells of the bacteria species. The cell wall binding properties are due to the hydrophobic and electron acceptor between the cell wall of inactive bacteria and the ochratoxin compound (Piotrowska 2014).

The elimination of three other mycotoxins, deoxynivalenol, fumonisins and zearalenone, was targeted with two bacterial strains, lactic acid and *Leuconostoc* bacteria. Both bacterial strains removed all three mycotoxins. The lactic acid bacteria remained highly efficient against all the mycotoxins as compared to the *Leuconostoc* strain (Niderkorn *et al.* 2007). *Lactobacillus casei* were found to reduce the concentration of DON. It has been shown that the activity of these bacteria is high in a liquid medium. Surface binding of mycotoxins with the cell wall of bacteria was identified as the mechanism of action of *Lactobacillus casei* (Sangsila *et al.* 2016). Another experiment (Taheur *et al.* 2017) was conducted on the reduction of mixed mycotoxins in food products. Milk with mycotoxins has been the subject of an experiment: *Lactobacillus* species such as kefir bacterial species (*Lactobacillus, Lactococcus, Streptococcus* and *Leuconostoc*), *Acetobacter* and *Kazachstania* spp. were used for the adsorption of the mycotoxins and the result showed that the kefir consortium had the highest efficiency for the adsorption and biotransformation of mycotoxins (Taheur *et al.* 2017).

7.3 Principles and Mechanisms Involved

The popular probiotic mechanisms of action can be divided into three main classes: gut microbial integration, adjustment of the immune response, and metabolic processes (Haukioja 2010). Three essential methods of probiotic activity have been described. The healthy native microflora limits the overgrowth of conceivably pathogenic flora in the gut. By hindering the ability of pathogens to grip, probiotics may directly affect various microorganisms. It has been reported that *Lactobacillus* species and *Bifidobacterium* repress a broad variety of colonizing pathogenic microscopic species by antagonistic actions against gastrointestinal microbes. In many cases, this principle is crucial for the prevention and treatment of contamination and the restoration of microbial harmony in the gut (Akbar *et al.* 2019; Karami *et al.* 2017).

The resultant system is characterized by the formation of antimicrobial agents, bacteriocins, organic acids and short-chain unsaturated fatty acids, and reduction of intestinal pH. All the formed compounds are responsible for disrupting the progress of other hazardous microbes such as foodborne microorganisms and other pathogens in the intestinal tract. The probiotic mechanism of effect is focused on microbial factors that evaluate a specific probiotic interaction and its feasible application for anticipation or medication of a particular disease by destruction of the target cell (Abatenh *et al.* 2018).

The third process is the stimulation of specific and non-specific T-cell defense and cytokine creation by boosting phagocytosis and IgA emission, adjusting T-cell responses, enhancing T helper type 1 reactions, and lowering Th2 responses (Karami 2017).

Almost all of the techniques by which microbes degrade toxins are a matter of great interest but are not very well established; some of them have been peer reviewed by researchers. Researchers have described the method of biodegradation of aflatoxin, with two sites, furofuran and the lactone ring, present on aflatoxin concerned for toxicity. Some microbes influence the stability of the two sites, which decreases the toxic effects of this toxin. It has also been revealed that aflatoxin can be degraded by attacking the coumarin molecules in the toxin. Bacterial species such as Rhodococcus, *Bacillus subtilis* and rumen fluid bacteria are the most frequently used biodegradation microbes. Biodegradation by these bacteria in food products such as milk, vegetable oil and maize has been demonstrated to be positive and highly healthy. Biodegradation is the best form of mycotoxin detoxification compared to physical and chemical detoxification (Khan *et al.* 2020).

Fungal species such as Mucor and *Gliocladium roseum* exhibit zearalenone (ZEA) detoxification capacity by converting the ZEA to ZEA-4-O-b-glucoside, a non-estrogenic product. Similarly, *Trichosporon mycotoxinivorans* has also been reported to degrade ZEA by breaking the ZEA macrocyclic ring at the C60 ketone group and converting it to hexanoic acid. Rhizopus species can also degrade ZEA completely. The hydroxyl group of DON may be oxidized and 3-keton-4-deoxynivalenol converted by any bacterial strain, which is less toxic than DON (Ji *et al.* 2016). Figure 7.2 shows the antifungal activities of lactic acid bacteria against fungi.

7.3.1 Control of Mycotoxins by Yeast

Yeasts may produce metabolites that have a significant suppressing effect on the expression of genes related to mycotoxin biosynthesis and inhibit the growth of filamentous fungi. The yeast *Pichia anomala* strain WRL-076 has been successfully tested for the reduction of aflatoxin contamination in tree nuts in California. It was reported that the strain produces a volatile compound identified as 2-phenylethanol, which can down regulate the gene responsible for aflatoxin production, resulting in a decrease in its production. It also affects other genes of *Aspergillus flavus* and alters the functionality of its sporing and growth (Hua *et al.* 2014).

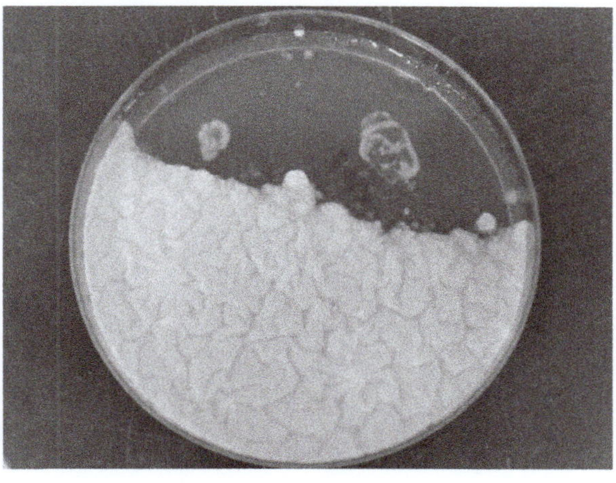

Figure 7.2 Antifungal activity of lactic acid bacteria against fungi.

The cell wall of yeast is able to adsorb many things from its environment. Viable cells, non-viable cells and cell wall products of probiotic yeasts with elevated adsorption capacity can reduce the bioactivity of toxins in foodstuffs. Yeast species are extremely diverse in their cell wall composition and, not surprisingly, in adsorption capacity. It has been reported that the cell wall components of yeast such as β-glucans, glucomannans and mannan-oligosaccharide help in mycotoxin adsorption. Aflatoxins, ZEA and ochratoxin have been usefully adsorbed using inactivated yeast and its cell wall components (Čolović *et al.* 2019). The ability to adsorb is dependent on both the yeast product and the mycotoxin shape. Toxin decontamination seems to be important for the structural integrity of the yeast cell wall, and non-viable cells (e.g. heat or acid treated) are typically more successful in their ability to adsorb. The beta-D-glucan content and its three-dimensional form in the cell wall have been shown to affect adsorption. Mycotoxin-detoxifying yeasts are known or are used as probiotics for livestock in the food and feed industry. There are also predictable and beneficial effects on organoleptic characteristics when decontaminated goods, such as wine, are intended for human consumption. (Petruzzi *et al.* 2015).

7.4 Conclusion and Future Prospects

Contamination by toxins of food and feed is a natural and common phenomenon. Different control methods have been applied for centuries with their associated pros and cons. Biological control is comparatively more acceptable for the application of toxin control by biodegradation and deactivation of active sites for the toxins using different microorganisms and their enzymes against particular toxins. The deployment of probiotic bacteria for this job has an edge over other microbes due to their human- and animal-friendly nature. Probiotic bacteria can safely be utilized against particular toxins as a protective culture in food and feed. The generally regarded as safe (GRAS) status of probiotics allows their use in food. The use of specific probiotics or consortia of probiotics against single and groups of toxins should now be the focus of research. This will help us to identify toxin-specific probiotics for toxin degradation and control in food and feed.

Acknowledgement

The authors acknowledge the financial support of ALP-PARC project No. AS 207 for this study.

References

Abatenh, E., Gizaw, B. and Tsegay, Z. (2018). Health benefits of probiotics. *J Bacteriol Infec Dis, 2018*, 2(1): 8–27.

Akbar, A. and Anal, A.K. (2014). Occurrence of Staphylococcus aureus and evaluation of anti-staphylococcal activity of Lactococcus lactis subsp. lactis in ready-to-eat poultry meat. *Annals of Microbiology*, 64(1): 131–138.

Akbar, A., Ali, I. and Anal, A.K. (2016). Industrial perspectives of lactic acid bacteria for biopreservation and food safety. *Journal of Animal & Plant Sciences*, 26(4).

Akbar, A., Sadiq, M.B., Ali, I., Anwar, M., Muhammad, N., Muhammad, J., Shafee, M., Ullah, S., Gul, Z., Qasim, S. and Ahmad, S. (2019). Lactococcus lactis subsp. lactis isolated from fermented milk products and its antimicrobial potential. *CyTA-Journal of Food*, 17(1): 214–220.

Bezerra, T.K.A., de Araujo, A.R.R., do Nascimento, E.S., de Matos Paz, J.E., Gadelha, C.A., Gadelha, T.S., Pacheco, M.T.B., do Egypto, R.D.C.R., de Oliveira, M.E.G. and Madruga, M.S. (2016). Proteolysis in goat "coalho" cheese supplemented with probiotic lactic acid bacteria. *Food Chemistry*, 196: 359–366.

Bordoloi, R. and Ganguly, S. (2014). Microbial toxin production: opportunists and true pathogens. *J Drug Metab Toxicol*, 5: e123.

Čolović, R., Puvača, N., Cheli, F., Avantaggiato, G., Greco, D., Đuragić, O., Kos, J. and Pinotti, L. (2019). Decontamination of mycotoxin-contaminated feedstuffs and compound feed. *Toxins*, 11(11): 617.

de Wit, P.J. (2013). Microbial toxins in the green world. *FEMS Microbiology Reviews*, 37(1): 1–2.

Del Prete, V., Rodriguez, H., Carrascosa, A.V., de las RIVAS, B.L.A.N.C.A., Garcia-Moruno, E. and Munoz, R. (2007). in vitro removal of ochratoxin A by wine lactic acid bacteria. *Journal of Food Protection*, 70(9): 2155–2160.

do Vale, A., Cabanes, D. and Sousa, S. (2016). Bacterial toxins as pathogen weapons against phagocytes. *Frontiers in Microbiology*, 7: 42.

Early, R. and Tamime, A.Y. (2017). Microbial toxins–an overview. *Microbial Toxins in Dairy Products*, 1.

El-Nezami, H., Mykkänen, H., Kankaanpää, P., Salminen, S. and Ahokas, J. (2000). Ability of Lactobacillus and Propionibacterium strains to remove aflatoxin B1 from the chicken duodenum. *Journal of Food Protection*, 63(4): 549–552.

Gratz, S., Mykkänen, H., Ouwehand, A.C., Juvonen, R., Salminen, S. and El-Nezami, H. (2004). Intestinal mucus alters the ability of probiotic bacteria to bind aflatoxin B1 in vitro. *Applied and Environmental Microbiology*, 70(10): 6306–6308.

Gratz, S., Wu, Q.K., El-Nezami, H., Juvonen, R.O., Mykkänen, H. and Turner, P.C. (2007). Lactobacillus rhamnosus strain GG reduces aflatoxin B1 transport, metabolism, and toxicity in Caco-2 cells. *Applied and Environmental Microbiology*, 73(12): 3958–3964.

Groopman, J.D., Egner, P.A., Schulze, K.J., Wu, L.S.F., Merrill, R., Mehra, S., Shamim, A.A., Ali, H., Shaikh, S., Gernand, A. and Khatry, S.K. (2014). Aflatoxin exposure during the first 1000 days of life in rural South Asia assessed by aflatoxin B1-lysine albumin biomarkers. *Food and Chemical Toxicology*, 74: 184–189.

Hardy, H., Harris, J., Lyon, E., Beal, J. and Foey, A.D. (2013). Probiotics, prebiotics and immunomodulation of gut mucosal defences: homeostasis and immunopathology. *Nutrients*, 5(6): 1869–1912.

Hathout, A.S., Mohamed, S.R., El-Nekeety, A.A., Hassan, N.S., Aly, S.E. and Abdel-Wahhab, M.A. (2011). Ability of Lactobacillus casei and Lactobacillus reuteri to protect against oxidative stress in rats fed aflatoxins-contaminated diet. *Toxicon*, 58(2): 179–186.

Haukioja, A. (2010). Probiotics and oral health. *European Journal of Dentistry*, 4(3): 348.

Hemaiswarya, S., Raja, R., Ravikumar, R. and Carvalho, I.S. (2013). Mechanism of action of probiotics. *Brazilian Archives of Biology and Technology*, 56(1): 113–119.

Hua, S.S.T., Beck, J.J., Sarreal, S.B.L. and Gee, W. (2014). The major volatile compound 2-phenylethanol from the biocontrol yeast, Pichia anomala, inhibits growth and expression of aflatoxin biosynthetic genes of Aspergillus flavus. *Mycotoxin Research*, 30(2): 71–78.

Ji, C., Fan, Y. and Zhao, L. (2016). Review on biological degradation of mycotoxins. *Animal Nutrition*, 2(3): 127–133.

Karami, A. (2017). Gaps in aquatic toxicological studies of microplastics. *Chemosphere*, 184: 841–848.

Karami, S., Roayaei, M., Hamzavi, H., Bahmani, M., Hassanzad-Azar, H., Leila, M. and Rafieian-Kopaei, M. (2017). Isolation and identification of probiotic Lactobacillus from local dairy and evaluating their antagonistic effect on pathogens. *International Journal of Pharmaceutical Investigation*, 7(3): 137.

Kataria, J., Li, N., Wynn, J.L. and Neu, J. (2009). Probiotic microbes: do they need to be alive to be beneficial? *Nutrition Reviews*, 67(9): 546–550.

Kechagia, M., Basoulis, D., Konstantopoulou, S., Dimitriadi, D., Gyftopoulou, K., Skarmoutsou, N. and Fakiri, E.M. (2013). Health benefits of probiotics: a review. *International Scholarly Research Notices*, 2013.

Khan, G.I., Akbar, A., Anwar, M., Shafee, M., Sadia, H., Razzaq, A. and Rehman, F.U. (2020). Eco-friendly bacterial biodegradation of mycotoxins. *Pure and Applied Biology*, 9(2): 1708–1717.

Koirala, S. and Anal, A.K. (2021). Probiotics-based foods and beverages as future foods and their overall safety and regulatory claims. *Future Foods*, 100013.

Kumaree, K.K., Akbar, A. and Anal, A.K. (2015). Bioencapsulation and application of Lactobacillus plantarum isolated from catfish gut as an antimicrobial agent and additive in fish feed pellets. *Annals of Microbiology*, 65(3): 1439–1445.

Lam, T.I., Tam, C.C., Stanker, L.H. and Cheng, L.W. (2016). Probiotic microorganisms inhibit epithelial cell internalization of botulinum neurotoxin serotype A. *Toxins*, 8(12): 377.

Mechoud, M.A., Juarez, G.E., de Valdez, G.F. and Rodriguez, A.V. (2012). Lactobacillus reuteri CRL 1098 and Lactobacillus acidophilus CRL 1014 differently reduce in vitro immunotoxic effect induced by Ochratoxin A. *Food and Chemical Toxicology*, 50(12): 4310–4315.

Niderkorn, V., Morgavi, D.P., Pujos, E., Tissandier, A. and Boudra, H. (2007). Screening of fermentative bacteria for their ability to bind and biotransform deoxynivalenol, zearalenone and fumonisins in an in vitro simulated corn silage model. *Food Additives and Contaminants*, 24(4): 406–415.

Oelschlaeger, T.A. (2010). Mechanisms of probiotic actions–a review. *International Journal of Medical Microbiology*, 300(1): 57–62.

Ohland, C.L. and MacNaughton, W.K. (2010). Probiotic bacteria and intestinal epithelial barrier function. *American Journal of Physiology-Gastrointestinal and Liver Physiology*, 298(6): G807–G819.

Petruzzi, L., Baiano, A., De Gianni, A., Sinigaglia, M., Corbo, M.R. and Bevilacqua, A. (2015). Differential adsorption of ochratoxin A and anthocyanins by inactivated yeasts and yeast cell walls during simulation of wine aging. *Toxins*, 7(10): 4350–4365.

Piotrowska, M. (2014). The adsorption of ochratoxin A by Lactobacillus species. *Toxins*, 6(9): 2826–2839.

Salminen, S., Nybom, S., Meriluoto, J., Collado, M.C., Vesterlund, S. and El-Nezami, H. (2010). Interaction of probiotics and pathogens—benefits to human health? *Current Opinion in Biotechnology*, 21(2): 157–167.

Sangsila, A., Faucet-Marquis, V., Pfohl-Leszkowicz, A. and Itsaranuwat, P. (2016). Detoxification of zearalenone by Lactobacillus pentosus strains. *Food Control*, 62: 187–192.

Settanni, L. and Corsetti, A. (2008). Application of bacteriocins in vegetable food biopreservation. *International Journal of Food Microbiology*, 121(2): 123–138.

Taheur, F.B., Fedhila, K., Chaieb, K., Kouidhi, B., Bakhrouf, A. and Abrunhosa, L. (2017). Adsorption of aflatoxin B1, zearalenone and ochratoxin A by microorganisms isolated from Kefir grains. *International Journal of Food Microbiology*, 251: 1–7.

Timmerman, H.M., Koning, C.J.M., Mulder, L., Rombouts, F.M. and Beynen, A.C. (2004). Monostrain, multistrain and multispecies probiotics—a comparison of functionality and efficacy. *International Journal of Food Microbiology*, 96(3): 219–233.

Vinderola, C.G. and Ritieni, A. (2014). Role of probiotics against mycotoxins and their deleterious effects. *Journal of Food Research*, 4: 10.5539/jfr.v4n1p10

Zain, M.E. (2011). Impact of mycotoxins on humans and animals. *Journal of Saudi Chemical Society*, 15(2): 129–144.

Zendo, T. (2013). Screening and characterization of novel bacteriocins from lactic acid bacteria. *Bioscience, Biotechnology, and Biochemistry*, 77(5): 893–899.

8

Potential of Probiotics as Alternative Sources for Antibiotics in Food Production Systems

Sarina Pradhan Thapa, Sushil Koirala and Anil Kumar Anal

Department of Food, Agriculture and Bioresources, School of Environment, Resources, and Development, Asian Institute of Technology, Pathumthani, Thailand

8.1 Introduction

The growing interest in a healthy lifestyle has prompted stakeholders in food systems to drive food safety as a major factor to ensure consumer safety. Numbers indicate that around 1 in 10 people fall ill every year due to the consumption of unsafe food, resulting in 420 000 fatalities (Thapa *et al.* 2020; WHO 2015). Today, foodborne illness has become one of the most serious public health problems around the world. In order to address this global challenge, the control of pathogenic microorganisms and other physical and chemical hazards in the "farm to fork" system is essential (Fung *et al.* 2018). The contamination of food can occur at any point in the food chain when proper measures and protocols are not followed, especially due to spoilage and pathogenic microorganisms (Akbar and Anal 2015). Hence, control measures have to be adhered to in order to ensure food safety (Anal *et al.* 2020). Conventional methods include the use of antibiotics, disinfectants and chemicals, which have done more harm than good such as the emergence of antimicrobial resistance (AMR), adverse effects on food systems, the environment and public health, low effectiveness and high cost (Anal 2019; Capita and Alonso-Calleja 2013; Fair and Tor 2014; Kraemer *et al.* 2019; Parsonage *et al.* 2017).

The unregulated use of antibiotics in the food supply chain continues to pose a global threat to public health. Antibiotics stop the growth of microorganisms and, in doing so, help to treat or prevent infections in humans and animals (Manyi-Loh *et al.* 2018). Since the discovery of penicillin in 1928, they have had a crucial role in human health by increasing life expectancy (Ventola 2015). In addition, it was discovered during the 1950s that a low-level dose of antibiotics in chicken feed had enormous production benefits. This strengthened the widespread use of antibiotics in animal feeds and replaced the cost-intensive treatment procedure, which resulted in almost 50% of all existing antibiotics are being used in veterinary applications (Hao *et al.* 2014). The global market of antimicrobial drugs was valued at USD 20.1 billion in 2010 and predicted to rise to USD 42.9 billion by

Probiotics, Prebiotics and Synbiotics: Technological Advancements Towards Safety and Industrial Applications, First Edition. Edited by Parmjit Singh Panesar and Anil Kumar Anal.

2025 (Fair and Tor 2014). The surge in the use of antibiotics is reflected in their benefits in increasing animal weight, efficiency of feed utilization and efficiency of reproduction, as well as decreasing morbidity and mortality. These benefits to animals and their producers are reflected in a decrease in the cost of the commodity to consumers. It has also been observed that almost half of the antibiotics used are not absorbed by animals and are thus released into the environment through feces, accumulating over a prolonged period of time and leaving residues (Chattopadhyay 2014; Marshall and Levy 2011). This is the consequence of the use of antibiotics as growth promoters and prophylactics, resulting in AMR. The impact of antibiotic residues on the ecosystem has been recognized as an international threat and significantly affects the food supply chain (Anal 2019). The importance of agricultural antibiotics as one of the reasons for the development and spread of antibiotic resistance is a matter of ongoing debate and controversy, with one prominent commentary asserting that "farming practices are largely to blame for the rise of antibiotic-resistant strains" (Thapa *et al.* 2020).

Numbers and data indicate alarming threats from antibiotic-resistant infections, which are responsible for more than half a million human deaths globally each year and this number is projected to reach 10 million in 2050 if the problem is not taken seriously worldwide. Having said that, the use of antibiotics in both humans and animals is projected to increase by 40% between now and 2030. The situation in developing countries is even worse (WHO 2020).

Developed countries are slowly phasing out antibiotics, investigating alternative strategies that are environmentally friendly and cost efficient. Probiotics are live beneficial microorganisms that confer positive effects on the human body when consumed in adequate amounts. The use of probiotics in treating animal infections in livestock agriculture has become more popular as indiscriminate use of antibiotics leads to the continuous emergence of new resistant strains of infectious diseases (Fair and Tor 2014; Hill *et al.* 2014; Manyi-Loh *et al.* 2018). Use of probiotics may help decrease the rate of development of antibiotic-resistant strains secondary to widespread and rampant antibiotic use. This prevents the transmission of the pathogens through food. As a result, probiotics have been postulated as an alternative approach to protect against pathogenic microorganisms for better healthcare and food safety (D'Orazio *et al.* 2015; Imperial and Ibana 2016; Kumaree *et al.* 2015; Muñoz-Atienza *et al.* 2013; Noomhorm *et al.* 2014; Ouwehand *et al.* 2016; Xiang *et al.* 2019).

8.2 Use of Antibiotics in the Food System

The World Health Organization (WHO) report on global surveillance of antibiotic resistance further points out the key linkages between use of antimicrobial drugs and resistance among pathogens (WHO 2014). The food chain is one of the key routes of entry of antibiotics into the human body. Antibiotic-resistant bacteria can enter the human body either by ingestion of food contaminated with antibiotics or plants treated with antibiotics (Figure 8.1). The WHO, the Food and Agriculture Organization of the United Nations (FAO) and the World Organization for Animal Health (OIE) consider AMR of zoonotic bacteria as a public health threat and recognize that resistance may be the consequence of

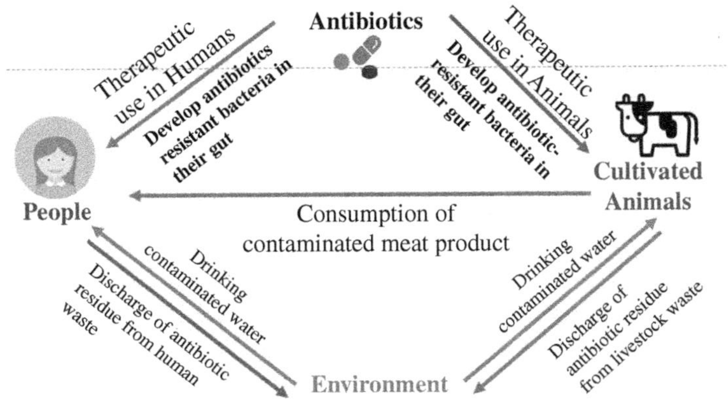

Figure 8.1 Occurrence and transmission of antibiotic resistance in bacteria via humans, animals and environment. *Source:* Thapa, S.P., Shrestha, S. and Anal, A.K. (2019). Addressing the antibiotic resistance and improving the food safety in food supply chain (farm-to-fork) in Southeast Asia. *Food Control*, 106809. doi:10.1016/j.foodcont.2019.106809.

the use of antibiotics in animal-derived food and may be transmitted to humans (Founou *et al.* 2016).

Antibiotics in animal feeds have been used to increase animal body weight and reproductive and feed utilization efficiency, and decrease morbidity and mortality. However, the relative impact of their application in food animals to human health is not well characterized (Marshall and Levy 2011). In plants, the use of antibiotics can be traced back to the nineteenth century in controlling bacterial diseases in fruit, vegetable and ornamental plants of high value. Among these, the most used are oxytetracycline and streptomycin, which are used to control fire blight in pears and apples and bacterial spot in peaches. Data published in 2009 in the United States show that 16 465 kg of active ingredients were applied to orchards, 0.12% of the total antibiotics used in animal husbandry (McManus *et al.* 2002). Animal manures contain high concentrations of residual antibiotics, which could disperse into agricultural soils and ultimately into the harvested vegetables. This poses a huge food safety risk, especially when consumers' eating preference is turning to eating raw salads (Cagri-Mehmetoglu 2018). Hence, rinsing, peeling or washing of such fruits and vegetables is highly recommended to reduce the residual impact of antibiotics along with control of pathogenic microorganisms (Bhilwadikar *et al.* 2019; Callejón *et al.* 2015; Herman *et al.* 2015; Olaimat and Holley 2012)

8.3 Classification and Mechanism of Use of Antibiotics

In order to reduce the indiscriminate use of antibiotics, the WHO has listed antimicrobials according to their importance in treating human health, in an effort to diminish the hazard of AMR (WHO 2017). The list includes critically important antimicrobials (CIAs: quinolones, macrolides and third- and fourth- generation cephalosporins), which are the antimicrobials of choice in treating *Salmonella* and *Campylobacter* infections. The use of

Table 8.1 Classification of antibiotics used in food animals.

Drug classification	Mode of action	Resistance mechanism	Reference
Sulfonamides, sulfadiazine	Bind and inhibit the enzyme responsible for synthesis of folate	Changes in dihydropteroate synthase (DHPS) enzyme Metabolic alteration	Sköld (2000)
Lincosamides, macrolides	Obstruct the formation of bacterial proteins	Modification of the ribosomal target by methylation or mutation and active efflux of the drug	Ungureanu (2010)
Tetracyclines	Prevent the production of bacterial protein	The ribosomal binding site and/or chromosomal mutations	Chopra and Roberts (2001)
Penicillin, β-lactamase sensitive, cephalosporins	Biosynthesis of the cell wall is blocked	Enzyme β-lactamase produced by bacteria causes hydrolysis of the antibiotic	Fernandes *et al.* (2013)
Quinolones, fluoroquinolones	Inhibition of DNA replication	Chromosomal mutation in the target enzyme DNA gyrase	Aldred *et al.* (2014)

Source: Adapted from Thapa, S.P., Shrestha, S. and Anal, A.K. (2019). Addressing the antibiotic resistance and improving the food safety in food supply chain (farm-to-fork) in Southeast Asia. *Food Control*, 106809. doi:10.1016/j.foodcont.2019.106809

antibiotics in food animals is classified as prophylactic and subtherapeutic (Table 8.1). Following the CIAs are the nine classes of antibiotics that are used during the lifecycle of food animals: (1) arsenicals, (2) polypeptides, (3) glycolipids, (4) tetracyclines, (5) elfamycins, (6) macrolides, (7) lincosamides, (8) polyethers, (9) β-lactams. The WHO, OIE and US Food and Drug Administration (FDA) stated that fluoroquinolones, third and fourth generation cephalosporins and macrolides were "critically important" antimicrobial agents (Scott *et al.* 2019).

Compared to animal use, the use of antibiotics in plants seems modest. Plant antibiotics are formulated in powder form with 17–20% active ingredient; solutions or suspensions with concentrations of 50–300 ppm are then applied in the form of mist. These are mainly used on high-value plants where the cost of the drug and its use can be compensated through the profits (Lillehoj *et al.* 2018). The most commonly used antibiotics in plants and animals are shown in Tables 8.1 and 8.2, respectively.

The commonly used antibiotics in plants, as shown in Table 8.2, are streptomycins, oxytetracyclines, gentamicins, oxolinic acid, penicillins and chloramphenicol.

8.4 Mechanism of Probiotic Action

According to the FAO and WHO, living microorganisms that provide benefit to the health of the human host when administered in suitable amounts are known as probiotics (Hill *et al.* 2014). Probiotics in food applications usually consist of lactic acid bacteria (LAB) (Kalhoro *et al.* 2019; Mathur *et al.* 2020). There are a few molds and yeasts that are also

Table 8.2 Classification of antibiotics used in plants adapted from different sources.

Drug classification	Mode of action	Resistance mechanism	Reference
Streptomycins	Inhibit the synthesis of protein by binding to the 30S ribosomal subunit	Chromosomal mutation, gene acquisition	Hyun *et al.* (2012)
Oxytetracyclines	Prevent the production of bacterial protein. Ribosomal translation is inhibited	Mutation within the binding sites of the ribosomes, chromosomal mutation	Chopra and Roberts (2001)
Gentamicins	Inhibition of translocation by binding to the 30S subunit of the bacterial RNA	Alterations in the ribosomal target, efflux pump activation	Garneau-Tsodikova and Labby (2016)
Oxolinic acid	Reversibly inhibit DNA synthesis	Efflux pump system is overexpressed. Mutation in DNA gyrase	Ruiz (2003)
Penicillins	Biosynthesis of the cell wall is blocked	Enzyme β-lactamase produced by bacteria causes hydrolysis of the antibiotic	Tenover (2006)
Chloramphenicol	Inhibits protein chain elongation	Inactivation of the enzyme, mutation of the target site	Fernández *et al.* (2012)

Source: Adapted from Thapa, S.P., Shrestha, S. and Anal, A K. (2019). Addressing the antibiotic resistance and improving the food safety in food supply chain (farm-to-fork) in Southeast Asia. *Food Control*, 106809. doi:10.1016/j.foodcont.2019.106809

being used as probiotics. Genera commonly used as probiotics include the bacteria *Lactobacillus, Bifidobacterium, Lactococcus, Carnobacterium, Enterococcus, Streptococcus, Pediococcus, Propionibacterium, Leuconostoc* and *Bacillus* species, *Saccharomyces* yeasts, and *Aspergillus* molds (Fijan 2014; Sornplang and Piyadeatsoontorn 2016).

Probiotics can be yeast or bacteria in live culture, heat treated or inactivated culture, or fermentation end-products as a result of incubation. In addition to this, for a probiotic to be designated for use in a food application, it has to be beneficial and safe to the host, capable of surviving the human gut environment such as low pH of the stomach, bile and organic acid and enzymes present in the intestines. Lastly, it should be stable under field conditions (Koirala and Anal 2021). A schematic representation for the qualification of a probiotic strain is shown in Figure 8.2.

Adhesion to the gut surface and colonization is an important prerequisite for probiotics, one that would facilitate the functional role of probiotics. Reduction of luminal pH, competitive inhibition against pathogens for adhesion sites and nutrition, production of antimicrobial substances, immunomodulation and toxin inactivation are some of the well-known mechanisms by which probiotics exert health benefits (do Carmo *et al.* 2020; Monteagudo-Mera *et al.* 2019; Plaza-Diaz *et al.* 2012, 2019; Yaqoob 2014). Furthermore, probiotics exerts other beneficial effects by enhancing the bioavailability of nutrients, stimulating food digestion, reducing the allergic response, reducing cholesterol, quorum sensing and contributing to reducing lactose intolerance. The production of antimicrobial

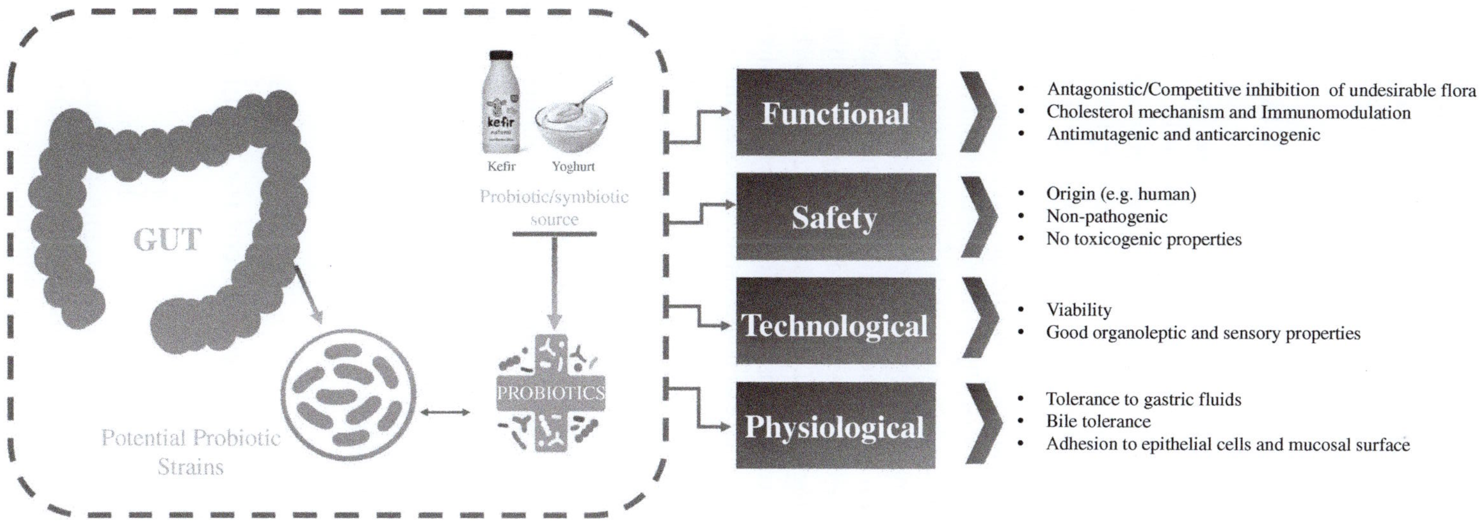

Figure 8.2 Criteria for selection of probiotic strains.

compounds, such as short chain fatty acids, hydrogen peroxide, nitric oxide and bacteriocins, has been proven to enhance the ability of probiotics to combat pathogens in the gastrointestinal tract (Bermudez-Brito *et al.* 2012; Brown 2011; Chapman *et al.* 2011; Goudarzi *et al.* 2014; Hemaiswarya *et al.* 2013; Kechagia *et al.* 2013; Syngai *et al.* 2016).

8.5 Probiotic Approach to Antibiotic Resistance

Good hygiene practices, feeding, transport prior to slaughter, and animal husbandry remain the conventional approach to prevent antibiotic resistance (Hedman *et al.* 2020). An innovative integrated approach by feeding probiotic supplements, maintaining a healthy intestinal ecosystem to improve food safety from farm to fork, is highly encouraged. By their nature, probiotics are an effective intervention strategy in preventing occurrence of zoonotic diseases, on a par with antibiotics (Ouwehand *et al.* 2016).

Probiotics are good bacteria whose significance is increasing as more and more studies prove their efficacy in vivo, especially in the prevention and treatment of cystic fibrosis, various cancers, urogenital infections, dental caries, periodontal diseases, irritable bowel syndrome (IBS) and oral malodor. Probiotics can help to restore beneficial bacteria when they are lost due to illness or treatment by antibiotics. In a nutshell, they help to balance beneficial and harmful bacteria to keep our body working like it should (Akbar *et al.,*, 2019; Gueimonde *et al.* 2013; Hempel *et al.* 2012; Macfarlane 2014; Ouwehand *et al.* 2014).

The cause of antibiotic resistance is the ability of bacteria to evolve via several biochemical aspects and spread resistance to non-resistant microbes. In a study by Alakomi *et al.* (2006), lactobacilli demonstrated susceptibility against the antimicrobial agents with an increase in the production of lactic acid. However, the supernatants of lactobacilli did not show any differences in minimal inhibitory concentration (MIC) values against the tested antibiotics (ampicillin, clavulanic acid and co-trimoxazole) for the *E. coli* isolates (Naderi *et al.* 2014). This study did not show any positive effect of probiotics against antibiotics, but the sensitivity of the results may have been affected by strain-dependent characteristics. In another study by Tannock *et al.* (2011), probiotic *E. coli* Nissle 1917 was evaluated for its ability to exclude quinolone-resistant *E. coli*. However, the study did not report such exclusion of the strains in the feces of elderly carriers during therapy as compared to placebo. However, the probiotic strains did not acquire any resistance during this randomized controlled trial. These observations show the uncertainty over whether probiotics can prevent or treat multidrug resistance.

8.6 Probiotics as Alternative Sources for Antibiotics: What Is Known So Far

The bacteriocins produced by probiotics can disrupt biofilms and decrease the amount of pathogenic bacteria at mucosal sites (Hills *et al.* 2019; Reid 2006). The reduction of pathogens and opportunistic microbes at the mucosal site can be supported by the administered probiotics by improving mucosal immunity. With the addition of probiotics, this can result in the eradication of the pathogenic organisms (Lin *et al.* 2015). Having said that, the real

Table 8.3 in vivo and ex vivo studies reporting the antimicrobial activity of probiotics.

Probiotic	Objective	Conclusion	Reference
Lactobacillus rhamnosus LGG	Milk fermented with LGG and placebo was administered to 281 children who attended day care centers	The risk of upper respiratory tract infections in children can be decreased by the administration of LGG	Hojsak *et al.* (2010)
Lactobacillus casei	in vivo study conducted in a murine model to compare the benefits of *L. casei*, a probiotic, alone and also in combination with antiprotozoal drugs against giardiasis	Oral administration of the combination therapy reduced *Giardia* infection significantly, proving that a blended approach can be a more effective therapy for recovery from gastrointestinal diseases	Shukla *et al.* (2013)
Bifidobacterium bifidum, *Lactobacillus acidophilus* HS101 and *Lactobacillus rhamnosus* HS111	A double-blind randomized study was conducted on 59 elderly denture wearers with *Candida* spp. in the oral cavity but without clinical symptoms	The combination of probiotic formulation was effective in decreasing *Candida* spp. in individuals	Ishikawa *et al.* (2015)
Bifidobacterium animalis subsp. *Lactis*	Yoghurt supplemented with *B. animalis,* a probiotic, was used for a periodontal health trial with 51 patients for 4 weeks. Randomized controlled study	A positive effect was seen with the use of yoghurt supplemented with *B. animalis* against the growth of bacterial plaque and other gingival inflammatory parameters	Kuru *et al.* (2017)
Lactobacillus paracasei	in vivo study. *G. mellonella* larvae infested with a toxic dose of *C. albicans* were inoculated with *L. paracasei* to treat *C. albicans* infection	*L. paracasei* was able to modulate the immune system of *G. mellonella* and protect against candidiasis	Rossoni *et al.* (2017)
Lactobacillus reuteri DSM 17938	*L. reuteri* was used to reduce inflammation in an ex vivo skin model, and in vitro to study the antimicrobial activity against the infectious agent on the skin	The probiotic was seen to reduce the inflammatory process and it also showed antimicrobial action against *S. aureus, Cutibacterium acnes, P. aeruginosa* and *S. pyogenes*	Khmaladze *et al.* (2019)

in vivo effect of probiotics in prevention of antibiotic-resistant infections has not been established yet, though major clinical agencies such as the US Centers for Disease Control and Prevention (CDC) have actively been doing the research (Corr *et al.* 2007). There is no conclusive evidence so far to elucidate the benefits and specific recommendations. Thus, with limited data and real-life applications, probiotics are a parallel treatment process to adjunct antibiotic infections. Although antibiotic resistance studies are limited to medical applications, it is important to increase our research on food animal production as well as aquaculture. The resistance genes are often mobile genetic elements and their pathway to the entire food ecosystem must be understood to make a correlation and apply intervention strategies. By doing so we can understand the resistance ecology, and targeted interventions to reduce the emergence, evolution and spread of antibiotic resistance will be more effective. Table 8.3 shows some of the studies reporting the antimicrobial activity of probiotics, hence enhancing their potential as an alternative source of antibiotics.

8.7 Conclusion and Future Prospects

Antimicrobial resistance presents a global public threat due to the rampant and uncontrolled use of antibiotics resulting in the emergence of resistant strains. Bacteria develop antibiotic resistance through several mechanisms and the genes are transferred to non-resistant bacteria through the DNA. The use of antibiotics in feed presents an indirect pathway for AMR in the food chain and thus poses a food safety threat. While conventional approaches using good animal husbandry are still in practice, probiotic application presents an innovative and sustainable solution as more studies prove its efficacy. Probiotics, through their production of bacteriocins and short chain fatty acids, limit the growth and survival of opportunistic and pathogenic bacteria and thus help to prevent antibiotic-resistant related infections. Thus, the application of probiotics as a potential alternative source in the feed and food chain will improve public health and we expect that the spread of antibiotic resistance might be reduced.

References

Akbar, A. and Anal, A.K. (2015). Isolation of Salmonella from ready-to-eat poultry meat and evaluation of its survival at low temperature, microwaving and simulated gastric fluids. *Journal of Food Science and Technology*, 52(5): 3051–3057.

Akbar, A., Sadiq, M.B., Ali, I., Anwar, M., Muhammad, N., Muhammad, J., Shafee, M., Ullah, S., Gul, Z. and Qasim, S. (2019). Lactococcus lactis subsp. lactis isolated from fermented milk products and its antimicrobial potential. *CyTA-Journal of Food*, 17(1): 214–220.

Alakomi, H.-L., Paananen, A., Suihko, M.-L., Helander, I. and Saarela, M. (2006). Weakening effect of cell permeabilizers on gram-negative bacteria causing biodeterioration. *Applied and Environmental Microbiology*, 72(7): 4695–4703.

Aldred, K.J., Kerns, R.J. and Osheroff, N. (2014). Mechanism of quinolone action and resistance. *Biochemistry*, 53(10): 1565–1574.

Anal, A.K. (2019). Quality ingredients and safety concerns for traditional fermented foods and beverages from Asia: A review. *Fermentation*, 5(1): 8.

Anal, A.K., Perpetuini, G., Petchkongkaew, A., Tan, R., Avallone, S., Tofalo, R., Van Nguyen, H., Chu-Ky, S., Ho, P.H. and Phan, T.T. (2020). Food safety risks in traditional fermented food from South-East Asia. *Food Control*, 109: 106922.

Bermudez-Brito, M., Plaza-Díaz, J., Muñoz-Quezada, S., Gómez-Llorente, C. and Gil, A. (2012). Probiotic mechanisms of action. *Annals of Nutrition and Metabolism*, 61(2): 160–174.

Bhilwadikar, T., Pounraj, S., Manivannan, S., Rastogi, N. and Negi, P. (2019). Decontamination of microorganisms and pesticides from fresh fruits and vegetables: A comprehensive review from common household processes to modern techniques. *Comprehensive Reviews in Food Science and Food Safety*, 18(4): 1003–1038.

Brown, M. (2011). Modes of action of probiotics: recent developments. *Journal of Animal and Veterinary Advances*, 10(14): 1895–1900.

Cagri-Mehmetoglu, A. (2018). Food safety challenges associated with traditional foods of Turkey. *Food Science and Technology*, 38(1): 1–12.

Callejón, R.M., Rodríguez-Naranjo, M.I., Ubeda, C., Hornedo-Ortega, R., Garcia-Parrilla, M.C. and Troncoso, A.M. (2015). Reported foodborne outbreaks due to fresh produce in the United States and European Union: trends and causes. *Foodborne Pathogens and Disease*, 12(1): 32–38.

Capita, R. and Alonso-Calleja, C. (2013). Antibiotic-resistant bacteria: a challenge for the food industry. *Critical Reviews in Food Science and Nutrition*, 53(1): 11–48.

Chapman, C., Gibson, G.R. and Rowland, I. (2011). Health benefits of probiotics: are mixtures more effective than single strains? *European Journal of Nutrition*, 50(1): 1–17.

Chattopadhyay, M.K. (2014). Use of antibiotics as feed additives: a burning question. *Frontiers in Microbiology*, 5: 334.

Chopra, I. and Roberts, M. (2001). Tetracycline antibiotics: mode of action, applications, molecular biology, and epidemiology of bacterial resistance. *Microbiology and Molecular Biology Reviews*, 65(2): 232–260.

Corr, S.C., Li, Y., Riedel, C.U., O'Toole, P.W., Hill, C. and Gahan, C.G. (2007). Bacteriocin production as a mechanism for the antiinfective activity of Lactobacillus salivarius UCC118. *Proceedings of the National Academy of Sciences*, 104(18): 7617–7621.

D'Orazio, G., Di Gennaro, P., Boccarusso, M., Presti, I., Bizzaro, G., Giardina, S., Michelotti, A., Labra, M. and La Ferla, B. (2015). Microencapsulation of new probiotic formulations for gastrointestinal delivery: in vitro study to assess viability and biological properties. *Applied Microbiology and Biotechnology*, 99(22): 9779–9789.

do Carmo, M.C.L., Martins, I.M., de Paula Menezes Barbosa, P., Macedo, G.A. and Macedo, J.A. (2020). Passiflora edulis extract effects on probiotic and pathogenic modulation for healthier microbiota. *Nutrire*, 45: 1–8.

Fair, R.J. and Tor, Y. (2014). Antibiotics and bacterial resistance in the 21st century. *Perspectives in Medicinal Chemistry*, 6: PMC. S14459.

Fernandes, R., Amador, P. and Prudêncio, C. (2013). β-Lactams: chemical structure, mode of action and mechanisms of resistance. *Reviews in Medical Microbiology*, 24(1): 7–17.

Fernández, M., Conde, S., de la Torre, J., Molina-Santiago, C., Ramos, J.-L. and Duque, E. (2012). Mechanisms of resistance to chloramphenicol in Pseudomonas putida KT2440. *Antimicrobial Agents and Chemotherapy*, 56(2): 1001–1009.

Fijan, S. (2014). Microorganisms with claimed probiotic properties: an overview of recent literature. *International Journal of Environmental Research and Public Health*, 11(5): 4745–4767.

Founou, L.L., Founou, R.C. and Essack, S.Y. (2016). Antibiotic resistance in the food chain: a developing country-perspective. *Frontiers in Microbiology*, 7: 1881.

Fung, F., Wang, H.-S. and Menon, S. (2018). Food safety in the 21st century. *Biomedical Journal*, 41(2): 88–95.

Garneau-Tsodikova, S. and Labby, K.J. (2016). Mechanisms of resistance to aminoglycoside antibiotics: overview and perspectives. *Medchemcomm*, 7(1): 11–27.

Goudarzi, M., Goudarzi, H. and Rashidan, M. (2014). Probiotics: an update on mechanisms of action and clinical applications. *Novelty in Biomedicine*, 2(1): 22–30.

Gueimonde, M., Sánchez, B., de Los Reyes-Gavilán, C.G. and Margolles, A. (2013). Antibiotic resistance in probiotic bacteria. *Frontiers in Microbiology*, 4: 202.

Hao, H., Cheng, G., Iqbal, Z., Ai, X., Hussain, H. I., Huang, L., Dai, M., Wang, Y., Liu, Z. and Yuan, Z. (2014). Benefits and risks of antimicrobial use in food-producing animals. *Frontiers in Microbiology*, 5: 288.

Hedman, H.D., Vasco, K.A. and Zhang, L. (2020). A review of antimicrobial resistance in poultry farming within low-resource settings. *Animals*, 10(8): 1264.

Hemaiswarya, S., Raja, R., Ravikumar, R. and Carvalho, I.S. (2013). Mechanism of action of probiotics. *Brazilian Archives of Biology and Technology*, 56(1): 113–119.

Hempel, S., Newberry, S.J., Maher, A.R., Wang, Z., Miles, J.N., Shanman, R., Johnsen, B. and Shekelle, P.G. (2012). Probiotics for the prevention and treatment of antibiotic-associated diarrhea: a systematic review and meta-analysis. *Jama*, 307(18): 1959–1969.

Herman, K., Hall, A. and Gould, L. (2015). Outbreaks attributed to fresh leafy vegetables, United States, 1973–2012. *Epidemiology & Infection*, 143(14): 3011–3021.

Hill, C., Guarner, F., Reid, G., Gibson, G.R., Merenstein, D.J., Pot, B., Morelli, L., Canani, R.B., Flint, H.J. and Salminen, S. (2014). Expert consensus document: The International Scientific Association for Probiotics and Prebiotics consensus statement on the scope and appropriate use of the term probiotic. *Nature Reviews Gastroenterology & Hepatology*, 11(8): 506.

Hills, R.D., Pontefract, B.A., Mishcon, H.R., Black, C.A., Sutton, S.C. and Theberge, C.R. (2019). Gut microbiome: profound implications for diet and disease. *Nutrients*, 11(7): 1613.

Hojsak, I., Snovak, N., Abdović, S., Szajewska, H., Mišak, Z. and Kolaček, S. (2010). Lactobacillus GG in the prevention of gastrointestinal and respiratory tract infections in children who attend day care centers: a randomized, double-blind, placebo-controlled trial. *Clinical Nutrition*, 29(3): 312–316.

Hyun, J.-W., Kim, H.-J., Yi, P.-H., Hwang, R.-Y. and Park, E.-W. (2012). Mode of action of streptomycin resistance in the citrus canker pathogen (Xanthomonas smithii subsp. citri) in Jeju Island. *Plant Pathol J*, 28(2): 207–211.

Imperial, I.C. and Ibana, J.A. (2016). Addressing the antibiotic resistance problem with probiotics: reducing the risk of its double-edged sword effect. *Frontiers in Microbiology*, 7: 1983.

Ishikawa, K.H., Mayer, M.P., Miyazima, T.Y., Matsubara, V.H., Silva, E.G., Paula, C.R., Campos, T.T. and Nakamae, A.E. (2015). A multispecies probiotic reduces oral Candida colonization in denture wearers. *Journal of Prosthodontics*, 24(3): 194–199.

Kalhoro, M.S., Visessanguan, W., Nguyen, L.T. and Anal, A.K. (2019). Probiotic potential of Lactobacillus paraplantarum BT-11 isolated from raw buffalo (Bubalus bubalis) milk and characterization of bacteriocin-like inhibitory substance produced. *Journal of Food Processing and Preservation*, 43(8): e14015.

Kechagia, M., Basoulis, D., Konstantopoulou, S., Dimitriadi, D., Gyftopoulou, K., Skarmoutsou, N. and Fakiri, E.M. (2013). Health benefits of probiotics: a review. *International Scholarly Research Notices*, 2013.

Khmaladze, I., Butler, É., Fabre, S. and Gillbro, J.M. (2019). Lactobacillus reuteri DSM 17938—A comparative study on the effect of probiotics and lysates on human skin. *Experimental Dermatology*, 28(7): 822–828.

Koirala, S. and Anal, A.K. (2021). Probiotics-based foods and beverages as future foods and their overall safety and regulatory claims. *Future Foods*: 100013.

Kraemer, S.A., Ramachandran, A. and Perron, G.G. (2019). Antibiotic pollution in the environment: from microbial ecology to public policy. *Microorganisms*, 7(6): 180.

Kumaree, K.K., Akbar, A. and Anal, A.K. (2015). Bioencapsulation and application of Lactobacillus plantarum isolated from catfish gut as an antimicrobial agent and additive in fish feed pellets. *Annals of Microbiology*, 65(3): 1439–1445.

Kuru, B.E., Laleman, I., Yalnızoğlu, T., Kuru, L. and Teughels, W. (2017). The influence of a Bifidobacterium animalis probiotic on gingival health: a randomized controlled clinical trial. *Journal of Periodontology*, 88(11): 1115–1123.

Lillehoj, H., Liu, Y., Calsamiglia, S., Fernandez-Miyakawa, M.E., Chi, F., Cravens, R.L., Oh, S. and Gay, C.G. (2018). Phytochemicals as antibiotic alternatives to promote growth and enhance host health. *Veterinary Research*, 49(1): 1–18.

Lin, X., Chen, X., Chen, Y., Jiang, W. and Chen, H. (2015). The effect of five probiotic lactobacilli strains on the growth and biofilm formation of S treptococcus mutans. *Oral Diseases*, 21(1): e128–e134.

Macfarlane, S. (2014). Antibiotic treatments and microbes in the gut. *Environmental Microbiology*, 16(4): 919–924.

Manyi-Loh, C., Mamphweli, S., Meyer, E. and Okoh, A. (2018). Antibiotic use in agriculture and its consequential resistance in environmental sources: potential public health implications. *Molecules*, 23(4): 795.

Marshall, B.M. and Levy, S.B. (2011). Food animals and antimicrobials: impacts on human health. *Clinical Microbiology Reviews*, 24(4): 718–733.

Mathur, H., Beresford, T.P. and Cotter, P.D. (2020). Health benefits of lactic acid bacteria (LAB) fermentates. *Nutrients*, 12(6): 1679.

McManus, P.S., Stockwell, V.O., Sundin, G.W. and Jones, A.L. (2002). Antibiotic use in plant agriculture. *Annual Review of Phytopathology*, 40(1): 443–465.

Monteagudo-Mera, A., Rastall, R.A., Gibson, G.R., Charalampopoulos, D. and Chatzifragkou, A. (2019). Adhesion mechanisms mediated by probiotics and prebiotics and their potential impact on human health. *Applied Microbiology and Biotechnology*, 103(16): 6463–6472.

Muñoz-Atienza, E., Gómez-Sala, B., Araújo, C., Campanero, C., Del Campo, R., Hernández, P.E., Herranz, C. and Cintas, L.M. (2013). Antimicrobial activity, antibiotic susceptibility and virulence factors of lactic acid bacteria of aquatic origin intended for use as probiotics in aquaculture. *BMC Microbiology*, 13(1): 1–22.

Naderi, A., Kasra-Kermanshahi, R., Gharavi, S., Fooladi, A.A.I., Alitappeh, M.A. and Saffarian, P. (2014). Study of antagonistic effects of Lactobacillus strains as probiotics on multi drug resistant (MDR) bacteria isolated from urinary tract infections (UTIs). *Iranian Journal of Basic Medical Sciences*, 17(3): 201.

Noomhorm, A., Ahmad, I. and Anal, A.K. (2014). *Functional Foods and Dietary Supplements: Processing Effects and Health Benefits*. John Wiley & Sons.

Olaimat, A.N. and Holley, R.A. (2012). Factors influencing the microbial safety of fresh produce: a review. *Food Microbiology*, 32(1): 1–19.

Ouwehand, A.C., DongLian, C., Weijian, X., Stewart, M., Ni, J., Stewart, T. and Miller, L.E. (2014). Probiotics reduce symptoms of antibiotic use in a hospital setting: a randomized dose response study. *Vaccine*, 32(4): 458–463.

Ouwehand, A.C., Forssten, S., Hibberd, A.A., Lyra, A. and Stahl, B. (2016). Probiotic approach to prevent antibiotic resistance. *Annals of Medicine*, 48(4): 246–255.

Parsonage, B., Hagglund, P.K., Keogh, L., Wheelhouse, N., Brown, R.E. and Dancer, S.J. (2017). Control of antimicrobial resistance requires an ethical approach. *Frontiers in Microbiology*, 8: 2124.

Plaza-Diaz, J., Muñoz-Quezada, S., Gomez-Llorente, C. and Gil, A. (2012). Probiotic mechanisms of action. *Ann Nutr Metab*, 61: 160–174.

Plaza-Diaz, J., Ruiz-Ojeda, F.J., Gil-Campos, M. and Gil, A. (2019). Mechanisms of action of probiotics. *Advances in Nutrition*, 10(suppl_1): S49–S66.

Reid, G. (2006). Probiotics to prevent the need for, and augment the use of, antibiotics. *Canadian Journal of Infectious Diseases and Medical Microbiology*, 17(5): 291–295.

Rossoni, R.D., Fuchs, B.B., De Barros, P.P., Velloso, M.d.S., Jorge, A.O.C., Junqueira, J.C. and Mylonakis, E. (2017). Lactobacillus paracasei modulates the immune system of Galleria mellonella and protects against Candida albicans infection. *PLoS ONE*, 12(3): e0173332.

Ruiz, J. (2003). Mechanisms of resistance to quinolones: target alterations, decreased accumulation and DNA gyrase protection. *Journal of Antimicrobial Chemotherapy*, 51(5): 1109–1117.

Scott, H.M., Acuff, G., Bergeron, G., Bourassa, M.W., Gill, J., Graham, D.W., Kahn, L.H., Morley, P.S., Salois, M.J. and Simjee, S. (2019). Critically important antibiotics: criteria and approaches for measuring and reducing their use in food animal agriculture. *Annals of the New York Academy of Sciences*, 1441(1): 8.

Shukla, G. Kaur, H. and Sharma, L. (2013). Comparative therapeutic effect of probiotic Lactobacillus casei alone and in conjunction with antiprotozoal drugs in murine giardiasis. *Parasitology Research*, 112(6): 2143–2149.

Sköld, O. (2000). Sulfonamide resistance: mechanisms and trends. *Drug Resistance Updates*, 3(3): 155–160.

Sornplang, P. and Piyadeatsoontorn, S. (2016). Probiotic isolates from unconventional sources: a review. *Journal of Animal Science and Technology*, 58(1): 1–11.

Syngai, G.G., Gopi, R., Bharali, R., Dey, S., Lakshmanan, G.A. and Ahmed, G. (2016). Probiotics-the versatile functional food ingredients. *Journal of Food Science and Technology*, 53(2): 921–933.

Tannock, G.W., Tiong, S., Priest, P., Munro, K., Taylor, C., Richardson, A. and Schultz, M. (2011). Testing probiotic strain Escherichia coli Nissle 1917 (Mutaflor) for its ability to reduce carriage of multidrug-resistant E. coli by elderly residents in long-term care facilities. *Journal of Medical Microbiology*, 60(3): 366–370.

Tenover, F.C. (2006). Mechanisms of antimicrobial resistance in bacteria. *The American Journal of Medicine*, 119(6): S3–S10.

Thapa, S.P., Shrestha, S. and Anal, A.K. (2020). Addressing the antibiotic resistance and improving the food safety in food supply chain (farm-to-fork) in Southeast Asia. *Food Control*, 108: 106809.

Ungureanu, V. (2010). Macrolides, lincosamides, streptogramines (MLS): mechanisms of action and resistance. *Bacteriologia, Virusologia, Parazitologia, Epidemiologia (Bucharest, Romania: 1990)*, 55(2): 131–138.

Ventola, C.L. (2015). The antibiotic resistance crisis: part 1: causes and threats. *Pharmacy and therapeutics*, 40(4): 277.

WHO (2014). Antimicrobial Resistance: Global Report on Surveillance. World Health Organization. https://apps.who.int/iris/bitstream/handle/10665/112642/9789241564748_eng.pdf?sequence=1 (accessed 26 January 2021).

WHO (2015). Global Action Plan on Antimicrobial Resistance. https://www.who.int/antimicrobial-resistance/publications/global-action-plan/en/ ().

WHO (2017). *WHO publishes list of bacteria for which new antibiotics are urgently needed.* https://www.who.int/news/item/27-02-2017-who-publishes-list-of-bacteria-for-which-new-antibiotics-are-urgently-needed (accessed 26 January 2021).

WHO (2020). *New report calls for urgent action to avert antimicrobial resistance crisis.* Retrieved 26 January 2021 from https://www.who.int/news/item/29-04-2019-new-report-calls-for-urgent-action-to-avert-antimicrobial-resistance-crisis (accessed 26 January 2021).

Xiang, H., Sun-Waterhouse, D., Waterhouse, G.I., Cui, C. and Ruan, Z. (2019). Fermentation-enabled wellness foods: A fresh perspective. *Food Science and Human Wellness*, 8(3): 203–243.

Yaqoob, P. (2014). Ageing, immunity and influenza: a role for probiotics? *Proceedings of the Nutrition Society*, 73(2): 309–317.

9

Probiotic Cereal-based Food and Beverages, their Production and Health Benefits

Sujitta Raungrusmee[1], *Simmi Ranjan Kumar*[2] *and Anil Kumar Anal*[2]

[1] *Program in Food, Nutrition and Dietetics, Department of Home Economics, Faculty of Agriculture, Kasetsart University, Bangkok, Thailand*
[2] *Food Engineering and Bioprocess Technology, Department of Food Agriculture and Bioresources, School of Environment and Resources, Asian Institute of Technology, Pathumthani, Thailand*

9.1 Introduction

Consumers embrace healthy, nutritious food that prevents disease with broader health benefits because of changes in food habits, living standards and health awareness. They are conscious of the vital role of food in welfare and prolongation of life, and laterally it helps in the prevention of non-communicable diseases. Due to consumers' increasing demands for healthy and nutritious food, the industry is also developing new functional products with nutraceutical properties (Anal 2019; Koirala and Anal 2021). Cereals are significant food sources, contributing nutrition for millions of years, and fermented food products from cereals are broadly beneficial to health. Moreover, cereal-based foods are an essential source of micronutrients, protein, fiber, energy and carbohydrates (El-Aidie *et al.* 2017). For functional food development, whole grains perform an essential role due to the many phytoestrogens, phytochemicals, phytic acids, phenolic compounds, antioxidants and sterols they contain. These whole grains also help the development of microorganisms such as lactic acid bacteria, providing hydrolytic enzymes and water (Mridula and Sharma 2015).

Probiotics are live microorganisms containing microbial food supplements that provide beneficial effects on consumers' health. These live microorganisms may release and produce substrate medium health-promoting compounds. Probiotic foods are mostly made of milk, but many fermented kinds of cereal are locally known to possess probiotic potential (Ukwuru and Ohaegbu 2018). Dairy-based probiotics are most widely available, but cereals can provide healthy alternatives for producing non-dairy innovative probiotic foods. Subsequently, they can solve several drawbacks related to fermented dairy products such as lactose intolerance, allergy and the effect on cholesterol levels. Lactose is the first crucial

Probiotics, Prebiotics and Synbiotics: Technological Advancements Towards Safety and Industrial Applications, First Edition. Edited by Parmjit Singh Panesar and Anil Kumar Anal.

carbohydrate that promotes the health of the neonate. Lactose intolerance is due to lack of lactase enzyme produced by the intestinal brush border, making it unable to hydrolyze lactose into digestible sugars to give energy. A total of 75% of the world's population is affected by lactose intolerance (Panghal *et al.* 2018). There is enormous demand from vegetarian consumers in both developing and developed countries and, due to this, a massive requirement for probiotic products from plants. Probiotic cereal-based food and beverages are excellent sources of bioactive and other health-promoting compounds such as vitamins and antioxidants. Cereal-based product features can be amplified by using different functional constituents. This chapter addresses the production and health benefits of cereal-based food and beverages with health properties.

9.2 Probiotics in Cereal-based Food and Beverages

Probiotic food products are conventionally dairy-based, incorporating a mixture of milk and fermented products. New products are focused on the probiotic capability of fermented cereal-based food and drinks as traditionally these have been a vital element of the diet. They are an abundant source of dietary fiber, protein, carbohydrates, vitamins, fructans and bioactive compounds. Moreover, lactose intolerance and veganism, coupled with the minimal cholesterol content, have compelled the recent recourse to non-dairy foods and drinks. Gradually, a whole-grain mixture became one of the most favored choices for a probiotic delivery medium. For that reason, formulation with whole-grain products providing fibers such as arabinoxylan, β-glucan, oligosaccharides, resistant starch and phytochemicals, as well as phenolic compounds, phytoestrogens, antioxidants, sterols and phytic acid, has thus been recommended to fulfill the prebiotic concept (Enujiugha and Badejo 2017).

Probiotic cereal-based food and beverages contain the live organism lactic acid bacteria family and health-enhancing food products. Probiotics can prevent and manage various kinds of infective and non-infective disorders. Probiotic cereal-based food and beverages play an essential role in the alleviation of gastrointestinal infections, antidiarrheal properties, reduction in serum cholesterol, antimutagenic properties, antimicrobial activity, immune system stimulation, anticarcinogenic properties and improvement in inflammatory bowel disease and lactose metabolism. In general, most probiotic strains that are defined and commercialized belong to the lactic acid bacteria (LAB) group, for example *Lactobacillus fermentum, L. plantarum, L. celibiosus, L. acidophilus, L. casei, L. pentosus* and *L. rhamnosus. Lactobacillus* spp. are Gram-positive, catalase-negative, non-sporing rods and cocci, usually non-motile when observed microscopically. Bifidobacteria are lactic acid producing bacteria that are phylogenetically distant but widely accepted in the LAB. The genus was discovered in 1889 and pronounced in the early 1900s by Tissier to be related with the feces, specifically those of breastfed infants in which *Bifidobacterium* spp., specifically *B. longum*, was found (Vasudha and Mishra 2013). While the yeasts that contribute to flavor enhancement are dominated mostly by *Saccharomyces cerevisiae* var. *boulardii*, *Candida* spp., *Kluyveromyces fragilis* (B0399), *Pichia* spp., *Hanseniaspora uvarum* and *Torulaspora delbrueckii* are the probiotic yeast species commercially accessible for human use. These yeasts are dominated mostly by *Candida* and *Saccharomyces cerevisiae* species, capable of producing enzymes such as phytase, lipase and esterase. Aroma and taste are determined by the action of esterase, while lipase plays a lipolytic role in fatty acids, which are flavor precursors. Phytase helps lower the phytic acids, which produce complexes with minerals, which negatively affects protein digestibility (Ukwuru and Ohaegbu 2018).

9.3 General Information about Probiotics

The Russian Nobel Laureate Elie Metchnikoff (1845–1916) first introduced the term "probiotic" and reported that the changes in the intestinal microbiome constitution with some beneficial bacteria could improve health and prolong life (Chugh and Kamal-Eldin 2020). In 1965, Lilly and Stilwell introduced the term "probiotics", which they defined as growth-promoting factors produced by microorganisms (Enujiugha and Badejo 2017).

Bifidobacterium and *Lactobacillus* spp., usually Gram-positive, round-ended rods, normally catalase negative, are the most common probiotics and occur in pairs of short or long chains. They are non-motile, non-flagellated and non-spore-forming, and the optimal growth temperature is 37 °C. They are intolerant to salt. Some strains, such as *L. casei*, tend to grow at an ideal pH of 6.5–7.0 at 30 °C. *L. acidophilus* is microaerophilic and capable of succeeding under aerobic conditions, while *Bifidobacterium* is anaerobic. Probiotic bacteria are categorized into three groups based on the type of fermentation product. The homofermentative probiotic bacteria include *L. acidophilus* and *L. helveticus*; the heterofermentation lactic acid bacteria include *L. brevis and L. reuteri*; and the facultative lactic acid bacteria comprise *L. casei* and *L. plantarum*.

Also, a diversity of beneficial compounds such as lactic acid, antimicrobials, hydrogen peroxide and various bacteriocins are developed by probiotics. Probiotics can also work with the host microflora and prevent the adhesion of microbial pathogens, viruses, bacteria and fungi (Song *et al.* 2012).

Probiotics are well defined by the FAO/WHO as live microorganisms in foods which at some levels may stabilize the gastrointestinal tract's microflora, thereby interacting with the host to produce health benefits. According to researchers, therapeutic amounts are given by populations of 10^6–10^7 colony forming units (CFU) CFU/g or CFU/mL, found in the final products by giving 10^8–10^9 CFUs a day per 100 g or 100 mL of food. The quantity of probiotics in the food at the point of intake should be ~10^6 CFU/mL (Enujiugha and Badejo 2017). For health benefits, each product should specify the daily required amount. *Bifidobacterium* and *Lactobacillus* are commonly used probiotics. *Bifidobacterium* colonizes the intestinal tracts of neonates from the day they are born and the population is changed by diet, age, stress and antibiotics. The effectiveness of this genus depends on its capability to inhabit the intestinal tract and control unwanted intestinal bacteria. In some of the isolated bifidobacteria, survivability and the adhesive factor are lacking. Lactobacilli are usually characterized as non-spore, catalase-negative, non-motile, Gram-positive microaerobic or strict anaerobic bacteria. Some species that use glucose as a carbon source then produce lactic and acetic acids (Enujiugha and Badejo 2017). *L. rhamnosus*, one of the broadly studied probiotics, shows promising results in reducing severity and duration of diarrhea.

9.4 Mechanism/Pathway for Probiotics in Cereal-based Food and Beverages

A probiotic is a collection of multiple mechanisms that prevent contamination and enhance immunity and provide improved nutritional value of food (Saulnier *et al.* 2009). A probiotic should have the capacity to persist under intestinal conditions such as acid pH, biliary salts and enzymes, etc. Apart from this, a probiotic should show stimulation of the immune system and antagonism against pathogens and, eventually, must have noticeable effects on the host's health.

Probiotics colonize and normalize perturbed intestinal microbial communities in children and adults. They can improve the host defense system in contradiction to pathogenic bacteria. The mucosal epithelial cell works as a barrier by inhibiting the adherence of the pathogens. It may be either enhancing the promotion of mucin production or reducing colonic permeability.

It also helps prevent pathogenic organisms and other toxic materials by decreasing intestinal permeability and mucin production. Saulnier *et al.* (2009) reported that surface-layer proteins present on *L. crispatus* and *L. helveticus* could stop adhesion of *Escherichia coli O157:H7* foodborne pathogens. Host immunity is boosted by host defensin production and mucosal antibody production by using probiotics. In immunomodulation, the surface proteins play an essential role. Probiotics can enhance immunity by increasing mucosal antibody synthesis, increasing pro-inflammatory cytokine expression, and increasing host defense production.

Probiotics produce an array of antimicrobial compounds against the growth of many foodborne pathogens. Generally, LAB produce short chain fatty acids (SCFAs) or organic acids, predominantly lactate and acetate, and this not only has immunomodulatory effects but also helps to decrease the pH by changing the colonic environment. It also boosts the mucosal morphology by decreasing translocation and binding to SCFAs, receptors on immune cells inside the gut lymphoid-associated tissue (GALT), and increased mucin production (Saulnier *et al.* 2009).

Bacteroidetes grow mainly on non-digestible polysaccharides, especially foods composed of cereals, legumes and vegetables. These bacteroidetes produce butyrate, which reduces the colon's inflammatory response (Karunaratne 2018). For colonocytes, butyrate is a leading energy source. Some individual receptors, for example G-protein coupled receptor 41(Gpr41), can bind to SCFAs. These receptors are robust controllers of the host energy balance, which affects gut microbiota. Proteins and peptides synthesized by probiotics are capable of inhibiting specific pathogenic strains. Several LAB can produce well-characterized inhibitory peptides. In contrast, some are not effective against antibiotics (class I), peptide bacteriocins (class II) and bacteriolysins (class III) (Saulnier *et al.* 2009). Bacteriocins can control growth of pathogens in the intestinal tract by generating pores in the targeted bacterial membrane and using these pores to apply bactericidal and bacteriostatic effects.

Bacteriocins also tend to decrease and avoid microbial degradation of the food and fermented products. *L. plantarum* and *L. casei* are isolated from fermented food products and contain bacteriocins that prevent and reduce specific pathogens spread by food (Nyanzi and Jooste 2012). Reuterin is an antibacterial agent produced by a probiotic, *L. reuteri*. It has a broad spectrum of activity against a diversity of pathogens, including bacteria, protozoa, fungi and viruses. These antimicrobial compounds also act as food preservatives or prophylactic agents against enteric infections. Moreover, probiotics are able to produce beneficial hydrogen peroxide.

The development by LAB of antimicrobial products that exhibit vigorous antagonistic behavior against food-contaminating microorganisms has been documented (Choi *et al.* 2018). Hydrogen peroxide, antifungal fatty acids, diacetyl, organic acids, bacteriocin-like, and phenyllactic acid bacteriocins are antimicrobial agents developed by LAB. Bacteriocins are antimicrobial small proteins or peptides that inhibit microorganisms of closely related species to the producer strain. Bacteriocins are associated with LAB and considered potential natural food preservatives that are preferable to chemical preservatives in fermented food products. Numerous bacteriocins produced by food-associated LAB have been identified and characterized, including diplococcin, nisin, acidophilin, plantaricins, bulgarican, lactacins and helvericins. Several bacteriocins are active against food-borne pathogens such as *Listeria monocytogenes, Staphylococcus aureus, Bacillus cereus* and *Clostridium difficile*. Nisin is one of the food preservatives widely accessible and is safe to use against food pathogens and spoilage agents, which are Gram positive.

Bacteriocins are primarily divided into three categories. Class I is composed of small heat-stable peptides and is defined as antibiotics due to thioether amino acids such as lanthionine. Nisin, lactocin and pediocin, formed by *L. lactis, L. sake* and *Pediococcus acidilactici*, are the bacteriocins in class I. Class II bacteriocins are non-modified, thin, hydrophobic, heat stable and composed of a single peptide, or two or more polypeptides. They are produced by *L. lactis, L. plantarum* and *Enterococcus faecium* and consist of lactococcin G, plantaricin S, plantaricin jk and enterococcin, respectively. Class III consists of abundant, hydrophilic, heat-labile proteins. Helveticin V-1829 and helveticin J developed by *L. helveticus* are examples of class III. Reuterin is a well-known antimicrobial agent similar to bacteriocin developed by *L. reuteri* with inhibitory activity against various bacteria, yeasts and molds. Plantaricin c is a bacteriocin developed primarily by *L. plantarum* that is active against a wide range of bacteria including *Streptococcus, Enterococcus, Lactobacillus, Clostridium* and *Bacillus* spp. (Kalui *et al.* 2010).

Probiotics block pathogens by producing bacteriocidal compounds and these compounds compete with toxins released by the pathogens on intestinal epithelium. As a protective response against pathogens, probiotics enhance barrier function and stimulate protective responses from intestinal epithelial cells. In human health, probiotics have beneficial effects such as modulation of the immune system. They also modulate inflammation induced by pathogens through Toll-like receptor-regulated signaling pathways and improve innate immunity. The *L. rhamnosus* GG-derived soluble protein, p40, has given promising results in preventing and treating oxazolone-induced colitis, acute colitis and dextran sulfate sodium (DSS)-induced intestinal injury. In mouse models of colitis, using p40 reduces intestinal epithelial apoptosis and interruption of barrier function in the colonic epithelium in an epidermal growth factor receptor-dependent manner. Additionally, p40 reduces keratinocyte chemoattractant, tumor necrosis factor (TNF), interferon (IFN)-γ production and IL-6. However, it is not effective against the expression of IL-17 in DSS-treated mice or IL-1β and IL-10, and it also does not affect the production of IL-13 in oxazolone-treated mice. These outcomes suggest that p40 performs a vital role in the Th1 immune response and innate immunity regulation (Yan and Polk 2011).

9.5 Types of Probiotic in Cereal-based Food and Beverages

Nowadays there is increased demand for nutritionally improved foods because their positive effects on human health are visible, especially in developed countries. Consumer expectations are also fulfilled by putting effort into designing products, specifically staple foods, with better health-promoting characteristics for the application of probiotic foods. Several studies have been done on both humans and animals. However, the addition of various probiotic strains does not change consumer perception and does not affect the product's flavor (Hekmat and Reid 2006) even though these products improved the balance of microbiota in the human body, giving physiological benefits to the host.

Due to the demand for functional bakery and new and innovative products like muffins, bread is prepared from wholegrain fermented oat flour to provide more nutritious protein, fiber, β-glucan and mineral content with improved palatability. Oat–wheat bread is naturally rich in β-glucan, though fermented oat–wheat bread is fermented using LAB, which improves digestibility and also provides health benefits by slow release of blood glucose, which leads to satiety and more organoleptic qualities compared to wheat bread (Ciesarová *et al.* 2014). Apart from this, sourdough from a wholegrain oat flour is produced by using the probiotic *L. plantarum*, which gives a gel consistency suitable for technological application and provides β-glucan and high fiber (Blažeková *et al.* 2015).

9.6 Traditional and Commercial Probiotic Cereal-based Foods and Beverages

Cereals are considered an essential source of food worldwide, contributing to human nutrition for millennia. Worldwide, the major cereal crops grown are rice, barley, wheat, maize, and others such as sorghum, oat, rye, triticale and millet. Besides these are pseudocereals such as amaranth, buckwheat and quinoa. In Asia and Africa, conventional fermented cereal-based products have been consumed from ancient times and are a rich source of probiotic microorganisms and prebiotic substances. Table 9.1 shows some traditional probiotic-based beverages and food.

9.6.1 Borde

In western and southern parts of Ethiopia, a traditional cereal-based fermented beverage known as borde is made from barley, millet, sorghum and wheat. Borde is a whitish-grey or brown opaque beverage with a sweet–sour taste. For conventional fermentation, people use a combination of lactobacilli and yeasts. Borde improves lactation and encourages mothers to drink after birth. It also improves constipation, malaria, abscesses and diarrhea (Abegaz *et al.* 2004).

Table 9.1 Conventional probiotic-based beverages and food.

Name of food and beverage	Source	Strain	Country	Reference
Borde	Maize, finger millet, tef	*L. acidophilus* *L. fermentum*	Ethiopia	Enujiugha and Badejo (2017)
Boza	Wheat, rye, millet, maize and other cereals	*L. plantarum* *L. acidophilus* *L. fermentum* *L. coprophilus* *Leuconostoc raffinolactis* *Leuconostoc mesenteroides* *L. brevis* *Saccharomyces cerevisiae* *Candida tropicalis* *C. glabrata* *Geotrichum penicillatum* *G. candidum*	Albania Turkey Bulgaria Romania	Blandino *et al.* (2003); Gotcheva *et al.* (2000)
Burukutu	Millet and sorghum	*Lactobacillus* spp. *Leuconostoc* spp. *Mesenteroides* *Acetobacter* spp. *Saccharomyces cerevisiae* *Rhodotorula glutinis* *Cryptococcus albidus* *Candida* spp. *Saccharomyces chevalieri*	Nigeria Benin Ghana	Blandino *et al.* (2003); Jimoh *et al.* (2012)

Bushera	Sorghum, millet	*L. brevis* *Streptococcus lactis* *Leuconostoc mesenteroides* *Lactococcus lactis*	Uganda	Enujiugha and Badejo (2017)
Chicha de jora	Maize	*L. plantarum* *L. fermentum* *Saccharomyces cerevisiae*	South America	Ray and Didier (2014)
Gowe	Sorghum	*L. fermentum* *Weissella confusa* *L. mucosae* *Pediococcus acidilactici*	Benin Republic	Enujiugha and Badejo (2017)
Kenkey/ kormi / kokoe / dorkunu	Maize, millet, sorghum	*L. plantarum* *L. fermentum* *L. brevis* *L. reuteri* *Pediococcus pentosaceus* *Candida krusei* *Saccharomyces cerevisiae*	African countries	Panghal *et al.* (2018)
Koko	Millet	*Weissella confusa* *L. fermentum* *L. salivarius* *Pediococcus* spp.	Northern Ghana	Lei and Jakobsen (2004)
Koozh	Rice, millet	*Weissella paramesenteroides* *L. plantarum* *L. fermentum*	South India	Panghal *et al.* (2018)

(*Continued*)

Table 9.1 (Continued)

Name of food and beverage	Source	Strain	Country	Reference
Kunun-zaki	Millet or sorghum	*L. plantarum* *L. pentosus* *L. celbiosus* *Leuconostoc mesenteroides* *Candida mycoderma* *Saccharomyces cerevisiae*	Nigeria	Amusa and Odunbaku (2009); Enujiugha and Badejo (2017); Nwachukwu *et al.* (2010)
Kvass	Rye, barley	*Lactobacillus casei* *Leuconostoc mesenteroides* *Saccharomyces cerevisiae*	Eastern Europe	Rigobelo (2012)
Kwete	Maize, millet	*L. brevis* *L. plantarum* *L. lactis*	Uganda	Enujiugha and Badejo (2017)
Mageu	Maize, wheat	*L. lactis* *L. fermentum*	South Africa	Enujiugha and Badejo (2017)
Mahewu	Corn meal, sorghum/millet malt	*L. lactis* *L. bulgaricus* *L. brevis*	Zimbabwe Arabian gulf	Blandino *et al.* (2003); Enujiugha and Badejo (2017); Gadaga *et al.* (1999)

Obiolo	Millet and sorghum	*L. fermentum* *L. plantarum* *L. acidophilus* *L. brevis* *L. rhamnosus* *Bifidobacterium longum* *Lactococcus lactis*	Nigeria	Achi (1990); Aka *et al.* (2014)
Ogi, akamu	Maize, sorghum, millet	*L. plantarum* *Streptococcus lactis* *L. fermentum*	Nigeria West Africa	Enujiugha and Badejo (2017)
Pito	Sorghum	*Pediococcus halophilus* *L. plantarum* *L. casei* *Saccharomyces cerevisiae* *Candida utilis* *Rhodotorula glutinis* *Candida pelliculosa* *Cryptococcus albidus* *Geotrichum candidum*	Nigeria Ghana	Jimoh *et al.* (2012); Orji *et al.* (2003)
Pozol	Maize	*Bacillus* spp. *Agrobacterium* spp.	Southeastern Mexico	Wacher *et al.* (2000)
Sobia	Wheat	*Lactobacillus* spp. *Leuconostoc* spp. *Pediococcus* spp. *Candida* spp.	Saudi Arabia	Gassem (2002)

(*Continued*)

Table 9.1 (Continued)

Name of food and beverage	Source	Strain	Country	Reference
Togwa	Maize, finger millet	*L. plantarum* *L. brevis* *L. fermentum* *L. cellobiosus* *Weissella confusa*	Tanzania Japan China	Enujiugha and Badejo (2017); Giraud *et al.* (1993); Panghal *et al.* (2018)
Uji	Maize, sorghum	*L. plantarum* *L. fermentum* *L. cellobiosus* *L. buchneri* *Pediococcus acidilactici* *Pediococcus pentosaceus* *L. rhamnosus* *Streptococcus thermophilus*	Kenya	Panghal *et al.* (2018)
Yosa	Oat bran	*L. acidophilus* LA5 *Bifidobacteria lactis* Bb12	Finland Scandinavian countries	Grumezescu and Holban (2019)

9.6.2 Boza

Boza is a very popular beverage in Turkey, Romania, Bulgaria and Albania. It is a mixture of rye, wheat, maize and sugar. Microflora analysis of Bulgarian boza confirms that it is mostly strains of LAB *Lactobacillus* spp. and yeast ratio of 2.4. The LAB isolated have been identified as *L. plantarum, L. acidophilus, L. fermentum, L. coprophilus, Leuconostoc raffinolactis, Leuconostoc mesenteroides* and *Lactobacillus brevis*. The yeasts isolated consist of *Candida tropicalis, Candida glabrata, Saccharomyces cerevisiae, Geotrichum penicillatum* and *Geotrichum candidum* (Blandino *et al.* 2003). Varieties of *L. fermentum* developed bacteriocins active against *L. casei, Escherichia coli, Pseudomonas aeruginosa*, and *Enterococcus faecalis, L. pentosus, L. paracasei,* and *L. rhamnosus* isolated from boza. The strains of *L. fermentum* and *L. plantarum* also exhibited antimicrobial activity and hindered Klebsiella pneumonia by developing bacteriocins (Enujiugha and Badejo 2017).

9.6.3 Burukutu

Burukutu is produced from millet sorghum and maize. Burukutu is the main drink consumed in the northern Guinea Savanna region of Nigeria, Benin Republic and Ghana. It is a brown-colored suspension with a vinegar-like favor, brewed from sorghum. The dominant microorganism during burukutu fermentation is yeast, mainly *Saccharomyces cerevisiae, Saccharomyces chevalieri, Candida tropicalis* and *Kloeckera apiculata, L plantarum, L. fermentum, L. pentosus, L. brevis, Pediococcus pentosaceus* and *L. mesenteroides*. Multifunction potentials of native yeasts from burukutu have been demonstrated in some studies. *Candida tropicalis* with lipase, esterase and phytase activities and probiotic potential was identified in burukutu (Shetty and Sarkar 2020).

9.6.4 Bushera

Bushera is one of the traditional drinks used by adults and children in the western region of Uganda. Germinated millets and sorghum were used as a raw material to ferment at room temperature (25–30 °C) for 1–6 days and from the bushera primarily five genera of LAB were isolated: *Lactococcus* spp., *Leuconostoc* spp., *Enterococcus* spp., *Streptococcus* spp. and *Lactobacillus* spp. (Vasudha and Mishra 2013). Bushera has many medical advantages including enhancing insusceptibility and the body's energy after fermentation. It is commercially manufactured by Multiline International, Nyendo, Uganda (Panghal *et al.* 2018).

9.6.5 Chicha de jora

Chicha de jora is generally made from yellow maize (jora). The predominant native yeasts and LAB are *Saccharomyces cerevisiae* and *L. fermentum* and *L. plantarum*. It has excellent cultural and medicinal value as the yeast provides riboflavin, thiamine and a wide variety of B vitamins. As probiotics, lactobacilli help reduce cholesterol, triglycerides and diarrhea, which is further useful in digestion and reduction of body weight (Ray and Didier 2014).

9.6.6 Gowe

In the Republic of Benin's metropolitan centers, gowe is a sour fermented beverage based on native sorghum. Gowe is a variation of non-malted and malted sorghum flour prepared by a starter culture of *Pediococcus acidilactici, Weissella confusa, L. fermentum, L. mucosae,* and *Pichia anomala* and *Kluyveromyces marxianus* yeasts by spontaneous fermentation (Enujiugha and Badejo 2017).

9.6.7 Kenky

Kenky is a probiotic product derived from millet, sorghum and maize and primarily eaten in Africa. Kenky grains are usually softened by soaking, followed by grinding and fermentation with *L. plantarum, L. fermentum, L. brevis, L. reuteri* and *Pediococcus pentosaceus*, (Nout 2009). The yeast that results during fermentation is *Candida krusei* and *Saccharomyces cerevisiae*. Kenky can be eaten immediately, ready to eat, and also has a good shelf-life (Panghal *et al.* 2018).

9.6.8 Koko

Many people in northern Ghana drink koko probiotic drinks regularly. Koko is prepared overnight by soaking pearl millet (*Pennisetum glaucum*), followed by wet-milling a mixture of spices such as ginger, garlic, chili pepper with the millet grains. The addition of water to the milled materials produces a dense slurry that is then sieved and fermented. After sedimentation for 2–3 h, the top-layer liquid is drained off, boiled for 1–2 h and eventually added to the bottom-layer sedimentation to the required consistency. *Weissella confusa* and *L. fermentum* were the dominant LAB isolated from koko, demonstrating a marked taxonomic heterogeneity at subspecies level between development stages and production sites, along with *L. salivarius* and *Pediococcus* spp. (Lei and Jakobsen 2004).

9.6.9 Koozh

Koozh is a fermented probiotic food product based on cereals, mainly rice and millet flour, originating from South India. *L. plantarum, Weissella paramesenteroides,* and *L. fermentum* are the varieties of LAB primarily used in koozh fermentation (Panghal *et al.* 2018).

9.6.10 Kunun-zaki

The traditional sour–sweet fermented cereal beverage kunun-zaki is very popular in Nigeria. The conventional production method involves steeping sorghum or millet followed by milling with pepper and ginger, then filtering and incomplete gelatinization followed by the addition of sugar and bottling. The LAB primarily involved are *Lactococcus lactis, L. plantarum* and *L. fermentum* (Nwachukwu *et al.* 2010).

9.6.11 Kvass

In Eastern Europe, kvass is a frequently consumed cereal-based beverage. It is prepared from the combination of barley malt liquor, rye flour, stale rye bread, rye and sucrose. The microorganisms primarily involved in kvass fermentation are *Leuconostoc mesenteroides, Saccharomyces cerevisiae* and *L. casei*. The presence of *L. casei* in kvass demonstrates the potential of cereal-based beverage as probiotic functional food (Rigobelo 2012).

9.6.12 Kwete

Kwete is a mixture of cereal-based beverages based on maize and malted millet flour. The count of *Lactococcus* spp. and *Lactobacillus* spp. varies from 5.40 to 7.36 log CFU/mL during fermentation. Maximum growth was observed for LAB between 24 and 48 h, and higher numbers of detectable *Lactobacillus* spp. were observed for fermentation at 72 h compared to *Lactococcus* spp. (Enujiugha and Badejo 2017).

9.6.13 Mageu

Mageu is a sour beverage made from boiled maize flour porridge of 8–10% solids (w/w) followed by wheat flour and LAB to initiate fermentation at 35 °C for 24 h. In mageu fermentation, the LAB cannot produce bacteriocins antagonistic to *Bacillus cereus* because of pH-lowering effects. The leading microorganisms engaged in the fermentation of mageu are *L. lactis* (Enujiugha and Badejo 2017).

9.6.14 Majewu

Majewu is a brew typically produced from cornmeal used in Africa and some countries in the Middle East. It is made from porridge made of maize mixed with water. The flour of sorghum, wheat, barley or millet malt is blended and prepared for fermentation. Majewu contains many nutritional components from the starch and phytochemicals. The microorganisms leading to mahewu's fermentation belong to *Lactococcus lactis* subsp. *lactis*. Industrial production is successfully carried out in Zimbabwe (Blandino *et al.* 2003).

9.6.15 Obiolo

Obiolo is a non-alcoholic drink prepared by fermentation of millet and sorghum in Nigeria. It is made from overnight-soaked millet and sorghum grains in water and then folded in banana leaves and set aside for 3 days for germination. The grain mixture is wet-milled and prepared into a slurry, then the slurry is blended with boiling water and the cooled mash sieved. The filtrate is boiled for 30 min with continuous stirring and then cooled and set aside for fermentation. The primary microorganisms involved in production of obiolo are *L. fermentum, L. plantarum, L. acidophilus, L. brevis, L. rhamnosus, Bifidobacterium longum* and *Lactococcus lactis* (Ukwuru and Ohaegbu 2018).

9.6.16 Ogi

Ogi is a fermented cereal porridge prepared using maize, sorghum or millet. It is considered as the essential food for infants in West Africa, and also for adults. In Nigeria, mothers give their babies ogi to drink, which helps treat diarrhea and abdominal discomfort.

L. plantarum is the predominant microorganism in ogi drink; also involved are *L. fermentum*, *Streptococcus lactis* and *Lactobacillus* spp. (Blandino *et al.* 2003). The nutritional qualities of ogi (such as phosphorus released from phytase) improve during fermentation; riboflavin and niacin contents also increase. Ogi is similar to yoghurt but has a sour flavor and a unique aroma different from other fermented products (Enujiugha and Badejo 2017).

9.6.17 Pito

Pito is the famous traditional drink of the western and middle belt region of Nigeria. Pito preparation comprises of soaking the cereal grains (sorghum, maize or a mixture of both) in water for 2 days, following by malting and resting for 5–6 days in a basket covered with moistened plantain leaves. The malted grains are then sun-dried before crushing. The malt flour is then mixed with water and boiled for 6–12 h. The resulting wash is cooled and later sieved, followed by overnight fermentation of the filtrate, which becomes slightly sour because of microbial action. It is cooked for 12 h and cooled again, and then the starter is added to the cooled concentrate and fermented for 12–24 h to get a dark brown liquid pito. The predominant microorganisms are *Pediococcus halophilus, L. plantarum, L. casei, Saccharomyces cerevisiae, Candida utilis, Rhodotorula glutinis, Candida pelliculosa, Cryptococcus albidus* and *Geotrichum candidum* (Ukwuru and Ohaegbu 2018).

9.6.18 Pozol

Pozol is one of the famous drinks of Southeastern Mexico. It is prepared using maize, which is cooked in 1% (w/v) lime solution, followed by washing and grinding to make a dough known as nixnatal (nixtamalization is a procedure wherein maize or other grains are soaked in lime water and cooked). The dough is then given a round shape wrapped in plantain leaves and placed for fermentation at room temperature for 1/2–4 days. After suspension of the fermented dough with water, the pozol is ready to drink. In nixtamalization, some fibers are not entirely solubilized and this sediment is found in the beverage. *Lactococcus lactis*, LAB and *Bacillus* spp. are among the microbes found in pozol. Meanwhie, *Bacillus* sp. *starin* CS93, which can be isolated from pozol, is effective against numerous Gram-positive and Gram-negative bacteria, yeast and molds. *Agrobacterium azotophilum* found in pozol has also been seen to have bacteriocidal, bacteriolytic and fungistatic activities (Enujiugha and Badejo 2017; Holzapfel 2014; Panghal *et al.* 2018; Rigobelo 2012).

9.6.19 Sobia

A fermented beverage prepared from wheat flour and malt flours known as sobia is commonly made in Saudi Arabia, specifically the western portion. Conventionally, sobia is made from malt and wheat flour suspended in water with a sweet–sour flavor (pH 3.44–4.0). Spices such as cardamom and cinnamon and sugar are added to the mixture and left to ferment at ambient temperature. Lactic acid bacteria consist of *L. cellobiosus, L. buchneri, L. plantarum, L. brevis, Pediococcus pentosaceus* and *L. delbrueckii* subsp. *delbrueckii*. Yeasts consist of *Saccharomyces cerevisiae, Candida tropicalis, Candida ciferrii, Candida guilliermondii, Candida lipolytica, Kloeckera japonica* and *Rhodotorula rubra* (Gassem 2002).

9.6.20 Togwa

Togwa is a probiotic product produced predominantly in Japan and China by the fermentation of a mixture of grains such as maize, sorghum and finger millet flour (Panghal *et al.* 2018). Togwa is cooked in water, then a seed culture (old togwa) and germinated cereal flour from grains are added after cooling to 35 °C. The microorganisms are *L. cellobiosus, Pediococcus pentosaceus, L, plantarum, L, brevis, L, fermentum, Weissella confusa, Saccharomyces cerevisiae, Issatchenkia orientalis, Candida tropicalis* and *Candida pelliculosa*. The organic acids include lactic, succinic, formic, pyruvic, citric, pyroglutamic, and uric acids during fermentation. Lactate was the primary acid and, increased dramatically over time. The volatile organic compounds were acetaldehyde, 2-methyl-propanal, 2-methyl-butanal, 3-methyl butanal, ethanol, 2-methyl-1-propanol, 2-methyl-1-butanol, 3-methyl-1-butanol, diacetyl and acetoin (Enujiugha and Badejo 2017).

9.6.21 Uji

Uji is a probiotic food that uses *L. fermentum, L. plantarum, L. cellobiosus, L. buchneri, Pediococcus acidilactici, Pediococcus pentosaceus, L. rhamnosus*, and *Streptococcus thermophilus* for fermentation in Kenya to make various combinations of maize and sorghum. First, for softening, grains are soaked, followed by grinding and fermentation. After that, uji is ready to serve as an infant food along with breastfeeding. The acidity of uji gives it an extended shelf-life and increases the safety of the product (Panghal *et al.* 2018).

9.6.22 Yosa

Yosa is a snack food made from oat bran cooked in water and fermented with *L. acidophilus* LA5 and *Bifidobacterium lactis* Bb12 (Grumezescu and Holban 2019). It is a domestic product of Finland and other Scandinavian countries. The mixture is then flavored with sucrose or fructose and fruit jam after fermentation. Yosa is similar in texture and taste to yoghurt but free of milk or other animal products (Blandino *et al.* 2003).

9.6.23 Commercially Available Cereal-based Functional Foods

Different kinds of cereal-based functional foods are available on the market worldwide. Some examples of commercially available products include Corny Active® cereal bars in Germany, Weetaflakes® whole-wheat breakfast cereal in France, Muesli® probiotic flakes in Portugal, fruit and probiotic yoghurt in Germany, whole-grain porridge in the UK and Vita Biosa® composed of aromatic herbs in Denmark (Montet and Ray 2016; Panghal *et al.* 2018). Other commercial cereal-based probiotic products are shown in Table 9.2.

GoodBelly, prepared with *L. plantarum* from oatmeal, was the first non-dairy probiotic drink on the US market in 2006 (Panghal *et al.* 2018). Grainfields Wholegrain liquid® is prepared from beans, seeds and grains, for example malted organic oats, maize, rice, alfalfa seed, pearl, barley, linseed, mung beans, rye, wheat and millets, and mainly fermented with *L. acidophilus, L. delbrueckii, Saccharomyces boulardii* and *Saccharomyces cerevisiae* (Grumezescu and Holban 2019).

Table 9.2 Commercially available cereal-based probiotic products.

Probiotic product	Probiotic microorganisms	Company
Avenly velle	*Lactobacillus* spp. *Bifidobacterium* spp.	Avenly Oy Ltd., Finland
Kefir soy	*Kluyveromyces marxianus* *Kluyveromyces lactis* *L. brevis* *L. kefir* *Leuconostoc mesenteroides* *L. helveticus*	Life way, Greece
Mucilon	*Bifidobacterium* spp.	Nestlé

Source: Adapted from Aspri, M., Papademas, P. and Tsaltas, D. (2020). Review on non-dairy probiotics and their use in non-dairy based products. *Fermentation*, 6: 30. https://doi.org/10.3390/fermentation6010030

Proviva is the first commercial oat-based probiotic beverage, and it has been made in Sweden by Skane Dairy since 1994. In this drink, malted barley is added with *L. plantarum,* and it contains approximately 5×10^{10} CFU/g. The fermented mixture is then mixed with a 5% concentration of different types of juices such as blackcurrant, blueberry, rosehip, tropical fruits and strawberry (Grumezescu and Holban 2019). The final product of Proviva contains approximately $5–10^{10}$ CFU/L of *L. plantarum* (Aspri *et al.* 2020).

Ricera is a practical rice-based probiotic foodstuff. The probiotic microorganisms *Bifidobacterium bifidum, Streptococcus thermophilus, L. acidophilus,* and *L. bulgaricus* are primarily used for the fermentation of this substance (Panghal *et al.* 2018).

Velli is a probiotic product with a mixture of oat bran and fruits fermented with probiotic bacteria such as *Bifidobacterium bifidum* and *L. acidophilus.* This product is readily available on the market with the name Velle Oats, St. Petersburg, Russia (Panghal *et al.* 2018).

The demand for probiotic cereal food and beverages has prompted efforts to develop new and innovative products. Cereals are rich sources of macronutrients, micronutrients, phytochemicals and antioxidants. Therefore many researchers are developing cereal-based probiotic food products.

Production of sourdough from wholegrain oat flour and specifically with *L. plantarum* gives a stable gel consistency suitable for technological application. It also provides β-glucan, high fiber with low energy value, and positive sensory acceptability (Blažeková *et al.* 2015). In comparison, β-glucan-rich wheat–oat bread fermentation with LAB increases digestibility, offering health benefits associated with reduced blood glucose release and greater subjective satiety. It results in an organoleptic consistency that is more desirable than wheat bread (Ciesarová *et al.* 2014).

Arora *et al.* (2010) formulated a probiotic food from germinated and non-germinated barley flour, whey powder and tomato pulp (2 : 1 : 1 w/w) fermented with 5% *L. acidophilus.* The cell count observed was higher (8.88 CFU/g) in the fermented mixture formulated from germinated flour than in the non-germinated barley-based mix. Combining germination and fermentation of indigenously developed food mixtures with probiotic microorganisms is a possible method for producing food products with improved nutritional content.

Chavan *et al.* (2018) investigated the effects of germinated and un-germinated barlely, ragi and moth bean with sugar, cardamom with distilled water, soymilk, almond milk and coconut milk on a non-probiotic drink using *L. acidophilus* as a probiotic culture. As the concentration of the drink mixture grew, the acidity, pH, probiotic count, antioxidant and polyphenols level increased. Trolox equivalent was found to be higher in the germinated probiotic drink. When compared to other probiotic drinks, the sensory acceptance scores for the coconut milk probiotic drink with a concentration of 4 g of drink mixture were good.

Rathore *et al.* (2012) chose and fermented mixed cereal flours of malt, barley and malt–barley with two probiotic strains: *L. plantarum* and *L. acidophilus*. The mixed and single cereal flour did not show any effect on the production of lactic acid. These results indicate that the functional and organoleptic properties could be modified by changing a substrate or inocula composition.

Panghal *et al.* (2018) fermented oat flour and honey with *L. plantarum* M-13. During development, they optimized the process, i.e. honey (3.0% w/v), oat flour (8.0% w/v) and incubation time (48 h). Optimization improved the viable cell count of *L. plantarum* M-13 from 14.4 log CFU/mL (unoptimized conditions) to 16.9 log CFU/mL, i.e. by 17.4%. Viability of *L. plantarum* M-13 was observed in probiotic fermented oat flour after 3 weeks of keeping at ambient temperature and in a chiller. Furthermore, lactic acid content was enhanced during storage, but sugar content was reduced. The product remained free from contamination by *Enterobacteriaceae*, although fungal and yeast contaminants were observed.

9.7 Health Benefits

Cereal is abundant in nutrients such as proteins, carbohydrates, vitamins, minerals, and many phytochemicals and other bioactive compounds, including sterols, phytoestrogens, phenolic compounds and antioxidants. Because cereals comprise water-soluble fiber (for example, β-glucan and arabinoxylane), oligosaccharides and resistant starch, they have been suggested to fulfill the prebiotic concept. Non-digestible carbohydrates of cereals accelerate the growth of *Bifidobacterium* spp. and *Lactobacillus* spp. present in the colon and act as a prebiotic, which helps the development of probiotics based functional foods (Kohajdová 2017). Regarding these functionalities and several health benefits, people are interested in consuming products containing probiotics.

Consumption of fermented or probiotic foods containing *Lactobacillus* spp. maintains healthy intestinal flora which is effective against disease-causing pathogens. Probiotic microorganisms have great potential to improve health by regulating the host's immune response, suppressing pathogens and competing with pathogens at adhesion sites. They also have significant potential for optimizing gut ecology, soothing duodenal disorders and refining nutrition. In fermented cereal-based foods, *Saccharomyces cerevisiae* and *Candida* spp. in particular play a vital role in flavor enhancement and produce enzymes such as esterase, phytase and lipase. Due to fatty acids, lipolytic activity acts as a precursor of flavor. In contrast, esterase activity promotes flavor and aroma, and phytase reduces phytic acid and forms complexes with minerals that adversely affect protein digestibility, and improves the immune system (Ukwuru and Ohaegbu 2018).

Probiotics modulate the immune system by different pathways, such as internal effects on active cells. They interact with Toll-like (TLR) receptors on epithelial cells, inducing cytokine secretion to inhibit apoptosis and improving the efficiency of epithelial cells. The immunomodulatory function of *L. casei* is predominantly dependent on TRL. Also, it hinders the development of colitis by inducing DSS with protective activity against myeloperoxidase and interleukin (IL)-12. Probiotics also enhance the immune system by hindering pro-inflammatory responses in epithelial cells. *L. rhamnosus* GG, which enhances the regeneration of epithelial cells and inhibits apoptosis, helps prolong the longevity of epithelial cellsby generating some factors by probiotics capable of preventing the operation of proteasomes in the intestine, ultimately inhibiting the NF-κB pathway and directly inducing certain cytoprotective proteins. *L. rhamnosus* GG is used in vivo to inhibit proapoptotic p38/mitogen-activated protein kinase by activating interferon, IL-1 or tumor necrosis factor α (TNF-α) and also increases the production of IgA, IgG and IgM by lymphocytes. Dendritic cells play an essential role in the early identification of bacterial infections and the production of IL-10 and TGF-β, which accelerate B-cell and T-cell production. Dendritic cells also cause the primary oral immune responses. Probiotics also modify these dendritic cells in the intestine (Zendeboodi *et al.* 2020).

Production of lactic acid in sourdough by fermentation of a cereal matrix helps interactions between gluten and starch. These interactions reduce starch accessibility and lower the glycemic index of these products. In a composite food matrix the cereal grains contain probiotic which is capable of hydrolyzing protein, reducing their toxicity and inflammatory effect. During fermentation, proteolysis of LAB leads to a progressive hydrolysis of native protein, resulting in an increase in peptides and free amino acid. Bread from sprouted and fermented flours indicated low starch availability and high protein digestibility in vitro; starch and protein digestibility were also improved by LAB in fermented sorghum flour (Tsafrakidou *et al.* 2020).

Additionally, probiotic bacteria can produce amino acids, small peptides, lactones, phenols and indoles, which help maintain energy balance, provide resistance to pathogens through immune signals, and contribute antioxidant by fermentation proteins. For the production of different metabolites, the aromatic amino acids act as a substrate that plays a crucial role in the decline of several malfunctions, for example tryptophan has an immunomodulatory effect, leading to a reduction of allergic reactions (Chugh and Kamal-Eldin 2020). The functions of LAB in foods are claimed by many but are still to be adequately verified. In fermented cereal products, *Lactobacillus* spp. are being used to reduce mycotoxins. There are many applications of different LAB in probiotic cereal foods: *L. casei* improves type 2 diabetes and also helps in reduction of recurrence of superficial bladder carcinoma in humans; *L. rhamnosus* helps in the reduction of dental caries; *Bifidobacterium longum* and *Lactobacillus* spp. are used in lowering low density lipoprotein and cholesterol; *Lactobacillus* spp. help in the inhibition of *Listeria monocytogenes* and *Clostridium* spp. The *Lactobacillus* species *L. plantarum* and *L. reuteri* are used as antifungal agents and as vehicles for drug delivery (Kalui *et al.* 2010).

Lactobacillus reuteri can decrease serum cholesterol associated with bile salt hydrolase activity by developing deconjugated bile acids that eventually co-precipitate with cholesterol and are excreted in the feces, influencing the metabolism of bile salt hosts. Probiotic microorganisms should have the potential to tolerate bile salt 0.3% (w/v) for 24 h and comfortably live in the stomach and intestine of the host (Ukwuru and Ohaegbu 2018). Also, *Bifidobacterium* spp. can suppress cholesterol development by producing an organic acid, propionic acid, which helps decrease circulating levels of blood lipids by reducing cholesterol synthesis. Also, the butyric acid provided by *L. plantarum* helps to deliver the colonocytes with energy. Bacteria also precisely extract cholesterol by binding to the cell surface during its development and absorbing it into the bacterial cell membrane (Karunaratne 2018).

Probiotics are live microbial feed supplements that help reduce pathogens in the gastrointestinal tract and improve intestinal microflora, which helps to prevent disease and to treat and prevent infantile viral diarrhea and antibiotic-associated diarrhea. Probiotic bacteria have the ability to suppress potentially harmful microorganisms in the gastrointestinal tract while also improving the balance in favor of beneficial microorganisms. In human clinical trials, *L. rhamnosus* GG (Valio) was effective against antibiotic-associated diarrhea (*Clostridium difficile*) and rotavirus diarrhea. For clinical effects, strains of *L. acidophilus*, *Bifidobacterium lactis*, *L. plantarum*, *L. reuteri*, *L. johnsonii* and *L. casei* Shirota show promising results (Ukwuru and Ohaegbu 2018). Cereal-based food and beverages have a synbiotic effect in the reduction of serum and hepatic cholesterol by which they decrease the ratio of low density lipoprotein (LDL) to high density lipoprotein (HDL) cholesterol, and also increase excretion of triglycerides, bile acids and cholesterol in feces of hyperlipidemic hamsters (Ciesarová *et al.* 2017).

These cereal-based probiotic foods and beverages can also reduce and control serum cholesterol by deconjugating conjugated bile acids, mainly by intestinal and fecal *Bifidobacterium* spp. and *Lactobacillus* spp. In the gut, enhancing the colonization of *Bifidobacterium* spp. and *Lactobacillus* spp. increases the production of deconjugated bile acid and promotes the enzyme bile salt hydrolase activity.

The feces excrete the deconjugated bile acids via the enterohepatic circulation because the gut cannot absorb the free unconjugated bile acid because of less solubility. For bile acid synthesis, the cholesterol intake demand increases to substitute the excreted bile acids, and in this way serum cholesterol is also reduced. Diabetes-associated and hypercholesterolemia-induced high blood pressure can be reduced by using probiotic. Cholesterol in plasma lipoprotein has been proposed as the preferred precursor for bile acid production in the liver, consequently probiotic is helpful for cholesterol level and can also improve insulin sensitivity. Improvement in insulin sensitivity partially affects insulin resistance and type 2 diabetes (Sivamaruthi *et al.* 2020). The following probiotic microorganism species cleave amide bonds by bile salt hydrolase: *L. plantarum*, *L. johnsonii*, *L. gasseri* and *L. acidophilus* and *Bifidobacterium* spp. (Zendeboodi *et al.* 2020). Viable and active probiotics which carry bile salt hydrolase can reduce cholesterol-related illness by enhancing the bile salt production.

Fermented cereal foods associated with different probiotic microorganisms can synthesize antimicrobial bioactive complexes such as short chain fatty acids, hydrogen peroxide and bacteriocins, boosting their biopreservative properties. However, short chain fatty acids are rich in antioxidants, affecting non-communicable diseases by suppressing the free radicals in the body. Reactive oxygen species are reactive to non-contagious conditions that damage lipids, proteins, DNA and carbohydrates. The gastrointestinal tract produces some reactive oxygen species: some are generated by chemical reactions of dietary components within the stomach, and some are present in food (Karunaratne 2018). Probiotics exert antimicrobial activity against pathogens by lowering pH, metabolizing toxic substances and agglutinating pathogens by producing mucus in the gut. Lactin B and acidolin compounds secreted by *L. acidophilus* inhibit the growth of lactobacilli and enteropathogenic organisms, respectively (Zendeboodi *et al.* 2020). Probiotics show a diverse range of antibiotic susceptibilities and resistance because probiotics were resistant to the inhibitors of the cell wall synthesis and neucleic acid synthesis. In an in vitro experiment, *L. plantarum*, *Candida rugosa* and *Candida lambica* strains were resistant to nine antibiotics: oxacillin, methicillin, cefotaxime, vancomycin, teicoplanin, tobramycin, kanamycin, trimethoprim-sulfamethoxazole, and nalidixic acid (Gotcheva *et al.* 2018).

Many pathogens are resistant to antibiotics. Methicillin (5 μg), oxacillin (1 μg), the second generation cephalosporin cefotaxime (30 μg), vancomycin (30 μg), teicoplanin (30 μg) and the glycopeptides were discovered to be resistant to the the bacteria growth by inhibiting bacterial cell wall synthesis and penicillinase resistant. Many LAB have vancomycin resistance as an intrinsic property that suggests it is resistant to antibiotic strain B_{25} but not resistant to third generation cephalosporins. However, chynolons and nalidixic acid and tobramycin (10 μg) and kanamycin (30 μg) showed nucleic acid synthesis inhibition. Some probiotic strains showed maximum resistance to nucleic acid synthesis, chynolons and nalidixic acid, and trimethoprim-sulfamethoxazole 1.25/23.75 mg. Some potential probiotics are useful as therapeutic treatment (Gotcheva *et al.* 2000; Ukwuru and Ohaegbu 2018).

In fermented products, shelf-life partially increases because of the presence of bacteriocins and antimicrobial peptides generated by LAB. Against the pathogens *Staphylococcus aureus, Bacillus cereus, Listeria monocytogenes, Escherichia coli* and *Enterococcus faecium*, *Pediococcus* sp. strain OF101 showed maximum antibacterial activity. In Africa, traditional fermented cereal products are consumed regularly, improving well-being and reducing diarrhea outbreaks in children by 40% (Tsafrakidou *et al.* 2020). According to the World Health Organization (WHO), in 1994, probiotics are considered to improve the immune defense system and reduce antibiotic resistance of commonly prescribed antibiotics. Probiotics can also suppress antibiotic-associated diarrhea and prevent gut infections. Probiotic preparations of *L. reuteri* have been found beneficial in the inhibition and treatment of antibiotic-associated diarrhea and infantile viral diarrhea (Kalui *et al.* 2010).

Lactose is an essential carbohydrate for strengthening the well-being of the neonate. In most babies, the intestinal enzyme lactase is maximal during the postnatal phase, decreasing with age. Among 2- to 12-year-old children there are two distinct groups: a "lactase-persistence" group, and a "lactase non-persistence" group. On this basis, lactose deficiency (insufficient amount of lactase enzyme for digesting lactose) may present from infancy to childhood. Cramps, gas production in the gastrointestinal tract, bloating, gastric pain, diarrhea, etc., are usually observed in lactose-intolerant people. Probiotics can reduce lactose intolerance symptoms. β-Galactosidase plays a vital role in lactose digestion and is released by probiotics in the small intestine (Panghal *et al.* 2018).

Probiotic bacteria can produce carbohydrate-digesting enzymes, which are lacking in human small and large intestines. The short chain fatty acids produced are mainly acetate, propionate and butyrate, produced by probiotic bacteria which have a variety of pathways to hydrolyze non-digestible carbohydrate into oligosaccharide and then monosaccharide under anaerobic conditions. Peroxisomes bind to the butyrate, increasing and activating receptor-γ (PPAR-γ), leading to β-oxidation and oxygen consumption. Apart from this, fermentation of butyrate provides 60–70% of the energy for brain cells, muscle and colon.

Oxygen is consumed by LAB, providing an anaerobic gut environment that is not suitable for pathogens. Short chain fatty acids, especially butyrate, show therapeutic effects against numerous diseases such as colon cancer, heart disease and inflammatory bowel disease because lower pH value changes gut microbiota composition and prevents overgrowth by pH-sensitive pathogenic bacteria, for example Enterobacteriaceae and clostridia (Den Besten *et al.* 2013). Short chain fatty acids are mediated by G-protein coupled receptors such as GPR43, which control power consumption. IL-10 with its immune-modulating properties is produced and triggered by binding of propionate and butyrate to the lymphocyte GPR43 receptor. Butyrate production plays an important role in the prevention of obesity, cancer and diabetes, (Chugh and Kamal-Eldin 2020).

Probiotic bacteria produce some vitamins not made by plants, such as B_{12} and vitamin K, to develop and establish beneficial bacteria in the gut. *L. reuteri* and *Propionibacterium shermanii* can produce useful metabolites, vitamin B_{12} and propionic acid (Karunaratne, 2018). Apart from B_{12}, B complex vitamins with folate and B_1 are produced by probiotic bacteria. *L. reuteri* produces cobalamin, whereas *Bifidobacterium* spp. can synthesize pyridoxine (vitamin B_6). *Escherichia coli* and *Bacillus subtilis* were found active in the production of riboflavin. Plants produce phylloquinone (vitamin K_1), and by converting this, bacteria can produce menaquinone (vitamin K_2). Hence, in humans, for the contribution of vitamin K status, the intestinal microflora plays an important role (Chugh and Kamal-Eldin 2020).

Probiotic bacteria induce the production of quorum-sensing molecules and exopolysaccharides (EPS) that help create biofilms that trigger the growth of beneficial bacteria in the gastrointestinal tract. EPS are linear high-molecular long-chain biopolymers bound to α-glycosidic and β-glycosidic bonds with homopolysaccharide side chains and/or heteropolysaccharides carbohydrate. EPS are produced by the action of glycan transferase and glycosyltransferase enzymes from sugar nucleotide precursors, and probiotic bacteria play an essential role in this process. Often formed by LAB, heteropolysaccharides consisting of different pentoses (D-arabinose, D-ribose, D-xylose), hexoses (D-glucose, D-galactose, D-mannose) or uronic acids (D-glucuronic acid, D-galacturonic acid) are capable of adhering to the intestinal cell membranes. LAB are able to modulate the composition in phenolic compounds and the inflammatory response by leading to the production of pro-inflammatory cytokines and to stimulate dendritic cell and other antigens presenting gene to Toll-like receptors (TLRs), consequently enhancing antioxidant and anti-inflammatory activity. Beside, EPS have been investigated because of their promising immune-modulating, cholesterol-lowering and anti-carcinogenic effects (Chugh and Kamal-Eldin 2020). EPS perform an essential role in creating biofilms, surface adhesion and cell recognition, facilitating the colonization of different ecosystems. These are the beneficial attributes of probiotics related to the gastrointestinal tract (Kalui *et al.* 2010).

Proglucagon is a hormone that reduces adiposity and regulates appetite, and probiotics are known to up-regulate expression of this hormone. Bacteroidetes and Firmicutes are specific microbes that are responsible for the development of diabetes and obesity. Lower bacterial diversity is found in obese than lean people. *Akkermansia muciniphila*-like bacteria have been shown to be more prevalent in healthy-weight than obese children. *L. casei* and *L. plantarum* were noted to be negatively associated with obesity, whereas *L. reuteri* is positively associated. In this way, a different *Lactobacillus* sp. beneficially affects the host. In addition to this, certain *Lactobacillus* spp. have an inhibitory activity effect on the hydrolysis of carbohydrates, they provide repressive activity and provide a mechanism for the management of diabetes (Karunaratne 2018).

Remarkably, the curative effects of the microbiota appear to extend beyond simple physical disorders and ease diseases involving cognitive defects. These include anxiety and mood disorders, along with autism and other neurodevelopmental disorders. The microbiota is thought to play an essential role in specific diseases via the gut–brain axis (Karunaratne 2018). Moreover, it has been reported by Zendeboodi *et al.* (2020) that probiotics termed "psychobiotic" regulate cognitive functions, learning processes and mood, in the same way as neurotransmitters and proteins. The generation of neurotransmitters such as serotonin, acetylcholine, γ-aminobutyric acid (GABA) and catecholamines is the possible pathway for the impact of probiotics on mental well-being. They allegedly modulate the hypothalamic–pituitary–adrenal axis in anti-inflammatory activities and stressful conditions. Some studies showed that the gut microbiota plays a vital part in cognitive development and brain behavior, thus improving brain-associated diseases by by stimulating immune cell recruitment into the brain, thus alleviating the progress of Alzheimer's disease (AD). Probiotic cells enhance brain health by developing neuropeptides and neurotransmitters, such as glucagon-like peptides and serotonin, modulating the enteric nervous system, such as the development of glial cells in the gut, hindering the release of α-synuclein from enteroendocrine cells in the gut caused dopaminergic neuron formation and alleviation of Parkinson's disease. Moreover, alteration and mediation of the sirtuin–1 pathway might inhibit amyloidogenesis and decrease Alzhimer's disease-type neuropathology.

Probiotics suppress gastrointestinal disorders' effect by reducing reactions to dietary allergens such as rhinitis, food allergies and atopic dermatitis. They change the composition of antigens, reducing the antigens' immunogenicity and intestinal permeability besides also inhibiting pro-inflammatory cytokine production, which is boosted in various allergic disorders. These cells control the immune system by developing anti-inflammatory cytokines or facilitating specific metabolites that impede the contiguity between intestinal mucosa and antigens. Also, probiotics produce short chain fatty acids, which increase peptide-1 glucagon-like (GLP-1). Also, the glucose-dependent insulinotropic polypeptide is responsible for the antiobesity activity of *Akkermansia muciniphila* (Zendeboodi *et al.*, 2020).

The decline of cereal allergenicity via the fermentation process is also significant. The autoimmune disease known as celiac disease is recognized in a genetically susceptible organism as an inflammatory disease of the upper small intestine, exacerbated predominantly by the ingestion of gluten-containing items. Gluten proteins from wheat and associated grains such as barley, rye and oats are widely known to be among the most important causes of allergy. Specifically, the pathway (IgE-dependent) that promotes cereal allergenicity involves low molecular glutenins, high molecular glutenins, gliadins (α, β, γ, ω) and albumin/globulin fractions. By degrading the respective antigenic epitopes, protein hydrolysis by endogenous or microbial proteases and peptidases during fermentation results in weakened allergic reactions. Based on their ability to hydrolyze gliadin fractions, *L. sanfranciscensis* 7A, *L. brevis* 14G, *L. alimentarius* 15M, and *L. hilgardii* 51B were used

(Di Cagno *et al.* 2002). Also, gluten disulfide bonds were diminished during the fermentation of sourdough by *Lactobacillus* spp., which further improved the enzymatic function of cereal proteases, thus enhancing the digestibility of gluten (Karunaratne 2018).

Osteoporosis is a condition of the bone that significantly affects quality of life. Novel, healthy and efficient methods for treating or avoiding osteoporosis associated with multiple factors and variables such as biological sex, age, illness and genetic history are challenging to establish. Oral probiotic supplementation may be an essential and safe alternative to avoid bone degradation in humans under different circumstances, including menopause and type 1 diabetes, and improve bone density in stable or mildly inflamed conditions. The prevention of osteoporosis happens by regulating absorption of minerals such as calcium, phosphorus and magnesium that are necessary for healthy bone.

9.8 Conclusion

In developed and developing countries, an inflated demand from the lactose-intolerant and vegan population is leading to the development of new probiotic non-diary functional beverages. Probiotic non-dairy foods are essential for consumers who do not like dairy products or are allergic to them. Recent trials have demonstrated the implementation of strains that are well suited to alternate matrices, and probiotic and prebiotic non-dairy products have an excellent marketing future. Cereals are rich in nutrients and have specific health benefits for the host's health. Cereals are an ideal substrate for fermentation by probiotic microorganisms such as LAB. The production of several probiotic products relies on probiotic microorganisms being single or mixed. Probiotics have positive implications for the host's gastrointestinal and respiratory system. Probiotics also impact human health by maintaining the host's health and progressively promoting and improving the balance of the intestinal flora. Fermented products based on cereals provide a promising source of prebiotic compounds containing different forms of soluble fibers such as galactooligosaccharides, resistant starch, fructooligosaccharides, β-glucans and arabinoxylans and their oligomeric products, phenolics and peptides, depending on the cereals used to ferment and produce the commodity. Traditional methods are still practiced in African, Asian and European countries to ferment cereals and produce beverages, gruels and porridge using different types of cereal grains such as maize, sorghum, millet, oats, barley, wheat and rye. Microorganisms involved in cereal probiotic foods are LAB and yeasts, which mostly belong to the genera *Lactobacillus, Lactococcus, Leuconostoc, Pediococcus* and *Bifidobacterium*. The yeasts are dominated by *Saccharomyces cerevisiae* and *Candida* species. Therefore, incorporating probiotic strains in cereal-based fermented foods is feasible and holds great promise for the present and the future.

References

Abegaz, K., Langsrud, T., Beyene, F. and Narvhus, J.A. (2004). The effects of technological modifications on the fermentation of borde, an Ethiopian traditional fermented cereal beverage. *Journal of Food Technology in Africa*, 9(1): 3–12.

Achi, O.K. (1990). Microbiology of 'obiolor': a Nigerian fermented non-alcoholic beverage. *Journal of Applied Bacteriology*, 69(3): 321–325.

Aka, S., Konan, G., Fokou, G., Dje, K.M. and Bonfoh, B. (2014). Review on African traditional cereal beverages. *American Journal of Research Communication*, 2(5): 103–153.

Amusa, N.A. and Odunbaku, O.A. (2009). Microbiological and nutritional quality of hawked kunun (a sorghum based non-alcoholic beverage) widely consumed in Nigeria. Pakistan Journal of Nutrition, 8(1): 20–25.

Anal, A.K. (2019). Quality ingredients and safety concerns for traditional fermented foods and beverages from Asia: A review. *Fermentation*, 5(1): 8.

Arora, S., Jood, S. and Khetarpaul, N. (2010). Effect of germination and probiotic fermentation On nutrient composition of barley based food mixtures. *Food Chemistry*, 119(2): 779–784.

Aspri, M., Papademas, P. and Tsaltas, D. (2020). Review on non-dairy probiotics and their use in non-dairy based products. *Fermentation*, 6(1): 30.

Blandino, A., Al-Aseeri, M.E., Pandiella, S.S., Cantero, D. and Webb, C. (2003). Cereal-based fermented foods and beverages. *Food Research International*, 36(6): 527–543.

Blažeková, L., Polakovičová, P., Mikušová, L., Kukurova, K., Saxa, V., Ciesarova, Z. and Šturdík, E. (2015). Development of innovative health beneficial bread using a fermented fibre-glucan product. *Czech Journal of Food Sciences*, 33(2): 118–125.

Chavan, M., Gat, Y., Harmalkar, M. and Waghmare, R. (2018). Development of non-dairy fermented probiotic drink based on germinated and ungerminated cereals and legume. *LWT-Food Science and Technology*, 91: 339–344.

Choi, A.R., Patra, J.K., Kim, W.J. and Kang, S.S. (2018). Antagonistic activities and probiotic potential of lactic acid bacteria derived from a plant-based fermented food. *Frontiers in Microbiology*, 9: 1963.

Chugh, B. and Kamal-Eldin, A. (2020). Bioactive compounds produced by probiotics in food products. *Current Opinion in Food Science*, 32: 76–82.

Ciesarová, Z., Kukurová, K., Mikušová, L., Basil, E., Polakovičová, P., Duchoňová, L., Vlček, M. and Šturdík, E. (2014). Nutritionally enhanced wheat-oat bread with reduced acrylamide level. *Quality Assurance and Safety of Crops & Foods*, 6(3): 327–334.

Ciesarová, Z., Mikušová, L., Magala, M., Kohajdová, Z. and Karovičová, J. (2017). Nonwheat cereal-fermented-derived products. In: *Fermented Foods in Health and Disease Prevention*, 417–432. Academic Press.

Den Besten, G., Van Eunen, K., Groen, A.K., Venema, K., Reijngoud, D.J. and Bakker, B.M. (2013). The role of short-chain fatty acids in the interplay between diet, gut microbiota, and host energy metabolism. *Journal of Lipid Research*, 54(9): 2325–2340.

Di Cagno, R., De Angelis, M., Lavermicocca, P., De Vincenzi, M., Giovannini, C., Faccia, M. and Gobbetti, M. (2002). Proteolysis by sourdough lactic acid bacteria: effects on wheat flour protein fractions and gliadin peptides involved in human cereal intolerance. *Applied and Environmental Microbiology*, 68(2): 623–633.

El-Aidie, S.A.A., El-Dieb, S.M., El-Nawawy, M., Emara, E. and Sobhy, H. (2017). Nutraceutical food based on cereal and probiotic fermented milk. *International Journal of Dairy Science*, 12: 377–384.

Enujiugha, V.N. and Badejo, A.A. (2017). Probiotic potentials of cereal-based beverages. *Critical Reviews in Food Science and Nutrition*, 57(4): 790–804.

Gadaga, T.H., Mutukumira, A.N., Narvhus, J.A. and Feresu, S.B. (1999). A review of Traditional fermented foods and beverages of Zimbabwe. *International Journal of Food Microbiology*, 53(1): 1–11.

Gassem, M.A. (2002). A microbiological study of Sobia: a fermented beverage in the Western province of Saudi Arabia. *World Journal of Microbiology and Biotechnology*, 18(3):173–177.

Giraud, E., Gosselin, L., Marin, B., Parada, J.L. and Raimbault, M. (1993). Purification and characterization of an extracellular amylase from Lactobacillus plantarum strain A6. *Journal of Applied Bacteriology*, 75(3): 276–282.

Gotcheva, V., Pandiella, S.S., Angelov, A., Roshkova, Z.G. and Webb, C. (2000). Microflora identification of the Bulgarian cereal-based fermented beverage boza. *Process Biochemistry*, 36(1-2): 127–130.

Gotcheva, V., Petrova, G., Petkova, M., Kuzmanova, Y. and Angelov, A. (2018). Molecular and in vitro assessment of some probiotic characteristics of amylolytic *Lactobacillus plantarum* strains from Bulgarian fermented products. *Engineering in Life Sciences*, 18(11): 820–830.

Grumezescu, A. and Holban, A.M. (eds) (2019). *Nutrients in Beverages: Volume 12: The Science of Beverages*. London: Elsevier.

Hekmat, S. and Reid, G. (2006). Sensory properties of probiotic yogurt is comparable to standard yogurt. *Nutrition research*, 26(4): 163–166.

Holzapfel, W. (ed.) (2014). *Advances in fermented foods and beverages: improving quality, technologies and health benefits*. London: Elsevier,.

Jimoh, S.O., Ado, S.A., Ameh, J.B., Whong, C.M. and Anglais, A.T.E. (2012). Characteristics and diversity of yeast in locally fermented beverages sold in Nigeria. *World J Eng Pure Appl Sci*, 2: 40.

Kalui, C.M., Mathara, J.M. and Kutima, P.M. (2010). Probiotic potential of spontaneously fermented cereal based foods–a review. *African Journal of Biotechnology*, 9(17): 2490–2498.

Karunaratne, A.M. (2018). Probiotic foods: benefits to the cereal based Sri Lankan diet. *Ceylon Journal of Science*, 47(2): 105–123.

Kohajdová, Z. (2017). Fermented cereal products. In: *Current Developments in Biotechnology and Bioengineering*, 91–117. Elsevier.

Koirala, S. and Anal, A.K. (2021). Probiotics-based foods and beverages as future foods and their overall safety and regulatory claims. *Future Foods*, 100013.

Lei, V. and Jakobsen, M. (2004). Microbiological characterization and probiotic potential of koko and koko sour water, African spontaneously fermented millet porridge and drink. *Journal of Applied Microbiology*, 96(2): 384–397.

Montet, D. and Ray, R.C. (eds) (2016). *Fermented Foods, Part I: Biochemistry and Biotechnology*. Florida: CRC Press.

Mridula, D. and Sharma, M. (2015). Development of non-dairy probiotic drink utilizing sprouted cereals, legume and soymilk. *LWT-Food Science and Technology*, 62(1): 482–487.

Nout, M.R. (2009). Rich nutrition from the poorest–cereal fermentations in Africa and Asia. *Food Microbiology*, 26(7): 685–692.

Nwachukwu, E., Achi, O.K. and Ijeoma, I.O. (2010). Lactic acid bacteria in fermentation of cereals for the production of indigenous Nigerian foods. *African Journal of Food Science and Technology*, 1(2): 21–26.

Nyanzi, R. and Jooste, P.J. (2012). Cereal-based functional foods. *Probiotics*, 161–197.

Orji, M.U., Mbata, T.I., Aniche, G.N. and Ahonkhai, I. (2003). The use of starter cultures to produce 'Pito', a Nigerian fermented alcoholic beverage. *World Journal of Microbiology and Biotechnology*, 19(7): 733–736.

Panghal, A., Janghu, S., Virkar, K., Gat, Y., Kumar, V. and Chhikara, N. (2018). Potential non-dairy probiotic products–A healthy approach. *Food Bioscience*, 21: 80–89.

Rathore, S., Salmerón, I. and Pandiella, S.S. (2012). Production of potentially probiotic beverages using single and mixed cereal substrates fermented with lactic acid bacteria cultures. *Food Microbiology*, 30(1): 239–244.

Ray, R.C. and Didier, M. (eds) (2014). *Microorganisms and Fermentation of Traditional Foods*. Florida: CRC Press.

Rigobelo, E. (ed.) (2012). *Probiotics*. Croatia: InTech.

Saulnier, D.M., Spinler, J.K., Gibson, G.R. and Versalovic, J. (2009). Mechanisms of probiosis and prebiosis: considerations for enhanced functional foods. *Current Opinion in Biotechnology*, 20(2): 135–141.

Shetty, K. and Sarkar, D. (eds) (2020). *Functional Foods and Biotechnology: Biotransformation and Analysis of Functional Foods and Ingredients*. Florida: CRC Press.

Sivamaruthi, B.S., Fern, L.A., Hj, D.S.N.R.P. and Chaiyasut, C. (2020). The influence of probiotics on bile acids in diseases and aging. *Biomedicine & Pharmacotherapy*, 128: 110310.

Song, D., Ibrahim, S. and Hayek, S. (2012). Recent application of probiotics in food and agricultural science. *Probiotics*, 10: 1–34.

Tsafrakidou, P., Michaelidou, A.M. and G Biliaderis, C. (2020). Fermented cereal-based products: nutritional aspects, possible impact on gut microbiota and health implications. *Foods*, 9(6): 734.

Ukwuru, M.U. and Ohaegbu, C.G. (2018). Local cereal fermented foods with probiotic potentials. *Research Journal of Food and Nutrition*, 2(1): 1–13.

Vasudha, S. and Mishra, H.N. (2013). Non dairy probiotic beverages. *International Food Research Journal*, 20(1): 7–15.

Wacher, C., Cañas, A., Bárzana, E., Lappe, P., Ulloa, M. and Owens, J.D. (2000). Microbiology of Indian and Mestizo pozol fermentations. *Food Microbiology*, 17(3): 251–256.

Yan, F. and Polk, D.B. (2011). Probiotics and immune health. *Current Opinion in Gastroenterology*, 27(6): 496.

Zendeboodi, F., Khorshidian, N., Mortazavian, A.M. and da Cruz, A.G. (2020). Probiotic: Conceptualization from a new approach. *Current Opinion in Food Science*, 32: 103–123.

10

Microencapsulation of Probiotics and its Potential Industrial Applications

Suwan Panjanapongchai, Chaichawin Chavapradit and Anil Kumar Anal

Food Engineering and Bioprocess Technology, Department of Food Agriculture and Bioresources, School of Environment and Resources, Asian Institute of Technology, Pathumthani, Thailand

10.1 Introduction

Over the past decade, there has been a global rise in research into the development of functional foods. Functional foods that provide an adequate amount of nutrients and positive health benefits to the consumer have become the center of attention for both researchers and industry (Doyon and Labrecque 2008). Several functional ingredients such as dietary fiber, vitamins, minerals, prebiotics, probiotics, fatty acids, and carotenoids have been incorporated in food products to enhance the bioactive properties and improve health benefits of the developed goods. These functional enhanced food products have been classified as the functional foods. The global functional foods market was estimated at around \$173.26 billion in 2019 (Precedence Research 2019). Health trends and the increasing demand for healthy products are tremendously encouraging the growth of the market.

With this rise in the functional food market, the exploration of functional ingredients has been conducted worldwide. One of the most promising functional ingredients to have been incorporated in several food products is probiotics. Probiotics are defined as living microorganisms that can provide the host with health benefits when administered in adequate amounts (Bielecka 2006).These beneficial living organisms have been utilized as the functional ingredient in dairy and food products such as yoghurt, sports drinks, baby foods, sugar-free confectionery and chewing gum (Misra *et al.* 2019).As the primary functional ingredients, the probiotic market size was estimated at around USD 49.4 billion in 2018. Moreover, annual growth expectation was predicted at over 7% (Grand view research, 2019). Lactic acid bacteria (LAB) such as *Lactobacillus* and *Bifidobacterium* are the Gram-positive bacteria that are widely utilized as probiotics (Fijan 2014). In addition, several LAB such as *Escherichia, Enterococcus, Streptococcus* and *Saccharomyces* that pass

Probiotics, Prebiotics and Synbiotics: Technological Advancements Towards Safety and Industrial Applications, First Edition. Edited by Parmjit Singh Panesar and Anil Kumar Anal.

the selective criteria are also labelled as probiotics (Merenstein, *et al.* 2017). The microbes in the human gastrointestinal tract play a crucial role in the development of the host immune system and have a long-term effect on preventing inflammatory diseases (Merenstein, Salminen and Team, 2017). The viable probiotics that colonize in the gastrointestinal tract effectively support the host. Their health benefits include reduction and inhibition of diarrhea, the enhancement of gastric microbial balance, rebuilding the microbiota, mitigation of lactose intolerance symptoms, inhibition of food allergies, and antimutagenic and immunomodulatory effects (Han *et al.* 2021).Therefore, routine intake of a probiotic supplement can adjust the host's microbial balance, resulting in the colonization of health-promoting bacteria that effectively enhance the health of the host and reduce the risk of potential diseases.

10.2 Why We Need Microencapsulation

The purpose of probiotic consumption is to colonize LAB bacteria in the host's gastrointestinal tract as the replacement for general gut bacteria (Han *et al.* 2021). Probiotics can only positively affect the host when they reach and colonize in the large intestine. Thus, an adequate number of probiotics must be administered to survive the harsh environmental conditions in the gastrointestinal tract. Due to the highly acidic conditions in the upper part of the human gut (pH 2), most viable probiotics are unable to survive and reach the target destination. As a result, no health benefit is acquired from probiotic consumption. Therefore, the recommended number of probiotic bacteria live in the food product should be 10^8–10^9 colony-forming units (CFU)/g or higher (Kechagia *et al.* 2013). The number of bacteria will be reduced during transportation in the gastrointestinal tract to around 10^6–10^7 CFU/g on reaching the colon. Moreover, the living cells may encounter several harsh environmental conditions such as heat, oxygen, pH and physical forces during industrialization processes and subsequent storage.

To protect the bacteria against severe environmental conditions and increase the survivability of probiotics in the gastrointestinal tract, microencapsulation techniques have been developed (Shori 2017). Microencapsulation techniques relate to entrapment of probiotic cells or active components in a polymer matrix or network, preventing the degradation of active compounds and enabling their delivery to a targeted destination (Singh *et al.* 2010). A control-release mechanism that controls the rate of release of the active compound is also included. Encapsulation of probiotics can effectively enhance the survivability of bacteria and protect them from the highly acidic conditions in the human gut, bile salts and other products of digestion that the probiotic must encounter during its transport through the gastrointestinal tract (Muthukumarasamy and Holley 2006). Moreover, processing conditions also significantly affect the survivability of the bacteria, and the entrapment layer from the encapsulation techniques acts as a protective barrier to protect the probiotics against extreme temperature and pH during food processing. The properties of the encapsulated product mostly depend on the chemical, physical and biological properties of the wall material used during production. Thus, the selection of wall materials is the crucial step which determines the outcome of the encapsulation. Generally, encapsulating polymers such as alginate, xanthan gum, starch, carrageenan, gelatin, chitosan and carboxymethyl cellulose that are recognized as safe can be utilized in food products due to the biocompatibility of these polymers (Abd El-Salam and El-Shibiny 2012). Protein-based polymers such as casein and whey protein have also been used as wall materials for the encapsulation process (Singh *et al.* 2010). pH-responsive materials are considered the most promising ingredients for probiotic encapsulation as the capsule created from these materials can swell and shrink depending on the environmental pH. pH-responsive material can shrink when faced with gastric acid, so the shrinking wall layer prevents contact between the acid and the entrapped compounds. However, when the capsule passes through the small and large intestine it will swell due to the shift of environmental pH, resulting in the release of probiotics in the small and large intestine (Shori 2017).

10.3 Encapsulation Techniques

10.3.1 Emulsion Technique

The emulsion techniques (Figure 10.1) are considered as one of the most researched encapsulation methods. The techniques relate to the immersion of one fluid into another immiscible fluid to create a harmonized miscible fluid (de Vos *et al.* 2010). The emulsion techniques can be utilized with the probiotic cells to entrap the cells in the liquid layer and increase the survivability of active cells when they pass through the gastrointestinal tract. The technique can be performed to encapsulate the probiotic cells inside small droplets of fluid and immerse them in another liquid layer, resulting in a stable probiotic-loaded emulsion. The interactions and association of continuous phases and dispersed phases are basic to emulsion technique. In depth, the cells are thoroughly dissolved in a water-based phase (discontinuous phase), which mixture is further added to an oil phase (continuous

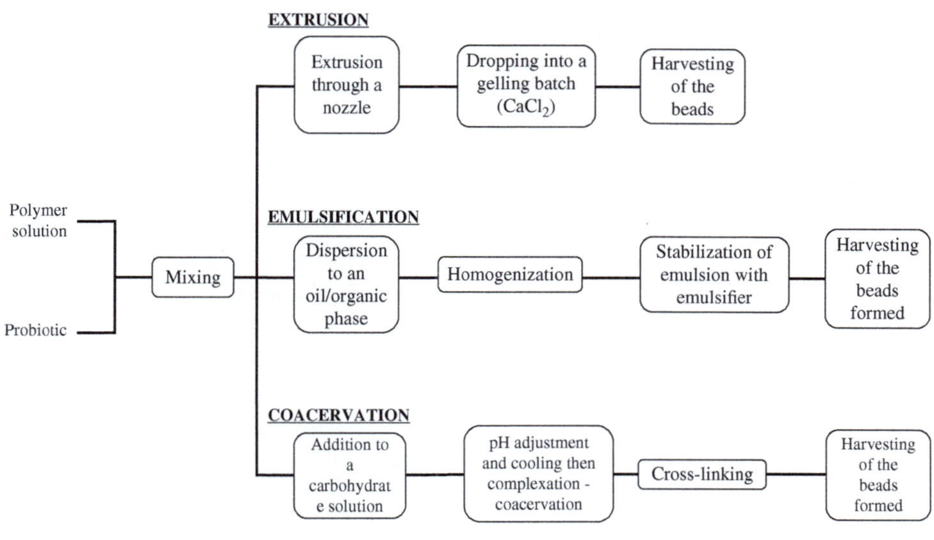

Figure 10.1 Chart of the extrusion, emulsion and coacervation processes.

phase). Then, these two phases are mixed by mechanical homogenization with the assistance of surfactant, forming a water-in-oil emulsion. The final harvests of this technique are separated in two ways: creation of a water-soluble biopolymer by insolubilization, or gel beads with organic phase by filtration or centrifugation. For water-soluble, the process depends on the properties of the supporting material used (Coghetto *et al. 2016*). The initial step can be cooling or adding a cross-linking agent such as alginate, carrageenan or pectin to the emulsion (Rathore *et al.* 2013). For continuous phase, an organic solvent is used for interfacial polymerization, which can improve the cells' productivity during fermentation. The emulsification technique can improve the thermal resistance properties of the microbeads by application of high-amylose starch (Khosravi Zanjani *et al.* 2018). The important substance in the emulsion technique is surfactant, which can reduce surface tension between coating matrix and beads (Burgain *et al.* 2011). A second coating can be added to the beads by soaking in additional polymer solution. In addition, the beads can be soaked with extra polymer solution for additional purposes such as improvement of protective and sensory characteristics. There are several factors that affect the size of the beads such as agitation speed, the concentration ratio between two phases, the cross-linking rate, and surfactant concentration (Rathore *et al.* 2013). This technique can be adapted easily to the industrial scale and obtains a high cell survival rate (Chen *et al.* 2007). The diameter of beads produced by this technique may be below 300 μm. Nevertheless, there are several disadvantages of this technique which are wide range in size and shape. Another disadvantage is the oil residues from the continuous phase on the particles' surface (Burgain *et al.* 2013).

10.3.2 Extrusion Technique

The extrusion methods are the traditional encapsulation techniques which have been widely researched. The method exploits the physical properties of an applied hydrocolloid to encapsulate the bioactive ingredients such as living probiotic cells and active compounds (see Figure 10.1) (Burgain *et al.* 2011). This technique is a basic process based on the driving force of the cell suspension through nozzles by droplet-generating devices (de Vos *et al.* 2010). The initial step is the mixing of probiotic cells with a biopolymer solution to form a suspension (Sagis 2015). The suspension is extruded through a nozzle to produce droplets that are dropped into a coagulate fluid (most generally a $CaCl_2$ solution). The ionic cross-linking between biopolymer and coagulate fluid forms gel beads as the cells are entrapped in a three-dimensional grid (Sagis 2015). The size and sphericity of the beads depend on conditions of the solution such as temperature, viscosity, flow rate and rpm of mixing. Other factors also affect the beads such as nozzle diameter, the distance between the nozzle and the coagulate fluid, and concentration of biopolymer (Rathore *et al.* 2013). The extrusion method can be applied in aerobic or anaerobic conditions. The advantages of this technique are that it is simple, easy to handle and low cost on a small scale. In addition, the sizes of beads produced by this technique are similar while in the emulsion technique they vary widely. However, the extrusion technique is difficult to apply at a large scale because of slow particle formation (Burgain *et al.* 2011). Multiple-nozzle systems and spinning disk atomizer techniques can be applied for the extrusion method at an industrial scale (de Vos *et al.* 2010).

10.3.3 Coacervation Technique

The coacervation technique is a process that separates colloid into two liquid portions. This process is divided into three parts: the formation of three immiscible phases, the deposition of the coating, and the solidification of the coating. The shell hardness can be enhanced by adding a cross-linker during the third step (see Figure 10.1) (Đorđević *et al.* 2014). Protein suspension is generally present in nature as the hydrocolloid substances that are suitable for the addition of probiotic cells. The difficulty of application depends on the number of biopolymers used during the formulation. For example, using one polymer is the most simple method: the polymer is adsorbed onto the interface between the suspension and the solvent. After suitable modification of the temperature and/or pH, it changes into an insoluble form called the "coacervate phase", which surrounds the suspended phase, and is deposited on it. The harvest of this method can be collected by centrifugation or filtration and spray drying.

Use of two or more biopolymers in the coacervation technique is called complex coacervation and involves electrostatic interactions of the two charged biopolymers in the solution. Adjustment of pH or the charge regulation mechanism leads to the formation of two separate liquid phases: a polymer-poor and a polymer-rich phase. Complex coacervation is supported by dilution, a property that differentiates this technique from other polymer phase-separation phenomena. Most general polymers used for the coacervation technique are protein as polycations and polysaccharides as polyanions (Ach *et al.* 2015). The selection of polymers depends on the requirement for special properties such as hydrophilic colloidal properties, water solubility and adequate charge density (Alvim and Grosso 2010). At the same pH value, the polysaccharide is combined into the protein–cells suspension when both: have the same charge. The changing pH can re-dissolve polymers from insoluble to soluble form. This reaction is reversible because of the ionic properties of the interactions between the polymers and the wall material of the beads. Consequently, the decreasing mechanical strength affects hardening of the polymers. In addition, this technique may be required to enhance the stability of the complex biopolymers. Heat treatment can improve the hardening properties of beads because of protein denaturation and the addition of a cross-linking agent (Zhang *et al.* 2012). Properties of the beads such as permeability and mechanical and thermal resistance can be modified by the cross-linking agents, which can be chemical or enzymatic (Alvim and Grosso 2010). The release rate of the beads depends on parameters during the cross-linking step such as hardening time, pH, temperature and cross-linker concentration (Zhang *et al.* 2012). There are several factors that affect coacervation such as the properties of the wall and core materials (molecular weight, conformation, charge density and composition), the percentage of total solid, and the dispersion conditions such as pressure, shearing force, temperature, pH and charge strength (Schmitt and Turgeon 2011). The advantages of coacervation are high cell load, high encapsulation efficiency and water immiscibility of beads, which can be optimal for controlling release of the beads. Furthermore, the technique can combine an extensive number of probiotic cells into a certain volume of the wall material. However, this method is quite expensive and complex because of the coacervation and hardening steps (Chavarri *et al.* 2012; Coghetto *et al.* 2016). Coacervation is also problematic to scale up, while an added drying process can be damaging to the cells (Chavarri *et al.* 2012).

10.3.4 Spray Drying

The best-known encapsulation technique is spray drying, which applies the principle of mass and heat transfer to develop the compact encapsulated beads (Figure 10.2) (Arslan *et al.* 2015). The process of spray drying is divided into three parts: mixing probiotics with wall material, using a nozzle to atomize the liquid mixture, and evaporation of water using hot air (Fang and Bhandari 2012; Sagis 2015). The wall material properties should increase protection of the cells from harsh conditions such as those in the gastrointestinal tract (Huang *et al.* 2016). The cyclone harvests dried particles by separation from the humid air (Fang and Bhandari 2012). There are various factors that impact the effectiveness of encapsulation such as characteristics of the probiotic (strain and growth phase), drying process (time, temperature and type of nozzle), wall material (type of material, concentration, type of stress applied: osmotic, oxidative or mechanical), the operational conditions (temperature and input rate) and the storage conditions (Zuidam and Nedovic 2010). Spray drying at high temperatures is damaging to living cells, while poor flow properties and membranes of high density on beads occur at low air temperature. In addition, adjustment of temperature facilitates inhomogeneous spraying (Dianawati *et al.* 2016). The survival rate of the probiotic can be increased by adding heat-protective agents such as granular starch, soluble fibers and trehalose, or lipophilic antioxidants (Ying *et al.* 2016). For instance, a second coating layer of the capsules can protect against the acid environment of the stomach and bile salts (Dianawati *et al.* 2016; Sagis 2015). Spray drying is the most economical microencapsulation method because it is a single unit process. Moreover, the products of the spray drying method are dry, low in bulk density, stable and have a long shelf-life. The method uses inexpensive equipment but has a high production rate and is also easy to scale up. Nevertheless, this method results in poor survival rate and low stability during storage because the hot air used in the spray drying process subjects the cells to extreme osmotic stress, causing significant loss of viability and activity (Her *et al.*, 2015; Huang *et al.* 2016). Moreover, as most of the microcapsules

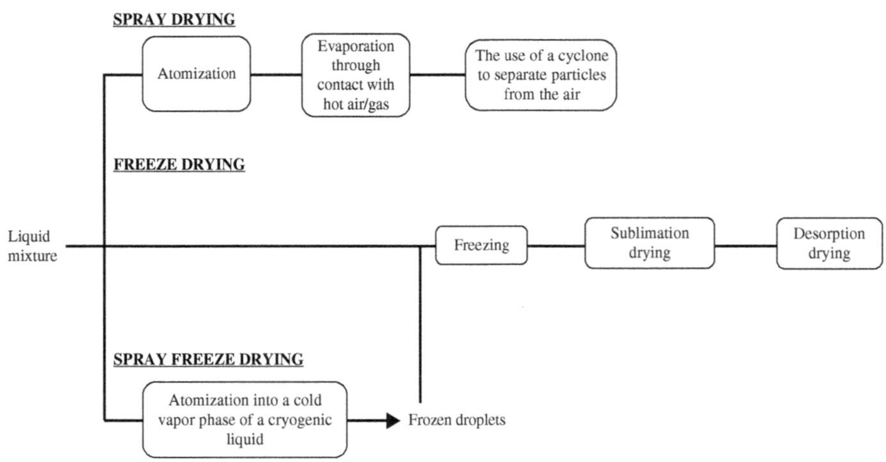

Figure 10.2 Comparative chart of spray drying, freeze drying, and spray freeze drying processes.

prepared by this method are water soluble, there is a danger of an early release of the probiotics that may limit their beneficial effects (Sagis 2015).

10.3.5 Ultrasonic Vacuum Spray Dryer

Spray drying causes oxidative and thermal stresses to cells or bioactive compounds during processing. These stresses can be reduced by ultrasonic vacuum spray drying. The application of an ultrasonic nozzle in a low temperature vacuum atmosphere can increase the viability of cells (Semyonov *et al.* 2011). Moreover, utilizing coating agents such as maltodextrin and trehalose can enhance the viability of cells (Martín *et al.* 2015).

10.3.6 Freeze Drying

Generally, bacterial cells are mostly susceptible to high temperature. The suitable drying method for these components is a low-temperature method, namely freeze drying, which is the preferred method for the encapsulation of bacterial cells. The method relates to the freezing and sublimation of water from a frozen state straight into the gas state, under vacuum to prevent any heating damage to the cells (see Figure 10.2) (Fang and Bhandari 2012; Her *et al.* 2015). However, freeze drying negatively affects the cell membrane (Nag and Das 2013). The solution to this is to use cryoprotectants such as polymers, sugars (maltodextrin, trehalose, fructose), milk, honey, alcohol sugar (sorbitol) and amino acid (glutamate) together with the probiotic (Dianawati *et al.* 2016). The concentration of cryoprotectant depends on strain of probiotic. Moreover, an immobilization technique can also increase the survival rate of probiotic cells (Dimitrellou *et al.* 2016). The freeze drying method requires long processing times and high capital and energy costs, which are the main disadvantage of this technique (Barbosa *et al.* 2015; Her *et al.* 2015).

10.3.7 Spray Freeze Drying

The combination of the spray and freeze drying methods is a new method, spray freeze drying, which can avoid side effects from heat during spray drying. The spray freeze drying process is divided into three steps. The first step is mixing of the wall material with probiotic cells. Second, the nozzle atomizes the mixture of wall material and cells into the cold vapor phase of a cryogenic liquid. The droplets freeze as they pass through the cold vapor chamber. Then, the final step related to the sublimation of the frozen water in droplet under pressure that remove all the existed water and leave only the dried form encapsulated bead. This brings about a dispersion of frozen droplets. The properties of droplets from the spray freeze drying method are different from those of the freeze-drying method. Consequently, the protectants in spray freeze drying are not same as in the freeze-drying method (Anandharamakrishnan and Ishwarya 2015; Her *et al.* 2015). The main advantage of spray freeze drying compared to spray drying is the precise control of the size of capsule and low environmental stress from heat for the active ingredients (Burgain *et al.* 2011). The encapsulation process duration of spray freeze drying is less than spray drying and freeze drying techniques because of higher heat transfers (Her *et al.* 2015). Nevertheless, this technique consumes more energy and is higher in cost than the spray drying technique (Burgain *et al.* 2011).

10.3.8 Spray Chilling

The principle of spray chilling is dissolution, emulsion or dispersion of a bioactive compound in a molten fat matrix. When the temperature of the air is below the melting point of the wall material, the nozzle atomizes the combination of wall material and probiotic cells, and when the droplets come into contact with cold air, they solidify as solid lipid microbeads (Figure 10.3) (Okuro *et al.* 2013; Pedroso *et al.* 2012). Fractionated vegetable oils with melting points between 32 and 42 °C are commonly used as the wall materials in spray chilling (Đorđević *et al.* 2014). Because lipids may be used as a substitute for biopolymers and polysaccharides, this technique for microencapsulating probiotics has a lot of potential. When the temperature exceeds the melting point of the carrier material, the core material is released, and the lipases in the intestines break down the lipid wall components, releasing the probiotics where they are needed. The release mechanism of probiotic cells depends on environmental temperature (i.e., the probiotic cells are released when environmental temperatures are higher than or equal to the melting point of the wall material). Moreover, the release mechanism also occurs in the gastrointestinal tract when lipases digest the lipid wall materials (Okuro *et al.* 2013). Spray chilling is possible to scale up to an industrial level because this method is the least expensive and has high yield. The size and morphology of the bead can facilitate the flow rate of the material, without spoiling the texture of the final food product (Martín *et al.* 2015). Nevertheless, this technique exhibits low cell load in encapsulation, as a significant number of probiotic cells are left over on the outer surface of the beads and are therefore exposed directly to the environment. Furthermore, the encapsulated probiotics must be carefully stored due to the characteristics of certain lipid materials such as the crystalline structure and polymorphic arrangement. These properties can lead to solidification and crystallization during storage and cause release of the probiotic (Pedroso *et al.* 2012).

10.3.9 Fluid Bed Coating

Fluid bed coating is a modification of the spray drying method. The coating agent is applied to solid particles during a fluidized bed process (Figure 10.4). The wall materials are sprayed by the nozzle when the probiotic cells are suspended in an air stream at certain temperature and humidity (de Vos *et al.* 2010; Nedovic *et al.* 2011). The hot air dried the aqueous medium from bottom of fluid bed. Moreover, the water activity of the powdered matrix are reduced to a desirable level (Nag and Das 2013). Water evaporation is affected by spraying speed, percentage of water in the medium, temperature, airflow, and humidity of the air

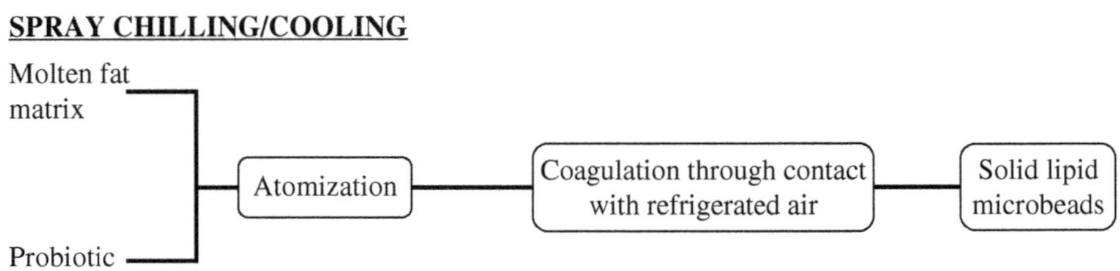

Figure 10.3 Spray chilling process.

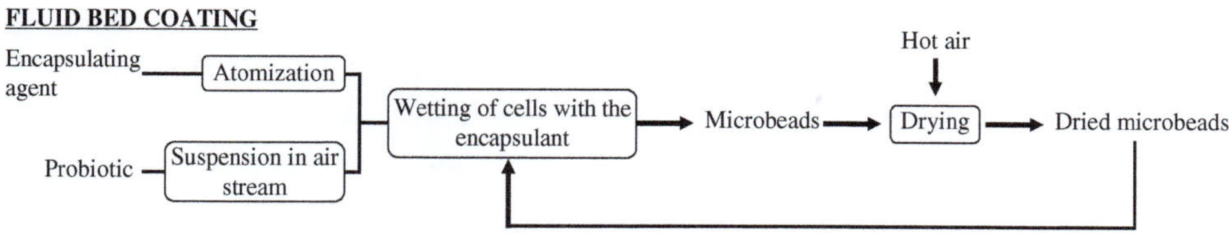

Figure 10.4 Fluid bed coating process.

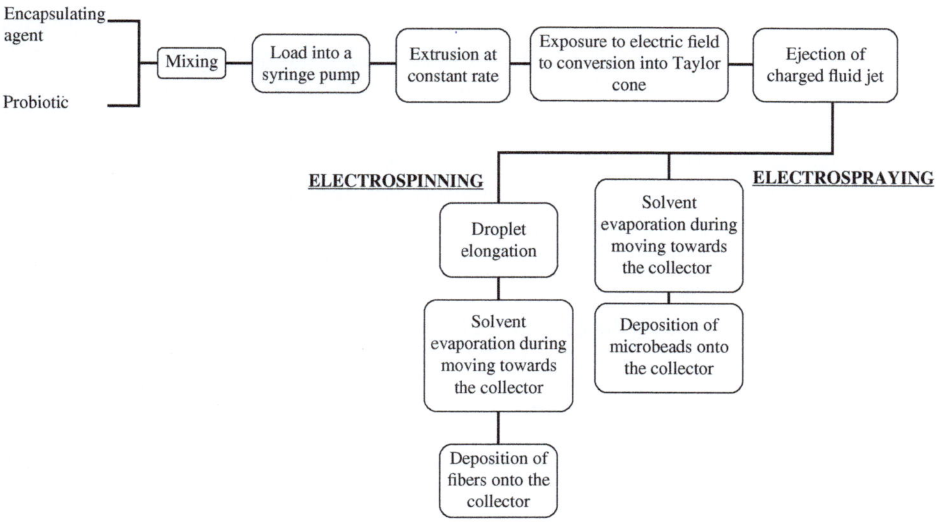

Figure 10.5 Comparative chart of electrospinning and electrospraying processes.

inlet (Đorđević *et al.* 2014). Several materials can be applied as encapsulating agents such as fats, proteins, carbohydrates, and gums (de Vos *et al.* 2010; Đorđević *et al.* 2014). When this technique is applied in a batch process, it has low energy consumption and causes mild heat damage to the cells (Nag and Das 2013). Besides, the temperature of this technique is controllable and it is easy to scale up or adapt to provide multilayer coatings (Martín *et al.* 2015). Uncontrolled aggregation of the beads is the main disadvantage of this technique because the material can coalesce when applied wet coated materials (Đorđević *et al.* 2014). This approach is also time consuming and hard to manage (Martín *et al.* 2015).

10.3.10 Electrospraying and Electrospinning

Electrospraying and electrospinning are electrohydrodynamic processes (Figure 10.5). The cell solution is atomized in a high-voltage electric field leading to the deposition of dry particles due to charged collector (Alehosseini *et al.* 2018; Gomez-Mascaraque *et al.* 2016). The voltage used in this method is approximately around 1–30 kV and is normally performed in indirect current mode (alternating current mode is also suitable) using a blunt-ended stainless steel needle or capillary, a syringe pump and a grounded collector which can be either a flat plate or a rotating drum (Anu Bhushani and Anandharamakrishnan 2014). The principle of electrospinning is that electrostatic forces draw a pendant droplet of the probiotic cell solution into a fine fiber which is then deposited on a grounded collector (Ghorani and Tucker 2015), while electrospraying is a process of liquid atomization by electrical forces. The extent of the molecular cohesion in the raw material of electrospinning and electrospraying differs. To control this parameter, the concentration of probiotic cells is adjusted to the appropriate level to reduce or increase the contact between wall material and microbial cells. In the case of low concentrations, the jet becomes destabilized and forms fine droplets (Ghorani and Tucker 2015). The droplets agglomerate and coagulate, which can prevent their dispersal as they are highly charged. Adding solvent evaporation compounds leads to contraction and solidification and finally the solid microparticles are deposited onto the collector (Anu Bhushani and Anandharamakrishnan 2014). Electrospraying and electrospinning are both easy, cost-effective, and adaptable processes (Anu Bhushani and Anandharamakrishnan 2014). The probiotic cells are not affected by the strong electric field (Đorđević *et al.* 2014). The system design, the parameter of the solution used and the operating conditions can adjust for appropriate final particle size at micron (>1 μm), submicron or nano (10–1000 nm). Moreover, both methods exhibit high encapsulation efficiency and a food-grade solvent can be used (Anu Bhushani and Anandharamakrishnan 2014). Nevertheless, dripping of the solution may occur when the process is not well optimized (Alehosseini *et al.* 2018; Gomez-Mascaraque *et al.* 2016).

10.3.11 Impinging Aerosol Technology

Impinging aerosol technology was applied (Sohail *et al.* 2011). Two aerosols are used in this method. The probiotic cells suspended in an alginate solution are injected at the top of a cylinder while at the bottom calcium chloride is injected. The average diameter of the cross-linked particles is less than 40 mm and they can be additionally spray dried or freeze dried (Sohail *et al.* 2012). The flow chart of this technology is presented in Figure 10.6. This technology is suitable for heat-sensitive materials. Furthermore, it has a high production yield, is a continuous process and results in products with small particle size (Sohail *et al.* 2012).

10.3.12 Hybridization method

The hybridization system (Figure 10.7) comprises of a high-speed rotor with blades, a stator and a powder recirculation circuit. The air stream is generated by a high-speed blade rotor. This allows the powder mixture to collide strongly. Subsequently, the ordered mixture is developed as probiotic cells are filmed on the surface of the encapsulating agent.

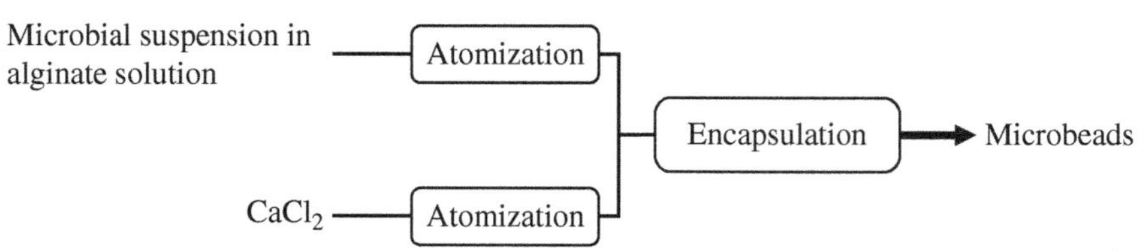

Figure 10.6 Impinging aerosol technology process.

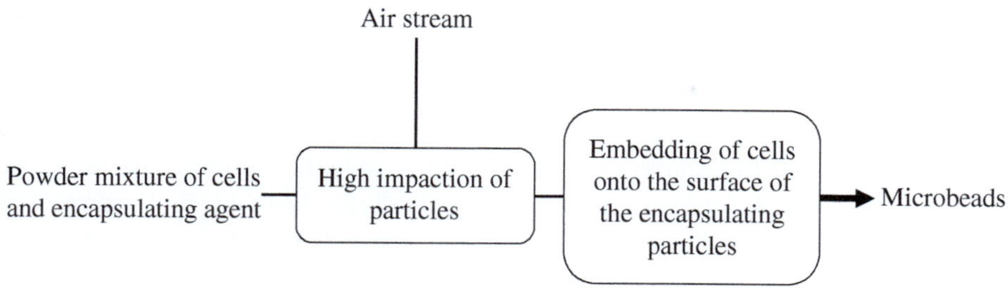

Figure 10.7 Hybridization process.

Prebiotic substances such as sorbitol, mannitol, lactulose, xylitol, inulin, fructooligosaccharides and raffinose have been shown to be suitable for this method. Hybridization is advantageous compared to other microencapsulation methods, including spray drying, because of high microencapsulation efficiency and the minimization of heat stress through its cooling system, which keeps temperatures below 30 °C (Ann *et al.* 2007).

10.4 Application of Probiotics in Food Matrices

Traditionally, probiotic microorganisms have been widely incorporated in food and beverage products, especially in dairy factories. Several dairy products such as milk, cheese, quark and fermented-base dairy products require the fermentation process from the microorganism (Saarela 2009). For production, most of the probiotic strains are selected based on both health benefits and growth conditions of the microorganisms (Maragkoudakis *et al.* 2006). This applies not only to dairy products; probiotic bacteria have also been broadly included in non-dairy food products and beverages such as meat, vegetables, fruits, juices, soft drink, bread and cereals (Shori 2015). During the industrial process, probiotics generally faced with harsh environmental conditions. For instance, microorganisms potentially encounter high temperature heating processes, acidic environments, high mechanical forces, and freezing and thawing processes. These severe processing conditions potentially damage and eliminate the microbial cells, resulting in the reduction of cells which ultimately leads to the loss of bioactive properties. Therefore, a protection process that helps to maintain the viability and functionality of the probiotic during industrial processing is essential. The encapsulation process has become the major tool for the food industry to address these issues. The information in the following paragraphs is related to specific industrial food products that utilize the encapsulation process to enhance the survivability of the microbial cells.

10.4.1 Dairy Products

10.4.1.1 Yoghurt

Yoghurt is the traditional fermented food product that was developed globally. The food was considered as the first probiotic carrier. Strains such as *S. thermophilus* and *Lb. bulgaricus* have conventionally been used as the starter culture for yoghurt production. These conventional cultures have also been co-cultured with probiotic bacteria such as *Lb. acidophilus* and *Bifidobacterium* spp. and incorporated in the encapsulation matrix (Zare *et al.* 2012). Evidently, free probiotic culture without encapsulation results in poor cell growth and survivability (Maragkoudakis *et al.* 2006). The probiotic culture when used alone for yoghurt production shows poor growth compared to the traditional bacteria. The acidic environment (pH 4.2–4.6) in the yoghurt is generally not favorable for the growth of probiotic cells, resulting in a low survival rate during storage (Chen *et al.* 2007). Thus, the probiotic culture has mostly been preferred as an additional culture after the fermentation process has finished. The growth of these probiotics potentially alters the taste and texture of the final yoghurt. During storage, the growth of probiotic bacteria significantly reduces the acidification, which leads to change in taste and textural properties of the yoghurt. Encapsulation techniques have been used to enhance the survivability of the probiotic cells and improve the texture of the product (Ribeiro *et al.* 2014). The effect of encapsulation on the survivability of the cells was conducted using *Lb. acidophilus* LA-5; the encapsulated cells showed a significantly higher survivability rate in yoghurt compared to the free cells. In addition, the encapsulated cells were also tested under gastrointestinal conditions. The results indicated that encapsulation potentially protects the probiotic bacteria from the acidic conditions, resulting in a higher number of cells being delivered in the large intestine (Ribeiro *et al.* 2014). However, the different wall materials and encapsulation techniques affect both physical and chemical properties of the developed encapsulated beads which further affect the sensory qualities and taste of the final yoghurt products. Encapsulation of probiotic cells using the combination of sodium alginate and Hi-Maize® starch effectively inhibited the syneresis and increased the viscosity of the yoghurt, these phenomena leading to better mouth feel in the final product. On the other hand, the encapsulated cells also produce undesirable grittiness in the final products (Kailasapathy 2006). An extrusion method was applied to encapsulate probiotic bacteria, and large-diameter hydrogel beads were developed. When the beads were incorporated in yoghurt, these micrometer sized beads were often tangible and offered inferior sensory characteristics. Similarly, encapsulation of *Lb. casei* using the combination of alginate and pectin polymers was conducted, and the combination of these polymeric materials exhibited higher protective ability compared with individual agents (Sandoval-Castilla *et al.* 2010). The optimized ratio between polymers provided the highest survivability in both yoghurt and a simulated gastrointestinal environment. Due to the unsuitable environmental conditions in yoghurt, several approaches have been conducted to enhance the survivability of probiotic cells. Agents such as whey protein concentrate and whey powders were added to the product so that these proteins could act as nutrient supplements for the probiotics (Maragkoudakis *et al.* 2006). However, the presence of acidic ingredients such as pulps and fruits is potentially harmful for the probiotic cells. These ingredients may also be contaminated with antimicrobial compounds which strongly affect the growth of the microbial cells (Shori 2015). Therefore, the milk proteins, which are inexpensive and plentiful, are preferable as the additive, as these proteins can enhance the viability of probiotics. The addition not only of protein, but also of cereals to the yoghurt can potentially enhance the growth of probiotic cells, the cereal acting as a source of nutrients. Prebiotic compounds such as inulin, lactulose and fiber are promising additives for yoghurt production, as the bacteria can fully utilize these ingredients as their nutrient sources.

10.4.1.2 Cheese

Cheese is one of the traditional fermented products which is available worldwide and also considered as a promising probiotic carrier. The lactic acid bacteria can be co-cultured with the starter culture for the cheese production (Shori 2015). The preferred type of cheese for use as the probiotic carrier is cheddar cheese due to its compatible environmental pH (5.5) with probiotic cells. In addition, the good buffering capacity and relatively high fat content in cheddar cheese can effectively prevent enzymatic degradation and acidic conditions during digestion (Burgain *et al.* 2011). Several studies have been conducted to observe the direct cultivation of probiotic cells in cheese products (Bezerra *et al.* 2017; Gomes de Oliveira *et al.* 2014;). When producing probiotic cheese, several factors such as processing conditions, cooking procedure, aerobic environment, and ripening and storage conditions have to be considered (Shori 2015). However, the survivability of the probiotic bacteria is significantly reduced during the ripening and storage steps due to the rise in acidity. In addition, the presence of the non-probiotic culture may negatively affect the growth of the probiotic. Thus, the microencapsulation process has been recommended to improve the survival rate of probiotic bacteria during the ripening periods (Demers-Mathieu *et al.* 2016), not only to increase probiotic survivability, but also to enhance the sensory properties and flavor of the cheese (Chen *et al.* 2007). The encapsulation of *B. bifidus* BB-12 and *Lb. acidophilus* LA-5 in white-brined cheese was conducted by (Özer *et al.* 2009). The result indicated that the encapsulation process significantly improves the cell viability. Moreover, the encapsulation also stimulates the formation of acetaldehyde and diacetyl compounds and increases long-chain fatty acid concentration. After encapsulation of *Lb. paracasei* using skim milk as the wall material and passage through the spray drying process, the encapsulated cells remained stable and viable after storage for 7 weeks under both room temperature and refrigeration. Microencapsulation of cells through rennet gelation of milk protein is also considered as an interesting approach for encapsulation (Beldarrain-Iznaga *et al.* 2020).

10.4.1.3 Desserts

Due to the globally rise in demand for healthy food and healthier products, the development of probiotic desserts has also been conducted (Shori 2015). Probiotic bacteria have been tested with several desserts such as chocolate mousse (Gul 2017) and chocolate (Possemiers *et al.* 2010). Chocolate-based dessert is generally rich in fat, and this composition encourages the use of probiotic bacteria. Moreover, creamy desserts mostly exhibit very high pH (more than 6), high moisture content and lack of competitive microbes. Therefore, these creamy desserts have become promising probiotic carriers (Valencia *et al.* 2016). Most of the probiotic cells can potentially survive in the dessert product; encapsulation has been developed to enhance the survivability of the probiotic when faced with the harsh environmental conditions of the gastrointestinal tract (Possemiers *et al.* 2010). Encapsulated probiotic cells incorporated in chocolate mousse exhibited higher survivability compared to free cells (Gul 2017). Probiotics have been tested with frozen dairy desserts, however several factors such as high acidity, osmotic pressure and freeze injury potentially hinder the use of these bacteria (Chen *et al.* 2007). In the case of ice cream, the environmental conditions such as high pH, high fat content and presence of milk in the product are very suitable for the growth of probiotic bacteria. However, the whipping-freezing step, oxygen toxicity and high redox values in the ice cream production process induce severe bacterial loss (Soukoulis *et al.* 2010). An encapsulation process can enhance the survival rate of the probiotic during ice cream production (Ranadheera *et al.* 2012). Moreover, the addition of prebiotic substances as one of the wall materials potentially enhances the viability of probiotic cells compared to free cells (Homayouni *et al.* 2007).

10.4.2 Non-dairy Products

Health trends in both food and beverage products are the driving force for the development of probiotic products. Currently, non-dairy products such as beverages, meat, baked goods and butter are being widely explored as potential probiotic carriers. However, unfavorable factors mostly arise from unsuitable growth environments such as highly acidic conditions, high oxygen levels and lack of carbon sources in these products. Therefore, the incorporation of probiotics in these non-dairy products is a challenge for the researcher.

10.4.2.1 Beverages

Due to the varying environmental conditions in beverages, a wide number of probiotics have been found to partially survive in them (Shori 2015). Microencapsulation has been carried out to enhance the availability of probiotic bacteria when exposed to unfavorable conditions. The extrusion process was performed with encapsulated *Lactobacillus casei*, *Lactobacillus acidophilus* and *Bifidobacterium lactis* BB-12; a herbal extract was included in the formula to enhance the survivability of the cells (Chaikham 2015). Encapsulated beads were incorporated in fruit juices, and the results indicated that the encapsulated cells exhibited higher cell viability after storage for 30 days. The combination of prebiotic compounds (inulin and galactooligosaccharides) and the extrusion process effectively increased the survivability of probiotic cells (Gandomi *et al.* 2016). Similarly, the combination of probiotic bacteria and prebiotic in the encapsulation process also enhanced the growth of probiotic cells in fruit juice (Krasaekoopt and Watcharapoka 2014). The encapsulated *Lb. plantarum* was tested in mango juices to observe the change of cell viability, and the results indicated that strong hydrogel beads developed from the combination of alginate and soy protein can withstand the pasteurization temperatures and protect the bacteria against gastric acids (Praepanitchai *et al.* 2019).

10.4.2.2 Meat Products

Probiotic bacteria have been utilized in meat products, especially fermented sausages (Pérez-Chabela *et al.* 2013). Meat is a favorable host for the cultivation of probiotic cells. The meat matrix potentially acts as a protective layer against gastric acids. In addition, the lack of heat treatment in sausage production also favors the growth of bacteria. Several microbes such as yeast, mold and bacteria can potentially be used in meat fermentation. However, the combination of probiotic cells with the conventional culture may alter the sensory properties and physiochemical properties of the product. Therefore, adjustment of the fermentation temperature is crucial and can potentially lead to positive sensory properties (Pasqualin Cavalheiro *et al.* 2015). Probiotic cells also impart antimicrobial properties to the meat, which ultimately decelerates spoilage of the meat. The encapsulation process is also recommended for meat production to protect the bacteria against some unfavorable conditions such as low pH, low moisture content and harmful curing agents (De Prisco and Mauriello 2016). Encapsulation of *Lb. reuteri* using the extrusion method was conducted (Muthukumarasamy and Holley 2006), and the developed bead was incorporated in fermented meat products. The results of this study indicated that encapsulated beads showed higher cell viability and no change in characteristics occurred.

10.4.2.3 Bakery Products

Utilization of probiotic bacteria in the bakery field is considered a new concept, and a limited amount of research has been conducted. Probiotics have been incorporated in bakery products such as biscuits, bread and cakes. The main hindrance, which significantly affects probiotic incorporation in bakery products, is the high baking temperature. In addition, alteration of chemical properties occurring from the change of pH, Maillard reaction and ethanol production also hinders the use of probiotics (De Prisco and Mauriello 2016). Directly incorporated probiotic bacteria in the product show negative results, as the cell count becomes significantly low after baking (Ahniyaz *et al.* 2014). However, the encapsulation process could be the solution for this issue. The combination of thermally resistant lactic acid bacteria with the encapsulation process is one promising formula for probiotic bakery products (Corona-Hernandez *et al.* 2013). There are several approaches to incorporating probiotics in bakery products. The probiotic cells can be applied on the surface of the products (Altamirano-Fortoul *et al.* 2012; Soukoulis *et al.* 2014), mixed with the dough (Seyedain-Ardabili et al. 2016), or added to the creams for pastries (Khosravi Zanjani *et al.* 2018). When an encapsulated probiotic strain was coated on the surface of partially baked breads, the survival rate of the bacteria was around 63% after baking. These results indicate that the microencapsulation process can act as a protective layer against the high temperature during baking (Altamirano-Fortoul *et al.* 2012). The addition of encapsulated probiotic cells to dough was conducted (Malmo *et al.* 2013); the results indicated that encapsulated cells exhibit a higher survival rate compared to free cells. However, the bacterial count was still low after baking. The combination of calcium alginate, chitosan and Hi-Maize® resistant starch using the emulsification and encapsulation process showed promising results, the bacterial count remaining high after the baking process (Seyedain-Ardabili *et al.* 2016). Lastly, encapsulation of probiotic in Hi-Maize® starch hydrogel beads and incorporation of the beads into cream prepared as cake filling showed promising results as this method exhibited high cell counts after heat treatments (Khosravi Zanjani *et al.* 2018).

References

ABD EL-SALAM, M. H. and EL-SHIBINY, S. (2012) 'Formation and potential uses of milk proteins as nano delivery vehicles for nutraceuticals: A review', *International Journal of Dairy Technology*, 65(1), pp. 13–21.

Ach, D., Stéphanie B., Vincent D., Jocelyne P., Guy B., Yves C. (2015) 'Influence of main whey protein components on the mechanism of complex coacervation with Acacia gum', *Colloids and Surfaces A: Physicochemical and Engineering Aspects*, 481, pp. 367–374.

Ahniyaz, A., A. G. (2014) *Microencapsulation in the Food Industry*. San Diego: Academic Press, pp. xix–xx.

Alehosseini, A. Behrouz G., Mahboobe S., Nick T. (2018) 'Principles of electrospraying: A new approach in protection of bioactive compounds in foods', *Critical Reviews in Food Science and Nutrition*. Taylor & Francis, 58(14), pp. 2346–2363.

Altamirano-Fortoul, R. *et al.* (2012) 'Viability of some probiotic coatings in bread and its effect on the crust mechanical properties', *Food Hydrocolloids. Elsevier Ltd*, 29(1), pp. 166–174.

Alvim, I. D. and Grosso, C. R. F. (2010) 'Microparticles obtained by complex coacervation: influence of the type of reticulation and the drying process on the release of the core material', *Ciência e Tecnologia de Alimentos*, 30(4), pp. 1069–1076.

Anandharamakrishnan, C. and Ishwarya, P. (2015) *Spray drying technique for food ingredient encapsulation*. Available at: http://onlinelibrary.wiley.com/book/10.1002/9781118863985.

Ann, E. Y., Kim, Y., Oh, S., Imm, J.-Y., Park, D.-J., Han, K. S. and Kim, S. H. (2007) 'Microencapsulation of Lactobacillus acidophilus ATCC 43121 with prebiotic substrates using a hybridisation system', *International Journal of Food Science & Technology*, 42(4), pp. 411–419.

Anu Bhushani, J. and Anandharamakrishnan, C. (2014) 'Electrospinning and electrospraying techniques: Potential food based applications', *Trends in Food Science and Technology*. Elsevier Ltd, 38(1), pp. 21–33.

Arslan, S., Mustafa E., Ismail T., and Ayhan T. (2015) 'Microencapsulation of probiotic Saccharomyces cerevisiae var: Boulardii with different wall materials by spray drying', *LWT - Food Science and Technology*. Elsevier Ltd, 63(1), pp. 685–690.

Barbosa, J., Ricardo V. C., Javier L.V., and Eva S. A. (2015) 'Comparison of spray drying, freeze drying and convective hot air drying for the production of a probiotic orange powder', *Journal of Functional Foods*. Elsevier Ltd, 17, pp. 340–351.

Beldarrain-Iznaga, T, Ricardo V. C.,Javier L., Eva S. A. (2020) 'Influence of multilayer microencapsulation on the viability of Lactobacillus casei using a combined double emulsion and ionic gelation approach', *Food and Bioproducts Processing*. Institution of Chemical Engineers, 124, pp. 57–71.

Bielecka, M. (2006) 'Probiotics in food', *Chemical and Functional Properties of Food Components, Third Edition*, pp. 413–426. Doyon, M. and Labrecque, J. A. (2008) 'Functional foods: A conceptual definition', *British Food Journal*, 110(11), pp. 1133–1149.

Burgain, J, Gaiani C., Linder M., and Scher J.. (2011) 'Encapsulation of probiotic living cells: From laboratory scale to industrial applications', *Journal of Food Engineering. Elsevier Ltd*, 104(4), pp. 467–483.

Burgain, J., C. Gaiani, G. Francius, A. M. Revol-Junelles, C. Cailliez-Grimal, S. Lebeer, H. L. P. Tytgat, J. Vanderleyden, J. Scher (2013) 'in vitro interactions between probiotic bacteria and milk proteins probed by atomic force microscopy', *Colloids and Surfaces B: Biointerfaces*. Elsevier B.V., 104(2013), pp. 153–162.

Chaikham, P. (2015) 'Stability of probiotics encapsulated with Thai herbal extracts in fruit juices and yoghurt during refrigerated storage', *Food Bioscience*. Elsevier, 12, pp. 61–66.

Chavarri, M., Maranon, I. and Carmen, M. (2012) 'Encapsulation Technology to Protect Probiotic Bacteria', *Probiotics*, (June 2014).

Chen, M.-J., Chen, K.-N. and Kuo, Y.-T. (2007). 'Optimal thermotolerance of Bifidobacterium bifidum in gellan–alginate microparticles', *Biotechnology and Bioengineering*. John Wiley & Sons, Ltd, 98(2), pp. 411–419.

Coghetto, C. C., Brinques, G. B. and Ayub, M. A. Z. (2016) 'Probiotics production and alternative encapsulation methodologies to improve their viabilities under adverse environmental conditions.', *International journal of food sciences and nutrition*. England, 67(8), pp. 929–943.

Corona-Hernandez, R. I., Emilio A. P., Jaime J. M., Alma R.., Laura. A. R., Abraham W. M. (2013) 'Structural Stability and Viability of Microencapsulated Probiotic Bacteria: A Review', *Comprehensive Reviews in Food Science and Food Safety*. John Wiley & Sons, Ltd, 12(6), pp. 614–628.

De Prisco, A. and Mauriello, G. (2016) 'Probiotication of foods: A focus on microencapsulation tool', *Trends in Food Science and Technology*. Elsevier Ltd, 48, pp. 27–39.

de Vos, P., Faas, M. M., Spasojevic, M. and Sikkema, J. (2010) 'Encapsulation for preservation of functionality and targeted delivery of bioactive food components', *International Dairy Journal*, 20(4), pp. 292–302.

Demers-Mathieu, V., St-Gelais, D., Audy, J., Laurin, É. and Fliss, I. (2016) 'Effect of the low-fat Cheddar cheese manufacturing process on the viability of Bifidobacterium animalis subsp. lactis, Lactobacillus rhamnosus, Lactobacillus paracasei/casei, and Lactobacillus plantarum isolates', *Journal of Functional Foods*, 24, pp. 327–337.

Dianawati, D., Mishra, V. and Shah, N. P. (2016) 'Survival of Microencapsulated Probiotic Bacteria after Processing and during Storage: A Review', *Critical Reviews in Food Science and Nutrition*. Taylor & Francis, 56(10), pp. 1685–1716.

Dimitrellou, D., Kandylis, P. and Kourkoutas, Y. (2016) 'Effect of cooling rate, freeze-drying, and storage on survival of free and immobilized Lactobacillus casei ATCC 393', *LWT - Food Science and Technology*. Elsevier eLtd, 69, pp. 468–473.

Đorđević, V. et al. (2014) Trends in Encapsulation Technologies for Delivery of Food Bioactive Compounds, *Food Engineering Reviews.*

Fang, Z. and Bhandari, B. (2012) '4 - Spray drying, freeze drying and related processes for food ingredient and nutraceutical encapsulation', in Garti, N. and McClements, D. J. B. T.-E. T. and D. S. for F. I. and N. (eds) *Woodhead Publishing Series in Food Science, Technology and Nutrition*. Woodhead Publishing, pp. 73–109.

Fijan, S. (2014) 'Microorganisms with claimed probiotic properties: An overview of recent literature', *International Journal of Environmental Research and Public Health*, 11(5), pp. 4745–4767.

Gandomi, H., Abbaszadeh, S., Misaghi, A., Bokaie, S. and Noori, N. (2016) 'Effect of chitosan-alginate encapsulation with inulin on survival of Lactobacillus rhamnosus GG during apple juice storage and under simulated gastrointestinal conditions', *LWT - Food Science and Technology*, 69, pp. 365–371.

Ghorani, B. and Tucker, N. (2015) 'Fundamentals of electrospinning as a novel delivery vehicle for bioactive compounds in food nanotechnology', *Food Hydrocolloids. Elsevier Ltd*, 51, pp. 227–240.

Gomes de Oliveira, M. E. *et al.* (2014) 'Addition of probiotic bacteria in a semi-hard goat cheese (coalho): Survival to simulated gastrointestinal conditions and inhibitory effect against pathogenic bacteria', *Food Research International. Elsevier Ltd*, 64, pp. 241–247.

Gomez-Mascaraque, L. G. *et al.* (2016) 'Optimization of electrospraying conditions for the microencapsulation of probiotics and evaluation of their resistance during storage and in-vitro digestion', *LWT - Food Science and Technology*, 69, pp. 438–446.

Grand view research (2019) Probiotics Market Size, Share & Trends Analysis Report By Product (Food & Beverages, Dietary Supplements), By Ingredient (Bacteria, Yeast), By End Use, By Distribution Channel, And Segment Forecasts, 2019 - 2025, *Grand View Research Inc.* Available at: https://www.grandviewresearch.com/industry-analysis/probiotics-market (Accessed: 26 July 2021).

Gul, O. (2017) 'Microencapsulation of Lactobacillus casei Shirota by spray drying using different combinations of wall materials and application for probiotic dairy dessert', *Journal of Food Processing and Preservation*. John Wiley & Sons, Ltd, 41(5), p. e13198.

Han, S. et al. (2021) 'Probiotic Gastrointestinal Transit and Colonization After Oral Administration: A Long Journey', *Frontiers in Cellular and Infection Microbiology*, 11(March), pp. 1–12.

Her, J. Y., Kim, M. S. and Lee, K. G. (2015) 'Preparation of probiotic powder by the spray freeze-drying method', *Journal of Food Engineering*. Elsevier Ltd, 150, pp. 70–74.

Homayouni, A., Ehsani, M. R., Azizi, A., Yarmand, M. S. and Razavi, S. H. (2007) 'Effect of lecithin and calcium chloride solution on the microencapsulation process yield of calcium alginate beads', *Iranian Polymer Journal (English Edition)*, 16(9), pp. 597–606.

Huang, S. et al. (2016) 'Double use of highly concentrated sweet whey to improve the biomass production and viability of spray-dried probiotic bacteria', *Journal of Functional Foods*, 23, pp. 453–463.

Kailasapathy, K. (2006) 'Survival of free and encapsulated probiotic bacteria and their effect on the sensory properties of yoghurt', *LWT - Food Science and Technology*, 39(10), pp. 1221–1227.

Khosravi Zanjani, M. A. *et al.* (2018) 'Promoting probiotics survival by microencapsualtion with hylon starch and genipin cross-linked coatings in simulated gastro-intestinal condition and heat treatment', *Iranian Journal of Pharmaceutical Research*, 17(2), pp. 753–766.

Krasaekoopt, W. and Watcharapoka, S. (2014) 'Effect of addition of inulin and galactooligosaccharide on the survival of microencapsulated probiotics in alginate beads coated with chitosan in simulated digestive system, yogurt and fruit juice', *LWT - Food Science and Technology*. Elsevier Ltd, 57(2), pp. 761–766.

Malmo, C., La Storia, A. and Mauriello, G. (2013) 'Microencapsulation of Lactobacillus reuteri DSM 17938 Cells Coated in Alginate Beads with Chitosan by Spray Drying to Use as a Probiotic Cell in a Chocolate Soufflé', *Food and Bioprocess Technology*, 6(3), pp. 795–805.

Maragkoudakis, P. A. *et al.* (2006) 'Production of traditional Greek yoghurt using Lactobacillus strains with probiotic potential as starter adjuncts', *International Dairy Journal*, 16(1), pp. 52–60.

Martín, M. J., Lara-Villoslada, F., Ruiz, M. A. and Morales, M. E. (2015) 'Microencapsulation of bacteria: A review of different technologies and their impact on the probiotic effects', *Innovative Food Science and Emerging Technologies*, 27, pp. 15–25.

Matilla, A. J. (2000) 'Ethylene in seed formation and germination', Seed Science Research Angel *J. Matilla Seed Science Research*, 10(10), pp. 111–126.

Merenstein, D., Salminen, S. and Team, W. G. O. R. (2017) 'World Gastroenterology Organisation Global Guidelines - Probiotics and prebiotics', *World Gastroenterology Organisation*, (February).

Misra, S., Mohanty, D. and Mohapatra, S. (2019) 'Applications of Probiotics as a Functional Ingredient in Food and Gut Health', *Journal of Food and Nutrition Research*, 7(3), pp. 213–223.

Muthukumarasamy, P. and Holley, R. A. (2006) 'Microbiological and sensory quality of dry fermented sausages containing alginate-microencapsulated Lactobacillus reuteri', *International Journal of Food Microbiology*, 111(2), pp. 164–169.

Nag, A. and Das, S. (2013) 'Improving ambient temperature stability of probiotics with stress adaptation and fluidized bed drying', *Journal of Functional Foods*, 5(1), pp. 170–177.

Nedovic, V., Kalusevic, A., Manojlovic, V., Levic, S. and Bugarski, B. (2011) 'An overview of encapsulation technologies for food applications', *Procedia Food Science*, 1, pp. 1806–1815.

Okuro, P. K., Thomazini, M., Balieiro, J. C. C., Liberal, R. D. C. O. and Fávaro-Trindade, C. S. (2013) 'Co- encapsulation of Lactobacillus acidophilus with inulin or polydextrose in solid lipid microparticles provides protection and improves stability', *Food Research International*, 53(1), pp. 96–103.

Özer, B., Kirmaci, H. A., Şenel, E., Atamer, M. and Hayaloğlu, A. (2009) 'Improving the viability of Bifidobacterium bifidum BB-12 and Lactobacillus acidophilus LA-5 in white-brined cheese by microencapsulation', *International Dairy Journal*, 19(1), pp. 22–29.

Pasqualin Cavalheiro, C., Ruiz-Capillas, C., Herrero, A. M., Jiménez-Colmenero, F., Ragagnin de Menezes, C. and Martins Fries, L. L. (2015) 'Application of probiotic delivery systems in meat products', *Trends in Food Science and Technology*, 46(1), pp. 120–131.

Pérez-Chabela, M. L., Lara-Labastida, R., Rodriguez-Huezo, E. and Totosaus, A. (2013) 'Effect of Spray Drying Encapsulation of Thermotolerant Lactic Acid Bacteria on Meat Batters Properties', *Food and Bioprocess Technology*, 6(6), pp. 1505–1515.

Possemiers, S., Marzorati, M., Verstraete, W. and Van de Wiele, T. (2010) 'Bacteria and chocolate: A successful combination for probiotic delivery', *International Journal of Food Microbiology*, 141(1–2), pp. 97–103.

Praepanitchai, O.-A., Noomhorm, A. and Anal, A. K. (2019) 'Survival and Behavior of Encapsulated Probiotics (*Lactobacillus plantarum*) in Calcium-Alginate-Soy Protein Isolate-Based Hydrogel Beads in Different Processing Conditions (pH and Temperature) and in Pasteurized Mango Juice', *BioMed Research International*. Edited by M. E. Potes. Hindawi, 2019, p. 9768152.

Precedence Research (2019) *Functional Food Market Size Worth Around USD 309 Bn by 2027, GlobeNewswire, Inc.* Available at: https://www.globenewswire.com/en/news-release/2020/11/20/2130656/0/en/Functional-Food-Market-Size-Worth-Around-USD-309-Bn-by-2027.html (Accessed: 26 July 2021).

Ranadheera, C. S. *et al.* (2012) 'in vitro analysis of gastrointestinal tolerance and intestinal cell adhesion of probiotics in goat's milk ice cream and yogurt', *Food Research International. Elsevier Ltd*, 49(2), pp. 619–625.

Rathore, S. *et al.* (2013) 'Microencapsulation of microbial cells', *Journal of Food Engineering*, 116(2), pp. 369–381.

Ribeiro, M. C. E. *et al.* (2014) 'Effect of microencapsulation of Lactobacillus acidophilus LA-5 on physicochemical, sensory and microbiological characteristics of stirred probiotic yoghurt', *Food Research International*. Elsevier Ltd, 66, pp. 424–431.

Saarela, M. (2009) 'Probiotics as ingredients in functional beverages', in *Functional and Speciality Beverage Technology*, pp. 55–70.

Sagis, L. M. C. (2015) 'Chapter 10 - Determination of Mechanical Properties of Microcapsules', in Sagis, L. M. C. (ed.) *Microencapsulation and Microspheres for Food Applications*. San Diego: Academic Press, pp. 195–205.

Sandoval-Castilla, O., Lobato-Calleros, C., García-Galindo, H. S., Alvarez-Ramírez, J. and Vernon-Carter, E. J. (2010) 'Textural properties of alginate-pectin beads and survivability of entrapped Lb. casei in simulated gastrointestinal conditions and in yoghurt', *Food Research International*, 43(1), pp. 111–117.

Schmitt, C. and Turgeon, S. L. (2011) 'Protein/polysaccharide complexes and coacervates in food systems', *Advances in Colloid and Interface Science*. Elseevier B.V., 167(1–2), pp. 63–70.

Semyonov, D., Ramon, O. and Shimoni, E. (2011) 'Using ultrasonic vacuum spray dryer to produce highly viable dry probiotics', *LWT - Food Science and Technology*. Elsevier Ltd, 44(9), pp. 1844–1852.

Seyedain-Ardabili, M., Sharifan, A. and Tarzi, B. G. (2016) 'The production of synbiotic bread by microencapsulation', *Food Technology and Biotechnology*, 54(1), pp. 52–59.

Shori, A. B. (2015) 'The potential applications of probiotics on dairy and non-dairy foods focusing on viability during storage', *Biocatalysis and Agricultural Biotechnology*, 4(4), pp. 423–431.

Shori, A. B. (2017) 'Microencapsulation Improved Probiotics Survival During Gastric Transit', *HAYATI Journal of Biosciences*, 24(1), pp. 1–5.

Singh, M. N., Hemant, K. S. Y., Ram, M. and Shivakumar, H. G. (2010) 'Microencapsulation: A promising technique for controlled drug delivery', *Research in pharmaceutical sciences*, 5(2), pp. 65–77.

Sohail, A., Turner, M. S., Coombes, A., Bostrom, T. and Bhandari, B. (2011) 'Survivability of probiotics encapsulated in alginate gel microbeads using a novel impinging aerosols method', *International Journal of Food Microbiology*, 145(1), pp. 162–168.

Soukoulis, C., Lyroni, E. and Tzia, C. (2010) 'Seensory profiling and hedonic judgement of probiotic ice cream as a function of hydrocolloids, yogurt and milk fat content', *LWT - Food Science and Technology*. Elsevier Ltd, 43(9), pp. 1351–1358.

Soukoulis, C., Yonekura, L., Gan, H. H., Behboudi-Jobbehdar, S., Parmenter, C. and Fisk, I. (2014) 'Probiotic edible films as a new strategy for developing functional bakery products: The case of pan bread', *Food Hydrocolloids*, 39, pp. 231–242.

Valencia, M. S., Salgado, S. M., Andrade, S. A. C., Padilha, V. M., Livera, A. V. S. and Stamford, T. L. M. (2016) 'Development of creamy milk chocolate dessert added with fructo-oligosaccharide and Lactobacillus paracasei subsp. paracasei LBC 81', *LWT - Food Science and Technology*, 69, pp. 104–109.

Ying, D. Y., Sanguansri, L., Weerakkody, R., Bull, M., Singh, T. K. and Augustin, M. A. (2016) 'Effect of encapsulant matrix on stability of microencapsulated probiotics', *Journal of Functional Foods*, 25, pp. 447–458.

Zare, F., Champagne, C. P., Simpson, B. K., Orsat, V. and Boye, J. I. (2012) 'Effect of the addition of pulse ingredients to milk on acid production by probiotic and yoghurt starter cultures', *LWT - Food Science and Technology*, 45(2), pp. 155–160.

Zhang, K., Zhang, H., Hu, X., Bao, S. and Huang, H. (2012) 'Synthesis and release studies of microalgal oil-containing microcapsules prepared by complex coacervation', *Colloids and Surfaces B: Biointerfaces*, 89(1), pp. 61–66.

Zuidam, N. and Nedovic, V. (2010) *Encapsulation Technologies for Active Food Ingredients and Food Processing, Encapsulation Technologies for Active Food Ingredients and Food Processing: ,:, ISBN 978-1-4419-1007-3. Springer-Verlag New York, 2010.*

11

Prebiotics and their Role in Functional Food Product Development

Divyani Panwar, Parmjit Singh Panesar and Anuradha Saini

Food Biotechnology Research Laboratory, Department of Food Engineering & Technology, Sant Longowal Institute of Engineering and Technology, Longowal, -148 106, Punjab, India

11.1 Introduction

For a long time, apart from the basic role of food to provide nutrients to humans for their necessary growth and development, some important aspects such as improvement of health and preventing diseases have been gaining importance. With the boosted interest of consumers in self-care and enhanced quality of life, research to understand the impact of interaction between the diet, gut and health has increased rapidly (Niva 2007; Rastall 2010). The human gut is known to be one of the most active metabolic organs containing a complex community of microorganisms or microbiota that affects the host's health (Holscher 2017). Moreover, it is a well-established fact that the gut microbiota maintains a synergetic relationship with the host and plays a critical role in various biological functions including utilization of nutrients, assistance in host digestion, strengthening of the immune system and protection against infectious pathogens (Bindels *et al.* 2015). However, certain undesirable changes/imbalance in patterns of gut microbiota known as dysbiosis are responsible for specific gastrointestinal and immune-mediated disorders such as celiac disease, Crohn's disease, obesity, liver diseases, multiple sclerosis, arthritis and cancer (Anadón *et al.* 2016).

This has led to the idea that deliberate manipulation in composition or metabolic activity of gut microbiota can be utilized as a therapeutic target to improve host health. As a consequence, utilization of functional foods and dietary supplements such as prebiotics, probiotics and synbiotics to regulate gut microbiota has gained interest, which has led to a brisk augmentation in the global market (de Preter and Verbeke 2014). The global market size for functional foods is currently estimated at USD 161.50 billion, and is predicted to rise to approximately USD 275.80 billion by the year 2025 (Figure 11.1). The chief leaders of the functional food market include the United States, Japan and Europe, whereas India, China and Latin America, along with some other Asian countries, are experiencing a high market growth rate (https://www.grandviewresearch.com/industry-analysis/functional-food-market/).

Probiotics, Prebiotics and Synbiotics: Technological Advancements Towards Safety and Industrial Applications, First Edition. Edited by Parmjit Singh Panesar and Anil Kumar Anal.

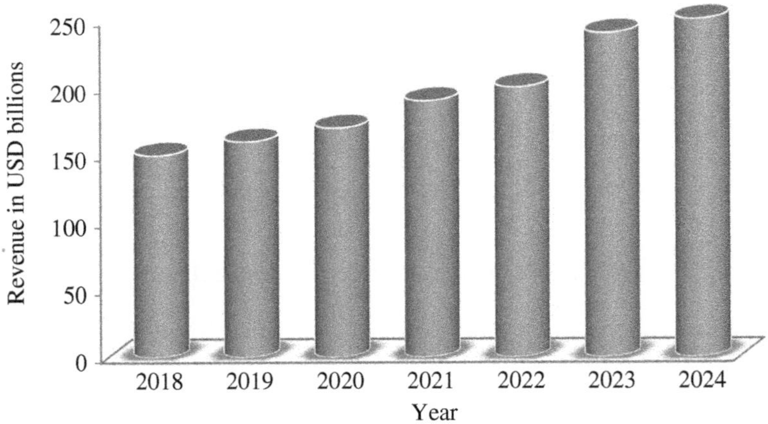

Figure 11.1 Global market size for functional food. *Source:* Adapted from Functional Foods Market Size, Share & Trends Analysis Report By Ingredient (Carotenoids, Prebiotics & Probiotics, Fatty Acids, Dietary Fibers), By Product, By Application, And Segment Forecasts, 2019-2025. Apr, 2019. https://www.grandviewresearch.com/industry-analysis/functional-food-market/

Amidst these functional products, prebiotics have engraved their own significant niche in the scientific community owing to their wide array of immunomodulatory, antioxidant, anticancer, and antihyperlipidemic therapeutic effects, among others (Patel and Goyal 2012). The term prebiotic was coined in 1995 by Gibson and Roberfroid and it was defined as a "non-digested food ingredient that, by selectively changing the activity and/or composition of single or a limited amount of bacteria residing in gastrointestinal tract, improves the host health". Since that time, fructooligosaccharides (FOS) and galactooligosaccharides (GOS) have been recognized to dominate the prebiotics category by stimulating the growth and activity of beneficial bacteria, especially *Bifidobacterium* and *Lactobacillus*, consequently inducing favorable effects on the composition of gut microbiota (Gibson *et al.* 2017). However, with advances in approaches for analysis of gut microbiota (microarray and sequencing), knowledge regarding its composition and additional metabolites affecting the microbial ecosystem has been enhanced. Moreover, it has been realized that the effect of prebiotics is not confined to specific microorganisms; rather a broad range of microorganisms is being affected by them (Collins and Reid 2016). Therefore, a new and revised definition of a prebiotic was proposed by Bindels *et al.* (2015) as "a non-digested ingredient that, by its fermentation in the human colon, modulates the activity and/or composition of gut microbiota, thereby improving the physiological health of host". It is noteworthy that fermentation of prebiotic products in the colon by gut microbiota produces certain metabolites including butyrate, propionate and acetate as major end-products. This subsequent production of short chain fatty acids (SCFAs) is reported to impart several physiological benefits to the host health such as improvement in intestinal function, regulation of the immune system and glucose metabolism, and absorption of minerals, as well as reduction in the risk of cancer, obesity and irritable bowel syndrome (Kaur and Panesar 2020).

However, it remains difficult to justify the criteria for prebiotics concerning stimulation of activity and growth of particular bacterial strains in the gut. Moreover, the in vitro/

in vivo fermentation or proliferation of a culture of particular bacterial strains is not considered as a prebiotic effect due to the lack of bacterial interaction with the gut (Roberfroid *et al.* 2010). Therefore, the consensus amongst researchers is to legitimize the continued use of the term "prebiotics" and derive absolute effective activity from it (Corrêa-Oliveira *et al.* 2016; Park *et al.* 2015). Over the past 20 years, the concept and definition of prebiotics have been refined several times and are in the forefront of research and scientific discussions worldwide (Table 11.1). This vagueness in the importance and potential therapeutic food applications of prebiotics has triggered an ample amount of research in areas of molecular biology and gastrointestinal microbiology in order to dig deeper into the concept. Keeping all this in view, this chapter is aimed to provide comprehensive information regarding prebiotics, their sources and methods of production, along with their health benefits and safety aspects.

11.2 Sources of Prebiotics: Classification and Characteristics

11.2.1 Characteristics of Prebiotics

Prebiotics are usually short chain, low molecular weight and non-digestible carbohydrates (oligosaccharides and polysaccharides). These compounds contain a complex backbone structure, having β-glycosidic bonds which resist them from being digested in the colon by colonic enzymes (Ashwini *et al.* 2019). Different types of food ingredients such as dietary fibers and different polysaccharides are predicted to have prebiotic effects, however not all of them are considered as prebiotics (Slavin 2013). Therefore, Wang (2009) defined a clear set of characteristics (Figure 11.2) required for a food ingredient to be considered as a prebiotic which includes:

1) Resistance of food to digestion in the upper area of intestinal tract and may reach the colon in an unaltered form.
2) Must be fermented selectively by colonic microflora.
3) Benefits host health by increased production of SCFAs along with reduction in colonic pH and nitrous end-products.
4) Must selectively stimulate the activity and/or growth of beneficial colonic microflora especially *Bifidobacterium* and *Lactobacillus*.
5) Must remain chemically and structurally stable and unaltered in all food processing conditions.

11.2.2 Classification of Prebiotics and their Sources

It is an established fact that the majority of prebiotics are known to be non-digestible carbohydrates having different molecular structures. Prebiotics are classified on the basis of their sources, type, substrate used for production, and structure (number of monomers) (Biswal *et al.* 2017). A classification of prebiotics, along with examples, is depicted in Figure 11.3. Prebiotics are usually present in natural sources (Table 11.2) including plant sources such as seeds, leeks, chicory, Jerusalem artichoke, legumes, beans, mustard, chickpeas, soybean, onion, bananas, berries, garlic, etc. and algal matrices such as seaweeds

Table 11.1 Evolution of the definition and concept of prebiotics.

Year	Definition of prebiotics	Foods considered as prebiotics	Changes made	Reference
1995	Non-digested food products that improve the host health by selectively stimulating the composition and/or activity of single or a limited group of bacteria residing in colon	FOS	–	Gibson and Roberfroid (1995)
2003	Non-digested ingredients that induce benefits to host physiology by selectively stimulating the growth and/or activity of a definite group of natural bacteria	Lactulose, TOS, FOS	Original definition has been extended to include other body sites along with the colon	Reid *et al.* (2003)
2004	Selectively fermented food compounds that confer specific changes in the activity and/or composition in the gastrointestinal microflora, thereby improving the host health	Lactulose, TOS, FOS, inulin	Original definition has been modified to include the gastrointestinal microflora	Gibson *et al.* (2004)
2007	Selectively fermented food compounds that confer specific changes in the activity and/or composition in the gut microflora, thereby improving the host health	TOS, inulin	No major changes were made in the original definition. However, specifically two oligosaccharides (tGOS and inulin) were considered as prebiotics	Roberfroid (2007)
2008	Non-viable food ingredients that benefit host health by modulating the gut microbiota	FOS, GOS, SOS, IMO, inulin, XOS, lactulose, dietary fibers, resistant starches, pyrodextrins and other non-digested oligosaccharides	Original definition has been changed by removing the limitation to the gastrointestinal tract. Moreover, according to the new definition, a prebiotic is not required to be fermented or metabolized by gut microflora, therefore it can be any substance that can modify the composition of gut microflora	Pineiro *et al.* (2008)
2010	Selectively fermented food compound that benefits human health by inducing specific changes in the activity and/or composition of gut microflora	Lactulose, inulin, TOS, polydextrose, lactosucrose, soybean oligosaccharides, IMO, glucans, XOS	This definition refers to prebiotics as fermented ingredients that specifically target the gastrointestinal tract	Gibson *et al.* (2010)
2015	Non-digestible ingredient that modulates the activity and/or composition of specific species present in gut and therefore confers beneficial effects to host health	Inulin, FOS, tGOS, human milk, resistant starch, pectin, whole grains, dietary fibers, other oligosaccharides	This definition has changed the original definition by replacing particular species by multiple consortia of gut microflora	Bindels *et al.* (2015)

FOS, fructooligosaccharides; GOS, galactooligosaccharides; IMO, isomaltooligosaccharides; SOS, soybean oligosaccharides; TOS, transgalactooligosaccharides; XOS, xylooligosaccharides.
Source: Adapted from Bindels, L.B., Delzenne, N.M., Cani, P.D. and Walter, J. (2015). Towards a more comprehensive concept for prebiotics. *Nature Reviews Gastroenterology & Hepatology*, 12(5): 303–310.

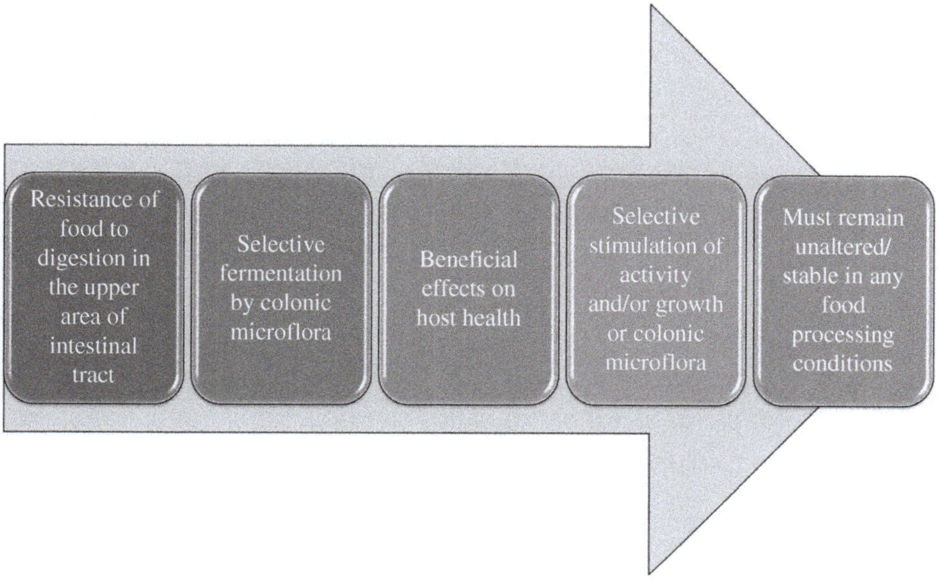

Figure 11.2 Criteria for selection of prebiotics. *Source:* Adapted from Markowiak P, Śliżewska K. (2017). Effects of probiotics, prebiotics, and synbiotics on human health. *Nutrients*, 9(9): 1021.

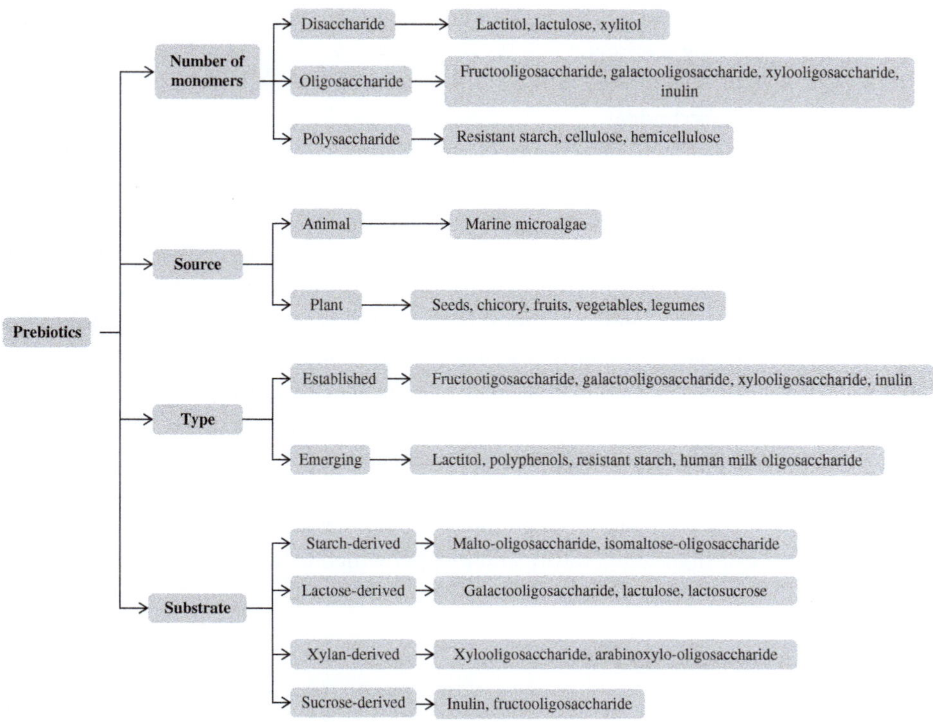

Figure 11.3 Classification of prebiotics along with suitable examples.

Table 11.2 Prebiotics and their sources.

Prebiotic	Sources
Galactooligosaccharides (GOS)	Milk (human, goat and cow)
Fructooligosaccharides (FOS)	Garlic, chicory, banana, barley, asparagus, Jerusalem artichoke, tomato, garlic
Xylooligosaccharides (XOS)	Fruits, vegetables, bamboo shoots, honey, milk, wheat bran
Lactulose	Milk
Isomaltulose	Sucrose
Isomaltooligosaccharides (IMO)	Potato, wheat, rice, barley, pulses
Soybean oligosaccharide	Soybean
Arabinoxylooligosaccharide (AXOS)	Brewer spent grain, wheat bran
Lactosucrose	Lactose
Inulin	Chicory, onion, Jerusalem artichoke, leeks, garlic, asparagus, banana
Resistant starch	Green banana, legumes, grains, raw potatoes, oats

Source: Adapted from Joshi, D., Roy, S. and Banerjee, S. (2018). Prebiotics. *Natural Products and Drug Discovery*, 507–523.

(Ashwini *et al.* 2019; Wang *et al.* 2019). Various prebiotics, along with their sources, are explained in the following sections.

11.2.2.1 Galactooligosaccharides

Galactooligosaccharides (GOS) are a group of carbohydrates consisting of two to eight saccharide units, with glucose at the reducing end along with galactose units linked together by β-glycosidic linkages (de Souza *et al.* 2015). They are usually found naturally in low concentrations in dairy products such as human milk (5–8 g/L), goat milk (0.25–0.30 g/L), ovine milk (0.02–0.04 g/L), and bovine milk (0.03–0.06 g/L) (Martinez-Ferez *et al.* 2006). Moreover, it is evident from previous literature that the structure of naturally occurring oligosaccharides in human breast milk resembles GOS, which is responsible for protecting infants from gastrointestinal pathogenic microorganisms and is therefore recognized as safe (Fischer and Kleinschmidt 2018). Therefore, GOS are often used as a supplement in infant foods with the purpose of imitating the beneficial effects of human milk oligosaccharides along with supporting the growth of beneficial bacteria *Lactobacillus* and *Bifidobacterium* (Bhatia *et al.* 2015; Sabater *et al.* 2016). Another characteristic of GOS is their high tolerance of high temperature and low pH which facilitates their incorporation as a supplement in a variety of food products (Vera *et al.* 2016).

11.2.2.2 Fructooligosaccharides

Fructooligosaccharides (FOS) are a mixture of oligosaccharides consisting of molecules of glucose linked to units of fructose by β-(1,2) glycosidic bonds having a degree of polymerization between 2 and 60 (Thamer and Penna 2005). FOS are naturally present in foods of vegetal origin such as wheat, chicory, Jerusalem artichokes, onion, asparagus, garlic and rye (Alander *et al.* 2001). Research studies have reported that FOS present in the gut are not digested but are fermented to produce SCFAs (propionate, butyrate and acetate), lactate and gas which stimulate the growth of *Lactobacillus* and *Bifidobacterium* and inhibit the growth of pathogenic microorganisms (Bornet *et al.* 2002; Hutkins *et al.* 2016). Moreover, FOS help in lowering cholesterol level and enhance bioabsorption of minerals such as calcium and magnesium (de la Rosa *et al.* 2019). FOS are reasonably sweet in taste and have almost identical functional and technological attributes to glucose and sucrose. In addition to this, FOS are known to have good solubility at room temperature which means they neither precipitate nor crystallize and also do not leave a sandy or dry mouth feel. Therefore, they can be successfully used as a sweetener in food products, for the development of "low-calorie products", which enables the expansion of their applications in the food and pharmaceutical sectors (de Souza *et al.* 2015; Flores-Maltos *et al.* 2016). Commercially, FOS are available on the market under names such as NutraFlora, Actilight, Meioligo and Neosugar (Bali *et al.* 2015).

11.2.2.3 Xylooligosaccharides

Xylooligosaccharides (XOS) are sugar oligomers consisting of xylose units linked together by β(1,4) glycosidic linkages with varying types and proportions of side groups such as 4-*O*-methyl derivative and α-D-glucopyranosyluronic acid. Usually two to ten xylose residues are involved in the formation of XOS and they can be classified as xylobiose, xylotriose, xylotetrose, etc., depending upon the number of units (Coelho *et al.* 2016). They are naturally found in fruits, vegetables, milk, bamboo shoots, corn cob and honey (Mohanty *et al.* 2018).

XOS have been reported to exhibit attractive physicochemical attributes including their crystalline structure, stability over a wide range of temperatures (up to 100 °C) and pH (2.5–8), non-carcinogenicity, high water activity and anti-freezing activity (de Souza *et al.* 2015). Also, XOS have a pleasant odor, possess no off taste, and their sweetness is equivalent to approximately 30% that of sucrose (Samanta *et al.* 2015). Therefore, XOS can be suitably incorporated into variety of food products as a fat replacer, emulsifier or stabilizer as well as in the development of low-calorie functional foods (Amorim *et al.* 2019). Furthermore, previous reports have suggested the role of XOS in stimulation of *Bifidobacterium* spp., thereby exhibiting beneficial effects on human health. XOS are also responsible for the suppression of pathogenic bacteria due to the generation of SCFAs, especially lactate (Carvalho *et al.* 2013). Research studies have also reported numerous biological properties of XOS such as antidiabetic, anti-inflammatory, anti-allergic, anticancer and reduction of oxidative stress, which have gained attention in the medical and pharmaceutical sectors (Amorim *et al.* 2020; Le *et al.* 2020; Lin *et al.* 2016; Long *et al.* 2019;).

11.2.2.4 Lactulose

Lactulose, chemically known as 4-*O*-β-D-galactopyranosyl-D-fructose, is a synthetic ketose disaccharide which is composed of two molecules of fructose and galactose joined together by β-(1,4) glycosidic linkage (Aït-Aissa and Aïder 2014; Panesar and Kumari 2011). These β-linkages are neither digested in the human gastrointestinal tract nor hydrolyzed by digestive enzymes, and therefore pass directly into the colon (Kaur and Panesar 2020). Studies have reported that consumption of lactulose resulted in significant growth of *Lactobacillus* and *Bifidobacterium* along with inhibition of pathogenic microorganisms (Mao *et al.* 2016; Zhai *et al.* 2018). For a long time lactulose has been used as a laxative which can be used for the treatment of constipation and hepatic encephalopathy (Panesar and Kumari 2011). Furthermore, lactulose is commercially available on the market in the form of a clear sweet yellow syrup and white sweet powder. It is highly soluble in alcohol and water and is stable at high temperatures and pH (Schumann 2002). Moreover, lactulose is reported to be sweeter than lactose and is therefore used as a sugar substitute for the development of low-calorie food products (Panesar and Kumari 2011).

11.2.2.5 Lactosucrose

Lactosucrose, chemically known as β-D-galactopyranosyl-(1,4)-α-D-glucopyranosyl-(1,2)--β-D-fructofuranoside, is a non-digestible trisaccharide consisting of glucose, fructose and galactose units (Fujita *et al.* 2009). It is usually manufactured by the transfructosylation process using levansucrase and fructofuranosidase enzymes, or through the process of transgalactosylation with β-D galactosidase enzyme, utilizing lactose and sucrose as substrates (Duarte *et al.* 2017). Clinical studies have reported that consumption of lactosucrose is linked with the increase in population of *Bifidobacterium* spp. in human feces along with reduction in numbers of fecal toxic microbes such as bacteroides and clostridia (Candela *et al.* 2010). In addition to this, lactosucrose demonstrates a high degree of laxative threshold and water-holding capacity, which is responsible for improvement in fecal formation, reduction in risk of diarrhea, and increased bowel peristalsis (Silvério *et al.* 2015). Furthermore, lactosucrose can be used in the food sector for the development of a variety of functional foods (Mu *et al.* 2013). However, lactosucrose is still not accepted completely as a prebiotic and further studies are required to prove that it fulfills all the required criteria to be considered as a prebiotic.

11.2.2.6 Inulin

Inulin is a non-digestible, naturally occurring storage polysaccharide belonging to the class of fructan that has been a part of the daily diet for a long time (Panesar *et al.* 2013). It is distributed widely in nature and is naturally found in leeks, Jerusalem artichoke, asparagus, chicory, onion, garlic and banana (Ashwini *et al.* 2019). Moreover, it has been estimated that an average American consumes approximately 1–4 g of inulin daily, whereas in Europe daily average consumption of inulin is estimated to be around 3–10 g (Bosscher 2009). Chemically, inulin is composed of fructosyl monomers linked by β-(2,1) linkage containing one glucose unit per molecule linked by α-(1,2) linkage (de Souza *et al.* 2015). Numerous studies have reported that consumption of inulin positively affects the metabolism of lipid, improves digestive health, increases nutrient absorption and reduces the risk of cancer and osteoporosis (Ahmed and Rashid 2019). Furthermore, inulin is extensively utilized in the food sector owing to its attractive technological properties such as moderate solubility in water, fat replacement, high stability, sugar replacement and texture modifier (Meyer *et al.* 2011).

11.2.2.7 Isomaltosoligosaccharides

Isomaltooligosaccharides (IMO) are oligosaccharides composed of glucose units linked together with α-D-(1,6) and sometimes α-D-(1,4) glycosidic linkages having a degree of polymerization ranging between three and six (Casci and Rastall 2006)). IMO are naturally present in soy sauce, sake, miso, honey and sugarcane juice (Mohanty *et al.* 2018). It has been observed that consumption of IMO significantly increases the population of *Bifidobacterium* spp. along with reduced risk of constipation and hyperlipidemia (Tung *et al.* 2018; Wu Y *et al.* 2017). Furthermore, IMO have attracted the interest of the food sector for the development of low-calorie functional foods due to their desirable attributes such as low sweetness, bulking properties and low viscosity (Chen *et al.* 2001; Panesar *et al.* 2013).

11.3 New and Tailored Prebiotics

A considerable number of clinical trials have exhibited a successful relationship between consumption of already established prebiotics such as GOS and FOS and improved host health (Guarino *et al.* 2020). However, with the growing demand for prebiotics, research efforts are being made to expand the existing collection of prebiotics having potential health benefits. Moreover, existing prebiotics can be tailored, either by modulating the length of saccharide chain and glycosidic linkages or by using a combination of different bioactives, in order to impart specific functional properties. It has been reported that these new prebiotics possess special linkages comprising of both fermentable sugar units and/or phytochemical substrates, which only some specific microbial species can cleave. These new and tailored prebiotics have been reported to beneficially modulate gut microbiota and impart health benefits; however, further investigation is required to understand and validate the underlying mechanism through well-designed clinical trials (Parkar *et al.* 2015). Some of the new and tailored prebiotics are discussed in subsequent sections.

11.3.1 Human Milk Oligosaccharides

Human milk oligosaccharides (HMO) are unconjugated carbohydrates found in ample quantities in human milk (Morozov *et al.* 2018). The amount and composition of HMO vary according to the genetic makeup and time of lactation of individual women, accounting for approximately 5–15 g of oligosaccharides per liter, and are ranked the third most abundant component in milk after lactose and lipids (Plaza-Díaz *et al.* 2018). Each HMO structure is based on a lactose backbone consisting of galactose and glucose further associated with units of fructose, *N*-acetylneuraminic acid, *N*-acetylglucosamine and sialic acid, thereby generating a myriad of more than 200 structures known to date (Ninonuevo *et al.* 2006). Owing to their complex structure, HMO resist digestion and hydrolysis in the gastrointestinal tract of an infant and reach the colon in an almost intact form (Rudloff *et al.* 2012). Moreover, they are known to impart prebiotic effects in the gut of an infant by stimulating the growth of beneficial intestinal bacteria and inhibiting the adhesion of pathogenic microorganisms such as *Escherichia coli*, *Pseudomonas aeruginosa*, *Campylobacter jejuni* and *Vibrio cholerae* to intestinal mucosa (Coppa *et al.* 2006; Weichert *et al.* 2013). They have also been recognized to modulate the developing microbiome and neonatal immunity in infants (Bering 2018). In addition to this, HMO also provide protection against various infectious diseases as they mimic the structure of viral receptors and inhibit their adherence to target cells, thereby preventing infections (Morozov *et al.* 2018). However, more efforts are still required for the large-scale industrial production of HMO with the ability to develop infant formulas with them that can mimic human breast milk.

11.3.2 Resistant Starch

Resistant starch is the fraction of starch that is resistant to digestion in the small intestine and reaches the colon in an intact form which is then fermented into SCFAs that are responsible for imparting prebiotic effects on the human body (Topping *et al.* 2003). It is composed of amylose possessing an α-D-(1,4) linkage and amylopectin possessing both α--D-(1,4) and α-D-(1,6) linkages (Fuentes-Zaragoza *et al.* 2011). Resistant starch is naturally present in bananas, lentils, oats, potatoes, beans, etc. (Adam-Perrot *et al.* 2009). Studies have shown that resistant starch is capable of influencing the composition of gut microbiota by generation of SCFAs which exert numerous physiological benefits on the host (Lordan *et al.* 2020). A study demonstrated that feeding mice with resistant starch promoted the production of SCFAs, modulated the gut microbiota by increasing growth of butyrate-producing bacteria (i.e. *Bifidobacterium*, *Lactobacillus*, *Clostridium*, *Ruminococcaceae* and *Lachnospiraceae*) and enhanced the absorption of minerals (iron, magnesium and iron) in intestine (Zeng *et al.* 2017). Moreover, consumption of resistant starch has been reported to exert antidiabetic and anti-inflammatory effects by improving insulin resistance and glucose tolerance as well as inhibiting the production of pro-inflammatory cytokines (Zhu *et al.* 2020).

11.3.3 Polyphenols

Polyphenols are non-nutritive, secondary metabolites extensively present in fruits, vegetables and various plant-derived products such as cereals, tea and coffee (Nazzaro *et al.* 2020). These compounds have gained much attention for a long time owing to their numerous health-promoting properties including protection against risk of inflammation, cancer, diabetes, cardiovascular diseases and neurodegenerative diseases such as Alzheimer's (Cueva *et al.* 2017). Polyphenols are basically consumed as a part of the food matrix (whole or processed), and it is estimated that a very small amount (5–10%) of total polyphenol is digested in the small intestine (Moorthy *et al.* 2020). The remaining portion reaches the colon in an undigested form where it is fermented by colonic microorganisms which generate large quantities of SCFAs that are responsible for exerting numerous health benefits in the host (Lin *et al.* 2019). Numerous clinical studies have reported the effects of interactions between polyphenol consumption and gut microbiota and their resulting health benefits (Moorthy *et al.* 2020; Tuohy *et al.* 2012). In one study, the prebiotic effects of blueberry polyphenols were demonstrated in obese mice and the authors concluded that daily consumption of polyphenols significantly modulated the gut microbiota and suppressed body weight gain by reducing the levels of cholesterol and triglyceride in feces (Jiao *et al.* 2019). Moreover, a recent study showed the ability of polyphenols from *Ocimum sanctum, Piper nigrum* and *Zingiber officinale* in treatment of inflammatory immune disorders (Babu *et al.* 2018). Polyphenols from apple have also been reported to have protective effects against cancer cells by inhibition of histone deacetylases in intestinal cells (Bordonaro *et al.* 2014). Given the numerous health benefits provided by polyphenols, they can be potentially included in the diet as novel prebiotics.

11.3.4 Soybean Oligosaccharides

Soybean oligosaccharides are low molecular weight, water-soluble carbohydrates that are mainly composed of raffinose and stachyose (Gibson *et al.* 2004). They are naturally present in large quantities in soybean (ranging from 100 to 150 g/kg of soy) and can be extracted directly without any enzymatic process (de Souza *et al.* 2015). The oligosaccharide extract is known to have a characteristically sweeter taste than sucrose and can therefore be used as a sugar replacer for the development of low-calorie foods. These oligosaccharides are resistant to digestion in the small intestine and reach the colon in unaltered form, where fermentation by colonic enzymes produces several prebiotic effects in human body such as reduced risk of cancer, osteoporosis and atherosclerosis (de Souza *et al.* 2015). In one study, the effect of feeding mice with soybean oligosaccharide was investigated and it was concluded that these oligosaccharides significantly modulated the gut microbiota and further increased the activity of immunoglobulins, T cells, NK cells and macrophages, thereby enhancing immunological function in mice (Ma *et al.* 2017). Moreover, a clinical study on women suffering from gestational diabetes demonstrated that daily consumption of soybean oligosaccharide significantly reduced oxidative stress and improved insulin resistance, thereby reducing the risk of diabetes (Fei *et al.* 2014). Despite having numerous health benefits, these oligosaccharides must be consumed in moderate doses as high doses can lead to intestinal discomfort and flatulence.

11.3.5 Lactitol

Lactitol is a type of sugar alcohol consisting of galactose and sorbitol, produced by catalytic hydrogenation of lactose (Martínez-Monteagudo *et al.* 2019). It is a sweet-tasting disaccharide that is commonly used as a sugar replacer in the development of low-calorie products (Olli *et al.* 2016). Since lactitol is not absorbed in the small intestine, it is fermented in the colon by colonic enzymes that generate SCFAs, thereby imparting numerous health benefits (Drakoularakou *et al.* 2007). In a study, oral administration of lactitol for 2 weeks significantly modulated the gut microbiota by increasing the population of *Bifidobacterium* which consequently acted as an osmotic laxative and alleviated the symptoms of constipation (Li *et al.* 2020). Moreover, lactitol combined with polydextrose, when orally administered in mice, successfully regulated body weight and postprandial metabolism by reducing levels of serum triglycerides (Olli *et al.* 2016).

11.3.6 Microbial Exopolysaccharides

Microbial exopolysaccharides (EPS) are high molecular weight polymers that are secreted during metabolic synthesis of microorganisms (Yildiz and Karatas 2018). For a long time, EPS secreted from lactic acid bacteria have received great attention owing to their generally recognized as safe (GRAS) status and numerous prebiotic effects on human health such as antitumor, antioxidant, cholesterol-lowering and immune-modulating activities (Li *et al.* 2019;

Morifuji *et al.* 2017; Van Hung *et al.* 2019). For example, EPS extracted from *Lactobacillus plantarum* successfully exhibited strong antitumor activity by inhibiting proliferation of HT-29 cells and inhibiting the formation of biofilm by pathogenic microorganisms such as *P. aeruginosa, Salmonella typhimurium* and *Staphylococcus aureus* (Liu *et al.* 2017). Another study investigated the effect of EPS from *Leuconostoc pseudomesenteroides* on mice and reported an increase in the population of *Bifidobacterium* after fecal fermentation and increased abundance of *Firmicutes* and *Oscillospira* in the microbiota of mouse cecum, suggesting that EPS might have potential benefits on the gut (Pan *et al.* 2020). EPS from lactic acid bacteria are also known to have significant applications in the food sector as natural additives such as stabilizer, gelling agent, texturizer and thickening agent (Mahdhi *et al.* 2017).

11.3.7 Seaweed Polysaccharides

Marine microalgae or seaweeds are one of the most abundantly found resources in the ocean (Zheng *et al.* 2020). Seaweed is an underexploited and sustainable crop that contains a rich diversity of structurally varied bioactive compounds, especially polysaccharides which have a wide array of biological activities such as antioxidant, anticoagulant, antiviral, anti-inflammatory and antidiabetic activities (Praveen *et al.* 2019). Therefore, polysaccharides from seaweed have attracted great interest for numerous therapeutic and industrial applications in the food, biotechnology and pharmaceutical sectors (Imbs *et al.* 2016). Seaweed algae are not digested in the small intestine and are subjected to fermentation in the colon by colonic microorganisms that release SCFAs, thereby exerting prebiotic effects on human health. Numerous in vitro and in vivo animal studies have been reported regarding prebiotic effects of seaweed algae; however, human studies still need to be explored (Conlon and Bird 2015). The fermentation ability of various major seaweed polysaccharides (laminaran, porphyran and ulvan) was demonstrated via microbial fermentability test and in vitro fecal fermentation and a growth in specific gut microorganisms (*Bifidobacterium, Lactobacillus* and *Bacteroides*) along with high levels of SCFAs (lactate, acetate and propionate) was observed which confirmed that these polysaccharides might have prebiotic effects on human gut (Seong *et al.* 2019). Similarly, an in vivo study in rats reported the prebiotic effects of *Ecklonia radiata* (brown seaweed) by generating high levels of SCFAs and reduced levels of phenol, *p*-cresol and pathogenic microorganisms (Charoensiddhi *et al.* 2017). However, further research is still required to understand the physicochemical properties of seaweed algae during its fermentation and mechanism of specific prebiotic effects.

11.4 Production Methods of Prebiotics

Prebiotics are naturally found in a large variety of food products and agricultural by-products, but in small quantities. Therefore, considering the increasing demands for prebiotics, they are now synthetically made in industries at a large scale. Furthermore, efforts are being made for the development of a sustainable, efficient, less expensive and more simple process for the production of prebiotics. Prebiotics are basically produced via two methods: biotechnological and chemical methods. Chemical prebiotic production involves the use of acids and solvents that degrade/hydrolyze the substrate. However, it has been reported that use of chemical methods leads to the formation of a complex mixture of products with a variety of linkages and structures and therefore lacks product specificity. Moreover, extreme conditions and long duration are required for these processes, which might result in degradation of the product (Torres *et al.* 2010). Therefore, taking into consideration these drawbacks of chemical methods, biotechnological routes, i.e. synthesis of prebiotics using enzymes, are increasingly preferred. The biotechnological method for the synthesis of the most commonly used prebiotics is discussed in the following sections and is described in Table 11.3.

11.4.1 Galactooligosaccharides

Galactooligosaccharides (GOS) are produced by transgalactosylation of the enzyme β-galactosidase using lactose as the substrate (Macfarlane 2010). The enzymatic process for their production is usually carried out in two steps: during the first step, the enzyme–galactosyl complex is formed and a glucose molecule is released; in the second step the galactose unit is transferred to a nucleophile, which is usually a carbohydrate instead of water (Zechel and Withers 2001). This method to produce GOS is a kinetically controlled process during which the hydrolysis of the substrate competes with the transgalactosylation activity. If the terminal galactosyl acceptor is water it results in the generation of glucose and galactose; however, if the acceptor is lactose it results in the formation of GOS (Splechtna *et al.* 2001).

It has been evident from various studies that the enzyme source, initial concentration of lactose, temperature, pH and reaction time have a significant effect on the structure, as well as degree of polymerization, of GOS. A high initial concentration of lactose is required for successful completion of the transgalactosylation reaction with high yields of GOS (Torres *et al.* 2010). In addition to this, high temperature (60 °C) has been observed to favor the rate of reaction, yields of GOS, stability of enzyme and solubility of lactose (Panesar *et al.* 2013). Moreover, reactor designs are considered to be one of the most important factors affecting the GOS production process. Different types of reactors have been reported for the production of GOS such as batch reactor, continuous reactor, fixed bed reactor, fluidized bed reactor, etc. Batch reactors are mainly used for GOS production, principally due to their ease of operation and reduced risk of contamination. However, product inhibition is a major constraint in this process. Therefore, continuous reactors are used to overcome the drawbacks of batch reactors as they facilitate continuous removal of galactose and glucose (Kaur and Panesar 2020).

Commercially, GOS are produced using β-galactosidase enzyme from different microorganisms such as *Aspergillus oryzae*, *Bacillus circulans*, *E. coli*, *Kluyveromyces marxianus*, *Aspergillus niger*, etc. High yields of GOS (24.2 g/L) have been synthesized using immobilized β-galactosidase enzyme from *B. circulans* in a continuous packed bed reactor operated at 45 °C (Rodriguez-Colinas *et al.* 2016). Similarly, the free form of β-galactosidase enzyme from *B. circulans* has been reported to continuously produce GOS in an enzyme membrane reactor at 50 °C (Cao *et al.* 2020). Besides lactose, whey has also been used for the production of GOS. For instance, conversion of whey into GOS has been reported using glass bead immobilized β-galactosidase enzyme from *A. oryzae* in a continuous packed bed reactor (Eskandarloo and Abbaspourrad 2018).

Table 11.3 Summary of enzymatic process for the production of different prebiotics.

Type of prebiotic	Enzyme used	Microbial source	Substrate	Type of fermentation process	Process conditions	Yield	Reference
FOS	Inulinase	*Saccharomyces cerevisiae*	Inulin	Shake flask fermentation	Substrate concentration 200 g/L; temperature 40 °C; time 24 h	0.9 g/g	Wang *et al.* (2016)
XOS	Xylanase	Xylanase and arabinofuranosidase	Kenaf stem	Enzymatic hydrolysis	Temperature 40 °C; pH 4.0; time 48 h	351.46 mg/g	Azelee *et al.* (2016)
GOS	β-Galactosidase	*Bacillus circulans*	Lactose	Continuous packed bed reactor	Substrate concentration 100 g/L; temperature 45 °C; time 48 h	24.2 g/L	Rodriguez-Colinas *et al.* (2016)
Lactulose	Cellobiose 2-epimerase	*Caldicellulosiruptor saccharolyticus*	Whey powder	Enzymatic membrane reactor	Substrate concentration 84.5 g/L; time 16 h; temperature 70 °C; enzyme concentration 7.5 U/mL	58.5%	Wu L *et al.* (2017)
FOS	–	*Aspergillus ibericus*	Sucrose	Shake flask fermentation	Temperature 37 °C; pH 6.2; time 38 h	0.64 g/g	Nobre *et al.* (2018)
GOS	β-Galactosidase	*Aspergillus oryzae*	Whey permeate	Packed bed reactor	Feed flow rate 0.5 mL/h; pH 5.2; temperature 60 °C	39.3%	Eskandarloo and Abbaspourrad (2018)
XOS	Xylanase	*Thermomyces lanuginosus*	Beechwood xylan	Mixing reactors	Time 24 h; pH 5.3; temperature 50 °C	9.18 mg/mL	Guido *et al.* (2019)
FOS	–	*Aspergillus oryzae*	Aguamiel sucrose	Glass reactor	Time 24 h	20.30 g/L	Muñiz-Márquez *et al.* (2019)
Lactulose	β-Galactosidase	*Aspergillus oryzae*	Fructose and lactose	Packed bed reactor	Temperature 50 °C; pH 4.5; fructose/lactose molar ratio 12	0.6 g/g	Guerrero *et al.* (2019)
GOS	β-Galactosidase	*Bacillus circulans*	Lactose	Enzyme membrane reactor	Temperature 50 °C; pH 6.0; substrate concentration 300 g/kg; flow rate 0.18 m^3/h	33%	Cao *et al.* (2020)
GOS	β-Galactosidase	*Klebsiella oxytoca*	Lactose	Shake flask fermentation	Substrate concentration 2.5 U/g; pH 7.0; temperature 40 °C; time 84 h	45.5% w/w	Huang *et al.* (2020)
Lactulose	β-Galactosidase	*Kluyveromyces lactis*	Cheese whey	–	Temperature 40 °C; pH 7.0	17.32 g/L	de Freitas *et al.* (2020)

FOS, fructooligosaccharides; GOS, galactooligosaccharides; XOS, xylooligosaccharides.

11.4.2 Fructooligosaccharides

Fructooligosaccharides (FOS) are usually produced by the enzymatic synthesis of β-fructofuranosidase (FFase) or fructosyltransferase (FTase) using sucrose or inulin as a substrate by the process of transfructosylation (de la Rosa *et al.* 2019). During this process the β-(2,1) glycosidic linkage of sucrose is hydrolyzed and the fructose unit is transferred to another moiety, especially FOS or sucrose (Flores-Maltos *et al.* 2016). The fructosylating enzymes responsible for production of FOS can be extracted from various microbial sources including yeast (*Candida* and *Kluyveromyces* spp.), bacteria (*Arthrobacter, Bacillus macerans, Lactobacillus reuteri* and *Zymomonas mobilis*) and fungus (*A. niger, A. japonicas, Aureobasidium pullulans, Penicillium* spp. and *Fusarium oxysporum*) (Panesar *et al.* 2013). Biotransformation of sucrose into FOS by a newly isolated strain of *A. ibericus* as whole cells through submerged state fermentation produced a high yield of FOS (118 g/L) at 30 °C and pH 6.2 (Nobre *et al.* 2018). Furthermore, FOS production (119 g/L) from sucrose has been successfully reported using immobilized cells of *Aureobasidium pullulans* and *Saccharomyces cerevisiae* in shake flask fermentation (Castro *et al.* 2019). Nowadays, agro-industrial by-products are being used as the substrate for the production of enzymes responsible for production of FOS. For instance, sugarcane bagasse has been successfully utilized as a substrate for the production of the enzymes fructosyltransferase and fructofuranosidase used for the synthesis of FOS (Ganaie *et al.* 2017; Guimarães *et al.* 2007). Similarly, FOS have been produced in a submerged state fermentation by three fungal strains (*A. niger* GH1, *A niger* PSH and *A. oryzae* DIA-MF) using aguamiel as a low-cost substrate (Muñiz-Márquez *et al.* 2019).

11.4.3 Xylooligosaccharides

Xylooligosaccharides (XOS) are commercially produced by hydrolysis of xylan using xylanase enzymes such as endoxylanase, β-D-xylosidases and esterases. It has been reported that enzymes having low xylanase or β-xylosidase activities are usually preferred in order to avoid product inhibition. Currently, XOS are produced from xylan present in lignocellulosic/agricultural residues (Panesar *et al.* 2013). However, xylan is usually present as a xylan–lignin complex which is not accessible by the enzymes. Therefore, a combination of pretreatment methods is applied on the biomass for the removal of lignin and cellulose, which further leads to higher yields of xylan (Brienzo *et al.* 2016). Different factors affecting the rate of enzymatic hydrolysis include the structure of the substrate, characteristics of the material and enzyme–substrate interactions. Heterogeneity of the substrate is another important factor affecting the process performance; therefore isolation of the polysaccharide of interest is required for better enzyme action (Moreira and Filho 2016). Numerous microorganisms have been used for the production of xylanase such as *Aspergillus, Clostridium, Trichoderma, Bacillus, Ruminococcus, Fibrobacter, Streptomyces,* etc. (Carvalho *et al.* 2013). Recently, the yeast *Pichia stipitis* has been successfully used for the production of xylanase (5536 U/g substrate) having the potential to hydrolyze xylan to XOS using a mixture of wheat bran and corn cob as the substrate in solid state fermentation at 50 °C (Ding *et al.* 2018). Furthermore, in a study, XOS have been successfully produced using an immobilized form of recombinant xylanase (XynA) isolated from *B. subtilis*

(Milessi *et al.* 2016). XOS production has also been reported from an enzyme combination of xylanase and arabinofuranosidase using a sulfuric acid/ionic liquid pretreated mixture of wheat straw and sugarcane bagasse as the substrate (Ávila *et al.* 2020). Investigation on utilization of novel microorganisms and substrates for xylanase production exhibiting high stability and activity is still in progress. Furthermore, efforts are being made for the development of a cost-effective process for large-scale production of XOS.

11.4.4 Lactulose

Lactulose is produced by the enzymatic activity of β-galactosidase and β-glycosidase utilizing fructose and lactose as substrate (Panesar and Kumari 2011; Wang *et al.* 2013). During this process, the lactose is hydrolyzed by the action of β-galactosidase to generate units of glucose and galactose to produce a galactosyl–enzyme complex. This step is then followed by transfer of the galactosyl unit to fructose, thereby generating lactulose via the transgalactosylation mechanism (Panesar and Kumari 2011; Wang *et al.* 2013). The enzyme for lactulose production can be isolated from various sources including microorganisms, animals and plants. However, the genera *Aspergillus* and *Kluyveromyces* are widely used microorganisms for β-galactosidase production used to synthesize lactulose (Guerrero and Wilson 2016). In order to achieve high yields of lactulose, excess quantities of fructose are added during the reaction process; however, significant amounts of unreacted fructose are left in the mixture. This issue can be solved by using a fed-batch system for the reaction due to its high compatibility with enzyme-catalyzed reactions having high substrate concentrations (Kaur and Panesar 2020). An optimal mutant of *Caldicellulosiruptor saccharolyticus* cellobiose 2-epimerase (*Cs*CE) has been successfully utilized for the production of lactulose with a high yield of 76% after four rounds of mutagenesis and screening (Shen *et al.* 2016). Furthermore, lactulose synthesis was reported from immobilized β-galactosidase isolated from *A. niger* in a continuous packed bed reactor and the maximum yield of 0.6 g/g was obtained at 50 °C temperature and 4.5 pH (Guerrero *et al.* 2019). Recently, whey has been recognized as a potential substrate for the production of lactulose. In a study, efficient production of lactulose has been reported from whey in an enzymatic membrane reactor by extracellularly expressing *Caldicellulosiruptor saccharolyticus* (*Cs*CE) in *Bacillus subtilis* (Wu L *et al.* 2017). Similarly, cheese whey has been successfully used as a substrate for the production of lactulose (17.32 g/L) using immobilized β-galactosidase isolated from *K. lactis* (de Freitas *et al.* 2020).

11.5 Mechanism of Action

Prebiotics are non-digestible carbohydrates that pass through the upper part of the gastrointestinal tract and reach the colon in an unaltered form. After reaching the colon, prebiotics interact with the good colonic microbes such as *Bifidobacterium* and *Lactobacillus* and are usually fermented by them which results in the production of SCFAs (acetate, propionate and butyrate) (Grajek *et al.* 2005). Production of SCFAs has been found to have a profound effect on host health as it reduces the pH of the colon and creates an environment that inhibits the growth of pathogenic microorganisms, thereby playing a major role in reducing the risk of several chronic diseases such as cancer, obesity and gastrointestinal infections (Sun and O'Riordan 2013). Furthermore, SCFAs exhibit antimicrobial properties, beneficially regulate the metabolic pathways, provide energy to cells, stimulate homeostasis by affecting the stability of colonic epithelium, as well as working as signaling molecules for specific receptors (Aachary and Prapulla 2011). SCFAs have also been reported to have several immunomodulatory properties such as producing pro-inflammatory cytokines (Parada Venegas *et al.* 2019; Van der Beek *et al.* 2017).

In addition to this, prebiotics have a wide array of benefits on human gut as they modulate the composition and activity of gut microflora, which subsequently enhances the absorption of nutrients and modifies bowel functions as well as improving lipid metabolism (Van Loo *et al.* 2005). This is probably due to the fact that utilization of SCFAs as an energy source by specific beneficial gut microorganisms can have a profound impact on the metabolism and composition of gut microbiota (Markowiak and Śliżewska 2017). Besides, prebiotics have been reported to increase the mucin level, which is responsible for improving the gut barrier function. Prebiotics consumption also leads to an increase in intestinal epithelial cells which provides a thicker coat of protection to the intestinal wall by secretion of mucus (Stoidis *et al.* 2011; Zhong *et al.* 2009). Therefore, through the production of antimicrobial substances and competition for nutrients and epithelial adhesion, the gut microbiota acts as a barrier for pathogenic microorganisms (Duncan 2013). Despite all the efforts made to understand the mechanism of action of prebiotics, the molecular mechanisms involved in this are still unclear. Moreover, due to differences in the chemical structures of prebiotics, efforts are required to understand their individual effect and health benefits. The mechanism of prebiotics is depicted in Figure 11.4.

11.6 Health Benefits of Prebiotics

Various scientific studies have reported a wide array of health benefits of prebiotics (Table 11.4) through generation of SCFAs as well as stimulating the growth of beneficial microorganisms (*Lactobacillus* and *Bifidobacterium*) which further inhibits the growth of pathogenic microorganisms (de Paulo Farias *et al.* 2019; Peredo-Lovillo *et al.* 2020). Some of the potential health benefits of prebiotics are discussed in subsequent sections.

11.6.1 Acute Gastroenteritis

Acute gastroenteritis is a type of intestinal infection that occurs when food or water infected with toxic microorganisms or their toxins is ingested. This disease is usually caused by such pathogens as *Clostridium perfringens*, *Campylobacter jejuni*, *Escherichia coli*, *Vibrio cholerae*, *Salmonella* and *Shigella* (Al-Sheraji *et al.* 2013). These pathogens colonize and grow in the intestine by utilizing and binding to the carbohydrates present in it and then infect the host. Moreover, the pathogens secrete toxins that contaminate the food even before it is consumed, and these subsequently disrupt the function of intestinal mucosa, thereby causing diarrhea, nausea, vomiting and abdominal pain (Joshi *et al.* 2018). Consumption of

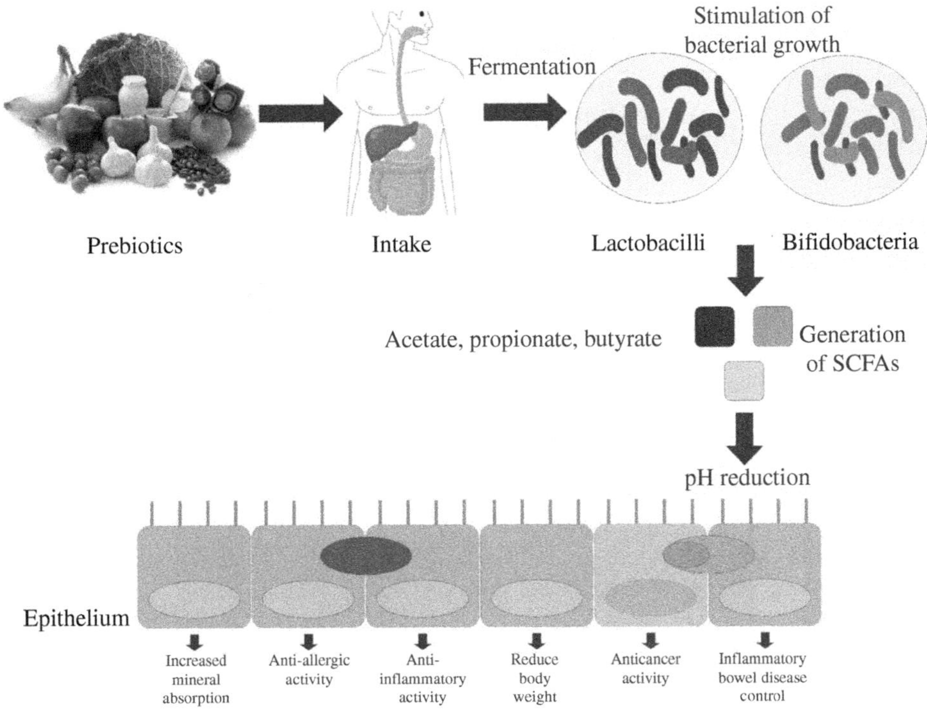

Figure 11.4 Mechanism of action of prebiotics. *Source:* Adapted from Biswal, P., Pal, A. and Das, A.P. (2017). Current trends and future prospective of prebiotics as therapeutic food. *Microbial Production of Food Ingredients and Additives*, 57–88. SCFAs, short chain fatty acids.

prebiotics reduces the risk of acute gastroenteritis by modulating the gut microflora (increased population of *Bifidobacterium* and *Lactobacillus*), and producing SCFAs which lower the pH of intestine, thereby providing protection from these pathogens (Vernazza *et al.* 2006). Moreover, prebiotics exhibit anti-adhesive properties as they compete for carbohydrates and acts as blocking agents to inhibit the binding of pathogens (Al-Sheraji *et al.* 2013). For example, daily supplementation of a combination of prebiotics (GOS and FOS) in a ratio of 9 : 1 to rats resulted in improvement in stool consistency and also reduced viral shedding significantly, thereby exhibiting protective action against acute gastroenteritis caused by rotavirus (Rigo-Adrover *et al.* 2017).

11.6.2 Reduction in Constipation

Constipation is one of the most common gastrointestinal disorders that affects individuals of all age groups. It is usually characterized by unsatisfactory and/or irregular bowel movements and hard or lumpy stool which becomes problematic to pass (Leser *et al.* 2015). Numerous factors responsible for this disorder include low water and fiber intake, stress, lack of physical activity, hormonal imbalance and consumption of antidepressants (Ahmad and Khalid 2018). For a long time, prebiotics have been used prominently for the treatment of constipation by generation of SCFAs that make the colon acidic, thereby leading to

Table 11.4 Applications of prebiotics for the treatment of various diseases.

Health benefit	Type of prebiotic	Experimental model	Outcomes of the study	Reference
	Combination of GOS and FOS	Suckling rat rotavirus infection model	Increased levels of SCFAs, decreased incidence of stools, improved stool consistency, significant reduction in viral shredding, improved immune system, reduced effects of rotavirus-induced gastroenteritis	Rigo-Adrover *et al.* (2017)
	GOS	Double-blind, controlled trial, formula-fed infants	Increased population of *Bifidobacterium*, improved immune system of host due to interaction of immune cells and host epithelium with colonic microbiota, reduced risk of infections	Nomayo *et al.* (2020)
Acute gastroenteritis				
Constipation	GOS	Randomized controlled trials	Increased stool frequency, improved stool consistency, ease of defecation and relief from abdominal pain and constipation	Yu *et al.* (2017)
	Inulin and lactitol	Randomized, double blinded, placebo-controlled clinical study	Reduced concentration of lipopolysaccharide, increased population of butyrate-producing bacteria (*Roseburia hominis*), reduced population of harmful bacteria (*Firmicutes* and *Clostridium*), improved frequency and consistency of stool	Chu *et al.* (2019)
	Lotus seed oligosaccharide	Mouse model	Decrease in appetite, reduced body weight gain, improved fecal water content, high SCFA production, improved intestinal peristalsis due to reduced time of defecation	Su *et al.* (2019)

(*Continued*)

Table 11.4 (Continued)

Health benefit	Type of prebiotic	Experimental model	Outcomes of the study	Reference
Anticancer activity	GOS and inulin	Wistar rats	Increased levels of cecum and fecal SCFAs in rats, reduced levels of ammonia, inhibition of aberrant crypt foci (ABF) formation, reduced concentration of tumor-promoting enzymes (β- glucosidase, azoreductase, nitroreductase, etc.)	Qamar *et al.* (2016)
	GOS derived from lactulose	Fischer 344 rats	Increase in cecum weight, modulation of gut microbiota, increased level of SCFAs, reduction in gut pro-inflammatory bacteria *Desulfovibrio*, significant reduction in tumor number and area, high anti-inflammatory properties	Fernández *et al.* (2018)
	FOS, resistant dextrin, XOS, and polydextrose	Randomized, double-blind, no treatment parallel control human clinical trial	Increased levels of IgM and IgG preoperatively, postoperative increased levels of IgG, IgA, total B lymphocytes and cytotoxic T cells. Modulation of gut microbiota by increased population of *Bifidobacterium* and reduced levels of *Bacteroides*	Xie *et al.* (2019)
Anti-obesity activity	Inulin	Double-blind, randomized, placebo-controlled human design	Increased fat oxidation, lower postprandial plasma free fatty acid concentrations, increased production of SCFAs, improvement in human metabolism	van der Beek *et al.* (2017)
	Inulin and GOS	in vitro	Increased population of *Bifidobacterium* and *Faecalibacterium*, increased levels of SCFAs, lower production rates of gas in fecal cultures, improved antioxidant property, and decreased inflammation	Nogacka *et al.* (2020)
	Polyphenols	Diet-induced obese mice	Improved glucose tolerance, insulin sensitivity, normal cholesterol, improved ratio of *Firmicutes/Bacteroidetes*, improved lipid metabolism, reduced expression of pro-inflammatory mediators and increased expression of mucin involved in maintenance of mucosal barrier	Diez-Echave *et al.* (2020)

Diabetes	Oligofructose-enriched inulin	Double-blinded, placebo-controlled design	Increase in anti-inflammatory cytokine IL-4, reduction in concentration of inflammatory cytokine IL-12 and IFN-γ, improved immune system, improved serum lipid and blood pressure profile	Dehghan *et al.* (2016)
	Raffinose	in vitro	Upregulation of IRβ/PI3K in adipocytes and skeletal muscle cells, increased glucose uptake, enhancement of autophosphorylation of Tyr-IRβ in insulin-resistant cells, upregulation of glycogen synthesis	Muthukumaran *et al.* (2018)
	Polysaccharides from acorn and sago	Mice	Increased levels of SCFAs, reduced expression of inflammatory genes such as IF-6, TNF-α and MCP-1, decreased insulin sensitivity and glucose intolerance	Ahmadi *et al.* (2019)
Enhanced mineral absorption	GOS	Sprague Dawley rats	Modulation of gut microbiota, increased absorption of calcium, magnesium, and iron	Maawia *et al.* (2016)
Lipid metabolism	β-Glucan	Randomized, double-blind, controlled, crossover design	Increased abundance of *Bifidobacterium*, reduced levels of plasma total cholesterol (TC) and low density lipopolysaccharide (LDL), improved bile acid and cholesterol binding ability	Connolly *et al.* (2016)
	Dietary fiber	High fat diet fed Wistar rats	Increased population of *Bifidobacterium,* increased SCFA levels, increased mucosal cell proliferation, inhibition of hepatic total lipids and triglyceride accumulation, rise in high density lipopolysaccharide (HDL) levels	Mateos-Aparicio *et al.* (2020)

FOS, fructooligosaccharides; GOS, galactooligosaccharides; IF, interferon; Ig, immunoglobulin; IL, interleukin; IR, insulin receptor; MCP-1, monocyte chemoattractant protein; PI3K, phosphatidylinositol-3 kinase, SCFAs, short chain fatty acids; TNF, tumor necrosis factor; XOS, xylooligosaccharides.

reduced absorption of ammonia in the mucosa. This large volume of ammonia present in the colon enables the activation of colonic peristalsis and transfer of water to the lower intestine, which increases the water content and bulk of stool (Chu *et al.* 2019; Macfarlane 2009). As a consequence, the transit time of digested food is decreased and intestinal motility is increased, which helps in treatment of constipation. Prebiotics including lactulose, lactitol, GOS and inulin, etc., are known to have a significant role in relieving symptoms of constipation and are therefore also known as laxatives. A randomized clinical study investigated the effect of prebiotics (consisting of inulin, lactitol and aloe vera gel) in adults (having stool frequency of maximum thrice a week), and an increase in fecal butyrate-producing bacteria, *Roseburia hominis*, and improvement in the frequency of stool was observed. Moreover, concentration of bacterial endotoxin lipopolysaccharide was significantly decreased, which helps in regulating intestinal motility (Chu *et al.* 2019).

11.6.3 Reduced Risk of Colon Cancer

Colon cancer is ranked as the third most common chronic disease among individuals and it represents a major public health issue. This disease is rapidly increasing due to severe changes in lifestyle and dietary habits of consumers including high consumption of alcohol, meat, fat and tobacco (Ahmad and Khalid 2018). Moreover, it is reported in individuals with a family history of colon cancer. It is well known that colon cancer arises due to generation of carcinogenic metabolites and toxins by some particular species of gut microflora which can lead to mutations in tissues and disruption of the heterozygous nature of tumor suppressor genes, thereby leading to activation of oncogenes (Ashwini *et al.* 2019). Therefore, gene–gut environment interaction and gut microbiota can have a considerable effect on the susceptibility and incidence of colon cancer (Sharma and Shukla 2016). Consumption of prebiotics has been reported to reduce the risk of colon cancer by stimulating the growth of *Bifidobacterium* and *Lactobacillus*, which inhibits the growth of carcinogens in human gut. Furthermore, generation of SCFAs after fermentation of prebiotic has been reported to exhibit anti-inflammatory effects on cancer cells and enhance the detoxification process (Rafter *et al.* 2007). For example, butyrate generated by GOS fermentation reduces metastasis and stimulates the process of apoptosis in colon cell lines (Wu *et al.* 2018). Furthermore, in a study, a mixture of the SCFAs acetate, butyrate and propionate was reported to provide therapeutic effects against colitis-associated colon cancer by limiting the expression of pro-inflammatory cytokines such as IL-6, TNF-α and IL-17 and inducing apoptosis in colon cancer cell lines (Tian *et al.* 2018). Prebiotics also reduce the risk of cancer by reducing the levels of indole and isovaleric acids, which are known to be markers of putrefaction (Ito *et al.* 1990).

11.6.4 Obesity

Obesity is a chronic disease characterized by the accumulation of excess fat in the body as a consequence of more energy being consumed than spent (Ejtahed *et al.* 2019). It is usually correlated with other chronic diseases including cardiovascular disorders, cancer, diabetes and hypertension (Klancic and Reimer 2020). Studies have shown that the gut microbiota plays an important role in obesity development. Therefore, consumption of prebiotics acts as a therapeutic alternative to reduce the risk of obesity (Shao *et al.* 2017). Prebiotics alter the populations of the gut microbiota involving reduction of pathogenic bacteria *Firmicutes* and *Bacteroidetes* along with increased growth of *Bifidobacterium* and *Lactobacillus*, which affects host appetite, glucose homeostasis and inflammation, thereby reducing the chances of obesity (Delgado and Tamashiro 2018; Diez-Echave *et al.* 2020; Zhang *et al.* 2020). Moreover, consumption of prebiotics is linked with increased secretion of energy-regulating hormones including glucagon-like peptide-1 (GLP-1), glucagon-like peptide-2 (GLP-2), oxyntomodulin (OXM), leptin, and peptide YY (PYY) along with a decreased proportion of orogenic hormones including ghrelin, which influences the regulation of metabolism, appetite and obesity (de Paulo Farias *et al.* 2019; Posovszky and Wabitsch 2015).

11.6.5 Diabetes

Type 2 diabetes mellitus is one of the major causes of deaths worldwide which are mainly linked with metabolic disturbances and abnormalities in the immune system (Dehghan *et al.* 2016). Consumption of prebiotics has been linked with reduced risk of diabetes as it can suppress the concentration of inflammatory cytokines including IL-6, IL-2 and interferons (Leylabadlo *et al.* 2020). In addition to this, prebiotics have been reported to significantly increase the anti-inflammatory cytokine IL-4, which further inhibits the production of tumor necrosis factor (TNF) and prostaglandin-2 as well as regulating the functions of T-helper cells, thereby reducing the risk of diabetes (Dehghan *et al.* 2016). Furthermore, prebiotic consumption can help reduce the risk of diabetes by ameliorating the glucose metabolism in the gut by modulating the gut microbiome–brain axis and increasing insulin resistance (Ahmadi *et al.* 2019).

11.6.6 Mineral Absorption

Minerals such as calcium, magnesium, potassium, iron, etc., are required for various biosynthetic pathways as well as for proper functioning of the human body (Ashwini *et al.* 2019). Prebiotics have been reported to improve absorption of minerals as the SCFAs generated can stimulate the binding sites of minerals and increase the absorption area in the gastrointestinal tract (Panesar *et al.* 2013). It has been reported by a clinical study that consumption of GOS for approximately 3–4 weeks improved the absorption of calcium, magnesium and iron. Similarly, oligofructose has also been shown to increase absorption of calcium by altering the gut microbiota and increasing the absorption area (Maawia *et al.* 2016).

11.6.7 Lipid Metabolism

For a long time, efforts have been made to improve lipid metabolism in humans as any abnormality in lipid metabolism is directly linked to several disorders including cardiovascular diseases, obesity and diabetes (Şanlidere Aloğlu *et al.* 2016). Prebiotics have received much attention in influencing lipid metabolism. Prebiotics have been reported to improve levels of serum triglyceride and cholesterol by modulating the synthesis of hepatic cholesterol in liver and inhibiting the synthesis of hepatic fatty acid and triacylglycerol (Yanık *et al.* 2013). Prebiotics such as GOS and fibers have been reported to exhibit excellent cholesterol-lowering ability. Moreover, FOS also exhibit hyperlipidemia as SCFAs generated by fermentation lead to inhibition of lipogenic enzymes in liver. Studies have shown that consumption of FOS and inulin exhibits significant improvement in levels of C-reactive protein, LDL cholesterol and total cholesterol (de Luis *et al.* 2011).

11.7 Safety Aspects of Prebiotics

Currently, prebiotics are considered among the most useful and consumed ingredients owing to their wide array of health benefits along with numerous industrial and commercial applications. One of the emerging applications of prebiotics is in the sector of food technology to be used as a supplement for the development of functional foods in order to maintain intestinal health (Wang 2009). Therefore, it has become important to understand the nature, role and safety aspects of prebiotics in the human body (Ashwini *et al.* 2019). Numerous in vivo and in vitro studies have been done on prebiotics and to date there have been no reports stating serious side effects after prebiotic consumption (Guarino *et al.* 2020).

Generally, prebiotics such as GOS, FOS and inulin have already established their Generally Recognized as Safe (GRAS) status and are widely used as supplements in food products (Biswal *et al.* 2017). However, consumer awareness towards selection of a particular prebiotic source and their safe level of dosage for consumption still need to be established (Ashwini *et al.* 2019). Another important point that must be considered for the safety evaluation of prebiotics includes the effect of inherent attributes of prebiotics on the ecology of the gut microflora (Hammes and Hertel 2002). Prebiotics should not adversely alter the composition of the gut microflora as this may lead to certain unfavorable health effects. For example, enhanced production of butyrate by gut microflora supports the growth of pathogenic bacteria, *Clostridium* spp. Therefore, research is required to select the most potent prebiotic with an aim to prevent the gut microflora from producing adverse effects on the host (Wang 2009). Another important criterion of a prebiotic is that it should be stable at a wide range of food processing parameters including pH and temperature, must not contain any impurities, should not be toxic, and must not alter the sensory attributes of the food product (Biswal *et al.* 2017). Therefore, more cytotoxic, mutagenic, pharmacokinetic and pharmacological studies are required to evaluate the toxicological information on prebiotics.

11.8 Global Status of Prebiotics

With increased consumer interest in health, and holistic medicine, demand for functional foods and dietary supplements has increased significantly (Panesar *et al.* 2018). Furthermore, rising concerns of customers regarding digestive health and chronic disorders such as obesity, diabetes and cardiovascular disease have resulted in growth of the functional food market globally (Kaur and Panesar 2020). In the past few years, prebiotics have gained focus among consumers and have been in the forefront among researchers and industrialists. As a consequence, the market for prebiotics has seen tremendous growth globally. In 2016, the worldwide market size of prebiotics was assessed to be approximately USD 3.34 billion and it is expected to rise to USD 7.90 billion by the year 2025. The global market of prebiotics has been forecasted to grow at a compound annual growth rate (CAGR) of 10%. In addition to this, the global demand for prebiotics was estimated to be around 623 kilotons in 2015 and is expected to grow at a CAGR of 8.0% by 2024 (https://www.grandviewresearch.com/industry-analysis/prebiotics-market).

The market for prebiotics can be classified according to geography, applications and ingredients. With regard to geographical areas, the market is basically divided into Europe, Asia Pacific, North America and the rest of the world. Of these, Europe dominates the global prebiotics market by holding a market share of approximately 40% which is expected to grow at a CAGR of 10.2% from 2016 to 2024 owing to elevated interest from the food and beverage industries. Furthermore, the prebiotic market in Asia Pacific countries including India, China and Japan has been anticipated to expand at a CAGR of 10.7% from 2016 to 2024 because of the high population, rise in chronic diseases and high demand for prebiotics. In addition to this, North America is expected to show a CAGR of 9.7% from 2016 to 2024. The market size for prebiotics in Australia, Brazil, Argentina and Chile is expected to witness high growth due to increase in demand for meat and dairy products along with the search for food-based medicine substitutes (https://www.grandviewresearch.com/industry-analysis/prebiotics-market).

1) With respect to applications, the prebiotic industry is separated into different sectors including food, beverages, animal feed and dietary supplements. The food and beverage sector includes bakery, meat, dairy, cereals and fermented food products which dominate the prebiotics market. Owing to the presence of health-promoting gut microorganisms in prebiotic food products along with high demand and ease of availability of beverages, especially dairy products, a significant increase in the prebiotics market is expected in upcoming years. Moreover, development of infant formulas including prebiotics is gaining much attention in order to provide complete nutrition, improve babies' gut health, enhance immunity and increase mineral absorption. Furthermore, rising consumer awareness towards protein consumption and growing concerns of older population regarding gut health have led to increased demand for dietary supplements which is also expected to boost the market size in future (https://www.adroitmarketresearch.com/industry-reports/prebiotics-market). Apart from human health, attention is also being given to improving the gut health of animals by fortifying animal feed with prebiotics; demand in the animal feed market in 2015 was witnessed to be USD 281.9 million and is expected to increase at a CAGR of 10.5% from 2016 to 2024.
2) Finally, with regard to the ingredients, FOS have received great attention and high demand in the food and beverage sector because of their ability to enhance the physical attributes of food along with their low caloric value. As a result, the FOS market is expected to anticipate growth to approximately USD 3.52 billion by 2024 (www.grandviewresearch.com). Production of FOS from sucrose accounted for approximately 50% of the total market share in 2015, followed by inulin-derived FOS which are

estimated to account for 40% of market share. Next to FOS, GOS are considered as the second most consumed prebiotics among consumers. In 2019, the market share of GOS was estimated around USD 600 million and is expected to increase at a CAGR of 6.2% by 2024 (www.erienewsnow.com). Moreover, the global market of lactulose was approximately USD 148 million in 2016 and is expected to expand to USD 180 million by 2024 (www.hexaresearch.com).

3) A large number of companies are involved in the manufacturing of prebiotics globally. Some of the major manufacturers of prebiotics include Abbott Laboratories, Yakult Honsha Co. Ltd., Kraft Foods Group, Cargill Inc., Solvay Pharmaceuticals, Bright Food Corporation, etc. Some commercially available prebiotics are Raftiline, Raftilose, Actlight, Beneo Oligofructose, Beneo Inulin, etc. Companies are currently working on the setting up of research and development for implementation of novel technological strategies to develop new products with improved health benefits (https://www.grandviewresearch.com/industry-analysis/prebiotics-market; Ashwini *et al.* 2019).

11.9 Conclusion and Future Prospects

The emerging interest regarding the relationship between diet and health has increased the necessity to understand the need for consumption of functional foods. Prebiotics are one such acknowledged functional food that imparts a wide array of health benefits to the host by modulating the growth or activity of gut microbiota. These compounds are naturally found in various plant and animal sources; however, to meet increased global demand, numerous efforts are being made for the development of sustainable and economic processes to produce them from different sources. Various processes such as chemical and enzymatic methods are being explored for the production of prebiotics at a large scale. However, enzymatic processes are currently gaining much focus due to the enhanced stability and activity of the final product. Furthermore, in order to develop a sustainable production process with low cost and to increase the variety of prebiotics, novel microbial sources and substrates such as agro-industrial biomass are currently being explored.

Recent trends have shown the utilization of prebiotics as functional ingredients for developing novel food products and supplements with more health-promoting effects. In addition, these compounds have also gained the attention of the pharmaceutical, health and chemistry sectors. Consumption of prebiotics has been recognized as safe for a long time, however limits for their safe human consumption still need to be established. In addition, strategically designed long-term clinical trials and metagenomic investigations are still needed to confirm the therapeutic claims made for prebiotics. Owing to the numerous health benefits of prebiotics, the global market is expected to grow exponentially in upcoming years; however, the regulatory bodies can play an important role among consumers in creating awareness regarding the usefulness, marketing and consumption of these ingredients.

References

Aachary, A.A. and Prapulla, S.G. (2011). Xylooligosaccharides (XOS) as an emerging prebiotic: microbial synthesis, utilization, structural characterization, bioactive properties, and applications. *Comprehensive Reviews in Food Science and Food Safety*, 10(1): 2–16.

Adam-Perrot, A., Gutton, L., Sanders, L., Bouvier, S., Combe, C., Van Den Abbeele, R., Potter, S. and Einerhand, A.W.C. (2009). Resistant starch and starch-derived oligosaccharides as prebiotics. *Paps*, 259.

Ahmad, A. and Khalid, S. (2018). Therapeutic aspects of probiotics and prebiotics. In: *Diet, Microbiome and Health*, Volume 11 (eds A.M. Holban and A.M. Grumezescu). Academic Press.

Ahmadi, S., Nagpal, R., Wang, S., Gagliano, J., Kitzman, D.W., Soleimanian-Zad, S., Sheikh-Zeinoddin, M., Read, R. and Yadav, H. (2019). Prebiotics from acorn and sago prevent high-fat-diet-induced insulin resistance via microbiome–gut–brain axis modulation. *The Journal of Nutritional Biochemistry*, 67: 1–13.

Ahmed, W. and Rashid, S. (2019). Functional and therapeutic potential of inulin: A comprehensive review. *Critical Reviews in Food Science and Nutrition*, 59(1): 1–13.

Aït-Aissa, A. and Aïder, M. (2014). Lactulose: production and use in functional food, medical and pharmaceutical applications. Practical and critical review. *International Journal of Food Science & Technology*, 49(5): 1245–1253.

Alander, M., Mättö, J., Kneifel, W., Johansson, M., Kögler, B., Crittenden, R., Mattila-Sandholm, T. and Saarela, M. (2001). Effect of galacto-oligosaccharide supplementation on human faecal microflora and on survival and persistence of *Bifidobacterium lactis* Bb-12 in the gastrointestinal tract. *International Dairy Journal*, 11(10): 817–825.

Al-Sheraji, S.H., Ismail, A., Manap, M.Y., Mustafa, S., Yusof, R.M. and Hassan, F.A. (2013). Prebiotics as functional foods: A review. *Journal of Functional Foods*, 5(4): 1542–1553.

Amorim, C., Silvério, S.C., Cardoso, B.B., Alves, J.I., Pereira, M.A. and Rodrigues, L.R. (2020). in vitro assessment of prebiotic properties of xylooligosaccharides produced by *Bacillus subtilis* 3610. *Carbohydrate Polymers*, 229: 115460.

Amorim, C., Silvério, S.C., Prather, K.L. and Rodrigues, L.R. (2019). From lignocellulosic residues to market: production and commercial potential of xylooligosaccharides. *Biotechnology Advances*, 37(7): 107397.

Anadón, A., Martínez-Larrañaga, M.R., Arés, I. and Martínez, M.A. (2016). Prebiotics and probiotics: An assessment of their safety and health benefits. *Probiotics, Prebiotics, and Synbiotics: Bioactive Foods in Health Promotion*, 1: 3.

Ashwini, A., Ramya, H.N., Ramkumar, C., Reddy, K.R., Kulkarni, R.V., Abinaya, V., Naveen, S. and Raghu, A.V. (2019). Reactive mechanism and the applications of bioactive prebiotics for human health. *Journal of Microbiological Methods*, 159: 128–137.

Ávila, P.F., Cairo, J.P.L.F., Damasio, A., Forte, M.B. and Goldbeck, R. (2020). Xylooligosaccharides production from a sugarcane biomass mixture: Effects of commercial enzyme combinations on bagasse/straw hydrolysis pretreated using different strategies. *Food Research International*, 128: 108702.

Azelee, N.I.W., Jahim, J.M., Ismail, A.F., Fuzi, S.F.Z.M., Rahman, R.A. and Illias, R.M. (2016). High xylooligosaccharides (XOS) production from pretreated kenaf stem by enzyme mixture hydrolysis. *Industrial Crops and Products*, 81: 11–19.

Babu, K.N., Hemalatha, R., Satyanarayana, U., Shujauddin, M., Himaja, N., Bhaskarachary, K. and Kumar, B.D. (2018). Phytochemicals, polyphenols, prebiotic effect of *Ocimum sanctum, Zingiber officinale, Piper nigrum* extracts. *Journal of Herbal Medicine*, 13: 42–51.

Bali, V., Panesar, P.S., Bera, M.B. and Panesar, R. (2015). Fructo-oligosaccharides: production, purification and potential applications. *Critical Reviews in Food Science and Nutrition*, 55(11): 1475–1490.

Bering, S.B. (2018). Human milk oligosaccharides to prevent gut dysfunction and necrotizing enterocolitis in preterm neonates. *Nutrients*, 10(10): 1461.

Bhatia, S., Prabhu, P.N., Benefiel, A.C., Miller, M.J., Chow, J., Davis, S.R. and Gaskins, H.R. (2015). Galacto-oligosaccharides may directly enhance intestinal barrier function through the modulation of goblet cells. *Molecular Nutrition & Food Research*, 59(3): 566–573.

Bindels, L.B., Delzenne, N.M., Cani, P.D. and Walter, J. (2015). Towards a more comprehensive concept for prebiotics. *Nature Reviews Gastroenterology & Hepatology*, 12(5): 303.

Biswal, P., Pal, A. and Das, A.P. (2017). Current trends and future prospective of prebiotics as therapeutic food. In: *Microbial Production of Food Ingredients and Additives*, Volume 5 (eds A.M. Holban and A.M. Grumezescu). Academic Press.

Bordonaro, M., Venema, K., Putri, A.K. and Lazarova, D. (2014). Approaches that ascertain the role of dietary compounds in colonic cancer cells. *World Journal of Gastrointestinal Oncology*, 6(1): 1.

Bornet, F.R.J., Brouns, F., Tashiro, Y. and Duvillier, V. (2002). Nutritional aspects of short-chain fructooligosaccharides: natural occurrence, chemistry, physiology and health implications. *Digestive and Liver Disease*, 34: S111–S120.

Bosscher, D. (2009). Fructan prebiotics derived from inulin. *Prebiotics and Probiotics Science and Technology*, 1: 163–206.

Brienzo, M., Carvalho, A.F.A., de Figueiredo, F.C. and de Oliva Neto, P. (2016). Sugarcane bagasse hemicellulose properties, extraction technologies and xylooligosaccharides production. *Food Waste: Practices, Management and Challenges*, 155–188.

Candela, M., Maccaferri, S., Turroni, S., Carnevali, P. and Brigidi, P. (2010). Functional intestinal microbiome, new frontiers in prebiotic design. *International Journal of Food Microbiology*, 140(2-3): 93–101.

Cao, T., Pázmándi, M., Galambos, I. and Kovács, Z. (2020). Continuous production of galacto-oligosaccharides by an enzyme membrane reactor utilizing free enzymes. *Membranes*, 10(9): 203.

Carvalho, A.F.A., de Oliva Neto, P., Da Silva, D.F. and Pastore, G.M. (2013). Xylo-oligosaccharides from lignocellulosic materials: chemical structure, health benefits and production by chemical and enzymatic hydrolysis. *Food Research International*, 51(1): 75–85.

Casci, T. and Rastall, R.A. (2006). Manufacture of prebiotic oligosaccharides. *Prebiotics: Development and Application*, 29–55.

Castro, C.C., Nobre, C., De Weireld, G. and Hantson, A.L. (2019). Microbial co-culturing strategies for fructo-oligosaccharide production. *New Biotechnology*, 51: 1–7.

Charoensiddhi, S., Conlon, M.A., Methacanon, P., Franco, C.M., Su, P. and Zhang, W. (2017). Gut health benefits of brown seaweed *Ecklonia radiata* and its polysaccharides demonstrated in vivo in a rat model. *Journal of Functional Foods*, 37: 676–684.

Chen, H.L., Lu, Y.H., Lin, J.J. and Ko, L.Y. (2001). Effects of isomalto-oligosaccharides on bowel functions and indicators of nutritional status in constipated elderly men. *Journal of the American College of Nutrition*, 20(1): 44–49.

Chu, J.R., Kang, S.Y., Kim, S.E., Lee, S.J., Lee, Y.C. and Sung, M.K. (2019). Prebiotic UG1601 mitigates constipation-related events in association with gut microbiota: A randomized placebo-controlled intervention study. *World Journal of Gastroenterology*, 25(40): 6129.

Coelho, E., Rocha, M.A.M., Moreira, A.S., Domingues, M.R.M. and Coimbra, M.A. (2016). Revisiting the structural features of arabinoxylans from brewers' spent grain. *Carbohydrate Polymers, 139*: 167–176.

Collins, S. and Reid, G. (2016). Distant site effects of ingested prebiotics. *Nutrients*, 8(9): 523.

Conlon, M.A. and Bird, A.R. (2015). The impact of diet and lifestyle on gut microbiota and human health. *Nutrients*, 7(1): 17–44.

Connolly, M.L., Tzounis, X., Tuohy, K.M. and Lovegrove, J.A. (2016). Hypocholesterolemic and prebiotic effects of a whole-grain oat-based granola breakfast cereal in a cardio-metabolic "at risk" population. *Frontiers in Microbiology*, 7: 1675.

Coppa, G.V., Zampini, L., Galeazzi, T., Facinelli, B., Ferrante, L., Capretti, R. and Orazio, G. (2006). Human milk oligosaccharides inhibit the adhesion to Caco-2 cells of diarrheal pathogens: *Escherichia coli, Vibrio cholerae*, and *Salmonella fyris*. *Pediatric Research*, 59(3): 377–382.

Corrêa-Oliveira, R., Fachi, J.L., Vieira, A., Sato, F.T. and Vinolo, M.A.R. (2016). Regulation of immune cell function by short-chain fatty acids. *Clinical & Translational Immunology*, 5(4): e73.

Cueva, C., Gil-Sánchez, I., Ayuda-Durán, B., González-Manzano, S., González-Paramás, A.M., Santos-Buelga, C., Bartolomé, B. and Moreno-Arribas, M. (2017). An integrated view of the effects of wine polyphenols and their relevant metabolites on gut and host health. *Molecules*, 22(1): 99.

de Freitas, M.D.F.M., Hortêncio, L.C., de Albuquerque, T.L., Rocha, M.V.P. and Gonçalves, L.R.B. (2020). Simultaneous hydrolysis of cheese whey and lactulose production catalyzed by β-galactosidase from *Kluyveromyces lactis* NRRL Y1564. *Bioprocess and Biosystems Engineering*, 43(4): 711–722.

de la Rosa, O., Flores-Gallegos, A.C., Muñíz-Marquez, D., Nobre, C., Contreras-Esquivel, J.C. and Aguilar, C.N. (2019). Fructooligosaccharides production from agro-wastes as alternative low-cost source. *Trends in Food Science & Technology*, 91: 139–146.

De Luis, D.A., De la Fuente, B., Izaola, O., Conde, R., Gutiérrez, S., Morillo, M. and Torres, C.T. (2011). Double blind randomized clinical trial controlled by placebo with an alpha linoleic acid and prebiotic enriched cookie on risk cardiovascular factor in obese patients. *Nutricion Hospitalaria*, 26(4): 827–833.

de Paulo Farias, D., de Araújo, F.F., Neri-Numa, I.A. and Pastore, G.M. (2019). Prebiotics: trends in food, health and technological applications. *Trends in Food Science & Technology*, 93: 23–35.

de Preter, V. and Verbeke, K. (2014). Functional aspects of prebiotics and the impact on human health. In: *Probiotics and Prebiotics: Current Research and Future Trends*, 1st edition (eds K. Venema and A.P. do Carmo). Norfolk, UK: Caister Academic Press.

de Souza, V.R., Menezes, C.C., Cunha, L.R., Pereira, P.A.P. and Pinto, U.M. (2015). Prebiotics: Technological aspects and human health. In: *Probiotics and Prebiotics: Current Research and*

Future Trends, 1st edition (eds K. Venema and A.P. do Carmo). Norfolk, UK: Caister Academic Press.

Dehghan, P., Farhangi, M.A., Tavakoli, F., Aliasgarzadeh, A. and Akbari, A.M. (2016). Impact of prebiotic supplementation on T-cell subsets and their related cytokines, anthropometric features and blood pressure in patients with type 2 diabetes mellitus: a randomized placebo-controlled trial. *Complementary Therapies in Medicine*, 24: 96–102.

Delgado, G.T.C. and Tamashiro, W.M.D.S.C. (2018). Role of prebiotics in regulation of microbiota and prevention of obesity. *Food Research International*, 113: 183–188.

Diez-Echave, P., Vezza, T., Rodríguez-Nogales, A., Ruiz-Malagón, A.J., Hidalgo-García, L., Garrido-Mesa, J., Molina-Tijeras, J.A., Romero, M., Robles-Vera, I., Pimentel-Moral, S. and Borras-Linares, I. (2020). The prebiotic properties of *Hibiscus sabdariffa* extract contribute to the beneficial effects in diet-induced obesity in mice. *Food Research International*, 127: 108722.

Ding, C., Li, M. and Hu, Y. (2018). High-activity production of xylanase by *Pichia stipitis*: purification, characterization, kinetic evaluation and xylooligosaccharides production. *International Journal of Biological Macromolecules*, 117: 72–77.

Drakoularakou, A., Hasselwander, O., Edinburgh, M. and Ouwehand, A. (2007). Lactitol, an emerging prebiotic: functional properties with a focus on digestive health. *Food Science and Technology Bulletin*, 3: 73–82.

Duarte, L.S., da Natividade Schöffer, J., Lorenzoni, A.S.G., Rodrigues, R.C., Rodrigues, E. and Hertz, P.F. (2017). A new bioprocess for the production of prebiotic lactosucrose by an immobilized β-galactosidase. *Process Biochemistry*, 55: 96–103.

Duncan, B. (2013). Prebiotics, probiotics, and health promotion: An overview. In: *Bioactive Food as Dietary Interventions for Liver and Gastrointestinal Disease: Bioactive Foods in Chronic Disease States*, 1st edition (eds R. Watson and V. Preedy). Academic Press.

Ejtahed, H.S., Angoorani, P., Soroush, A.R., Atlasi, R., Hasani-Ranjbar, S., Mortazavian, A.M. and Larijani, B. (2019). Probiotics supplementation for the obesity management; A systematic review of animal studies and clinical trials. *Journal of Functional Foods*, 52: 228–242.

Eskandarloo, H. and Abbaspourrad, A. (2018). Production of galacto-oligosaccharides from whey permeate using β-galactosidase immobilized on functionalized glass beads. *Food Chemistry*, 251: 115–124.

Fei, B.B., Ling, L., Hua, C. and Ren, S.Y. (2014). Effects of soybean oligosaccharides on antioxidant enzyme activities and insulin resistance in pregnant women with gestational diabetes mellitus. *Food Chemistry*, 158: 429–432.

Fernández, J., Moreno, F.J., Olano, A., Clemente, A., Villar, C.J. and Lombó, F. (2018). A Galacto-oligosaccharides preparation derived from lactulose protects against colorectal cancer development in an animal model. *Frontiers in Microbiology*, 9: 2004.

Fischer, C. and Kleinschmidt, T. (2018). Synthesis of galactooligosaccharides in milk and whey: a review. *Comprehensive Reviews in Food Science and Food Safety*, 17(3): 678–697.

Flores-Maltos, D.A., Mussatto, S.I., Contreras-Esquivel, J.C., Rodríguez-Herrera, R., Teixeira, J.A. and Aguilar, C.N. (2016). Biotechnological production and application of fructooligosaccharides. *Critical Reviews in Biotechnology*, 36(2): 259–267.

Fuentes-Zaragoza, E., Sánchez-Zapata, E., Sendra, E., Sayas, E., Navarro, C., Fernández-López, J. and Pérez-Alvarez, J.A. (2011). Resistant starch as prebiotic: A review. *Starch-Stärke*, 63(7): 406–415.

Fujita, K., Ito, T. and Kishino, E. (2009). Characteristics and applications of lactosucrose. In: *Proceedings of the Research Society of Japan Sugar Refineries' Technologists*, 57, Research Society of Japan Sugar Refineries' Technologists: 13–21.

Ganaie, M.A., Soni, H., Naikoo, G.A., Oliveira, L.T.S., Rawat, H.K., Mehta, P.K. and Narain, N. (2017). Screening of low cost agricultural wastes to maximize the fructosyltransferase production and its applicability in generation of fructooligosaccharides by solid state fermentation. *International Biodeterioration & Biodegradation*, 118: 19–26.

Gibson, G.R. and Roberfroid, M.B. (1995). Dietary modulation of the human colonic microbiota: introducing the concept of prebiotics. *The Journal of Nutrition*, 125(6): 1401–1412.

Gibson, G.R., Hutkins, R., Sanders, M.E., Prescott, S.L., Reimer, R.A., Salminen, S.J., Scott, K., Stanton, C., Swanson, K.S., Cani, P.D. and Verbeke, K. (2017). Expert consensus document: The International Scientific Association for Probiotics and Prebiotics (ISAPP) consensus statement on the definition and scope of prebiotics. *Nature Reviews Gastroenterology & Hepatology*, 14(8): 491.

Gibson, G.R., Probert, H.M., Van Loo, J., Rastall, R.A. and Roberfroid, M.B. (2004). Dietary modulation of the human colonic microbiota: updating the concept of prebiotics. *Nutrition Research Reviews*, 17(2): 259–275.

Gibson, G.R., Scott, K.P., Rastall, R.A., Tuohy, K.M., Hotchkiss, A., Dubert-Ferrandon, A., Gareau, M., Murphy, E.F., Saulnier, D., Loh, G., Macfarlane, S., Delzenne, N., Ringel, Y., Kozianowski, G., Dickmann, R., Lenoir-Wijnkoop, I., Walker, C., and Buddington, R. (2010). Dietary prebiotics: current status and new definition. *Food Science and Technology Bulletin: Functional Foods*, 7(1): 1–19.

Grajek, W., Olejnik, A. and Sip, A. (2005). Probiotics, prebiotics and antioxidants as functional foods. *Acta Biochimica Polonica*, 52(3): 665–671.

Guarino, M.P.L., Altomare, A., Emerenziani, S., Di Rosa, C., Ribolsi, M., Balestrieri, P., Iovino, P., Rocchi, G. and Cicala, M. (2020). Mechanisms of action of prebiotics and their effects on gastro-intestinal disorders in adults. *Nutrients*, 12(4): 1037.

Guerrero, C. and Wilson, L. (2016). Enzymatic production of lactulose. In: *Lactose-derived Prebiotics: A Process Perspective*, 1st edition (eds A. Illanes, C. Guerrero, C. Vera, L. Wilson, R. Conejeros and F. Scott). Academic Press.

Guerrero, C., Valdivia, F., Ubilla, C., Ramírez, N., Gómez, M., Aburto, C., Vera, C. and Illanes, A. (2019). Continuous enzymatic synthesis of lactulose in packed-bed reactor with immobilized *Aspergillus oryzae* β-galactosidase. *Bioresource Technology*, 278: 296–302.

Guido, E.S., Silveira, J.T. and Kalil, S.J. (2019). Enzymatic production of xylooligosaccharides from beechwood xylan: effect of xylanase preparation on carbohydrate profile of the hydrolysates. *International Food Research Journal*, 26(2).

Guimarães, L.H.S., Terenzi, H.F., de Moraes, M.D.L.T. and Jorge, J.A. (2007). Production and characterization of a thermostable extracellular β-D-fructofuranosidase produced by *Aspergillus ochraceus* with agroindustrial residues as carbon sources. *Enzyme and Microbial Technology*, 42(1): 52–57.

Hammes, W.P. and Hertel, C. (2002). Research approaches for pre-and probiotics: challenges and outlook. *Food Research International*, 35(2-3): 165–170.

Holscher, H.D. (2017). Dietary fiber and prebiotics and the gastrointestinal microbiota. *Gut Microbes*, 8(2): 172–184.

Huang, J., Zhu, S., Zhao, L., Chen, L., Du, M., Zhang, C. and Yang, S.T. (2020). A novel β-galactosidase from *Klebsiella oxytoca* ZJUH1705 for efficient production of galacto-oligosaccharides from lactose. *Applied Microbiology and Biotechnology*, 104: 6161–6172.

Hutkins, R.W., Krumbeck, J.A., Bindels, L.B., Cani, P.D., Fahey Jr, G., Goh, Y.J., Hamaker, B., Martens, E.C., Mills, D.A., Rastal, R.A. and Vaughan, E. (2016). Prebiotics: why definitions matter. *Current Opinion in Biotechnology*, 37, 1–7.

Imbs, T.I., Ermakova, S.P., Malyarenko, O.S., Isakov, V.V. and Zvyagintseva, T.N. (2016). Structural elucidation of polysaccharide fractions from the brown alga *Coccophora langsdorfii* and in vitro investigation of their anticancer activity. *Carbohydrate Polymers*, 135: 162–168.

Ito, M., Deguchi, Y., Miyamori, A., Matsumoto, K., Kikuchi, H., Matsumoto, K., Kobayashi, Y., Yajima, T. and Kan, T. (1990). Effects of administration of galactooligosaccharides on the human faecal microflora, stool weight and abdominal sensation. *Microbial Ecology in Health and Disease*, 3(6): 285–292.

Jiao, X., Wang, Y., Lin, Y., Lang, Y., Li, E., Zhang, X., Zhang, Q., Feng, Y., Meng, X. and Li, B. (2019). Blueberry polyphenols extract as a potential prebiotic with anti-obesity effects on C57BL/6 J mice by modulating the gut microbiota. *The Journal of Nutritional Biochemistry*, 64: 88–100.

Joshi, D., Roy, S. and Banerjee, S. (2018). Prebiotics: a functional food in health and disease. In: *Natural Products and Drug Discovery*, 1st edition (eds S.C. Mandal, V. Mandal and T. Konishi). Elsevier.

Kaur, R. and Panesar, P.S. (2020). Enzyme systems for high-value biomolecule production. In: *Biomass, Biofuels, Biochemicals*, 1st edition (eds A. Pandey, S.V. Mohan, J. Chang, P. Hallenbeck and C. Larroche). Elsevier.

Klancic, T. and Reimer, R.A. (2020). Gut microbiota and obesity: Impact of antibiotics and prebiotics and potential for musculoskeletal health. *Journal of Sport and Health Science*, 9(2): 110–118.

Le, B., Ngoc, A.P.T. and Yang, S.H. (2020). Synbiotic fermented soymilk with *Weissella cibaria* FB069 and xylooligosaccharides prevents proliferation in human colon cancer cells. *Journal of Applied Microbiology*, 128(5): 1486–1496.

Leser, T.D., Gottlieb, C.T. and Johansen, E. (2015). Bifidobacteria–regulators of intestinal homeostasis. In: *Probiotics and Prebiotics: Current Research and Future Trends*, 1st edition (eds K. Venema and A.P. do Carmo). Norfolk, UK: Caister Academic Press.

Leylabadlo, H.E., Sanaie, S., Heravi, F.S., Ahmadian, Z. and Ghotaslou, R. (2020). From role of gut microbiota to microbial-based therapies in type 2-diabetes. *Infection, Genetics and Evolution*, 81:104268.

Li, B., Du, P., Smith, E.E., Wang, S., Jiao, Y., Guo, L., Huo, G. and Liu, F. (2019). in vitro and in vivo evaluation of an exopolysaccharide produced by *Lactobacillus helveticus* KLDS1. 8701 for the alleviative effect on oxidative stress. *Food & Function*, 10(3): 1707–1717.

Li, X.Q., Zhang, X.M., Wu, X., Lan, Y., Xu, L., Meng, X.C. and Li, J.N. (2020). Beneficial effects of lactitol on the composition of gut microbiota in constipated patients. *Journal of Digestive Diseases*, 21(8): 445–453.

Lin, S., Wang, Z., Lam, K.L., Zeng, S., Tan, B.K. and Hu, J. (2019). Role of intestinal microecology in the regulation of energy metabolism by dietary polyphenols and their metabolites. *Food & Nutrition Research*, 63.

Lin, S.H., Chou, L.M., Chien, Y.W., Chang, J.S. and Lin, C.I. (2016). Prebiotic effects of xylooligosaccharides on the improvement of microbiota balance in human subjects. *Gastroenterology Research and Practice*, 2016: 5789232.

Liu, Z., Zhang, Z., Qiu, L., Zhang, F., Xu, X., Wei, H. and Tao, X. (2017). Characterization and bioactivities of the exopolysaccharide from a probiotic strain of *Lactobacillus plantarum* WLPL04. *Journal of Dairy Science*, 100(9): 6895–6905.

Long, J., Yang, J., Henning, S.M., Woo, S.L., Hsu, M., Chan, B., Heber, D. and Li, Z. (2019). Xylooligosaccharide supplementation decreases visceral fat accumulation and modulates cecum microbiome in mice. *Journal of Functional Foods*, 52, 138–146.

Lordan, C., Thapa, D., Ross, R.P. and Cotter, P.D. (2020). Potential for enriching next-generation health-promoting gut bacteria through prebiotics and other dietary components. *Gut Microbes*, 11(1): 1–20.

Ma, Y., Wu, X., Giovanni, V. and Meng, X. (2017). Effects of soybean oligosaccharides on intestinal microbial communities and immune modulation in mice. *Saudi Journal of Biological Sciences*, 24(1): 114–121.

Maawia, K., Iqbal, S., Qamar, T.R. and Rafiq, P. (2016). Production of impure prebiotic galacto-oligosaccharides and their effect on calcium, magnesium, iron and zinc absorption in Sprague-Dawley rats. *PharmaNutrition*, 4(4): 154–160.

Macfarlane, H.S.S. (2009). Mechanisms of prebiotic impact on health. In: *Prebiotics and Probiotics Science and Technology*, Volume 1 (eds D. Charalampopoulos and R.A. Rastall). New York, NY: Springer.

Macfarlane, S. (2010). Prebiotics in the gastrointestinal tract. In: *Bioactive Foods in Promoting Health*, 1st edition (eds R.S. Watson and V.R. Preedy). Academic Press.

Mahdhi, A., Leban, N., Chakroun, I., Chaouch, M.A., Hafsa, J., Fdhila, K., Mahdouani, K. and Majdoub, H. (2017). Extracellular polysaccharide derived from potential probiotic strain with antioxidant and antibacterial activities as a prebiotic agent to control pathogenic bacterial biofilm formation. *Microbial Pathogenesis*, 109: 214–220.

Mao, B., Li, D., Ai, C., Zhao, J., Zhang, H. and Chen, W. (2016). Lactulose differently modulates the composition of luminal and mucosal microbiota in C57BL/6J mice. *Journal of Agricultural and Food Chemistry*, 64(31): 6240–6247.

Markowiak, P. and Śliżewska, K. (2017). Effects of probiotics, prebiotics, and synbiotics on human health. *Nutrients*, 9(9): 1021.

Martinez-Ferez, A., Rudloff, S., Guadix, A., Henkel, C.A., Pohlentz, G., Boza, J.J., Guadix, E.M. and Kunz, C. (2006). Goats' milk as a natural source of lactose-derived oligosaccharides: Isolation by membrane technology. *International Dairy Journal*, 16(2): 173–181.

Martínez-Monteagudo, S.I., Enteshari, M. and Metzger, L. (2019). Lactitol: Production, properties, and applications. *Trends in Food Science & Technology*, 83: 181–191.

Mateos-Aparicio, I., de la Peña, R.J., Pérez-Cózar, M.L., Rupérez, P., Redondo-Cuenca, A. and Villanueva-Suárez, M.J. (2020). Apple by-product dietary fibre exhibits potential prebiotic and hypolipidemic effectsin high-fat fed Wistar rats. *Bioactive Carbohydrates and Dietary Fibre*, 100219.

Meyer, D., Bayarri, S., Tárrega, A. and Costell, E. (2011). Inulin as texture modifier in dairy products. *Food Hydrocolloids*, 25(8): 1881–1890.

Milessi, T.S., Kopp, W., Rojas, M.J., Manrich, A., Baptista-Neto, A., Tardioli, P.W., Giordano, R.C., Fernandez-Lafuente, R., Guisan, J.M. and Giordano, R.L. (2016). Immobilization and stabilization of an endoxylanase from *Bacillus subtilis* (XynA) for xylooligosaccharides (XOs) production. *Catalysis Today*, 259: 130–139.

Mohanty, D., Misra, S., Mohapatra, S. and Sahu, P.S. (2018). Prebiotics and synbiotics: Recent concepts in nutrition. *Food Bioscience*, 26: 152–160.

Moorthy, M., Chaiyakunapruk, N., Jacob, S.A. and Palanisamy, U.D. (2020). Prebiotic potential of polyphenols, its effect on gut microbiota and anthropometric/clinical markers: A systematic review of randomised controlled trials. *Trends in Food Science & Technology*, 99: 634–649.

Moreira, L.R.S. and Filho E.X.F. (2016). Insights into the mechanism of enzymatic hydrolysis of xylan. *Applied Microbiology and Biotechnology*, 100(12): 5205–5214.

Morifuji, M., Kitade, M., Fukasawa, T., Yamaji, T. and Ichihashi, M. (2017). Exopolysaccharides isolated from milk fermented with lactic acid bacteria prevent ultraviolet-induced skin damage in hairless mice. *International Journal of Molecular Sciences*, 18(1): 146.

Morozov, V., Hansman, G., Hanisch, F.G., Schroten, H. and Kunz, C. (2018). Human milk oligosaccharides as promising antivirals. *Molecular Nutrition & Food Research*, 62(6): 1700679.

Mu, W., Chen, Q., Wang, X., Zhang, T. and Jiang, B. (2013). Current studies on physiological functions and biological production of lactosucrose. *Applied Microbiology and Biotechnology*, 97(16): 7073–7080.

Muñiz-Márquez, D.B., Teixeira, J.A., Mussatto, S.I., Contreras-Esquivel, J.C., Rodríguez-Herrera, R. and Aguilar, C.N. (2019). Fructo-oligosaccharides (FOS) production by fungal submerged culture using aguamiel as a low-cost by-product. *LWT*, 102: 75–79.

Muthukumaran, P., Thiyagarajan, G., Babu, R.A. and Lakshmi, B.S. (2018). Raffinose from *Costus speciosus* attenuates lipid synthesis through modulation of PPARs/SREBP1c and improves insulin sensitivity through PI3K/AKT. *Chemico-Biological Interactions*, 284, 80–89.

Nazzaro, F., Fratianni, F., De Feo, V., Battistelli, A., Da Cruz, A.G. and Coppola, R. (2020). Polyphenols, the new frontiers of prebiotics. *Advances in Food and Nutrition Research*, 94: 35–89.

Ninonuevo, M.R., Park, Y., Yin, H., Zhang, J., Ward, R.E., Clowers, B.H., German, J.B., Freeman, S.L., Killeen, K., Grimm, R. and Lebrilla, C.B. (2006). A strategy for annotating the human milk glycome. *Journal of Agricultural and Food Chemistry*, 54(20): 7471–7480.

Niva, M. (2007). 'All foods affect health': understandings of functional foods and healthy eating among health-oriented Finns. *Appetite*, 48(3): 384–393.

Nobre, C., Alves Filho, E.G., Fernandes, F.A., Brito, E.S., Rodrigues, S., Teixeira, J.A. and Rodrigues, L.R. (2018). Production of fructo-oligosaccharides by *Aspergillus ibericus* and their chemical characterization. *LWT*, 89: 58–64.

Nogacka, A.M., Salazar, N., Arboleya, S., Ruas-Madiedo, P., Mancabelli, L., Suarez, A., Martinez-Faedo, C., Ventura, M., Tochio, T., Hirano, K. and Endo, A. (2020). in vitro evaluation of different prebiotics on the modulation of gut microbiota composition and function in morbid obese and normal-weight subjects. *International Journal of Molecular Sciences*, 21(3): 906.

Nomayo, A., Schwiertz, A., Rossi, R., Timme, K., Foster, J., Zelenka, R., Tvrdik, J. and Jochum, F. (2020). Infant formula with cow's milk fat and prebiotics affects intestinal flora, but not the incidence of infections during infancy in a double-blind randomized controlled trial. *Molecular and Cellular Pediatrics*, 7(1): 1–12.

Olli, K., Saarinen, M.T., Forssten, S.D., Madetoja, M., Herzig, K.H. and Tiihonen, K. (2016). Independent and combined effects of lactitol, polydextrose, and *Bacteroides thetaiotaomicron* on postprandial metabolism and body weight in rats fed a high-fat diet. *Frontiers in Nutrition*, 3: 15.

Pan, L., Han, Y. and Zhou, Z. (2020). in vitro prebiotic activities of exopolysaccharide from *Leuconostoc pseudomesenteroides* XG5 and its effect on the gut microbiota of mice. *Journal of Functional Foods*, 67: 103853.

Panesar, P.S. and Kumari, S. (2011). Lactulose: production, purification and potential applications. *Biotechnology Advances*, 29(6): 940–948.

Panesar, P.S., Kaur, R., Singh, R.S. and Kennedy, J.F. (2018). Biocatalytic strategies in the production of galacto-oligosaccharides and its global status. *International Journal of Biological Macromolecules*, 111: 667–679.

Panesar, P.S., Kumari, S. and Panesar, R. (2013). Biotechnological approaches for the production of prebiotics and their potential applications. *Critical Reviews in Biotechnology*, 33(4): 345–364.

Parada Venegas, D., De la Fuente, M.K., Landskron, G., González, M.J., Quera, R., Dijkstra, G., Harmsen, H.J., Faber, K.N. and Hermoso, M.A. (2019). Short chain fatty acids (SCFAs)-mediated gut epithelial and immune regulation and its relevance for inflammatory bowel diseases. *Frontiers in Immunology*, 102: 77.

Park, J., Kim, M., Kang, S.G., Jannasch, A.H., Cooper, B., Patterson, J. and Kim, C.H. (2015). Short-chain fatty acids induce both effector and regulatory T cells by suppression of histone deacetylases and regulation of the mTOR–S6K pathway. *Mucosal Immunology*, 8(1): 80–93.

Parkar, S.G., Blatchford, P.A., Kim, C.C., Rosendale, D.I. and Ansell, J. (2015). New and tailored prebiotics: Established applications. In: *Probiotics and Prebiotics: Current Research and Future Trends*, 1st edition (eds K. Venema and A.P. do Carmo). Norfolk, UK: Caister Academic Press.

Patel, S. and Goyal, A. (2012). The current trends and future perspectives of prebiotics research: a review. *3 Biotech*, 2(2): 115–125.

Peredo-Lovillo, A., Romero-Luna, H.E. and Jiménez-Fernández, M. (2020). Health promoting microbial metabolites produced by gut microbiota after prebiotics metabolism. *Food Research International*, 109473.

Pineiro, M., Asp, N.G., Reid, G., Macfarlane, S., Morelli, L., Brunser, O. and Tuohy, K. (2008). FAO Technical meeting on prebiotics. *Journal of Clinical Gastroenterology*, 42: S156–S159.

Plaza-Díaz, J., Fontana, L. and Gil, A. (2018). Human milk oligosaccharides and immune system development. *Nutrients*, 10(8): 1038.

Posovszky, C. and Wabitsch, M. (2015). Regulation of appetite, satiation, and body weight by enteroendocrine cells. Part 2: therapeutic potential of enteroendocrine cells in the treatment of obesity. *Hormone Research in Paediatrics*, 83(1): 11–18.

Praveen, M.A., Parvathy, K.K., Balasubramanian, P. and Jayabalan, R. (2019). An overview of extraction and purification techniques of seaweed dietary fibers for immunomodulation on gut microbiota. *Trends in Food Science & Technology*, 92: 46–64.

Qamar, T.R., Syed, F., Nasir, M., Rehman, H., Zahid, M.N., Liu, R.H. and Iqbal, S. (2016). Novel combination of prebiotics galacto-oligosaccharides and inulin-inhibited aberrant crypt foci formation and biomarkers of colon cancer in wistar rats. *Nutrients*, 8(8): 465.

Rafter, J., Bennett, M., Caderni, G., Clune, Y., Hughes, R., Karlsson, P.C., Klinder, A., O'Riordan, M., O'Sullivan, G.C., Pool-Zobel, B. and Rechkemmer, G. (2007). Dietary synbiotics reduce cancer risk factors in polypectomized and colon cancer patients. *The American Journal of Clinical Nutrition*, 85(2): 488–496.

Rastall, R.A. (2010). Functional oligosaccharides: application and manufacture. *Annual Review of Food Science and Technology*, 1: 305–339.

Reid, G., Sanders, M.E., Gaskins, H.R., Gibson, G.R., Mercenier, A., Rastall, R., Roberfroid, M., Rowland, I., Cherbut, C. and Klaenhammer, T.R. (2003). New scientific paradigms for probiotics and prebiotics. *Journal of Clinical Gastroenterology*, 37(2): 105–118.

Rigo-Adrover, M., Saldaña-Ruíz, S., Van Limpt, K., Knipping, K., Garssen, J., Knol, J., Franch, A., Castell, M. and Pérez-Cano, F.J. (2017). A combination of scGOS/lcFOS with *Bifidobacterium breve* M-16V protects suckling rats from rotavirus gastroenteritis. *European Journal of Nutrition*, 56(4): 1657–1670.

Roberfroid, M. (2007). Prebiotics: the concept revisited. *The Journal of Nutrition*, 137(3): 830S–837S.

Roberfroid, M., Gibson, G.R., Hoyles, L., McCartney, A.L., Rastall, R., Rowland, I., Wolvers, D., Watzl, B., Szajewska, H., Stahl, B. and Guarner, F. (2010). Prebiotic effects: metabolic and health benefits. *British Journal of Nutrition*, 104(S2): S1–S63.

Rodriguez-Colinas, B., Fernandez-Arrojo, L., Santos-Moriano, P., Ballesteros, A.O. and Plou, F.J. (2016). Continuous packed bed reactor with immobilized β-galactosidase for production of galactooligosaccharides (GOS). *Catalysts*, 6(12): 189.

Rudloff, S., Pohlentz, G., Borsch, C., Lentze, M.J. and Kunz, C. (2012). Urinary excretion of in vivo 13 C-labelled milk oligosaccharides in breastfed infants. *British Journal of Nutrition*, 107(7): 957–963.

Sabater, C., Prodanov, M., Olano, A., Corzo, N. and Montilla, A. (2016). Quantification of prebiotics in commercial infant formulas. *Food Chemistry*, 194: 6–11.

Samanta, A.K., Jayapal, N., Jayaram, C., Roy, S., Kolte, A.P., Senani, S. and Sridhar, M. (2015). Xylooligosaccharides as prebiotics from agricultural by-products: production and applications. *Bioactive Carbohydrates and Dietary Fibre*, 5(1), 62–71.

Şanlidere Aloğlu, H., Demir Özer, E. and Öner, Z. (2016). Assimilation of cholesterol and probiotic characterisation of yeast strains isolated from raw milk and fermented foods. *International Journal of Dairy Technology*, 69(1): 63–70.

Schumann, C. (2002). Medical, nutritional and technological properties of lactulose. *An update. European Journal of Nutrition*, 41(1): i17–i25.

Seong, H., Bae, J.H., Seo, J.S., Kim, S.A., Kim, T.J. and Han, N.S. (2019). Comparative analysis of prebiotic effects of seaweed polysaccharides laminaran, porphyran, and ulvan using in vitro human fecal fermentation. *Journal of Functional Foods*, 57: 408–416.

Shao, A., Campbell, W.W., Chen, C.O., Mittendorfer, B., Rivas, D.A. and Griffiths, J.C. (2017). The emerging global phenomenon of sarcopenic obesity: Role of functional foods; a conference report. *Journal of Functional Foods*, 33: 244–250.

Sharma, M. and Shukla, G. (2016). Metabiotics: one step ahead of probiotics; an insight into mechanisms involved in anticancerous effect in colorectal cancer. *Frontiers in Microbiology*, 7: 1940.

Shen, Q., Zhang, Y., Yang, R., Pan, S., Dong, J., Fan, Y. and Han, L. (2016). Enhancement of isomerization activity and lactulose production of cellobiose 2-epimerase from *Caldicellulosiruptor saccharolyticus*. *Food Chemistry*, 207: 60–67.

Silvério, S.C., Macedo, E.A., Teixeira, J.A. and Rodrigues, L.R. (2015). Perspectives on the biotechnological production and potential applications of lactosucrose: A review. *Journal of Functional Foods*, 19: 74–90.

Slavin, J. (2013). Fiber and prebiotics: mechanisms and health benefits. *Nutrients*, 5(4): 1417–1435.

Splechtna, B., Petzelbauer, I., Baminger, U., Haltrich, D., Kulbe, K.D. and Nidetzky, B. (2001). Production of a lactose-free galacto-oligosaccharide mixture by using selective enzymatic oxidation of lactose into lactobionic acid. *Enzyme and Microbial Technology*, 29(6-7): 434–440.

Stoidis, C.N., Misiakos, E.P., Patapis, P., Fotiadis, C.I. and Spyropoulos, B.G. (2011). Potential benefits of pro-and prebiotics on intestinal mucosal immunity and intestinal barrier in short bowel syndrome. *Nutrition Research Reviews*, 24(1): 21–30.

Su, H., Chen, J., Miao, S., Deng, K., Liu, J., Zeng, S., Zheng, B. and Lu, X. (2019). Lotus seed oligosaccharides at various dosages with prebiotic activity regulate gut microbiota and relieve constipation in mice. *Food and Chemical Toxicology*, 134: 110838.

Sun, Y. and O'Riordan, M.X. (2013). Regulation of bacterial pathogenesis by intestinal short-chain fatty acids. In: *Advances in Applied Microbiology*, 1st edition (eds S. Sariaslani and G.M. Gadd), 85. Academic Press.

Thamer, K.G. and Penna, A.L.B. (2005). Effect of whey, sugar and frutooligosacharides on the probiotic lactic acid bacteria population in fermented beverages. *Revista Brasileira de Ciências Farmacêuticas*, 41(3): 393–400.

Tian, Y., Xu, Q., Sun, L., Ye, Y. and Ji, G. (2018). Short-chain fatty acids administration is protective in colitis-associated colorectal cancer development. *The Journal of Nutritional Biochemistry*, 57: 103–109.

Topping, D.L., Fukushima, M. and Bird, A.R. (2003). Resistant starch as a prebiotic and synbiotic: state of the art. *Proceedings of the Nutrition Society*, 62(1): 171–176.

Torres, D.P., Gonçalves, M.D.P.F., Teixeira, J.A. and Rodrigues, L.R. (2010). Galacto-oligosaccharides: production, properties, applications, and significance as prebiotics. *Comprehensive Reviews in Food Science and Food Safety*, 9(5): 438–454.

Tung, T.Y., Yang, C.L., Chuang, C.L., Lin, C.C. and Chen, J.Y. (2018). Isomalto-oligosaccharides improve constipation in peritoneal dialysis patients-a randomized, double-blind, placebo-controlled trial. *Acta Nephrologica*, 32(4): 171–176.

Tuohy, K.M., Conterno, L., Gasperotti, M. and Viola, R. (2012). Up-regulating the human intestinal microbiome using whole plant foods, polyphenols, and/or fiber. *Journal of Agricultural and Food Chemistry*, 60(36): 8776–8782.

van der Beek, C.M., Dejong, C.H., Troost, F.J., Masclee, A.A. and Lenaerts, K. (2017). Role of short-chain fatty acids in colonic inflammation, carcinogenesis, and mucosal protection and healing. *Nutrition Reviews*, 75(4): 286–305.

Van Hung, T., Wanatanbe, J., Yonejima, Y., Hisa, K., Yamamoto, Y. and Suzuki, T. (2019). Exopolysaccharides from *Leuconostoc mesenteroides* attenuate chronic kidney disease in mice by protecting the intestinal barrier. *Journal of Functional Foods*, 52: 276–283.

Van Loo, J., Clune, Y., Bennett, M. and Collins, J.K. (2005). The SYNCAN project: goals, set-up, first results and settings of the human intervention study. *British Journal of Nutrition*, 93(S1): S91–S98.

Vera, C., Córdova, A., Aburto, C., Guerrero, C., Suárez, S. and Illanes, A. (2016). Synthesis and purification of galacto-oligosaccharides: state of the art. *World Journal of Microbiology and Biotechnology*, 32(12): 197.

Vernazza, C.L., Rabiu, B.A. and Gibson, G.R. (2006). Human colonic microbiology and the role of dietary intervention: introduction to prebiotics. In: *Prebiotics: Development and Application*, 1st edition (eds G.R. Gibson and R.A. Rastall). John Wiley and Sons, Ltd.

Wang, D., Li, F.L. and Wang, S.A. (2016). Engineering a natural Saccharomyces cerevisiae strain for ethanol production from inulin by consolidated bioprocessing. *Biotechnology for Biofuels*, 9(1): 1–11.

Wang, H., Yang, R., Hua, X., Zhao, W. and Zhang, W. (2013). Enzymatic production of lactulose and 1-lactulose: current state and perspectives. *Applied Microbiology and Biotechnology*, 97(14): 6167–6180.

Wang, Y. (2009). Prebiotics: Present and future in food science and technology. *Food Research International*, 42(1): 8–12.

Wang, Y., Guo, Q., Goff, H.D. and LaPointe, G. (2019). Oligosaccharides: structure, function and application. In: *Encyclopedia of Food Chemistry*, 1st edition (eds L. Melton, F. Shahidi and P. Varelis). Academic Press.

Weichert, S., Jennewein, S., Hüfner, E., Weiss, C., Borkowski, J., Putze, J. and Schroten, H. (2013). Bioengineered 2′-fucosyllactose and 3-fucosyllactose inhibit the adhesion of *Pseudomonas aeruginosa* and enteric pathogens to human intestinal and respiratory cell lines. *Nutrition Research*, 33(10): 831–838.

Wu, L., Xu, C., Li, S., Liang, J., Xu, H. and Xu, Z. (2017). Efficient production of lactulose from whey powder by cellobiose 2-epimerase in an enzymatic membrane reactor. *Bioresource Technology*, 233: 305–312.

Wu, X., Wu, Y., He, L., Wu, L., Wang, X. and Liu, Z. (2018). Effects of the intestinal microbial metabolite butyrate on the development of colorectal cancer. *Journal of Cancer*, 9(14): 2510.

Wu, Y., Pan, L., Shang, Q.H., Ma, X.K., Long, S.F., Xu, Y.T. and Piao, X.S. (2017). Effects of isomalto-oligosaccharides as potential prebiotics on performance, immune function and gut microbiota in weaned pigs. *Animal Feed Science and Technology*, 230: 126–135.

Xie, X., He, Y., Li, H., Yu, D., Na, L., Sun, T., Zhang, D., Shi, X., Xia, Y., Jiang, T. and Rong, S. (2019). Effects of prebiotics on immunologic indicators and intestinal microbiota structure in perioperative colorectal cancer patients. *Nutrition*, 61: 132–142.

Yang, J., Summanen, P.H., Henning, S.M., Hsu, M., Lam, H.M., Huang, J., Tseng, C.H., Dowd, S.E., Finegold, S.M., Heber, D. and Li, Z. (2015). Xylooligosaccharide supplementation alters gut bacteria in both healthy and prediabetic adults: a pilot study. *Frontiers in Physiology*, 6: 216.

Yanık, D.K., Erbağcı, A.B. and Göğüş, F. (2013). Probiotics and prebiotics in lipid metabolism. In: *Probiotics and Prebiotics in Food, Nutrition and Health*, 1st edition (eds S. Otles). Boca Raton, FL: CRC Press.

Yildiz, H. and Karatas, N. (2018). Microbial exopolysaccharides: resources and bioactive properties. *Process Biochemistry*, 72: 41–46.

Yu, T., Zheng, Y.P., Tan, J.C., Xiong, W.J., Wang, Y. and Lin, L. (2017). Effects of prebiotics and synbiotics on functional constipation. *The American Journal of the Medical Sciences*, 353(3): 282–292.

Zechel, D.L. and Withers, S.G. (2001). Dissection of nucleophilic and acid–base catalysis in glycosidases. *Current Opinion in Chemical Biology*, 5(6): 643–649.

Zeng, H., Huang, C., Lin, S., Zheng, M., Chen, C., Zheng, B. and Zhang, Y. (2017). Lotus seed resistant starch regulates gut microbiota and increases short-chain fatty acids production and mineral absorption in mice. *Journal of Agricultural and Food Chemistry*, 65(42): 9217–9225.

Zhai, S., Zhu, L., Qin, S. and Li, L. (2018). Effect of lactulose intervention on gut microbiota and short chain fatty acid composition of C57 BL/6J mice. *MicrobiologyOpen*, 7(6): e00612.

Zhang, C., Abdo, A.A.A., Kaddour, B., Wu, Q., Xin, L., Li, X., Fan, G. and Teng, C. (2020). Xylan-oligosaccharides ameliorate high fat diet induced obesity and glucose intolerance and modulate plasma lipid profile and gut microbiota in mice. *Journal of Functional Foods*, 64: 103622.

Zheng, L.X., Chen, X.Q. and Cheong, K.L. (2020). Current trends in marine algae polysaccharides: The digestive tract, microbial catabolism, and prebiotic potential. *International Journal of Biological Macromolecules*, 151: 344–354.

Zhong, Y., Cai, D., Cai, W., Geng, S., Chen, L. and Han, T. (2009). Protective effect of galactooligosaccharide-supplemented enteral nutrition on intestinal barrier function in rats with severe acute pancreatitis. *Clinical Nutrition*, 28(5): 575–580.

Zhu, Y., Dong, L., Huang, L., Shi, Z., Dong, J., Yao, Y. and Shen, R. (2020). Effects of oat β-glucan, oat resistant starch, and the whole oat flour on insulin resistance, inflammation, and gut microbiota in high-fat-diet-induced type 2 diabetic rats. *Journal of Functional Foods*, 69: 103939.

12

Galactooligosaccharides as Potential Prebiotics

Rupinder Kaur and Parmjit Singh Panesar

Food Biotechnology Research Laboratory, Department of Food Engineering & Technology, Sant Longowal Institute of Engineering and Technology, Longowal-148 106, Punjab, India

12.1 Introduction

With the augmentation in research about the relationship between human health and diet there has been a tremendous increase in consumer preference for healthier food, especially functional foods, over the past decade (Davis *et al.* 2010). The term functional foods was coined as "Foods for Specified Health Use" in Japan in 1991. They consist of those food ingredients that are consumed in the daily diet and have a beneficial impact on the host besides providing nutrition (Grajek *et al.* 2005). According to the statistics, the market size in 2018 was expected to be USD 150 million, and was further anticipated to increase to USD 250 million in the future (Patel and Goyal 2012).

Prebiotics have received immense attention owing to their diverse health benefits. They are defined as the "non-digestible food ingredients that stimulate the activity and/or growth of the colonic microflora, thus demonstrating various physiological effects on the body" (Gibson and Roberfroid 1995). As per the International Scientific Association for Probiotics and Prebiotics (ISAPP) guidelines, a food can be considered a prebiotic only if it meets certain criteria, such as resistance to enzymatic hydrolysis, ability to ferment and selective growth of colonic microbes (Gibson *et al.* 2017). Therefore, non-digestible oligosaccharides (NDOs) are considered as prebiotics because they are known to exhibit both physiological as well as physiochemical properties similar to those of prebiotics (Roberfroid and Slavin 2000). However, only small numbers of NDOs are considered as prebiotics, such as fructooligosaccharides (FOS), lactulose, isomaltooligosaccharides (IMO), galactooligosaccharides (GOS), tagatose, etc.

Of these, GOS are of primary interest due to various clinical benefits for both immune and digestive systems. Moreover, having similarities with human milk oligosaccharides (HMO), GOS have gained the interest of researchers worldwide (Sangwan *et al.* 2011).

Probiotics, Prebiotics and Synbiotics: Technological Advancements Towards Safety and Industrial Applications, First Edition. Edited by Parmjit Singh Panesar and Anil Kumar Anal.

In view of their nutritional and economic importance, this chapter explains various aspects of GOS: chemical structure, properties, technological strategies for production, applications in various sectors and global demand.

12.2 Galactooligosaccharides

Galactooligosaccharides are a class of lactose-derived oligosaccharides constituting of two to eight or even more monosaccharide units with the terminal glucose unit linked to the galactose units via β-glycosidic linkages, as represented in Figure 12.1 (Tzortzis and Vulevic 2009). Due to the presence of these β-bonds, GOS are known to resist hydrolysis in the upper intestinal tract and thus reach the colon as a whole molecule, wherein they

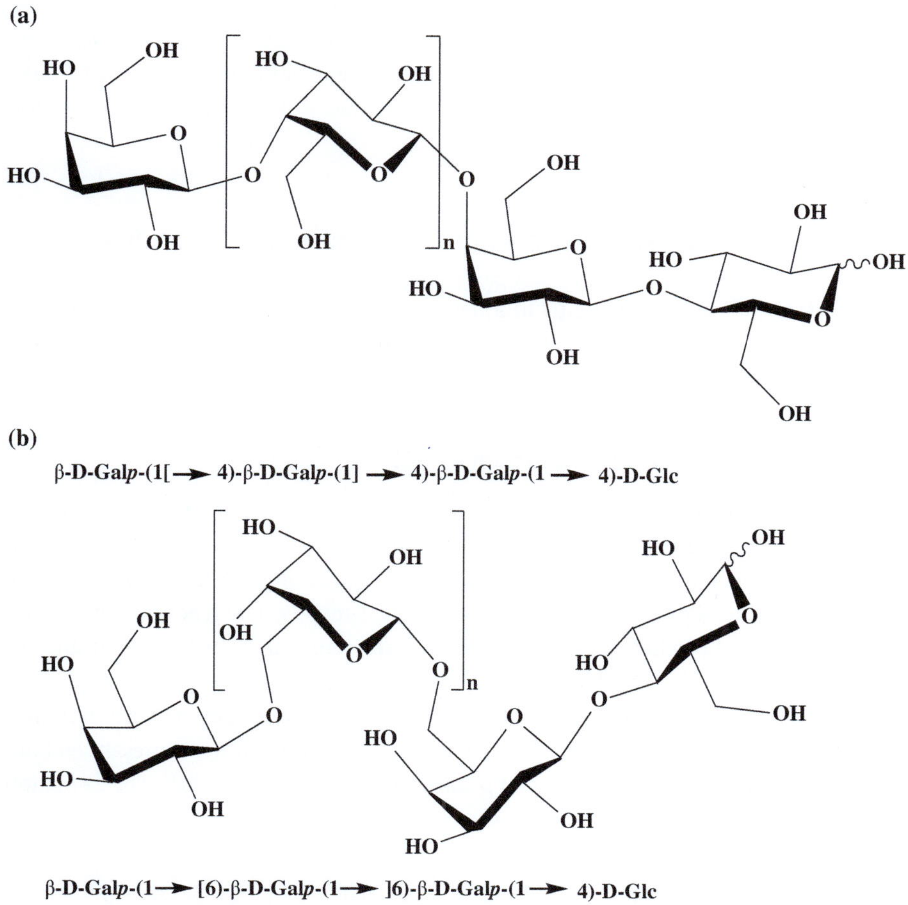

Figure 12.1 Structure of galactooligosaccharides: (a) β(1-4) bond; (b) β(1-6) bond. *Sources:* Adapted from Mannucci, F. (2009) Enzymatic Synthesis of Galactooligosaccharides From Whey Permeate. M. Phil Thesis. Technological University Dublin; Panesar, P.S., Kaur, R., Singh, R.S. and Kennedy, J.F. (2018). Biocatalytic strategies in the production of galacto-oligosaccharides and its global status. *International Journal of Biological Macromolecules*, 111: 667–679.

perform various physiological roles such as growth and cellular differentiation of colonic epithelial cells, synthesis of short chain fatty acids, lipid and carbohydrate metabolism and energy transduction in colonocytes. These functions are further associated with varied health-related activities such as protection against infection, reduction in the number of pathogenic microbiota, enhancement of mineral absorption and improvement in the normal functioning of the gut (van den Broek *et al.* 2008).

Apart from aforementioned, owing to various other properties, such as stability at high temperature as well as low pH conditions that differentiate them from other prebiotics and facilitate their use in various food products, GOS have received immense recognition from researchers worldwide in the last few years (Czermark *et al.* 2004). Moreover, having structural similarity with HMO, they have the potential to be used as a prebiotic supplement in infant formulas (Bode 2009).

GOS are naturally present in breast as well as cows milk, fruits and vegetables and various other sources, but the concentration is quite low (Angus *et al.* 2005). Moreover, commercially available GOS contain ample quantities of galactose and unreacted lactose that are unsuitable for lactose-intolerant people as well as diabetic patients (Cheng *et al.* 2006). In order to meet the ever-growing demand from consumers, large-scale production has become a necessity.

12.3 Technologies for Synthesis of Galactooligosaccharides

Both chemical as well as enzymatic techniques have been proposed for the synthesis of GOS, each having their own merits and demerits. Technological aspects of the production of GOS are discussed in detail in the subsequent sections.

12.3.1 Chemical Technique for Production of GOS

A chemical process for GOS production involves the formation of glycosidic bonds through the linkage of two polyfunctional groups. This linkage occurs via the displacement of the nucleophile of the leaving group (X) that is attached to the anomeric carbon by an alkoxy group of an alcohol ROH or any partially protected sugar moiety. The reaction is catalyzed by an activator, preferably a Lewis acid that facilitates the removal of the leaving group "X" as represented in Figure 12.2 (Nicolaou and Mitchell 2001).

The success of the reaction depends upon several factors such as reactivity between the donor as well as the acceptor molecule, action of the promoter, types of substituents present on both the sugar molecules and the formation of α- or β- anomeric forms (Garegg 2004). The formation

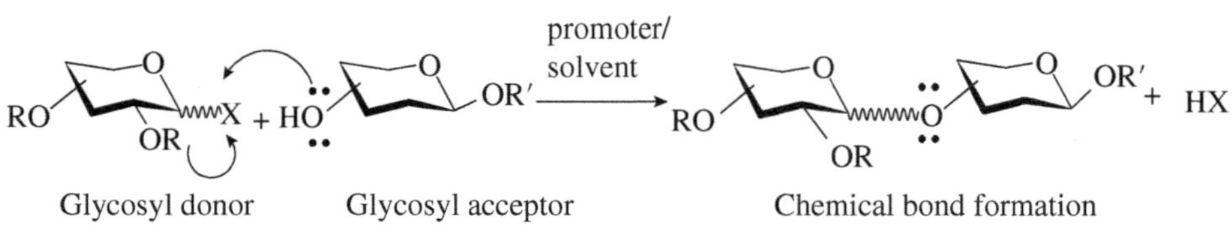

Figure 12.2 Generalized mechanism of galactooligosaccharide formation.

of either an α- or β-anomeric form depends upon the type and nature of the group at the C2 position. The displacement of the nucleophile by a glycosyl acceptor would lead to the formation of β-anomeric glycosidic linkage (Figure 12.3). However, if an O-acyl group is present at the C2 position, a dioxolenium cation intermediate is formed after the removal of the leaving group "X" due to the participation of the acyl group as the neighboring group (pathway b in Figure 12.3). The application of solvent also has a profound effect on the stereoselectivity.

The process for GOS production by a chemical technique is strenuous because it requires hydroxyl differentiation between the carbohydrate molecules to ensure protection and deprotection of the groups during the synthesis, making it a tedious and difficult process. Apart from this, multiple steps are required for the modification at any specific position. In addition, the utilization of large amounts of chemicals and massive generation of toxic compounds makes the process uneconomical and also limits its scalability (Weijers *et al.* 2008).

12.3.2 Enzymatic Production of GOS

To circumvent the problems associated with chemical synthesis, enzyme-catalyzed reactions have emerged as an alternative and promising strategy in terms of feasibility, economy and eco-friendliness as compared to the chemical one. The enzymes involved in the

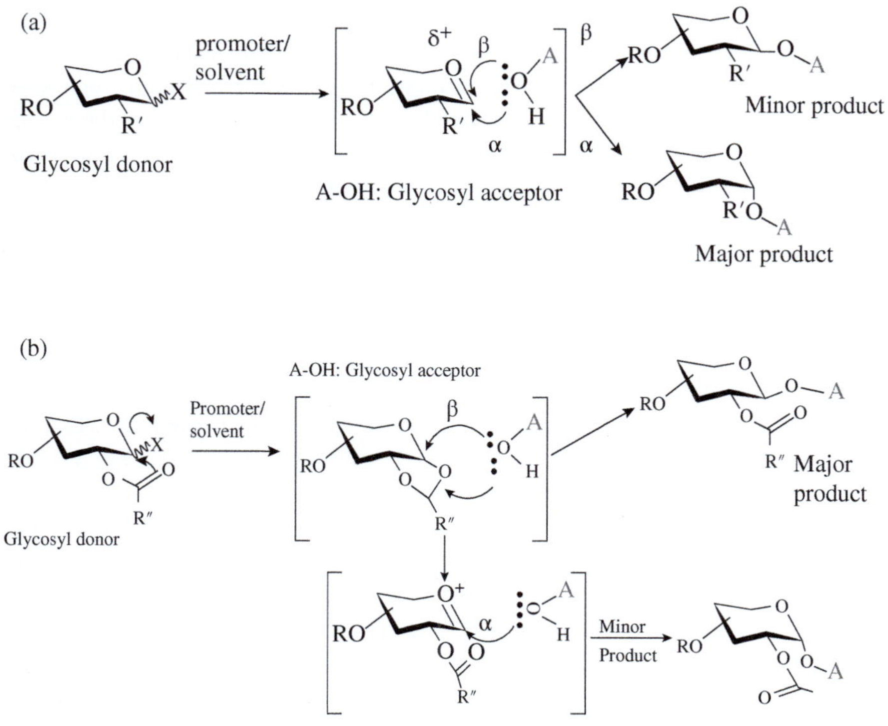

Figure 12.3 Synthesis of galactooligosaccharide: (a) without participation of the neighboring group; (b) with participation of the neighboring group. R": non-participating group; CO-R": participating group. *Source:* Weijers, C.A.G.M., Franssen, M.C.R. and Visser, G.M. (2008). Glycosyltransferase-catalyzed synthesis of bioactive oligosaccharides. *Biotechnology Advances*, 26(5): 436–456. doi:10.1016/j.biotechadv.2008.05.001.

glycoside formation belong to the families of glycosidases and glycotransferases (Weijers *et al.* 2008).

12.3.2.1 Glycosyltransferases

Glycosyltransferases (E.C. 2.4) catalyze the transfer of the sugar moiety from the donor molecule to the acceptor compound that lead to the formation of most of the cell-surface glycoconjugates with the formation of glycosidic linkages (Schuman *et al.* 2007). The carbohydrates acting as glycosyl donors are activated by one of the following methods: (i) addition of nucleoside mono- or di-phosphate, resulting in the formation of a nucleotide sugar; (ii) non-activated in the form of sucrose- or starch-derived oligosaccharides; and (iii) direct phosphorylation, thus leading to the production of sugar phosphate. Depending upon the types of carbohydrates, glycosyltransferases are classified into two groups: Leloir and non-Leloir (Coutinho *et al.* 2003).

Non-Leloir enzymes that use a phosphorylated donor generally catalyze the formation of *N*-acetylglucosaminyl linkages having α- or β-glucose-1-phosphate linkages. Similarly, those enzymes that utilize sucrose are also classed as non-Leloir groups. Since sucrose can donate only glucose and fructose molecules, the glycosyltransferases are known as glucosyltransferase (transfer of glucose) or fructosyltransferase (transfer of fructose), thus forming glucan and fructans, respectively (Seibel *et al.* 2006). In contrast to the non-Leloir enzymes, Leloir enzymes catalyze the transfer of monosaccharide that has been activated by kinase and further activated with nucleoside 5′-triphosphate to yield nucleotide-activated sugar (Ohtsubo and Marth 2006). Although these enzymes are highly regioselective, stereoselective and efficient, their industrial applications are limited by their price, availability and, most importantly, the use of particular sugar molecules (Torres *et al.* 2010). Therefore, in recent times enzymes belonging to the glycosidase family are being used for GOS production. These enzymes are less stereoselective compared to the glycosyltransferases, but they are readily available and do not have the requirement for nucleotide sugars, thereby leading to the development of an economic production strategy.

12.3.2.2 Glycosidases

Glycoside hydrolases or glycosidases (E.C. 3.2.1) are known for catalyzing the breakage of glycosidic linkage. The enzymes have gained immense attention due to their robust nature, easy availability and tolerance to various organic solvents, coupled with the use of inexpensive carbohydrate molecules as glycosyl donors (Faijes and Planas 2007).

Among them, β-galactosidase (3.2.1.23), commonly called lactase, is one of the important enzymes that have been widely used for the production of GOS. As per the information in CAZy database, it has been classed under the GH2 family; however, those belonging to thermophiles, halophiles or psychrophiles belong to the GH42 family (www.cazy.org). Lactases of multigene plants, fungi as well as some of the archae are classed under GH35 and GH1, respectively (Tanthanuch *et al.* 2008). β-Galactosidase is known for its ability to catalyze hydrolysis and the transgalactosylation reaction, thus having tremendous applications in various food and pharmaceutical sectors (Otieno 2010).

The structural conformation of β-galactosidase is a tetramer with four identical subunits comprised respectively of 1023 amino acids, which further join together to form five structural domains as depicted in Figure 12.4. Among these five domains, one constitutes a

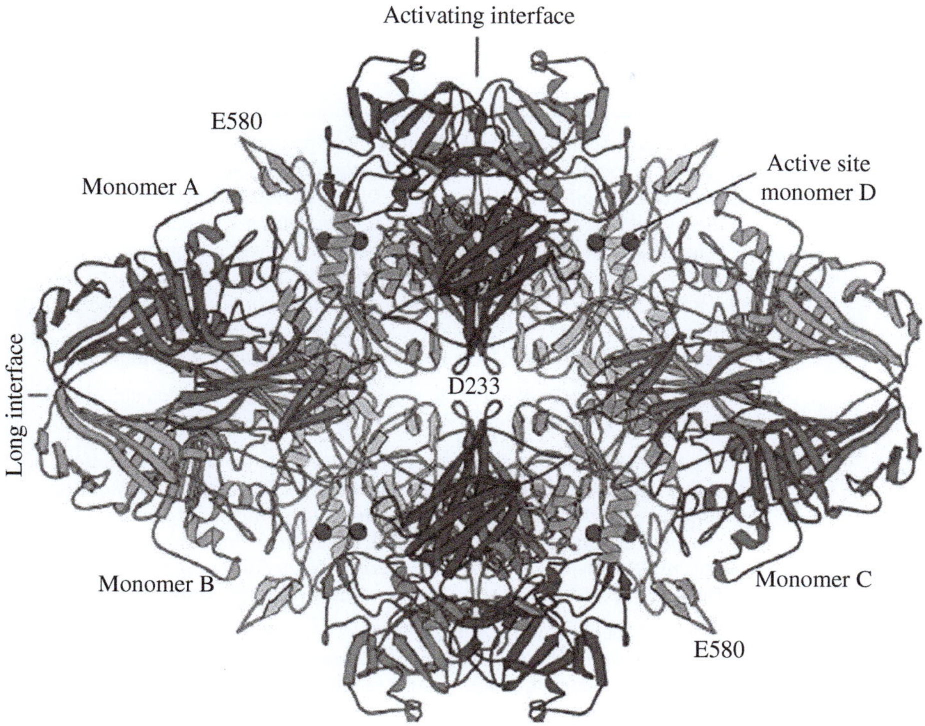

Figure 12.4 Structure of β-galactosidase. Domains in different colors: domain 1, blue; domain 2, green; domain 3, yellow; domain 4, cyan; domain 5, red. Lighter and darker shades differentiate the same domains in different subunits. The metal cations in each of the four active sites are depicted in spheres: green, Na^+; blue, Mg^{2+}. *Source:* Juers, D.H., Jacobson, R.H., Wigley, D., Zhang, X.-J., Huber, R.E., Tronrud, D.E. and Matthews, B.W. (2000). High resolution refinement of β-galactosidase in a new crystal form reveals multiple metal-binding sites and provides a structural basis for α-complementation. *Protein Science*, 9(9): 1685–1699.

triose phosphate isomerase (TIM)-type barrel, also known as central domain, that serves as an active site and is further composed of tetramer units; disruption of this unit results in the loss of enzyme activity (Corral *et al.* 2006; Huber *et al.* 1976).

Lactase is ubiquitous in nature and can be obtained from various sources, such as animals, plants and microorganisms (Table 12.1); however, the characteristics of the enzyme vary markedly with the source (Haider and Husain 2007).

12.4 Biotechnological Strategies for Biotransformation of GOS

Lactase from various sources, such as *Lactobacillus, Bacillus, Rhodotorula, Kluyveromyces, Sterigmatomyces* as well as *Aspergillus,* has been widely explored as a potential biocatalyst for the biotransformation of lactose to GOS, having significant applications in the food and pharmaceutical sectors (Otieno 2010; Rehman 2009). β-Galactosidase identifies not only

Table 12.1 Sources of β-galactosidase.

Microorganisms	Sources
Bacteria	*Alicyclobacillus acidocaldarius, Arthrobacter* spp., *Bacillus acidocaldarius, B. circulans, B. coagulans, B. subtilis, B. megaterium, B. stearothermophilus, Bifidobacterium bifidum, B. longum, B. infantis, Clostridium acetobutylicum, C. thermosulfurogens, Escherichia coli, Lactobacillus acidophilus, L. bulgaricus, L. helveticus, L. lactis, L. sporogens, L. delbrueckii, L. kefiranofaciens, Leuconostoc citrovorum, Pediococcus acidilacti, P. pento, Propionibacterium shermanii, Streptococcus cremoris, S. lactis, S. thermophilus, Pseudomonas fluorescens, Sulfolobus solfataricus, Xanthomonas campestris, Thermoanaerobacter* spp., *Thermus rubus, T. aquaticus, T. thermophilus*
Yeast	*Kluyveromyces fragilis, K. lactis, K. marxianus, Candida pseudotropicalis, C. utilis, C. kefyr, C. muscorum, Bullera singularis, Pichia* spp., *Torula* spp.
Fungus	*Alternaria alternata, A. palmi, Aspergillus oryzae, A. carbonarius, A. niger, A. foetidis, A. fonsecaeus, A. tubingensis. A. alliaceus, Aureobasidium pullulans, Fusarium moniliforme, F. oxysporum, Rhizomucor miehei, R. pusillus, Neurospora crassa, Paecilomyces variotii, Penicillium chrysogenum, P. conescens, Rhizobium meliloti, Trichoderma reesei, Saccharopolyspora rectivirgula, Sporotrichum* spp., *Streptomyces violaceus, Beauveria bassiana*
Plants	Peaches, apricots, almonds, apples, tomato, Japanese pear, coffee, alfalfa seeds, papaya, strawberry, avocado, nasturtium seeds, muskmelon, kiwifruit, mango, barley, cowpea, kidney beans, radish, carrot, lupin, rice shoots, kefir grains, tips of wild roses
Animals	Snails, intestine of dogs, calves, sheep, goats, rats, mice, bulls and boars, brain and skin tissue

Source: Adapted from Nagy Z, Kiss T, Szentirmai A, Biró S. Beta-galactosidase of Penicillium chrysogenum: production, purification, and characterization of the enzyme. Protein Expr Purif. 2001 Feb;21(1):24–9; el-Gindy A. Production, partial purification and some properties of beta-galactosidase from Aspergillus carbonarius. Folia Microbiol (Praha). 2003;48(5):581–4; Panesar, Parmjit & Kumari, Dr. Shweta & Panesar, Reeba. (2010). Potential Applications of Immobilized β-Galactosidase in Food Processing Industries. Enzyme research. 2010. 473137; Husain, Q. (2010). β Galactosidases and their potential applications: A review. Critical reviews in biotechnology. 30. 41-62; Aqib S, Akram A, Halim SA, Tassaduq R. Sources of β-galactosidase and its applications in food industry. 3 Biotech. 2017 May;7(1):79. doi: 10.1007/s13205-017-0645-5. Epub 2017 May 12.

the glucose–glucose bond, but also the glucose–galactose bond, and catalyzes the transfer of the galactose moiety to an acceptor molecule having a hydroxyl group.

The enzymatic process for the biotransformation of lactose to GOS is a two-step process and the mechanism has been represented in Figure 12.5.

The first step of the reaction involves the development of an enzyme–galactosyl complex, which is an irreversible reaction. In the second step, the galactose molecule is transferred to sugar, leading to the production of GOS. The whole process is kinetically controlled, whereby hydrolysis and the transgalactosylation reaction compete with each other and the terminal acceptor determines the end-products of the reaction. For example, if the acceptor is a water molecule, then the reaction leads towards the production of monosaccharides. On the other hand, if a sugar molecule is present as the galactose acceptor, the reaction proceeds towards the production of GOS (Boon *et al.* 2000).

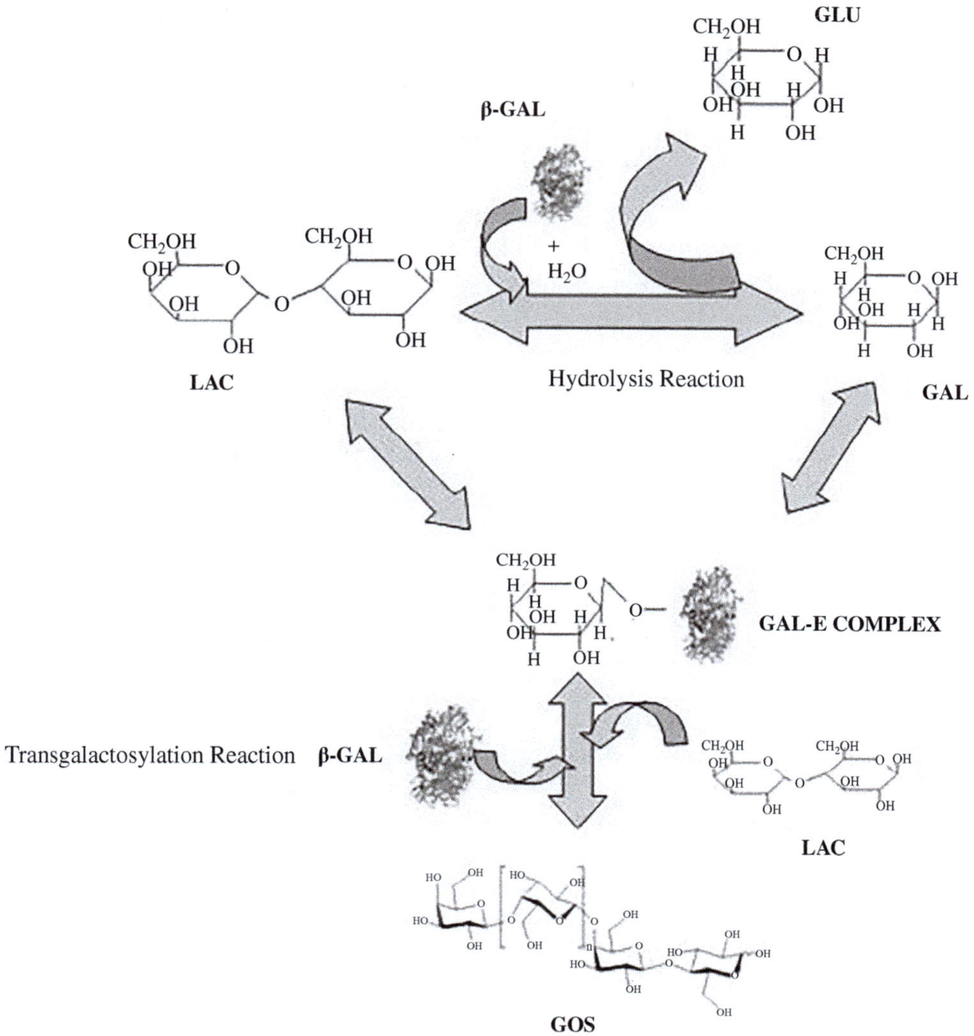

Figure 12.5 Reaction mechanism of β-galactosidase for the production of galactooligosaccharides. GAL, galactose; β-Gal, β-galactosidase; GAL-E, galactose–enzyme complex; GLU, glucose; GOS, galactooligosaccharides; LAC, lactose.

12.4.1 Factors Affecting GOS Production

Several factors have a significant impact not only on the yield of GOS, but also on the structure of GOS in terms of saccharide composition, glycosidic linkages and degree of polymerization. The major parameters include enzyme source, initial concentration of substrate, preferably lactose, reaction time and temperature (Otieno 2010).

Substrate concentration or lactose concentration is one of the important factors that influence the yield of GOS. A high concentration of lactose favors the transgalactosylation reaction because a higher substrate concentrate competes with water for the formation of the end-product. On the other hand, a lower concentration of lactose facilitates the hydrolysis reaction, thereby resulting in the production of galactose and glucose (Vera *et al.* 2011). Two approaches, the equilibrium and the kinetic approaches, have been studied in order to promote GOS production. The former approach favors GOS production through a high substrate concentration with a sufficient enzyme to substrate ratio in the reaction medium (Otieno 2010), whereas the other method works by increasing the kinetic variables that stimulate a favorable rate of product formation (Adamczak *et al.* 2009).

Besides this, the source of β-galactosidase also has a profound effect on the product formation as different species vary in their capability for building glycosidic linkages, which leads to structural variability of GOS. For instance, enzyme from *A. oryzae* produces β-(1-6) as well as β-(1-3) linked GOS, whereas enzymes from *K. lactis* mainly produce GOS with β-(1-3) glycosidic linkages (Albayrak and Yang 2002). Similarly, lactase from *Lactobacillus* spp. synthesizes GOS with β-(1-6) as well as β-(1-3) glycosidic linkage (Nguyen *et al.* 2012), yet lactase from *B. circulans* produces β-(1-4) linked GOS (Rodriguez-Colinas *et al.* 2014). In terms of structure of GOS, β-galactosidase from *B. circulans* is known to synthesize tetra- and pentasaccharides, whereas that of *A. oryzae* generally synthesizes trisaccharides with small amounts of tetrasaccharides. Similarly, tri- and tetrasaccharides are the main form synthesized by yeast, especially *Kluyveromyces* spp. (Boon *et al.* 2000). Apart from this, the enzyme also affects the yield of GOS and the rate of lactose converted during the reaction, which indicates the amount of substrate (lactose) utilized during GOS production. Lactose conversion is of prime importance both in terms of nutritional and technological significance. Besides the source of enzyme, process parameters such as initial substrate concentration, temperature, pH and presence of inhibitors or activators affect the enzyme activity and further influence the GOS yield (Manucci 2009).

Temperature has a profound impact on the reaction rate and enzyme stability as well as solubility of lactose. However, at an elevated temperature, denaturation of the enzyme is the major issue (Vera *et al.* 2012). During the past decade, attention has shifted towards the use of thermostable enzymes during the transgalactosylation reaction (Chen *et al.* 2008; Hatzinikolaou *et al.* 2005). Thermostable enzymes can result in maximum GOS yields, given that a higher temperature favors a higher reaction rate and greater lactose solubility and stimulates equilibrium towards the transgalactosylation reaction (Haki and Rakshit 2003).

In the initial stages of reactions, the transgalactosylation reaction is favored as it leads to a high amount of GOS. However, with the increase in yield, the concentration of lactose in the reaction mixture reduces. As the reaction proceeds, GOS level decreases, whereas the amount of monosaccharides, such as glucose and galactose, increases. Therefore, duration of the reaction is also a crucial factor; as the point at which maximum yield is obtained is reached, the reaction must be halted (Torres *et al.* 2010).

In terms of pH, reports have indicated 6–7 as the optimum range during the reaction (Park *et al.* 2008). However, the optimum pH value differs with the enzyme source (Gosling *et al.* 2010). For example, lactase from *A. oryzae* exhibits maximum activity in acid conditions. However, Mano and co-workers (2019) have stated that the catalytic properties of this enzyme are influenced by the initial concentration of lactose present in the reaction mixture rather than pH.

Apart from the aforementioned aspects, some other factors have also been reported to influence the production of GOS (Vera *et al.* 2016). Non-conventional substrates, such as organic solvents in aqueous phase, have also been investigated for synthesis of GOS (Bednarski and Kulikowska 2007). Further, dicotyl sodium sulfosuccinate and isooctane in a reverse micelle system led to an increase in yield to 55% from 31% (Chen *et al.* 2001). The higher yield in the biphasic system may be attributed to the separation of the final product from the enzyme and inhibitors. Despite the reported higher yields, scaling up of this process is hampered by a decrease in the rate of reaction and enzyme stability, and higher cost of production (Dong *et al.* 2015).

Moreover, configuration of the reactor during GOS production also affects the yield and the structure. Generally, product inhibition is most profound when the reaction is carried out in a batch reactor in contrast to a continuous one where the products and the by-products are continuously removed during the reaction (Das *et al.* 2011). Although these reactors are cost-effective and higher yields are obtained, when designing the reactor certain points have to be considered such as flow rate and the total residence time in the reactor (Kaur and Panesar 2020).

Several biotechnological strategies, such as whole cells, free enzymes and immobilized enzymes have been explored throughout the years for the production of GOS (Table 12.2). Novel approaches have also been explored to improve the yield, either by using recombinant enzymes or through protein engineering. The various production strategies are discussed in the following sections.

12.4.2 Production of GOS using Whole Cells

Varied species of bacteria, yeast and fungus having elevated enzyme activity have been used as potential catalysts during production. The utilization of whole cells is advantageous with reference to the availability and economics of the process. However, the permeability barrier of the cell envelope is the major issue that results in low reaction rate and, further, lower yields. Therefore, to circumvent this issue, permeabilization of the cells has to be carried out (Kumari *et al.* 2013).

A comparative study undertaken by Rodriguez-Colinas *et al.* (2011) compared *K. lactis* cells with the two commercial yeast enzymes Lactozym 3000 L HP G and Maxilact LGX 5000. With a 400 g/L initial lactose concentration, whole cells were able to synthesize 177 g/L of GOS as compared to 160 g/L and 154 g/L for Lactozym 3000 L HP G and Maxilact LGX 5000, respectively. The properties of the enzyme, temperature and duration of the reaction had a strong influence on the yield. Although enzyme concentration had an impact on the duration of the reaction, it did not affect the yield.

A consortium of microbes, *Sporobolomyces singularis* MTCC 5491 and yeast isolate NUTIDY007, was examined for their transgalactosylation potential, which indicated a maximum yield of 10.9 g/L/h with a purity of approximately 85% under optimal reaction conditions during continuous production in a reactor equipped with a microfiltration membrane system (Saravanan *et al.* 2017). Similarly, a process was developed for the production of GOS from a sugar reaction mixture using *Saccharomyces lactis* followed by *K. lactis* var. *lactis,* which resulted in purity of about 65% (Srivastava and Mishra 2019). The mixture of microbes during biotransformation is intended to overcome two hurdles, purity of the enzyme and purification of the final product, thereby leading to the development of a cost-effective technique.

Table 12.2 Enzymatic techniques for the production of GOS.

Types of biocatalyst	Source	Reaction parameters						Reference
		ILC	Enzyme concentration	pH	Temp. (°C)	Time	Yield	
Whole cells	*Pediococcus acidilactici*	30%	2.75 IU	7.0	47.5	–	–	Chanalia *et al.* (2018)
	Pantoea anthophila Bac 55.2	400 g/L	15 U/mL	7.5	50	24 h	136 g/L	Yañez-Ñeco *et al.* (2017)
	P. anthophila Bac 69.1						145 g/L	
	Sporobolomyces singularis and yeast isolate (NUTIDY007)	25%	7%		30	60 h	65%	Saravanan *et al.* (2017)
	Tetradesmus obliquus	50 g/L	1×10^6 cells/mL	6.8	21	21 days	4.4 g/L	Suwal *et al.* (2019)
	Propionibacterium acidipropionici LET 120	30%	1.3 U/mL	6.5	45	24 h	26.8%	Sabater *et al.* (2019)
	Klebsiella oxytoca ZJUH1705	40%	2.5 U/g lactose	7.0	40	48 h	45.5 ± 2.3%	Huang *et al.* (2020)
	Lactobacillus delbrueckii subsp. *bulgaricus*	300 g/L	1.3 U/mL	6.5	45	24 h	38.1%	Fara *et al.* (2020)
	K. lactis	400 g/L	1.2 U/mL	6.8	40	6 h	177 g/L	Rodriguez-Colinas *et al.* (2011)

Free enzymes	*Aspergillus lacticoffeatus*	300 g/L	5 mL	4.5	37	30 h	6.3 g/L	Cardoso *et al.* (2017)
	Lactobacillus delbrueckii	40%	/mL	7	40	–	40%	Gomaa (2018)
	L. reuteri						35%	
	Pediococcus acidilactici	30%	2.75 U	7	47.5	–	–	Chanalia *et al.* (2018)
	A. oryzae and *K. lactis*	200 g/L	50 UONPG/g lactose	6.5	45	3 h 20 min	33.1%	Fischer and Kleinschmidt (2018)
	A. oryzae + glucose oxidase + catalase	200 g/L	–	4.5	–	4 h	54.1 ± 1.9 g/L	Fischer and Kleinschmidt (2019)
	K. lactis (HA-Lactase 5200) + glucose oxidase	15 mL	1.7 U/mL		40–45	–	–	Rico-Rodríguez *et al.* (2020)
	L. leichmannii 313	600 mM	100 µL	–	37	4 h	–	Deng *et al.* (2020)
	A. oryzae	50%	20 U/g	4.5	50	25 min	25.1%	Wang *et al.* (2020)
	K. lactis (Lactozym 3000 L HP G)	400 g/L	1.5 U/mL	7.0	40	–	160 g/L	Rodriguez-Colinas *et al.* (2011)
	K. lactis (Maxilact LGX 5000)						154 g/L	
	A. oryzae	40%	0.05%	4.5	50	4 h	23%	Jenab *et al.* (2018)

(*Continued*)

Table 12.2 (Continued)

Types of biocatalyst	Source	Reaction parameters					Yield	Reference
		ILC	Enzyme concentration	pH	Temp. (°C)	Time		
Recombinant enzyme/cells	*A. oryzae*	60%	–	4.5	40	7 h	59.8 ± 0.3%	Gao *et al.* (2019)
	Marinomonas sp. BSi20414	480 mM	3.5 U	7.0	40	5 h	–	Ding *et al.* (2018)
	Bifidobacterium longum RD 47	36%	–	8.5	45	140 min	268.3 g/L	Oh *et al.* (2017)
	Yarrowia lipolytica CGMCC7326	500 g/L	5 mg/mL	5.5	60	6 h	160 g/L	An *et al.* (2016)
	Paenibacillus barengoltzii	350 g/L	5 U/mL	7.5	40	8 h	47.9%	Liu *et al.* (2017)
	Thermotoga naphthophila RKU-10	0.2 mM	4 mg/mL	7.0	75	24 h	207.63 mM	Yang *et al.* (2017)
	E. coli	40%	2 U	8.0	50	8 h	64.53 ± 2.85 g/L	Liu *et al.* (2019)
	Alteromonas sp. QD01	5 mg/mL	100 μL	8.0	40	360 min	–	Li *et al.* (2020)

Immobilized enzyme/cells	*A. aculeatus*	250 g/L	–	6.5	59	24 h	20.2%	González-Delgado *et al.* (2018)
	A. oryzae	40%	–	4.5	40		23.3%	Aburto *et al.* (2018)
	A. oryzae	300 g/L	0.499 g	5.0	35	45 min	24.4 kg/kg lactose	Adamíková *et al.* (2019)
	K. lactis					48 h		Gennari *et al.* (2019)
	A. aculeatus	–	–	4.5	60	–	–	Nguyen *et al.* (2019)
	Bacillus circulans	100 g/L		5.5	45	48 h	24.2 g/L	Rodriguez-Colinas *et al.* (2016)
	A. oryzae and *K. marxianus*	300 g/L	0.08 mg/mL	4.5	30	30 h	71.7 g/L	Tokošová *et al.* (2016)
	B. circulans	300 g/L	3 spheres/mL	3	30	8 h	30.79 g/L	Duarte *et al.* (2017)
	Bifidobacterium bifidum NCIMB 41171	43%	10U/g lactose	6.5	55	–	42–44%	Osman *et al.* (2014)
	A. oryzae	1.17 mol/L	–	3.5	30	7 days	31%	Sass and Jördening (2020)
	K. lactis and *A. oryzae*	165 mM	–	–	–	48 h	–	Todea *et al.* (2020)

12.4.3 Production of GOS using Free Enzyme

A wide array of enzymes obtained from a variety of microbial sources has been explored for the biotransformation of lactose to GOS, the commercially important sources being *B. circulans, K. fragilis, K. lactis, A. oryzae* and *A. niger*. Biotransformation of lactose was carried out at pH 4.5 using 400 g/L lactose (Carević *et al.* 2016). The duration of GOS synthesis represents the formation of trisaccharides, tetrasaccharides and overall GOS that is aligned in three steps. The first stage involves the production of trisaccharides, which is followed by the production of tetrasaccharide in the second stage. Although production of tetrasaccharide in the second stage becomes prominent, the concentration of trisaccharide still increases in this time period. The third stage of the reaction, where all the trisaccharides have been converted to tetrasaccharide, results in the overall GOS yield. The overall duration of the reaction was about 150 min, after which there was onset of the hydrolysis reaction and a depletion in the GOS concentration was observed. The effect of various process parameters such as lactose concentration, enzyme concentration, pH and temperature was investigated during the transgalactosylation reaction carried out by lactase from *A. oryzae* (Jenab *et al.* 2018) and indicated that the yield of GOS increased from 7 to 23% with an increase in the lactose concentration from 5 to 40%, trisaccharides being the major product accounting for almost 78% of the total GOS.

Several blends of commercial β-galactosidases such as Maxilact LGI 5000 Nola Fit 5500, Maxilact A4 MG and Saphera 2600 L were explored to achieve higher yields of GOS (Botvynko *et al.* 2019). The combination of Nola Fit 5500 and Maxilact LGI 5000 led to a yield of 105 g/L, while Maxilact LGI 5000 along with Maxilact A4 MG resulted in maximum GOS yield of 1411 g/L. Lactase from the novel bacterium *Paracoccus marcusii* was investigated for its transgalactosylation capability, resulting in a yield of 45 g/L GOS under optimal conditions at 50 °C for 24 h (Kalathinathan and Muthukaliannan 2020).

Apart from lactose, whey as a source of lactose has also been extensively studied to minimize the cost of production. The effect of the reactor configuration (batch and recycle membrane reactor) during the reaction revealed greater efficiency of the recycle membrane reactor, as yield was enhanced by 33% in contrast to the batch reactor using lactase from *B. circulans* and whey as a substrate (Das *et al.* 2011). Further, enzymes from *K. lactis* and *A. oryzae* have been investigated for their efficiency in the biotransformation reaction using both sweet as well as acid whey as substrate. The study demonstrated that both the enzymes were highly efficient and led to yields of about 10.56 ± 0.59% and 11.32 ± 0.59%, respectively, from acid whey (Fischer and Kleinschmidt 2015).

Although various reports are available on the utilization of enzymes from varied sources for GOS production, further optimization of the reaction conditions by using statistical methods and immobilization of the enzymes can improve the efficiency of enzymes during reaction.

12.4.4 Production of GOS using Immobilized Enzyme

Production of GOS using an immobilized enzyme is preferred in respect of enzyme stability, reusability and process economy. In addition to this, continuous production and ease of enzyme separation are the other factors that add to the advantages of the immobilized enzyme (Panesar *et al.* 2010).

β-Galactosidase from *B. circulans,* immobilized to aldehyde-activated agarose beads, indicated tremendous stability after 14 cycles at 45 °C during the biotransformation reaction in a packed bed reactor (Rodriguez-Colinas *et al.* 2016). A concentration of about 24.2 g/L was obtained after 48 h using 100 g/L lactose with 48.6% lactose conversion. Similarly, continuous flow packed bed reactors have been used for the enzymatic conversion of whey permeate to GOS (Eskandarloo and Abbaspourrad 2018). It had been demonstrated that yield increased with reduction in the flow rate of the substrate. This may be due to the prolonged reaction time and deliberate reaction between the substrate and the enzyme (Ansari and Husain 2010).

Besides the traditional matrices and methods, other novel matrices such as electrospun nanofibers have also been investigated for the immobilization of lactase and further used for the production of GOS. Chemically modified electrospun polystyrene nanofibers have been used as potential carriers for the immobilization of lactase and subsequently used for GOS production in an in-house fabricated recirculating column reactor system (Misson *et al.* 2020). Approximately, 145 g/L yield of GOS was obtained at the feed rate of 6 mL/min. Nanofibers are made using an electrospinning device and their size varies from nanometers to few micrometers. They are considered a promising enzyme carrier due to their outstanding characteristics in terms of high porosity and interconnectivity that diminishes the resistance of mass transfer. In addition, the high surface area to mass ratio allows greater enzyme-loading capacity, which provides vast opportunities for nanofiber application in the bioreactor.

12.4.5 Improvement in GOS Production

Over the past decade, β-galactosidase has gained immense attention for the biotransformation of GOS. Nevertheless, low productivity is one of the major issues in the recent era. The principal method to solve this issue is to mine for new β-galactosidase varieties or to modify enzyme genes, either by genetic or protein engineering, to obtain a high-quality β-galactosidase with good tolerance and thermostable features that can further help to achieve higher GOS yields. Thermostability is an important requirement for the industrial application of enzymes owing to the numerous benefits such as reduction in the risk of contamination, enhanced reaction velocity, prolonged half-lives, decreased product inhibition and improvement in the substrate solubility (Ding *et al.* 2018; Park and Oh 2010;). Thus, recombinant thermostable β-galactosidase has become the recent area of research for the production of GOS.

Lactase from *Marinomonas* sp. BSi 20414 overexpressed in *E. coli* revealed maximum yield having β-(1-3) linkages that exhibited good bifidogenic factor in contrast to β-(1-6) and β-(1-4) linkage (Ding *et al.* 2018). Similarly, the lactase-encoding gene galA, isolated from *Alteromonas* sp. ANT48 and expressed in *E. coli*, was reported by Li *et al.* (2019) for the production of GOS. This enzyme depicted maximum stability and resulted in maximum GOS yield of 30.9%, where about 90.6% of lactose was hydrolyzed within 15 min at 40 °C. Two single mutants (N140C and W806F) and one double mutant (N140C/W806F) from *A. oryzae* were developed and the yields were compared (Gao *et al.* 2019). The highest yield (59.8%) was obtained from the N140C/W806F mutant followed by N140C (50.7%) and W806F (49.6), whereas a yield of about 35.7% was obtained from wild strain. The mechanism behind the enhanced biocatalytic activity of the N140C mutant may be due to the destruction of the galactose bond, which further might have affected the preference for sugar as the terminal acceptor rather than water. Similarly, the higher transgalactosylation activity of W806F might perhaps be due to the increase in the hydrophobic nature at the active site. Further, the activity of N140C/W806F could be the result of the mutual impact of two individual mutants, thus leading to the higher yields.

Another approach, surface display technology, was proposed by An *et al.* (2016), in which the enzyme was attached on the surface of the *Yarrowia lipolytica* strain. Using this technique, maximum yield of 160 g/L GOS was reported within 6 h from 500 g/L lactose at pH 5.5 and 60 °C. The mechanism underlying this technique may be the N-glycosylation of the enzyme displayed on the surface of the strain that led to higher concentrations of the product even at higher temperature, thus proving to be an efficient strategy to improve the productivity of GOS.

Protein engineering has also proved to be a robust method to refine the transgalactosylation ability of β-galactosidase. In general, three strategies are used, either alone or in combination: error-prone polymerase chain reaction (ep PCR) based "directed evolution" (Arab-Jaziri *et al.* 2013); multiple sequence alignment as well as conserved residue analysis based "property grafting" (Gao *et al.* 2019); and "rational design" (Durand *et al.* 2016). Thermostability of the enzyme from *K. lactis* was improved through the rational method by insertion of disulfide units between the enzyme subunits (Rico-Díaz *et al.* 2017). Similarly, using this technique, two mutants (R116C/T270C and R116C/T270C/G818C) were developed that showed better catalytic as well as thermal stability in contrast to the native one. Further, R116C/T270C/G818C had better transgalactosylation activity than the other and thus resulted in maximum yield within 2 h at lower enzyme concentration. Another strategy, known as double hydrophobic amino acid scanning, was proposed that resulted in the development of two mutants C510V and H512I, which were further evaluated for their transgalactosylation activity (Qin *et al.* 2019). When compared, both mutants resulted in higher yields in a shorter reaction time (59.1% at 10 h for C510V and 51.5% at 2 h for H512I), whereas a yield of 45.3% was achieved from native enzyme after 16 h.

Although every strategy has successful applications, certain limitations also exist. Since there is no thorough screening method, identification of the clones through a random mutagenesis library is extremely tiresome and time-consuming (Bissaro *et al.* 2015). In the case of the property grafting technique, at least one homolog possessing elevated catalytic property is a prerequisite (Zeuner *et al.* 2019). On the other hand, in the case of other techniques, the residues may be similar to those of the homolog, thereby making the process useless. In the case of rational design, the major drawback lies in the acquisition of the crystal structures leading to inadequate success rates. Thus, new strategies need to be developed to attain higher productivity.

12.5 Global Status of GOS

Among all the prebiotics, GOS has the largest market share after fructooligosaccharides. Rising demand for prebiotic dietary supplements, potential health applications and nutritional needs of the elderly are some of the prime factors for the sudden rise in the GOS market. Another significant factor contributing to GOS market size is the rise in chronic diseases in both developed and developing countries, which has urged several industries to invest in research and technological innovations for the development of GOS having both nutritional and functional properties. Furthermore, demand for GOS in infant formulas globally has also boosted the worldwide market for GOS (Panesar *et al.* 2018). Another factor aiding the world market is the rise in the demand for novel functional foods by addition of GOS into diverse products such as bread, yoghurt and butter as well as other food products. According to statistical data, the worldwide GOS market is anticipated to rise to USD 1622.28 million by 2026 from USD 768.38 million in 2018 at a compound annual growth rate (CAGR) of 9.79% (https://www.qyresearch.com). GOS are manufactured in the form of syrup and powders; the syrup division led the global market with a growth of 52.38% in 2018 and is foreseen to enhance around 59% by 2028.

In a geographical context, the global lead players are North America and Europe followed by Africa, the Middle East, South America, Asia Pacific and others (Figure 12.6). Of these, in 2018, Europe contributed the largest market share of about USD 387.80 million (https://www.globenewswire.com), followed by Asia Pacific, which is expected to witness rapid growth in the market at a CAGR of 11.4% from 2019 to 2025 (https://www.businesswire.com).

The key market players are Clasado Biosciences, Friesland Campina, Yakult Honsha Co., Nissin Sugar Co., Ingredion, Snow Brand Milk Products, Lactose (India) Limited, Kowa Europe GmbH, Samyang and many others (Table 12.3). Production of GOS is mainly carried out either in the powder or in the syrup form and several manufacturers have employed novel strategies for the development of GOS-incorporated functional foods with the aim not only of meeting the demands of the population, but also exerting various health beneficial properties (https://www.businesswire.com; www.grandviewresearch.com). For example, King-Prebiotics GOS-570-S, GOS content of 57% in liquid form is widely used in the food and beverage sector in formulated milk products, liquid milk, dietary supplements and beverages (https://www.adroitmarketresearch.com).

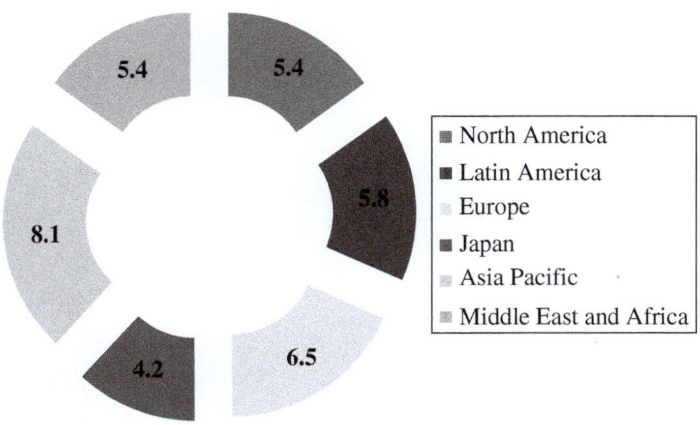

Figure 12.6 Galactooligosaccharide market worldwide on the basis of CAGR (%). *Source:* Data from Galacto Oligosaccharides Market Forecast, Trend Analysis & Competition Tracking - Global Market insights 2018 to 2028, Sep-2018. https://www.factmr.com/report/1707/galacto-oligosaccharides-market

Table 12.3 Commercially available galactooligosaccharides.

Serial number	Brand name	Type	Manufacturer
1	Oligomate 55 N	Syrup	Yakult Honsha Co. Ltd., Japan
2	Oligomate 55 P	Powder	
3	Cup-Oligo H70	Liquid	Nissin Sugar Co. Ltd., Japan
4	Cup-Oligo P	Powder	
5	Vivinal GOS	Syrup	Friesland Campina Domo, Netherlands
6	Vivinal GOS Easy drying syrup	Syrup	
7	Vivinal GOS	Powder	
8	Vivinal GOS Powder WPC	Powder	
9	Vivinal GOS Powder Maltodextrin	Powder	
10	Bimuno	Powder	Clasado Biosciences Ltd, UK
11	Bimuno	Syrup	
12	Promovita	–	Dairy Crest limited, UK
13	BIOLIGO GL 5700 IMF	Syrup	Ingredion Inc., Korea
14	Euoligo	–	Quantum Hi-Tech Biological Co. Ltd., China
15	GOS-270-P	–	New Francisco Biotechnology Corporation, China
16	GOS-700-P	Powder	
17	GOS-800-P		
18	GOS-900-P		
19	GOS-1000-P		
20	GOS-570-S	Syrup	
21	Profile GOS	–	Kerry Group, Ireland
22	GOS	Powder and syrup	Baoling Bao Biology, China
23	Galactomune	Powder	Klaire Labs, USA
24	Purimune	–	Corn Products International Inc., USA
25	GOS	–	Lactose India Ltd., India

12.6 Applications of GOS as Prebiotics

GOS are considered as one of the most important prebiotics owing to their enormous nutritional as well as health benefits. In general, two mechanisms have been proposed by which GOS impart health benefits on the host. First is the fermentation of GOS in the colon by health-beneficial microbes, such as lactic acid bacteria and bifidobacteria, which inhibit the growth of the pathogenic microflora in the gut, thereby reducing various infections.

The second involves the production of short chain fatty acids (SCFAs), which is the result of fermentation of GOS and bacterial metabolism. SCFAs exhibit several favorable activities such as reduction in risk of cancer, enhancement of the immune system, increase in mineral absorption and many more (Sangwan *et al.* 2011).

GOS act in the host in an indirect way, as there is proliferation of a selected group of microbes, which brings alterations in the gut microbiome. Moreover, new interactions are established both within the microflora and between the different groups or species of prokaryotic microorganisms. Besides this, interactions are also present between the prokaryotes and the eukaryotes of the colonic wall, such as epithelium. Due to the various interactions among the microbes, there are alterations in the colon and body functions, thereby reducing the risk of diseases (Gibson and Roberfroid 2008). Thus, the potential health benefits that are direct effects of GOS bring about the most substantial changes. The potential health benefits of GOS (Figure 12.7) are discussed in detail in the following sections.

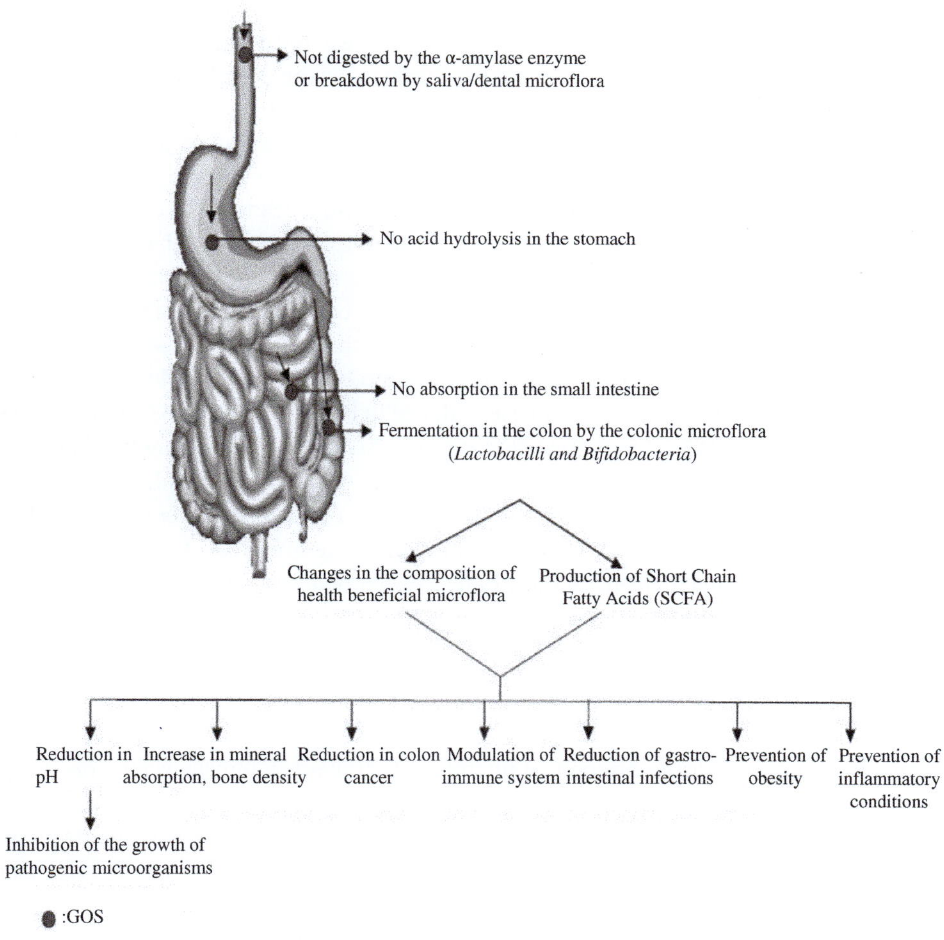

Figure 12.7 Health applications of galactooligosaccharides (GOS).

12.6.1 Stimulation of Health-promoting Bacteria

The intestinal microbial population has a positive impact on the host by preventing the adherence and invasion of pathogenic bacteria. Moreover, these organisms are also responsible for the modulation of the immune system (Berg 1996). The intestinal population varies not only between individuals, but also in the different sections of the gastrointestinal tract (Tannock 1995). Therefore, owing to the important role of the intestinal microflora in human health, several studies are being carried out to modify the composition and activity of these microorganisms. GOS have been widely recognized as a prebiotic ingredient that enhances the growth of colonic microflora as it gets fermented and produces SCFAs (Lamsal 2012).

The in vitro fermentation potential of Bimuno GOS (contains approximately 65% GOS) on the composition of colonic microflora and their metabolites was investigated through in situ hybridization and ^{1}H nuclear magnetic resonance (NMR) as well as gas chromatography analysis, respectively (Grimaldi *et al.* 2016). The results indicated that Bimuno GOS had significant prebiotic activity in terms of high numbers of bifidobacteria in the gut after 8 h of fermentation. Further, there was an increase in SCFAs, especially acetate, as compared to butyrate and propionate concentrations, which may be due to the decrease in the concentrations of mono- and disaccharides that could have influenced the overall experiments.

An investigation was conducted by Arnold and co-workers (2018) in order to evaluate the mechanism of GOS metabolism by *Lactobacillus rhamnosus* strains of intestinal origin (AMC143, AMC010) and one strain of dairy origin (Lc705). The observation of this study led to the hypothesis that variability in the gut microflora leads to fluctuation in the response and that the genotypic and phenotypic differences of the microbe influence the metabolism of GOS in gut. Although these strains had overall identity of more than 95%, their carbohydrate preferences varied. For instance, the Lc705 strain had a preference for lactose over trisaccharides and only metabolized trisaccharides in the absence of lactose despite the overexpression of *lac3* operon in this strain, which was vital in utilization of GOS by AMC143. Similarly, *lac2* operon was induced in both AMC010 and Lc705, but was not regulated in AMC143. This suggested that the Lc705 strain will only metabolize GOS when the lactose content in the medium is diminished. On the other hand, AMC010 was incapable of metabolizing GOS even in the absence of lactose. In contrast to this, AMC143 was able to break down GOS even in the presence of lactose. Despite this variation in carbohydrate metabolism, all the strains showed preference towards the trisaccharides rather than tetra- or longer oligosaccharides.

12.6.2 Modulation of Immune System

Mammalian intestine hosts a diversity of microflora that plays an indispensable role in the maintenance of intestinal morphology, digestion and absorption of nutrients, prevention of diseases and modulation of immunity (Hooper *et al.* 2012; Yu *et al.* 2018). The structure and function of the immune system develops immediately after birth, which is accompanied by colonization of the gut microflora (Schokker *et al.* 2014).

The change in the composition, metabolism and function of ileal microflora after the application of GOS in the neonatal piglet model revealed a subsequent increase in *Lactobacillus* and reduction in abundance of *E. coli* cells (Tian *et al.* 2019). This further led to enhancement in the concentration of SCFAs and lactate. In addition, the endocrine peptides (IGF-1, EGF, GLP-1 and GLP-2) that are responsible for the various functions, such as proliferation, differentiation and apoptosis, of the intestinal epithelial cells were also produced by the microflora. The main mechanism might be that the SCFAs produced after the fermentation of GOS might have activated the GPR41 and GPR43 that led to the synthesis of these peptides (Miyamoto *et al.* 2016; Nøhr *et al.* 2013). Further, intrusion of GOS boosted the mRNA expression of IL-10, and also led to the secretion of antimicrobial peptides PBD-1 and PBD-3.

In a similar study, intervention of GOS in newborn piglets revealed an increase in the concentrations of acetate, butyrate and other SCFAs in the gut on the eighth day that was further increased on day 21 (Wang *et al.* 2019). A higher SCFA concentration enhanced the concentration of the cytokine IL-10 and the barrier proteins Claudin-1 and ZO-1 by regulating the phosphorylation of NF-κB and activating the AMP-activated protein kinase (AMPK) signaling pathway. Previous studies indicate that SCFAs enter the cell through diffusion and active transport (Hung and Suzuki 2018). This leads to the suppression of NF-κB activity by inhibiting IκB degradation (Meijer *et al.* 2010)

12.6.3 Enhancement of Mineral Absorption

In the past few years, micronutrient deficiencies are of growing concern not only in developing but also in developed countries. Deficiency of these nutrients causes adverse health effects such as osteoporosis or other problems like reduced hemoglobin during pregnancy or anemia. To date, several strategies have been explored such as biofortification, supplementation and reduction of antinutritional components in foods, yet bioavailability of minerals has been the biggest issue. Various factors have been reported that affect the absorption of minerals in the body, some of which include their availability, intestinal ecosystem and expression of proteins that help in binding and absorption (Scholz-Ahrens *et al.* 2001). Numerous prebiotics, especially GOS, have been investigated to improve the conditions for absorption and enhance the bioavailability of these essential minerals in the body (Weaver *et al.* 2014).

Sprague Dawley rats fed with doses of GOS (5 g/100 g) significantly improved the absorption of calcium (34.55–39.33%), magnesium (51.22–58.05%) and iron (31.58–39.21%), whereas there was no impact on the absorption of zinc during 3–4 weeks (Maawia *et al.* 2016). Similarly, a FOS/GOS mixture was fed to osteopenic rats and the prebiotic potential was determined over a span for 45 days, which indicated that feeding the rats with this mixture subsequently increased the absorption of calcium, phosphorus (P) and magnesium (Seijo *et al.* 2018). Although phosphate ions are more rapidly circulated than calcium ions, the absorption of phosphorus increased with the increase in consumption of the prebiotic mixture, and a similar phenomenon was observed for calcium absorption, indicating the similarity between the metabolism of calcium and phosphorus. Several studies indicate that SCFAs produced during fermentation, especially butyrate, act as a source of energy that controls the growth and differentiation of the cells (Scholz-Ahrens *et al.* 2001). Moreover, they lower the pH, which helps in the ionization of minerals and increase in gut epithelial cells. This further enhances the surface area and facilitates the absorption of minerals that is necessary for bone health (Scholz-Ahrens and Schrezenmeir 2007).

Daily consumption of GOS for about 3–4 weeks in order to enhance iron absorption in Kenyan infants (Paganini *et al.* 2017) and iron-depleted young women (Jeroense *et al.* 2019) was investigated, which indicated an increase in iron absorption by 62% and 61%, respectively. Scientific methods have been reported to describe the correlation between GOS consumption and iron absorption. One possible reason is the fermentation of GOS by *lactobacilli* and *bifidobacteria* to SCFAs that lead to reduction in the colonic pH, which boosts the breakdown of iron and availability for uptake by the divalent metal transporter 1 (Bertelsen *et al.* 2016). Other possibilities may be due to an increase in the expression of genes (Marciano *et al.* 2015), changes in the colonic mucosal structure (Lobo *et al.* 2014; Yasuda *et al.* 2009) and reduced circulating hepcidin (Marciano *et al.* 2015).

12.6.4 Reduction in the Risk of Colon Cancer

Colorectal cancer (CRC) is one of the foremost causes of death in humans, irrespective of gender, worldwide (Siegel *et al.* 2011). Various factors are responsible, the most significant being family history, age, presence of pre-carcinogens (Watson and Collins 2011), inflammatory bowel diseases, low intake of fruits and vegetables, higher consumption of processed as well as red meat (Bastide *et al.* 2011; Khan *et al.* 2010) and hereditary genetic factors (Van Engeland *et al.* 2011). Cancer development is the result of a variety of pathological changes, which may range from aberrant crypt foci (ACF) to malignant tumors. ACF can be induced chemically or with 1,2-dimethylhydrazine dihydrochloride (DMH) or azoxymethane (AOM; Gupta and Schoen 2009). In the last decade, several studies have been conducted and research is still being carried out to evaluate the role of prebiotics in the preclusion of cancer (Tanaka 2009).

Studies to evaluate the protective role of GOS alone (Qamar *et al.* 2017) or in the combination of GOS and inulin (Qamar *et al.* 2016) against the various biomarkers of colon cancer including enzymes, SCFAs and ACF in a rodent model induced with DMH have been carried out. The results indicated that the combination of GOS and inulin inhibited the production of ACF and also provided resistance against DMH-induced body weight loss, besides enhancing the levels of cecal and fecal SCFAs (Qamar *et al.* 2016). Further, the prebiotic mixture reduced the levels of enzymes (β-glucuronidase, β-glucosidase, azoreductase and nitroreductase) significantly; these enzymes play the most important role in the onset of cancer. The reduction in ACF may be due to the changes in the gut microflora and increased concentrations of SCFA (Aachary *et al.* 2015). Among all the SCFAs, butyrate is one of the major factors in preventing colon cancer owing to its multiple roles, such as absorption of minerals, cell growth and differentiation, intestinal barrier function (Daly *et al.* 2005) and immunomodulatory properties (Vinolo *et al.* 2011). Moreover, higher concentrations of butyrate have also been reported to diminish ammonia-mediated toxicity in the colon (De Preter *et al.* 2007; Geboes *et al.* 2006).

Similarly, the antitumor effect of GOS-Lu (GOS derived from lactulose) was studied in an animal model that indicated that colon tumors (induced by dextran sulfate sodium [DSS]/AOM) were reduced to about 57.5%, which may be attributed to the higher levels of SCFAs, especially propionate, in the gut (Fernández *et al.* 2018).

12.6.5 Inflammatory Bowel Disease

Inflammatory bowel disease (IBD) or acute gastroenteritis (GIT) is caused by alterations in the colonic microflora that can also result in the development of ulcerative colitis (UC) and Crohn's disease (CD) (Cummings *et al.* 2003; Cummings and Jewell 2005). The exact reasons for the occurrence of IBD or UC are unknown, but some suggest that it may be due to genetic susceptibility, intestinal microflora or immune factors (Manichanh *et al.* 2012).

in vitro experiments on human colon epithelial cells (FHC) revealed that GOS prevented the release of pro-inflammatory cytokines, including IL-1β, IFN-γ and TNF-α (Sun *et al.* 2019). Further, in vivo and in vitro studies demonstrated that GOS have an anticolitis effect that is achieved by up-regulating miR-19b. Another study also indicated that miR-19b may attack TNF-α and curb the development of UC (Zhou *et al.* 2013). Further, animal experiments have reported that GOS could significantly reduce DSS-induced colonic inflammation and also attenuate the secretion of IL-33, IL-13, IL-6, and IL-8 as well as mRNA expression in the colon via the NF-κB signaling pathway that led to the suppression of colitis in the mice (Chu *et al.* 2020).

12.7 Conclusion and Future Prospects

The increase in scientific advances as well as awareness among the population about a healthy lifestyle has led to an upsurge in the demand for functional foods. Of these, prebiotics, especially galactooligosaccharides, is one such acclaimed candidate that has gained massive attention from researchers worldwide on account of the diverse functional and nutritional properties. Various methods and techniques have been investigated over the years for the production of GOS. Nevertheless, due to the techno-economic benefits, enzymatic production of GOS is preferred at the industrial scale over the chemical one. Although various enzymes have been tested for their transgalactosylation activity, β-galactosidase is the preferred enzyme. Diverse biotechnological strategies have been proposed for the biotransformation reaction using the versatile biocatalyst β-galactosidase. Despite this, there is a need for novel microbial sources capable of producing elevated levels of enzyme or enzyme that can survive harsh reaction conditions. To circumvent the latter problem, genetic modification of the microbe or protein engineering of the enzyme can be carried out to enhance its transgalactosylation activity. Although various techniques have been proposed, novel techniques still need to be developed to surmount the existing limitations. Besides this, the development of cost-effective strategies not only for enzyme production but also for the production of GOS is the need of the hour; this can be achieved by using various agro-industrial wastes that can economize the whole process.

GOS are known to impart varied health beneficial activities in the host, and thus have significant applications in food as well as pharmaceutical sectors. Furthermore, considering their different physiological characteristics, GOS have a significant role in the development of functional foods. Even though various scientific evidence is available on the health beneficial properties of GOS, certain barriers remain regarding stability as well as bioavailability in the host and the mechanism. Thus, there is a need for an advanced study to understand the underlying mechanism behind the action of GOS through the development of various tools and techniques such as genomics, proteomics, ohmic strategies, in vitro studies and so on.

References

Aachary, A.A., Gobinath, D., Srinivasan, K. and Prapulla, S.G. (2015). Protective effect of xylooligosaccharides from corncob on 1, 2-dimethylhydrazine induced colon cancer in rats. *Bioactive Carbohydrates and Dietary Fibre*, 5(2): 146–152.

Aburto, C., Guerrero, C., Vera, C., Wilson, L. and Illanes, A. (2018). Co-immobilized β-galactosidase and *Saccharomyces cerevisiae* cells for the simultaneous synthesis and purification of galacto-oligosaccharides. *Enzyme and Microbial Technology*, 118: 102–108.

Adamczak, M., Charubin, D. and Bednarski, W. (2009). Influence of reaction medium composition on enzymatic synthesis of galactooligosaccharides and lactulose from lactose concentrates prepared from whey permeate. *Chemical Papers*, 63(2): 111–116.

Adamíková, J., Antošová, M. and Polakovič, M. (2019). A Method of early phase selection of carrier for *Aspergillus oryzae* β-galactosidase immobilization for galactooligosaccharides production. *Biotechnology Journal*, 14(3): 1800120.

Albayrak, N. and Yang, S.T. (2002). Production of galacto-oligosaccharides from lactose by *Aspergillus oryzae* β-galactosidase immobilized on cotton cloth. *Biotechnology and Bioengineering*, 77(1): 8–19.

An, J., Zhang, L., Li, L., Liu, D., Cheng, H., Wang, H., Nawaz, M.Z., Cheng, H. and Deng, Z. (2016). An alternative approach to synthesizing galactooligosaccharides by cell-surface display of β-galactosidase on *Yarrowia lipolytica*. *Journal of Agricultural and Food Chemistry*, 64(19): 3819–3827.

Angus, F., Smart, S., and Shortt. C. (2005). Prebiotic ingredients with emphasis on galacto-oligosaccharides and fructooligosaccharides. In: *Probiotic Dairy Products* (ed. A.Y. Tamime). Oxford: Blackwell Publishing Ltd.

Ansari, S.A. and Husain, Q. (2010). Lactose hydrolysis by β galactosidase immobilized on concanavalin A-cellulose in batch and continuous mode. *Journal of Molecular Catalysis B: Enzymatic*, 63(1-2): 68–74.

Aqib, S., Akram, A., Halim, S.A. and Tassaduq R. (2017). Sources of β-galactosidase and its applications in food industry. *3 Biotech*, 7(1):79.

Arab-Jaziri, F., Bissaro, B., Dion, M., Saurel, O., Harrison, D., Ferreira, F., Milon, A., Tellier, C., Fauré, R. and O'Donohue, M.J. (2013). Engineering transglycosidase activity into a GH51 α-l-arabinofuranosidase. *New Biotechnology*, 30(5): 536–544.

Arnold, J.W., Simpson, J.B., Roach, J., Bruno-Barcena, J.M. and Azcarate-Peril, M.A. (2018). Prebiotics for lactose intolerance: Variability in galacto-oligosaccharide utilization by intestinal *Lactobacillus rhamnosus*. *Nutrients*, 10(10): 1517, doi:10.3390/nu10101517.

Bastide, N.M., Pierre, F.H. and Corpet, D.E. (2011). Heme iron from meat and risk of colorectal cancer: a meta-analysis and a review of the mechanisms involved. *Cancer Prevention Research*, 4(2): 177–184.

Bednarski, W. and Kulikowska, A. (2007). Influence of two-phase system composition on biocatalytic properties of β-galactosidase preparations. *Chemical Papers*, 61(5): 364–369.

Berg, R.D. (1996). The indigenous gastrointestinal microflora. *Trends in Microbiology*, 4(11): 430–435.

Bertelsen, R.J., Jensen, E.T. and Ringel-Kulka, T. (2016). Use of probiotics and prebiotics in infant feeding. *Best Practice and Research Clinical Gastroenterology*, 30(1): 39–48.

Bissaro, B., Durand, J., Biarnés, X., Planas, A., Monsan, P., O'Donohue, M.J. and Fauré, R. (2015). Molecular design of non-Leloir furanose-transferring enzymes from an α-L-arabinofuranosidase: a rationale for the engineering of evolved transglycosylases. *ACS Catalysis*, 5(8): 4598–4611.

Bode, L. (2009). Human milk oligosaccharides: prebiotics and beyond. *Nutrition Reviews*, 67(suppl_2): S183–S191.

Boon, M.A., Janssen, A.E.M. and Van't Riet, K. (2000). Effect of temperature and enzyme origin on the enzymatic synthesis of oligosaccharides. *Enzyme and Microbial Technology*, 26(2-4): 271–281.

Botvynko, A., Bednářová, A., Henke, S., Shakhno, N. and Čurda, L. (2019). Production of galactooligosaccharides using various combinations of the commercial β-galactosidases. *Biochemical and Biophysical Research Communications*, 517(4): 762–766.

Cardoso, B.B., Silvério, S.C., Abrunhosa, L., Teixeira, J.A. and Rodrigues, L.R. (2017). β-galactosidase from *Aspergillus lacticoffeatus*: A promising biocatalyst for the synthesis of novel prebiotics. *International Journal of Food Microbiology*, 257: 67–74.

Carević, M., Bezbradica, D., Banjanac, K., Milivojevic, A., Fanuel, M., Rogniaux, H., Ropartz, D. and Velickovic, D. (2016). Structural elucidation of enzymatically synthesized galacto-oligosaccharides using ion-mobility spectrometry–tandem mass spectrometry. *Journal of Agricultural and Food Chemistry*, 64(18): 3609–3615.

Chanalia, P., Gandhi, D., Attri, P. and Dhanda, S. (2018). Purification and characterization of β-galactosidase from probiotic *Pediococcus acidilactici* and its use in milk lactose hydrolysis and galactooligosaccharide synthesis. *Bioorganic Chemistry*, 77: 176–189.

Chen, S.X., Wei, D.Z. and Hu, Z.H. (2001). Synthesis of galacto-oligosaccharides in AOT/isooctane reverse micelles by β-galactosidase. *Journal of Molecular Catalysis B: Enzymatic*, 16(2): 109–114.

Chen, W., Chen, H., Xia, Y., Zhao, J., Tian, F. and Zhang, H. (2008). Production, purification, and characterization of a potential thermostable galactosidase for milk lactose hydrolysis from *Bacillus stearothermophilus*. *Journal of Dairy Science*, 91(5): 1751–1758.

Cheng, C.C., Yu, M.C., Cheng, T.C., Sheu, D.C., Duan, K.J. and Tai, W.L. (2006). Production of high-content galacto-oligosaccharide by enzyme catalysis and fermentation with *Kluyveromyces marxianus*. *Biotechnology Letters*, 28(11): 793–797.

Chu, H., Tao, X., Sun, Z., Hao, W. and Wei, X. (2020). Galactooligosaccharides protects against DSS-induced murine colitis through regulating intestinal flora and inhibiting NF-κB pathway. *Life Sciences*, 242: 17220, https://doi.org/10.1016/j.lfs.2019.117220

Corral, J.M., Bañuelos, O., Adrio, J.L. and Velasco, J. (2006). Cloning and characterization of a β-galactosidase encoding region in *Lactobacillus coryniformis* CECT 5711. *Applied Microbiology and Biotechnology*, 73(3): 640–646.

Coutinho, P.M., Deleury, E., Davies, G.J. and Henrissat, B. (2003). An evolving hierarchical family classification for glycosyltransferases. *Journal of Molecular Biology*, 328(2): 307–317.

Cummings, F.J. and Jewell, D.P. (2005). Clinical implications of inflammatory bowel disease genetics on phenotype. *Inflammatory Bowel Diseases*, 11(1): 56–61.

Cummings, J.H., Macfarlane, G.T. and Macfarlane, S. (2003). Intestinal bacteria and ulcerative colitis. *Current Issues in Intestinal Microbiology*, 4(1): 9–20.

Czermak, P., Ebrahimi, M., Grau, K., Netz, S., Sawatzki, G. and Pfromm, P.H. (2004). Membrane-assisted enzymatic production of galactosyl-oligosaccharides from lactose in a continuous process. *Journal of Membrane Science*, 232(1-2): 85–91.

Daly, K., Cuff, M.A., Fung, F. and Shirazi-Beechey, S.P. (2005). The importance of colonic butyrate transport to the regulation of genes associated with colonic tissue homoeostasis. *Biochemical Society Transactions*, 33: 733–735.

Das, R., Sen, D., Sarkar, A., Bhattacharyya, S. and Bhattacharjee, C. (2011). A comparative study on the production of galacto-oligosaccharide from whey permeate in recycle membrane reactor and in enzymatic batch reactor. *Industrial and Engineering Chemistry Research*, 50(2): 806–816.

Davis, L.M.G., Martinez, I., Walter, J. and Hutkins, R. (2010). A dose dependent impact of prebiotic galactooligosaccharides on the intestinal microbiota of healthy adults. *International Journal of Food Microbiology*, 144(2): 285–292.

De Preter, V., Vanhoutte, T., Huys, G., Swings, J., De Vuyst, L., Rutgeerts, P. and Verbeke, K. (2007). Effects of Lactobacillus casei Shirota, Bifidobacterium breve, and oligofructose-enriched inulin on colonic nitrogen-protein metabolism in healthy humans. *American Journal of Physiology-Gastrointestinal and Liver Physiology*, 292(1): G358–G368.

Deng, Y., Xu, M., Ji, D. and Agyei, D. (2020). Optimization of β-galactosidase Production by Batch Cultures of *Lactobacillus leichmannii* 313 (ATCC 7830™). *Fermentation*, 6(1): 27, doi:10.3390/fermentation6010027.

Ding, H., Zhou, L., Zeng, Q., Yu, Y. and Chen, B. (2018). Heterologous expression of a thermostable β-1, 3-galactosidase and its potential in synthesis of galactooligosaccharides. *Marine Drugs*, 16(11): 415.

Dong, Y., Sun, Y., Chen, Y. and Wu, W. (2015). Determination of lactose solubility in organic-aqueous biphasic system. *Journal of Chinese Institute of Food Science and Technology*, 15: 262–267.

Duarte, L.S., da Natividade Schöffer, J., Lorenzoni, A.S.G., Rodrigues, R.C., Rodrigues, E. and Hertz, P.F. (2017). A new bioprocess for the production of prebiotic lactosucrose by an immobilized β-galactosidase. *Process Biochemistry*, 55: 96–103.

Durand, J., Biarnés, X., Watterlot, L., Bonzom, C., Borsenberger, V., Planas, A., Bozonnet, S., O'Donohue, M.J. and Fauré, R. (2016). A single point mutation alters the transglycosylation/hydrolysis partition, significantly enhancing the synthetic capability of an endo-glycoceramidase. *ACS Catalysis*, 6(12): 8264–8275.

El-Gindy, A. (2003). Production, partial purification and some properties of β-galactosidase from *Aspergillus carbonarius*. *Folia Microbiologica*, 48(5): 581.

Eskandarloo, H. and Abbaspourrad, A. (2018). Production of galacto-oligosaccharides from whey permeate using β-galactosidase immobilized on functionalized glass beads. *Food Chemistry*, 251: 115–124.

Faijes, M. and Planas, A. (2007). in vitro synthesis of artificial polysaccharides by glycosidases and glycosynthases. *Carbohydrate Research*, 342(12-13): 1581–1594.

Fara, A., Sabater, C., Palacios, J., Requena, T., Montilla, A. and Zárate, G. (2020). Prebiotic galactooligosaccharides production from lactose and lactulose by *Lactobacillus delbrueckii* subsp. *bulgaricus* CRL450. *Food and Function*, 11(7): 5875–5886.

Fernández, J., Moreno, F.J., Olano, A., Clemente, A., Villar, C.J. and Lombó, F. (2018). A galacto-oligosaccharides preparation derived from lactulose protects against colorectal cancer development in an animal model. *Frontiers in Microbiology*, 9: 2004, doi: 10.3389/fmicb.2018.02004

Fischer, C. and Kleinschmidt, T. (2015). Synthesis of galactooligosaccharides using sweet and acid whey as a substrate. *International Dairy Journal*, 48: 15–22.

Fischer, C. and Kleinschmidt, T. (2018). Combination of two β-galactosidases during the synthesis of galactooligosaccharides may enhance yield and structural diversity. *Biochemical and Biophysical Research Communications*, 506(1): 211–215.

Fischer, C. and Kleinschmidt, T. (2019). Effect of glucose depletion during the synthesis of galactooligosaccharides using a trienzymatic system. *Enzyme and Microbial Technology*, 121: 45–50.

Gao, X., Wu, J. and Wu, D. (2019). Rational design of the beta-galactosidase from *Aspergillus oryzae* to improve galactooligosaccharide production. *Food chemistry*, 286: 362–367.

Garegg, P.J. (2004). Synthesis and reactions of glycosides. *Advances in Carbohydrate Chemistry and Biochemistry*, 59: 69–134.

Geboes, K.P., De Hertogh, G., De Preter, V., Luypaerts, A., Bammens, B., Evenepoel, P., Ghoos, Y., Geboes, K., Rutgeerts, P. and Verbeke, K. (2006). The influence of inulin on the absorption of nitrogen and the production of metabolites of protein fermentation in the colon. *British Journal of Nutrition*, 96(6): 1078–1086.

Gennari, A., Mobayed, F.H., Catto, A.L., Benvenutti, E.V., Volpato, G. and de Souza, C.F.V. (2019). *Kluyveromyces lactis* β-galactosidase immobilized on collagen: catalytic stability on batch and packed-bed reactor hydrolysis. *Reaction Kinetics, Mechanisms and Catalysis*, 127(2): 583–599.

Gibson, G.R. and Roberfroid, M. (2008). *Handbook of Prebiotics*. Boca Raton, FL: CRC Press.

Gibson, G.R. and Roberfroid, M.B. (1995). Dietary modulation of the human colonic microbiota: introducing the concept of prebiotics. *The Journal of Nutrition*, 125(6): 1401–1412.

Gibson, G.R., Hutkins, R., Sanders, M.E., Prescott, S.L., Reimer, R.A., Salminen, S.J., Scott, K., Stanton, C., Swanson, K.S., Cani, P.D. and Verbeke, K. (2017). Expert consensus document: The International Scientific Association for Probiotics and Prebiotics (ISAPP) consensus statement on the definition and scope of prebiotics. *Nature Reviews Gastroenterology and Hepatology*, 14(8): 491–502.

Gomaa, E.Z. (2018). β-galactosidase from *Lactobacillus delbrueckii* and *Lactobacillus reuteri*: Optimization, characterization and formation of galactooligosaccharides. *Indian Journal of Biotechnology*, 17(3): 407–415.

González-Delgado, I., Segura, Y., Martín, A., López-Muñoz, M.J. and Morales, G. (2018). β-galactosidase covalent immobilization over large-pore mesoporous silica supports for the production of high galacto-oligosaccharides (GOS). *Microporous and Mesoporous Materials*, 257: 51–61.

Gosling, A., Stevens, G.W., Barber, A.R., Kentish, S.E. and Gras, S.L. (2010). Recent advances refining galactooligosaccharide production from lactose. *Food Chemistry*, 121(2): 307–318.

Grajek, W., Olejnik, A. and Sip, A. (2005). Probiotics, prebiotics and antioxidants as functional foods. *Acta Biochimica Polonica*, 52(3): 665–671.

Grimaldi, R., Swann, J.R., Vulevic, J., Gibson, G.R. and Costabile, A. (2016). Fermentation properties and potential prebiotic activity of Bimuno® galacto-oligosaccharide (65% galacto-oligosaccharide content) on in vitro gut microbiota parameters. *British Journal of Nutrition*, 116(3): 480–486.

Gupta, A.K. and Schoen, R.E. (2009). Aberrant crypt foci: are they intermediate endpoints of colon carcinogenesis in humans? *Current Opinion in Gastroenterology*, 25(1): 59–65.

Haider, T. and Husain, Q. (2007). Calcium alginate entrapped preparations of *Aspergillus oryzae* β galactosidase: its stability and applications in the hydrolysis of lactose. *International Journal of Biological Macromolecules*, 41(1): 72–80.

Haki, G.D. and Rakshit, S.K. (2003). Developments in industrially important thermostable enzymes: A review. *Bioresource Technology*, 89(1): 17–34.

Hatzinikolaou, D.G., Katsifas, E., Mamma, D., Karagouni, A.D., Christakopoulos, P. and Kekos, D. (2005). Modeling of the simultaneous hydrolysis–ultrafiltration of whey permeate by a thermostable β-galactosidase from *Aspergillus niger*. *Biochemical Engineering Journal*, 24(2): 161–172.

Hooper, L.V., Littman, D.R. and Macpherson, A.J. (2012). Interactions between the microbiota and the immune system. *Science*, 336(6086): 1268–1273.

https://www.adroitmarketresearch.com/industry-reports/galacto-oligosaccharides-gos-market (accessed 23 July 2021).

https://www.businesswire.com/news/home/20190620005476/en/Global-Galacto-oligosaccharides-GOS-Market-Reach-1.58-Billion (accessed 23 July 2021).

https://www.factmr.com/report/1707/galacto-oligosaccharides-market (accessed 23 July 2021).

https://www.globenewswire.com/news-release/2019/07/08/1879622/0/en/Global-Galacto-Oligosaccharide-GOS-Market-is-Expected-to-Reach-USD-1-622-28-Million-by-2026-Fior-Markets.html (accessed 23 July 2021).

https://www.grandviewresearch.com/industry-analysis/prebiotics-market (accessed 23 July 2021).

https://www.qyresearch.com/index/detail/1087497/global-galactooligosaccharides-gos-market (accessed 23 July 2021).

Huang, J., Zhu, S., Zhao, L., Chen, L., Du, M., Zhang, C. and Yang, S.T. (2020). A novel β-galactosidase from *Klebsiella oxytoca* ZJUH1705 for efficient production of galacto-oligosaccharides from lactose. *Applied Microbiology and Biotechnology*, 104: 6161–6172.

Huber, R.E., Kurz, G. and Wallenfels, K. (1976). A quantitation of the factors which affect the hydrolase and transgalactosylase activities of β-galactosidase (*E. coli*) on lactose. *Biochemistry*, 15(9): 1994–2001.

Hung, T.V. and Suzuki, T. (2018). Short-chain fatty acids suppress inflammatory reactions in Caco-2 cells and mouse colons. *Journal of Agricultural and Food Chemistry*, 66(1): 108–117.

Husain, Q. (2010). β Galactosidases and their potential applications: a review. *Critical Reviews in Biotechnology*, 30(1): 41–62.

Jenab, E., Omidghane, M., Mussone, P., Armada, D.H., Cartmell, J. and Montemagno, C. (2018). Enzymatic conversion of lactose into galacto-oligosaccharides: The effect of process parameters, kinetics, foam architecture, and product characterization. *Journal of Food Engineering*, 222: 63–72.

Jeroense, F.M., Michel, L., Zeder, C., Herter-Aeberli, I. and Zimmermann, M.B. (2019). Consumption of galacto-oligosaccharides increases iron absorption from ferrous fumarate: a stable iron isotope study in iron-depleted young women. *The Journal of Nutrition*, 149(5): 738–746.

Juers, D.H., Jacobson, R.H., Wigley, D., Zhang, X.J., Huber, R.E., Tronrud, D.E. and Matthews, B.W. (2000). High resolution refinement of β-galactosidase in a new crystal form reveals multiple metal-binding sites and provides a structural basis for α-complementation. *Protein Science*, 9(9): 1685–1699.

Kalathinathan, P. and Muthukaliannan, G.K. (2020). A statistical approach for enhanced production of β-galactosidase from *Paracoccus* sp. and synthesis of galacto-oligosaccharides. *Folia Microbiologica*, 65(5): 811–822.

Kaur, R. and Panesar, P.S. (2020). Enzyme systems for high-value biomolecule production. In: *Biomass, Biofuels, Biochemicals* (eds S.P. Singh, A. Pandey, R.R. Singhania, C. Larroche and Z. Li). Elsevier.

Khan, N., Afaq, F. and Mukhtar, H. (2010). Lifestyle as risk factor for cancer: Evidence from human studies. *Cancer Letters*, 293(2): 133–143.

Kumari, S., Panesar, P.S., Bera, M.B. and Panesar, R. (2013). Permeabilization of a newly isolated *Kluyveromyces* sp. for the preparation of whole cell biocatalysts with β-galactosidase activity. *International Journal of Food Science and Nutrition*, 2(1): 22–26.

Lamsal, B.P. (2012). Production, health aspects and potential food uses of dairy prebiotic galactooligosaccharides. *Journal of the Science of Food and Agriculture*, 92(10): 2020–2028.

Li, D., Li, S., Wu, Y., Jin, M., Zhou, Y., Wang, Y., Chen, X. and Han, Y. (2020). Cloning and characterization of a new β-galactosidase from *Alteromonas* sp. QD01 and its potential in synthesis of galacto-oligosaccharides. *Marine Drugs*, 18(6): 312, doi:10.3390/md18060312.

Li, S., Zhu, X. and Xing, M. (2019). A new β-galactosidase from the antarctic bacterium *Alteromonas* sp. ANT48 and its potential in formation of prebiotic galacto-oligosaccharides. *Marine Drugs*, 17(11): 599, doi: 10.3390/md17110599.

Liu, P., Wang, W., Zhao, J. and Wei, D. (2019). Screening novel β-galactosidases from a sequence-based metagenome and characterization of an alkaline β-galactosidase for the enzymatic synthesis of galactooligosaccharides. *Protein Expression and Purification*, 155: 104–111.

Liu, Y., Chen, Z., Jiang, Z., Yan, Q. and Yang, S. (2017). Biochemical characterization of a novel β-galactosidase from *Paenibacillus barengoltzii* suitable for lactose hydrolysis and galactooligosaccharides synthesis. *International Journal of Biological Macromolecules*, 104: 1055–1063.

Lobo, A.R., Gaievski, E.H., De Carli, E., Alvares, E.P. and Colli, C. (2014). Fructo-oligosaccharides and iron bioavailability in anaemic rats: the effects on iron species distribution, ferroportin-1 expression, crypt bifurcation and crypt cell proliferation in the caecum. *British Journal of Nutrition*, 112(8): 1286–1295.

Maawia, K., Iqbal, S., Qamar, T.R. and Rafiq, P. (2016). Production of impure prebiotic galacto-oligosaccharides and their effect on calcium, magnesium, iron and zinc absorption in Sprague-Dawley rats. *PharmaNutrition*, 4(4): 154–160.

Manichanh, C., Borruel, N., Casellas, F. and Guarner, F. (2012). The gut microbiota in IBD. *Nature Reviews Gastroenterology and Hepatology*, 9(10): 599–608.

Mano, M.C.R., Paulino, B.N. and Pastore, G.M. (2019). Whey permeate as the raw material in galacto-oligosaccharide synthesis using commercial enzymes. *Food Research International*, 124: 78–85.

Manucci, F. (2009). Enzymatic synthesis of galactooligosaccharides from whey permeate. M.Phil Thesis, Dublin Institute of Technology.

Marciano, R., Santamarina, A.B., de Santana, A.A., Silva, M.D.L.C., Amancio, O.M.S., Oyama, L.M. and de Morais, M.B. (2015). Effects of prebiotic supplementation on the expression of proteins regulating iron absorption in anaemic growing rats. *British Journal of Nutrition*, 113(6): 901–908.

Meijer, K., de Vos, P. and Priebe, M.G. (2010). Butyrate and other short-chain fatty acids as modulators of immunity: what relevance for health? *Current Opinion in Clinical Nutrition and Metabolic Care*, 13(6): 715–721.

Misson, M., Jin, B., Dai, S. and Zhang, H. (2020). Interfacial biocatalytic performance of nanofiber-supported β-galactosidase for production of galacto-oligosaccharides. *Catalysts*, 10(1): 81.

Miyamoto, J., Hasegawa, S., Kasubuchi, M., Ichimura, A., Nakajima, A. and Kimura, I. (2016). Nutritional signaling via free fatty acid receptors. *International journal of molecular sciences*, 17(4): 450.

Nagy, Z., Kiss, T., Szentirmai, A. and Biró, S. (2001). β-Galactosidase of *Penicillium chrysogenum*: production, purification, and characterization of the enzyme. *Protein Expression and Purification*, 21(1): 24–29.

Nguyen, T.T., Nguyen, H.A., Arreola, S.L., Mlynek, G., Djinović-Carugo, K., Mathiesen, G., Nguyen, T.H. and Haltrich, D. (2012). Homodimeric β-galactosidase from *Lactobacillus delbrueckii* subsp. *bulgaricus* DSM 20081: expression in *Lactobacillus plantarum* and biochemical characterization. *Journal of Agricultural and Food Chemistry*, 60(7): 1713–1721.

Nguyen, V.D., Styevkó, G., Madaras, E., Haktanirlar, G., Tran, A.T., Bujna, E., Dam, M.S. and Nguyen, Q.D. (2019). Immobilization of β-galactosidase on chitosan-coated magnetic nanoparticles and its application for synthesis of lactulose-based galactooligosaccharides. *Process Biochemistry*, 84: 30–38.

Nicolaou, K.C. and Mitchell, H.J. (2001). Adventures in carbohydrate chemistry: new synthetic technologies, chemical synthesis, molecular design, and chemical biology. *Angewandte Chemie International Edition*, 40(9): 1576–1624.

Nøhr, M.K., Pedersen, M.H., Gille, A., Egerod, K.L., Engelstoft, M.S., Husted, A.S., Sichlau, R.M., Grunddal, K.V., Seier Poulsen, S., Han, S. and Jones, R.M. (2013). GPR41/FFAR3 and GPR43/FFAR2 as cosensors for short-chain fatty acids in enteroendocrine cells vs FFAR3 in enteric neurons and FFAR2 in enteric leukocytes. *Endocrinology*, 154(10): 3552–3564.

Oh, S.Y., Youn, S.Y., Park, M.S., Kim, H.G., Baek, N.I., Li, Z. and Ji, G.E. (2017). Synthesis of β-galactooligosaccharide using bifidobacterial β-galactosidase purified from recombinant *Escherichia coli*. *Journal of Microbiology and Biotechnology*, 27(8): 1392–1400.

Ohtsubo, K. and Marth, J.D. (2006). Glycosylation in cellular mechanisms of health and disease. *Cell*, 126(5): 855–867.

Osman, A., Symeou, S., Trisse, V., Watson, K.A., Tzortzis, G. and Charalampopoulos, D. (2014). Synthesis of prebiotic galactooligosaccharides from lactose using bifidobacterial β-galactosidase (BbgIV) immobilised on DEAE-Cellulose, Q-Sepharose and amino-ethyl agarose. *Biochemical Engineering Journal*, 82: 188–199.

Otieno, D.O. (2010). Synthesis of β-galactooligosaccharides from lactose using microbial β-galactosidases. *Comprehensive Reviews in Food Science and Food Safety*, 9(5): 471–482.

Paganini, D., Uyoga, M.A., Cercamondi, C.I., Moretti, D., Mwasi, E., Schwab, C., Bechtler, S., Mutuku, F.M., Galetti, V., Lacroix, C. and Karanja, S. (2017). Consumption of galacto-oligosaccharides increases iron absorption from a micronutrient powder containing ferrous fumarate and sodium iron EDTA: a stable-isotope study in Kenyan infants. *The American Journal of Clinical Nutrition*, 106(4): 1020–1031.

Panesar, P.S., Kaur, R., Singh, R.S. and Kennedy, J.F. (2018). Biocatalytic strategies in the production of galacto-oligosaccharides and its global status. *International Journal of Biological Macromolecules*, 111: 667–679.

Panesar, P.S., Kumari, S. and Panesar, R. (2010). Potential applications of immobilized β-galactosidase in food processing industries. *Enzyme Research*, 2010: 1–16.

Park, A.R. and Oh, D.K. (2010). Galacto-oligosaccharide production using microbial β-galactosidase: current state and perspectives. *Applied Microbiology and Biotechnology*, 85(5): 1279–1286.

Park, H.Y., Kim, H.J., Lee, J.K., Kim, D. and Oh, D.K. (2008). Galactooligosaccharide production by a thermostable β-galactosidase from *Sulfolobus solfataricus*. *World Journal of Microbiology and Biotechnology*, 24(8): 1553–1558.

Patel, S. and Goyal, A. (2012). The current trends and future perspectives of prebiotics research: a review. *3 Biotech*, 2(2): 115–125.

Qamar, T.R., Iqbal, S., Syed, F., Nasir, M., Rehman, H., Iqbal, M.A. and Liu, R.H. (2017). Impact of novel prebiotic galacto-oligosaccharides on various biomarkers of colorectal cancer in wister rats. *International Journal of Molecular Sciences*, 18(9): 1785.

Qamar, T.R., Syed, F., Nasir, M., Rehman, H., Zahid, M.N., Liu, R.H. and Iqbal, S. (2016). Novel combination of prebiotics galacto-oligosaccharides and inulin-inhibited aberrant crypt foci formation and biomarkers of colon cancer in wistar rats. *Nutrients*, 8(8): 465.

Qin, Z., Li, S., Huang, X., Kong, W., Yang, X., Zhang, S., Cao, L. and Liu, Y. (2019). Improving galactooligosaccharide synthesis efficiency of β-galactosidase Bgal1-3 by reshaping the active site with an intelligent hydrophobic amino acid scanning. *Journal of Agricultural and Food Chemistry*, 67(40): 11158–11166.

Rehman, S.U. (2009). Reduced lactose and lactose-free dairy products. *Advanced Dairy Chemistry*, 3: 98–104.

Rico-Díaz, A., Ramírez-Escudero, M., Vizoso-Vázquez, Á., Cerdán, M.E., Becerra, M. and Sanz-Aparicio, J. (2017). Structural features of *Aspergillus niger* β-galactosidase define its activity against glycoside linkages. *The FEBS Journal*, 284(12): 1815–1829.

Rico-Rodríguez, F., Villamiel, M., Ruiz-Aceituno, L., Serrato, J.C. and Montilla, A. (2020). Effect of the lactose source on the ultrasound-assisted enzymatic production of galactooligosaccharides and gluconic acid. *Ultrasonics Sonochemistry*, 67: 104945, https://doi.org/10.1016/j.ultsonch.2019.104945

Roberfroid, M. and Slavin, J. (2000). Nondigestible oligosaccharides. *Critical Reviews in Food Science and Nutrition*, 40(6): 461–480.

Rodriguez-Colinas, B., de Abreu, M.A., Fernandez-Arrojo, L., de Beer, R., Poveda, A., Jimenez-Barbero, J., Haltrich, D., Ballesteros Olmo, A.O., Fernandez-Lobato, M. and Plou, F.J. (2011). Production of galacto-oligosaccharides by the β-galactosidase from *Kluyveromyces lactis*:

Comparative analysis of permeabilized cells versus soluble enzyme. *Journal of Agricultural and food Chemistry*, 59(19): 10477–10484.

Rodriguez-Colinas, B., Fernandez-Arrojo, L., Ballesteros, A.O. and Plou, F.J. (2014). Galactooligosaccharides formation during enzymatic hydrolysis of lactose: Towards a prebiotic-enriched milk. *Food Chemistry*, 145: 388–394.

Rodriguez-Colinas, B., Fernandez-Arrojo, L., Santos-Moriano, P., Ballesteros, A.O. and Plou, F.J. (2016). Continuous packed bed reactor with immobilized β-galactosidase for production of galactooligosaccharides (GOS). *Catalysts*, 6(12): 189.

Sabater, C., Fara, A., Palacios, J., Corzo, N., Requena, T., Montilla, A. and Zárate, G. (2019). Synthesis of prebiotic galactooligosaccharides from lactose and lactulose by dairy propionibacteria. *Food Microbiology*, 77: 93–105.

Sangwan, V., Tomar, S.K., Singh, R.R.B., Singh, A.K. and Ali, B. (2011). Galactooligosaccharides: novel components of designer foods. *Journal of Food Science*, 76(4): R103–R111.

Saqib, S., Akram, A., Halim, S.A. and Tassaduq, R. (2017). Sources of β-galactosidase and its applications in food industry. *3 Biotech*, 7(1): 79.

Saravanan, R., Shubethar, S., Narayanan, S., Jain, M., Lade, S., Jadhav, D., Maheswaran, P., Avalakki, U.K. and Dubey, A.K. (2017). A novel process for the production of high-purity galactooligosaccharides (GOS) using consortium of microbes. *Preparative Biochemistry and Biotechnology*, 47(3): 245–253.

Sass, A.C. and Jördening, H.J. (2020). Immobilization of β-Galactosidase From *Aspergillus oryzae* on electrospun gelatin nanofiber mats for the production of galactooligosaccharides. *Applied Biochemistry and Biotechnology*, 191: 1155–1170.

Schokker, D., Zhang, J., Zhang, L.L., Vastenhouw, S.A., Heilig, H.G., Smidt, H., Rebel, J.M. and Smits, M.A. (2014). Early-life environmental variation affects intestinal microbiota and immune development in new-born piglets. *PloS ONE*, 9(6): e100040.

Scholz-Ahrens, K.E. and Schrezenmeir, J. (2007). Inulin and oligofructose and mineral metabolism: the evidence from animal trials. *The Journal of Nutrition*, 137(11): 2513S–2523S.

Scholz-Ahrens, K.E., Schaafsma, G., van den Heuvel, E.G. and Schrezenmeir, J. (2001). Effects of prebiotics on mineral metabolism. *The American Journal of Clinical Nutrition*, 73(2): 459s–464s.

Schuman, B., Alfaro, J.A. and Evans, S.V. (2007). Glycosyltransferase structure and function. In: *Bioactive Conformation I. Topics in Current Chemistry*. Berlin: Springer.

Seibel, J., Beine, R., Moraru, R., Behringer, C. and Buchholz, K. (2006). A new pathway for the synthesis of oligosaccharides by the use of non-Leloir glycosyltransferases. *Biocatalysis and Biotransformation*, 24(1-2): 157–165.

Seijo, M., Bryk, G., Coronel, M.Z., Bonanno, M., Río, M.E., de Portela, M.L.P.M. and Zeni, S.N. (2018). Effect of adding a galacto-oligosaccharides/fructo-oligosaccharides (GOS/FOS®) mixture to a normal and low calcium diet, on calcium absorption and bone health in ovariectomy-induced osteopenic rats. *Calcified Tissue International*, 104(3): 301–312.

Siegel, R., Ward, E., Brawley, O. and Jemal, A. (2011). The impact of eliminating socioeconomic and racial disparities on premature cancer deaths. *CA:A Cancer Journal for Clinicians*, 61(4): 212–236.

Srivastava, A. and Mishra, S. (2019). Enrichment and evaluation of galacto-oligosaccharides produced by whole cell treatment of sugar reaction mixture. *Molecular Biology Reports*, 46(1): 1181–1188.

Sun, J., Liang, W., Yang, X., Li, Q. and Zhang, G. (2019). Cytoprotective effects of galacto-oligosaccharides on colon epithelial cells via up-regulating miR-19b. *Life Sciences*, 231: 116589, https://doi.org/10.1016/j.lfs.2019.116589

Suwal, S., Bentahar, J., Marciniak, A., Beaulieu, L., Deschênes, J.S. and Doyen, A. (2019). Evidence of the production of galactooligosaccharide from whey permeate by the microalgae *Tetradesmus obliquus*. *Algal Research*, 39: 101470.

Tanaka, T. (2009). Colorectal carcinogenesis: Review of human and experimental animal studies. *Journal of Carcinogenesis*, 8: 5.

Tannock, G.W. (1995). *Normal Microflora: An Introduction to Microbes Inhabiting the Human Body*. Springer Science and Business Media.

Tanthanuch, W., Chantarangsee, M., Maneesan, J. and Ketudat-Cairns, J. (2008). Genomic and expression analysis of glycosyl hydrolase family 35 genes from rice (*Oryza sativa* L.). *BMC Plant Biology*, 8(1): 84.

Tian, S., Wang, J., Yu, H., Wang, J. and Zhu, W. (2019). Changes in ileal microbial composition and microbial metabolism by an early-life galacto-oligosaccharides intervention in a neonatal porcine model. *Nutrients*, 11(8): 1753, doi:10.3390/nu11081753

Todea, A., Benea, I.C., Bîtcan, I., Péter, F., Klébert, S., Feczkó, T., Károly, Z. and Biró, E. (2020). One-pot biocatalytic conversion of lactose to gluconic acid and galacto-oligosaccharides using immobilized β-galactosidase and glucose oxidase. *Catalysis Today*, https://doi.org/10.1016/j.cattod.2020.06.090

Tokošová, S., Hronská, H. and Rosenberg, M. (2016). Production of high-content galacto-oligosaccharides mixture using β-galactosidase and *Kluyveromyces marxianus* entrapped in polyvinylalcohol gel. *Chemical Papers*, 70(11): 1445–1451.

Torres, D.P., Gonçalves, M.D.P.F., Teixeira, J.A. and Rodrigues, L.R. (2010). Galacto-oligosaccharides: production, properties, applications, and significance as prebiotics. *Comprehensive Reviews in Food Science and Food Safety*, 9(5): 438–454.

Tzortzis, G. and Vulevic, J. (2009). Galacto-oligosaccharide prebiotics. In: *Prebiotics and Probiotics: Science and Technology* (eds D. Charalampopoulos and R.A. Rastall). New York: Springer.

van den Broek, L.A., Hinz, S.W., Beldman, G., Vincken, J.P. and Voragen, A.G. (2008). Bifidobacterium carbohydrases – their role in breakdown and synthesis of (potential) prebiotics. *Molecular Nutrition and Food Research*, 52(1): 146–163.

Van Engeland, M., Derks, S., Smits, K.M., Meijer, G.A. and Herman, J.G. (2011). Colorectal cancer epigenetics: complex simplicity. *Journal of Clinical Oncology*, 29(10): 1382–1391.

Vera, C., Córdova, A., Aburto, C., Guerrero, C., Suárez, S. and Illanes, A. (2016). Synthesis and purification of galacto-oligosaccharides: state of the art. *World Journal of Microbiology and Biotechnology*, 32(12): 197.

Vera, C., Guerrero, C. and Illanes, A. (2011). Determination of the transgalactosylation activity of *Aspergillus oryzae* β-galactosidase: effect of pH, temperature, and galactose and glucose concentrations. *Carbohydrate Research*, 346(6): 745–752.

Vera, C., Guerrero, C., Conejeros, R. and Illanes, A. (2012). Synthesis of galacto-oligosaccharides by β-galactosidase from *Aspergillus oryzae* using partially dissolved and supersaturated solution of lactose. *Enzyme and Microbial Technology*, 50(3): 188–194.

Vinolo, M.A., Rodrigues, H.G., Nachbar, R.T. and Curi, R. (2011). Regulation of inflammation by short chain fatty acids. *Nutrients*, 3(10): 858–876.

Wang, G., Zhu, J., Liu, L., Yaqoob, M.U., Pei, X., Tao, W., Xiao, Z., Sun, W. and Wang, M. (2020). Optimization for galactooligosaccharides synthesis: A potential alternative for gut health and immunity. *Life Sciences*, 245: 117353.

Wang, Y., Gong, L., Wu, Y.P., Cui, Z.W., Wang, Y.Q., Huang, Y., Zhang, X.P. and Li, W.F. (2019). Oral administration of *Lactobacillus rhamnosus* GG to newborn piglets augments gut barrier function in pre-weaning piglets. *Journal of Zhejiang University-SCIENCE B*, 20(2): 180–192.

Watson, A.J. and Collins, P.D. (2011). Colon cancer: a civilization disorder. *Digestive Diseases*, 29(2): 222–228.

Weaver, C.M. (2014). Bioactive foods and ingredients for health. *Advances in Nutrition*, 5(3): 306S–311S.

Weijers, C.A., Franssen, M.C. and Visser, G.M. (2008). Glycosyltransferase-catalyzed synthesis of bioactive oligosaccharides. *Biotechnology Advances*, 26(5): 436–456.

Yañez-Ñeco, C.V., Rodriguez-Colinas, B., Amaya-Delgado, L., Ballesteros, A.O., Gschaedler, A., Plou, F.J. and Arrizon, J. (2017). Galactooligosaccharide production from *Pantoea anthophila* strains isolated from "Tejuino", a Mexican traditional fermented beverage. *Catalysts*, 7(8): 242.

Yang, J., Wang, Q., Zhou, Y., Li, J., Gao, R. and Guo, Z., 2017. Engineering *T. naphthophila* β-glucosidase for enhanced synthesis of galactooligosaccharides by site-directed mutagenesis. *Biochemical Engineering Journal*, 127: 1–8.

Yasuda, K., Dawson, H.D., Wasmuth, E.V., Roneker, C.A., Chen, C., Urban, J.F., Welch, R.M., Miller, D.D. and Lei, X.G. (2009). Supplemental dietary inulin influences expression of iron and inflammation related genes in young pigs. *The Journal of Nutrition*, 139(11): 2018–2023.

Yu, M., Mu, C., Zhang, C., Yang, Y., Su, Y. and Zhu, W. (2018). Marked response in microbial community and metabolism in the ileum and cecum of suckling piglets after early antibiotics exposure. *Frontiers in Microbiology*, 9: 1166.

Zeuner, B., Teze, D., Muschiol, J. and Meyer, A.S. (2019). Synthesis of human milk oligosaccharides: Protein engineering strategies for improved enzymatic transglycosylation. *Molecules*, 24(11): 2033.

Zhou, P., Chen, B., Hu, P. and Sun, Y. (2013). Role of miR-19a in ulcerative colitis in mice. *Nan Fang Yi Ke Da Xue Xue Bao*, 33(9): 1325–1328.

13

Fructooligosaccharides as Prebiotics, their Metabolism, and Health Benefits

Orlando de la Rosa[1], Adriana C. Flores-Gallegos[1], Juan A. Ascacio-Valdés[1], Leonardo Sepúlveda[1], Julio C. Montáñez[2], and Cristóbal N. Aguilar[1]

[1]Bioprocesses & Bioproducts Research Group, Food Research Department, School of Chemistry, Universidad Autónoma de Coahuila, Saltillo, 25280, Coahuila, Mexico
[2]Laboratory of Chemical Engineering, School of Chemistry, Universidad Autónoma de Coahuila, Saltillo, 25280, Coahuila, México

13.1 Introduction

Nowadays, people's lifestyles have a strong impact on health. Several factors, such as stress, reduced sleep time, lack of exercise time and bad eating habits, have led to the increase of diseases. On the other hand, people are aware of this problem and, with the concern to have a longer and healthier life, it has led to a consumer consciousness of the type of food and nutrients they look for in a food product. Interest in improving health through food products with added benefits for humans has grown, leading to an increased demand for healthier products. That tendency has captured the attention of food technologists to satisfy consumer demands; new products are being developed that attend not only to nutritional requirements but also health-promoting properties that may help prevent lifestyle-related diseases.

13.2 Chemical Structure and Sources

FOS belong to the fructan family [α-D-glucopyranoside-(1-2)-]-p,D-fructofuranosyl-[(1-2)-P-D-fructofuranosyl] which have different degrees of polymerization (DP) between two and more than 60. The short chain FOS (scFOS), are chemically composed of a series of fructosyl moieties (F) linked to the β-(2-1) position of a sucrose molecule (Chen *et al.* 2014;); on the other side, single terminal glucose (G) is linked by an α-(1,2) linkage. Short chain FOS have between two and four fructose units with degrees of polymerization between three and five, having an average DP of 4.8. The formula GFn indicates the degree of polymerization by the amount of fructose that is present bound to glucose (Niness 1999). Short chain FOS comprise mainly 1-kestose (GF2)

Probiotics, Prebiotics and Synbiotics: Technological Advancements Towards Safety and Industrial Applications, First Edition. Edited by Parmjit Singh Panesar and Anil Kumar Anal.

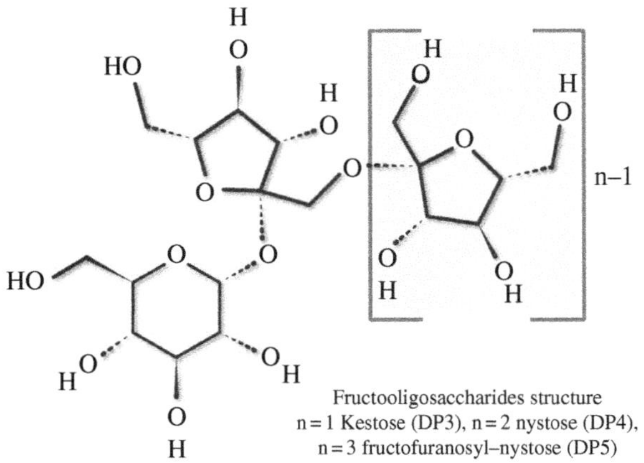

Figure 13.1 FOS structure and general formula. n = 1–3 fructosyl units.

(molecular formula: $C_{18}H_{32}O_{16}$), 1-nystose (GF3) (molecular formula: $C_{24}H_{42}O_{21}$) and 1-β-fructofuranosyl-nystose (GF4) (molecular formula: $C_{30}H_{52}O_{26}$) and their molecular weight is 505, 666, and 828, respectively, the average molecular weight for scFOS being 700. FOS structures are illustrated in Figure 13.1.

FOS are naturally present in various families of plants as storage oligosaccharides (Li *et al.* 2014). Among the most consumed and popular sources are garlic (*Allium sativum*) and onion (*Allium cepa*) which belong to the family Liliaceae and contain a good quantity of FOS (Benkeblia 2013; Kumar *et al.* 2015). FOS in onion have osmotic-regulating activity when bulbing starts (Darbyshire and Henry 1978). Roots are also a source of these oligosaccharides; burdock root (*Arctium lappa* L.) usually contains abundant amounts of FOS, usually considered as its main bioactive components (Corradini *et al.* 2013; Li *et al.* 2013). In yacon root (*Smallanthus sonchifolius* Poepp. And Endl.) FOS are present in high amounts in the tissue (~60–70%, dry basis) (Corradini *et al.* 2013; Fernández *et al.* 2013; Pedreschi *et al.* 2003). Chicory roots (*Cichorium intybus* L.) and bulbs of Jerusalem artichoke (*Helianthus tuberosus*) are also well known for their FOS presence (Bornet *et al.* 2002; Courtin *et al.* 2009; Durieux *et al.* 2001; Kovács *et al.* 2014). FOS presence has been reported in other crops and foods such as wheat, rye and barley, in fruits like banana, tomatoes, and other sources like honey and agave syrup (Bornet *et al.* 2002; Muñiz-Márquez *et al.* 2015).

FOS concentration in some plants and fruits was analyzed by Campbell *et al.* (1997). In this study, 25 samples were analyzed for FOS content; among them, 20 showed detectable levels of FOS. FOS content in fruits ranged from 0.1 to 0.2 mg/g in 12 of 20 of the fruits with FOS presence. Ripe bananas showed the highest FOS concentration, which was as high as 2.0 mg/g FOS. For vegetables, six vegetables contained 0.1–0.2 mg/g FOS, and in other 16 vegetables FOS content ranged from 0.3 to 58.4 mg/g FOS.

13.3 Prebiotic Concept

Gibson and Roberfroid (1995) introduced the concept of prebiotics, referring to them as "those compounds that are non-digestible food ingredients that beneficially affect the host by selectively stimulating the growth and/or activity of one or a limited number of bacterial species already resident in the colon, and thus attempt to improve host health". The attempt to improve host health refers to health modulation via fermentation products of the increased population of the beneficial colonic microbiota. In that first definition, FOS were included in the classification of prebiotics.

Later the concept was updated by Gibson *et al.* (2004) because of the need to clarify between some carbohydrates classified as dietary fiber. Not all of them had the effects necessary to be claimed as prebiotics. In order to establish a clear criterion for prebiotic classification, Gibson *et al.* proposed some premises that a compound has to fulfill to be considered as prebiotic. Those premises should be demonstrated scientifically and are the following:

1) No hydrolysis or absorption in the upper part of the digestive system (mouth, stomach, small intestine).
2) Selectively fermented by certain desired populations of the intestinal microbiota.
3) Stimulates the growth selectively and/or activity of intestinal bacteria associated with health benefits.

The third premise, concerning the selective stimulation of growth and/or activity of bacteria, is the most difficult to fulfill. Indeed, it requires anaerobic sampling followed by a reliable and quantitative microbiological analysis of a wide variety of bacterial genera.

Reporting fermentation in pure cultures of single microbial strains or an increase in a limited number of bacterial genera in complex mixtures of bacteria (for example, fecal slurries) either in vitro or in vivo cannot confirm a prebiotic effect. Therefore, a decision was taken to build upon the current prebiotic status and define a niche for "dietary prebiotics", defining a dietary prebiotic as "a selectively fermented ingredient that results in specific changes in the composition and/or activity of the gastrointestinal microbiota, thus conferring benefit(s) upon host health".

At first, the definition was more specific for lactobacilli and bifidobacteria genera, because those are among the species that are present in greater quantity in human microbiota, but a debate arose based on extending the range of inclusion of more microorganisms with beneficial effects to the host.

According to the "ingredients", any dietary material that is non-digestible and enters the large intestine was claimed as a candidate prebiotic (Gibson *et al.* 2010). These include polysaccharide-type carbohydrates such as resistant starch and dietary fiber, as well as proteins and lipids. The compounds claimed as accepted prebiotics are those "ingredients" that shift to the colon and then are selectively fermented or promote specific changes such as non-digestible oligosaccharides (NDOs), which have been proved to be selectively fermented by specific bacterial populations (most likely bifidobacteria) (Al-Sheraji *et al.* 2013). Among oligosaccharides, different degrees of polymerization can claim different prebiotic or functional effects. FOS are among the compounds that have been considered prebiotics since the first definition was published and remained considered in the classification through all the definition changes. As previously mentioned in Section 13.2, FOS belong to the fructan family, in which FOS have lower DP, having different prebiotic activity compared to longer DP fructans (time of fermentation). Microbiota changes after fermentable fiber ingestion do not guarantee beneficial health impact, so not all fermentable compounds fulfill prebiotic criteria (Bindels *et al.* 2015; Valcheva and Dieleman 2016). In the case of FOS, the end components of its metabolism are short chain fatty acids (SCFAs), which have been proved to exert beneficial effects on the host. The SCFAs commonly produced are acetic acid, propionic acid and butyric acid, which are used by the host organism as an energy source or promote other activities that benefit host health (Al-Sheraji *et al.* 2013; Gibson and Roberfroid 1995; Gibson *et al.* 2004, 2010;). Prebiotics are non-digestible food ingredients that have a specific stimulatory effect upon selected populations of gut bacteria (Rastall and Gibson 2014).

13.4 Health-promoting Properties

Fructooligosaccharides have attracted special attention among the prebiotics because of their health-promoting properties and their food industry applications. FOS are reported to have immunomodulatory activity generated by the gut microbiota enhancement (Choque Delgado *et al.* 2011; Hemarajata and Versalovic 2013; Kumar *et al.* 2015). FOS represent low calorie ingestion because they resist hydrolysis by digestive enzymes and are not used as an energy source in the body. FOS can be included in a wide variety of products such as functional foods and pharmacological products. They play an important role in reduction of cholesterol, triglycerides and phospholipids, and improving mineral absorption such as calcium and magnesium in the intestine (Adriano *et al.* 2019; van den Heuvel *et al.* 2009; Wang *et al.* 2010; Yen *et al.* 2011).

13.4.1 Prebiotic Activity

Prebiotics can restore the intestinal balance even after the disturbance caused by diseases such as diarrhea, stress, antibiotics and other drugs. FOS stand out for their multiple health-promoting properties in addition to being non-digestible by humans but fermentable by specific human gastrointestinal microbiota, promoting the growth and activity of specific microbial groups. The capacity of FOS to reduce chronic diseases such as colon cancer, ulcerative colitis, intestinal cancer, cardiovascular diseases and obesity has been reported (de Cossío *et al.* 2016; Serrano-Villar *et al.* 2017; Valcheva and Dieleman 2016; Vieira De Almeida *et al.* 2019). This is mainly the result of the activity of the microbial groups enhanced by FOS, due in part to the fact that they resist digestion by digestive enzymes and gastric juices, which allows them to reach the intestine and colon where they act as fermentable substrates for populations of probiotic bacteria, which act synergistically between microbial groups that produce metabolites such as SCFAs (butyrate, propionate, etc.) that are known for their anticancer effect (Kahouli *et al.* 2013; Koirala and Anal 2021; Serban 2014; Vieira De Almeida *et al.* 2019; Xie *et al.* 2019).

13.4.2 Influence of Gut Microbiome

To understand all the benefits to the host related to prebiotic consumption, epigenetics is of great importance because it can explain how prebiotic structures and the metabolites produced or derived from microbiota can act on signaling cell pathways and epigenetic control. As we know, our intestinal microbiota is composed of trillions of microorganisms that have been provided since birth in the first contact with our mother and through the ingestion of breast milk (Mohajeri *et al.* 2018). This microbiota is influenced and submitted to changes during our early childhood, moderated by nutrition and the environment during our development (Paul *et al.* 2019). Being modified by those factors, our microbiota is unique and presents differences between individuals (Martínez *et al.* 2018). The way our microbiota interacts with our genome has attracted attention in the need to understand and prevent chronic diseases (Schmidt *et al.* 2018). The collective genomes of our microbiota are termed the "microbiome" (Butler *et al.* 2019), and it has a crucial role in metabolism as it carries out several metabolic activities such as catabolism and bioconversion of compounds related to metabolism that reach distant organs and systems (Baliou *et al.* 2019; Salvucci 2019; Young 2017).

As mentioned earlier, the gut microbiota takes part in the metabolism of SCFAs, but other compounds are also produced such as branched chain fatty acids (BCFAs), branched-chain amino acids (BCAAs), biogenic amines, vitamins, bile acids (BAs), and xenobiotics (Sen and Orešič 2019). These take part in distinct functions such as regulation of the immune system, modulation of cellular growth and maintenance of barrier function (Salvucci 2019).

Given the importance of the intestinal microbiota in the host's health, it is vitally important to maintain the balance and diversity of these microbial populations. This balance can be interrupted by poor diets or habits that cause changes in these populations, which can lead to a predisposition to various diseases (Baliou *et al.* 2019; Martínez *et al.* 2018).

Through the consumption of prebiotics such as FOS, it is feasible to alter the balance of gut microbiota towards the production of metabolites or modulating bacterial population size, which can lead to recovery of host health (Mohajeri *et al.* 2018). As a consequence of the changes in host-beneficial microbiota modulated by prebiotics, SCFAs are produced (mainly acetate, propionate and butyrate) (Joseph *et al.* 2019; Nawaz *et al.* 2018; Neri-Numa and Pastore 2020). These compounds are absorbed briefly in the large intestine; their metabolism leads to modulation of the phenotype and function of colonic epithelial cells, macrophages, neutrophils and dendritic cells which make a significant impact in several immunological functions (Daguet *et al.* 2016; Nawaz *et al.* 2018; Serban 2014). The fermentation of prebiotics not only impacts host health directly; when the activity of microbiota is shifted, very diverse chain effects can be displayed as a consequence of what is called "cross-feeding". This term refers to the assimilation of products derived from the metabolic activity of a group of microorganisms by other specific microorganisms. It has been proved that *Eubacterium hallii* can be benefited by cross-feeding on lactate generated by *Bifidobacterium adolescentis* initially enhanced by FOS production (Belenguer *et al.* 2006). Similar activity has been reported for *B. longum* as it was capable of degrading arabinoxylan oligosaccharides leading to an increase of acetate which in turn is transformed to butyrate by a different bacterial population, eliciting cross-feeding between bacterial populations (Rivière *et al.* 2015).

Recently, scFOS along with anthocyanin were used to modulate intestinal microbiota in obese patients. The FOS–anthocyanin blend was administered for an 8-week period and the trial evidenced that the intake of the anthocyanin–prebiotic blend enhanced the Bacteroidetes population and lowered the Firmicutes count (Hester *et al.* 2018).

FOS stand out among prebiotics because of the ability to enhance/promote the activity of certain bacterial populations. Several studies, among them in vitro studies, in vivo studies in animal models and also clinical trials, have proved their prebiotic activity. Geigerová *et al.* (2017) evaluated FOS among other commercial prebiotics as a supplement to improve the survival of bifidobacteria in the intestine of calves. First, in vitro utilization of different prebiotics by *Bifidobacterium animalis* ssp. *animalis* (two strains), *B. choerinum*, *B. thermophilum*, and *B. longum* ssp. *suis* was investigated. Then FOS and GOS (the substrates with the highest specific growth rates) were tested in vivo. FOS were able to improve the survival of bifidobacteria passing through the digestive tract with counts of more than 10^7 CFU/g. Also, bifidobacteria showed a preference for short chain FOS compared to inulin as a substrate for growth.

Prebiotics have been able to restore the balance of microbiota after antibiotics, but their use as an alternative to antibiotics has also been tested. Shang *et al.* (2018) studied the dietary effect of FOS supplementation as an alternative to antibiotics on ileal mucosa and digesta microbiota in broiler chickens. The study was carried out for 21 days and included three dietary treatments: (i) positive control (PC), a normal diet containing antibiotics (virginiamycin and monensin); (ii) negative control (NC), a normal diet without antibiotics; and (iii) NC + FOS, an NC normal diet supplemented with 0.5% of FOS. Ileal mucosa and digesta were collected and subjected to 16S rRNA-based next-generation sequencing. Supplementation with FOS resulted in a more diverse microbiota in the ileal mucosa when compared with PC and NC groups. Microorganisms that have pathogenic properties such as *Helicobacter* and *Desulfovibrio* were reduced significantly in the NC + FOS group compared to the NC group in the ileal mucosa. The resulting modulation of gut microbiota by a FOS-supplemented diet favors chicken health and could be used as an alternative method to replace antibiotic growth promoters (AGPs).

Gut microbiota balance in the elderly is more susceptible than in younger people because of lifestyle conditions. Dietary supplementation of FOS has been suggested to restore and regularize the gut microbiota in older people. The impact of FOS along with nucleosides (NS), and yeast extract (YE) supplementation on the microbiota population from older people was assessed. NS, YE and FOS tested separately and combined at different proportion levels enhanced the population number of bacterial species producing butyrate, lactobacilli and bifidobacteria. It was observed that FOS and YE accumulatively elevated butyrate and decreased propionate. This was attributed to the butyrogenic effect of FOS (Doo *et al.* 2019).

Prebiotic activity of FOS has continuously been tested not only with commercial preparations but also with plant extracts or blends that have FOS among their components. *Agave salmiana* is a vegetal species with naturally occurring FOS in its leaves and its fluid, called "aguamiel", which is fermented by wild microorganisms including lactic acid bacteria to produce pulque. The ability of FOS in *A. salmiana* powder in the specific stimulation of probiotic bacteria was tested compared to commercial prebiotic products. FOS present in *A. salmiana*, among other components, supported the growth of probiotic bacteria in almost the same stimulation as Inulin Orafti GR. *Lactobacillus acidophilus* was the strain that showed the best growth with *A. salmiana* powder, decreased the final pH value to the lowest level and produced the highest concentration of lactate (Martinez-Gutierrez *et al.* 2017). As discussed in the previous section, Jerusalem artichoke is one of the natural sources of FOS and evaluation of its prebiotic effect is of great interest. Elaheh *et al.* (2016) investigated and compared the prebiotic effect in vitro on the survivability and activity of

Bifidobacterium bifidum and Escherichia coli of Jerusalem artichoke fructans compared to a high molecular weight fraction of chicory-derived inulin. Jerusalem artichoke tuber FOS showed potential to be used as a prebiotic component as FOS improved the growth of *Bifidobacterium bifidum* significantly compared to the control. Prebiotic effect of FOS from burdock roots has also been tested. Moro *et al.* (2018) attempted to use FOS and the phenolic compounds of burdock root flour as an ingredient for prebiotic cookies.

Prebiotics play a key role in stimulating the production of desirable proteins in probiotic strains. This has been evidenced by Comerlato *et al.* (2020), where FOS and GOS were evaluated for their specific influence of protein stimulation related to their metabolism by *Enterococcus durans* LAB18S. The results of this trial showed that both FOS and GOS were used as a carbon source by *E. durans* LAB18S, up-regulating the production of proteins associated with intestinal mucosa adhesion, carbohydrate and nitrogen metabolism, and stress response. Stimulation of the production of proteins related to amino acid metabolism and energy conversion was also observed with FOS as substrate.

The success of prebiotics in promoting health benefits is not due to stimulating the growth of beneficial probiotics but also helping to reduce pathogenic bacteria. In a recent study, Anand *et al.* (2018) evaluated the prebiotics FOS, inulin and maltodextrin for their effect on aggregation characteristics of the strain *Lactobacillus rhamnosus* NCDC 298. The trial comprised of evaluating the capacity to mitigate adhesive capacity of the enterotoxigenic strain *E. coli* (ETEC) subsequent to the evaluation of the symbiotic effect of virulence of ETEC to intestinal cell lines HT-29. FOS enhanced autoaggregation and co-aggregation characteristics of *L. rhamnosus* NCDC 298 with ETEC. FOS and inulin were found to have the best adherence inhibition percentage. FOS promoted the adhesion of *L. rhamnosus* NCDC 298, exhibiting also properties that inhibited the virulence capacity of ETEC. In another study, in vitro resistance of commercial FOS and xylooligosaccharides (XOS) to gastric enzymes was assayed, along with in vitro growth of probiotic *Bifidobacterium*, *Lactobacillus* and pathogenic *Salmonella*. Assays proved that FOS and XOS are resistant to gastric tract acidity and enzymes. Growth experiments showed that *L. acidophilus* and *B. lactis* can use FOS as substrate. For *Salmonella typhimurium*, absence of growth was observed in the cultures with oligosaccharides in 4 h, demonstrating prebiotic specificity for probiotic bacteria (de Figueiredo *et al.* 2020). Other recent studies have reported successful FOS stimulation of different bacterial populations such as *Bifidobacterium* and *Lactobacillus* strains, Prevotellaceae, Tannerellaceae, *Faecalibacterium prausnitzii* and *Torulaspora delbrueckii* (Bersaneti *et al.* 2019; Duysburgh *et al.* 2019; Freire *et al.* 2017; Nobre *et al.* 2018a; Speranza *et al.* 2018; Verruck *et al.* 2017).

13.4.3 Prevention against Colon Cancer and Immunomodulation

Since colon cancer prevention with FOS consumption is strongly associated with the immunological response, FOS immunomodulation and ability to prevent colon cancer is reviewed in this section. Colorectal cancer (CRC) is characterized by genetic and epigenetic alterations along with infiltration of inflammatory cell malignant and stromal cells. Malignant cell infiltration can be induced by changes in the microenvironment and generate the formation of tumors, as well as metastasis. CRC is strongly related to chronic inflammation and therefore it could be prevented by stimulating the microenvironment that favors anti-inflammatory activity. As reviewed in the previous sections, prebiotics such as FOS can influence the activity or proliferation of specific bacterial populations that keep the microbiota in balance. The most common end-products of FOS fermentation by gut microbiota are SCFAs, among them butyrate and propionate. Butyrate is employed as a source of energy for colon epithelial cells and can induce cell differentiation and proliferation in the intestine; it also presents mechanisms of inhibition of cancer cells, adenomas and carcinomas in the colon and promotes cell apoptosis in these, helping to prevent the formation of tumors (Al-Sheraji *et al.* 2013; Gomes *et al.* 2014; Moreno *et al.* 2017; Serban 2014). Furthermore, butyrate contributes to the reduction of toxicity of chemotherapy drugs against CRC (Chen *et al.* 2016). SCFAs can cross the intestinal epithelium and reach the lamina propria, directly shaping mucosal immune responses (Koh *et al.* 2016; Vieira De Almeida *et al.* 2019). Under SCFA stimulation, the CD4+ effector T cells increase T-bet and IFN-γ expression and can exert beneficial effects depending on SCFA concentration. These effects are regulated by the expression of differentiation markers (alkaline phosphatase), glutathione-S-transferase, and other response genes, as well as the suppression of 2-cyclooxygenase expression. Anti-inflammatory capacity has been reported for propionate in colon cancer cells (Serban 2014).

Besides the direct effects of SCFAs against colon cancer, the proliferation of probiotics induced by FOS can unchain a series of immune responses beneficial for cancer prevention, such as improving epithelial gut barrier function by inducing the secretion of anticarcinogenic and antioxidant molecules and by activating mononuclear cells, lymphocytes and enhancing IgA production (Chen *et al.* 2016; Le Bourgot *et al.* 2016; Liu *et al.* 2017; Xie *et al.* 2019). The increase in probiotic populations also reduces the expression of specific Toll-like receptors (TLRs), which improves epithelial barrier resistance (Jia *et al.* 2019; Serban 2014; Vieira De Almeida *et al.* 2019) and activates phagocytes, which contribute to maintain a vigilance state against tumor formation, especially in the early stages (Delcenserie *et al.* 2008; Vieira De Almeida *et al.* 2019).

It is important to point out that the beneficial effects of probiotics against cancer are based on early administration. To prevent early phases of colorectal cancer (CRC), different effects of probiotics could result in advanced phases depending on specific probiotic strains (Vieira De Almeida *et al.* 2019).

The administration of symbiotic mixtures has proved to have promising benefits as a potential therapeutic strategy against cancer. In a study, a symbiotic mixture (FOS together with *B. lactis* Bb12 and *L. rhamnosus* GG) proved to be successful in decreasing *Clostridium perfringens* bacterial populations and promoting the growth of *Bifidobacterium* and *Lactobacillus*, consequently lowering the cytotoxicity of fecal water on colonic cells (Chen *et al.* 2016). In another study, a symbiotic mixture of oligofructose plus *B. infantum, L. acidophilus, B. bifidum* and maltodextrin enhanced the expression of intestinal ZO-1, MUC2 and TLR2 and reduced the expression of COX-2 and TLR4 in rats (Kuugbee *et al.* 2016).

In a recent study, the effects of prebiotic consumption on immunomodulation and gut microbiota in perioperative patients with CRC were investigated. The experiment was a randomized, double-blind, no-treatment parallel control clinical trial involving 140 perioperative patients. The oral administration of prebiotics resulted in significant effects on immunological indices in both the preoperative and postoperative periods but in different ways. In the preoperative period, prebiotics increased serum levels of IgG, IgM and transferrin; in the postoperative period, they enhanced levels of IgG, IgA, suppressor/cytotoxic T cells, and total B lymphocytes (Xie *et al.* 2019). Other studies have evidenced immune stimulation after FOS inclusion in animal diets (Azimirad *et al.* 2016; Jia *et al.* 2019; Paz *et al.* 2019).

13.4.4 Impact on Obesity

Among benefits related to FOS intake, their prebiotic nature and soluble fiber have the ability to impact obesity. FOS intake can help to reduce food and energy consumption in people with obesity, resulting in weight loss and health improvement. This is because, thanks to their ability to resist hydrolysis and digestion by human digestive enzymes and gastric acid, they represent almost no caloric intake. Also, the fermentation of these prebiotics by beneficial microbiota results in immune regulation leading to anti-inflammatory effects, improvement of intestinal permeability and better metabolism. Prebiotics also influence metabolism by regulating intestinal anorectic hormones, such as tyrosine, tyrosine peptide, glucagon-1 peptide and leptin, and reducing levels of orogenic hormones such as ghrelin (Anal *et al.* 2021).

Yacon syrup rich in FOS was evaluated for its effect on postprandial levels of insulin, glucose and triglycerides. The clinical trial consisted of 40 patients: 20 with grade I obesity, and 20 normal weight. The normal weight group were administered 40 g of placebo plus their breakfast; patients with obesity received their breakfast and additionally 40 g of yacon syrup (containing 14 g of FOS). Blood samples were taken after 15, 30, 45, 60, 90 and 120 min. Results showed lower glucose and insulin concentration after consumption of yacon syrup in comparison to placebo after 30 min. Postprandial decrease of glucose and insulin levels following yacon syrup rich in FOS was confirmed (Adriano *et al.* 2019).

In a study conducted by Dehghan *et al.* (2014), 52 patients with type 2 diabetes were given a dose of 10 g of oligofructose plus inulin per day. A decrease in plasma glucose levels and reduction in glycosylated hemoglobin levels were found.

13.4.5 Effects on Serum Lipid and Cholesterol Concentrations

Lipid and cholesterol concentration in the host can also be influenced following prebiotic intake. Al-Sheraji *et al.* (2013) reported that there are several possible mechanisms by which prebiotics may lower cholesterol, such as: (i) increased viscosity in the upper intestinal tract may act as a physical barrier and decrease the re-absorption of fats; (ii) reduced cecal pH lowers solubility of bile acids and lipid absorption; (iii) altered hepatic triacylglycerol synthesis leads to a decrease in serum (LDL-C) cholesterol concentration; (iv) fermentation end-products of prebiotics such as propionate reach the liver by the portal vein and inhibit cholesterol pathways by the inhibition of HMG-CoA reductase; (v) reduced serum insulin and glucose occasioned by prebiotic intake stimulate the production of lipogenic enzymes.

Zhou *et al.* (2018) studied the effects of prebiotic inclusion in the diet on the neonatal characteristics of pregnant sows, and the results showed enhanced serum lipid profiles, a higher tolerance to glucose and good resistance to insulin. Also, an increase in the levels of propionate and butyrate during pregnancy was observed, along with an increase in fecal bile acid excretion and calcium digestibility. Several reports provided evidence that FOS decreases the de novo synthesis of triglycerides in the liver. The reduction in triglycerides, total cholesterol (TC) and LDL-C can reduce the risks of cardiovascular diseases (Jameson *et al.* 2014).

13.4.6 Improving Mineral Adsorption

Several studies report that FOS also enhance the absorption of minerals, increase bone density and prevent osteopenia (Arjmandi *et al.* 2010; Hooshmand *et al.* 2010; Kuugbee *et al.* 2016; Wang *et al.* 2010). Mineral absorption and bioavailability can be influenced by the cecal environment. This environment is modified when FOS are fermented and SCFAs and organic acids are produced. The presence of these compounds lowers the luminal pH in the large intestine and modifies ion speciation, enhancing mineral solubility in the luminal fluid and facilitating the transfer of ions. Also, the improved gut absorptive area caused by cell vitality is involved in enhanced mineral absorption (Arjmandi *et al.* 2010; Chen *et al.* 2016; Hooshmand *et al.* 2010). Roberfroid (2002) reported an increase in the apparent absorption of calcium after the administration of 15 g per day of oligofructose or 40 g per day of inulin. Improvement in magnesium absorption after FOS intake has also been observed (Al Sheraji *et al.* 2013; Bornet *et al.* 2002). Beneficial effects produced in the host derived from FOS intake are illustrated in Figure 13.2 and Table 13.1.

13.5 FOS Production

FOS are produced by biosynthesis or by hydrolysis using sucrose as substrate or inulin respectively. For the synthesis, enzymes such as β-fructofuranosidase (FFase; 3.2.1.26) and fructosyltransferase (FTase; 2.4.1.9) are applied to catalyze sucrose bioconversion into

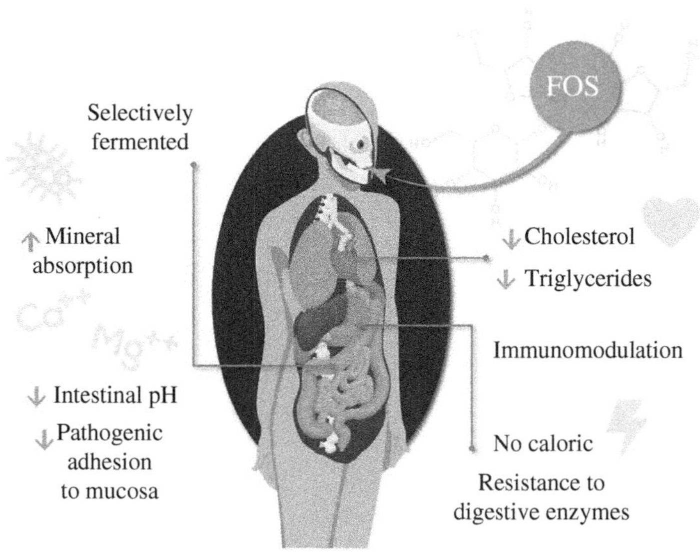

Figure 13.2 Beneficial effects produced in the host by fructooligosaccharide (FOS) intake.

Table 13.1 Evaluation of FOS beneficial effects by different in vitro, in vivo and clinical trials.

Dose/prebiotic	Model	Beneficial effect	Reference
Prebiotic activity			
scGOS/lcFOS plus fermented milk	Mixture of FOS and fermented milk administered to rats, T= 21 days	↓ Diarrhea symptomatology; protective effect against rotavirus infection	Rigo-Adrover *et al.* (2019)
Orafti® inulin-type fructans	Healthy infants (n = 209), prebiotic administration, T= 24 weeks	↑ Population of *Bifidobacterium* ↑ Resistant gut microbiota population ↑Immunomodulation	Soldi *et al.* (2019)
FOS	Broiler chickens (n = 180) 3 dietary treatments from d1 to 21	↑ Diverse microbiota ↓Pathogenic *Helicobacter* and *Desulfovibrio*	Shang *et al.* (2018)
Obesity and diabetes			
FOS-enriched inulin	52 Diabetic women 10 g/day 8 weeks	↓ Fasting glucose, ↓ glycosylated Hb, ↓ IL-6, ↓ TNF-α, ↓ LPS	Dehghan *et al.* (2014)
FOS + *L. acidophilus*, *B. bifidum*	20 Adults with type 2 diabetes, 50–60 years old, 30-day period	↑ HDLeC, ↓ glycemia	Moroti *et al.* (2012)
Capsule containing: 100 mg FOS + *L. acidophilus*, *L. casei*, *L. rhamnosus*, *L. bulgaricus*, *B. brevis*, *B. longum*	54 Adults with type 2 diabetes, 35–70 years old, 8 weeks	↓ hs-CRP, ↑ GSH, ↓ fasting glucose	Asemi *et al.* (2013)
scGOS/lcFOS	Prebiotic blend or synbiotics + *B. breve* M-16V) postnatal (PN) day 42, mice C57BL/6 J, 8 weeks	Synbiotics ↑ protect against diet- induced obesity in adult mice	Mischke *et al.* (2018)
scFOS	48 axenic C57BL/6J mice. Diet: containing 10% of scFOS for 7 weeks	↑*Bifidobacterium* and *Clostridium coccoides* ↓ Insulinemia	Respondek *et al.* (2013)
Mineral absorption			
Dried plum (DP) polyphenols + FOS	180 3-month-old female ovariectomized (Ovx) rats with osteoporosis	Diets supplemented with 5% FOS + 7.5% DP ↓ Bone mineral density loss ↓Calcium loss	Arjmandi *et al.* (2010)
Genistin + FOS	48 ovariectomized (OVX) female rats	Combination: genistin-rich isoflavones diet + 5% FOS ↑ Bone mineral density	Hooshmand *et al.* (2010)

(*Continued*)

Table 13.1 (Continued)

Dose/prebiotic	Model	Beneficial effect	Reference
FOS	60 Kun-Ming mice were fed diets to evaluate the effects of FOS and phytic acid	FOS ↑ absorption rate of calcium, iron and magnesium	Wang *et al.* (2010)
scFOS	10 g/day, 36 days. Administered to female adolescents	↑ Magnesium and vitamin D absorption	van den Heuvel *et al.* (2009)

FOS, fructooligosaccharides; GOS, galactooligosaccharides; GSH, growth stimulating hormone; HDLeC, human dermal lymphatic endothelial cells; hs-CRP, high-sensitivity C-reactive protein; IL, interleukin; lc, long chain; LPS, lipopolysaccharide; sc, short chain; TNF, tumor necrosis factor.
Sources: Based on Rigo-Adrover *et al.* (2019); Soldi *et al.* (2019); Shang *et al.* (2018).

FOS. These enzymes possess hydrolysis and transfructosylation activity, as they act on sucrose by cleaving β-1,2 linkages and transfer the fructosyl moiety to an acceptor molecule, which could be sucrose or another FOS; glucose is released as a by-product (Ganaie *et al.* 2014; Sangeetha *et al.* 2005). FOS synthesis could also lead to production of neo-FOS in which fructosyl moieties are linked at the β(2–6) position of sucrose, forming neokestose and 6-kestose, respectively (Linde *et al.* 2012; Ning *et al.* 2010; Sheu *et al.* 2013a; Zambelli *et al.* 2014). FOS production by hydrolysis is performed by inulinases such as exoinulinase (2,1-β-D-fructan fructohydrolase, EC 3.2.1.80), which acts on the non-reducing β(2,1) end of inulin, cleaving fructose, and endoinulinases (2,1-β-D-fructan-fructan hydrolase, EC, 3.2.1.7) which act on internal linkages of inulin (Mutanda *et al.* 2014; Rawat *et al.* 2015; Singh *et al.* 2017). FOS mixtures obtained by synthesis and hydrolysis can present several differences such as different length of fructooligosaccharides (usually oligosaccharides obtained by hydrolysis are larger) and not all the oligosaccharides have the same terminal glucose (depending on the type of inulinases) (Mutanda *et al.* 2014).

These enzymes are produced by several microbial sources such as bacteria, yeasts and fungi and depending on this microbial source a wide variety of FOS types, yields and enzyme activity can be exhibited. Bacterial sources such as *B. amyloliquefaciens* (Li *et al.* 2015; Tian and Karboune 2012; Tian *et al.* 2014) are reported to produce levan-type FOS. Yeast sources such as *Xanthophyllomyces* and *Rhodotorula* can produce neo-FOS (Alvarado-Huallanco and Maugeri Filho 2011; Gimeno-Pérez *et al.* 2015; Hernalsteens and Maugeri 2008; Ning *et al.* 2012; Sheu *et al.* 2013a; Soares *et al.* 2014). Fungal strains that are the most reported for FOS production report mainly *Aspergillus* species such as *A. oryzae* (Muñiz-Márquez *et al.* 2016; 2019), *A. japonicus* (Mussatto and Teixeira 2010; Mussatto *et al.* 2013; Sheu *et al.* 2013b), *A. ibericus* (Nobre *et al.* 2018b, 2018c), and other fungi such as *Aureobasidium pullulans* (Castro *et al.* 2017, 2019) and *Penicillium* (Nascimento *et al.* 2016; Nobre *et al.* 2019; Zambelli *et al.* 2014).

13.5.1 FOS Formation Kinetics

As mentioned previously, FOS synthesis is mediated by a series of hydrolysis and transfructosylation reactions that depend on the amount of substrate and enzyme, enzyme source and grade of purity of the enzyme, among other process conditions. Therefore, several authors have studied FOS formation kinetics and have proposed several equations that explain the mechanism of FOS synthesis (Alvarado-Huallanco and Maugeri Filho 2011; Ganaie *et al.* 2014; Khandekar *et al.* 2014; Romano *et al.* 2016; Vega and Zuniga-Hansen 2014). Although differences are displayed between enzymes, the main mechanism remains very similar and is explained in a general way as follows.

At the beginning of the reaction, the availability of sucrose (GF) is high. The reaction is displaced to the production of kestose (GF2), with liberation of glucose (G). Equation 1 will exemplify two molecules of sucrose (GF) that act as fructose donors and acceptors for the formation of one molecule of glucose (G) and one molecule of 1-kestose (GF2), where the substrate sucrose (GF) binds with enzyme (E) to form enzyme–sucrose complex (E-GF). Equations collectively represent the hydrolysis of E-GF to glucose (G) and fructose (F) via the formation of enzyme–fructose complex (E-F) and then the enzyme transfers the fructosyl group to another sucrose (GF) molecule to form kestose (GF2) (Equation 1). Once the GF concentration is lower than GF2, GF2 acts as both fructosyl donor and acceptor to produce nystose (GF3). A high concentration of kestose (GF2) needs to be present in the media to act as donor and acceptor of fructosyl units so in Equation 2 we will exemplify nystose (GF3) formation parting from two kestose (GF2) molecules. As a result, and considering that GF had been mostly consumed, GF2 is no longer produced but GF3 is synthesized. At first, the enzyme binds to a GF2 molecule (E-GF2) to hydrolyze and cleave a fructosyl group (E-F), then the enzyme transfers the fructosyl group to another GF2 acting as acceptor, forming GF3. In the case of GF4 formation, the steps to be followed are the same: when enough GF3 has accumulated in the media, it can act as donor and acceptor to form GF4. GF4 production is strongly determined by initial sucrose concentration and reaction time, as higher efficiency of production is achieved at lower initial concentrations of sucrose and prolonged reaction times.

Equations:

1) Formation of kestose (GF2):

$$\mathrm{GF + E + GF \leftrightarrow E - GF + GF \leftrightarrow E - F + GF + G \leftrightarrow GF2 + G + E}$$

2) Formation of nystose (GF3):

$$\mathrm{GF2 + GF2 + E \leftrightarrow E - GF2 + GF2 \leftrightarrow GF + GF2 + E - F \leftrightarrow GF + GF3 + E}$$

3) Formation of 1-FN (GF4):

$$\mathrm{GF3 + GF3 + E \leftrightarrow E - GF3 + GF3 \leftrightarrow GF2 + GF3 + E - F \leftrightarrow GF2 + GF4 + E}$$

4) * Hydrolysis:

$$\mathrm{E + GF \leftrightarrow E - GF \leftrightarrow E - G + F \leftrightarrow G + F + E}$$

On the contrary, at higher initial concentrations of sucrose, GF2 is synthesized at a greater proportion and takes more time to displace the reaction to GF3 synthesis. Therefore, GF3 production is less efficient (in terms of yield) and if there is not a high enough concentration of GF3, consequently the production of GF4 production is less efficient. This indicates that the production of GF4 is determined by the kinetics of synthesis of GF2 and GF3. As long as these reactions occur, glucose that is liberated in the reaction mixture can act as an enzyme inhibitor, generating more hydrolysis (Equation 4).

Hydrolysis can occur at all steps of synthesis and it is reported that hydrolysis/transfer ratio is highly influenced by initial sucrose concentration (Alvarado-Huallanco and Maugeri Filho 2011; Ganaie *et al.* 2014; Khandekar *et al.* 2014; Kralj *et al.* 2018; Romano *et al.* 2016; Vega and Zuniga-Hansen 2014). Hydrolysis predominates over transfructosylation activity at lower sucrose concentrations (Khandekar *et al.* 2014). FFase possesses hydrolytic activity in low sucrose concentration and transfructosylating activity in high sucrose concentration (Ganaie *et al.* 2014). In addition, high sucrose concentrations may also exclude H_2O from entering the active site, thereby also directing enzymes towards increased transfructosylation activity and reduced hydrolytic activity (Kralj *et al.* 2018). The inhibitory effects of glucose and fructose were studied by Alvarado-Huallanco and Maugeri Filho (2011). They tested concentrations of fructose and glucose from 5 to 20% (w/v), using sucrose, 1-kestose and nystose as substrates. Glucose showed a competitive inhibitory effect on sucrose, 1-kestose and nystose uptake. In the case of fructose, it only exhibited an inhibitory effect at concentrations above 50%, which was considered negligible since the fructose concentration in the reaction mixture never reached such a value and therefore the actual impact on the kinetics of the reaction was considered insignificant. Romano *et al.* (2016) evaluated the effect of initial sucrose concentration at different reaction times and found that, at lower sucrose concentrations, the maximum yield of FOS was reached faster (after 1.5 h of reaction time) and after that FOS yield decreased. FOS produced at lower sucrose concentrations were kestose (GF2), nystose (GF3) and 1-FN (GF4); besides FOS, maximum glucose yield was also higher at lower concentrations of sucrose. On the contrary, at high concentrations of sucrose (40% and 60% w/v), the maximum FOS yield is reached after a longer reaction time and was then stable for the remainder of the 6 h reaction time. The analysis of yield of GF2, GF3 and GF4 in the course of the reactions revealed that GF4 was not produced at high sucrose concentration. Statistical comparisons revealed no significant differences for the maximum FOS yield ($P > 0.05$) achieved in each condition of synthesis.

13.5.2 Biotechnological Production of FOS

FOS are synthesized conventionally with purified enzymes, achieving good fermentation yields. However, the use of microorganisms containing the respective enzymes without needing the enzyme production and purification steps has also been employed recently with great success. In the following sections, we will review and discuss both FOS production processes in depth.

In FOS production, the yield, purity and productivity are the key points on which the efficiency of the process is evaluated. Comparison between FOS enzymatic synthesis is usually about enzymatic activity, FOS production, variety of FOS produced, amounts of glucose, fructose and sucrose residual in the media, and FOS yield, which is the most important because it determines how well the enzyme bioconverts sucrose to FOS under the evaluated conditions. As mentioned previously, every enzyme has a different hydrolysis/transfer ratio, which means some enzymes will bioconvert sucrose into FOS more efficiently, leaving fewer residual sugars such as unreacted sucrose, fructose and glucose produced by hydrolysis. On the other hand, an enzyme with higher hydrolyzing activity could lead to deficient FOS synthesis and more residual sugars present in the media, resulting in a FOS mixture with low purity. Purity is strongly related to FOS yield; a better FOS yield represents a higher percentage of FOS in the mixture meaning a lower amount of mono- and disaccharides and, consequently, higher FOS purity. FOS yield is calculated as the amount of FOS produced by the amount of initial sucrose present in the media and is usually represented as g FOS/g sucrose. FOS purity is calculated as the amount of FOS divided into the amount of the other carbohydrates present in the mixture and is usually represented as FOS%.

The maximum theoretical yield for FOS produced by microbial FTases is around 55–60% based on the initial sucrose concentration (Sangeetha *et al.* 2005).

FOS research usually progresses in the following stages. First, strains with the potential to produce FTases or FFases are isolated and evaluated. Next, the enzymes of selected strains are evaluated for the best conditions in which they can achieve high production yields. In this step different enzyme purities are tested under different reaction conditions and FOS production kinetics are developed with the enzyme of interest. This is followed by optimization of the process: at this point FOS are produced at good conversion yield. For FOS purification, research is focused on removing residual sugars by employing different purification strategies. The final stage is prebiotic evaluation. Some researchers evaluate their FOS mixtures produced in vitro with probiotic strains simulating gastrointestinal conditions and in vivo with animal models hoping to obtain beneficial effects or improve the health of a sick individual.

13.5.3 Enzymatic Synthesis

As discussed earlier, enzymatic synthesis of FOS is carried out with fructosyltransferase (FTase) and β-fructofuranosidase (FFase) enzymes. These enzymes are produced by several microorganisms and can be intracellular or extracellular; also, a microorganism can produce several FTases or FFases with different activities and production yields. To evaluate the capacity of a strain to produce β-fructofuranosidase or fructosyltransferase, enzymatic reactions are performed to estimate the strain's FOS synthesis ability. Commonly, to estimate the enzymatic activity of a strain takes multiple steps to determine if the strain is capable of producing high FFase or FTase activity, which may not be feasible for screening a wide range of strains. Zhang *et al.* (2019) worked on the development of a plate chromogenic assay that forms pink coloration around colonies that exhibit FFase activity. It is based on two enzymes (glucose oxidase and peroxidase) that react with glucose released from the hydrolysis of sucrose. The authors evaluated the method on the screening of an *Aspergillus niger* ATCC 20611 mutant library and the positive strains for FFase production were evaluated for FOS production. The resulting positive strains were then confirmed by thin-layer chromatography (TLC) to possess the highest FFase activity, proving that this technique is suitable for fungal strains.

Enzyme preparation is often carried out by fermentation with mediums rich in sucrose (between 50 and 200 g/L of sucrose). Enzyme preparation can be performed either by submerged fermentation (SmF) or by solid state fermentation (SSF) with working pH around

5.5, and growing temperatures between 25 and 30 °C. On the other hand, enzymatic activity is performed in saturated sucrose solutions (between 100 and 600 g/L) with buffered pH around 5.5 and optimal temperatures between 50 and 60 °C.

Yang *et al.* (2016) reported the expression of FTase from *A. niger* YZ59 in *Pichia pastoris* GS115 reaching 1020.0 U/mL of enzymatic activity at an optimum pH and temperature of 5.5 and 55 °C respectively. Xu *et al.* (2014) reported optimal enzymatic activity for a neokestose-producing β-fructofuranosidase at pH 5.5 and 60 °C using sucrose solution (500 g/L) with a total FOS production of 224.7 g/L.

Enzyme immobilization is often reported to improve stability and reusability of enzymes. Chen *et al.* (2014) tested the immobilization of β-fructofuranosidase on chitosan-coated magnetic nanoparticles to produce FOS. After ten batches, the immobilized enzyme retained 55% of its initial activity, having a maximum FOS yield of 0.59 g FOS/g sucrose using a 500 g/L sucrose solution at an optimal pH of 5.5 and temperature of 60 °C.

There are some commercial enzyme preparations that can be employed for FOS synthesis. Vega-Paulino and Zuñiga-Hansen (2012) evaluated the transfructosylation activity of 25 commercial enzyme preparations used in the food industry and obtained FOS production yields between 0.58 and 0.62 g FOS/g sucrose after 6 h of reaction time. Pectinex Ultra SP-L, Rohapect CM, Vis-cozyme L and Pectinex Smash exhibited the highest transfrustosylation/hydrolysis ratio. Lorenzoni *et al.* (2014) worked on the partial purification and immobilization of the commercial enzyme preparation Viscozyme L. The enzyme was immobilized on glutaraldehyde-activated chitosan particles which allowed it to be reused 50 times (100 min per batch at 50 °C and pH 5.5), resulting in an average yield of 0.55 g FOS/g sucrose.

13.5.4 Whole Cell/One-step Fermentation

Whole cell fermentation involves the production and activity of the enzyme in a single-step process (Fernández *et al.* 2004). The whole cell fermentation process presents several advantages: (i) the enzyme purification step is avoided as a result of the use of whole cells containing the enzymes; (ii) better efficiency can be achieved as the enzymes are more secure in the cells and are most resistant to temperature and pH changes; (iii) cells can be used repeatedly, avoiding an immobilization process (Zeng *et al.* 2016). A study evaluating whole cells of *A. niger* 6640 demonstrated that is possible to synthesize FOS by whole cell fermentation, obtaining a FOS yield of 50.21% (Liu *et al.* 2012). Nobre *et al.* (2018b) reported the use of *Aspergillus ibericus* whole cells for FOS production, obtaining excellent results after process optimization (temperature and pH) with production yields of 0.53 g FOS/g sucrose in flask fermentation and 0.64 g FOS/g sucrose at bioreactor scale. High yields of FOS production utilizing whole cells have also been reported by Dominguez *et al.* (2012) and Nobre *et al.* (2016) who each obtained yields of 0.63 g FOS/g sucrose. Results obtained recently by whole cell fermentations point to this strategy as having potential to develop for FOS commercial production as it presents some advantages over enzymatic synthesis (currently used for commercial production of FOS).

13.5.5 Agro-industrial Residues and Bioresources Employed for FOS Production

In the search to develop low-cost processes but also to find a use for discarded agro-wastes or to exploit low-cost bioresources, several researchers have focused on the development of strategies to produce FOS in high yields without the use of just sucrose solutions or defined synthetic media. These bioresources and agro-wastes are commonly a complex mixture of carbohydrates, proteins and minerals that can be useful for the growth of microorganisms and production of FOS-producing enzymes. Among the substrates reported for FOS production are sources rich in sucrose such as sugar cane and sugar beet molasses, spent osmotic solutions, aguamiel and syrups (Coetzee *et al.* 2020; de la Rosa *et al.* 2019; Dorta *et al.* 2006; Ghazi *et al.* 2006; Muñiz-Márquez *et al.* 2016; 2018; Ruiz *et al.* 2014; Shin *et al.* 2004;) and sources rich in nutrients or with desired properties for FOS production by solid state fermentation such as banana leaf and peel, sugar cane bagasse, coffee pulp and coffee silverskin, and apple pomace, among others (Dapper *et al.* 2016; de la Rosa *et al.* 2019; Ganaie *et al.* 2017; Gnaneshwar Goud *et al.* 2013; Mussatto *et al.* 2013; Patil *et al.* 2011).

13.6 FOS Purification

One of the challenges in the production of FOS is that after the fermentation there remains a mixture of sugars with the presence of monosaccharides, disaccharides and FOS, decreasing the prebiotic activity of the product. Due to that the product has a low purity, containing about 50–60% FOS, 30–40% glucose and 10–20% sucrose. Therefore, the product requires a further purification process so that it can be considered prebiotic and incorporated into commercial dietetic products that are healthy and suitable for diabetic patients.

Different techniques and strategies have been reported for the removal of di- and monosaccharides in the medium. Some techniques are used for low volumes and others for large-scale separation, and commonly a combination of different downstream techniques is used to improve FOS purity.

13.6.1 Nanofiltration

Nanofiltration has proved successful at laboratory scale for purification. Kuhn *et al.* (2010) reported the use of nanofiltration for the purification of FOS obtained by enzymatic synthesis from cane molasses. The process included two nanofiltration steps with the same membrane: the first step consisted of a diafiltration and concentration process, and the second consisted of nanofiltration of the permeate, resulting in FOS purities over 90% with 80% yield.

13.6.2 Activated Charcoal

Another technique that has given excellent results is the employment of activated charcoal, which is less expensive than chromatography resins and has good adsorption capacity for sugars of different molecular weight (Kovács *et al.* 2014; Nobre *et al.* 2015). Kuhn and Filho

(2010) reported the use of an activated charcoal fixed bed column for the purification of a FOS mixture obtained by enzymatic synthesis. The effects of ethanol concentration and temperature were analyzed using a central composite design. A good separation coefficient was obtained between glucose and FOS and between fructose and FOS (3.99 ± 0.07 and 2.89 ± 0.36, respectively) with ethanol concentration of 15% (v/v) as eluent and temperature of 50 °C. FOS purification could be obtained up to 80% and 97.8% of product recovery. Nevertheless, the purification could not achieve a good separation between FOS and sucrose. The use of activated charcoal was also reported by Nobre *et al.* (2012). In this study the aim was to improve FOS purity from a fermented mixture in which the other purpose was desalting the medium. Different gradients of ethanol/water were evaluated and optimized for the best desorption and separation of sugars from the fermentation broth. The process allowed removal of up to 93% (w/w) of the monosaccharides with water elution and recovery of 74.5% (w/w) of the FOS with a purity of 92.9% (w/w) with ethanol solutions from 10 to 40% (v/v). The use of activated charcoal was also reported for the purification of a FOS fermentation mixture produced by *Penicillium citreonigrum* URM 4459, achieving a purity of the FOS mixture up to 92% (w/w) (Nobre *et al.* 2019). In summary, process simplicity and effective purification of FOS mixtures make activated charcoal one of the best strategies for FOS purification.

13.6.3 Microbial Treatments

Microbial treatments present another alternative for purification of FOS mixtures. These can be classified as successive fermentation and co-culture in which usually two different microorganisms are employed, a FOS producer strain and another strain capable of using the small saccharides as substrates and also incapable of hydrolyzing FOS in the mixture (Castro *et al.* 2019; Nobre *et al.* 2016, 2018c). In the case of successive fermentation, FOS are first synthesized by the producer strain and the microorganism is removed at the end of the fermentation to proceed to a second fermentation performed by the second strain that is capable of improving FOS purity of the mixture, which usually contains fructose, glucose, unreacted sucrose and FOS. Co-culture is performed with the two microorganisms acting at the same time in a mixed culture. In this case an advantage is that only one fermentation is carried out, but more factors need to be taken into account such as compatibility between strains, enough nutrients in the media (sometimes strains require different nutrients and the media have to be optimized), growing pH for both strains, and also to ensure that strains do not compete for sucrose because that affects FOS yield. Nobre *et al.* (2016) evaluated both types of microbial treatment, co-culture and successive fermentation. In this study *Aureobasidium pullulans* was used as the FOS producer strain and *Saccharomyces cerevisiae* to purify the FOS mixture. Successive fermentation was more favorable for FOS purification as it was able to reach 81.6 ± 0.8% (w/w) FOS purity. In co-culture, the strain *S. cerevisiae* demanded different nutrients than *A. pullulans* as it was unable to grow in the FOS production medium, so the medium was optimized to meet the needs of both strains. FOS yield was also affected as invertase activity from *S. cerevisiae* could compete with the fungi for sucrose, decreasing the sucrose concentration available for FOS production. To overcome sucrose competitivity between strains, Nobre *et al.* (2018c) proposed the use of *S. cerevisiae* YIL162W, a genetically modified strain incapable of hydrolyzing sucrose, in co-culture with *A. ibericus* (the FOS producer). The process was optimized to ensure the best broth composition, inoculation conditions, temperature and pH. Co-culture was performed successfully as it led to purities in the FOS mixtures of 97.4 ± 0.2% (w/w) in flasks and 93.8 ± 0.7% (w/w) in a bioreactor. The use of microbial treatments employing immobilized cells has been reported by Lu *et al.* (2013), Sheu *et al.* (2013b) and Castro *et al.* (2019), obtaining purities of 98.2%, 80.1% and 67.0% (w/w) respectively, employing the strains *Pichia heimii*, *Wickerhamomyces anomalus* and *S. cerevisiae*. The use of microbial treatments offers a good alternative to improve purities of FOS mixtures and has great potential to develop through the employment of strains able to deplete small saccharides to produce other value-added compounds.

13.7 New Developments in Food

Development of functional foods has led to the inclusion of FOS in formulations, not only for their prebiotic activity but also for their technological properties as they add desirable textures to creams, ice creams, yoghurts and beverages.

Speranza *et al.* (2018) developed a functional fresh cream cheese with prebiotics (FOS, inulin and lactulose) and *B. animalis* subsp. *lactis* DSM 10140 or *Lactobacillus reuteri* DSM 20016. At the in vitro stage FOS proved to be able to protect *Lb. reuteri* DSM 20016 and were added to the cheese formulation along with lactulose, resulting in maintaining cell viability above the recommended level during 28 days of storage at 4 °C and also presenting good sensory characteristics.

Functional desserts have also been developed with the addition of FOS. In a study, Valencia *et al.* (2016) developed creamy milk chocolate desserts containing *Lactobacillus paracasei* subsp. *paracasei* LBC 81 and FOS, obtaining formulations with good sensory attributes and maintaining the viability of *L. paracasei* in 8 log CFU/g during 28 days of storage. Balthazar *et al.* (2017) assessed the effects of the inclusion of several prebiotics (including FOS) to replace fat in non-fat sheep milk ice cream. Prebiotic addition significantly decreased the melting time and temperature and increased the white intensity and glass transition temperature.

The use of FOS in fermented beverages from maize and rice with the probiotic strains *Lactobacillus plantarum* CCMA 0743, *Torulaspora delbrueckii* CCMA 0235 and *Lactobacillus acidophilus* LACA 4 was evaluated (Freire *et al.* 2017). FOS concentration of 50 g/L favored the growth of *L. acidophilus* LACA 4 and maintained cell viability of 10^7 CFU/mL after 28 days of storage at 4 °C. The beverages also showed good acceptability by more than 50% of consumers.

Other uses of prebiotics in food matrices such as edible coatings, dehydrated apple, papaya nectar and yoghurts have also been reported (Bambace *et al.* 2019; Braga and Conti-Silva 2015; Delgado-Fernández *et al.* 2019; González-Herrera *et al.* 2016).

13.8 Conclusion

The importance of FOS lies in their ability to impact and improve host health via modulation of intestinal microbiota and the immune system. Regular intake unchains a series of benefits, reducing the risk of chronic diseases such as colon cancer, diabetes and osteoporosis, among others. A series of techniques have been developed to improve FOS production yields to satisfy industry needs for FOS in terms of volume of production, low-cost processes and purer FOS products with less mono- and disaccharides in FOS mixtures, improving their scope of use in industry. However, there is still a need to develop large-scale processes that involve simpler and less expensive fermentation techniques, exploiting low-cost substrates and sources for FOS synthesis.

Acknowledgements

Orlando D. de la Rosa acknowledges CONACYT for the financial support during the PhD program in Food Science and Technology (CVU 860996) offered by the Autonomous University of Coahuila, Mexico.

References

Adriano, L.S., Dionísio, A.P., Abreu, F.A.P. de, Carioca, A.A.F., Zocolo, G.J., Wurlitzer, N.J., Pinto, C. de O., de Oliveira, A.C. and Sampaio, H.A. de C. (2019). Yacon syrup reduces postprandial glycemic response to breakfast: A randomized, crossover, double-blind clinical trial. *Food Research International*, 126: 108682.

Al-Sheraji, S.H., Ismail, A., Manap, M.Y., Mustafa, S., Yusof, R.M. and Hassan, F.A., (2013). Prebiotics as functional foods: A review. *Journal of Functional Foods*, 5: 1542–1553.

Alvarado-Huallanco, M.B. and Maugeri Filho, F. (2011) Kinetic studies and modelling of the production of fructooligosaccharides by fructosyltransferase from Rhodotorula sp. *Catalysis Science and Technology*, 1: 1043–1050.

Anal, A.K., Koirala, S. and Shrestha, S. (2021). Gut microbiome and their possible roles in combating mycotoxins. In: *Mycotoxins in Food and Beverages*, 213–235. CRC Press.

Anand, S., Mandal, S., Singh, K.S., Patil, P. and Tomar, S.K. (2018). Synbiotic combination of Lactobacillus rhamnosus NCDC 298 and short chain fructooligosaccharides prevents enterotoxigenic Escherichia coli infection. *Lwt – Food Science and Technology*, 98: 329–334.

Arjmandi, B.H., Johnson, C.D., Campbell, S.C., Hooshmand, S., Chai, S.C. and Akhter, M.P. (2010). Combining fructooligosaccharide and dried plum has the greatest effect on restoring bone mineral density among select functional foods and bioactive compounds. *Journal of Medicinal Food*. 13: 312–319.

Asemi, Z., Zare, Z., Shakeri, H., Sabihi, S.S. and Esmaillzadeh, A. (2013). Effect of multispecies probiotic supplements on metabolic profiles, hs-CRP, and oxidative stress in patients with type 2 diabetes. *Annals of Nutrition and Metabolism*, 63: 1–9.

Azimirad, M., Meshkini, S., Ahmadifard, N. and Hoseinifar, S.H. (2016). The effects of feeding with synbiotic (Pediococcus acidilactici and fructooligosaccharide) enriched adult Artemia on skin mucus immune responses, stress resistance, intestinal microbiota and performance of angelfish (Pterophyllum scalare). *Fish and Shellfish Immunology*, 54: 516–522.

Baliou, S., Adamaki, M., Spandidos, D.A., Kyriakopoulos, A.M., Christodoulou, I. and Zoumpourlis, V. (2019). The microbiome, its molecular mechanisms and its potential as a therapeutic strategy against colorectal carcinogenesis (Review). *World Academy of Sciences Journal*, 1: 3–19.

Balthazar, C.F., Silva, H.L.A., Cavalcanti, R.N., Esmerino, E.A., Cappato, L.P., Abud, Y.K.D., Moraes, J., Andrade, M.M., Freitas, M.Q., Sant'Anna, C., Raices, R.S.L., Silva, M.C. and Cruz, A.G. (2017). Prebiotics addition in sheep milk ice cream: A rheological, microstructural and sensory study. *Journal of Functional Foods*, 35: 564–573.

Bambace, M.F., Alvarez, M.V. and Moreira, M. del R. (2019). Novel functional blueberries: Fructo-oligosaccharides and probiotic lactobacilli incorporated into alginate edible coatings. *Food Research International*, 122: 653–660.

Belenguer, A., Duncan, S.H., Calder, A.G., Holtrop, G., Louis, P., Lobley, G.E. and Flint, H.J. (2006). Two routes of metabolic cross-feeding between *Bifidobacterium adolescentis* and butyrate-producing anaerobes from the human gut. *Applied and Environmental Microbiology*, 72: 3593–3599.

Benkeblia, N. (2013). Fructooligosaccharides and fructans analysis in plants and food crops. *Journal of Chromatography A*, 131: 54–61.

Bersaneti, G.T., Garcia, S., Mali, S. and Pedrine Colabone Celligoi, M.A. (2019). Evaluation of the prebiotic activities of edible starch films with the addition of nystose from Bacillus subtilis natto. *Lwt*, 116: 108502.

Bindels, L.B., Delzenne, N.M., Cani, P.D. and Walter, J. (2015). Towards a more comprehensive concept for prebiotics. *Nature Reviews Gastroenterology & Hepatology*, 12: 303–310.

Bornet, F.R.J., Brouns, F., Tashiro, Y. and Duvillier, V. (2002). Nutritional aspects of short-chain fructooligosaccharides: Natural occurrence, chemistry, physiology and health implications. *Digestive and Liver Disease*, 34(Suppl 2): S111–S120.

Braga, H.F. and Conti-Silva, A.C. (2015). Papaya nectar formulated with prebiotics: Chemical characterization and sensory acceptability. *LWT - Food Science and Technology*, 62: 854–860.

Butler, M.I., Cryan, J.F. and Dinan, T.G. (2019). Man and the microbiome: A new theory of everything? *Annual Review of Clinical Psychology*, 15: 371–398.

Campbell, J.M., Bauer, L.L., Fahey, G.C., Hogarth, A.J.C.L., Wolf, B.W. and Hunter, D.E. (1997). Selected fructooligosaccharide (1-kestose, nystose, and 1F-β-fructofuranosylnystose) composition of foods and feeds. *Journal of Agricultural and Food Chemistry*, 45: 3076–3082.

Castro, C.C., Nobre, C., Duprez, M.E., De Weireld, G. and Hantson, A.L. (2017). Screening and selection of potential carriers to immobilize Aureobasidium pullulans cells for fructo-oligosaccharides production. *Biochemical Engineering Journal*, 118: 82–90.

Castro, C.C., Nobre, C., De Weireld, G. and Hantson, A-L. (2019). Microbial co-culturing strategies for fructo-oligosaccharide production. *New Biotechnology*, 51: 1–7.

Chen, G., Li, C. and Chen, K. (2016). Fructooligosaccharides: A review on their mechanisms of action and effects. *Studies in Natural Products Chemistry*, 48: 209–229.

Chen, S.C., Sheu, D.C. and Duan, K.J. (2014). Production of fructooligosaccharides using β-fructofuranosidase immobilized onto chitosan-coated magnetic nanoparticles. *Journal of the Taiwan Institute of Chemical Engineers*, 45: 1105–1110.

Choque Delgado, G.T., da Silva Cunha Tamashiro, W.M., Maróstica, M.R. Jr., Moreno, Y.M.F., Pastore, G.M. (2011). The putative effects of prebiotics as immunomodulatory agents. *Food Research International*, 44: 3167–3173.

Coetzee, G., van Rensburg, E. and Görgens, J.F. (2020). Evaluation of the performance of an engineered β-fructofuranosidase from Aspergillus fijiensis to produce short-chain fructooligosaccharides from industrial sugar streams. *Biocatalysis and Agricultural Biotechnology*, 23: 101484.

Comerlato, C.B., Ritter, A.C., Miyamoto, K.N. and Brandelli, A. (2020). Proteomic study of Enterococcus durans LAB18S growing on prebiotic oligosaccharides. *Food Microbiology*, 89: 103430.

Corradini, C., Lantano, C. and Cavazza, A. (2013). Innovative analytical tools to characterize prebiotic carbohydrates of functional food interest. *Analytical and Bioanalytical Chemistry*, 405: 4591–4605.

Courtin, C.M., Swennen, K., Verjans, P. and Delcour, J.A. (2009). Heat and pH stability of prebiotic arabinoxylooligosaccharides, xylooligosaccharides and fructooligosaccharides. *Food Chemistry*, 112: 831–837.

Daguet, D., Pinheiro, I., Verhelst, A., Possemiers, S. and Marzorati, M. (2016). Arabinogalactan and fructooligosaccharides improve the gut barrier function in distinct areas of the colon in the Simulator of the Human Intestinal Microbial Ecosystem. *Journal of Functional Foods*, 20: 369–379.

Dapper, T.B., Arfelli, V. C., Henn, C., Simões, M. A. R., dos Santos, M. F., Della Torre, C. L., da Conceição Silva, J.L., Simão, R.D.C.A.G. and Kadowaki, M.K. (2016). β-Fructofuranosidase production by Aspergillus versicolor isolated from Atlantic forest and grown on apple pomace. *African Journal of Microbiology Research*, 10(25): 938–948.

Darbyshire, B. and Henry, R.J. (1978). The distribution of fructans in onions. *New Phytologist*, 81: 29–34.

de Cossío, L.F., Fourrier, C., Sauvant, J., Everard, A., Capuron, L., Cani, P.D., Layé, S. and Castanon, N. (2016). Impact of prebiotics on metabolic and behavioral alterations in a mouse model of metabolic syndrome. *Brain, Behavior, and Immunity*, 64: 33–49.

de Figueiredo, F. C., de Barros Ranke, F. F. and de Oliva-Neto, P. (2020). Evaluation of xylooligosaccharides and fructooligosaccharides on digestive enzymes hydrolysis and as a nutrient for different probiotics and Salmonella typhimurium. *Lwt*, 118: 108761.

de la Rosa, O., Flores-Gallegos, A. C., Muñíz-Marquez, D., Nobre, C., Contreras-Esquivel, J. C. and Aguilar, C. N. (2019). Fructooligosaccharides production from agro-wastes as alternative low-cost source. *Trends in Food Science & Technology*, 91: 139–146.

Dehghan, P., Pourghassem Gargari, B. and Asghari Jafar-abadi, M. (2014). Oligofructose-enriched inulin improves some inflammatory markers and metabolic endotoxemia in women with type 2 diabetes mellitus: A randomized controlled clinical trial. *Nutrition*, 30: 418–423.

Delcenserie, V., Martel, D., Lamoureux, M., Amiot, J., Boutin, Y. and Roy, D. (2008). Immunomodulatory effects of probiotics in the intestinal tract. *Current Issues in Molecular Biology*, 10: 37–54.

Delgado-Fernández, P., Corzo, N., Olano, A., Hernández-Hernández, O. and Moreno, F.J. (2019). Effect of selected prebiotics on the growth of lactic acid bacteria and physicochemical properties of yoghurts. *International Dairy Journal*, 89: 77–85.

Dominguez, A., Nobre, C., Rodrigues, L.R., Peres, A.M., Torres, D., Rocha, I., Lima, N. and Teixeira, J. (2012). New improved method for fructooligosaccharides production by Aureobasidium pullulans. *Carbohydrate Polymers*, 89: 1174–1179.

Doo, E. H., Schwab, C., Chassard, C. and Lacroix, C. (2019). Cumulative effect of yeast extract and fructooligosaccharide supplementation on composition and metabolic activity of elderly colonic microbiota in vitro. *Journal of Functional Foods.*, 52: 43–53.

Dorta, C., Cruz, R., de Oliva-Neto, P. and Moura, D.J.C. (2006). Sugarcane molasses and yeast powder used in the Fructooligosaccharides production by Aspergillus japonicus -FCL 119T and Aspergillus niger ATCC 20611. *Journal of Industrial Microbiology and Biotechnology*, 33: 1003–1009.

Durieux, A., Fougnies, C., Jacobs, H. and Simon, J.P. (2001). Metabolism of chicory fructooligosaccharides by bifidobacteria. *Biotechnology Letters*, 23: 1523–1527.

Duysburgh, C., Van den Abbeele, P., Krishnan, K., Bayne, T.F. and Marzorati, M. (2019). A synbiotic concept containing spore-forming Bacillus strains and a prebiotic fiber blend consistently enhanced metabolic activity by modulation of the gut microbiome in vitro. *International Journal of Pharmaceutics: X*, 1: 100021.

Elaheh, M., Ali, M.S., Elnaz, M. and Ladan, N. (2016). Prebiotic effect of Jerusalem artichoke (Helianthus tuberosus) fructans on the growth performance of Bifidobacterium bifidum and Escherichia coli. *Asian Pacific Journal of Tropical Disease*, 6: 385–389.

Fernández, E.C., Rajchl, A., Lachman, J., Čížková, H., Kvasnička, F., Kotíková, Z., Milella, L. and Voldřich, M. (2013). Impact of yacon landraces cultivated in the Czech Republic and their ploidy on the short- and long-chain fructooligosaccharides content in tuberous roots. *LWT - Food Science and Technology*, 54: 80–86.

Fernández, R.C., Maresma, B.G., Juárez, A. and Martínez, J. (2004). Production of fructooligosaccharides by β-fructofuranosidase from Aspergillus sp 27H. *Journal of Chemical Technology and Biotechnology*, 79: 268–272.

Freire, A.L., Ramos, C.L. and Schwan, R.F. (2017). Effect of symbiotic interaction between a fructooligosaccharide and probiotic on the kinetic fermentation and chemical profile of maize blended rice beverages. *Food Research International*, 100: 698–707.

Ganaie, M.A., Lateef, A. and Gupta, U.S. (2014). Enzymatic trends of fructooligosaccharides production by microorganisms. *Applied Biochemistry and Biotechnology*, 172: 2143–2159.

Ganaie, M.A., Soni, H., Naikoo, G.A., Santos Oliveira, L.T., Rawat, H.K., Mehta, P.K. and Narain, N. (2017). Screening of low cost agricultural wastes to maximize the fructosyltransferase production and its applicability in generation of fructooligosaccharides by solid state fermentation. *International Biodeterioration & Biodegradation*, 118: 19–26.

Geigerová, M., Bunešová, V., Vlková, E., Salmonová, H. and Rada, V. (2017). Selection of prebiotic oligosaccharides suitable for synbiotic use in calves. *Animal Feed Science and Technology*, 229: 73–78.

Ghazi, I., Fernandez-Arrojo, L., Gomez De Segura, A., Alcalde, M., Plou, F.J. and Ballesteros, A. (2006). Beet sugar syrup and molasses as low-cost feedstock for the enzymatic production of fructo-oligosaccharides. *Journal of Agricultural and Food Chemistry*, 54: 2964–2968.

Gibson, G.R. and Roberfroid, M.B. (1995). Dietary modulation of the human colonic microbiota: introducing the concept of prebiotics. *The Journal of Nutrition*, 125: 1401–1412.

Gibson, G.R., Probert, H.M., Loo, J. Van, Rastall, R.A. and Roberfroid, M.B. (2004). Dietary modulation of the human colonic microbiota: updating the concept of prebiotics. *Nutrition Research Reviews*, 17: 259.

Gibson, G.R., Scott, K.P., Rastall, R.A., Tuohy, K.M., Hotchkiss, A., Dubert-Ferrandon, A., Gareau, M., Murphy, E.F., Saulnier, D., Loh, G., Macfarlane, S., Delzenne, N., Ringel, Y., Kozianowski, G., Dickmann, R., Lenoir-Wijnkook, I., Walker, C. and Buddington, R. (2010). Dietary prebiotics: current status and new definition. *Food Science and Technology Bulletin: Functional Foods*, 7: 1–19.

Gimeno-Pérez, M., Linde, D., Fernández-Arrojo, L., Plou, F.J. and Fernández-Lobato, M. (2015). Heterologous overproduction of β-fructofuranosidase from yeast Xanthophyllomyces dendrorhous, an enzyme producing prebiotic sugars. *Applied Microbiology and Biotechnology*, 99: 3459–3467.

Gnaneshwar Goud, K., Chaitanya, K. and Reddy, G. (2013). Enhanced production of β-d-fructofuranosidase by Saccharomyces cerevisiae using agro-industrial wastes as substrates. *Biocatalysis and Agricultural Biotechnology*, 2: 385–392.

Gomes, A.C., Bueno, A.A., de Souza, R.G.M. and Mota, J.F. (2014). Gut microbiota, probiotics and diabetes. *Nutrition Journal*, 13: 60.

González-Herrera, S.M., Rutiaga-Quiñones, O.M., Aguilar, C.N., Ochoa-Martínez, L.A., Contreras-Esquivel, J C., López, M.G. and Rodríguez-Herrera, R. (2016). Dehydrated apple matrix supplemented with agave fructans, inulin, and oligofructose. *LWT - Food Science and Technology*, 65: 1059–1065.

Hemarajata, P. and Versalovic, J. (2013). Effects of probiotics on gut microbiota: Mechanisms of intestinal immunomodulation and neuromodulation. *Therapeutic Advances in Gastroenterology*, 6: 39–51.

Hernalsteens, S. and Maugeri, F. (2008). Purification and characterisation of a fructosyltransferase from Rhodotorula sp. *Applied Microbiology and Biotechnology*, 79: 589–596.

Hester, S.N., Mastaloudis, A., Gray, R., Antony, J.M., Evans, M. and Wood, S.M. (2018). Efficacy of an anthocyanin and prebiotic blend on intestinal environment in obese male and female subjects. *Journal of Nutrition and Metabolism*, 2018: 7497260.

Hooshmand, S, Juma, S. and Arjmandi, B.H. (2010). Combination of genistin and fructooligosaccharides prevents bone loss in ovarian hormone deficiency. *Journal of Medicinal Food*. 13: 320–325.

Jameson, K., Zhang, Q., Zhao, C., Ramey, D.R., Tershakovec, A.M., Gutkin, S.W. and Marrett, E. (2014). Total and low-density lipoprotein cholesterol in high-risk patients treated with atorvastatin monotherapy in the United Kingdom: analysis of a primary-care database. *Current Medical Research and Opinion*, 30: 655–665.

Jia, E., Zheng, X., Cheng, H., Liu, J., Li, X., Jiang, G., Liu, W. and Zhang, D. (2019). Dietary fructooligosaccharide can mitigate the negative effects of immunity on Chinese mitten crab fed a high level of plant protein diet. *Fish and Shellfish Immunology*, 84: 100–107.

Joseph, N., Vasodavan, K., Saipudin, N.A., Yusof, B.N.M., Kumar, S. and Nordin, S.A. (2019). Gut microbiota and short-chain fatty acids (SCFAs) profiles of normal and overweight school children in Selangor after probiotics administration. *Journal of Functional Foods*, 57: 103–111.

Kahouli, I., Tomaro-Duchesneau, C. and Prakash, S. (2013). Probiotics in colorectal cancer (CRC) with emphasis on mechanisms of action and current perspectives. *Journal of Medical Microbiology*, 62: 1107–1123.

Khandekar, D.C., Palai, T., Agarwal, A. and Bhattacharya, P.K. (2014). Kinetics of sucrose conversion to fructo-oligosaccharides using enzyme (invertase) under free condition. *Bioprocess and Biosystems Engineering*, 37: 2529–2537.

Koh, A., De Vadder, F., Kovatcheva-Datchary, P. and Bäckhed, F. (2016). From dietary fiber to host physiology: Short-chain fatty acids as key bacterial metabolites. *Cell*, 165: 1332–1345.

Koirala, S. and Anal, A.K. (2021). Probiotics-based foods and beverages as future foods and their overall safety and regulatory claims. *Future Foods*, 100013.

Kovács, Z., Benjamins, E., Grau, K., Ur Rehman, A., Ebrahimi, M. and Czermak, P. (2014). Recent developments in manufacturing oligosaccharides with prebiotic functions. *Advances in Biochemical Engineering/Biotechnology*, 143: 257–295.

Kralj, S., Leeflang, C., Sierra, E.I., Kempiński, B., Alkan, V. and Kolkman, M. (2018). Synthesis of fructooligosaccharides (FosA) and inulin (InuO) by GH68 fructosyltransferases from Bacillus agaradhaerens strain WDG185. *Carbohydrate Polymers*, 179: 350–359.

Kuhn, R.C. and Filho, F.M. (2010). Purification of fructooligosaccharides in an activated charcoal fixed bed column. *New Biotechnology*, 27: 862–869.

Kuhn, R.C., Maugeri Filho, F., Silva, V., Palacio, L., Hernández, A. and Prádanos, P. (2010). Mass transfer and transport during purification of fructooligosaccharides by nanofiltration. *Journal of Membrane Science*, 365: 356–365.

Kumar, V.P., Prashanth, K.V.H. and Venkatesh, Y.P. (2015). Structural analyses and immunomodulatory properties of fructo-oligosaccharides from onion (Allium cepa). *Carbohydrate Polymers*, 117: 115–122.

Kuugbee, E.D., Shang, X., Gamallat, Y., Bamba, D., Awadasseid, A., Suliman, M.A., Zang, S., Ma, Y., Chiwala, G., Xin, Y. and Shang, D. (2016). Structural change in microbiota by a probiotic cocktail enhances the gut barrier and reduces cancer via TLR2 signaling in a rat model of colon cancer. *Digestive Diseases and Sciences*, 61: 2908–2920.

Le Bourgot, C., Ferret-Bernard, S., Blat, S., Apper, E. and Le Huërou-Luron, I. (2016). Short-chain fructooligosaccharide supplementation during gestation and lactation or after weaning differentially impacts pig growth and IgA response to influenza vaccination. *Journal of Functional Foods*, 24: 307–315.

Li, J., Liu, X., Zhou, B., Zhao, J. and Li, S. (2013). Determination of fructooligosaccharides in burdock using HPLC and microwave-assisted extraction. *Journal of Agricultural and Food Chemistry*, 61: 5888–5892.

Li, J., Hu, D., Zong, W., Lv, G., Zhao, J. and Li, S. (2014). Determination of inulin-type fructooligosaccharides in edible plants by high-performance liquid chromatography with charged aerosol detector. *Journal of Agricultural and Food Chemistry*, 62: 7707–7713.

Li, M., Seo, S. and Karboune, S. (2015). Bacillus amyloliquefaciens levansucrase-catalyzed the synthesis of fructooligosaccharides, oligolevan and levan in maple syrup-based reaction systems. *Carbohydrate Polymers*, 133: 203–212.

Linde, D., Rodríguez-Colinas, B., Estévez, M., Poveda, A., Plou, F.J. and Fernández Lobato, M. (2012). Analysis of neofructooligosaccharides production mediated by the extracellular β-fructofuranosidase from Xanthophyllomyces dendrorhous. *Bioresource Technology*, 109: 123–130.

Liu, D.M., Zhou, K., Fan, M. et al. (2012). Preparation method of fructooligosaccharides using whole-cell biotransformated by a newly strain A. niger 6640. China Patent, ZL201210531671.1. 2012-12-11.

Liu, Y., Gibson, G.R. and Walton, G.E. (2017). A three-stage continuous culture approach to study the impact of probiotics, prebiotics and fat intake on faecal microbiota relevant to an over 60 s population. *Journal of Functional Foods*, 32: 238–247.

Lopez, M.G., Mancilla-Margalli, N.A. and Mendoza-Diaz, G. (2003). Molecular structures of fructans from Agave tequilana Weber var. azul. *Journal of Agricultural and Food Chemistry*, 51: 7835–7840.

Lorenzoni, A.S.G., Aydos, L.F., Klein, M.P., Rodrigues, R.C. and Hertz, P.F. (2014). Fructooligosaccharides synthesis by highly stable immobilized β-fructofuranosidase from Aspergillus aculeatus. *Carbohydrate Polymers*, 103: 193–197.

Lu, L., Wu, J., Song, D., Zhao, H., Gu, G., Guo, Y., Lan, J. and Xiao, M. (2013). Purification of fructooligosaccharides by immobilized yeast cells and identification of ethyl β-d-fructofuranoside as a novel glycoside formed during the process. *Bioresource Technology*, 132: 365–369.

Martinez-Gutierrez, F., Ratering, S., Juárez-Flores, B., Godinez-Hernandez, C., Geissler-Plaum, R., Prell, F., Zorn, H., Czermak, P. and Schnell, S. (2017). Potential use of Agave salmiana as a prebiotic that stimulates the growth of probiotic bacteria. *Lwt*, 84: 151–159.

Martínez, I., Maldonado-Gomez, M.X., Gomes-Neto, J.C., Kittana, H., Ding, H., Schmaltz, R., Joglekar, P., Cardona, R.J., Marsteller, N.L., Kembel, S.W., Benson, A.K., Peterson, D.A., Ramer-Tait, A.E. and Walter, J. (2018). Experimental evaluation of the importance of colonization history in early-life gut microbiota assembly. *eLife*, 7: 1–26.

Mischke, M., Arora, T., Tims, S., Engels, E., Sommer, N., van Limpt, K., Baars, A., Oozeer, R., Oosting, A., Bäckhed, F. and Knol, J. (2018). Specific synbiotics in early life protect against diet-induced obesity in adult mice. *Diabetes, Obesity and Metabolism*, 20: 1408–1418.

Mohajeri, M.H., Brummer, R.J.M., Rastall, R.A., Weersma, R.K., Harmsen, H.J.M., Faas, M. and Eggersdorfer, M. (2018). The role of the microbiome for human health: from basic science to clinical applications. *European Journal of Nutrition*, 57: 1–14.

Moreno, F.J., Corzo, N., Montilla, A., Villamiel, M. and Olano, A. (2017). Current state and latest advances in the concept, production and functionality of prebiotic oligosaccharides. *Current Opinion in Food Science*, 13: 50–55.

Moro, T.M.A., Celegatti, C.M., Pereira, A.P.A., Lopes, A.S., Barbin, D.F., Pastore, G.M. and Clerici, M.T.P.S. (2018): Use of burdock root flour as a prebiotic ingredient in cookies. *Lwt*, 90: 540–546.

Moroti, C., Souza Magri, L., De Rezende Costa, M., Cavallini, D.C.U. and Sivieri, K. (2012). Effect of the consumption of a new symbiotic shake on glycemia and cholesterol levels in elderly people with type 2 diabetes mellitus. *Lipids in Health and Disease*, 11: 1–8.

Muñiz-Márquez, D.B., Contreras, J.C., Rodríguez, R., Mussatto, S.I., Wong-Paz, J.E., Teixeira, J. A. and Aguilar, C.N. (2015). Influence of thermal effect on sugars composition of Mexican Agave syrup. *CyTA - Journal of Food*, 1–6.

Muñiz-Márquez, D.B., Contreras, J.C., Rodríguez, R., Mussatto, S.I., Teixeira, J.A. and Aguilar, C.N. (2016). Enhancement of fructosyltransferase and fructooligosaccharides production by A. oryzae DIA-MF in solid-state fermentation using aguamiel as culture medium. *Bioresource Technology*, 213: 276–282.

Muñiz-Márquez, D.B., Teixeira, J.A., Mussatto, S.I., Contreras-Esquivel, J.C., Rodríguez-Herrera, R. and Aguilar, C.N. (2019). Fructo-oligosaccharides (FOS) production by fungal submerged culture using aguamiel as a low-cost by-product. *LWT-Food Science and Technology*, 102: 75–79.

Mussatto, S.I. and Teixeira, J.A. (2010). Increase in the fructooligosaccharides yield and productivity by solid-state fermentation with Aspergillus japonicus using agro-industrial residues as support and nutrient source. *Biochemical Engineering Journal*, 53: 154–157.

Mussatto, S.I., Ballesteros, L.F., Martins, S., Maltos, D.A.F., Aguilar, C.N. and Teixeira, J.A. (2013). Maximization of fructooligosaccharides and β-fructofuranosidase production by Aspergillus japonicus under solid-state fermentation conditions. *Food and Bioprocess Technology*, 6: 2128–2134.

Mutanda, T., Mokoena, M.P., Olaniran, A.O., Wilhelmi, B.S. and Whiteley, C.G. (2014). Microbial enzymatic production and applications of short-chain fructooligosaccharides and inulooligosaccharides: Recent advances and current perspectives. *Journal of Industrial Microbiology and Biotechnology*, 41: 893–906.

Nascimento, A.K.C., Nobre, C., Cavalcanti, M.T.H., Teixeira, J.A. and Porto, A.L.F. (2016). Screening of fungi from the genus Penicillium for production of β-fructofuranosidase and enzymatic synthesis of fructooligosaccharides. *Journal of Molecular Catalysis B: Enzymatic*, 134: 70–78.

Nawaz, A., Bakhsh javaid, A., Irshad, S., Hoseinifar, S.H. and Xiong, H. (2018). The functionality of prebiotics as immunostimulant: Evidences from trials on terrestrial and aquatic animals. *Fish and Shellfish Immunology*, 76: 272–278.

Neri-Numa, I.A. and Pastore, G.M. (2020). Novel insights into prebiotic properties on human health: A review. *Food Research International*, 131: 108973.

Niness, K.R. (1999). Inulin and oligofructose: what are they? *The Journal of Nutrition*, 129: 1402S–1406S.

Ning, Y., Wang, J., Chen, J., Yang, N., Jin, Z. and Xu, X. (2010). Production of neo-fructooligosaccharides using free-whole-cell biotransformation by Xanthophyllomyces dendrorhous. *Bioresource Technology*, 101: 7472–7478.

Ning, Y., Li, Q., Chen, F., Yang, N., Jin, Z. and Xu, X. (2012). Low-cost production of 6G-fructofuranosidase with high value-added astaxanthin by Xanthophyllomyces dendrorhous. *Bioresource Technology*, 104: 660–667.

Nobre, C., Teixeira, J.A. and Rodrigues, L.R. (2012). Fructo-oligosaccharides purification from a fermentative broth using an activated charcoal column. *New Biotechnology*, 29: 395–401.

Nobre, C., Teixeira, J.A. and Rodrigues, L.R. (2015). New trends and technological challenges in the industrial production and purification of fructo-oligosaccharides. *Critical Reviews in Food Science and Nutrition*, 55: 1444–1455.

Nobre, C., Castro, C.C., Hantson, A.L., Teixeira, J.A., De Weireld, G. and Rodrigues, L.R. (2016). Strategies for the production of high-content fructo-oligosaccharides through the removal of small saccharides by co-culture or successive fermentation with yeast. *Carbohydrate Polymers*, 136: 274–281.

Nobre, C., Sousa, S.C., Silva, S.P., Pinheiro, A.C., Coelho, E., Vicente, A.A., Gomes, A.M.P., Coimbra, M.A., Teixeira, J.A. and Rodrigues, L.R. (2018a). in vitro digestibility and fermentability of fructo-oligosaccharides produced by Aspergillus ibericus. *Journal of Functional Foods*, 46: 278–287.

Nobre, C., Alves Filho, E.G., Fernandes, F.A.N., Brito, E.S., Rodrigues, S., Teixeira, J.A. and Rodrigues, L.R. (2018b). Production of fructo-oligosaccharides by Aspergillus ibericus and their chemical characterization. *LWT - Food Science and Technology*, 89: 58–64.

Nobre, C., Gonçalves, D.A., Teixeira, J.A. and Rodrigues, L.R. (2018c). One-step co-culture fermentation strategy to produce high-content fructo-oligosaccharides. *Carbohydrate Polymers*, 201: 31–38.

Nobre, C., do Nascimento, A.K.C., Silva, S.P., Coelho, E., Coimbra, M.A., Cavalcanti, M.T.H., Teixeira, J.A. and Porto, A.L.F. (2019). Process development for the production of prebiotic fructo-oligosaccharides by penicillium citreonigrum. *Bioresource Technology*, 282: 464–474.

Patil, P.R., Reddy, G.S.N. and Sulochana, M.B. (2011). Production, optimization and characterization of β-fructofuranosidase by Chrysonilia sitophila PSSF84 — A novel source. *Indian Journal of Biotechnology* 10: 56–64.

Paul, H.A., Collins, K.H., Nicolucci, A.C., Urbanski, S.J., Hart, D.A., Vogel, H.J. and Reimer, R.A. (2019). Maternal prebiotic supplementation reduces fatty liver development in offspring through altered microbial and metabolomic profiles in rats. *FASEB Journal*, 33: 5153–5167.

Paz, A. de L., da Silva, J.M., da Silva, K.M.M. and Val, A.L. (2019). Protective effects of the fructooligosaccharide on the growth performance, hematology, immunology indicators and survival of tambaqui (Colossoma macropomum, Characiformes: Serrasalmidae) infected by Aeromonas hydrophila. *Aquaculture Reports*, 15: 100222.

Pedreschi, R., Campos, D., Noratto, G., Chirinos, R. and Cisneros-Zevallos, L. (2003). Andean yacon root (Smallanthus sonchifolius Poepp. Endl) fructooligosaccharides as a potential novel source of prebiotics. *Journal of Agricultural and Food Chemistry*, 51: 5278–5284.

Rastall, R.A. and Gibson, G.R. (2014). Recent developments in prebiotics to selectively impact beneficial microbes and promote intestinal health. *Current Opinion in Biotechnology*, 32C: 42–46.

Rawat, H.K., Ganaie, M.A. and Kango, N. (2015). Production of inulinase, fructosyltransferase and sucrase from fungi on low-value inulin-rich substrates and their use in generation of fructose and fructo-oligosaccharides. *Antonie van Leeuwenhoek, International Journal of General and Molecular Microbiology*, 107: 799–811.

Respondek, F., Gerard, P., Bossis, M., Boschat, L., Bruneau, A., Rabot, S., Wagner, A. and Martin, J.C. (2013). Short-chain fructo-oligosaccharides modulate intestinal microbiota and metabolic parameters of humanized gnotobiotic diet induced obesity mice. *PLoS ONE*, 8: e71026.

Rigo-Adrover, M.D.M., Knipping, K., Garssen, J., van Limpt, K., Knol, J., Franch, À., Castell, M., Rodríguez-Lagunas, M.J. and Pérez-Cano, F.J. (2019). Prevention of rotavirus diarrhea in suckling rats by a specific fermented milk concentrate with prebiotic mixture. *Nutrients*, 11: 189.

Rivière, A., Gagnon, M., Weckx, S., Roy, D. and De Vuyst, L. (2015). Mutual cross-feeding interactions between Bifidobacterium longum subsp. longum NCC2705 and Eubacterium rectale ATCC 33656 explain the bifidogenic and butyrogenic effects of arabinoxylan oligosaccharides. *Applied and Environmental Microbiology*, 81: 7767–7781.

Roberfroid, M. (2002). Functional food concept and its application to prebiotics. *Digestive and Liver Disease*, 34: S105–S110.

Romano, N., Santos, M., Mobili, P., Vega, R. and Gómez-Zavaglia, A. (2016). Effect of sucrose concentration on the composition of enzymatically synthesized short-chain fructo-oligosaccharides as determined by FTIR and multivariate analysis. *Food Chemistry*, 202: 467–475.

Ruiz, Y., Klotz, B., Serrato, J., Guio, F., Bohórquez, J. and Sánchez, O.F. (2014). Use of spent osmotic solutions for the production of fructooligosaccharides by Aspergillus oryzae N74. *Food Science and Technology International*, 20: 365–372.

Salvucci, E. (2019). The human-microbiome superorganism and its modulation to restore health. *International Journal of Food Sciences and Nutrition*, 70: 781–795.

Sangeetha, P.T., Ramesh, M.N. and Prapulla, S.G. (2005). Recent trends in the microbial production, analysis and application of fructooligosaccharides. *Trends in Food Science and Technology*, 16: 442–457.

Schmidt, T.S.B., Raes, J. and Bork, P. (2018). The human gut microbiome: From association to modulation. *Cell*, 172: 1198–1215.

Sen, P. and Orešič, M. (2019). Metabolic modeling of human gut microbiota on a genome scale: An overview. *Metabolites*, 9: 22.

Serban, D.E. (2014). Gastrointestinal cancers: Influence of gut microbiota, probiotics and prebiotics. *Cancer Lett*, 345: 258–270.

Serrano-Villar, S., Vázquez-Castellanos, J.F., Vallejo, A., Latorre, A., Sainz, T., Ferrando-Martínez, S., Rojo, D., Martínez-Botas, J., Del Romero, J., Madrid, N., Leal, M., Mosele, J.I., Motilva, M.J., Barbas, C., Ferrer, M., Moya, A., Moreno, S., Gosalbes, M.J. and Estrada, V. (2017). The effects of prebiotics on microbial dysbiosis, butyrate production and immunity in HIV-infected subjects. *Mucosal Immunology*, 10: 1279–1293.

Shang, Y., Kumar, S., Thippareddi, H. and Kim, W.K. (2018). Effect of dietary fructooligosaccharide (FOS) supplementation on ileal microbiota in broiler chickens. *Poultry Science*, 97: 3622–3634.

Sheu, D.C., Chang, J.Y., Chen, Y.J. and Lee, C.W. (2013a). Production of high-purity neofructooligosaccharides by culture of Xanthophyllomyces dendrorhous. *Bioresource Technology*, 132: 432–435.

Sheu, D.C., Chang, J.Y., Wang, C.Y., Wu, C.T. and Huang, C.J. (2013b). Continuous production of high-purity fructooligosaccharides and ethanol by immobilized Aspergillus japonicus and Pichia heimii. *Bioprocess and Biosystems Engineering*, 36: 1745–1751.

Shin, H.T., Baig, S.Y., Lee, S.W., Suh, D.S., Kwon, S.T., Lim, Y.B. and Lee, J.H. (2004). Production of fructo-oligosaccharides from molasses by Aureobasidium pullulans cells. *Bioresour Technol*, 93: 59–62.

Singh, R.S., Chauhan, K. and Kennedy, J.F. (2017). A panorama of bacterial inulinases: Production, purification, characterization and industrial applications. *International Journal of Biological Macromolecules*, 96: 312–322.

Soares, M.B.A.H., Rodrigues, M.I. and Maugeri-Filho, F. (2014). Modelling, simulation and factorial design as tools for the in silico process optimisation of fructooligosaccharide production by immobilised fructosyltransferase in a basket reactor. *Biocatalysis and Biotransformation*, 32: 84–92.

Soldi, S., Vasileiadis, S., Lohner, S., Uggeri, F., Puglisi, E., Molinari, P., Donner, E., Sieland, C., Decsi, T., Sailer, M. and Theis, S. (2019). Prebiotic supplementation over a cold season and during antibiotic treatment specifically modulates the gut microbiota composition of 3-6 year-old children. *Beneficial Microbes*, 10: 253–263.

Speranza, B., Campaniello, D., Monacis, N., Bevilacqua, A., Sinigaglia, M. and Corbo, M.R. (2018). Functional cream cheese supplemented with Bifidobacterium animalis subsp. lactis DSM 10140 and Lactobacillus reuteri DSM 20016 and prebiotics. *Food Microbiology*, 72: 16–22.

Tian, F. and Karboune, S. (2012). Enzymatic synthesis of fructooligosaccharides by levansucrase from Bacillus amyloliquefaciens: Specificity, kinetics, and product characterization. *Journal of Molecular Catalysis B: Enzymatic*, 82: 71–79.

Tian, F., Karboune, S. and Hill, A. (2014). Synthesis of fructooligosaccharides and oligolevans by the combined use of levansucrase and endo-inulinase in one-step bi-enzymatic system. *Innovative Food Science and Emerging Technologies*, 22: 230–238.

Valcheva, R. and Dieleman, L.A. (2016). Prebiotics: Definition and protective mechanisms. *Best Practice and Research: Clinical Gastroenterology*, 30: 27–37.

Valencia, M.S., Salgado, S.M., Andrade, S.A.C., Padilha, V.M., Livera, A.V.S. and Stamford, T.L.M. (2016). Development of creamy milk chocolate dessert added with fructo-oligosaccharide and Lactobacillus paracasei subsp. paracasei LBC 81. *LWT - Food Science and Technology*, 69: 104–109.

van den Heuvel, E.G.H.M., Muijs, T., Brouns, F. and Hendriks, H.F.J. (2009). Short-chain fructo-oligosaccharides improve magnesium absorption in adolescent girls with a low calcium intake. *Nutrition Research*, 29: 229–237.

Vega-Paulino, R.J. and Zuñiga-Hansen, M.E. (2012). Potential application of commercial enzyme preparations for industrial production of short-chain fructooligosaccharides. *Journal of Molecular Catalysis B: Enzymatic*, 76: 44–51.

Vega, R. and Zuniga-Hansen, M.E. (2014). A new mechanism and kinetic model for the enzymatic synthesis of short-chain fructooligosaccharides from sucrose. *Biochemical Engineering Journal*, 82: 158–165.

Verruck, S., de Carvalho, M.W., de Liz, G.R., Amante, E.R., Vieira, C.R.W., Amboni, R.D. de M.C. and Prudencio, E.S. (2017). Survival of Bifidobacterium BB-12 microencapsulated with full-fat goat's milk and prebiotics when exposed to simulated gastrointestinal conditions and thermal treatments. *Small Ruminant Research*, 153: 48–56.

Vieira De Almeida, C., Rodrigues de Camargo, M., Russo, E. and Amedei, A. (2019). Role of diet and gut microbiota on colorectal cancer immunomodulation. *World J Gastroenterol*, 9327: 151–162.

Wang, Y., Zeng, T., Wang, S-e., Wang, W., Wang, Q. and Yu, H.X. (2010). Fructo-oligosaccharides enhance the mineral absorption and counteract the adverse effects of phytic acid in mice. *Nutrition*. 26: 305–311.

Xie, X., He, Y., Li, H., Yu, D., Na, L., Sun, T., Zhang, D., Shi, X., Xia, Y., Jiang, T., Rong, S., Yang, S., Ma, X. and Xu, G. (2019). Effects of prebiotics on immunologic indicators and intestinal microbiota structure in perioperative colorectal cancer patients. *Nutrition*, 61: 132–142.

Xu, Q., Zheng, X., Huang, M., Wu, M., Yan, Y., Pan, J., Yang, Q., Duan, C.J., Liu, J.L. and Feng, J.X. (2014). Purification and biochemical characterization of a novel β-fructofuranosidase from Penicillium oxalicum with transfructosylating activity producing neokestose. *Process Biochemistry*, 50: 1237–1246.

Yang, H., Wang, Y., Zhang, L. and Shen, W. (2016). Heterologous expression and enzymatic characterization of fructosyltransferase from Aspergillus niger in Pichia pastoris. *New Biotechnology*, 33: 164–170.

Yen, C.H., Kuo, Y.W., Tseng, Y.H., Lee, M.C. and Chen, H.L. (2011). Beneficial effects of fructo-oligosaccharides supplementation on fecal bifidobacteria and index of peroxidation status in constipated nursing-home residents – A placebo-controlled, diet-controlled trial. *Nutrition*, 27: 323–328.

Young, V.B. (2017). The role of the microbiome in human health and disease: An introduction for clinicians. *BMJ (Online)*, 356:j831.

Zambelli, P., Fernandez-Arrojo, L., Romano, D., Santos-Moriano, P., Gimeno-Perez, M., Poveda, A., Gandolfi, R., Fernández-Lobato, M., Molinari, F. and Plou, F.J. (2014). Production of fructooligosaccharides by mycelium-bound transfructosylation activity present in Cladosporium cladosporioides and Penicilium sizovae. *Process Biochemistry*, 49: 2174–2180.

Zeng, X.A., Zhou, K., Liu, D–m., Brennan, C.S., Brennan, M., Zhou, J–s. and Yu, S–j. (2016). Preparation of fructooligosaccharides using Aspergillus niger 6640 whole-cell as catalyst for bio-transformation. *LWT - Food Science and Technology*, 65: 1072–1079.

Zhang, J., Wang, L., Luan, C., Liu, G., Liu, J. and Zhong, Y. (2019). Establishment of a rapid and effective plate chromogenic assay for screening of Aspergillus species with high β-fructofuranosidase activity for fructooligosaccharides production. *Journal of Microbiological Methods*, 166: 105740.

Zhou, P., Wang, Y., Li, S., Zhao, Y., Deng, K., Chao, D., Jin, C., Zhuo, Y., Che, L., Li, J., Lin, Y., Xu, S., Feng, B., Fang, Z. and Wu, D. (2018). Effects of prebiotic inulin addition to low- or high-fat diet on maternal metabolic status and neonatal traits of offspring in a pregnant sow model. *Journal of Functional Foods*, 48: 125–133.

14

Lactulose: Production and Potential Applications

Shweta Kumari[1], *Parmjit Singh Panesar*[2], *Divyani Panwar*[2] *and Gisha Singla*[2]

[1] *Department of Biochemical Engineering & Biotechnology, Indian Institute of Technology, Hauz Khas, New Delhi-110016, India*
[2] *Food Biotechnology Research Laboratory, Department of Food Engineering & Technology, Sant Longowal Institute of Engineering and Technology, Longowal-148 106, Punjab, India*

14.1 Introduction

The disaccharide lactulose (4-O-β-D-galactopyranosyl-D-fructofuranose) is a non-digestible compound made up of two monosaccharides, fructose and galactose, bonded together with a β-1,4-glycosidic bond. It is a "bifidus factor", which is produced by lactose isomerization. The β-glycosidic linkage present in lactulose is not hydrolyzed by digestive enzymes and the ingested lactulose is directly passed through the colon in an unaltered form (Ruttloff *et al.* 1967). It is generally utilized by a large number of probiotic bacteria such as *Bifidobacterium* spp., present in human intestine (Figure 14.1) (Tamura *et al.* 1993). Due to its prebiotic property, it induces the growth of healthy gut bacteria such as bifidobacteria and lactobacilli (Table 14.1) and also inhibits the growth of pathogenic bacteria such as *Salmonella* (Aider and de Halleux 2007; Panesar *et al.* 2009).

14.2 Structure and Properties

Lactulose is a non-digestible synthetic isomer made up of two monomers, galactose and fructose. The structural and physicochemical properties of lactulose are shown in Table 14.2. Lactulose is predominantly found in a variety of isomeric forms including α- or β-pyranose, α- or β-furanose, and acyclic forms. Among these, α-furanose β-pyranose and β-furanose isomers are mainly formed during the currently available methods of lactulose production at different ratios, but the presence of α-pyranose has not been reported (Aït-Aissa and Aider 2014a).

Lactulose syrup available commercially is a clear yellow and odorless sweet syrup containing about 80% solid contents (Schumann 2002). Moreover, pure lactulose is commercially available in white crystalline form and is made up of anhydride and trihydrate structures

Probiotics, Prebiotics and Synbiotics: Technological Advancements Towards Safety and Industrial Applications, First Edition. Edited by Parmjit Singh Panesar and Anil Kumar Anal.

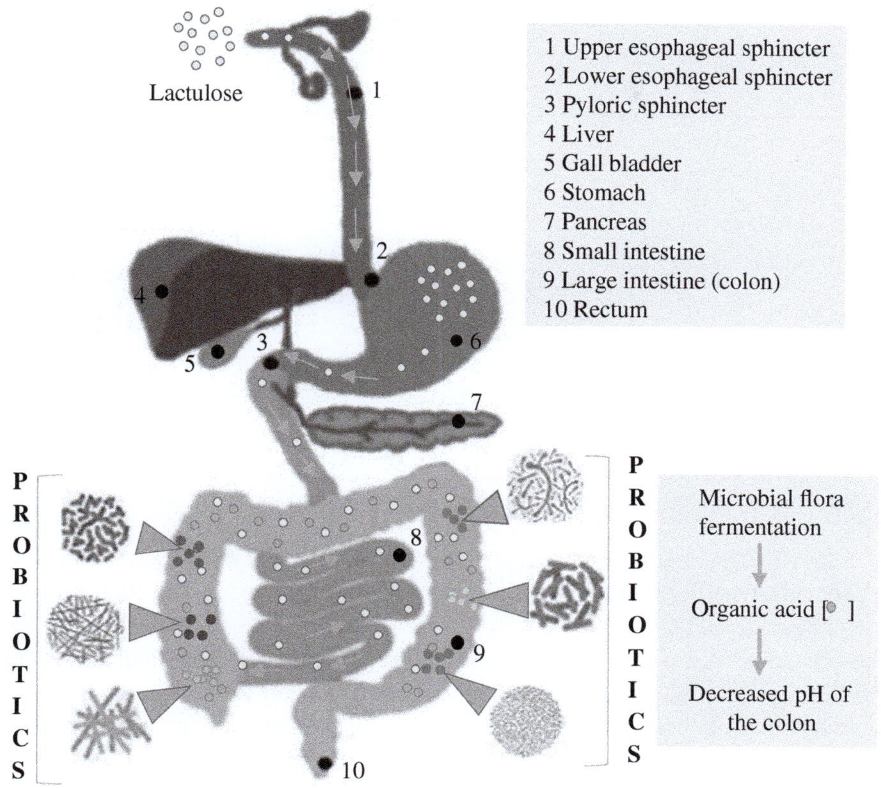

Figure 14.1 Diagrammatic representation of lactulose-based delivery system. *Source:* Based on Tamura, Y., Mizota, T., Shimamura, S. and Tomita, M. (1993). Lactulose and its application to the food and pharmaceutical industries. *Bulletin of the International Dairy Federation*, 289: 43–53.

Table 14.1 Intestinal microflora that can grow on lactulose.

Microorganism
Bacteroides fragilis C-2
Bacteroides vulgatus E 1
Bifidobacterium adolescentis ATCC 15705
Bifidobacterium bifidum S 28
Bifidobacterium breve S1
Bifidobacterium infantis S12
Bifidobacterium longum E 194
Clostridium perfringens ATCC 13124
Clostridium ramosum ATCC 13937
Escherichia coli No. 28
Lactobacillus acidophilus ATCC 4356
Lactobacillus casei 8138
Lactobacillus salivarius ATCC 11741
Streptococcus faecalis ATCC 19434

Source: Modified from Panesar, P.S. and Kumari, S. (2011). Lactulose: Production, purification and potential applications. *Biotechnology Advances*, 29(6): 940–948.

Table 14.2 Structure and physicochemical properties of lactulose.

Structure	Properties
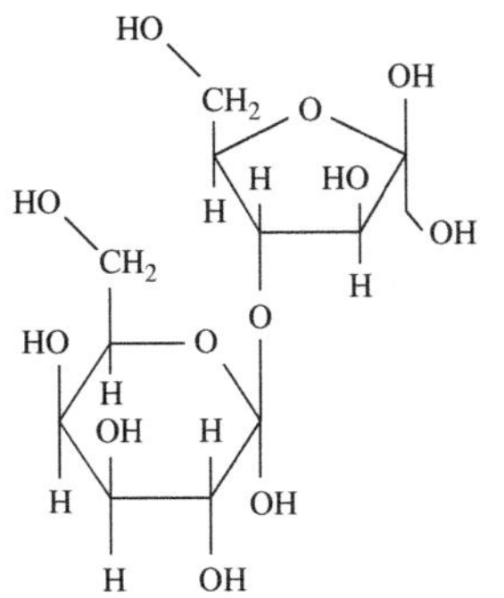	• Empirical formula: $C_{12}H_{22}O_{11}$ • Molecular weight (g/mole): 342.3 • Melting point (°C): 168.5–170 • Specific rotation $[\alpha]_D^{20}$ at 589 nm: -51.5 °C • Sweetness: 0.48–0.62 (relative to sucrose) • 1.5 (sweeter than lactose) • Water solubility: 76.4% (w/w) at 30 °C • 86.0% (w/w) at 90 °C • Methanol solubility: 25.4 (g/L) at 30 °C

Sources: Based on Schumann (2002); Playne and Crittenden (2009); Nooshkam and Madadlou (2016a).

(Seki and Saito 2012). Numerous procedures for the purification and separation of lactulose after the isomerization reaction are available and increase the cost of the final product (Panesar and Kumari 2011).

Lactulose can be used in a range of foods as a bifidus factor or as a functional ingredient since it also possesses various properties that are beneficial for consumers' health. It can be added as a sugar substitute, sweetener for diabetics, in dairy desserts, infant milk powders, beverages, and bakery products, and in various liquids or dried food formulations which are normally prepared for the elderly population (Crittenden and Playne 1996; Strohmaier 1998; Tamura *et al.* 1993). Lactulose is also known for a variety of favorable properties such as water solubility, browning behavior, and flavor-enhancing properties, which impart desirable effects in food products. Besides, being a prebiotic, it has also been used to enhance the survival of probiotic strains present in yoghurt (Tabatabaie and Mortazavi 2008). Moreover, owing to its high stability under acidic and thermal conditions, lactulose has also proved to be a useful additive, especially in fruit juices (Seki and Saito 2012).

14.3 Lactulose Production

Lactulose is mainly produced by the process of lactose isomerization when the glucose residue is regrouped to the molecule of fructose (Kochetkov and Bochkov 1967). Different methods such as chemical, biotechnological and electro-activation pathways can be used for the synthesis of lactulose (Figure 14.2). Depending upon the method used for its preparation, a variety of catalysts such as alkalis, complex reagents or enzymes can be employed in the isomerization of lactose. Moreover, lactulose can also be synthesized using the electro-activation method. The catalyst must have the properties of being economical, non-toxic, safe and environmentally friendly besides being easily separated from the reaction mixture. Thus, biotechnological methods have various environmental and technological benefits over chemical methods. Information on the work carried out on different methods (chemical, enzymatic and electro-activation) used for lactulose production is tabulated in Table 14.3a–c and details are discussed in the following sections.

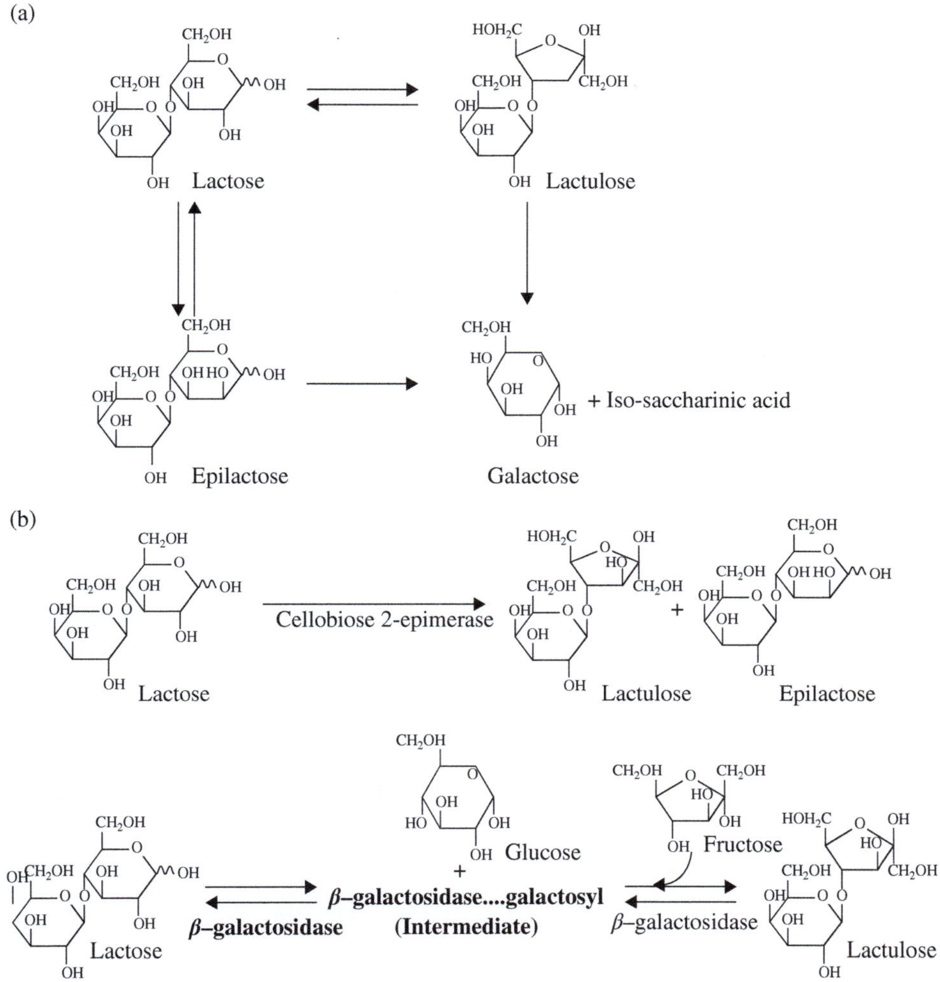

Figure 14.2 Schematic representation of (a) alkaline isomerization of lactose and (b) enzymatic synthesis of lactulose using β-galactosidase and cellobiose 2-epimerase. *Sources:* Based on Montilla *et al.* 2005; Silvério *et al.* 2016.

14.3.1 Chemical Methods

The chemical isomerization of lactose to lactulose exclusively takes place through the Lobry de Bruyn–Alberda van Ekenstein (LA) rearrangement, which is carried out by using catalyzing processes (Aider and de Halleux 2007). In the presence of an alkaline catalyst, the transformation of the glucose moiety in lactose into fructose takes place via an intermediate enolization. The chemical methods normally resulted in a low yield of lactulose along with the appearance of a brownish color due to the occurrence of side reactions that lead to unwanted products. Thus, expensive steps for separation and purification are required for the removal of these unwanted products (Panesar and Kumari 2011). Chemical catalysts used in the synthesis of lactulose are discussed under three categories, namely alkaline homogeneous catalysts, complex reagents and natural catalysts.

Table 14.3a Lactulose production using chemical catalysts.

Chemical catalyst	Temperature (°C)	pH	Incubation time (h)	Y lactulose/ lactose (%)	Reference
Alkaline agents					
Calcium hydroxide (lactose)	35	–	36	~30	Montgomery and Hudson (1930)
Sodium hydroxide (lactose)	70	11	0.25	27	Zokaee *et al* (2002)
Sodium hydroxide, ultrasound at 70% of amplitude (lactose)	60	10.6	1	24	Corzo-Martínez *et al.* (2014)
Sodium hydroxide, microwave-assisted; 600 W power (lactose)	100	9	0.02	10.9	Nooshkam and Madadlou (2016a)
Complex reagents					
Boric acid with triethylamine (lactose)	70	11	4	87	Hicks and Parrish (1980)
Sodium aluminate	50–70	4.5–8.0	0.5–1	–	U.S. Patent No 4957564 (1990)
Boric acid	70	11	2	~75	Kozempel and Kurantz (1994)
Sodium aluminate (lactose)	60	12	0.83	85.45	Wang *et al.* (2017)
Natural catalysts					
Sepiolite with alkaline ions (milk permeate)	90	–	2.5	20	Villamiel *et al.* (2002)
Egg shell (milk permeate)	98	–	1	1.18	Montilla *et al.* (2005)
(whey permeate)	98		2.5	16.1	Corzo-Martínez *et al.* (2013)
(milk permeate)	97		1	17.3	Nooshkam and Madadlou (2016b)
Oyster shell, limestone (milk permeate)	96	–	2	18–21	Paseephol *et al.* (2008)

Sources: Based on Montgomery and Hudson (1930); Zokaee *et al.* (2002); Corzo-Martínez *et al.* (2014); Nooshkam and Madadlou (2016a).

1) *Alkaline homogeneous catalysts* have been used as catalysts for the synthesis of lactulose. The catalysts employed under this category are tertiary amines, sodium hydroxide, calcium hydroxide, potassium hydroxide, sodium aluminate, borates, magnesium oxide, potassium carbonate, etc. (Zokaee *et al.* 2002). Zeolites and sepiolites also have been projected as heterogeneous catalysts (Villamiel *et al.* 2002). By using these catalysts, about 20–33% of lactulose was produced at a reaction temperature of 70–100 °C within a few hours. However, with further increase in the reaction time, a significant reduction in

Table 14.3b Lactulose production using free and immobilized cells.

Enzyme catalyst	Form of enzyme	Temperature (°C)	pH	Incubation time (h)	Lactose/fructose (%, w/w)	Y lactulose/ lactose (%)	Productivity (g/L/ h)	Reference
β-galactosidase								
Saccharomyces fragilis	Free	37	7.2	–	12/20	7.5	–	Vaheri and Kaupinnen (1978)
Kluyveromyces lactis	Permeabilized cells	60	7.0	3	40/20	–	6.8	Lee *et al.* (2004)
Aspergillus oryzae	Free	37	5	–	15/5	30	–	Mayer *et al.* (2004)
Sulfolobus solfataricus	Free (recombinant)	80	6.0	6	40/20	–	8.3	Kim *et al.* (2006)
A. oryzae	Free	40	6.5	–	20/15	–	–	Adamczak *et al.* (2009)
K. lactis	Immobilized	47	7.5	–	20/20	9.6	–	Song *et al.* (2013b)
K. lactis	Free	40	6.7	–	9–12/25–30	20	–	Khatami *et al.* (2014)
A. oryzae	Free	50	4.5	–	2.1/47.9	31	–	Guerrero *et al.* (2015)
	Immobilized	50	4.5	–	2.1/47.9	25.4	–	
K. lactis	Free	50	7.0	2	15/30	–	11.3	de Albuquerque *et al.* (2018)
β-glycosidase								
Pyrococcus furiosus	Free (recombinant)	75	5.0	–	2.62/20.7	47.06	–	Mayer *et al.* (2004)
	Immobilized (recombinant)	75	5.0	–	2.62/20.7	43	–	Mayer *et al.* (2010)
Cellobiose 2-epimerase	-							
Caldicellulosiruptor saccharolyticus	Free	80	7.5	–	70	58	–	Kim and Oh (2012)
	Free	50	–	24	48.5	57.7	–	Rentschler *et al.* (2015)
		8	–	72	48.5	56.7	–	
	Free (recombinant)	80	7.0	–	20	58.5	–	Wu *et al.* (2017)

Sources: Based on Vaheri and Kaupinnen (1978); Lee *et al.* (2004).

Table 14.3c Production of lactulose by electro-isomerization.

Electro-isomerization	Temperature (°C)	pH	Incubation time (h)	Y lactulose/ lactose (%)	Reference
200 mA current intensity (lactose)	23	14	1	25	Aider and Gimenez-Vidal (2012)
(whey)	23	12.5	1	10	
300 mA current intensity, Na_2SO_4 (lactose)	10	9–10.5	0.5	32.5	Aït-Aissa and Aïder (2014b)
400 mA current intensity, Na_2SO_4 (whey)	10	11	0.67	35	Kareb *et al.* (2016)
900 mA current intensity (lactose)	22	11.27	0.67	38	Karim and Aide (2020)

Sources: Based on Aider and Gimenez-Vidal (2012); Aït-Aissa and Aïder (2014b); Kareb *et al.* (2016).

the concentration of lactulose was observed, which is probably due to the degradation of lactulose into galactose and other undesirable compounds (Schuster-Wolff-Bühring *et al.* 2010). It has been reported that microwave radiation created rapid heat due to interaction with polar and ionic molecules (Rodríguez *et al.* 2015). Therefore, the microwave heating method (at 600 W for 60 s) has been found effective in decreasing the lactose to lactulose isomerization time (Nooshkam and Madadlou 2016a).

2) *Complex reagents* such as borates and aluminates under alkaline pH result in the formation of insoluble, stable complexes with ketoses like lactulose, which can shift in reaction equilibrium towards lactulose synthesis, with minimum thermal degradation of lactulose. However, the need for the removal of aluminate and borate is the major problem in this process from an industrial standpoint (Carobbi and Innocenti 1990; Krumbbloz and Dorscheid 1991; Zokaee *et al.* 2002). Sweet cheese whey ultrafiltrate has also been utilized for the synthesis of lactulose and a good isomerization yield (80%) was observed with sodium hydroxide/triethylamine (Hicks *et al.* 1984). Using sodium hydroxide and borate, an isomerization yield of 78% has also been achieved from lactose (Kozempel and Kurantz 1994). Besides this, sodium aluminate, as well as a combination of boric acid and sodium hydroxide, has also been employed in lactulose synthesis. An isomerization yield of 75–80% was observed using this catalyst combination after a reaction period of 120 min (Zokaee *et al.* 2002)
3) *Natural catalysts* such as egg shell, sepiolites, oyster shell and limestone are considered easily available heterogeneous catalysts, which helps in the reduction of waste production (Schuster-Wolff-Bühring *et al.* 2010). Egg shell has been successfully utilized for the isomerization of milk whey lactose (Montilla *et al.* 2005). A yield of 18–21% lactulose from milk permeate using calcium carbonate-based catalysts has been obtained (Paseephol *et al.* 2008). The isomerization of milk ultrafiltration permeate using egg shell powder as a catalyst has resulted in the conversion of 17% of whey lactose to lactulose (Nooshkam and Madadlou 2016a).

14.3.2 Biotechnological Methods

Different biotechnological strategies (enzymatic, whole cells) have also been developed for the synthesis of lactulose, as detailed in the following sections.

14.3.2.1 Enzymatic Methods

Enzymatic methods have been widely employed for the synthesis of lactulose.

14.3.2.1.1 Enzyme Used

Lactulose synthesis has been done with different enzymes including β-galactosidase, β-glycosidase and cellobiose 2-epimerase. The enzyme β-galactosidase is a well-known biocatalyst having transgalactosylation activity and has been used for the production of lactulose and galactooligosaccharides (Panesar *et al.* 2006, 2010). A variety of sources such as microorganisms, plants and animals have been reported for the production of this enzyme, however, its properties differ significantly according to the sources. Among these sources, microbial β-galactosidases have gained much interest because of various advantages offered by microorganisms over other sources (Panesar *et al.* 2006). Besides, this enzyme has been used in free as well as immobilized form in the production of lactulose.

β-Glycosidases (also known as glycoside hydrolases or glycosyl hydrolases) are the enzymes that hydrolyze the glycosidic bonds in β-D-glucosides and oligosaccharides, with release of glucose (Cox *et al.* 2000). Glycosidases are generally available from natural sources such as microorganisms or fungus cultures, plant cells and animal cells.

Another enzyme, cellobiose 2-epimerase, is a unique enzyme that can convert lactose into epilactose and lactulose, which are the epimeric and isomeric forms, respectively. Epilactose and lactulose are functional food materials that have significant economic value in dairy industries (Chen *et al.* 2018).

14.3.2.1.2 Methods used for the Production of Lactulose

Enzymatic production of lactulose can be carried out by using a free enzyme or an immobilized enzyme.

Lactulose Production Using Free Enzyme The synthesis of lactulose using β-galactosidase enzyme obtained from *Saccharomyces fragilis* DSM 70344 and fructose as acceptor was first reported by Vaheri and Kaupinnen (1978). Amongst different microbial sources such as *Kluyveromyces fragilis, Aspergillus oryzae, Escherichia coli* and *Kluyveromyces lactis* used for the production of β-galactosidases, the highest lactulose yield was observed with β-galactosidase obtained from *K. lactis* (Lee *et al.* 2004).

The enzymatic transgalactosylation of lactose along with lactulose production has been reported using β-galactosidase obtained from *Aspergillus oryzae* and the hyperthermostable *Pyrococcus furiosus* β-glycosidase (Mayer *et al.* 2004). The lactulose productivities were higher (46 mmol/L) with *P. furiosus* β-glycosidase as compared to *A. oryzae* β-galactosidase (30 mmol/L).

In another study, cloning of a gene for thermostable β-galactosidase obtained from *Sulfolobus solfataricus* and its expression in *E. coli* was carried out and it was further employed in the production of lactulose (Kim *et al.* 2006). The selection of method for preparation of β-galactosidase, concentration of substrate, and ratio of fructose and lactose are the major factors that affect the enzymatic synthesis of galactooligosaccharide and lactulose (Adamczak *et al.* 2009).

Cellobiose 2-epimerase (isolated from thermophilic *Caldicellulosiruptor saccharolyticus*) has been used for lactulose production along with borate to increase the yield of lactulose. The studies have resulted in significant increase in lactulose yield (up to 51%), however processing costs also increased due to the complex purification steps (Kim *et al.* 2013).

The commercial β-galactosidase DSM Maxilact®5000 has also been used for the preparation of 1-lactulose and lactulose using fructose as substrate and the maximum yield of 1-lactulose and lactulose was found to be approximately 22 and 8 g/L, respectively, under optimal conditions (Hua *et al.* 2013). Synthesis of lactulose utilizing β-galactosidase obtained from *K. lactis* in two aqueous and non-conventional media resulted in the highest lactose conversion rate to lactulose at a lactose concentration of 9–12% (w/w) and fructose concentration of 25–30% (w/w) (Khatami *et al.* 2014). Further, the addition of acetone decreased lactulose yield, whereas an increase in lactulose yield (up to 20%) was observed after addition of tri-ethyl phosphate (up to 30% w/w).

Lactulose production was performed through lactose conversion by a thermophilic cellobiose 2-epimerase obtained from *Caldicellulosiruptor saccharolyticus*. The transformation of milk lactose (48.5 ± 2.1 g/L) resulted in a final yield of 57.7% (28.0 g/L) lactulose after 24 h at 50 °C, whereas 56.7% (27.5 g/L) lactulose was obtained after 72 h at 8 °C (Rentschler *et al.* 2015).

The influence of operating conditions (agitation, pH, molar ratio of lactose to fructose, hydraulic residence time) using *K. lactis* β-galactosidase was also investigated in terms of lactulose concentration, productivity and selectivity (Sitanggang *et al.* 2015). The maximum lactulose concentration was observed at 350 rpm, pH 6.8 and a molar ratio of 1 : 2 (lactose to fructose ratio). With a further increase in this ratio, synthesis of galactooligosaccharides was promoted rather than lactulose. In long-term operation, at a molar ratio of 1 : 2 (lactose to fructose) and hydraulic residence time of 9 h, a mean constant lactulose concentration of 14.51 ± 0.07 g/L was reached between 23 and 32 h. The production of lactulose by *K. lactis* β-galactosidase using cheese whey as feedstock has also been studied (de Albuquerque *et al.* 2018). The optimal conditions for lactulose production using free β-galactosidase were lactose/fructose ratio of 15 : 30% (w/v), total initial concentration of lactose and fructose of 200 g/L, pH 7 at temperature 50 °C with the addition of 0.01% (w/v) Mg^{2+}. Under these optimal conditions, a maximum lactulose production of 22.6 g/L with a productivity of 11.3 g (L/h) was reported in 2 h.

Recently, the effect of concentration of lactose and fructose as well as enzymatic activities of two commercially available β-galactosidases (Enzeco and Lactozym) has also been investigated (Schmidt *et al.* 2020a). The optimal feed composition was observed as 1.28 or 0.74 mol/kg fructose and 0.17 or 0.19 mol/kg lactose with an enzymatic activity of 2.0 or 2.8 μkat/kg for acid or sweet whey to yield optimal concentration of lactulose. Further, seven commercial β-galactosidases have also been tested with reference to their ability for the production of lactulose in sweet and acid whey UF-permeates (Schmidt *et al.* 2020b). Three enzyme preparations, Enzeco (pH 6.0), Biolactase (pH 6.5) and Lactozym (pH 6.0), were identified as having high lactulose yields of 0.27, 0.21 and 0.21, respectively.

The commercial preparation of *Bacillus circulans* β-galactosidase was also assessed in the production of lactulose. The best results were obtained at lactose mass ratio and fructose of 20, with a yield of 0.54, productivity of 0.043 g/h mg/enz, and selectivity of 30.9 for lactulose synthesis. Yields achieved with *Bacillus circulans* β-galactosidase were higher than enzymes of other origins at comparable conditions (Aburto *et al.* 2020).

Lactulose Production Using Immobilized Enzyme Commercial enzymes are very expensive and the soluble enzymes have to be discarded after a single use, which makes the whole process uneconomical. To overcome this problem, enzymes can be coupled with a suitable support material through the process of immobilization. Immobilized β-galactosidase may offer several advantages over soluble β-galactosidase such as reusability, high yield, high reactor productivity, better thermal stability and easy separation or purification, and continuous operation is easy (Kishore *et al.* 2012). Immobilization is a technical process whereby biocatalysts are bound to or entrapped within solid supports, resulting in a heterogeneous immobilized enzyme system. Traditionally, the enzyme has been immobilized by various methods such as adsorption, covalent bonding, entrapment and cross-linking, as shown in Figure 14.3 (Nguyen and Kim 2017).

The synthesis of lactulose using β-galactosidase obtained from *E. coli* immobilized on Eupergit was first carried out by Ajisaka *et al.* (1987). Lactulose yield of 3.3 g/L was observed along with the formation of a new disaccharide (1-lactulose). Solutions of galactose and fructose circulated through columns containing β-galactosidases obtained from *A. oryzae* and *E. coli* as well as activated carbons have also been employed to enhance lactulose production (Ajisaka *et al.* 1988). A considerable increase in lactulose production was observed with a conversion yield of 11.3% after 24 h with β-galactosidase from *E. coli*.

Furthermore, lactulose synthesis has been successfully carried out by a dual-enzymatic method (immobilized glucose isomerase and immobilized lactase) in a two-phase organic aqueous medium using lactose and fructose as the raw materials. Immobilized lactase was prepared by cross-linking the free lactase into Fe_3O_4-chitosan magnetic microspheres (Hua *et al.* 2010). In another study, a process for the continuous enzymatic production of lactulose was developed using both free and immobilized β-glycosidase from *P. furiosus* (Mayer *et al.* 2010).

Studies on the effect of galactose, glucose and fructose on β-galactosidase activity on hydrolysis of whey lactose and lactulose synthesis have indicated that galactose and glucose have strong inhibitory effects on the transgalactosylation reaction when compared with lactose hydrolysis (Song *et al.* 2013b). Additionally, 19.1 g/L of lactulose was observed in a continuous

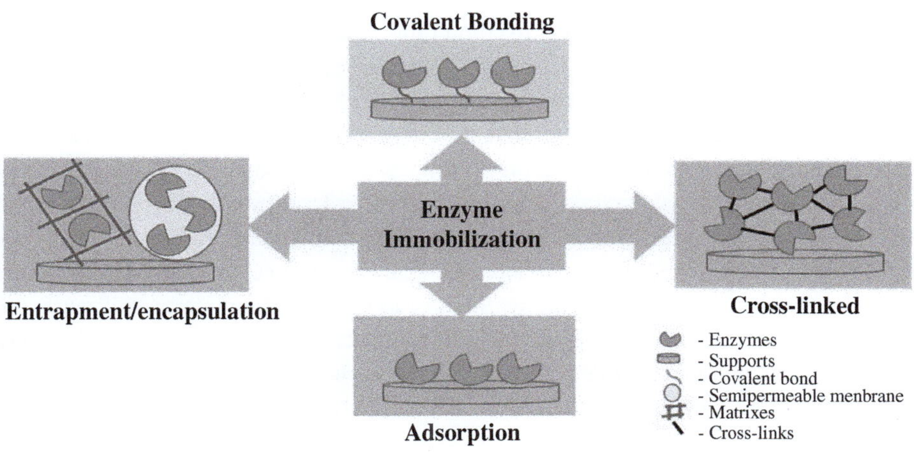

Figure 14.3 Different methods of enzyme immobilization. *Source:* Nguyen, H.H. and Kim, M. (2017). An overview of techniques in enzyme immobilization. *Applied Science and Convergence Technology,* 26(6): 157–163.

packed-bed reactor using immobilized β-galactosidase, and the catalytic activity of the immobilized β-galactosidase was retained up to 52.9% after 10 recycles. In other studies, immobilized β-galactosidase and glucose isomerase on silica gels were used for lactulose production from whey lactose, and lactulose with a yield of 7.68 g/L was produced under optimal reaction conditions (Song *et al.* 2013a).

The enzymatic production of lactulose by immobilized *K. lactis* β-galactosidase using cheese whey as feedstock has also been reported (Song *et al.* 2013b). Immobilization of β-galactosidase on chitosan activated with glutaraldehyde was carried for the synthesis of lactulose from cheese whey, which resulted in maximum production of 17.3 g/L lactulose (de Albuquerque *et al.* 2018).

Synthesis of lactulose from fructose and lactose in a continuous packed-bed reactor operation was carried out with glyoxyl–agarose immobilized *A. oryzae* β-galactosidase. A maximum lactulose yield of 0.6 g/g was observed with 50% w/w total sugars, flow rate of 15 mL/min, fructose : lactose molar ratio of 12, biocatalyst-inert packing material mass ratio of 1 : 8 g/g and pH 4.5 at 50 °C (Guerrero *et al.* 2019). Lactulose production was also carried out using immobilized β-galactosidase obtained from *A. oryzae* cross-linked aggregates. Lactulose synthesis was performed in both batch and repeated-batch operation with 50% w/w total sugars, 200 IUH/g of enzyme, fructose : lactose molar ratio of 8, pH 4.5 at 50 °C. Lactulose yields of 0.19 g/g and 0.24 g/g were observed for fructose to lactose molar ratio of 4 mol/mol and 8 mol/mol with selectivities of 3.3 mol/mol and 6.6 mol/mol, respectively, for aggregation and cross-linking, obtaining catalysts by ethanol and propanol precipitation (Guerrero *et al.* 2020).

14.3.2.2 Whole Cell Biocatalysts for Lactulose Production

The enzyme cost in lactulose production is a major hindrance in commercialization of the enzymatic process. To overcome this problem, several attempts have been made in order to develop an economical process. For this purpose, the utilization of intracellular β-galactosidase as a whole cell biocatalyst has been found to be an efficient way to reduce enzyme production cost, since no purification step is required, which can result in the development of a cost-effective process. Although whole cells offer numerous advantages over purified enzymes, however, the permeability barrier for substrates and products due to the cell envelope may result in lower reaction rates. Therefore, to reduce this permeability barrier of whole cell biocatalysts, permeabilized yeast cells with high activities can be a good choice for the enzymatic reaction (Panesar *et al.* 2006).

Among the different β-galactosidases tested, the enzyme from *K. lactis* showed highest lactulose productivity. Optimization of reaction conditions for the production of lactulose using permeabilized yeast cells was carried out and an increase in lactulose concentration (1.3- and 2.1-fold) was observed using permeabilized cells when compared to untreated cells (Lee *et al.* 2004). Wang *et al.* (2015) reported cellobiose 2-epimerase from *C. saccharolyticus* to be the most efficient enzyme for the enzymatic synthesis of lactulose. Ethanol-permeabilized *E. coli* cells containing *C. saccharolyticus* cellobiose 2-epimerase were used as biocatalysts for lactulose production, and maximum lactulose production was observed under optimized conditions.

Lactulose production using immobilized cells containing thermostable cellobiose 2-epimerase has also been successfully carried out. A process was developed for lactulose production using cellobiose 2-epimerase and screened improved mutant enzymes from a library generated by an error-prone polymerase chain reaction (PCR) technique (Park *et al.* 2016). A 1.3-fold increase in lactulose conversion yield was observed as compared to that of wild-type cellobiose 2-epimerase. The immobilized cell beads were found to be more stable after continuous cycles and retained up to 80% of their original enzyme activity after four cycles.

14.3.3 Electro-activation Method

This method of lactulose synthesis is an electrocatalytic method and is also considered as a safe and environmentally friendly green technology as it utilizes no reagents. It is generally used to generate high alkaline conditions in the reaction medium used for the isomerization of lactose to lactulose (Aider and Gimenez-Vidal 2012; Aït-Aissa and Aïder 2014b). In this approach to lactulose synthesis, the reaction is performed in an electrolysis reactor that consists of two electrodes kept in an electrolytic solution which further conducts the ions after an external electric field is applied (Aider and Gimenez-Vidal 2012). In another report on the electro-activation method, the reactor had three compartments (cathodic, anodic and central) wherein the cathodic compartment contained a lactose solution, and the central and anodic compartment contained an electrolyte solution. Furthermore, the anion and cation exchange membranes connected the central part to other compartments, whereas the electro-isomerization reaction was carried out in the cathodic compartment (Aït-Aissa and Aider 2013). As the process of isomerization needs an alkaline medium as proton acceptor, this was generated at the cathode interface through water electrolysis. The lactose solutions of 5 and 10% were then subjected to electric fields of 100 and 200 mA at an ambient temperature for 60 min, and lactulose yield of 25% was attained with no epilactose production (Aider and Gimenez-Vidal 2012). Additionally, a lactose to lactulose conversion yield of 35% was achieved by applying a cheese whey based lactose (7% w/v) to an electric field of 400 mA at 10 °C for 40 min (Kareb *et al.* 2016).

The electro-activation approach for lactulose synthesis was also applied using high current intensity (900 mA) in a 10% lactose solution for 40 min to achieve highest yield (Karim and Aider 2020). A higher lactulose yield of 38% was achieved in the electro-activation approach within a short reaction period as compared to that of chemical isomerization. In view of this result, it was suggested that the electro-activation approach may be a good alternative in future to enhance lactulose production from lactose with fewer demineralization and purification steps.

14.4 Techniques for the Analysis of Lactulose

The analysis of lactulose in the reaction mixture is also a very important step in the process. The analytical technique to determine the level of lactulose should be simple, rapid and precise. Various methodologies have been developed for the determination of lactulose including gas–liquid chromatography (GC), gas chromatography–mass spectrometry (GC-MS), thin-layer chromatography (TLC), high-performance liquid chromatography (HPLC), liquid chromatography–mass spectrometry (LC-MS), nuclear magnetic resonance (NMR) and other related techniques such as capillary electrophoresis, spectroscopic method and flow analysis methods (Adhikari *et al.* 1991; Celli *et al.* 1995; Fleming *et al.* 1990; Jayalakshmi *et al.* 2009; Lee *et al.* 2004; Martinez-Castro and Olano 1981; Mayer *et al.* 1996; Montero *et al.* 2004; Rodriguez *et al.* 2009).

Nowadays, HPLC with refractive index (RI) detector has become the most preferred technique for the identification and quantification of lactulose (Zimmer *et al.* 2017). The quantification of lactulose has been performed using HPLC equipped with a column containing NH_2 as ionic form containing a mixture of acetonitrile and water as mobile phase (Adamczak *et al.* 2009; Wang *et al.* 2017).

14.5 Applications of Lactulose

Lactulose has been found to be effective for the treatment of many medical disorders. In addition to this, lactulose has also been used in many food products as a prebiotic ingredient/additive for intestinal regulation. The applications of lactulose in both food and health sectors are summarized in Figure 14.4.

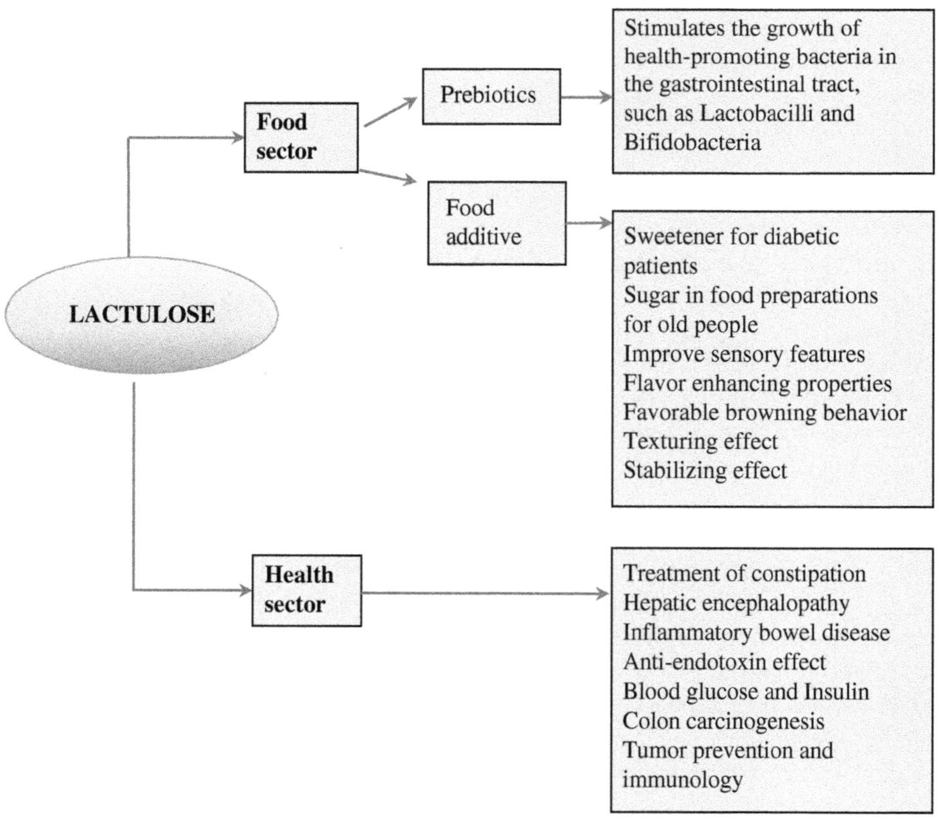

Figure 14.4 Potential applications of lactulose. *Sources:* Based on Tamura *et al.* 1993; Crittenden and Playne 1996; Battermann 1997; Strohmaier 1998; Schumann 2002.

14.5.1 Food Sectors

Lactulose as a bifidus factor or functional ingredient can be applied in a wide variety of food products, especially for intestinal regulation, as discussed in the following sections.

14.5.1.1 Lactulose as a Bifidus Factor

Prebiotics are non-digestible food ingredients that have a potential role in stimulating the activity and/or growth of various health-promoting microflora to proliferate significantly in the colon of the host (Panesar *et al.* 2013). Due to its prebiotic potential, lactulose is neither absorbed nor metabolized in the upper portion of the digestive tract (stomach and small intestine) and is broken down by the bacteria that live in the lower part of the gut. Lactulose as a substrate stimulates the growth of health-promoting bacteria in the gastrointestinal tract, such as lactobacilli and bifidobacteria. These health-beneficial intestinal bacteria that ferment lactulose into short chain fatty acids result in lower pH of intestine, which further leads to inhibition of the growth of potentially harmful bacteria such as *E. coli*, *Bacteroides* and clostridia (Ait-Aissa and Aider 2014a). Furthermore, owing to the prebiotic properties of lactulose, it is also responsible for enhancement of the survival rate of probiotic strains present in yoghurt (Tabatabaie and Mortazavi 2008). Several studies have revealed increased stability of *Bifidobacterium* spp. and *Lactobacillus* spp., which are able to survive for a longer time in the presence of lactulose. Another study also concluded that the use of lactulose as a prebiotic improves the quality of skimmed milk fermented by *Lactobacillus acidophilus*, *Lactobacillus rhamnosus*, *Lactobacillus bulgaricus* and *B. lactis* in co-culture with *Streptococcus thermophilus* (Pinheiro De Souza Oliveira *et al.* 2011).

14.5.1.2 Lactulose as a Functional Additive

Lactulose is known for numerous attributes such as high water solubility, favorable browning behavior and flavor-enhancing properties, which are desirable for food products. In addition to providing useful modifications in foods' flavor and physicochemical characteristics, lactulose also possesses various properties that are beneficial for the health of consumers. Moreover, it can be added as a sugar replacer in beverages, confectionery and bakery products, infant milk powders and dairy products, as well as in products generally designed for customers with diabetics (Crittenden and Playne 1996; Seki and Saito 2012; Strohmaier 1998; Tamura *et al.* 1993). Apart from this, lactulose has also been used in fortifying fruit juices and other acidic foods due to its high thermal stability at low pH (Seki and Saito 2012).

14.5.2 Health Sectors

In health sectors, lactulose can be used for an extensive range of applications such as relief in constipation, hepatic encephalopathy and liver diseases, prevention of tumors, control of blood sugar level, etc. (Schumann 2002). It can also be applied in the diagnosis of colonic disorders through a breath hydrogen test (Simren and Stotzer 2006).

14.5.2.1 Salmonella Carriers

Salmonella is a major enteric Gram-negative pathogen that colonizes the intestinal tract. Oral administration of lactulose induces a drop in the pH of the colon, which reduces the survival rate of *Salmonella* spp. Moreover, the ability of lactulose to act as a prebiotic in non-typhoid *Salmonella* carriers has also been reported (Hoffmann 1975). Lactulose therapy helps to reduce the population of fecal *Shigella and Salmonella* spp. as well as lowering the occurrence of urinary tract and respiratory infections (Liao *et al.* 1994).

14.5.2.2 Constipation and Hepatic Encephalopathy

Lactulose is used for the treatment of constipation in all age groups, from infants to the elderly, owing to its laxative effects, safety and efficacy profile (Ait-Aissa and Aider 2014a). In the colon, intestinal microflora can metabolize lactulose into its active components that help to draw water into the colon, which softens the stool and makes it easier to pass. Lactulose is widely used in the treatment of hepatic encephalopathy by drawing ammonia from the blood into the colon (Foster *et al.* 2010; Paik *et al.* 2005; Sharma *et al.* 2009).

14.5.2.3 Anti-endotoxin Effects

Preoperative administration of lactulose has been reported to prevent several endotoxin-dependent complexities such as renal dysfunction (Özçelik *et al.* 1997; Pain *et al.* 1991). Moreover, the anti-endotoxin effect exhibited by lactulose is known for preventing several metabolic diseases including exocrine pancreatic dysfunction, hepatorenal syndrome, hypercholesterolemia and diabetes mellitus (Kramer 1988; Liao and Florin 1995; Mack *et al.* 1992; Tabatabaie *et al.* 1997; Yelich *et al.* 1992). In another study, the role of lactulose in prevention of systemic endotoxemia was also investigated in patients with obstructive jaundice (Koutelidakis *et al.* 2003).

14.5.2.4 Colon Carcinogenesis

The etiology of colon cancer is linked to the generation of various toxins and metabolites during the many biochemical processes occurring in the mucosa, lumen and tissues of the large intestine. Therefore, the colonic microflora and numerous metabolic products generated by them may increase the incidence of carcinoma of colon. Probiotic health-promoting bacteria and prebiotics such as lactulose may help in reducing the risk of colonic carcinoma (Wollowski *et al.* 2001).

14.5.2.5 Inflammatory Bowel Disease

The consumption of lactulose may help to prevent systemic endotoxemia of colonic origin. Therefore, lactulose is also utilized for the treatment of inflammatory bowel diseases because bacteria and their endotoxins play a vital role in the development of this syndrome. The oral administration of lactulose in obstructive jaundice can prevent systemic endotoxemia and its subsequent inflammatory response (Koutelidakis *et al.* 2003). The hydrolysis of lactulose by gastrointestinal tract bacteria produces a significant quantity of endogenous hydrogen that acts as an indirect antioxidant, thereby providing protection against dextran sulfate sodium (DSS)-induced colitis, reducing oxidative stress and ameliorating the symptoms of inflammatory bowel disease (Chen *et al.* 2011).

14.5.2.6 Tumor Prevention and Immunology

Numerous studies on tumor prevention are being carried out worldwide and bifidobacteria showed exceptional efficacy in the prevention of tumor. The consumption of lactulose has been reported to increase the population of bifidobacteria that further enhances the immunological and antitumor effects (Schumann 1997, 2002). Lactulose is also used for preoperative oral treatment for the prevention of complications in patients undergoing surgery for obstructive jaundice (Greve *et al.* 1990).

14.5.2.7 Blood Glucose and Insulin

Lactulose is a poorly absorbed disaccharide, having an important role for reducing insulin and blood glucose levels (Bianchi *et al.* 1994). In another study, it was suggested that endotoxins reduce the production of insulin in the pancreas and that therefore lactulose also functions as an antidiabetic agent (Cornell 1985).

14.5.2.8 Diagnostic Applications

Lactulose has diagnostic applications and can be applied for identifying colonic disorders through a breath hydrogen test, which involves oral administration of a single dose of lactulose and measurement of exhaled hydrogen during the following hours. The formation of hydrogen in the gut is due to bacterial metabolism of lactulose. The extent of exhalation and production of hydrogen determines colonization of microflora as well as colonic transit time (Simren and Stotzer 2006; Yu *et al.* 2011). The other function of the lactulose breath test is to identify the excessive proliferation of bacteria in the small intestine. During this, lactulose is metabolized by bacterial flora in large intestine and the rate of exhaled hydrogen becomes faster than that of the healthy population (Nucera *et al.* 2005).

14.6 Future Developments

In recent years, with the growing interest in functional foods, lactulose has become a potential candidate for numerous commercial applications in the health and food sectors. Lactulose is known for a wide array of health applications in treating various disorders. In the food industry, lactulose is utilized as a bifidus factor and a prebiotic food additive for fortifying and enrichment purposes. Apart from its potential applications, lactulose offers excellent and scientifically tested multifunctional properties, which make it a potential candidate to be used as a delivery system in future. With the growing interest of consumers in high nutrition values and a healthy diet, the concept of functional foods is of growing importance. The ability to use lactulose for micro/nano-encapsulation processes can also be applied in the food and pharmaceutical sectors. Further, the utilization of lactulose for the nano-encapsulation and delivery of bioactive material is promising.

14.7 Conclusion

Lactulose is a non-digestible disaccharide with prebiotic activities that is significantly used as a potential component of a functional diet. It is known for a wide array of applications in the health and food sectors. As a potent prebiotic, it enhances the growth of beneficial gut microflora as well as neutralizing harmful species. Moreover, due to its health-promoting attributes, it is considered as a promising component to be added as a potential supplement into a variety of food products. In the health sector, it is also used as a potential therapeutic agent for the treatment of severe chronic disorders. Among different methods used for the production of lactulose, biotechnological methods have various environmental and technological benefits over chemical methods. Enzymatic bioconversion of lactose to lactulose is eco-friendly and product purification by enzyme immobilization is easy and simple. Furthermore, use of permeabilized whole cells as a biocatalyst can also improve the economics of the process.

References

Aburto, C., Guerrero, C., Vera, C. and Illanes, A. (2020). Improvement in the yield and selectivity of lactulose synthesis with *Bacillus circulans* β-galactosidase. *LWT - Food Science and Technology*, 118: 108746.

Adamczak, M., Charubin, D. and Bednarski, W. (2009). Influence of reaction medium composition on enzymatic synthesis of galactooligosaccharides and lactulose from lactose concentrates prepared from whey permeate. *Chemical Papers*, 6: 111–116.

Adhikari, A.K., Sahai, O. and Mathur, O.N. (1991). A rapid spectrophotometric method for quantitative determination of lactulose in heated milk and milk products. *Lait*, 71: 555–564.

Aider, M. and de Halleux, D. (2007). Isomerization of lactose and lactulose production: review. *Trends in Food Science and Technology*, 18: 356–364.

Aider, M. and Gimenez-Vidal, M. (2012). Lactulose synthesis by electro-isomerization of lactose: Effect of lactose concentration and electric current density. *Innovative Food Science and Emerging Technologies*, 16: 163–170.

Aït-Aissa, A. and Aıder, M. (2013). Lactose isomerization into lactulose in an electro-activation reactor and high-performance liquid chromatography (HPLC) monitoring of the process. *Journal of Food Engineering*, 119: 115–124.

Aït-Aissa, A. and Aider, M. (2014a). Lactulose: production and use in functional food, medical and pharmaceutical applications. Practical and critical review. *International Journal of Food Science and Technology*, 49: 1245–1253

Aït-Aissa, A. and Aïder, M. (2014b). Lactose electroisomerization into lactulose: Effect of the electrode material, active membrane surface area-to-electrode surface area ratio, and interelectrode-membrane distance. *Journal of Dairy Science*, 97(8): 4811–4823.

Ajisaka, K., Fujimoto, H. and Nishida, H. (1988). Enzymic synthesis of disaccharides by use of the reversed hydrolysis activity of β-D-galactosidases. *Carbohydrate Research*, 180(1): 35–42.

Ajisaka, K., Nishida, H. and Fujimoto, H. (1987). Use of an activated carbon column for the synthesis of disaccharides by use of a reversed hydrolysis activity of β-galactosidase. *Biotechnology Letters*, 9(6): 387–392.

Battermann W. (1997). Lactulose powder – main technological properties and its relevance in functional food. Internal Report Solvay Deutschland GmbH. Report no. AWTLAC.

Bianchi, G.P., De Mitri, M.S., Bugianesi, E., Abbiati, R., Fabbri, A. and Marchesini, G. (1994). Lowering effects of a preparation containing fibres and lactulose on glucose and insulin levels in obesity. *Italian Journal of Gastroenterology*, 26: 174–178.

Carobbi, R. and Innocenti, F. (1990). Process for preparing lactulose from lactose by epimerisation with sodium aluminate. European patent 0320670.

Celli, M., D'Eufemia, P., Dommarco, R., Finocchiaro, R., Aprigliano, D., Martino, F., Cardi, E. and Giardini, O. (1995). Rapid gas-chromatographic assay of lactulose and mannitol for estimating intestinal permeability. *Clinical Chemistry*, 41(5): 752–756.

Chen, Q., Xiao, Y., Zhang, W., Zhang, T., Bo Jiang, B., Stressler, T., Fischer, L. and Mu, W. (2018). Current research on cellobiose 2-epimerase: Enzymatic properties, mechanistic insights, and potential applications in the dairy industry. *Trends in Food Science and Technology*, 82: 167–176.

Chen, X., Zuo, Q., Hai, Y. and Sun, X.J. (2011). Lactulose: An indirect antioxidant ameliorating inflammatory bowel disease by increasing hydrogen production. *Medical Hypotheses*, 76, 325–327.

Cornell, R.P. (1985). Endogenous gut-derived bacterial endotoxin tonically primes pancreatic secretion of insulin in normal rats. *Diabetes*, 34: 1253–1259.

Corzo-Martínez, M., Copoví, P., Olano, A., Moreno, F.J. and Montilla, A. (2013). Synthesis of prebiotic carbohydrates derived from cheese whey permeate by a combined process of isomerisation and transgalactosylation. *Journal of the Science of Food and Agriculture*, 93(7): 1591–1597.

Corzo-Martínez, M., Montilla, A., Megías-Pérez, R., Olano, A., Javier Moreno, F. and Villamiel, M. (2014). Impact of high-intensity ultrasound on the formation of lactulose and Maillard reaction glycoconjugates. *Food Chemistry*, 157: 186–192.

Cox, M., Lehninger, A.L. and Nelson, D.R. (2000). In: *Lehninger Principles of Biochemistry*, 306–308. New York: Worth Publishers. ISBN 1-57259-931-936.

Crittenden, R.G. and Playne, M.J. (1996). Production, properties and applications of food-grade oligosaccharides. *Trends in Food Science and Technology*, 7: 353–361.

de Albuquerque, T.L., Gomes, S.D.L., D'Almeida, A.P., Fernandez-Lafuente, R., Gonçalves, L.R.B., and Rocha, M.V.P. (2018). Immobilization of β-galactosidase in glutaraldehyde-chitosan and its application to the synthesis of lactulose using cheese whey as feedstock. *Process Biochemistry*, 73: 65–73.

Fleming, S.C., Kapembwa, M.S., Laker, M.F., Levin, G.E. and Griffin, G.E. (1990). Rapid and simultaneous determination of lactulose and mannitol in urine, by HPLC with pulsed amperometric detection, for use in studies of intestinal permeability. *Clinical Chemistry*, 36: 797–799.

Foster, K.J., Lin, S. and Turck, C.J. (2010). Current and emerging strategies for treating hepatic encephalopathy. *Critical Care Nursing Clinics North America*, 22: 341–350.

Gonçalvesa, L.R.B. and Rochaa, M.V.P. (2004). Immobilization of β-galactosidase in glutaraldehyde-chitosan and its application to the synthesis of lactulose using cheese whey as feedstock. *Applied Microbiology Biotechnology*, 64(6): 787–793.

Greve, J.W., Gouma, D.J., Leeuwen, P.A.M. and Buurman, W.A. (1990). Lactulose inhibits endotoxin induced tumour necrosis factor production by monocytes. *An in vitro study. Gut*, 31: 198–203.

Guerrero, C., Aburto, C., Súarez, S., Vera, C. and Illanes, A. (2020). Improvements in the production of *Aspergillus oryzae* β-galactosidase crosslinked aggregates and their use in repeated-batch synthesis of lactulose. *International Journal of Biological Macromolecules*, 142: 452–462.

Guerrero, C., Valdiviaa, F., Ubillaa, C., Ramíreza, N., Gómeza, M., Aburtoa, C., Verab, C. and Illanesa, A. (2019). Continuous enzymatic synthesis of lactulose in packed-bed reactor with immobilized *Aspergillus oryzae* β-galactosidase. *Bioresource Technology*, 278: 296–302.

Guerrero, C., Vera, C., Araya, E., Conejeros, R., and Illanes, A. (2015). Repeated-batch operation for the synthesis of lactulose with β-galactosidase immobilized by aggregation and crosslinking. *Bioresource Technology*, 190: 122–131.

Hicks, K.B. and Parrish, F.W. (1980). A new method for the preparation of lactulose from lactose. *Carbohydrate Research*, 82: 393–397.

Hicks, K.B., Raupp, D.L., and Smith, P.W. (1984). Preparation and purification of lactulose from sweet cheese whey ultrafiltrate. *Journal of Agricultural and Food Chemistry*, 32(2): 288–292.

Hoffmann, K. (1975). Behandlung von gesunden Salmonellen-ausscheidern mit lactulose. *Deutsche Medizinische Wochenschrift*, 100: 1429–1431.

Hua, X., Yang, R., Shen, Q., Ye, F., Zhang, W. and Zhao, W. (2013). Production of 1-lactulose and lactulose using commercial β-galactosidase from *Kluyveromyces lactis* in the presence of fructose. *Food Chemistry*, 137: 1–7.

Hua, X., Yang, R., Zhang, W., Fei, Y., Jin, Z. and Jiang, B. (2010). Dual-enzymatic synthesis of lactulose in organic-aqueous two-phase media. *Food Research International*, 43: 716–722.

Jayalakshmi, K., Ghoshal, U.C., Kumar, S., Misra, A., Roy, R. and Khetrapal, C.L. (2009). Assessment of small intestinal permeability using ^{1}H-NMR spectroscopy. *Journal of Gastrointestinal and Liver Diseases*, 18: 27–32.

Kareb, O., Champagne, C.P. and Aïder, M. (2016). Contribution to the production of lactulose-rich whey by in situ electro-isomerization of lactose and effect on whey proteins after electro-activation as confirmed by matrix-assisted laser desorption/ionization time-of-flight-mass spectrometry and sodium dodecyl sulfate-polyacrylamide gel electrophoresis. *Journal of Dairy Science*, 99(4): 2552–2570.

Karim, A. and Aider, M. (2020). Sustainable electroisomerization of lactose into lactulose and comparison with the chemical isomerization at equivalent solution alkalinity. *ACS Omega*, 5: 2318–2333.

Khatami, S., Ashtiani, F. Z., Bonakdarpour, B. and Mehrdad, M. (2014). The enzymatic production of lactulose via transglycosylation in conventional and non-conventional media. *International Dairy Journal*, 34(1): 74–79.

Kim, Y.S. and Oh, D.K. (2012). Lactulose production from lactose as a single substrate by a thermostable cellobiose 2-epimerase from *Caldicellulosiruptor saccharolyticus. Bioresource Technology*, 104: 668–672.

Kim, Y.S., Kim, J.E., and Oh, D.K. (2013). Borate enhances the production of lactulose from lactose by cellobiose 2-epimerase from Caldicellulosiruptor saccharolyticus. *Bioresource Technology*, 128: 809–812.

Kim, Y.S., Parkand, C.S. and Oh, D.K. (2006). Lactulose production from lactose and fructose by a thermostable β-galactosidase from *Sulfolobus solfataricus. Enzyme and Microbial Technology*, 39: 903–908.

Kishore, D., Talat, M., Srivastava, O.N. and Kayastha, A.M. (2012). Immobilization of β-galactosidase onto functionalized graphene nano-sheets using response surface methodology and its analytical applications. *PLoS ONE*, 7(7): e40708.

Kochetkov, N.K. and Bochkov, A.F. (1967). In: *Chemistry of Carbohydrates*, 672. Moscow.

Koutelidakis, I., Papaziogas, B., Giamarellos-Bourboulis, E.J., Makris, J, Pavlidis, T., Giamarellou, H. and Papaziogas, T. (2003). Systemic endotoxaemia following obstructive jaundice: the role of lactulose. *Journal of Surgical Research*, 113: 243–247.

Kozempel, M., and Kurantz, M. (1994). A continuous reactor system for production of lactulose. *Journal of Chemical Technology and Biotechnology*, 59(3): 265–269.

Kramer, H.J. (1988) Therapie des hepatorenalen syndroms. *Deutsche Medizinisch Wochenschrift*, 113: 561–564.

Krumbbloz, R.E. and Dorscheid, M.G. (1991). Method of manufacturing lactulose. European patent 0375040.

Lee, Y.J., Kim, C.S. and Oh, D.K. (2004). Lactulose production by β-galactosidase in permeabilized cells of *Kluyveromyces lactis*. *Applied Microbiology and Biotechnology*, 64: 787–793.

Liao, W. and Florin, C.H. (1995). Endotoxin, cytokines and hyperlipidemia. *Scandinavian Journal of Gastroenterology*, 28: 97–103.

Liao, W., Cui, X.S., Jin, X.Y. and Florén, C.H. (1994). Lactulose – a potential drug for the treatment of inflammatory bowel disease. *Medical Hypotheses*, 43: 234–238.

Mack, D.R., Flick, J.A., Durie, P.R., Rosentein, B.J., Ellis, L.E. and Perman, J.A. (1992). Correlation of intestinal lactulose permeability with exocrine pancreatic dysfunction. *Journal of Pediatrics*, 120: 696–701.

Martinez-Castro, I. and Olano, A. (1981). Ready detection of small amount of lactulose in dairy products by thin-layer chromatography. *Chromatographia*, 14: 11–12.

Mayer, J., Conrad, J., Klaiber, I., Lutz-Wahl, S., Beifuss, U. and Fischer, L. (2004). Enzymatic production and complete nuclear magnetic resonance assignment of the sugar lactulose. *Journal of Agricultural and Food Chemistry*, 52(23): 6983–6990.

Mayer, J., Kranz, B. and Fischer, L. (2010). Continuous production of lactulose by immobilized thermostable β-glycosidase from *Pyrococcus furiosus*. *Journal of Biotechnology*, 145(4): 387–393.

Mayer, M., Genrich, M., Künnecke, W. and Bilitewski, U. (1996). Automated determination of lactulose in milk using an enzyme reactor and flow analysis with integrated dialysis. *Analytica Chimica Acta*, 324: 37–45.

Montero, C.M., Dodero, M.C., Sánchez, D.A. and Barroso, C.G. (2004). Analysis of low molecular weight carbohydrates in food and beverages: a review. *Chromatographia*, 59: 15–30.

Montgomery, E.M. and Hudson, C.S. (1930). Relations between rotating power and structure in the sugar group. Synthesis of new disaccharide ketoses from lactose. *Journal of the American Chemical Society*, 52: 2101–2111.

Montilla, A., Castillo, M.D., Sanz, M.L. and Olano, A. (2005). Egg shell as catalyst of lactose isomerization to lactulose. *Food Chemistry*, 90: 883–890.

Nguyen, H.H. and Kim, M. (2017). An overview of techniques in enzyme immobilization. *Applied Science and Convergence Technology*, 26(6): 157–163.

Nooshkam, M. and Madadlou, A. (2016a). Microwave-assisted isomerisation of lactose to lactulose and Maillard conjugation of lactulose and lactose with whey proteins and peptides. *Food Chemistry*, 200: 1–9.

Nooshkam, M., and Madadlou, A. (2016b). Maillard conjugation of lactulose with potentially bioactive peptides. *Food Chemistry*, 192: 831–836.

Nucera, G., Gabrielli, M., Lupascu, A., Lauritano, E.C., Santoliquido, A., Cremonini, F., Cammarota, G., Tondi, P., Pola, P., Gasbarrini, G. and Gasbarrini, A. (2005). Abnormal breath tests to lactose, fructose and sorbitol in irritable bowel syndrome may be explained by small intestinal bacterial overgrowth. *Alimentary Pharmacology and Therapeutics*, 21, 1391–1395.

Özçelik, M.F., Pekmezci, S., Altinli, E., Eroglu, C., Göksel, S. and Göksoy, E. (1997). Lactulose to prevent translocation in biliary obstruction. *Digestive Surgery*, 14: 267–271.

Paik, Y.H., Lee, K.S. and Han, K.H. (2005). Comparison of rifaximin and lactulose for the treatment of hepatic encephalopathy: a prospective randomized study. *Yonsei Medical Journal*, 46: 399–407.

Pain, J.A., Cahill, C.J., Gilbert, J.M., Johnson, C.D., Trapnell, J.E. and Bailey, M.E. (1991). Prevention of postoperative dysfunction in patients with obstructive jaundice: a multicentre study of bile salts and lactulose. *British Journal of Surgery*, 78: 467–469.

Panesar, P.S. and Kumari, S. (2011). Lactulose: Production, purification and potential applications. *Biotechnology Advances*, 29(6): 940–948.

Panesar, P.S., Kaur, G., Panesar, R. and Bera, M.B. (2009). Synbiotics: potential dietary supplements in functional foods. UK: FST Bulletin, Food Science Central, IFIS Publishing.

Panesar, P.S., Kumari, S., and Panesar, R. (2010). Potential applications of immobilized β-galactosidase in food processing industries. *Enzyme Research*, 2010: 1–15.

Panesar, P.S., Kumari, S. and Panesar, R. (2013). Biotechnological approaches for the production of prebiotics and their potential applications. *Critical Review in Biotechnology*, 33: 345–354.

Panesar, P.S., Panesar, R., Singh, R.S., Kennedy, J.F. and Kumar, H. (2006). Microbial production, immobilization and applications of β-D-galactosidase. *Journal of Chemical Technology and Biotechnology*, 81: 530–543.

Park, A.-R., Koo, B.-S., Kim, J.-S. and Kim, E.-J. (2016). Lactulose production using immobilized cells including *Thermostable Cellobiose* 2-epimerase. *Korean Journal of Microbiology and Biotechnology*, 44(4): 504–511.

Paseephol, T., Small, D.M., and Sherkat, F. (2008). Lactulose production from milk concentration permeate using calcium carbonate-based catalysts. *Food Chemistry*, 111(2): 283–290.

Pinheiro De Souza Oliveira, R., Rodrigues Florence, A.C., Perego, P., Nogueira De Oliveira, M. and Converti, A. (2011). Use of lactulose as prebiotic and its influence on the growth, acidification profile and viable counts of different probiotics in fermented skim milk. *International Journal of Food Microbiology*, 145: 22–27.

Playne, M.J. and Crittenden, R.G. (2009). Galacto-oligosaccharide and other products derived from lactose. In: *Advanced Dairy Chemistry: Lactose, Water, Salts and Major Constituents* (ed. P.L.H. McSweeney and P.F. Fox), 3rd edition, volume 3, 155.

Rentschler, E., Schuh, K., Krewinkel, M., Baur, C., Claaßen, W., Meyer, S., Kuschel, B., Stressler, T. and Fischer, L. (2015). Enzymatic production of lactulose and epilactose in milk. *Journal of Dairy Science*, 98: 6767–6775.

Rodríguez, A.M., Prieto, P., de la, Hoz, Díaz-Ortiz, A., Martín, D.R. and Garcíab, J.I. (2015). Influence of polarity and activation energy in microwave–assisted organic synthesis (MAOS), *Chemistry Open*, 4(3): 308–317.

Rodriguez, H., Suchodolski, J.S., Berghoff, N. and Steiner, J.M. (2009). Development and analytic validation of a gas chromatography–mass spectrometry method for the measurement of sugar probes in canine serum. *American Journal of Veterinary Research*, 70: 320–329.

Ruttloff, H., Taufel, A., Krause, W., Haenel, H. and Taufel, K. (1967). Enzymatic hydrolysis of galacto-oligosaccharides in the human and animal intestine with particular regard to *L. bifidus*. Behavior of lactulose in the intestine. *Nahrung*, 11: 39–46.

Schmidt, C.M., Balinger, F., Conrad, J., Günther, J., Beifuss, U. and Hinrichs, J. (2020a). Enzymatic generation of lactulose in sweet and acid whey: Optimization of feed composition and structural elucidation of 1-lactulose. *Food Chemistry*, 305: 125481.

Schmidt, C.M., Nedele, A.-K. and Hinrichs, J. (2020b). Enzymatic generation of lactulose in sweet and acid whey: Feasibility study for the scale up towards robust processing. *Food and Bioproducts Processing*, 119: 329–336.

Schumann, C. (1997). Die immunologischen Effekte der Lactulose. *Notabene Medici*, 27: 288–290.

Schumann, C. (2002). Medical, nutritional and technological properties of lactulose. An update. *European Journal of Nutrition*, 41: 17–25.

Schuster-Wolff-Bühring, R., Fischer, L. and Hinrichs, J. (2010). Production and physiological action of the disaccharide lactulose. *International Dairy Journal*, 20(11): 731–741.

Seki, N., and Saito, H. (2012). Lactose as a source for lactulose and other functional lactose derivatives. *International Dairy Journal*, 22(2): 110–115.

Sharma, B.C., Sharma, P., Agrawal, A. and Sarin, S.K. (2009). Secondary prophylaxis of hepatic encephalopathy: An open-label randomized controlled trial of lactulose versus placebo. *Gastroenterology*, 137: 885–891.

Silvério, S.C., Macedo, E.A., Teixeira, J.A. and Rodrigues, L.R. (2016). Biocatalytic approaches using lactulose: end product compared with substrate. *Comprehensive Reviews in Food Science and Food Safety*, 15: 878–896.

Simren, M. and Stotzer, P.O. (2006). Use and abuse of hydrogen breath tests. *Gut.* 55: 291–303.

Sitanggang, A. B., Drews, A., and Kraume, M. (2015). Influences of operating conditions on continuous lactulose synthesis in an enzymatic membrane reactor system: a basis prior to long-term operation. *Journal of Biotechnology*, 203: 89–96.

Song, Y.S., Lee, H.U., Park, C. and Kim, S.W. (2013a). Optimization of lactulose synthesis from whey lactose by immobilized β-galactosidase and glucose isomerase. *Carbohydrate Research*, 22: 1–5.

Song, Y.S., Lee, H.U., Park, C. and Kim, S.W. (2013b). Batch and continuous synthesis of lactulose from whey lactose by immobilized β-galactosidase. *Food Chemistry*, 136(2): 689–694.

Strohmaier, W. (1998). Lactulose: status of health-related applications. *International Dairy Federation*, 9804: 262–271.

Tabatabaie, F. and Mortazavi, A. (2008). Influence of lactulose on the survival of probiotic strains in yoghurt. *World Applied Sciences Journal*, 3: 88–90.

Tabatabaie, T., Kotake, Y., Wallis, G., Jacob, J.M. and Floyd, RA. (1997). Spin trapping agent phenyl-Ntert-butylnitrone protects against the onset of drug-induced insulin-dependent diabetes mellitus. *FEBS Letters*, 407: 148–152.

Tamura, Y., Mizota, T., Shimamura, S. and Tomita, M. (1993). Lactulose and its application to the food and pharmaceutical industries. *Bulletin of the International Dairy Federation*, 289: 43–53.

U.S. Patent No 4957564. Process for preparing lactulose from lactose by epimerization with sodium aluminate. 1990.

Vaheri, M. and Kaupinnen, V. (1978). The formation of lactulose (4-O-β-galactopyranosylfructose) by β-galactosidase. *Acta Pharmaceutica Fennica*, 87: 75–83.

Villamiel, M., Corzo, N., Foda, M. I., Montes, F. and Olano, A. (2002). Lactulose formation catalysed by alkaline-substituted sepiolites in milk permeate. *Food Chemistry*, 76(1): 7–11.

Wang, M., Gasmalla, M. A., Tessema, H. A., Hua, X., and Yang, R. (2017). Lactulose production from efficient isomerization of lactose catalyzed by recyclable sodium aluminate. *Food Chemistry*, 233, 151–158.

Wang, M., Yang, R., Hua, X., Shen, Q., Zhang, W. and Zhao, W. (2015). Lactulose production from lactose by recombinant cellobiose 2-epimerase in permeabilised *Escherichia coli* cells. *International Journal of Food Science and Technology*, 50: 1625–1631.

Wollowski, I., Rechkammer, G. and Pool-Zobel, B.L. (2001). Protective role of probiotics and prebiotics in colon cancer. *American Journal of Clinical Nutrition*, 73: 451–455.

Wu, L., Xu, C., Li, S., Liang, J., Xu, H., and Xu, Z. (2017). Efficient production of lactulose from whey powder by cellobiose 2-epimerase in an enzymatic membrane reactor. *Bioresource Technology*, 233: 305–312.

Yelich, M.R., Schieber, C.K., Umporowicz, D.M. and Filkins, J.R. (1992). Polymyxin-B suppresses endotoxin-induced insulin hypersecretion in pancreatic islets. *Circulatory Shock*, 38: 85–90.

Yu, D., Chesseman, E. and Vanner S. (2011). Combined oro-caecal scintigraphy and lactulose hydrogen breath testing demonstrate that breath testing detects oro-caecal transit, not small intestinal bacterial overgrowth in patients with IBS. *Gut*, 60: 334–340.

Zimmer, F.C., Gohara, A.K., De Souza, A.H.P., Matsushita, M., De Souza, N.E. and Rodrigues, A.C. (2017). Obtainment, quantification and use of lactulose as a functional food – a review. *Food Science and Technology*, 37(4): 515–521.

Zokaee, F., Kaghazchi, T., Zare, A. and Soleimani, M. (2002). Isomerisation of lactose to lactulose – study and comparison of three catalytic systems. *Process Biochemistry*, 37: 629–635.

15

Isomaltooligosaccharides as Prebiotics and their Health Benefits

Waraporn Sorndech

Expert Centre of Innovative Health Food (InnoFood), Thailand Institute of Scientific and Technological Research (TISTR), 35 M.3 Technopolis, Khlong Ha, Khlong Luang, Pathumthani, 12120, Thailand

15.1 Isomaltooligosaccharide Structure, Properties and Market Trends

Oligosaccharides are glucose polymer segments composed of two to ten glucose residues (Gänzle and Follador 2012). They are commonly used as a sweetener in beverages, desserts, bakery products, etc. However, most oligosaccharides such as maltodextrin still quickly increase blood sugar level and calorie intake after consumption which is not good for a high level of consumption. Nowadays, consumers are educated in calorie counting and ways to prepare healthy foods, hence functional food ingredients have attracted increasing interest. Slowly-digestible starch (SDS) and oligosaccharide are classified as the starch and starch-derivative fractions which are completely hydrolyzed to glucose after incubation for 20–120 min using a human emulation digestive enzyme system (Englyst *et al.* 2018). SDS is important due to its ability to extend digestion and glucose release in the small intestine. This phenomenon can reduce the glycemic response and slow down the rise in blood glucose level (Zhang and Hamaker 2009). IMO are starch derivatives that consist of α-glucans less than DP 10. They are commonly linked together by α-1,4 and α-1,1, or α-1,2, or α-1,3 or α-1,6 glucosidic linkages. IMO are normally produced from starch by enzymatic modification. Briefly, starch structure is composed of α-D-glucose molecules which are covalently linked by *O*-glucosidic bonds. The ratio of amylose and amylopectin, the two main components of starch, varies depending on the starch source and type. Normally, most starch molecules contain approximately 20–30% of amylose content and 70–80% of amylopectin content. The molecular weights of amylose range from 10^5 to 10^6 Da with DP ranging from 500 to 5000. The major linkages of amylose are considered to be linear, consisting of α-1,4 glucosidic linkages with a small amount of α-1,6 glucosidic linkages as reported by Hizukuri *et al.* (1981). Molecular weights of amylopectin range from 10^7 to 10^9 Da and it contains approximately 5% of α-1,6 glucosidic linkages, leading to the short, α-1,4 glucosidic linkages that occur in a bimodal distribution of A chains (DP approximately 12), B chains (DP approximately 45) and C chain, which is the backbone chain of starch. Starch is the abundant carbohydrate source which is

Probiotics, Prebiotics and Synbiotics: Technological Advancements Towards Safety and Industrial Applications, First Edition. Edited by Parmjit Singh Panesar and Anil Kumar Anal.

delivered as an energy source for life. The nutritional quality of starch is affected by its structure, source and processing. It is also used as animal feed, fuel, and in the paper and textile industry, etc. Regarding the structure of starch, it is easily converted to IMO by enzymatic modification. Typically, starch is liquefied using glycosidase enzymes (EC 3.2.1) such as α-amylase and pullulanase, and then the liquefied starch is converted by β-amylase to produce maltose. In the final step, transferase enzymes convert the liquefied starch to produce IMO due to the high specificity of the α-1,6 glucosidic linkage formation. The rapid expansion in the development of novel IMO structures has occurred because of their functional properties. Several degrees of polymerization of IMO were produced by involving new enzyme activities and their structures are detailed in the following sections (Figure 15.1).

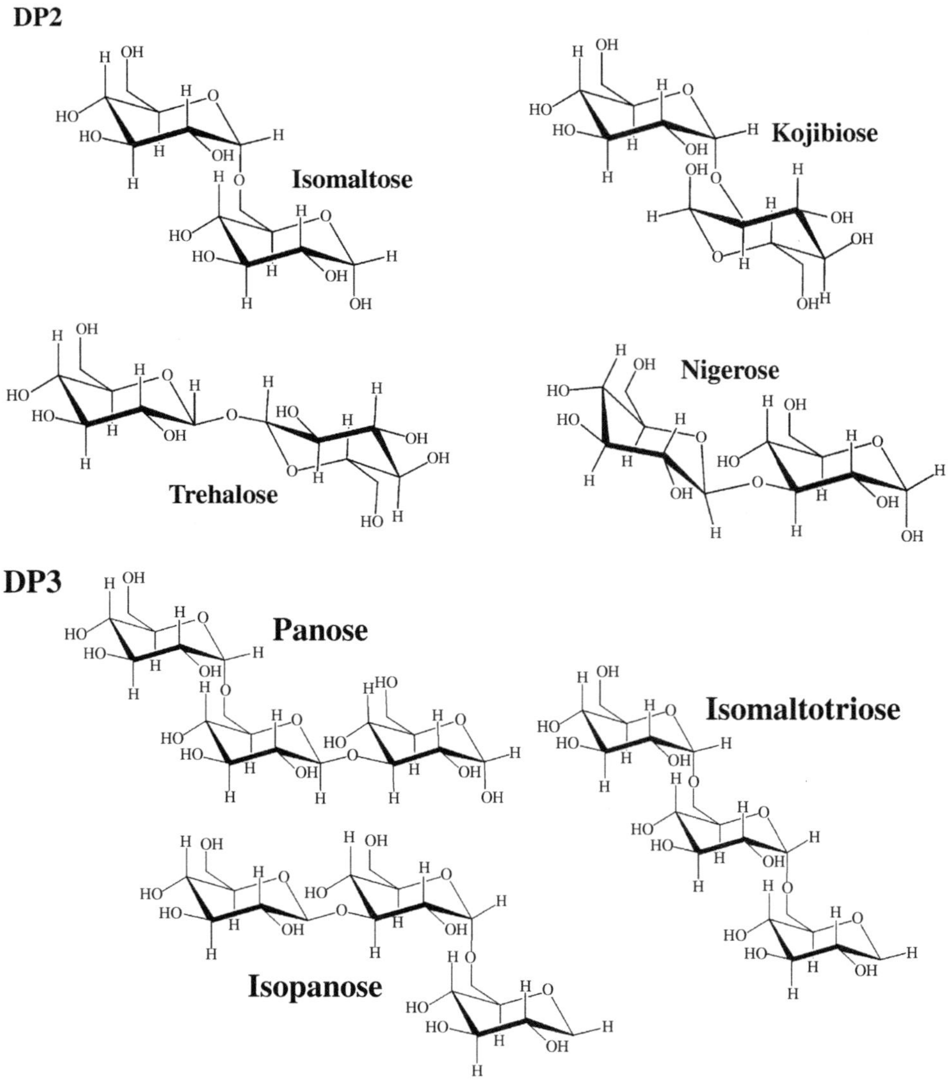

Figure 15.1 IMO chemical structures. *Sources:* Based on Song *et al.* (2020); Fujimoto *et al.* (2017); Rudeekulthamrong *et al.* (2013); Sorndech *et al.* (2018).

DP≥4

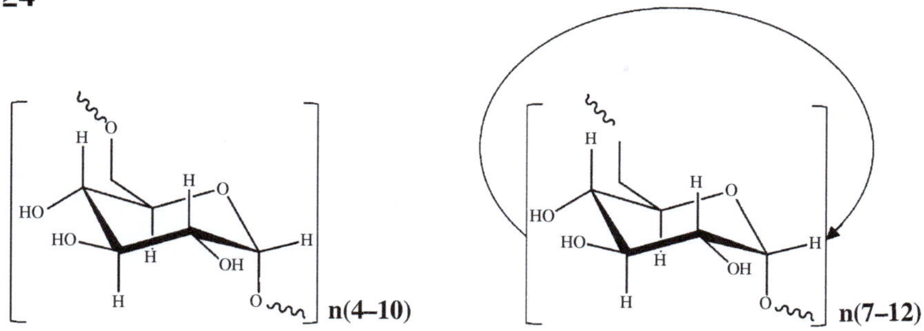

Long-chain IMOs **Cyclo-IMOs**

Figure 15.1 (Continued)

DP2-IMO Trehalose, kojibiose, nigerose and isomaltose represent the DP2-IMO which are linked by α-1,1, or α-1,2, or α-1,3 or α-1,6 glucosidic linkages, respectively. The most well-known IMO in the DP2-group is isomaltose, which is categorized as an isomer of maltose. The difference between these disaccharide structures is the type of glucosidic linkage that joins these two glucose units. In maltose, the glucose monomers are linked together by an α-1,4 glucosidic linkage, whereas isomaltose structure consists of α-1,6 glucosidic linkages. Isomaltose is classified as a reducing sugar because an open-chain structure can be formed with its functional group acting as a reducing agent. Isomaltose can be hydrolyzed by isomaltase (SI, EC 3.2.1.10) and releases two glucose subunits during amylolytic enzyme digestion in the small intestine.

DP3-IMO Isomaltotriose, panose and isopanose are classified as DP3-IMO. Isomaltotriose is composed of three glucose monomers attached together by two α-1,6 glucosidic linkages and can be partially hydrolyzed by isomaltase in the small intestine. Moreover, the remaining isomaltotriose, which is transferred to the large intestine, is preferentially metabolized by *Bifidobacterium breve* as an energy source better than isomaltose (Hu *et al.* 2013). According to Zhang *et al.* (2019), the recombinant α-glucosidase of *Geobacillus* spp. provided high hydrolysis mechanism on α-1,4 glucosidic linkages and high transglucosylation activity, and maltose is efficiently converted to IMO with 37% yield of isomaltose, isomaltotriose and panose.

DP ≥4: Long Chain IMO Linear IMO with DP ≥4 are widely developed nowadays because the long chain IMO provide good potential sources of prebiotics as compared with short chain IMO. Amylomaltase and transglucosidase were combined to produce long chains IMO as reported by Rudeekulthamrong *et al.* (2013). Amylomaltase could catalyze the disproportionation reaction from maltose to maltoheptaose substrates while glucose could not be used as a substrate. These data correspond to those of Terada *et al.* (1999) who reported that amylomaltase can catalyze the transglycosylation reaction of larger molecules (maltotetraose and maltopentaose) better than smaller molecules (maltose and maltotriose), yielding IMO from DP 2 to DP 6. Moreover, dextransucrase of *Leuconostoc mesenteroides* was used to convert sucrose and maltose to produce long chain IMOs (Lee *et al.* 2008). The results showed that long chain IMO were produced ranging from DP 3 to DP 9 with 70–90% yields, respectively. The long chain IMO are desirable due to their longer persistence in the colon as reported by Lee *et al.* (2008) and Kaulpiboon *et al.* (2015). Overall, long chain IMO are attracting interest due to their digestion property in the small intestine, where short chain IMO are absorbed better than long chain IMO.

DP ≥4: Cyclo-IMO

Cyclo-IMO are cyclic glucose polymer chains consisting of α-1,4 and α-1,6 glucosidic bonds. They are claimed to prevent tooth decay, as reported by Kobayashi *et al.* (1995). Cyclo-IMO with DP 7–17 were found in a *Paenibacillus* sp. cell culture in which dextran was used as a carbon source (Fujimoto *et al.* 2017). Hence, *Paenibacillus* sp. 598K cycloisomaltooligosaccharide glucanotransferase has been widely studied for cyclo-IMO production. The cycloisomaltooligosaccharide glucanotransferase catalyzes the transglucosylation of dextran molecules to produce cyclo-IMO with DP ≥7 (Suzuki *et al.* 2012) and it also catalyzes the disproportionation, coupling and hydrolytic reactions of dextran. The cyclo-IMO show high water solubility and have an internal cavity in their structure, hence they have high potential to form complexes with other components such as drugs and can therefore be used as an encapsulated compound like cyclodextrin. This property of cyclo-IMO can be used in a wide range of applications, including drugs carrier, cosmetic products, encapsulation materials for food and household cleaning products (Funane *et al.* 2007).

15.1.1 IMO: Global Patent Trend

IMO production processes have been developed in recent years because IMO show great potential to improve the physiochemical quality of various types of food due to their solubility in water, bulking property, low viscosity, low sweetness, mild taste and the fact that they are classified as a fermentable sugar. IMO are used in various kinds of beverage, drink and dairy products, mainly for sucrose replacement and slow glucose release and to provide suitable organoleptic properties. In bakery products, IMO provide a compatible source of soluble dietary fibers or prebiotics for positive digestive effects. Moreover, with regard to the key features of food and beverages, IMOs have no aftertaste, which makes them suitable for use as fat and sucrose replacers. In addition, consumers wanting a modern healthy lifestyle are increasing in number, and detailed information on food product composition, especially confectionery, is needed for this kind of consumer. IMO are used in the formulation of confectionery products such as cocoa, candy, chocolate and breath-freshening microsweets, which are claimed to be sugar-free and with health benefits, and are widespread in the market to meet consumer requirements. As regards intellectual property, Figure 15.2 examines the current IMO patent trends, which are related to demand and supply in addition to the recent developments. The values obtained are correlated with the primary inputs of the key stakeholders in the IMOs value chain and were obtained from The Lens. The patent document count of IMO has increased since 2000 and continues to do so.

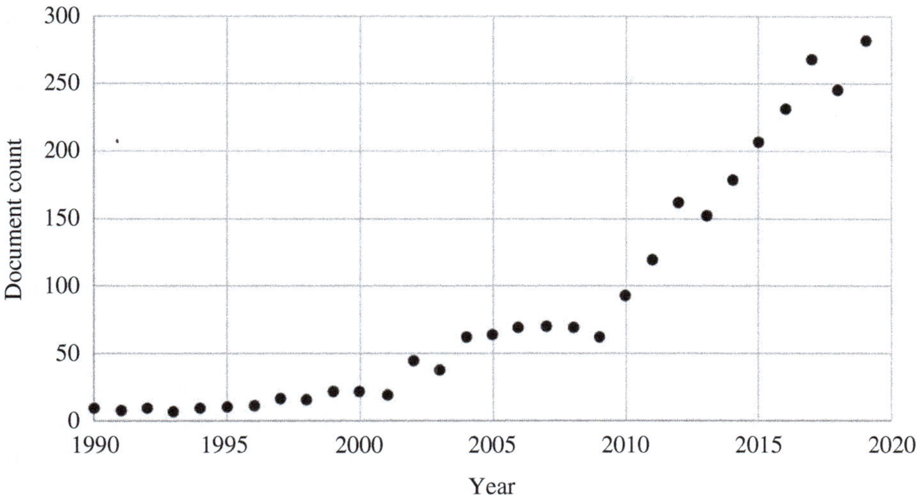

Figure 15.2 Patented isomaltooligosaccharides. *Source:* Based on data extracted from https://www.lens.org/

15.2 Production

Nowadays, enzymatic modification of starch to generate desirable properties for food is gaining interest as an environmentally friendly, clean and safe technology compared to chemical modification (Sorndech *et al.* 2015). Small amounts of IMO occur naturally and they are found in beer, honey, nectar and fermented food (Tungland and Meyer 2002). The high market demand for products containing IMO makes it impossible to harvest sufficient naturally occurring IMO for commercial use. Pilot or industrial-scale extraction of IMO from natural sources is not economically feasible. Hence, commercial IMO are instead produced by modification of starch, typically using enzymatic modification methods.

15.2.1 Enzymatic Production

Glucosyltransferase enzymes play an important role in IMO production. Basically, glucanotransferase is classified in the group EC 2.4 and normally catalyzes the formation of α-1,1 (e.g. trehalase), α-1,4 (e.g. amylomaltase) and α-1,6 (e.g. branching enzyme and transglucosidase) glucan chain transfer to a new position in the acceptor starch chains. For IMO production, starch is normally converted to soluble small molecules by hydrolase enzymes (e.g. α-amylase and glucoamylase). This process, called saccharification, occurs by hydrolysis or hydrolysis and is followed by the transglycosylation process. The best-known glucanotransferase used as a main enzyme for IMO production is α-transglucosidase (TGase, EC 2.4.1.24, GH31, 1,4-α-D-glucan: 1,4-α-D-glucan [D-glucose] 6-α-D-glucosyltransferase). TGase is widely found in animals, plants and several microorganisms. This enzyme catalyzes the hydrolytic and transfer reactions of glucosyl residues from the non-reducing ends of maltose molecules to form α-1,6 glucosidic linkages of glucose and maltose to generate isomaltose, isomaltotriose, panose or other higher DP oligosaccharides. Moreover, this enzyme also transfers non-reducing glucosyl residues to the α-1,2 and α-1,3 glucosidic linkages of glucose to form kojibiose and nigerose respectively or back to α-1,4 glucosidic linkages to form maltose. For the conventional procedure, TGase is combined with α-amylase, β-amylase, maltogenic α-amylase and pullulanase to produce IMOs (Lee *et al.* 2002). The resulting IMO have been used as functional food and beverage ingredients in several products (Do *et al.* 2012) such as desserts, fillings, bakery, confectionery, sauces, baby food, etc.

Normally, IMO production from starch consists of several process steps including liquefaction, saccharification and purification (Dobruchowska *et al.* 2012). This production procedure requires at least four or five types of enzyme to attain the desired IMO composition. Growing health concern worldwide is one of the drivers of the growth of the global IMO market. IMO market revenue is continuously increasing and IMO have been launched widely at academic, research institutional and industrial levels to demonstrate the possibilities for alternative and efficient production methods to produce high yields of IMO. These processes usually involve new enzyme types which contribute to more efficient production technologies as described in the following sections.

The common approach for IMO production involves starch (i.e. corn starch, rice starch, cassava starch and soluble starch) as the general raw material, followed by enzymatic transglucosylation as the catalytic procedure. However, several types of raw material have been tested for IMO production (i.e. disaccharides, maltooligosaccharides puffed rice flour and dextran), as presented in Table 15.1. The main enzyme classifications used for IMO production are within the glucanotransferases and hydrolases. These enzyme categories have been utilized in various manufacturing protocols for the production of IMO from disaccharides, dextran, flour, starch and starch derivatives (Table 15.1). Recombinant enzyme technology showed significantly improved IMO production (Rudeekulthamrong *et al.* 2013) and reduced some problems in IMO production, principally the generation of high-glycemic sugar, mainly glucose.

15.2.1.1 Enzymatic Technologies for Formation of Various IMO Structures

The use of enzymes in the food industry is gaining more attention. Enzyme utilization in the food industry includes starch processing at the industrial scale (syrups), bakery industry, food flavoring industry, beverage and milk production industry, fruit juice industry and meat-processing industry. In the case of IMO, combined enzyme systems are normally used as a common method for IMO DP 2–7 production. The enzymes used in combined systems are those from the glycosidases group (EC 3.2.1), such as α-amylase (EC 3.2.1.1), β-amylase (EC 3.2.1.2), dextranase (EC 3.2.1.11), α-glucosidase (EC3.2.1.20), pullulanase (EC 3.2.1.41) and maltogenic amylase (EC 3.2.1.133), and from the hexosyltransferases group (EC 2.4.1), such as dextransucrase (EC 2.4.1.5), branching enzyme (EC 2.4.1.18), α-transglucosidase (EC 2.4.1.24), amylomaltase (EC 2.4.1.25) and cycloisomaltooligosaccharides glucanotransferase (EC 2.4.1.248). The enzymatic modification of starch to produce IMO has proved useful at the industrial scale due to its potential for food and medical applications as it consists of a biocompatible, environmentally friendly, minimal waste and uncomplicated process. Table 15.1 presents an overview of the substrates and enzymes used in production of various IMO structures. Several types of disaccharides, oligosaccharides, starch, flour and other polysaccharides (i.e. dextran) were used as substrates for IMO production to obtain IMO DP 2–7, long chain IMO and cyclo-IMO.

Table 15.1 Substrates and enzymes used for formation of various IMO structures.

IMO Products	Substrate	Enzyme	References
Isomaltose, isomaltotriose and panose		Amylomaltase (EC 2.4.1.25) and maltogenic α-amylase (EC 2.4.1.24)	Lee *et al.* (2002)
	Sucrose	Dextransucrase (EC 2.4.1.5)	Song *et al.* (2020)
	Maltose	Immobilized α-glucosidase (EC3.2.1.20)	Wang *et al.* (2017)
	Corn starch	Recombinant *Bacillus naganoensis* pullulanase, α-amylase, β-amylase and α-transglucosidase (EC 2.4.1.24)	Niu *et al.* (2017)
IMO DP 2–7	Puffed rice flour	Maltogenic amylase (EC 3.2.1.133), pullulanase (EC 3.2.1.41) and transglucosidase (EC 2.1.2.24)	Lee *et al.* (2018)
	Corn starch	Immobilized β-amylase, pullulanase, fungal α-amylase and thermostable α-glucosidase	Chen *et al.* (2018)
	Rice starch	α-amylase and transglucosidase (EC 2.4.1.24)	Plongbunjong *et al.* (2017)
	Cassava starch	α-amylase, β-amylase, branching enzyme and α-transglucosidase	Sorndech *et al.* (2017)
	Rice starch and cassava starch	α-amylase, β-amylase, pullulanase and α-transglucosidase (EC 2.4.1.24)	Saman *et al.* (2019)
	Soluble starch	α-amylase and α-glucosidase	Basu *et al.* (2016)
Long IMO	Maltotriose	Amylomaltase (EC 2.4.1.25) and α-transglucosidase (EC 2.4.1.24)	Rudeekulthamrong *et al.* (2013)
	Tapioca starch	Amylomaltase (EC 2.4.1.25) and α-transglucosidase (EC 2.4.1.24)	Kaulpiboon *et al.* (2015)
	Dextran	Engineered dextranase (EC 3.2.1.11)	Klahan *et al.* (2018)
	Maltopentaose, or isomaltopentaose, or commercialized maltodextrins	Thermostable *Thermoanaerobacter thermocopriae* cycloisomaltooligosaccharide glucanotransferase (EC 2.4.1.248)	Yang *et al.* (2019)
	Sucrose and maltose	Dextransucrase (EC 2.4.1.5)	Lee *et al.* (2008)
	Sucrose and maltose	Dextransucrase (EC 2.4.1.5)	Shi *et al.* (2016)
Cyclo-IMO	Dextran	Cycloisomaltooligosaccharides glucanotransferase (EC 2.4.1.248)	Kawamoto *et al.* (2001)
	Dextran	Endo-dextranases (EC 3.2.1.11)	Kim *et al.* (2012)
	Dextran	Cycloisomaltooligosaccharides glucanotransferase (EC 2.4.1.248)	Suzuki *et al.* (2012)
	Dextran	Cycloisomaltooligosaccharides glucanotransferase (EC 2.4.1.248)	Oguma *et al.* (2014)
	Dextran	Cycloisomaltooligosaccharides glucanotransferase (EC 2.4.1.248)	Fujimoto *et al.* (2017)
*O*4-branched dextrans and reuteran-like structure	Sucrose	Mutant dextransucrase from *Lactobacillus reuteri* TMW 1.106 (EC 2.4.1.5)	Münkel *et al.* (2020)

Sources: Based on Lee *et al.* (2002); Song *et al.* (2019); Wang *et al.* (2017).

All the enzymatic technologies previously detailed provide new and high efficiency to generate DP 2–3 IMO (isomaltose, isomaltotriose, panose and isopanose). Nonetheless, other types of IMO are consistently produced, including long chain and cyclo-IMO, as characterized in Table 15.1. Long chain and cyclo-IMO may be claimed as prebiotic ingredients. Some researchers reported that long chain IMO can be produced using a combination of two enzymes, amylomaltase and α-transglucosidase (Kaulpiboon *et al.* 2015; Rudeekulthamrong *et al.* 2013). Moreover, the action of cyclo-isomaltooligosaccharide glucanotransferase was previously demonstrated to produce cyclo-IMO from dextran substrate (Fujimoto *et al.* 2017; Oguma *et al.* 2014; Suzuki *et al.* 2014). A novel approach for increasing the dietary fiber content of IMO was recently established and reported by Song *et al.* (2020). Normal corn starch was converted to produce IMO by liquefaction and saccharification processes. The obtained IMO and sucrose were mixed and further converted by dextransucrase. The soluble dietary fiber content in the modified IMO was significantly increased when using 10% sucrose and 20% IMO as substrates. Overall, various new processes for high-efficiency production of IMO have been investigated and they are under research and development. Several of these processes have high potential for up-scaling to industrial production.

15.2.1.2 Production Strategies

The key driver for IMO production strategies is demand in the functional food and beverages sector due to growing awareness of the health benefits. Worldwide, soluble dietary fiber is being developed as a use for adjusted starches. According to the current analysis, the global dietary fiber market is expected to continuously increase in the next few years. Hence, IMO production adjustment is one of the most important keys for the industrial-scale production. Glucose is the major by-product in IMO production. Various strategies are used for glucose reduction or elimination such as microbial fermentation, enzyme genetic engineering, enzyme immobilization, use of enzyme cocktails, etc.

15.3 Technological Developments

15.3.1 Microbial Fermentation and Enzyme Genetic Engineering

Bioconversion processes have been widely investigated, such as that of using whole bacterial cells in biocatalysis for starch or flour conversion to IMO. This technique is typified by cell-bound α-glucosidase of *Microbacterium* sp. which was used for maltose conversion to IMO, establishing a 24% conversion efficiency (Ojha *et al.* 2015). Solid state fermentation is an alternative method that has been used to produce IMO. Glutinous rice and rice bran were converted to IMO using *Aspergillus oryzae* TISTR 3102 and TISTR 3222. The α-glucosidase activity was monitored during incubation and the results showed that panose and isomaltotriose were mostly found after fermentation. Moreover, amylomaltase and maltogenic α-amylase were simultaneously overexpressed in *Escherichia coli*. The synergistic mode of action of these two enzymes provided an increase in IMO content up to 68%, which was 15% higher than that of a conventional procedure. The use of an enzyme fusion technique is an interesting approach for IMO production. Endo-dextranase and dextransucrase were engineered to generate a fusion enzyme (Kim *et al.* 2009). This approach demonstrated greater efficiency compared to use of separate enzymes and resulted in more than 30-fold IMO yields. Moreover, an engineered dextranase from *Streptococcus mutans* was reported to enhance the production of long chain IMO (DP >5) from dextran substrate (Klahan *et al.* 2018). Thus, microbial fermentation and enzyme genetic engineering have provided an effective IMO production process for the industrial scale.

15.3.2 Enzyme Immobilization

Immobilization of enzymes has also been investigated to increase IMO production yields and to prevent the inactivation of the enzyme after the end of the process. The combination of alginate–chitosan–calcium phosphate hybrid carriers was created out in order to immobilize α-transglucosidase. The results showed that enzyme activity could be retained up to 60% of its initial activity after 15 repeated cycles, which significantly lowered the production cost (Zhang *et al.* 2009). In addition, Bertrand *et al.* (2014) demonstrated an endodextranase immobilized using an epoxy resin. The enzyme displayed high stability and the remaining enzymatic activity was 78% after 78 days. Enzyme membrane reactors have also been developed. This approach was used for α-glucosidase, which was fixed between two sheets of ultrafiltration membrane, allowing IMOs to diffuse through the membrane, and reaching IMO yields of 58.1% (Zhang *et al.* 2010). Moreover, immobilization of cycloisomaltooligosaccharide glucanotransferase was applied in the production of cyclo-IMO from dextran. The data revealed that the immobilized enzyme was less thermostable than the non-immobilized one (Kawamoto *et al.* 2001).

15.3.3 Enzyme Cocktails

Simultaneous saccharification and transglucosylation or use of an enzyme cocktail is a recent development in which IMO were produced from several types of substrate such as starch, flour, and oligosaccharides using combinations of glucosyl-hydrolases and transferases (Niu *et al.* 2017; Sorndech *et al.* 2017). The benefits of enzyme cocktails are increasing IMO production efficiency, obtaining a wider range of different IMO structure, reduction of enzyme content and simple-step liquefaction/saccharification operations.

15.3.4 Glucose, Fructose and Linear Oligosaccharide Elimination

One major drawback of the production of IMO by enzymatic modification is that the pre-existing glucose still remains in the system which can adversely affect the commercial value of IMO. Hence, various methods have been tested for elimination of glucose. Membrane filtration and chromatographic methods were reported as methods for reduction of glucose and oligosaccharides (Crittenden and Playne 1996). This idea is consistent with that of Goulas *et al.* (2002), who used cross-flow nanofiltration for the removal of glucose from the system. Immobilized *Zymomonas mobilis* cells have also been used for the glucose, fructose and sucrose removal process (Crittenden and Playne 2002). Glucose oxidase and catalase were considered for elimination of glucose during the IMO production process because these two enzymes provided a shorter reaction time and generated fewer by-products at the end of the conversion process, as reported by Zhao *et al.* (2018).

15.4 Health Benefits of IMO

Nowadays, an important aspect of people's health consciousness is an increased awareness of avoiding high-carbohydrate food. Prebiotics from carbohydrate-based molecules constitute alternative healthy food ingredients. An updated definition of a prebiotic coined by The International Scientific Association for Probiotics and Prebiotics (ISAPP) is "a substrate that is selectively utilized by host microorganisms conferring a health benefit". This definition of prebiotics is related to that of probiotics, which are "live micro-organisms which, when administered in adequate amounts, confer a health benefit on the host" (FAO/WHO 2001). Healthy lifestyle and dietary components are the most importance factors in protection and prevention of various kinds of disease. Relationships between lifestyle and diet have been reported (Kromhout *et al.* 2002). Consumers seek alternative carbohydrate-based prebiotics, and various kinds of them are utilized as functional food ingredients such as fructooligosaccharides (FOS), galactooligosaccharides (GOS), arabinoxylooligosaccharides (AXOS), pectin-derived oligosaccharides (POS) and IMO. IMO are a mixture of branched maltooligosaccharides (MOS), classified as functional food ingredients with prebiotic potential. IMO are composed predominantly of a series of α-1,1, α-1,2, α-1,3 and α-1,6 linked sugars such as isomaltose, panose, isomaltotriose, isomaltotetraose, isomaltopentaose, nigerose, kojibiose and higher branched oligosaccharides (DP ≤10) (Ketabi *et al.* 2011; Koleva *et al.* 2014). They are partially resistant to digestion by amylolytic enzymes in the digestive tract and are claimed as prebiotic substances (Roberfroid 2007). Some reports suggest that the caloric value of IMO is 1.5–2.0 kcal/g depending on their structure (Nakanishi *et al.* 2006). IMO have been reported to generally meet the criteria for prebiotics, which are (i) resistance to gastric acidity and amylolytic enzymes in the digestive system and (ii)) fermentation by intestinal microbiota and selective stimulation of the growth and activity of some desirable intestinal bacteria. IMO are utilized as alternative low-calorie sweeteners in food and beverage products as their caloric content is 1.5–2.0 kcal/g, which is approximately 75% lower than that of maltose (Ketabi *et al.* 2011). The relative sweetness level of IMO is approximately 60% lower than that of sucrose (Health Canada 2012; Ketabi *et al.* 2011).

Beneficial health effects of IMO consumption have been reported by in vitro, animal and human studies. In in vitro investigations, IMO fermentation normally promotes bifidobacteria and lactobacilli and inhibits growth of *Clostridium* (*histolyticum* subgroup) and *Bacteroides* (Sorndech *et al.* 2019). However, the data relating to the bifidogenic effects of IMO are not consistent when compared to other typical oligosaccharides, such as inulin or FOS (Zhang *et al.* 2010), due to their internal structures. IMO stimulated bowel movement, improved gut function and fecal excretion, and decreased total cholesterol levels in an animal study (Candela *et al.* 2010), which is related to the study of Wang *et al.* (2017), who reported that IMO has the ability to be involved in the repair damage system of ileal epithelial cells in a rat model. This suggested that IMO can help to reduce the effects of irritable bowel syndrome (IBS). IMO also have great therapeutic potential in the management of inflammatory bowel disease (IBD). Moreover, IMO have been used as a dietary supplement to support animal health. A mixture of probiotic and IMO significantly improved the intestinal microbiota of broiler chickens and their growth performance and reduced mortality (Tarabees *et al.* 2019). In livestock, the supplementation of IMO and *Bacillus* spp. during the perinatal period can improve the lactational performance of gestating sows (Gu *et al.* 2019). In human studies, the effect of long-term consumption of IMO supplementation on fecal microbiota, bowel function and nutritional status in constipated elderly people was investigated. After 4 weeks of IMO consumption, the fecal bifidobacteria, lactobacilli and *Bacteroides* counts were significantly increased and clostridia count was decreased. Moreover, the plasma total cholesterol and low density lipoprotein cholesterol (LDL) levels were lower as compared to the placebo group (Yen *et al.* 2011). In addition, IMO showed the ability to improve gastroesophageal reflux symptoms, as reported by Selling *et al.* (2018).

Although IMO have prebiotic properties they are partially digested by enzymes such as the intestinal brush border enzymes, which are maltase-glucoamylase (MGAM) and sucrase-isomaltase (SI) (Lin *et al.* 2012). The glucose content of IMO can be released and some studies report that IMO are classified as caloric sweeteners due to an increase in glycemic and insulinemic response and incretin hormone secretion in healthy adults (Gourineni *et al.* 2018; Subhan *et al.* 2020). The short chain IMO are generally partially hydrolyzed by amylolytic enzymes in the small intestine (Kaneko *et al.* 1994) and contribute to reduction of blood glucose level, but the prebiotic properties may not remain. Long chain IMO can be more resistant to degradation by amylolytic enzymes. Long chain IMO have been displayed to provide more effective stimulation of the growth and activities of bifidobacteria and lactobacilli than short chain IMO (Kaulpiboon *et al.* 2015). In reality, IMO are not eaten in isolation as a food source, and the food matrix can affect glycemic responses and insulin secretion to IMO. Consumption of IMO with starchy food may lead to an increase in the hydrolysis rate of brush border enzymes and would likely increase the glycemic response; food products containing IMO, whey protein and fat provided a lower glucose release as compared to the sample that used dextrose instead of IMO as a control (Grubic *et al.* 2018). This food matrix approach can be linked to the correlation between food containing IMO and their slow digestion properties. Slowly digestible oligosaccharide is important due to its ability to extend digestion and glucose release in the small intestine. This phenomenon can reduce the glycemic response and slow down the rise in blood glucose level (Zhang and Hamaker 2009). The gut feedback and glycemic response is affected by food components and the interaction of food components with the gastrointestinal tract. A slow glucose release leads to an improvement of blood glucose level over an extended time period and the activities of the gastrointestinal tract such as release of gut hormones and neurohormonal negative feedback mechanisms. When slowly digestible oligosaccharides reach the ileum, a part of the small intestine, the brush border α-glucosidase enzymes of maltase-glucoamylase (MGAM) and sucrase-isomaltase (SI) digest starch for glucose liberation. The released glucose content can stimulate the secretion of glucagon-like peptide 1 (GLP1) and peptide YY (PYY) hormone, indicating coordination between the mechanisms of α-glucosidase and hormone secretion. The regulatory effect of starch digestion can be expressed in the term of sugar sensing, which refers to glucose-sensing mechanisms such as the activity of pancreatic α-amylase, brush border enzymes, sodium/glucose cotransporter 1 (SGLT-1) and type 1 G-protein-coupled receptors (T1R) (Zhang *et al.* 2015). Moreover, the short chain fatty acids from good colon microbiota fermentation also stimulate the secretion of those hormones, resulting in reduction of gastric emptying rate and food intake (Lee *et al.* 2013). The mechanism of action of low glycemic index and fiber foods in the gastrointestinal tract is composed of multiple processes (Rivellese *et al.* 2012). Slowly digestible oligosaccharides can increase hypothalamic signals of satiety and thus decrease food intake. Their health benefits have been reported in in vitro and in vivo studies. IMO can stimulate the secretion of gut incretin hormones (Wachters-Hagedoorn *et al.* 2006), are also recommended for the prevention of diabetes (Wolever 2003), decrease the risk of cardiovascular diseases (Stenvers *et al.* 2014), improve the metabolic profile, particularly in lower postprandial insulinemia (Grubic *et al.* 2018), increase the impact of satiety-influencing factors (Benton and Nabb 2003), decrease the risk of colon and breast cancer (Jenkins *et al.* 2008), lower levels of circulating triacylglycerols (Petrova and Petrov 2017) and also can be utilized as source of energy for the athlete (Grubic *et al.* 2019).

15.5 Conclusion

Personal health and well-being has long been a focus of attention. Many modified starches were commercialized in the market in response to consumer demand. In food industrial applications, consumer demand for functional food ingredient prebiotics, such as IMO, have continuously increased in recent years. IMO show high potential for application in a wide variety of foods and beverages. The goal of any ingredient's demand and supply process is to get as close to consumer demand as possible. For this reason, food entrepreneurs provide the propulsion to develop IMO production technologies in order to reduce cost, increase IMO production capacity and investigate their health-promoting benefits for commercialization and marketing. Development of enzymatic technology to improve IMO production has provided an increase in IMO yields and been helpful in creating the diversity of IMO structures. The functional properties of IMO are founded on the fact that their digestion is delayed and some part of their structure can be classified as a slowly digestible oligosaccharide. Some IMO result in a reduction and flattening of blood glucose levels. Finally, the amylolytic-tolerant fraction of the IMO becomes an energy source for colonic bacteria, producing some desirable metabolites that improve the gastrointestinal tract's health. These data can be used as the guide for developments in IMO manufacturing to support a budding multi-niche IMO market. All production technologies used to produce IMO nowadays can produce various IMO structures that can serve different customers' needs.

References

Basu, A., Mutturi, S. and Prapulla, S.G. (2016). Production of isomaltooligosaccharides (IMO) using simultaneous saccharification and transglucosylation from starch and sustainable sources. *Process Biochemistry*, 51(10): 1464–1471.

Benton, D. and Nabb, S. (2003). Carbohydrate, memory, and mood. *Nutrition Reviews*, 61(5): 61–67.

Bertrand, E., Pierre, G., Delattre, C., Gardarin, C., Bridiau, N., Maugard, T. et al. (2014). Dextranase immobilization on epoxy CIM® disk for the production of isomaltooligosaccharides from dextran. *Carbohydrate Polymers*, 111: 707–713.

Candela, M., Maccaferri, S., Turroni, S., Carnevali, P. and Brigidi, P. (2010). Functional intestinal microbiome, new frontiers in prebiotic design. *International Journal of Food Microbiology*, 140(2): 93–101.

Chen, P., Xu, R., Wang, J., Wu, Z., Yan, L., Zhao, W., Liu, Y., Ma, W., Shi, X. and Li, H. (2018). Starch biotransformation into isomaltooligosaccharides using thermostable alpha-glucosidase from *Geobacillus stearothermophilus*. *PeerJ*, 6: e5086.

Crittenden, R.G. and Playne, M.J. (1996). Production, properties and applications of food-grade oligosaccharides. *Trends in Food Science and Technology*, 7(11): 353–361.

Crittenden, R. and Playne, M. (2002). Purification of food-grade oligosaccharides using immobilised cells of *Zymomonas mobilis*. *Applied Microbiology and Biotechnology*, 58(3): 297–302.

Do, H.V., Lee, E.J., Park, J.H., Park, K.H., Shim, J.Y., Mun, S. and Kim, Y.R. (2012). Structural and physicochemical properties of starch gels prepared from partially modified starches using *Thermus aquaticus* 4-α-glucanotransferase. *Carbohydrate Polymers*, 87(4): 2455–2463.

Dobruchowska, J.M., Gerwig, G.J., Kralj, S., Grijpstra, P., Leemhuis, H., Dijkhuizen, L. et al. (2012). Structural characterization of linear isomalto-/malto-oligomer products synthesized by the novel GTFB 4,6-α-glucanotransferase enzyme from Lactobacillus reuteri 121. *Glycobiology*, 22(4): 517–528.

Englyst, K., Goux, A., Meynier, A., Quigley, M., Englyst, H., Brack, O. and Vinoy, S. (2018). Inter-laboratory validation of the starch digestibility method for determination of rapidly digestible and slowly digestible starch. *Food Chemistry*, 245: 1183–1189.

FAO/WHO (2001). Joint FAO/WHO Expert Consultation on evaluation of health and nutritional properties of probiotics in food including powder milk with live lactic acid bacteria. Cordoba, Argentina, October 2001.

Fujimoto, Z., Kishine, N., Suzuki, N., Suzuki, R., Mizushima, D., Momma, M., Kimura, K. and Funane, K. (2017). Isomaltooligosaccharide-binding structure of *Paenibacillus* sp. 598K cycloisomaltooligosaccharide glucanotransferase. *Bioscience Reports*, 37(2): BSR20170253.

Funane, K., Terasawa, K., Mizuno, Y., Ono, H., Miyagi, T., Gibu, S. et al. (2007). A novel cyclic isomaltooligosaccharide (cycloisomaltodecaose, CI-10) produced by Bacillus circulans T-3040 displays remarkable inclusion ability compared with cyclodextrins. *Journal of Biotechnology*, 130(2): 188–192.

Gänzle, M. and Follador, R. (2012). Metabolism of oligosaccharides and starch in lactobacilli: A review. *Frontiers in Microbiology*, 3(340).

Goulas, A.K., Kapasakalidis, P.G., Sinclair, H.R., Rastall, R.A. and Grandison, A.S. (2002). Purification of oligosaccharides by nanofiltration. *Journal of Membrane Science*, 209(1): 321–335.

Gourineni, V., Stewart, M.L., Icoz, D., and Zimmer, J.P. (2018). Gastrointestinal tolerance and glycemic response of isomaltooligosaccharides in healthy adults. *Nutrients*, 10(3): 301.

Grubic, T.J., Kreider, R.B., Sowinski, R.J., Dalton, R.L., Favot, C.J., Greenwood, M., Earnest, C.P., Reyes, A. and Rasmussen, C. (2018). Glycemic and insulinemic response to ingestion of a novel food bar containing whey protein and isomalto-oligosaccharides. *Austin Journal of Nutrition and Food Sciences*, 6(1): 1099.

Grubic, T.J., Sowinski, R.J., Nevares, B.E., Jenkins, V.M., Williamson, S.L., Reyes, A. G., Rasmussen, C., Greenwood, M., Murano, P.S., Earnest, C.P. and Kreider, R.B. (2019). Comparison of ingesting a food bar containing whey protein and isomalto-oligosaccharides to carbohydrate on performance and recovery from an acute bout of resistance-exercise and sprint conditioning: an open label, randomized, counterbalanced, crossover pilot study. *Journal of the International Society of Sports Nutrition*, 16(1): 1–17.

Gu, X.L., Song, Z.H., Li, H., Wu, S., Wu, S.S., Ding, Y.N., He, X., Yin, Y.L. and Fan, Z.Y. (2019). Effects of dietary isomaltooligosaccharide and Bacillus spp. supplementation during perinatal period on lactational performance, blood metabolites, and milk composition of sows. *Journal of the Science of Food and Agriculture*, 99(13): 5646–5653.

Health Canada (2012). Novel Food Information – Isomalto-oligosaccharide (VitaFiber™). Food and Nutrition [serial on the Internet]. https://www.canada.ca/en/health-canada/services/food-nutrition/genetically-modified-foods-other-novel-foods/approved-products/isomalto-oligosaccharide-vitafiber-trade.html (accessed 23 July 2021).

Hizukuri, S., Takeda, Y., Yasuda, M. and Suzuki, A. (1981). Multi-branched nature of amylose and the action of debranching enzymes. *Carbohydrate Research*, 94(2): 205–213.

Hu, Y., Ketabi, A., Buchko, A. and Gänzle, M.G. (2013). Metabolism of isomalto-oligosaccharides by *Lactobacillus reuteri* and bifidobacteria. *Letters in Applied Microbiology*, 57(2): 108–114.

Jenkins, D.A., Kendall, C.C., McKeown-Eyssen, G., Josse, R.G., Silverberg, J., Booth, G.L., Vidgen, E., Josse, A.R., Nguyen, T.H., Corrigan, S., Banach, M.S., Ares, S., Mitchell, S., Emam, A., Augustin, L.S., Parker, T.L. and Leiter, L.A. (2008). Effect of a low–glycemic index or a high–cereal fiber diet on type 2 diabetes: A randomized trial. *Journal of the American Medical Association*, 300(23): 2742–2753.

Kaneko, T., Kohmoto, T., Kikuchi, H., Shiota, M., Iino, H. and Mitsuoka, T. (1994). Effects of isomaltooligosaccharides with different degrees of polymerization on human fecal bifidobactcria. *Bioscience, Biotechnology, and Biochemistry*, 58(12): 2288–2290.

Kaulpiboon, J., Rudeekulthamrong, P., Watanasatitarpa, S., Ito, K. and Pongsawasdi, P. (2015). Synthesis of long-chain isomaltooligosaccharides from tapioca starch and an in vitro investigation of their prebiotic properties. *Journal of Molecular Catalysis B: Enzymatic*, 120: 127–135.

Kawamoto, H., Oguma, T., Sekine, H. and Kobayashi, M. (2001). Immobilization of cycloiso-maltooligosaccharide glucanotransferase for the production of cycloisomaltooligosaccharides from dextran. *Enzyme and Microbial Technology*, 28(6): 515–521.

Ketabi, A., Dieleman, L.A. and Gänzle, M.G. (2011). Influence of isomalto-oligosaccharides on intestinal microbiota in rats. *Journal of Applied Microbiology*, 110(5): 1297–1306.

Kim, Y.-M., Kiso, Y., Muraki, T., Kang, M.-S., Nakai, H., Saburi, W., Lang, W., Kang, H.-K., Okuyama, M., Mori, H., Suzuki, R., Funane, K., Suzuki, N., Momma, M., Fujimoto, Z., Oguma, T., Kobayashi, M., Kim, D. and Kimura, A. (2012). Novel dextranase catalyzing cycloisomaltooligosaccharide-formation and identification of catalytic amino acids and their functions using chemical rescue approach. *Journal of Biological Chemistry*, 2012: 1–16.

Kim, Y.-M., Seo, M.-Y., Kang, H.-K., Atsuo, K. and Kim, D. (2009). Construction of a fusion enzyme of dextransucrase and dextranase: Application for one-step synthesis of isomalto-oligosaccharides. *Enzyme and Microbial Technology*, 44(3), 159–164.

Klahan, P., Okuyama, M., Jinnai, K., Ma, M., Kikuchi, A., Kumagai, Y., Tagami, T. and Kimura, A. (2018). Engineered dextranase from *Streptococcus mutans* enhances the production of longer isomaltooligosaccharides. *Bioscience, Biotechnology, and Biochemistry*, 82(9): 1480–1487.

Kobayashi, M., Funane, K. and Oguma, T. (1995). Inhibition of dextran and mutan synthesis by cycloisomaltooligosaccharides. *Bioscience, Biotechnology, and Biochemistry*, 59(10): 1861–1865.

Koleva, P., Ketabi, A., Valcheva, R., Gänzle, M.G. and Dieleman, L.A. (2014). Chemically defined diet alters the protective properties of fructo-oligosaccharides and isomalto-oligosaccharides in HLA-B27 transgenic rats. *PLoS ONE*, 9(11): 111717.

Kromhout, D., Menotti, A., Kesteloot, H. and Sans, S. (2002). Prevention of coronary heart disease by diet and lifestyle: Evidence from prospective cross-cultural, cohort, and intervention studies. *Circulation*, 105(7): 893–898.

Lee, B.H., Bello-Pérez, L.A., Lin, A.H.M., Kim, C.Y. and Hamaker, B.R. (2013). Importance of location of digestion and colonic fermentation of starch related to its quality. *Cereal Chemistry Journal*, 90(4): 335–343.

Lee, E.B., Kim, H.-Y., Han, G.J. and Park, B.-R. (2018). Preparation of isomaltooligosaccharides using puffed rice flour and evaluation of physicochemical properties. *Korean Journal of Food Preservation*, 25(2): 229–236.

Lee, H.-S., Auh, J.-H., Yoon, H.-G., Kim, M.-J., Park, J.-H., Hong, S.-S. et al. (2002). Cooperative action of α-glucanotransferase and maltogenic amylase for an improved process of isomaltooligosaccharide (IMO) production. *Journal of Agricultural and Food Chemistry*, 50(10): 2812–2817.

Lee, M.S., Cho, S.K., Eom, H.J., Kim, S.Y., Kim, T.J. and Han, N.S. (2008). Optimized substrate concentrations for production of long-chain isomaltooligosaccharides using dextransucrase of *Leuconostoc mesenteroides* B-512F. *Journal of Microbiology and Biotechnology*, 18(6): 1141–1145.

Lin, A. H.-M., Nichols, B.L., Quezada-Calvillo, R., Avery, S.E., Sim, L., Rose, D.R., Naim, H.Y. and Hamaker, B.R. (2012). Unexpected high digestion rate of cooked starch by the Ct-maltase-glucoamylase small intestine mucosal α-glucosidase subunit. *PloS ONE*, 7(5): e35473.

Münkel, F., Fischer, A. and Wefers, D. (2020). Structural characterization of mixed-linkage α-glucans produced by mutants of *Lactobacillus reuteri* TMW 1.106 dextransucrase. *Carbohydrate Polymers*, 231: 115697.

Nakanishi, T., Nomura, S. and Takeda, Y. (2006). An improved method for the quantitative analysis of commercial isomaltooligosaccharide products using the calibration curve of standard reagents. *Journal of Applied Glycoscience*, 53(3): 215–222.

Niu, D., Qiao, J., Li, P., Tian, K., Liu, X., Singh, S. et al. (2017). Highly efficient enzymatic preparation of isomalto-oligosaccharides from starch using an enzyme cocktail. *Electronic Journal of Biotechnology*, 26: 46–51.

Oguma, T., Kitao, S. and Kobayashi, M. (2014). Purification and characterization of cycloisomaltooligosaccharide glucanotransferase and cloning of *cit* from *Bacillus circulans* U-155. *Journal of Applied Glycoscience*, 61(4): 93–97.

Ojha, S., Mishra, S. and Chand, S. (2015). Production of isomalto-oligosaccharides by cell bound α-glucosidase of Microbacterium sp. *LWT - Food Science and Technology*, 60(1): 486–494.

Petrova, P. and Petrov, K. (2017). Prebiotic–probiotic relationship: The genetic fundamentals of polysaccharides conversion by Bifidobacterium and Lactobacillus genera. Chapter 7 in: *Food Bioconversion* (ed. A.M. Grumezescu and A.M. Holban), 237–278). Academic Press.

Plongbunjong, V., Graidist, P., Knudsen, K.E.B. and Wichienchot, S. (2017). Isomaltooligosaccharide synthesised from rice starch and its prebiotic properties in vitro. *International Journal of Food Science and Technology*, 52(12): 2589–2595.

Rivellese, A.A., Giacco, R. and Costabile, G. (2012). Dietary carbohydrates for diabetics. *Current Atherosclerosis Reports*, 14: 563–569.

Roberfroid, M. (2007). Prebiotics: The concept revisited. *The Journal of Nutrition*, 137(3): 830–837.

Rudeekulthamrong, P., Sawasdee, K. and Kaulpiboon, J. (2013). Production of long-chain isomaltooligosaccharides from maltotriose using the thermostable amylomaltase and transglucosidase enzymes. *Biotechnology and Bioprocess Engineering*, 18(4): 778–786.

Saman, P., Kuancha, C., Chaiongkarn, A., Moonmangmee, S. and Fungsin, B. (2019). Isomalto-oligosaccharides production from rice flour and cassava starch. *Journal of Food Science and Agricultural Technology*, 5: 188–192.

Selling, J., Swann, P., Madsen, L.R., II and Oswald, J. (2018). Improvement in gastroesophageal reflux symptoms from a food-grade maltosyl-isomaltooligosaccharide soluble fiber supplement: A case series. *Integrative Medicine (Boulder)*, 17(5): 40–42.

Shi, Q., Hou, Y., Juvonen, M.K., Tuomainen, P.M.S., Kajala, I., Shukla, S. and Tenkanen, T.M. (2016). Optimization of isomaltooligosaccharide size distribution by acceptor reaction of *Weissella confusa* dextransucrase and characterization of novel α-(1→2)-branched isomaltooligosaccharides. *Journal of Agricultural and Food Chemistry*, 64(16): 3276–3286.

Song, J. Y., Kim, Y.-M., Lee, B.-H. and Yoo, S.-H. (2020). Increasing the dietary fiber contents in isomaltooligosaccharides by dextransucrase reaction with sucrose as a glucosyl donor. *Carbohydrate Polymers*, 230: 115607.

Sorndech, W., Meier, S., Jansson, A.M., Sagnelli, D., Hindsgaul, O., Tongta, S. and Blennow, A. (2015). Synergistic amylomaltase and branching enzyme catalysis to suppress cassava starch digestibility. *Carbohydrate Polymers*, 132: 409–418.

Sorndech, W., Nakorn, K. N., Tongta, S. and Blennow, A. (2018). Isomalto-oligosaccharides: Recent insights in production technology and their use for food and medical applications. *LWT*, 95: 135–142.

Sorndech, W., Rodtong, S., Blennow, A. and Tongta, S. (2019). Impact of resistant maltodextrins and resistant starch on human gut microbiota and organic acids production. *Starch - Stärke*, 71(5-6): 1800231.

Sorndech, W., Sagnelli, D., Blennow, A. and Tongta, S. (2017). Combination of amylase and transferase catalysis to improve IMO compositions and productivity. *LWT - Food Science and Technology*, 79: 479–486.

Stenvers, D.J., Schouten, L.J., Jurgens, J., Endert, E., Kalsbeek, A., Fliers, E. and Bisschop, P.H. (2014). Breakfast replacement with a low-glycaemic response liquid formula in patients with type 2 diabetes: A randomised clinical trial. *British Journal of Nutrition*, 112(04): 504–512.

Subhan, F.B., Hashemi, Z., Archundia Herrera, M.C., Turner, K., Windeler, S., Gänzle, M. G. and Chan, C.B. (2020). Ingestion of isomalto-oligosaccharides stimulates insulin and incretin hormone secretion in healthy adults. *Journal of Functional Foods*, 65: 103730.

Suzuki, R., Terasawa, K., Kimura, K., Fujimoto, Z., Momma, M., Kobayashi, M., Kimura, A. and Funane, K. (2012). Biochemical characterization of a novel cycloisomaltooligosaccharide glucanotransferase from *Paenibacillus* sp. 598K. *Biochimica et Biophysica Acta (BBA) - Proteins and Proteomics*, 1824(7): 919–924.

Tarabees, R., Gafar, K.M., El-Sayed, M.S., Shehata, A.A. and Ahmed, M. (2019). Effects of dietary supplementation of probiotic mix and prebiotic on growth performance, cecal microbiota composition, and protection against Escherichia coli O78 in broiler chickens. *Probiotics and Antimicrobial Proteins*, 11(3): 981–989.

Terada, Y., Fujii, K., Takaha, T. and Okada, S. (1999). Thermus aquaticus ATCC 33923 amylomaltase gene cloning and expression and enzyme characterization: production of cycloamylose. *Applied and Environmental Microbiology*, 65(3): 910–915.

Tungland, B.C. and Meyer, D. (2002). Nondigestible oligo- and polysaccharides (dietary fiber): Their physiology and role in human health and food. *Comprehensive Reviews in Food Science and Food Safety*, 1(3): 90–109.

Wachters-Hagedoorn, R.E., Priebe, M.G., Heimweg, J.A.J., Heiner, A.M., Englyst, K.N., Holst, J.J. and Vonk, R.J. (2006). The rate of intestinal glucose absorption is correlated with plasma glucose-dependent insulinotropic polypeptide concentrations in healthy men. *The Journal of Nutrition*, 136(6): 1511–1516.

Wang, W., Xin, H., Fang, X., Dou, H., Liu, F., Huang, D., Han, S., Fei, G., Zhu, L., Zha, S., Zhang, H. and Ke, M. (2017). Isomalto-oligosaccharides ameliorate visceral hyperalgesia with repair damage of ileal epithelial ultrastructure in rats. *PloS ONE*, 12(4): e0175276.

Wolever, T.M.S. (2003). Carbohydrate and the regulation of blood glucose and metabolism. *Nutrition Reviews*, 61(5): 40–48.

Yang, S.-J., Choi, S.-J., Park, B.-R. and Kim, Y.-M. (2019). Thermostable CITase from *Thermoanaerobacter thermocopriae* shows negative cooperativity. *Biotechnology Letters*, 41(4): 625–632.

Yen, C.-H., Tseng, Y.-H., Kuo, Y.-W., Lee, M.-C. and Chen, H.-L. (2011). Long-term supplementation of isomalto-oligosaccharides improved colonic microflora profile, bowel function, and blood cholesterol levels in constipated elderly people—A placebo-controlled, diet-controlled trial. *Nutrition*, 27(4): 445–450.

Zhang, F., Wang, W., Bah, F.B.M., Song, C., Zhou, Y., Ji, L. and Yuan, Y. (2019). Heterologous expression of a thermostable α-glucosidase from *Geobacillus* sp. strain HTA-462 by *Escherichia coli* and its potential application for isomaltose–oligosaccharide synthesis. *Molecules*, 24(7): 1413.

Zhang, G. and Hamaker, B.R. (2009). Slowly digestible starch: Concept, mechanism, and proposed extended glycemic index. *Critical Reviews in Food Science and Nutrition*, 49(10): 852–867.

Zhang, G., Hasek, L.Y., Lee, B.H. and Hamaker, B.R. (2015). Gut feedback mechanisms and food intake: a physiological approach to slow carbohydrate bioavailability. *Food and Function*, 6(4): 1072–1089.

Zhang, L., Jiang, Y., Jiang, Z., Sun, X., Shi, J., Cheng, W. et al. (2009). Immobilized transglucosidase in biomimetic polymer–inorganic hybrid capsules for efficient conversion of maltose to isomaltooligosaccharides. *Biochemical Engineering Journal*, 46(2): 186–192.

Zhang, L., Su, Y., Zheng, Y., Jiang, Z., Shi, J., Zhu, Y. and Jiang, Y. (2010). Sandwich-structured enzyme membrane reactor for efficient conversion of maltose into isomaltooligosaccharides. *Bioresource Technology*, 101(23): 9144–9149.

Zhao, B., Zhou, L., Ma, L., He, Y., Gao, J., Li, D. and Jiang, Y. (2018). Co-immobilization of glucose oxidase and catalase in silica inverse opals for glucose removal from commercial isomaltooligosaccharide. *International Journal of Biological Macromolecules*, 107: 2034–2043.

16

Starch and its Derivatives as Potential Source of Prebiotics

Yudi Pranoto

Department of Food and Agricultural Product Technology, Faculty of Agricultural Technology, Universitas Gadjah Mada, Jl. Flora No. 1, Bulaksumur, Yogyakarta, 55281, Indonesia

16.1 Introduction

Around the globe, starch is established as the main energy contributor for humans. It is presented as a reserve polysaccharide produced in the amyloplasts of plants (in roots, cereals, tubers and rhizomes) as oval, round, lenticular or polyhedral, ogival or elongated to flat discrete granules, with diameter sizes ranging from sub-microns to more than 100 μm (Bertoft 2017; Jane *et al.* 1994).

Starch granules are basically composed of two polyglucans, amylose and amylopectin. The molecular arrangement of the former is relatively simple, consisting of glucose units linked through α-(1,4) linkages into long polysaccharide chains with low numbers of α-(1,6) branches. The latter, amylopectin, has a similar primary structure, but with relatively shorter polysaccharide chains and numerous α-(1,6) branches (Bertoft 2017).

The major component of most starch granules is amylopectin, whereas the minor one is amylose, which usually constitutes 15–30% of the starch. However, in some plant carbohydrates, exceptions may exist. With the endosperm's waxy character in waxy cereals, waxy starches have very little or no amylose. Another exception can also be found in starches obtained from genetically modified plants, containing 50–80% amylose (Bertoft 2017; Collona and Mercier 1985). A recent report discovered that an engineered barley starch contained almost 100% amylose (Carciofi *et al.* 2012).

When the starch reaches the small intestine in human digestion, α-amylases, glucoamylase and sucrase-isomaltase break down or hydrolyze the starches to yield free glucose followed by absorption (Nugent 2005); however, some typical starches found in our food are not readily broken down by enzymes and absorbed in our small intestine. Those typical starches are well known as resistant starch (RS) (Raungrusmee *et al.* 2020). RS can occur in all starchy foods and, as a human food source, it has a long history. RS comprises the portion of starch that can resist the digestive enzymes in the small intestine and hence reach the colon. RS consists of an extensive range of materials and several different types

Probiotics, Prebiotics and Synbiotics: Technological Advancements Towards Safety and Industrial Applications, First Edition. Edited by Parmjit Singh Panesar and Anil Kumar Anal.

(RS1 to RS5). Its great nutritional interest is linked to its physiological effects, comparable to those of dietary fiber. The steady intake of certain highly fermentable dietary fiber subgroups causes gut-associated immune and microbiota modulation, besides significant short chain fatty acid (SCFA) production. Therefore, RS is considered prebiotic, and it is also not absorbed in the intestine of the human digestion system (Fuentes-Zaragoza *et al.* 2011). Amongst the diverse physiological functions of RS, its prebiotic effect is the most attractive.

Improvement of microflora and colonic health, lower glycemic index, treatment of diabetes, attenuation of blood cholesterol levels, decreased bile stone development, enhanced mineral absorption and ability to enhance fat oxidation are among the list of health benefits of RS. Some factors affect the RS content in foods, namely, the characters of native starch, processing techniques and storage temperature. In the market, commercial preparations of RS are yet available. Technically, RS can be prepared through different methods, by chemical, physical and enzymatic modifications. Food industries employ these RS preparation methods to produce a food constituent that reduces the products' caloric content and enhances their textural and sensory characteristics (Raigond *et al.* 2017). This chapter highlights the potential of RS as a novel prebiotic, its health benefits and its prospective applications in the food industry area.

16.2 Starch Digestion

Starch plays a role as the main energy-generating source for humans. The digestibility of the starch is credited to the association of several determinants such as plant source, granule size, amylose/amylopectin ratio, degree of crystallinity, degree of molecular interaction between components, length of amylose chain and existence of amylose–lipid complexes in the starch (Cummings and Englyst 1995). Lipids or fatty acids are particularly interacted with amylose to form complexes, thereby reducing starch digestibility. Because of those complex formations, enzymatic hydrolysis by amylase is inhibited (Taylor *et al.* 2015).

As the action of chewing, or mastication, crushes the lumps of food into more diminutive particles in the oral cavity, the digestion of carbohydrates (starches) immediately occurs (Wrolstad 2012). The greater ratio of surface area to volume of the chewed food particle compared to the original size provides a sufficient coating of saliva secreted by the salivary glands in response to mastication. Having a pH of 6.8 and mostly constituted of water, roughly 1% of saliva is a combination of enzymes and electrolytes. α-Amylase, which plays a role in the hydrolysis of starch by non-sequentially breaking down the $\alpha(1 \rightarrow 4)$ linkages in starch molecules, is known as one of the enzymes.

When the food particle size is small enough and it is adequately mixed and coated in saliva, it will continue to move through the pharynx and esophagus into the stomach. The presence of hydrochloric acid (HCl) creates a very low pH, around 1.0, in the stomach environment. The acidic conditions eventually deactivate the α-amylase from the mouth saliva and therefore no more enzymatic digestion of carbohydrates happens in the stomach (Jackson and Mclaughlin 2009). Meanwhile, the enzymatic breakdown of proteins and lipids is started by the presence of other digestive enzymes, namely proteases and lipases, respectively.

Food digestion continues as the chyme, a mixture of partially digested food, enzymes and acids, proceeds from the stomach to the duodenum, the first section of the small intestine. In this section, the pH starts to increase to around 7.8 due to the pancreas and gall bladder secretions, allowing α-amylase introduced from the small intestine's epithelial cell lining to function. Therefore, the enzymatic hydrolysis or breakdown of starch advances, producing varying lengths of smaller and shorter carbohydrate chains, namely dextrin and maltose. Other pancreatic enzymes, particularly maltase, function to cleave the α(1→4) linkage of maltose as α-amylase cannot break down the molecules completely. The glucose resulting from this digestive process is absorbed through the small intestine wall into the bloodstream via several complex pathways (Björck 2006; Sullivan 2020).

In general, free glucose resulting from the digestible starches that have been hydrolyzed or broken down by enzymes is eventually absorbed in the small intestine (Nugent 2005). The degree and rate of carbohydrate digestion in the human body are greatly dependent on the chain length, the number of glycosidic bonds present, and their form. Glucose, maltose, fructose and other small molecule carbohydrates, often found in sweet-tasting foods such as confectionery, cake and fruits, are digested and absorbed quickly because they require little to no enzymatic digestion. On the other hand, larger or more complex carbohydrates such as oligosaccharides and starch necessitate more complex digestion and take longer to be digested.

Determined by their rate and extent of digestibility by the enzymes, three groups of starches can be listed, as follows (Sajilata *et al.* 2006; Sullivan 2020):

1) *Rapidly digestible starch (RDS).* Amorphous and dispersed starches dominate this starch group. RDS is commonly available in large quantities in starchy foods processed under heat and moisture, such as potatoes, cookies and bread. RDS can be chemically measured by converting starch by enzymatic digestion into glucose units within 20 min of reaction. Some studies correlate RDS to the glycemic index (GI) of food.
2) *Slowly digestible starch (SDS).* This type of starch is supposed to be entirely digested in the small intestine. However, for certain reasons, the digestion process occurs slowly and takes longer than RDS. High SDS foods are associated with low GI, bringing health benefits. Amorphous starch that is physically inaccessible and raw starch with a type A and type C crystalline structure, such as cereals and type B starch, are included in this starch group. SDS measurement is conducted using enzymatic digestion as starch samples are converted to glucose molecules after 120 min of reaction.
3) *Resistant starch (RS).* This group consists of the starch fraction that resists hydrolysis in the small intestine after 120 min of being consumed. In other words, the fraction of dietary starch escaping digestion in the small intestine is described as RS. Because the starch reaches the large intestine, it may be available to be fermented by the gut microflora. The amount of RS can be obtained by deducting the difference between total starch (TS) taken from a homogenized and chemically treated sample, and the sum of RDS and SDS fraction, extracted from non-homogenized samples by enzymatic digestion, as described by the following equation:

$$\mathrm{RS} = \mathrm{TS} \quad \left(\mathrm{RDS} + \mathrm{SDS}\right)$$

The physical form of seeds and grains, plant genotype, interaction between starch and other components, processing methods (milling, cooking, annealing, autoclaving, high-pressure treatment, extrusion, irradiation), storage period and conditions, and other factors determine starch digestibility. Insufficient grinding of a food rich in starches could reduce the digestibility of the starch. Also, the degree of digestibility of a starch is influenced by the types of plant sources, structural compactness and other matrices surrounding the starch granules. For instance, the starch digestibility of food made from barley flakes could increase from 83.5% to 99.1% by choosing the same materials but in a milled form. The insufficient chewing of whole canned beans, generating rather large particle sizes, showed low starch digestibility of 64.1%. This kind of RS (lately known as RS1) has been incorporated in various conventional foods due to its stability in most processing methods. Nevertheless, like fine milling, some processing steps can damage the plant cell or tissue structure's integrity, thus significantly reducing the RS1 content (Li 2018).

16.3 Starch as a Probiotic Food Source

The human gut microbiota is populated densely by various kinds of bacteria, up to 10^{14} bacterial cells. Amongst the parts of the human gastrointestinal tract colonized by bacteria, the large intestine has the largest population. Carbohydrate fermentation and degradation pathways are usually the main functions of the gut microbiota. The fraction of the ingested food arriving at the large intestine is known to contain the complex polysaccharides that are resistant to digestion by the host enzymes. Various kinds of complex glycans, including undigestible polysaccharides, as well as monosaccharides, and disaccharides that are not fully absorbed in the upper part of the gastrointestinal tract due to overconsumption or lack of complete digestion, along with endogenous substrates, namely glycoproteins, are then accessible for the colonic microbiota metabolism (Chassard and Lacroix 2013).

Most colonic microbiotas are recognized as saccharolytic bacteria, and several known bacterial groups such as *Bacteroides, Eubacterium*, *Bifidobacterium* and *Escherichia* can ferment starch. *Bifidobacterium* and *Clostridium butyricum* species are effective starch-utilizing bacteria as proven *in vitro* (Brown *et al.* 1998). From the average total anaerobic count of a subject sample containing starch-hydrolyzing bacteria, the amylolytic count average was around 56%. The amylolytic isolates were dominated by bifidobacteria (58%) and bacteroides (18%), while butyrivibrios and fusobacteria made up about 10% of starch-hydrolyzing bacteria. More studies on pure cultures of starch-hydrolyzing bacteria discovered that the amylolytic enzymes of bifidobacteria and *Bacteroides* were cell associated. This discovery provided further evidence that both bacteria were accountable for the amylolytic activities detected in washed cell fecal fractions (Macfarlane and Englyst 1986).

For carbohydrate digestion, enzymes (amylases and glucoamylases) are secreted to degrade the starch completely. Meanwhile, in the upper part of the gastrointestinal tract, non-starch polysaccharides (NSPs), such as polysaccharides from plant cell walls (cellulose, lignin, hemicellulose) and plant stored polysaccharides (oligosaccharides and pectin), are not digested. Furthermore, they can undergo fermentation in the large intestine by the colonic microbiota. These gut microorganisms degrade and ferment complex polysaccharides; however, undigested lignin and cellulose are unsuccessfully fermented in some individual cases. The fibrinolytic organism degradation is mainly accountable for fiber fermentation and involves certain anaerobic enzymes produced by gut microbes. These microbes were members of the predominant groups such as *Roseburia* (fermenting resistant starch, oligosaccharides and xylan), *Bacteroides* (fermenting resistant starch, xylan), *Ruminococcus* (fermenting resistant starch, cellulose), or *Bifidobacterium* (fermenting oligosaccharides) (Chassard and Lacroix 2013). Since resistant starch (RS) moves almost undigested through the small intestine, it behaves as a food source for the growth of probiotic microorganisms. Therefore, the incorporation of RS in probiotic substances to support the growth of beneficial microorganisms, such as *Bifidobacterium*, has been proposed (Sajilata *et al.* 2006).

Potential probiotic traits have been investigated in some bacteria and yeasts, especially *Lactobacillus* and *Bifidobacterium*. Both Gram-positive and lactic acid-producing genera have been used for thousands of years in human food history, for food preservation through fermentation, and they are conclusively distinguished as "generally recognized as safe" (GRAS). They are also the dominant microbiota residents in the intestine in humans and animals (de Vrese and Schrezenmeir 2008). The bacteria can have dual benefits by acting as agents for food fermentation and providing health advantages in consuming fermented food (Guarner *et al.* 2011). Other species listed as probiotics are the genera of *Lactococcus, Propionibacterium, Enterococcus* and *Saccharomyces* (e.g. *S. cerevisiae* and *S. boulardii*), primarily because of their proven health-promoting impacts (Terpou *et al.* 2019).

Recent studies have been carried out by including RS in probiotic compositions to facilitate beneficial microorganisms like *Bifidobacterium*. The proliferation of *Bifidobacterium* in the intestinal tract of pigs consuming high-amylose starch containing RS indicated its potential benefit in acting as a prebiotic in humans. Brown *et al.* (1998) noticed that yoghurt to which RS was added maintained viable counts of *Bifidobacterium* over several weeks, which was lacking in yoghurt prepared without RS. It has been shown that RS modifies the human gut microflora by stimulating lactic acid bacteria (Lilia-Baby *et al.* 2015). The amount of butyrate and the numbers of *Lactobacillus* and *Bifidobacterium* in the large intestine could be increased by ingesting retrograded high-amylose starch (Birt *et al.* 2013). Therefore, the effect gut bacteria on human health is already well known, namely their impact on nutritional acquisition, immune capacity, controlling appetite and positively influencing disorders such as mental disorder, obesity and linked metabolic impairment.

16.4 Resistant Starch as a Novel Prebiotic

Resistant starch is defined as the fraction of starch and starch products that withstands digestive processes when traveling throughout the gastrointestinal tract (Nugent 2005). Others described RS as the fraction of starch that is not broken down into D-glucose in the small intestine within 120 min of being consumed; thus, it is readily available for fermentation in the colon (Tharanathan 2002).

Based on its structure or mechanism in withstanding digestion, RS has been grouped into five general subtypes, namely RS1–RS5, as reported by Fuentes-Zaragoza *et al.* (2011), Birt *et al.* (2013) and Li (2018), which are described as follows.

1) RS1 is classified as the starches that are physically inaccessible to enzymatic digestion due to their entrapment within the food matrix, namely proteins, cell wall materials and other

physical barriers in whole or partly milled grains, tubers and seeds. A good example of RS1 is the RS in pasta. The compact protein matrix of pasta has been reported to be responsible for its higher RS content than other wheat products. Grinding, milling and protease hydrolysis that can destroy the physical barriers in foods certainly reduce the RS1 content.

2) RS2 incorporates native, unprocessed starch granules with B- or C-type polymorphs, namely those found in raw potatoes, unripe banana starches, and high-amylose maize starches, whose granule crystallinity makes them resistant to enzymatic hydrolysis. A disadvantage of RS2 for food applications is that its RS content decreases substantially after thermal processing. A particular type of RS2 called HAM (high-amylose maize starch) is uniquely stable to most cooking operations because of long-chain double-helical crystallites.
3) RS3 refers to retrograded or crystalline non-granular starch formed after cooking, like the starch found in cooked and cooled potatoes, bread crusts, cornflakes and retrograded high maize starch. RS3 refers to non-granular starch-derived materials that resist digestion. During food processing, in most cases in which heat and moisture are involved, RS1 and RS2 can be destroyed, but RS3 can be formed. During retrogradation, the two polymer chains reassociate to form double helices stabilized by hydrogen bonds, making the structure more resistant to enzymatic hydrolysis. Linear amylose molecules are preferred for the formation of RS3 because they retrograde faster and form more resistant crystallites than amylopectin.

   Storey *et al.* (2007) classified a soluble polysaccharide called "retrograded resistant maltodextrins" as type 3 RS. They are derived from starch that is processed to rearrange or hydrolyze starch molecules purposefully, and subsequent retrogradation, to render them soluble and resistant to digestion. This process results in the formation of indigestible crystallites that have a molecular similarity to type RS3 but with a smaller degree of polymerization and a lower molecular weight, converting a portion of the normal α1,4-glucose linkages to random 1,2-, 1,3-, and 1,4-α or β linkages.
4) RS4 includes starches that undergo chemical modification, namely esterification, etherification or cross-linking. RS4 is further grouped into subcategories based on its solubility in water and the experimental protocols used for analyses. Chemical modifications reduce the digestion of starch by forming steric hindrances at the sites of enzymatic action. For example, octenyl succinic anhydride modification of starch introduces hydrophobic octenyl succinate (OS) groups into starch molecules, which interfere with starch binding by amylolytic enzymes. Cross-linking of starch is another effective approach to prepare RS4.
5) RS5 can be formed from high-amylose starches that form a complex with lipid. These amylose–lipid complexes require higher temperatures for gelatinization and are more susceptible to retrograde. In general, the structure and amount of starch–lipid in foods depend on their botanical sources. Also, RS5, a polysaccharide that consists of water-insoluble linear poly α-1,4-glucan that is not susceptible to degradation by α-amylases. Also, poly α-1,4 D-glucans promote the formation of SCFAs, particularly butyrate, in the colon and are thus suitable for use as nutritional supplements for the prevention of colorectal diseases.

   RS5 has been proposed to have two different components. The first component involves amylose–lipid complexes, which is a single helical structure formed between amylose

Table 16.1 Type of RS, food sources and rate of digestion.

RS type	Explanation	Food sources	Rate of digestion
RS1	Physically inaccessible to enzymatic digestion	Whole-kernel or coarsely ground grain products (e.g. seeds, legumes and bread)	Slow
RS2	Unprocessed resistant granules with type B crystallinity	Green bananas, ginkgo starch, raw potatoes, high-amylose maize	Very slow
RS3	Retrograded starch	Starchy foods that undergo cooking and cooling for example rice, potatoes, cornflakes, pasta, bread (especially stale bread),	Slow
RS4	Starches that are processed through chemical modification	Food comprising starches that undergo chemical modification, for instance cross-linked starch and octenyl succinate (e.g. some commercially produced cakes and breads)	Resist hydrolysis
RS5	Amylose–lipid complexes	Foods comprising naturally or artificially occurring amylose–lipid complexes, for instance bread containing fat as an ingredient or stearic acid-complexed high-amylose starch, respectively	Slow

Sources: Based on Raigond *et al.* (2017); Homayouni *et al.* (2013); Lockyer and Nugent (2017).

and lipids. The second component is resistant maltodextrin, which is obtained by subjecting native starch to sequential applications of pyroconversion and enzymatic hydrolysis. Resistant maltodextrins are non-sweet low molecular weight compounds containing the native α-(1→4), α-(1→6) bonds, β-(1→2), β-(1→3) bonds, and levoglucosan. They have similar characteristics to dietary fiber. However, mostly RS5 is described as amylose–lipid complexes.

A summary of RS types, their brief explanation, food sources and digestion rate is presented in Table 16.1.

Furthermore, Sharma et al. (2008) have classified food sources and their range of RS content as presented in Table 16.2.

RS is not technically a fiber but a type of starch that acts like prebiotic fiber. It resists stomach digestion, passes through the small intestines, and arrives in the large intestine completely intact. The bacteria feed on RS and produce an SCFA, butyrate, which provides exceptional benefits over other prebiotics. RS keeps our gut cells healthy, reducing inflammation and bowel cancer risk because it acts as a medium for probiotics growth and, therefore, is called a "prebiotic".

The description of a prebiotic is "non-digestible food ingredients that beneficially affect the host by selectively stimulating the growth and (or) activity of one or a limited number of bacterial species already resident in the colon, and, thus, attempt to improve host health" (Gibson *et al.* 2017). Fructooligosaccharides (FOS) are commonly known as one of the best

Table 16.2 Categories of food sources and their RS content.

Category	RS content (% dry matter)	Food materials
Negligible	<1.0	Wheat flour, pasta, boiled rice (hot), boiled potato (hot), breakfast cereals containing a high proportion of bran
Low	1.0–2.5	Breads, biscuits, pasta, boiled potato (cooled), boiled rice (cooled), breakfast cereals
Intermediate	2.5–5.0	Extruded legumes, fried potatoes, breakfast cereals (rice crispies, cornflakes)
High	5.0–15.0	Peas, raw rice, cooked legumes (lentils, beans, chickpeas), autoclaved and cooled starches (potato, wheat, maize), cooked and frozen starchy foods
Very high	>15.0	Unripe banana, raw legumes, raw potatoes, amylo-maize, retrograded amylose

Source: Data from Sharma *et al.* (2008).

prebiotics; however, some other carbohydrates have also been discovered to be prebiotic candidates. Davani-Davari *et al.* (2019) classified the prebiotics into five types: (i) fructan; (ii) galactooligosaccharides; (iii) starch and glucose-derived oligosaccharides; (iv) other saccharides; and (v) non-carbohydrate oligosaccharides.

Prebiotics are used to facilitate the well-being of beneficial microbiota in the gut called probiotics. Prebiotics include non-digestible oligosaccharides with numerous favorable influences on the gastrointestinal system. These health advantages are delivered by selectively facilitating the growth or activity of specific bacteria. Common prebiotics are dietary fibers (DF), comprising inulin, oligosaccharides and RS. Because prebiotics are important in preventing certain diseases, they have become an attractive area of research. DF are described as an arrangement of 10 or more glucose units forming carbohydrate polymers. In the digestive system, they are hardly broken down by endogenous enzymes. Nevertheless, their important trait is their ability to be used by beneficial gut microbiota, known as probiotics. This may lead to improved beneficial bacteria growth and increased fecal bulk; consequently, fibrous substances have prebiotic effects (Homayouni *et al.* 2013).

On the other hand, it is not easy to establish the appropriateness of RS to be considered a prebiotic candidate due to the wide variety of starches included. In general, to be fully recognized as prebiotic, an RS must satisfy certain requirements:

- Survive the acidic conditions in the stomach and withstand enzymatic digestion by mammalian enzymes and gastrointestinal absorption.
- Be able to be fermented and metabolized by beneficial colonic microorganisms.
- Selectively promote activity and/or growth of one or several gut microbiota species that improve the host's health and well-being (Lockyer and Nugent 2017; Zaman and Sarbini 2016).

Table 16.3 Evaluation method to measure the prebiotic potential of resistant starch.

Parameter	In vitro evaluation	In vivo evaluation
Survive acidic conditions in the stomach, withstand digestion by mammalian enzymes and gastrointestinal absorption	Simulate gastrointestinal conditions by pretreatment of the starch sample in resisting several acids and mammalian enzymes	Weighing the starch recovery in feces of rat Performing gastrointestinal tract intubation in anesthetized rats Administering the sample orally followed by direct recovery of undigested fragments in the distal ileum
Able to be fermented and metabolized by beneficial colonic microorganisms	Batch or continuous fermentation of starch sample inoculated by fecal bacteria	Animal model: feeding rats with prebiotic for a certain period, then terminating the animals to obtain their colon to be used in subsequent analysis Indirect method: regularly collecting the air breathed at intervals to investigate the concentration of gases, i.e. hydrogen Direct method: measuring the sample recovery through animal feces
Selectively promote the activity and/or growth of one or a certain gut microbiota species that improve the host's health and well-being	Similar to the above-mentioned analysis, followed by further analysis involving bacteria enumeration, e.g. fluorescent in situ hybridization (FISH) and culture-dependent methodology	Similar to the above-mentioned analysis, followed by further analysis involving bacteria enumeration, e.g. fluorescent in situ hybridization (FISH) and culture-dependent methodology

A method to evaluate the potential of RS as a prebiotic for some food sources is described in Table 16.3.

The probable applications of RS as prebiotic ingredients in functional food formulations can be summarized as:

- Fermentable substrates for the growth of probiotic microbiota, particularly lactobacilli and bifidobacteria.
- Dietary supplements promoting several advantageous physiological effects.
- Encapsulation materials for probiotic bacteria in order to improve their stability (Fuentes-Zaragoza *et al.* 2011).

As RS almost completely passes through the small intestine, it is classified as a type of fiber. Thus it would be expected to provide benefits to gut health, specifically in the large intestine where RS is fermented and releases SCFAs (formate, acetate, propionate, butyrate and valerate), a smaller number of organic acids (lactate and succinate), gases (methane, hydrogen and carbon dioxide) and alcohols (methanol and ethanol). This process involves several vital bacterial groups such as amylolytic gut bacteria (including Bacteroidetes, Firmicutes and Actinobacteria), which facilitate amylose breakdown, butyrogenic Archaea (including *Eubacterium rectale*), which are involved in the production of butyrate, and methanogenic Archaea, which are needed for methane production. On the whole, the research into the effects of RS on gut health has focused on endpoints, for instance SCFAs, gas production, and bacterial composition (Li 2018).

Rising health consciousness and increasing demand for functional foods from consumers are steering food manufacturers globally to develop innovations in food products with health advantages. Science has discovered that dietary fiber has a beneficial role in attenuation and prevention of some chronic disorders. Therefore, consumers' awareness regarding the consumption of dietary fiber and its healthy role has been raised, and products based on fiber-enriched cereal have been gaining in popularity. There is a considerable increase in the advancement of slowly digestible carbohydrates due to the awareness of foods with low GI value and to manage diabetes, obesity and the risk of cardiovascular disease (Fuentes-Zaragoza *et al.* 2010). Nutritional influences of RS in foods have become interesting because its physiological effects are comparable to those of dietary fiber such as increased laxation, lower postprandial glucose response, decreased risk of developing digestive tract cancers, decreased blood lipid levels, and potentially involvement in the prevention of gallstone development. Scientific interest in RS in the last decades has mostly been due to its capability to generate a large amount of butyrate in the colon. Investigations have been conducted regarding the effect of butyrate on cell metabolism, differentiation and growth, as well as the effect on the inhibition mechanism of colon tumor development through several factors that underlie the initiation, progression and growth of tumors (Fuentes-Zaragoza *et al.* 2011).

The role of RS as a medium for probiotic microorganisms had been suspected because RS almost entirely passes through the small intestine. In *in vitro* studies, an RS-supplemented diet has been shown to increase lactobacilli, bifidobacteria, staphylococci and streptococci significantly. It also reduces the population of enterobacteria and governs microbial enzyme metabolism in the colon (Tabibloghmany and Ehsandoost 2014). Silvi *et al.* (1999) studied the result of RS consumption on the human gut and observed that RS modifies the human gut microflora by stimulating lactic acid bacteria.

The role of RS in gut microbiota was elicited by facilitating the growth of *Lactobacillus,* enhancing the growth of bifidobacteria in rats, and stabilizing bifidobacteria in acidic conditions and bile acid in the gastrointestinal tract. Furthermore, an intervention with an RS-rich diet might significantly improve bifidobacteria, lactobacilli and streptococci, lower the number of enterobacteria, and govern microbial enzyme metabolism in the colon of experimental rodents. Laboratory studies on pigs and humans have discovered a time-dependent shift in fecal and SCFA profiles in large bowel, demonstrating advantageous synergy of probiotic bacteria with the RS. A study reported that high-amylose maize starch (HAM RS2) had the ability to maintain the viability of probiotic bacteria. Improved fecal *Bifidobacterium* count in rodents after treatment with the diet containing HAM starch demonstrated that *Bifidobacterium* used most of the ingested HAM RS2 (Ashwar *et al.* 2016).

Apart from intrinsic states of starch (e.g. granular structure, crystallinity, the proportion of amylose to amylopectin) affecting RS formation, processing factors also alter RS content and formation in processed food. Birt *et al.* (2013) reported that the prebiotic effect did not appear to be restricted to a high portion of amylose starches, but that chemically modified starches (i.e. RS4) are also efficient. Furthermore, the authors reported that the total number of starches arriving at the colon is essential; however, the prebiotic characteristics were also critically circumscribed by the chemical and physical properties of RS. Based on *in vitro* studies, it was considered that bifidobacteria could stick to starches modified by acylation, octenylsuccinylation, carboxymethylation and succinylation (Brown *et al.* 1998). This chemically modified starch probably results in type RS4.

Some processes, such as extrusion cooking, pasta production, baking and autoclaving, influence starch gelatinization and retrogradation, and eventually affect the amount of RS in the final food product. Studies in cornflakes, puffed breakfast cereals, and snacks have reported the influence of extrusion on the RS content. For instance, the formation of RS3 (especially retrograded starch amylose) in dehulled barley flours was usually determined by the extrusion process at various moisture contents, heats and screw speeds. The extrusion parameters could enhance starch depolymerization, gelatinization, retrogradation and recrystallization that contributed to higher RS contents in extruded barley. Adjusting moisture content and temperature in employing a single-screw extruder to optimize starch gelatinization, with feed moisture at 20% and a mass temperature of 150 °C could create the optimum RS content. The extrusion process led to starch depolymerization through the shear stress of the screw, which eventually facilitated the formation of RS. Even after leaving the extruder, RS formation in the extruded materials continued through retrogradation and recrystallization of the starch (Birt *et al.* 2013). For potatoes that are chilled after the heating process, the digestibility of the starch changes, and these phenomena may be considered as having nutritional importance. Chilling after cooking the potato would profoundly transform starch digestibility: the content of rapidly digested starch (RDS) declines; the content of slowly digested starch (SDS) improves markedly; and the proportion of RS rises. The improvement in RS content indicates that the input of non-digested polysaccharides (dietary fiber) into the colon is markedly elevated, which means the process of chilling cooked potato could be a procedure to obtain dietary fiber. Moreover, it also contains a type of RS that exhibited a role as a prebiotic (Fuentes-Zaragoza *et al.* 2010).

Processing and chemical modification of RS was observed in one of the traditional rice dishes in Indonesia, containing a mixture of rice and coconut milk. Nine rice varieties with different amylose content were processed with cooling-reheating and then coconut milk, including several fatty acids, were added. It was found that higher amylose content correlated with higher RS as well. Treatment by cooling-reheating significantly increased RS content from 1.25 to 3.42% (nearly three times). In addition, coconut milk increased RS content from 1.25 to 5.35% (nearly five times). So cooked rice, processed with a cooling-reheating step and coconut milk addition, results in higher RS than freshly cooked rice (Anugrahati *et al.* 2015). Acetylation of arenga starch with butyric anhydride led to an increase in the RS value of treated starch. Butyrylation modified hydrophilic hydroxyl groups in the starch into more hydrophobic butyryl groups, leading to greater resistance against enzymatic digestion. The RS of native starch (5.69%) was raised to 11.72–12.94% by butyrylation (Rahim *et al.* 2012).

Fermentation using lactic acid bacteria (LAB) combined with autoclaving-cooling has been employed to increase the RS of taro starch. Taro chips were first fermented by a mixed culture of *Lactobacillus plantarum* D-240 and *Leuconostoc mesenteroides* SU-LS 67 (1 : 1) at 37 °C for 18 h, and subsequently were further autoclaved (121 °C, 15 min) and cooled (4 °C, 24 h). The chips were then dried (70 °C, 16 h), milled and sieved (80 mesh) to obtain the modified flour. The results showed that fermentation followed by one cycle of autoclaving-cooling increased the RS content 2.8-fold (from 4.13 to 11.45%) compared with control without fermentation. Fermentation of taro chips could reduce the number of autoclaving-cooling cycles to only one. The modified taro flour demonstrated better prebiotic effect, prebiotic index and activity than control (Setiarto *et al.* 2018).

When utilized as a prebiotic ingredient, RS offers advantages over a commercial prebiotic like inulin. The starch sources are abundantly available, obtained from food-producing plants with varying RS value for easy selection. Technically, it is possible to enhance RS content in foods by manipulating processing conditions such as cooking temperature, heating duration, pH, heating and cooling cycles, freezing and drying, and chemical and enzymatic modifications.

16.5 Health Benefits

The starch source, composition, other constituents in the material, and processing techniques affect nutritional characteristics of starch-based foods. Starch-based foods supply around 60–70% of total energy expended by most people globally, according to the food guide pyramid, which advocates an intake of starch-based foods of around 6–11 servings per day. Thus, the role of starch in human nutrition is indisputable (Homayouni *et al.* 2013).

The functional properties of RS, besides its implied health benefits, offer a way to improve total DF in nutritional intake through regularly consumed foods. DF are described as carbohydrate polymers with 10 or more glucose units that cannot be broken down by endogenous enzymes (McCleary *et al.* 2012). Since numerous digestive impairments are caused by inadequate or inappropriate diet, increasing indigestible carbohydrates is important in improving the diet. Among various DF, RS has roughly half of the calorific value (8 kJ/g) of digestible starch (15 kJ/g) (Khoozani *et al.* 2019).

RS consumption of around 20 g/day is suggested to achieve beneficial health impacts. However, dietary consumption of RS is assumed to differ considerably around the world. The ingestion of RS in developing countries with high starch consumption rates is estimated to range from approximately 30 to 40 g/day (Sajilata *et al.* 2006).

Several physiological benefits have been revealed when RS is included in the diet. Apart from its immediate effect on reducing GI, most health effects of RS have been attributed to its prebiotic properties (Khoozani *et al.* 2019). In other words, there is an universal agreement that there are two main advantages of including RS in the diet: (i) a decreased glycemic response as well as physiological responses following the glycemic response; and (ii) the production of SCFAs from RS fermentation in the colon, and physiological responses following the existence of SCFAs in the colon (BeMiller 2020).

RS is reported as one of the most plentiful dietary sources of non-digestible carbohydrates and can be as vital as non-starch polysaccharides (NSP) in favoring large bowel health and avoiding inflammatory bowel diseases and colorectal cancer, but has less

Table 16.4 Physiological effects and health benefits of resistant starch.

Health benefits	Implied physiological effects
Preventing diabetes	Management of glycemic and insulinemic responses
Preventing cardiovascular disease, lipid metabolism syndrome, cholesterol and triglycerides	Attenuation of blood lipid profile
Prevention of colorectal cancer, ulcerative colitis, inflammatory bowel disease, diverticulitis and constipation	Better bowel health
Colonic health	Prebiotic effect and culture support
Avoiding obesity	Enhancing satiety and lowering energy consumption
Improved mineral and calcium absorption, avoidance of osteoporosis,	Increased micronutrient absorption

Sources: Based on Fuentes-Zaragoza *et al.* (2010); Tabibloghmany and Ehsandoost (2014); Homayouni *et al.* (2013).

influence on glucose and lipid metabolism (Nugent 2005). Dietary fiber, as well as RS with low calorific value, brings numerous health advantages such as lowering blood glucose and cholesterol, and improving laxation.

Several physiological effects of RS and the health benefits that have been proven are listed in Table 16.4. The physiological characteristics, and hence the potential health benefits, of RS can vary broadly based on the project conditions and variations in the sources, types and dose of RS ingested (Nugent 2005).

RS consumption can prevent obesity because it has lower energy intake due to its low-calorie value, causing the feeling of fullness and hence lessening the desire to eat. RS can decrease the duration of rotavirus diarrhea by enhancing the action of probiotics. Other impacts of RS intake are avoiding constipation, improving excretion frequency and fecal bulk, reducing production of mutagenic compounds and decreasing pH and ammonia levels in the colon (Homayouni *et al.* 2013). Production of SCFAs in the large bowel that causes enhanced absorption of calcium and magnesium is another effect of RS.

Some studies have discovered a positive impact of RS intake on development of colorectal cancer. Colonic microbiota, especially *Bifidobacterium bifidum* sp., ferment RS into SCFAs. The presence of acetic, propionic and butyric acids leads to reduced environmental pH, thereby inhibiting the proliferation of carcinomatous cells (Khoozani *et al.* 2019). Similarly, the production of SCFAs (acetic, propionic and butyric acid) through RS fermentation triggered by anaerobic bacteria can lower the lumen pH, creating an environment less vulnerable to the formation of cancerous tumors (Khalili and Amini 2014). Generally speaking, the indirect effects of RS intake are predominantly due to the activity of probiotic microbiota (Khoozani *et al.* 2019).

16.5.1 Hypoglycemic Effects

Different factors, namely the native environment of the starch granule, the amylose/amylopectin ratio, gelatinization of starch, moisture content and heating temperature of the processed foods, might influence the GI of starchy foods. Thus, the factors determining the GI values are in agreement with those influencing formation of RS. Using glucose as a reference, GI was found to vary from 10 for starch in legumes to close to 100 in particular potato, breakfast cereal and rice commodities. Therefore, RS could decrease the extent of digestion of food that contains them. The characteristic of slow digestion of RS results in its application in controlled glucose release (Sajilata *et al.* 2006), and thus lessened insulin response and greater possibilities to utilize stored fat (Nugent 2005). This is obviously vital for people with diabetes and has led to main developments in dietary guidance for such patients (Fuentes-Zaragoza *et al.* 2010; Tabibloghmany and Ehsandoost 2014).

Hypoglycemia occurs as an accompanying disorder in patients with diabetes mellitus and possibly in other illnesses. Foods loaded with RS have a slow metabolism speed. This RS characteristic is crucial in type 2 diabetes because of its deliberate glucose release rate and metabolism duration. The starch's durability to digestive enzymes, namely isoamylase, α-amylase and pullulanase, is the reason for lessened postprandial blood glucose and insulin response. With RS, diets containing high SDS are also good for improving the health of diabetics, and even people without diabetes. Entire grains rich in dietary fibers are a valid representation of low GI food, as the glucose is released at a slow rate. The method of processing can decrease starch digestibility and improve the RS and SDS value in cereal grains, promoting the nutritional significance of cereal grains (Raigond *et al.* 2017).

Digestion of RS occurs 5–7 h after intake, as opposed to regularly processed starch which is digested immediately. Digestion time over 5–7 h causes a decrease of postprandial insulinemia and glycemia and extends the feeling of fullness, thus reducing exaggerated appetite. Based on a clinical study employing a commercial RS3 product, the peak of blood glucose level was observed to be significantly less than that of other carbohydrate samples, namely simple sugars, oligosaccharides and regular starch. Positive impacts were usually detected immediately (in the first 2–8 h) after intake. RS could be an alternative to diabetes prevention by lessening the postprandial insulin response, increasing insulin responsiveness, decreasing postprandial glucose response, and suspending insulin resistance development (Homayouni *et al.* 2013). A bar containing RS3 reduced postprandial blood glucose and offers enhanced metabolic control in type 2 diabetes (Sajilata *et al.* 2006). RS must be consumed as at least 14% of the total starch in the diet to bring any positive impact to glycemic or insulinemic responses (Nugent 2005).

In addition, an investigation to produce different glucose responses in RS4 (chemically modified starches) was conducted. The impact of two test diets comprising β-cyclodextrin-enriched potato starch (2–3%) and 1–2% acetylated potato starch was tested in humans. The former was observed to lower blood glucose levels. This might be due to the distal absorption of β-cyclodextrin in the intestines or prolonged gastric emptying (Sharma *et al.* 2008).

16.5.2 Hypocholesterolemic Effects

Hypocholesterolemic impacts of RS have been extensively proven. The increase in cecal size and the cecal pool of SCFAs in rats treated with RS-containing diets (25% raw potato) was notable along with SCFA absorption and decreased triglyceride and plasma cholesterol levels. There were also decreased cholesterol concentrations in every lipoprotein fraction, notably HDL1, and reduced triglyceride (TG) concentrations in TG-rich lipoprotein fractions (Sajilata *et al.* 2006). From studies in rodents, reductions in a variety of lipid metabolism measures were recognized, and RS appeared to have a particular effect on lipid metabolism, comprising total lipids, total cholesterol, very low density lipoproteins (VLDL), low density lipoproteins (LDL), intermediate density lipoproteins (IDL), high density lipoproteins (HDL), TGs and TG-rich lipoproteins (Nugent 2005).

Starches derived from beans decreased serum total cholesterol and VLDL, IDL and LDL cholesterol, and improved the cecal concentration of SCFAs (particularly butyric acid) and the excretion of fecal neutral sterol. Diets comprising cassava starch extruded with 9.9% oat fiber or cassava starch extruded with 9.7% RS were fed to hamsters and both showed hypocholesterolemic effects, implying their potential incorporation in foods to promote cardiovascular health. According to several studies, RS intake might reduce serum cholesterol levels in rodents fed with a cholesterol-free diet (Fuentes-Zaragoza *et al.* 2010).

Several previous clinical researches suggested that RS effectively lowered plasma triglyceride and cholesterol levels. However, some studies have recorded contrasting results regarding the effect of RS on total human cholesterol, therefore, further investigations are needed to obtain a better understanding of the effect of RS on human cholesterol metabolism (Ashwar *et al.* 2016; Fuentes-Zaragoza *et al.* 2010; Nugent 2005).

16.5.3 Prevention of Colon Cancer

Fermentation by the colonic microbiota may be the reason for most health effects of RS. The production of SCFAs by probiotics provides protection against susceptibility to cancerous tumor growth (Fuentes-Zaragoza *et al.* 2011). There is an indication that butyrate may lessen the chance of cancerous transformation in cells. Studies in cecum of rodents treated with RS diets have shown increased fecal bulking and decreased fecal pH, along with increased SCFA production. All of these are correlated with a reduced occurrence of colon cancer. It has been inferred that the effect was due to ingestion of soluble dietary fiber (Sharma *et al.* 2008; Tharanathan 2002). An *in vitro* study using human fecal inocula demonstrated that dietary fiber and RS were fermented in the large bowel, yielding a large amount of butyric acid or salts (Sajilata *et al.* 2006). Butyrate is one of the dominant energy sources for large intestine epithelial cells and hinders the harmful alteration of those cells *in vitro*. Therefore, easily fermentable RS fractions in particular are exceptional in colon cancer prevention. Several studies have mentioned that butyrates potentially had an inhibitory influence on the growth and proliferation of tumor cells *in vitro* by arresting one of the cell cycle (G1) phases (Sharma *et al.* 2008). Earlier studies on the impact of RS on the colonic setting and genotoxic-induced apoptosis (controlled cell death) had exhibited that intake of RS2 from high-amylose maize (HAM) triggered increased levels of cell apoptosis in an animal model that was treated with azoxymethane. Giving an RS2-rich diet to the rodents improved apoptosis by approximately 30% (Ashwar *et al.* 2016).

Combining RS with an insoluble dietary fiber, for example wheat bran, results in significantly higher SCFA levels, especially butyrate, which was detected in the feces. When RS was blended with a soluble fiber, namely psyllium (*Plantago ovata*), the site of RS fermentation was shifted more distally in rat intestines. Most tumors grow in the distal colon, so it may be of additional advantage for cancer prevention if fermentation of RS occurred at that site (Fuentes-Zaragoza *et al.* 2010).

Recently, inhibition of colonic aberrant crypt foci (ACF) formation was observed in RS dose-dependently, only when the starch was present during the development phase to a genotoxic carcinogen in the middle and distal colon, indicating that treatment with RS may delay growth and/or the progress of neoplastic lesions in the colon. Hence, colon tumorigenesis may be highly treatable with dietary management. Adult patients who have colonic preneoplastic lesions might be helped by consumption of dietary RS. This hints at the suitability of RS as a preventive agent for persons vulnerable to developing colon cancer (Fuentes-Zaragoza *et al.* 2010).

16.5.4 Prebiotic Effect

RS performs partly as a prebiotic and partly as a synbiotic agent. A prebiotic is defined as a non-digestible food component that positively influences the host by selectively promoting the growth and/or the actions of probiotics in the gastrointestinal tract. RS passes almost entirely undigested through the small intestine and can therefore act as a substrate for the growth and viability of probiotic organisms. The viability of probiotic microorganisms in the colon can be sustained by RS ingestion. RS functions by shielding some of the ingested microorganisms on their way to the colon and amplifying the initial levels of probiotic bacteria as soon as they reach the colon. Examples of ordinary prebiotics are inulin and oligofructose that are available naturally in several fruits and vegetables, namely chicory, Jerusalem artichokes, leeks, onions, garlic, wheat and bananas. Recently, the prebiotic attributes of RS have been extensively investigated. RS enhanced the proliferation of bifidobacteria in the gastrointestinal tract of experimental rodents, stimulated the growth of *Lactobacillus*, and improved the endurance of bifidobacteria in a solution containing acidic buffer or bile acid. A diet rich in RS significantly improved the populations of lactobacilli, streptococci and bifidobacteria, reduced the numbers of enterobacteria, and restored the colon's microbial enzyme metabolism in rats (Ashwar *et al.* 2016; Fuentes-Zaragoza *et al.* 2010; Tabibloghmany and Ehsandoost 2014).

Several laboratory studies on pigs and humans have discovered a time-dependent transformation in SCFA profiles of the fecal and large bowel, implying potential synergy of RS with the ingested microorganisms. Compared with all other dietary fibers, RS offers a high portion of butyrate production and hence is very valuable for human health. Being a source of butyrate in the colon, RS counters the risk of developing colorectal cancer. Butyrate functions as a substrate for epithelial cells and hinders mutagenesis of these cells *in vitro*. The rate of RS fermentation defines the location of SCFA production in the colon. RS can also be advantageous for adults with colonic lesions. In general, RS has the capability to reduce the possibility of several food-related disorders and develop human well-being (Raigond *et al.* 2017).

16.5.5 Preventing Obesity

In line with the function of preventing obesity, a role for RS has also been reported for weight reduction or fat accumulation. Overconsumption of calories leads to the widespread occurrence of obesity, and innovative approaches are necessary to lessen calorie consumption. One prospective dietary recommendation is to improve the intake of DF, which has been correlated with prolonged satiety and reduction of body mass index (BMI). DF is defined as a varied carbohydrate group varying widely in its physical and chemical attributes. As a result, a similar influence on satiety or body weight might not be found in all fiber sources. RS offers several of the advantages of dietary fiber; thus, it may potentially help with weight management, although sufficient proof has not been gathered. Some evidence from animal studies recommends that substituting rapidly digestible starch (RDS) with RS decreases body weight. In diet-induced obese rats, a diet high in RS lowered body weight by 40%. However, the diet comprised 23.4% RS, which may not be feasible in human diets. Another study treating rats with a diet including 4%, 8%, or 16% RS observed that applying a diet with more than 8% RS decreased adiposity compared to the control with 0%. Furthermore, for every 4% increase in RS, energy consumption was diminished by 9.8 kJ/day. This calls for long-term investigations on the impact of increasing RS intake on body weight in humans (Birt *et al.* 2013).

Despite the shortage of long-term investigations, there are many arguments to consider utilizing RS in weight management. First, because RS contains fewer calories, substituting RDS with RS lowers the diet's calorie density. Several investigations have noticed that lowering the diet's calorie density improves satiety and weight loss. Second, including RS in a meal might enhance feelings of fullness. Even though fiber consumption has been correlated with improved satiety, the influence of RS on satiety is ambiguous. In a clinical study, consuming bread loaded with RS triggered greater satiety approximately 70 and 120 min after consumption, in contrast to white bread (Tabibloghmany and Ehsandoost 2014). The few investigations conducted in humans have exhibited confusing contrasts. Third, RS may affect body weight by raising the energy expenditure of fat oxidation. Changing RDS for RS may stimulate fat mobilization as a consequence of a decrease in insulin secretion. However, at present there is little proof to back up this hypothesis, and some studies have been unable to demonstrate that RS enhances energy consumption or fat burning (Birt *et al.* 2013). Another report demonstrated that by replacing 5.4% of the total dietary carbohydrates with RS, postprandial lipid oxidation was markedly increased, demonstrating a function of RS in reducing fat buildup in the long term (Sajilata *et al.* 2006). It was suggested that consuming an RS-rich diet considerably improved the mobilization and utilization of stored fat because of lower insulin secretion. Decreased levels of body fat and the building of lean body mass have been demonstrated in consumption of HAM RS2. Noticeable shifts in the body fat arrangement happened more specifically, with decreased epididymal and retroperitoneal fat with an RS-rich diet. SCFAs, namely acetic, propionic and butyric acids, are recorded to hinder adipose tissue lipolysis. In the liver, acetate was suggested to hinder glycogenolysis, with the effects of sparing carbohydrates and improving fat burning (Ashwar *et al.* 2016).

16.5.6 Reduction of Gallstone Formation

Resistant starch has been reported to prevent gallstone formation (Ashwar *et al.* 2016). Digestible starch plays a role in gallstone formation via greater secretion of insulin, leading to cholesterol synthesis and eventually to gallstone formation. RS is observed to lower the occurrence of gallstones. The incidence of gallstone formation is lower in Southern India, where people consume whole grains, as compared to Northern India where flour is consumed. This is because the starch digestibility in rice and wheat is increased by milling to flour. Notably, RS dietary consumption is two- to four-fold less in the United States, Australia and Europe as compared to countries consuming high-starch diets, namely China and India. This might be reflected in the lower number of gallstone cases in the latter countries (Raigond *et al.* 2017; Sajilata *et al.* 2006; Tabibloghmany and Ehsandoost 2014).

16.5.7 Mineral Absorption

Several studies demonstrated that RS could positively affect the intestinal absorption of minerals in humans and animals. Rats fed with an RS-rich diet exhibited improved ileal absorption of minerals, namely calcium, zinc, magnesium, iron and copper. RS improved the absorption of calcium; however, absorption of other minerals was not altered in humans. A study on the apparent absorption of minerals such as calcium, iron, phosphorus and zinc along with RS and digestible starches showed that an RS-loaded diet essentially improved the apparent absorption of iron and calcium, in contrast to the fully digestible starch (Ashwar *et al.* 2016). RS might therefore have a beneficial influence on the absorption of intestinal iron and calcium (Sajilata *et al.* 2006). Increased magnesium and calcium absorption was reported in rats; the absorption mechanism was through increased mineral solubility in the cecum and/or large intestine. Treating rats with a raw potato starch diet improved starch fermentation in the distal part of the digestive tract, leading to enhanced absorption of zinc, calcium, magnesium and copper due to cecal acidification and hypertrophy of the cecal wall (Raigond *et al.* 2017). For a fair understanding of the health impact of RS, it is essential to know that the intake of large volumes of RS may result in undesirable effects on gastrointestinal function. These undesirable effects involve borborygmi (sound of intestinal gas movement), bloating, colic, flatulence and more watery feces. Overall, the advantages of RS intake outweigh any gastrointestinal unease (Tabibloghmany and Ehsandoost 2014).

16.6 Future Applications

There is considerable interest in RS for its implied health advantages and functional characteristics. In contrast to traditional fiber, RS has the upper hand with its bland flavor and fine particles that make combining several food commodities possible with good consumer acceptance and better palatability. RS has fiber-like characteristics and performs positive physiological functions in humans, which may protect us from developing some diseases. Foods with high RS levels result in lower calories and lower glycemic loads, which are important considerations for the weight-conscious and diabetics. A varied range of uses having nutraceutical impacts was made feasible through several commercially available RS formulations (Rai *et al.* 2019).

Aside from the inherent health benefits, another positive advantage of RS is its minimal influence on the organoleptic characteristics of food, in comparison with conventional sources of fiber, namely fruits, whole grains or bran. The excellent physicochemical characteristics of RS, namely viscosity, gel formation, swelling capacity and excellent water-binding capability, make it beneficial in various meal products (Ashwar et al. 2016; Fuentes-Zaragoza *et al.* 2010).

As opposed to conventional DF, RS displays enhanced eating qualities, such as developing crispiness, decreasing oil absorption in fried foods, and even acting as a component in the microencapsulation of probiotics. The unusual features of RS, such as its natural sources, white color, fine particle size, bland taste, decreased water-holding capacity (WHC) and excellent water-binding capacity (WBC) compared to conventional fibers, good extrusion qualities (GEQ) and high gelatinization temperature (HGT), recommend it as an important ingredient in varied types of functional foods. RS is available in the form of water-soluble or water-insoluble starches. This attribute profoundly affects the possible applications in food preparation (Homayouni *et al.* 2013).

It was considered that processing conditions such as temperature, moisture, pH, pressure, autoclaving, freezing, and storage conditions might influence the formation of some types of RS, particularly RS3. However RS3 endured heating, even during frying, so its presence improved the total DF in fried battered products. In the frying process, RS3 played a role as a shield against fat absorption and limited moisture loss. Based on its structural characteristics, amylose may possess higher WBC than natural starch. This attribute, combined with lower WHC in RS, tends to reduce water activity (a_W) and extend the shelf-life of products. In the freezing process of dairy products such as ice cream, lower a_W might hinder the formation of ice crystals and gritty texture.

An overview of the technological benefits of RS has been presented by Homayouni *et al.* (2013), as seen in Figure 16.1.

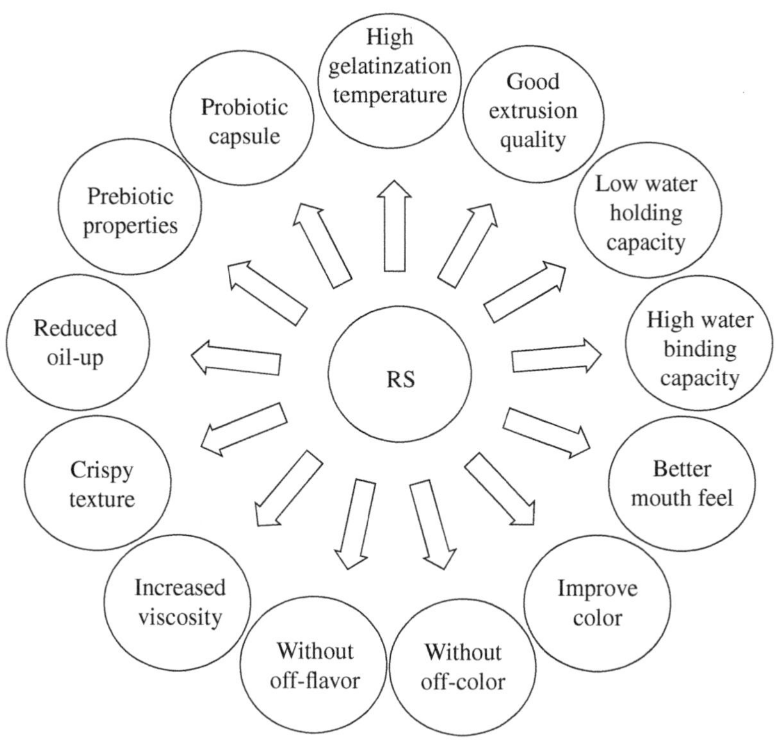

Figure 16.1 Functionality attributes of resistant starch (RS). *Source:* Data from Homayouni *et al.* (2013).

RS is specifically appropriate for industrial application in low and intermediate moisture foods based on grain as an insoluble product. The physical characteristics of RS, such as its low WHC, allow it to be a functional ingredient that offers excellent qualities in processing, such as crispness, expansion and refined texture of the finished product (Khalili and Amini 2014; Sajilata *et al.* 2006). Inclusion of RS as a fiber source in some bakery products, namely bread and breakfast cereals, is possible. The amount of RS used to substitute flour is determined by the starch being utilized, the intended product, the intended fiber content, and, in some cases, the desired structure–function requirements. From a quality viewpoint, some products are more susceptible to flour substitution than others. For instance, bread and rolls, which normally exhibit a bland taste, are low in fat and need the least amount of gluten for structure; the highest flour substitution is usually 10–20% without marked alteration of the texture (Sajilata *et al.* 2006). Some studies of applications of RS in several food products are described in the following sections.

16.6.1 Cheese

Several investigations regarding the possibility of producing a low-fat cheese comprising RS have been conducted. The cheese was supplemented with RS to enhance the health benefits, rather than to replace the more expensive casein (Li 2018).

Low-fat cheese products were introduced by the cheese industry in the 1990s. Mozzarella cheese is a common ingredient in pizza and usually comprises around 20–27% of fat. One experimental study demonstrated that the addition of Novelose® 330 (RS3) or Novelose® 240 (RS2) in mozzarella lowered the fat content up to 50%, with acceptable functional properties. The hardness of the cheese was proportionally enhanced with higher RS addition. RS3 was reported to be more effective than RS2. With increasing addition of RS2, the product's cohesiveness was proportionally enhanced; however, a similar phenomenon was not observed in RS3. It was possible to replace dry matter with RS up to 43.2% in cheeses with 52–60% moisture content while keeping the intended functional attribute. The addition of RS exhibited a homogeneous and smooth texture without obvious moisture loss. A type of RS2, known as Hi-Maize® 240, was also applied to increase crispness in simulated heated expanded cheese. A functional cheese was successfully produced with the fat content substituted with 15.3% Hi-Maize® 240 (Homayouni *et al.* 2013; Li 2018).

RS was claimed to physically entrap H_2O molecules inside the cheese matrix. The functional properties, water activity (a_w), and moisture sorption changes in artificial cheese supplemented with RS2 have been investigated. The moisture of cheese remained stable (58%), while the RS2 content increased from 8.9 to 18.2%. With the raised level of RS2, cohesiveness and hardness exhibited no significant increase, excluding the 12.9% level. Changing starch content from 8.9 to 12.9% led to the decrease of a_w from 0.986 to 0.978, although higher RS content had no notable effect on a_w. Lastly, the increase in RS2 concentration did not affect the sorption behavior of artificial cheese. In conclusion, RS2 of 18% did not affect the cheese texture and overall acceptability while having health benefits for customers (Khalili and Amini 2014).

16.6.2 Pasta Products

During extrusion cooking of dried pasta fortified with 15% RS, slight and almost no effect on dough handling and rheology were perceived (Li 2018). RS2 improved the attributes of the finished product in pasta formulation. Pasta supplemented with RS4 had increased textural properties; however, pasta enriched with 5% bran certainly had altered cooking attributes, while supplementation with RS2 up to 10% had no undesirable effect. Raising the pasta's RS2 content caused a notable reduction in yellow color and minimal shift in the redness, with no observable effect in the brightness. The color of pasta substituted with 50% of RS2 appeared lighter than all the other formulated pasta products. No effect on sensory attributes was observed in pasta with RS supplementation up to 20%, for instance firmness, slipperiness, rubberiness, chewiness, and floury mouth feel, in contrast to the regular pasta. Furthermore, the substitution of 20% RS2 reduced *in vitro* digestibility. The characteristics of pasta dough enriched with RS2 and RS3 (in the concentration of 10% and 20% substitution with semolina) have been studied. The result showed that the more RS was supplemented, the weaker the dough would become. This might be explained by RS competition with the semolina for hydration and its low WHC. Considering these phenomena, the appearance of a functional pasta would be one of the most important variables for good sales of the products (Homayouni *et al.* 2013; Khalili and Amini 2014).

16.6.3 Battered Fried Products

RS3 is more stable at high temperatures than the other RS types. Considering that color is one of the important characteristics of fried battered foods representing the optimum time to monitor frying, this product's desired color is light golden brown. The higher RS3 concentration led to a notable improvement in the desired color. The principal mechanisms for the desired color were caramelization and the Maillard reaction. The sensory evaluation of battered fried products substituted with 20% RS exhibited a notable increase in the batter crust's hardness and fragility. Consumer acceptance scores on color, flavor, crispiness, oiliness and overall acceptability were no less than 5, indicating that all the formulations (10% RS3, 20% RS3, no-RS3 added) were satisfactory. In another report by Sanz *et al.* (2008), a comparison of substitution by RS2 (Hi-Maize® 260) and RS3 (Novelose® 330) in a fried battered food on rheological properties and consumer acceptability of the batter was accomplished. The report revealed that RS3 established a darkened color than both control and RS2. The test panel gave RS2 the highest scores on acceptability compared to RS3 and the control. Thus, adding RS3 may enhance the color and nutritional values of the final products (Homayouni *et al.* 2013).

16.6.4 Bakery Products

Dietary fiber is frequently supplemented in bread, but high-fiber bread would possess some undesirable characteristics, namely decreased loaf volume, poor mouth feel, darkened color and reduced flavor. These undesirable characteristics might hinder RS application. An investigation into the effect of several fiber sources, such as wheat fiber, oat fiber, cellulose, two commercially available RS with 23% (Hylon® VII) and 40% DF (Novelose® 260) and a mixture of oat fiber with Novelose® 260 on bread attributes was conducted. The flour fortified with two RS sources had similar water absorption capacity to that of control, while notably high water absorption capacity was observed in flours added with wheat fiber, oat fiber and cellulose. Accordingly, the low water absorption capacity of RS exhibited a less undesirable influence on dough rheology and resembled the control dough. Bread fortification with 40% RS demonstrated larger loaf size and better cell arrangement in comparison to conventional fibers (Ashwar *et al.* 2016).

The incorporation of RS3 and RS2 increased the bread firmness by 10 and 20% after 7 days of storage, respectively. Furthermore, RS content improved markedly with the supplementation with both types of RS. The outcomes exhibited that after up to 4 days of storage in ambient, refrigeration and freezing temperatures, the crumb and whole bread's RS content increased and later declined. The reduction in RS might have been due to a reverse in retrogradation of amylopectin, change of amylopectin crystals or starch unavailability. This resulted from the formation of starch–lipid complexes or starch–protein, which could be attributed to the development of RS5. The enrichment of bread with RS may result in functional bread formulation with health benefits for customers (Homayouni *et al.* 2013; Khalili and Amini 2014).

16.6.5 Baked Goods

Resistant starch is included in many forms of baked goods, namely in batter systems in cakes, brownies or muffins. Trials exhibited that RS functions as a texture modifier, imparting desirable tenderness or crispness characteristics to the crumb (Sajilata *et al.* 2006). RS3 was applied as a replacer of low-calorie flour in bakehouse goods, in which it showed baking attributes such as golden-brown color, surface cracking, cookie spread and delightful aroma similar to those obtained with control wheat flour (Ashwar *et al.* 2016).

The quality of sponge cakes was improved by substituting 30% of flour with RS3 and RS4, while for obtaining yellow layer cake, the substitution level reached up to 12.5%. Loaf cakes substituted with 40% TDF evaluated 24 h after baking by a sensory panel test showed the best results in tenderness, flavor, moisture perception and grittiness. Short dough biscuits made by substituting a portion of wheat flour with RS-loaded ingredients exhibited improvement in breaking strength and crumbliness. Fortification level of 20–40% RS content did not decrease the initial perception of consumers towards biscuits organoleptically. The report showed that RS could be utilized for the improvement of fiber-rich biscuits without influencing their overall characteristics (Ashwar *et al.* 2016).

A type III enzyme-RS with a melting point of at least 140 °C can be utilized as a flour replacer in low-calorie baked goods. The final product showed baking properties (cookie spread, golden brown color, surface cracking, delightful aroma) equal to those obtained utilizing regular wheat flour (Li 2018; Sajilata *et al.* 2006).

16.6.6 Microencapsulation of Probiotics

Sultana *et al.* (2000) studied the survival of probiotics encapsulated by alginate–starch gel in yoghurt during storage at 4 °C over a period of 8 weeks. They reported that adding 2% RS2 (Hi-Maize® 260) to the alginate mix revealed an improvement in *Lactobacillus casei* population from 4×10^8 to 3.1×10^{11} CFU/g. However, the addition of 4% RS2 did not increase the efficiency of encapsulation. In 8 weeks of storage, a one log decrease was shown in strains of both *Lactobacillus acidophilus* and *Bifidobacterium infantis* when kept as free cultures, while encapsulated cells presented a 0.5 log decline. This demonstrated the beneficial function of RS2 (Sultana *et al.* 2000). Similar outcomes were exhibited in the observation of *Bifidobacterium animalis* and *Lactobacillus rhamnosus* viability (Ziar *et al.* 2012). There were no significant changes in bacterial number observed after 4 weeks of yoghurt refrigeration. In addition, in simulated gastrointestinal conditions, the viability of encapsulated cells was markedly greater than that of free cells. Furthermore, in a *Bifidobacterium animalis* microencapsulated sample, pH values did not alter significantly from day 1 to 28; on the contrary, in yoghurt with encapsulated *Lactobacillus rhamnosus*, a notable reduction in pH was attained from day 7 (Ziar *et al.* 2012).

Homayouni *et al.* (2008) investigated the viability of *Lactobacillus casei* and *Bifidobacterium lactis* during ice cream storage at −20 °C for 180 days. The study observed that microencapsulation of the probiotics with a mixture of 2% starch–calcium alginate was notably improved at the level of 30%, compared to the control. Additionally, the assessment of texture, color and taste revealed that adding encapsulated probiotics did not affect the sensory characteristics of non-fermented synbiotic ice cream (Homayouni *et al.* 2008). Thus, microencapsulation is the best prebiotic–probiotic symbiosis model. Encapsulation is frequently defined as a means to protect probiotics against unfavorable environmental conditions (Khalili and Amini 2014). RS has also been applied with other substances to enhance viability of encapsulated bacteria in yoghurt, ice cream and cheese. Certainly, the use of type 2 RS has offered solutions to several technological difficulties, such as thermal stabilization, controlled release of bioactive components, and prolonged shelf-life of delicate substances (Homayouni *et al.* 2013).

It is beneficial to begin with a native starch with high amylose content in RS commercial development. Almost all patented practices are determined by the tendency of high-amylose starch to retrograde, or develop highly crystalline areas, resistant to enzymatic hydrolysis. High-amylose maize starches require high gelatinization temperatures, needing temperatures that are usually not attained in the traditional cooking process (154–171°C) before the granules are entirely broken down. These starches offer a chance to modify RS content in the final products (Sajilata *et al.* 2006). However, the RS naturally existing in food varieties may lose its endurance to digestion during the processing step, namely boiling. Therefore, the use of commercially produced RS that can resist processing conditions to a certain degree would allow products to be designed with an improved degree of TDF.

Three kinds of RS (RS1, RS2 and RS3) are commercially obtainable as ingredients to be incorporated in processed foods.

1) Raw high-amylose starches (mostly from maize): Hylon® VII and Novelose® 240.
2) Retrograded high-amylose starches (mostly from maize): Novelose® 330.
3) Retrograded maltodextrins (from high-amylose starch for CrystaLean®, or tapioca starch for C*Actistar).

In 1993, Hi-Maize® was the first commercial RS launched in Australia. This product is a completely native granular form of starch originally comprising higher than 80% amylose and 42% RS. Since then, it has been developed to provide a TDF of approximately 60%. It is classified as RS and utilized in numerous products such as biscuits, nutrition bars, dairy products, bread and other bakery goods (Sajilata *et al.* 2006). Other commercial sources of RS, for example Novelose® 240 and Novelose® 260 (thermally modified RS 2), Novelose® 330 (RS 3, National Starch and Chemicals Co., Bridgewater, New Jersey, USA), CrystaLean® (retrograded RS Opta Food ingredients, Inc., Bedford, Massachusetts, USA), C*Actistar (Cerestar Food and Pharma specialties), Nutriose FB (Roquette, Freres, France), and Amylomaize VII (Cerestar Inc., Hammond, Indiana, USA) are now available to improve the TDF content in the product and offer other functional attributes (Sajilata *et al.* 2006).

As opposed to common sources of RS (potatoes, legumes, bananas), commercially produced types are more appropriate under several conditions of processing and storage. The amount of RS2 in green bananas reduces as the fruit ripens, whereas Hi-Maize® (RS2) does not experience these problems. Amongst the most valuable advancements in RS is Novelose®. This starch is available in different TDF levels. The newest product, Novelose® 260, contains a TDF of 60%, allowing food producers to offer products with a "source of high fiber" or "rich in fiber" label. The introduction of Novelose® 260 marks a start in developing physiologically functional ingredients, presenting fiber in daily foods without disturbing a pleasurable eating experience. Unlike other sources of fibers, namely rice, oat or wheat bran, Novelose® with a particle size of approximately 10–15 μm has a neutral flavor and white color, facilitating its inclusion in a diversity of food products without changing their color or flavor. It also continues to be resistant after moderate food processing. A fiber source like wheat bran also includes oil and fat, which can experience rancidity, so some components utilized to improve fiber content have a limited shelf-life due to the appearance of an "off taste" (Sharma *et al.* 2008).

The functional properties of RS and its possible physiological advantages offer the prospect of improving the diet's DF content through conventional foods. Nevertheless, processing steps, particularly those involving heat, may reduce the RS content of both naturally containing RS and RS-enriched products. In this regard, researchers have begun to seek methods to improve the amount of RS or make it more resistant against processing conditions (Khoozani *et al.* 2019). Several procedures have been introduced to provide RS-rich products, such as hydrothermal treatments and annealing, partial gelatinization and recrystallization, autoclaving, temperature-cycled retrogradation, pullulanase debranching, acetylation and oxidation, phosphorylation and hydroxypropylation, and citric acid modification (Ashwar *et al.* 2016).

16.7 Production of RS-rich Ingredients

Khoozani *et al.* (2019) reported three main methods to provide RS-rich powdered ingredients, physical, chemical and enzymatic, as described as follows.

1) *Physical procedures*. The major physical method is through recurring heating-cooling cycles, which leads to the rearrangement of linear chains of starch into a different form that endures hydrolysis by digestive enzymes (Raungrusmee and Anal 2019). Disaggregation and fracture of amylose and amylopectin happen when a dispersion of high-amylose starch undergoes heating, eventually causing the occurrence of shorter

linear chains. For the subsequent process, cooling down the chains leads to the development of denser double-helical aggregates that are more resistant to hydrolysis. The RS resulting from this method is more resistant to heating and can be utilized for food product fortification as functional ingredients (Khoozani *et al.* 2019).

2) *Chemical procedures.* The alteration of starch granules induced by chemical methods can be carried out by acetylation, esterification, oxidation, lintnerization, hydroxypropylation, phosphorylation or combinations of these techniques. In these methods, the chemicals hinder the enzymes from binding starch correctly. For example, free hydroxyl groups available on the starch's glucose units can be esterified with acetyl groups, acetic anhydride commonly being used. In the oxidation process, certain reagents, namely hydrogen peroxide, oxygen, sodium hypochlorite, periodate and ozone, are commonly used, resulting in carbonyl and carboxylic groups that hinder the starch digestive enzymes. For hydroxypropylation, propylene oxide is widely employed in high alkaline conditions. In this way, the esterified propylene is employed to free hydroxy groups from the starch structure, producing a bulky structure which cannot be digested by digestive enzymes. Lintnerization is described as the process of treating starch with mineral acid, mainly with hydrochloric acid. Disrupting amorphous parts of starch and acid treatment results in a higher fraction of crystalline portion, which is more difficult for enzymes to access (Khoozani *et al.* 2019).
3) *Enzymatic procedures.* Focusing on debranching the α-1-6 amylopectin bonds by pullulanase and isoamylase, enzymatic procedures begin reordering the structure in the following retrogradation step. Other enzymes such as α- and β-amylase are utilized to hydrolyze amorphous parts of the starch and provide a firmly packed crystalline structure. Accordingly, debranching enzymes are employed to hydrolyze the amylopectin branch, giving a higher portion of linear parts. In this way, following retrogradation there is a higher amount of RS3 with double-helical structures stabilized by hydrogen bonds. However, some process parameters such as pH, temperature, time and pH of reaction need to be precisely regulated to achieve maximum enzyme performance (Khoozani *et al.* 2019).

To obtain optimal RS value, it is common to adjust processing conditions such as heating temperature and time, pH, heating and cooling cycles, freezing and drying. Therefore, the number of commercially ready RS products allows for an extensive range of purposes with functional impacts (Sajilata *et al.* 2006). Various techniques can also be introduced to result in specific RS characteristics (Setiarto *et al.* 2018).

Future improvements of RS have bestowed a huge opportunity, particularly for artificial starch derivatives with numerous alterations, even though the difficulty of obtaining legal approval for applying novel starch derivatives in food formulations is still debatable. Although previous reports have studied the effect of alterations on the physicochemical, structural and functional attributes of starches, comprehensive exploration and understanding of these starches' properties is necessary, which would assist their application in manufacturing food (Ashwar *et al.* 2016).

More efforts are necessary to produce RS that is stable to heat treatment through processing. Although various health advantages of consuming RS have been reported, additional studies are needed to develop RS products with favorable characteristics to provide specific health advantages, such as lowering the GI and improving blood health. Even though some figures have been suggested for specific health benefits, it is very difficult to recommend a figure for RS consumption for universal health benefit (Raigond *et al.* 2017). A study reported that RS intake has declined over the last few decades, probably because of the elevated consumption of low-fiber foods and fast foods. Observing this tendency, food experts have produced some RS- or dietary fiber-rich products that are readily obtainable. RS is considered fitting for fortification of ready-to-eat cereals, pasta, snacks, noodles, fried foods and baked foods. Those products can be branded directly as "starch conferring additional nutraceutical benefits" (Raigond *et al.* 2017).

16.8 Conclusion

Many foods enriched with fiber have been progressively improved to increase fiber in the dietary intake. Announced as a recently known source of fiber, resistant starch (RS) is categorized as a fiber constituent that is partially or completely fermented in the colon, providing numerous advantageous impacts on human health, and is an ideal DF with several nutritive benefits. RS potentially functions as a prebiotic, based on current and forthcoming investigations undertaken on the role of RS in influencing the gut microbiota. Its capability to result in large quantities of butyrate all along the colon is of distinct interest. As a functional fiber, the unique properties of RS, that is, fine particle size, bland flavor, high gelatinization temperature, good extrusion and film-forming qualities, and decreased water-holding characteristics, allow varied food formulation products, conceivably with upgraded sensory attributes. In contrast to conventional fiber-rich products, RS demonstrates increased crispness and expansion in some products, with better mouth feel, color and flavor than products prepared with conventional insoluble fibers.

Current knowledge demonstrates a big hurdle for plant breeders and food technologists to optimize the techno-functional characteristics of RS in foods. In various food items, positive outcomes were observed in RS applications, bringing hope for more healthy products with good texture. Possessing inherent physiological advantages, RS may have the capability to function as a nutritional ingredient to improve foods to be healthier and more appetizing. Another important topic needing to be approached is establishing standard measures to determine prebiotic properties via *in vitro* and/or *in vivo* evaluations, which is complicated by the variety of RS sources. Along with the increased demand for prebiotics, the development of RS could meet this challenge.

Practically, it is possible to enhance RS by using several physical, chemical and enzymatic modifications. However, the various techniques used to measure RS with notable variances in sample preparation, enzymes used, and the verification of experimental conditions that simulate the gastrointestinal environment could lead to ambiguity in RS determination. Therefore, some specific general method for RS measurement is needed. Furthermore, appropriately devised and controlled investigations to determine the effects of RS on human glucose and lipid glucose metabolism, over more extended time periods, are also needed. Therefore, the effect of RS consumption by humans still needs to be more deeply investigated to provide an accurate picture of its health benefits.

References

Anugrahati, N.A., Pranoto, Y., Marsono, Y. and Marseno, D.W. (2015). *In vitro* digestibility of Indonesian cooked rice treated with cooling-reheating process and coconut milk addition. *International Research Journal of Biological Sciences*, 4(12): 34–39.

Ashwar, B.A., Gani, A., Shah, A., Wani, I.A. and Masoodi, F.A. (2016). Preparation, health benefits and applications of resistant starch – a review. *Starch/Stärke*, 68(3-4): 287–301.

BeMiller, J.N. (2020). Resistant starch. In: *Science and Technology of Fibers in Food Systems* (ed. J. Welti-Chanes, S.O. Serna-Saldívar, O. Campanella and V. Tejada-Ortigoza), 153–183. Cham: Springer.

Bertoft, E. (2017). Understanding starch structure: recent progress. *Agronomy*, 7(3): 56.

Birt, D.F., Boylston, T., Hendrich, S., Jane, J.-L., Hollis, J., Li, L. et al. (2013). Resistant starch: Promise for improving human health. *Advances in Nutrition*, 4(6): 587–601.

Björck, I. (2006). Starch: Nutritional aspects. In: *Carbohydrate in Foods, Second Edition* (ed. A. Eliasson), 471–521. Boca Raton, FL: CRC Press.

Brown, I.L., Wang, X., Topping, D.L., Playne, M.J. and Conway P.L. (1998). High amylose maize starch as a versatile prebiotic for use with probiotic bacteria. *Food Australia*, 50(12): 603–610.

Carciofi, M., Blennow, A., Jensen, S.L., Shaik, S.S., Henriksen, A., Buléon, A. et al. (2012). Concerted suppression of all starch branching enzyme genes in barley produces amylose-only starch granules. *BMC Plant Biology*, 12: 223–238.

Chassard, C. and Lacroix, C., (2013). Carbohydrates and the human gut microbiota. *Current Opinion in Clinical Nutrition and Metabolic Care*, 16: 453–460.

Collona, P. and Mercier, C. (1985). Gelatinization and melting of maize and pea starches with normal and high-amylose. *Phytochemistry*, 24(8): 1667–1674.

Cummings, J.H. and Englyst, H.N. (1995). Gastrointestinal effects of food carbohydrate. *The American Journal of Clinical Nutrition*, 61(4): 938S–945S.

Davani-Davari, D., Negahdaripour, M., Karimzadeh, I., Seifan, M., Mohkam, M., Masoumi, S.J. et al. (2019). Prebiotics: Definition, types, sources, mechanisms, and clinical applications. *Foods*, 8(3): 92.

de Vrese, M. and Schrezenmeir, J. (2008). Probiotics, prebiotics, and synbiotics. *Advances in Biochemical Engineering/Biotechnology*, 111: 1-66.

Fuentes-Zaragoza, E., Riquelme-Navarrete, M.J., Sánchez-Zapata, E. and Pérez-Álvarez, J.A. (2010). Resistant starch as functional ingredient: A review. *Food Research International*, 43: 931–942.

Fuentes-Zaragoza, E., Sánchez-Zapata, E., Sendra, E., Sayas, E., Navarro, C., Fernández-López, J. and Pérez-Alvarez J.A. (2011). Resistant starch as prebiotic: A review. *Starch/Starke*, Volume 63: 406–415.

Gibson, G.R., Hutkins, R., Sanders, M.E., Prescott, S.L., Reimer, R.A., Salminen, S.J. and Reid, G. (2017). Expert consensus document: The International Scientific Association for Probiotics and Prebiotics (ISAPP) consensus statement on the definition and scope of prebiotics. *Nature Reviews Gastroenterology & Hepatology*, 14(8): 491–502.

Guarner, F. et al. (2011). *World Gastroenterology Organisation Global Guidelines-Probiotics and Prebiotics*. Milwaukee: World Gastroenterology Organisation.

Homayouni, A., Azizi, A., Ehsani, M.R., Yarmand, M.S. and Razavi, S.H. (2008). Effect of microencapsulation and resistant starch on the probiotic survival and sensory properties of synbiotic ice cream. *Food Chemistry*, 111(1): 50–55.

Homayouni, A., Amini, A., Keshtiban, A.K., Mortazavian, A.M., Esazadeh, K. and Pourmoradian, S. (2013). Resistant starch in food industry: A changing outlook for consumer and producer. *Starch/Stärke*, 65: 1–13.

Jackson, A.D. and Mclaughlin, J. (2009). Digestion and absorption. *Surgery (Oxford)*, 27(6): 231–236.

Jane, J.-L., Kasemsuwan, T., Leas, S., Zobel, H. and Robyt J.F. (1994). Anthology of starch granule morphology by scanning electron microscopy. *Starch/Starke*, 46: 121–129.

Khalili, L. and Amini, A. (2014). Resistant starch in food industry. In: *Polysaccharides: Bioactivity and Biotechnology* (ed. K.G. Ramawat and J. Mérillon), 663–673. Switzerland: Springer, Cham.

Khoozani, A.A., Birch, J. and Bekhit, A.E.-D. (2019). Resistant starch preparation methods. In: *Encyclopedia of Food Chemistry* (ed.L. Melton, F. Shahidi and P. Varelis), 390–394. New York: Elsevier.

Li, Z. (2018). Resistant starch and its applications. In: *Functional Starch and Applications in Food* (ed. Z. Jin), 63–90. Singapore: Springer.

Lilia-Baby, Suman, K.T., Krishnan, S. and Indira, V. (2015). Physiological effect of resistant starch. *International Journal of Current Research*, 7(12): 23529–23536.

Lockyer, S. and Nugent, A.P. (2017). Health effects of resistant starch. *Nutrition Bulletin*, 42(1): 10–41.

Macfarlane, G.T. and Englyst, H.N. (1986). Starch utilization by the human large intestinal microflora. *Journal of Applied Bacteriology*, 60: 195–201.

McCleary, B.V., DeVries, J.W., Rader, J.I., Cohen, G., Prosky, L., Mugford, D.C. et al. (2012). Determination of insoluble, soluble, and total dietary fiber (CODEX definition) by enzymatic-gravimetric method and liquid chromatography: collaborative study. *Journal of AOAC International*, 95(3): 824–844.

Nugent, A.P. (2005). Health properties of resistant starch. *British Nutrition Foundation, Nutrition Bulletin*, 30: 27–54.

Rahim, A., Haryadi, Cahyanto, M.N. and Pranoto, Y. (2012). Characteristics of butyrylated arenga starch prepared at different reaction time and butyric anhydride concentration. *International Food Research Journal*, 19(4): 1655–1660.

Rai, A.K., Singh, N., Rani, R. and Shingh, S. (2019). Resistant starch and its health benefits. *Trends in Biosciences*, 12(2): 905–908.

Raigond, P., Dutt, S. and Singh, B. (2017). Resistant starch in food. In: *Bioactive Molecules in Food* (ed. J. Mérillon and K.G. Ramawat), 1–33. New York: Elsevier, Cham.

Raungrusmee, S. and Anal, A.K. (2019). Effects of lintnerization, autoclaving, and freeze-thaw treatments on resistant starch formation and functional properties of Pathumthani 80 rice starch. *Foods*, 8: 558.

Raungrusmee, S., Shrestha, S., Sadiq, M.B. and Anal, A.K. (2020). Influence of resistant starch, xanthan gum, inulin and defatted rice bran on the physicochemical, functional and sensory properties of low glycemic gluten-free noodles. *LWT*, 126: 109279.

Sajilata, M.G., Singhal, R.S. and Kulkarni, P.R. (2006). Resistant starch – A review. *Comprehensive Reviews in Food Science and Food Safety*, 5(1): 1–17.

Sanz, T., Salvador, A. and Fiszman, S.M. (2008). Resistant starch (RS) in battered fried products: Functionality and high-fibre benefit. *Food Hydrocolloids*, 22: 543–549.

Setiarto, R.H., Jenie, B.S.L., Faridah, D.N., Saskiawan, I. and Sulistiani (2018). Effect of lactic acid bacteria fermentation and autoclaving-cooling for resistant starch and prebiotic properties of modified taro flour. *International Food Research Journal*, 25(4): 1691–1697.

Sharma, A., Yadav, S.B. and Ritika (2008). Resistant starch: Physiological roles and food applications. *Food Reviews International*, 24(2): 193–234.

Silvi, S., Rumney, C.J., Cresci, A. and Rowland, I.R. (1999). Resistant starch modifies gut microflora and microbial metabolism in human flora-associated rats inoculated with faeces from Italian and UK donors. *Journal of Applied Microbiology*, 86(3): 521–530.

Storey, D., Lee, A., Bornet, F. and Brouns, F. (2007). Gastrointestinal responses following acute and medium term intake of retrograded resistant maltodextrins, classified as type 3 resistant starch. *European Journal of Clinical Nutrition*, 61: 1262–1270.

Sullivan, W.R. (2020). Resistant starch. In: *Chemical Properties of Starch* (ed. M. Emeje), 1–10. London: IntechOpen.

Sultana, K., Godward, G., Reynolds, N., Arumugaswamy, R., Peiris, P. and Kailasapathy, K. (2000). Encapsulation of probiotic bacteria with alginate–starch and evaluation of survival in simulated gastrointestinal conditions and in yoghurt. *International Journal of Food Microbiology*, 62(1-2): 47–55.

Tabibloghmany, F.S. and Ehsandoost, E. (2014). Investigation of nutritional and functional properties of resistant starch in food industry: A review. *International Journal of Recent Research and Review*, VII(I): 27–44.

Taylor, J.R.N., Emmambux, N.N. and Kruger, J. (2015). Developments in modulating glycaemic response in starchy cereal foods. *Starch/Stärke*, 67: 79–89.

Terpou, A., Papadaki, A., Lappa, I.K., Kachrimanidou, V., Bosnea, L.A. and Kopsahelis, N. (2019). Probiotics in food systems: Significance and emerging strategies towards improved viability and delivery of enhanced beneficial value. *Nutrients*, 11(7): 1591.

Tharanathan, R.N., (2002). Food-derived carbohydrates — structural complexity and functional diversity. *Critical Reviews in Biotechnology*, 22(1): 65–84.

Wrolstad, R.E., (2012). Nutritional roles of carbohydrates. In: *Food Carbohydrate Chemistry* (ed. R.E. Wrolstad), 147–164. United Kingdom: Wiley-Blackwell.

Zaman, S.A. and Sarbini, S.R., (2016). The potential of resistant starch as a prebiotic. *Critical Reviews in Biotechnoogy*, 36(3): 578–584.

Ziar, H., Gerard, P. and Riazi, A. (2012). Calcium alginate-resistant starch mixed gel improved the survival of Bifidobacterium animalis subsp. lactis Bb12 and Lactobacillus rhamnosus LBRE-LSAS in yogurt and simulated gastrointestinal conditions. *International Journal of Food Science and Technology*, 47(7):1421–1429.

17

Gut Microbiome as Potential Source for Prevention of Metabolic-Related Diseases

Nuntarat Boonlao, Krisha Pant and Anil Kumar Anal

Food Engineering and Bioprocess Technology, Department of Food Agriculture and Bioresources, School of Environment and Resources, Asian Institute of Technology, Pathumthani, Thailand

17.1 Introduction

There has been a rapidly increasing incidence of obesity and related diseases such as type 2 diabetes mellitus (T2DM), cardiovascular disease and non-alcoholic fatty liver disease (NAFLD). The gut microbiome acts as a significant metabolic and endocrine organ contributing to disease development or targeted treatment (Skelly *et al.* 2019). The gut microbiome comprises bacteria, viruses, fungi and protozoa, with a total of 10^{14} or 100 trillion microbes present in the human gut (Warmbrunn *et al.* 2020). The human gut microbiome consists mainly of two phyla, Bacteroidetes and Firmicutes, while Actinobacteria, Proteobacteria and Verrucomicrobia are less common (Dannenberg *et al.* 2020). The gut microbiota performs several functions in the human body, including the breakdown of ingested food to provide nutrients, and particularly fermentation of complex polysaccharides to produce short chain fatty acids (SCFAs), which play a role in host metabolism (Rastelli *et al.* 2018). In addition, the types of diet have been known to strongly influence the composition of the gut microbiota. The diversity of the gut microbiome and the balance in its composition promote human health (Vallianou *et al.* 2019). Change in the variety and structure of the gut microbiome is referred to as dysbiosis, a phenomenon that affects metabolic activities, resulting in obesity and associated diseases (Faith *et al.* 2013). This chapter reviews the composition of the gut microbiome and the interaction between the gut microbiome and host metabolism regulation. The role of the gut microbiome on the incidence of related metabolic diseases is also represented. Furthermore, the modulation of the gut microbiome and possible mechanisms of action by the gut microbiome for targeted prevention of metabolic diseases are mentioned.

Probiotics, Prebiotics and Synbiotics: Technological Advancements Towards Safety and Industrial Applications, First Edition. Edited by Parmjit Singh Panesar and Anil Kumar Anal.

17.2 Gut Microbiome and Host Interaction

Although the hypothesis that 100 trillion bacteria inhabit the mammalian gut has been challenged, it is undeniable that hundreds to thousands of bacteria directly and indirectly impart functionality in the host (Huttenhower *et al.* 2012). The majority of the gut microbiome is anaerobic in nature which makes the bacteria difficult to culture in vitro and hence only 30% of the gut microbiome has been cultured till now. The main reason behind that has been suggested to be lack of information on the optimal conditions for the growth of these microbes (Fraher *et al.* 2012).

17.2.1 Microbial Composition and Colonization

The diversity of microorganisms in the gut is divided into three phyla: Bacteroidetes (e.g. *Porphyromonas*, *Prevotella*, etc.), Firmicutes (e.g. *Ruminococcus*, *Clostridium*, *Eubacteria*, etc.) and Actinobacteria (*Bifidobacterium*). Bacteroidetes and Firmicutes constitute up to 90% of the total microbial count (Eckburg *et al.* 2005). Also, *Lactobacillus*, *Streptococcus* and *Escherichia coli* (*E. coli*) are present in small numbers. Genomic analysis of these bacteria suggested that Bacteroidetes and Firmicutes phyla are the dominant microbes in the gastrointestinal tract. A great deal of research has been done on the effect of pathogenic microbes such as *Streptococcus pyogenes*, *Bordetella pertussis*, *Corynebacterium diphtheriae*, *Clostridium tetani*, *Salmonella typhimurium* and *Vibrio cholerae* in humans and their effects on the gastrointestinal tract. The effect of non-pathogenic microbes has also been studied to a certain extent.

The first contact with microorganisms like *Lactobacillus*, *Prevotella*, *Sneathia*, *Staphylococcus*, *Corynebacterium* and *Propionibacterium* spp., in humans takes place during birth through the oral and nasopharyngeal membrane as well as skin and gut which continues to build up communities in the stomach, especially during the first month of birth (Dominguez-Bello *et al.* 2010). The microbial colony grows competitively during the first year in the gut and then after that, during the second and third year, the microbes in the gut microbiome start to resemble those in the adult (Bokulich *et al.* 2016). This variation is largely dependent on the individual, through breast milk and solid food intake throughout the first years of life (Huttenhower *et al.* 2012). The development of the intestinal microbiome depends heavily on diet, breastfeeding often favoring bacterial diversity with *Lactobacillus*, *Staphylococcus*, *Megasphaera* and a class of Actinobacteria, vastly different from that of formula feeding where the growth of Clostridiales and phylum Proteobacteria can be observed. In addition to the diet pattern during infancy, application of antibiotics, host genetics, age, lifestyle, hygiene factors, allergen contact, diets, consumption of pro- or prebiotics, and infections have an impact (Sommer and Bäckhed 2013). These core microbes are similar in most individuals; differences often arise from the relative abundance and species composition (Wostmann *et al.* 1983).

After the inoculation of the microbes, the concentration of the bacteria increases throughout the length of the gastrointestinal tract, the stomach harboring only 10^1 bacteria per gram. The content increases throughout the duodenum (10^3/g), jejunum (10^4/g), ileum (10^7/g) and colon (10^{12}/g) (Sekirov *et al.* 2010). Aside from the gastrointestinal tract location, the microbiome's concentration also depends on the characteristics of the lumen and epithelium of the intestine itself. The ability of the microbiome to adhere to the intestinal surface depends on the attachment ability to the mucosa of the epithelium produced by goblet cells. Goblet cells produce specialized glycosylated proteins, also known as mucins, which primarily work as a barrier between the microbiome and epithelial cells and act as a carbon source for the attachable microbiome (Juge 2012). These mucins have an inner denser layer and an outer loosely adherent layer, the denser layer acting as a very efficient barrier against pathogenic microbes while allowing epithelial microbes to isolate and thrive in the outer layers such as *Clostridium*, *Lactobacillus* or *Enterococcus* (Juge 2012). In contrast to the selective presence of microbes due to mucin, a variety of microorganisms can be found in the feces, including *Bacteroides, Bifidobacterium, Streptococcus, Enterobacteriaceae, Enterococcus, Clostridium, Lactobacillus and Ruminococcus* (Sekirov *et al.* 2010). As an exception to the usual lack of attachment of pathogens, microorganisms such as *Helicobacter pylori, Clostridium jejuni* and noroviruses were found to adhere to the mucus.

17.2.2 Non-bacterial Growth in the Intestine

In addition to the bacterial colony formation in the intestine, growth of archaea, virome (bacteriophage, mammalian viruses and the endogenous retroviruses), unicellular eukaryotes, fungi and also multicellular helminthic worms can be observed. Although not as extensively studied as the bacteria, it has been predicted that they also have a functional role in maintaining the physiology of the body (Norman *et al.* 2015). As for the viruses, significant patterns may be observed in the case of inflammatory bowel diseases. The same applies for fungi, which constitutes only 0.2–0.3% of the total microbiota and mainly includes the genera *Aspergillus, Candida*, *Cryptococcus* and *Penicillium*, alterations in which can be observed in both inflammatory bowel diseases and irritable bowel diseases (Sokol *et al.* 2017). As for the bacteriophages, it has been observed that they are capable of affecting the survival, reproduction, composition and functionality of their bacterial hosts (Manrique *et al.* 2016).

17.2.3 Next Generation Probiotics

The traditional probiotics have a variable and extensive history of use. In addition, several other strictly anaerobic strains have been identified and characterized for their application in intestinal integrity and homeostasis (Lin *et al.* 2019) through the use of 16S ribosomal RNA (rRNA) gene and shotgun metagenomic sequencing (Chang *et al.* 2019). To overcome the traditional effects of bacteremia, which was observed in trials based on the administration of lactobacillus probiotics in patients in intensive care units (Yelin *et al.* 2019), next generation probiotics (NGP) have been explored to some extent for their use as drugs to target specific diseases (Abid and Koh 2019). The traditional probiotics target general intestinal health; in contrast, NGP have been developed to target specific diseases (Kaklamanos *et al.* 2019) as immunotherapeutic agents, specifically in cancer therapy and immune therapy (Langella *et al.* 2019). Some of the major NGP isolated from feces are *Faecalibacterium prausnitzii* (extremely oxygen sensitive) (Martín *et al.* 2017), *Prevotella copri* (improve prebiotic syndrome) (Li *et al.* 2010), *Christensenella minuta* (Lukiw 2016), *Parabacteroides goldsteinii* (relieves prediabetes syndrome and liver inflammation) (Gopalakrishnan *et al.* 2018), *Akkermansia muciniphila* (mucin-degrading microbe) (Everard *et al.* 2014), *Bacteroides fragilis* and *Bacteroides uniformis* (primary colonizers of the gut) (Wexler 2007), *Eubacterium hallii* (butyrate-producing anaerobe) (Engels *et al.* 2016), *Clostridium butyricum* (authorized novel food ingredient) (Shang *et al.* 2016), *Bacteroides xylanisolvens* (Sears 2005) and members of the clostridia clusters IV, XIVa and XVIII (El Hage *et al.* 2017). Further information on their effect and site of action is provided in Table 17.1. Another group of important group of NGP are fructophilic lactic acid bacteria (FLAB), named for their ability to metabolize fructose as opposed to glucose by lactic acid bacteria (LAB), a traditional probiotic. These FLAB are present in fructose-rich products such as wine, flower, fruits and cocoa beans, and also in the gastrointestinal tracts of the animals and insects (bees, giant ants, tropical fruit flies and bumblebees) that consume these products. *Fructobacillus fructosus*, *F. pseudoficulneus*, *F. ficulneus*, *F. durionis* and *F. tropaeoli* are the five major species of fructose-hydrolyzing bacteria (Endo *et al.* 2015).

Even though the complexity of the probiotics makes it difficult to understand the host–probiotic interaction, it has been understood that the probiotics play a functional role in the host's body (El Hage *et al.* 2017). Traditional probiotics help maintain gut health by regulating metabolic diseases, especially diseases related to leaky gut syndrome (Foster and Neufeld 2013). The NGP instigate the enhancing of a healthy epithelial layer, increasing the concentration of IgA and bile production, and finally increasing the production of antimicrobial peptides (Olveira and González-Molero 2016). Furthermore, due to the lack of specificity of the traditional probiotics in metabolic diseases, the importance of the NGP increases exponentially (Bottacini *et al.* 2017).

17.2.4 Host Cell and Microbes – Symbiotic Relationship

The microbes attach to the host cells through the mucin in the epithelium of the intestine. The host and the microbes have a symbiotic relationship, the host gaining metabolites, vitamins and protection against pathogens, and the microbes using complex polysaccharides also known as "microbiota accessible carbohydrates" (MAC) (Pistollato *et al.* 2016) as a carbon source for growth (Rajoka *et al.* 2017). This interaction is observed through various pathways; as observed in germ-free mice, the microbes increased the immunity in the intestine through Toll-like receptor (TLR) expression (Bäckhed *et al.* 2005), antigen-presenting cells, differentiated T cells, and lymphoid follicles (Belkaid and Hand 2014). In addition, systemic immunity was also found to be effected through increased splenic CD4+ T cells and systemic antibody expression (Noverr and Huffnagle 2004).

17.3 Gut Microbes and Diet Interaction

Post-inoculation of the microbes at birth and the type and composition of the diet play a major role in dictating the microbes' diversity and dominancy in the gut. Changes in the gut microbiome can be observed just 24 h after changing major components in the diet such as conversion to a plant-based or animal-based diet, and immediate conversion to 48 h after reverting to the previous diet (David *et al.* 2014). Macronutrients such as carbohydrate, protein and fat in the diet directly affect the number and type of microbes favored inside the gut. Diet affects the host system's health by regulating and modulating the microbes in the gut (Rajoka *et al.* 2017), as can be further observed in Table 17.2.

Table 17.1 Next generation probiotics (NGP) and their effects in the body.

Serial number	NGP	Isolated from	Effects	Site of action/ energy source	References
1.	*Akkermansia muciniphila*	Clinical blood infection	Maintain host metabolism, anticancer immunoefficacy and immunity Pasteurized bacteria. Prevent obesity and insulin resistance	Mucin-carbon, nitrogen and energy source	Bárcena *et al.* (2019); Dubourg *et al.* (2017); Zhai *et al.* (2019); Plovier *et al.* (2017)
2.	*Bacteroides* species *B. fragilis, B. xylanisolvens, Prevotella copri*	–	Produce capsular polysaccharides Modulate neuroinflammation Prevent viral encephalitides	–	Yang *et al.* (2011); De Vadder *et al.* (2016)
3.	*Christensenella minuta*	Feces	Modulate metabolism Reduce obesity Potential pathogen – use limited	–	Yang *et al.* (2018)
4.	*Clostridium* species *C. acetobutylicum, C. beijerinckii, C. butyricum, C. cellulolyticum, C. ljungdahlii*	–	Maintain homeostasis Prevent diarrhea in patients with chemotherapy treating lung cancer, modulation of inflammatory response	Cellulose and sugars	Dash *et al.* (2016); Uzal *et al.* (2018)
5.	Eggerthellaceae species *Gordonibacter urolithinfaciens, Gordonibacter pamelaeae*	Feces	Modulation of inflammatory and neurological response, anticarcinogenic, cardioprotective	Transformation of ellagic acid (source: walnuts, berries) into urolithins metabolites	Selma *et al.* (2017)
6.	*Faecalibacterium prausnitzii*	–	Gut environment maintained, positive modulation of regulatory T cells, promote immune checkpoint blockade (ICB) therapy, therapeutic treatment for cancer patients	Ferments glucose into short chain fatty acids	Wrzosek *et al.* (2013); Sedwick (2014)
7.	*Parabacteroides goldsteinii*	Blood from patient with abdominal infection	Prevent obesity, modulate inflammatory response and insulin sensitivity	–	Wu *et al.* (2019); Awadel-Kariem *et al.* (2010)
8.	Lactic acid bacteria *Pediococcus pentosaceus*	–	Reduction of cholesterol in blood Antimicrobial agent production and food preservative	End product: lactic acid	Syakila *et al.* (2019)

Sources: Based on Bárcena *et al.* (2019); Dubourg *et al.* (2017); Zhai *et al.* (2019); Plovier *et al.* (2017).

Table 17.2 Interaction between diet components and gut microbes.

Serial number	Dietary component	Relevant sources	Observation	Affecting gut microbiome	Reference
1.	Polyphenol	Catechins, flavonols, flavones, anthocyanins, proanthocyanidins and phenolic acids	Enrichment of gut microbiome	*Bifidobacterium* and *Lactobacillus*	Cuervo *et al.* (2016); Cabral *et al.* (2019)
2.	Proteins	High beef diet	Increased number	*Bacteroides* and *Clostridium*	Hentges *et al.* (1977)
		Whey and pea protein extract	Increased SCFA levels	*Bifidobacterium* and *Lactobacillus*	Dominika *et al.* (2011)
		High protein/low carbohydrate	Reduced SCFAs (butyrate)	*Roseburia* and *Eubacterium rectale*	Russell *et al.* (2011)
3.	Carbohydrate	Plant-based polysaccharides	Significant increase in number	*Firmicutes, Xylanibacter, Bacteroidetes* and *Prevotella*	Parvin *et al.* (2015)
		Glucose, fructose, and sucrose	Reduced	*Bifidobacterium, Bacteroides*	Eid *et al.* (2014)
		Artificial sweeteners	Increased Reduced	*Bacteroides,* *Lactobacillus reuteri*	Suez *et al.* (2014)
4.	Fibers/ complex polysaccharide/ prebiotics	Whole grain and wheat bran	Energy source for microbial growth	*Bifidobacterium* and *Lactobacillus*	Respondek *et al.* (2008)
		Resistant starch and whole grain barley		*Prevotella and Xylanibacter*	Schnorr *et al.* (2014)
5.	Fat	High saturated fat diet	Reduced total anaerobic microflora	*Bacteroides, Lactobacillus intestinalis*	Wu *et al.* (2011)
		Low saturated fat	Increased number in feces	*Bifidobacterium*	Fava *et al.* (2013)
		High unsaturated fat from salmon	No change in microflora	–	Urwin *et al.* (2014)

AOS, arabino-oligosaccharides; FOS, fructo-oligosaccharides; SCFAs, short chain fatty acids.*Sources:* Based on Cuervo *et al.* (2016); Cabral *et al.* (2019).

17.3.1 Carbohydrate

While the majority of the ingested carbohydrate is hydrolyzed by enzymes in the upper gastrointestinal tract, 20–60 g of ingested carbohydrates reach the colon, subsequently being broken down by enzymes and bacteria in the colon and converted to beneficial metabolites for the host cells (Flint *et al.* 2012). A higher carbohydrate diet has been linked with the enrichment of *Prevotella* genus, and a high protein and fat diet with the enrichment of *Bacteroidetes* microbial species in the gut. These microbes, upon interaction with such a diet, produce the SCFAs acetate and butyrate. Further, the products of degradation include amino acids which occurs at the end of the colon through proteolytic enzymes. Lactose was also found to increase the concentration of SCFAs in the feces in contrast to research that points out lactose to be a possible irritant in the gastrointestinal tract (Francavilla *et al.* 2012). In contrast to glucose, sucrose and fructose, a high concentration of artificial sweeteners induced glucose intolerance through gut metabolism. The biomarkers for this induction were found to be increased concentration of *Bacteroides* and reduced *Lactobacillus reuteri* in the gut colony (Suez *et al.* 2014). Based on the gut microbiome, it has been hypothesized that the consumption of artificial sweeteners could be more detrimental to health than that of sucrose, fructose and glucose (Singh *et al.* 2017). It has been predicted that up to 10% of the energy from the total dietary intake is dependent on the gut microbiome in humans. Some of the carbohydrate-active enzymes (CAZymes), which include glycoside hydrolases and carbohydrates esterases and are responsible for the breakdown of polysaccharides in mammals, can also be found in the bacteria and a few in eukaryotes (Flint *et al.* 2012).

17.3.2 Proteins

Proteins in the diet have also been found to regulate the gut microbiome, hence directly controlling the severity of diseases like colitis. Whey protein intake consisting of bioactive compounds such as lactoferrin and glycomacropeptide (cheese whey), was found to relieve symptoms like chronic inflammation of the large intestine (Daddaoua *et al.* 2005). The whey also contained other amino acids such as threonine, cysteine, serine and, to a lesser extent proline, which are also a vital constituent of the mucin in the gastrointestinal tract (Sprong *et al.* 2010). In addition, feeding the protein isolated from whey cheese having constituents such as cysteine or threonine to rats significantly increased the number of bifidobacteria and lactobacilli and decreased Clostridiaceae in the feces, hence increasing beneficial bacteria and decreasing harmful bacteria (Guerville and Boudry 2016). A high protein and low carbohydrate diet reduced the concentration of *Roseburia* and *Eubacterium rectale* in intestines and decreased concentration of SCFAs such as butyrate.

17.3.3 Complex Carbohydrate/Fibers

The fiber in the diet goes through the gastrointestinal tract, finally passing the small intestine and reaching the colon where it is digested by bacteria and converted to the SCFAs acetate and butyrate. Sources of fiber include soybeans, inulin, unrefined wheat and barley and raw oats. Non-digestible polysaccharides like insulin, starch and oligosaccharides go through this digestion whereas others like cellulose are excreted unaltered. These digestive products from bacteria act as a carbon source for probiotics such as *Lactobacillus* and *Bifidobacterium* and are commonly known as prebiotics, which are responsible for the growth of bacteria (Respondek *et al.* 2008). These compounds also produce a notable shift in the metabolic and immune systems. Intake of non-digestible carbohydrates present in food has been proven to reduce pro-inflammatory cytokine IL-6, insulin resistance and peak post-prandial glucose. The concentration and composition of macronutrients in the diet has been found to directly influence gut microbial concentration and growth (Martínez *et al.* 2013).

17.3.4 Fat

A diet consisting of high fat and low fiber results in a lower number of pathogenic bacteria and a large amount of beneficial microbes, such as *Prevotella* and *Xylanibacter*, the opposite of which is true for low fat and high fiber diet (Schnorr *et al.* 2014).

17.3.5 Probiotics

The ingestible microorganisms from fermented food and vegetables have been proven to have a regulatory and treatment effect on intestinal metabolism and bowel diseases respectively (Shen *et al.* 2014). These microorganisms have been collectively referred to as probiotics and have been a vital component of the diet. The probiotic strains *Bifidobacterium* and/or *Lactobacillus* were found to alter concentration of high density lipoprotein (HDL) cholesterol, triglycerides, total cholesterol, low density lipoprotein cholesterol, very low density lipoprotein cholesterol (Rajkumar *et al.* 2014) and sensitivity to insulin. Furthermore, consequent reduction in the concentrations of pathogenic bacteria, *E. coli* and *H. pylori* (Yang and Sheu 2012), which adhere to the epithelial tissue was also observed.

17.3.6 Phenolic Compounds

The intake of phenolic compounds such as catechins, flavonols, flavones, anthocyanins, proanthocyanidins and foods rich in phenolic acids such as fruits, seeds, vegetables, tea, cocoa products and wine (Pérez-Jiménez *et al.* 2010) has been found to alter the intestinal flora by enriching the bacterial genera such as *Bifidobacterium* and *Lactobacillus* (Cuervo *et al.* 2016) and reducing enteropathogens such as *Staphylococcus aureus, Salmonella typhimurium* (Parkar *et al.* 2008) and pathogenic *Clostridium* species (Druart *et al.* 2014).

The mounting evidence that the diet directly and indirectly affects overall body health through the immune system and metabolism suggests that the rise of irregularities such as obesity, psoriasis, autism and mood disorders may result from lack of modulation in the diet (Mangiola *et al.* 2016). Specifically, segmented filamentous bacteria have been known to enhance the Th17 response, promoting autoimmune arthritis (Ivanov *et al.* 2009). The effect of LAB and *Bifidobacterium* can be observed as declining responses of T effector-mediated inflammation and rising expression of anti-inflammatory T regulatory cells according to research done in mice (Kwon *et al.* 2010). In the presence of metabolic disorders such as obesity and diabetes, intestinal dysbiosis could be observed as compared to the healthy gut (Karlsson *et al.* 2013b).

17.4 Gut Microbiome and Metabolism Regulation

In addition to the hydrolyzation of macromolecules by the gut microbiome, post attachment of the microbes to the intestine epithelium, these microbes show protection against enteropathogens and ferment undigested compounds in the colon, producing SCFAs and some vitamins (Cabral *et al.* 2019). A study in the digesta of mice showed that the bacterial mass present was found to increase the thickness of the mucus and that mice that had a thin mucus layer in their gastrointestinal tract showed lower resistance to enteric infections (Sommer and Bäckhed 2013). In contrast, these microbes were also found to have a deleterious effect aided by the degradation of the amino acids (Cabral *et al.* 2019).

17.4.1 Gut Microbiome and Brain

The relationship between gut host organisms and brain functions has been established as a vital nerve response. In order to maintain homeostasis in the body, during stress, the hypothalamic–pituitary–adrenal axis and sympathetic nervous system are activated (Tsigos and Chrousos 2002). An interesting observation was made in the gut microbiome altered using probiotics and antibiotics during the pregnancy of both humans and rodents (Sharon *et al.* 2016). The offspring were found to be vulnerable to alteration in brain, neurological and immune development. The following are the possible pathways and metabolites by which gut microbiome and brain interact and regulation occurs.

17.4.1.1 Neural Pathways

The gut microbiome has been observed to play a role in the maintenance of homeostasis during stress responses (Sudo 2019). Different nerve endings such as vagus nerve and spinal afferent nerve were found to respond to the central nervous system and finally the brain through the lumen of the intestine. The expression of c-fos in the hypothalamus was found to respond immediately after the oral administration of *B. infantis* in germ-free mice (Sudo *et al.* 2004). This response could be partially repressed by the administration of capsaicin (Sudo 2012) and granisetron, which is an antagonist for serotonin type 3 receptors. This experiment concluded that the serotonin produced by the enterochromaffin cells acts as an antagonistic serotonin type 3 receptor in the sites where nerve endings are sensitive for capsaicin, which generates a response in the brain (Sudo 2016). These enterochromaffin cells can bridge the brain and gut microbiome by binding microbial products and secreting serotonin (Reigstad *et al.* 2015). It has also been demonstrated that vagal sensory neurons in the gut are linked to striatal dopamine release, demonstrating that the gut nerval affinities and responses affect brain function through the nervous system (Han *et al.* 2018)The negative alteration of these vagal sensory neurons has been discovered to result in psychiatric and depressive disorders, including autism spectrum disorders (ASD) and affective disorders (Foster and Neufeld 2013). In case of the major depressive disorders, the presence of Enterobacteriaceae and *Alistipes* in the gut was found to be increased and that of *Faecalibacterium* was found to be decreased. This negative correlation between severity of depression and *Faecalibacterium* shows us that major depressive symptoms are associated with the decrease in beneficial bacteria and increase in detrimental bacteria in the gut (Jiang H *et al.* 2015). The gut microbiome has been found to interact with the central nervous system through three distinct channels in the human body: nervous, endocrine, and immune signaling. Alterations in the gut–brain–nervous system were related to nervous disorders such as multiple sclerosis (MS), Parkinson's disease, fibromyalgia and chronic pain syndrome (Martin *et al.* 2018). The central nervous system interacts with the brain through metabolites, translocation of the gut microbiome and endotoxin translocation from the gut to the nervous system (Dalile *et al.* 2019).

17.4.1.2 Metabolites

It has already been established that SCFAs (acetate, propionate and butyrate) are produced by the gut microbiome through the anaerobic fermentation of complex polysaccharides (Høverstad and Midtvedt 1986). Depending upon the fiber content of the diet, concentration and diversity of microbiomes and gut transit time, 500–600 mmol/day of SCFAs are produced in the human gut (Macfarlane and Macfarlane 2003). Furthermore, although the presence of these metabolites in the brain itself is analytically very low in concentration, they can be found in human cerebrospinal fluid in concentration ranges of 0–171 μM for acetate, 0–6 μM for propionate, and 0–2.8 μM for butyrate (Silva *et al.* 2020). These metabolites act as a source of carbon for microbe growth and further epithelial proliferation, mucus secretion, and water and mineral absorption in the host cells of the gastrointestinal tract (Kasubuchi *et al.* 2015). Growing evidence suggests that, in addition to their basic function, these metabolites also possess neuroactive properties.

Furthermore, the bacterial population and its metabolites have been found to alter the neurotransmitter precursors and can even produce their own set of neurotransmitters such as γ-aminobutyric acid, serotonin, dopamine and noradrenaline (Sherwin *et al.* 2018). These metabolites can directly influence brain function and neuroglial cells located throughout the brain and nervous system also known as microglia (Browning *et al.* 2017).

17.4.2 Gut Microbiome and Immune System

In the interaction between the gut microbiome and immune system, common pathways involved are the epithelial cells and gut associated lymphoid tissue (GALT) (Hooper *et al.* 2012). The lymphoid tissue is situated in the basal layer of intestinal tissues, covered by epithelial tissue and mucin. This protected layer is called the lamina propria and is a part of the lymphatic circulation system in mammals. The lymphatic circulation houses immune cells comprising macrophages, mast cells and plasma cells throughout the body. Specific to the intestine, this system comprises Peyer's patches, which consist of isolated lymphoid tissue, which further consists of β cells, T cells and dendritic cells (Mowat 2003). This interaction helps the immune system to separate beneficial and harmful components in a very basic way.

17.4.3 Gut and Regulation of Metabolism

It has been established that in metabolic diseases such as obesity and type 2 diabetes, the composition of microbial flora in the gut is quite different as compared to healthy people (Kootte *et al.* 2017). Among other modulations in bacterial diversity, the most common change was observed for SCFAs such as butyrate producing bacteria in the gut (Sanna *et al.* 2019). In accordance with that, SCFAs can bind to the G protein-coupled receptors (GPCR), also known as free fatty acids receptors, FFAR2 and FFAR3. The effects of this binding depend upon the cells on which these receptors are expressed. For example, for enteroendocrine cells, modulation of glucagon-like peptides (GLP) can be observed (Silva *et al.* 2020), whereas for pancreatic cells, increased insulin secretion can be observed (Puddu *et al.* 2014), which ultimately effects the presence of metabolic disorders (De Vadder *et al.* 2014). Orexigenic neurons, which express neuropeptide Y in the hypothalamus, have been known to be suppressed by the activation of these FFAR receptors (Li Z *et al.* 2018), finally contributing to modulation of the sleep–wake cycle (circadian rhythm) and control of appetite (Torres-Fuentes *et al.* 2019). Recent experiments in mice show that this can be further manipulated by the administration of butyrate-producing probiotics that work by raising GLP-1 and pro-opiomelanocortin expressed by the hypothalamus (Barrea *et al.* 2019).

17.4.4 Gut Microbiome and COVID-19

With the physical, economical and sociological effects of COVID-19, it is undeniable that the virus has an extensive research importance. It was established that, out of all the physical effects, the virus causes major lung infection by binding to the angiotensin converting enzyme (ACE) 2 receptors, which are present in the alveolar epithelial cells of the lungs. Further investigation showed that the intestinal epithelial cells, especially enterocytes, also showed similar expression of ACE2 receptors. In addition, it was discovered that COVID virus RNA could be found in the feces of infected patients, providing a window to hypothesize the interaction between the gut and the virus (Dhar and Mohanty 2020).

17.5 Role of Gut Microbiome on Metabolic Diseases

The alteration of gut microbiota has been considered to be a key factor for the development of metabolic diseases. The gut microbiota is recognized as an endocrine organ involving molecular cross-talk, restoration of energy homeostasis and stimulation of the immune system of the host. Diet, lifestyle and diseases trigger alterations in the composition of the gut microbiome. The alteration of gut microbiome composition/diversity related to negative effects is called dysbiosis (Figure 17.1), and it dramatically changes the symbiotic relationship between the gut microbiome and the host. This alteration causes development of metabolic diseases. The gut microbiota particularly contributes to metabolic diseases through stimulation of low-grade inflammation (Boulangé *et al.* 2016). Several mechanisms have been proposed as a link between the gut microbiota and metabolic disorders.

17.5.1 Gut Barrier and Inflammation

The intestinal epithelial monolayer acts as a barrier between the organism and the external environment. In a healthy individual, the intestinal barrier allows the passage of water, nutrients and bioactive compounds, while it blocks the access of harmful substances (e.g. bacterial and dietary antigens) (Groschwitz and Hogan 2009). The gut microbiota has a

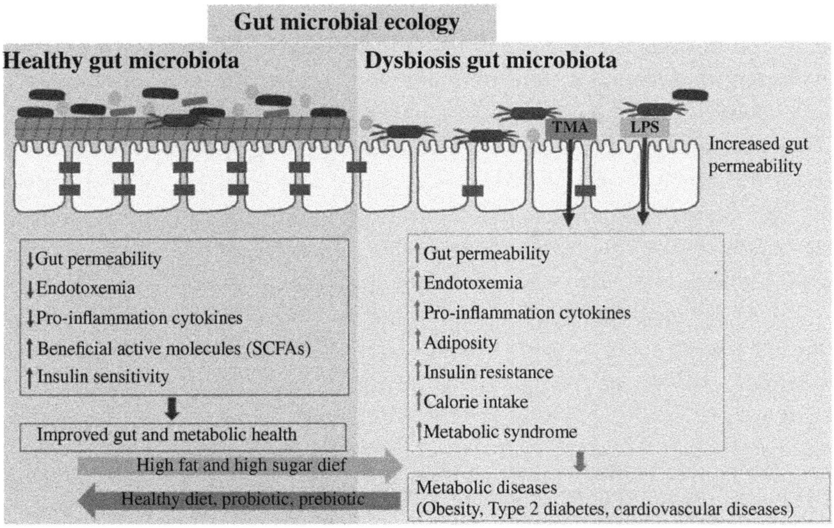

Figure 17.1 Impact of gut microbial ecology on the metabolic health of the host. LPS, lipopolysaccharide: SCFA, short chain fatty acids; TMA, trimethylamine.

variety of mechanisms to regulate intestinal integrity. Dendritic cells eliminate microbial antigens from the gut lumen, activate immune cells and induce the secretion of mucus, antimicrobial peptide and IgA (Wang *et al.* 2020). Gut microorganisms can also produce metabolites such as secondary bile acid and aryl hydrocarbon receptor agonist, which indirectly support gut barrier function (Natividad *et al.* 2018). The endogenous factors of the host also impact on gut barrier integrity. For example, the level of insulin in the blood regulates the secretion of mucus (Wei *et al.* 2012).

The gut microbiome is regulated by environmental and host factors (dietary, diarrhea, genetic, etc.). These factors may induce the expression of lipopolysaccharide (LPS), promote Toll-like receptor (TLR) signaling, disintegrate the mucus layer causing endotoxemia, generate pro-atherogenic trimethylamine or some other process and basically cause metabolic disorders (Wang *et al.* 2020). One of the significant indicators of obesity and related diseases is chronic low-grade inflammation and insulin resistance (Gregor and Hotamisligil 2011). Obesity is considered to be a pro-inflammatory state in which the level of pro-inflammatory cytokines such as TNF-α, IL-6, angiotensin II, leptin, resistin and plasminogen activator inhibitor 1 increases in adipose tissue and in the immune cells (Asghar and Sheikh 2017; Makki *et al.* 2013). Low-grade chronic inflammation in obesity is induced by immune cells. Indeed, immune cells are also a main factor contributing to the pathogenesis of insulin resistance resulting in type 2 diabetes.

LPS, known as endotoxins, are structural components that are found as a major constituent of the outer cell membrane of Gram-negative bacteria. LPS are composed of three main compartments: o-antigen (made up of repeated oligosaccharide units), a core oligosaccharide, and lipid A. Lipid A in particular contributes to LPS toxicity (Gomes *et al.* 2017). On the other hand, a normal level of LPS presence in the intestine does not cause any harmful effects to the host (Geurts *et al.* 2014).

LPS is associated with the initiation of inflammation-related pathways, increasing the onset of several chronic diseases such as obesity and type 2 diabetes (Creely *et al.* 2007). Administration of a diet high in fat and cholesterol has been shown to increase intestinal permeability, leading to LPS translocation into the circulatory system. This induces the state of metabolic endotoxemia (Moreira *et al.* 2012). LPS can enter the body either by crossing the mucus layer through the leakage of intestinal tight junctions or by combining with chylomicron (a lipoprotein responsible for absorption of dietary triglycerides and cholesterol) (Boulangé *et al.* 2016).

The elevated LPS level causes inflammation by interacting with Toll-like receptor (TLR)-4 (De La Serre *et al.* 2010). The interaction between LPS and TLR4 of the host promotes the expression of downstream pro-inflammatory factors including interleukin (IL)-6 and tumor necrosis factor (TNF)-α, which further contribute to tissue inflammation. In the liver, LPS encourages inflammation that contributes to increased hepatic insulin resistance and lipogenesis. In adipose tissue, inflammation contributes to insulin resistance, resulting in the development of diabetes. The intercellular tight junction is important in the maintenance of gut barrier integrity. This gut barrier integrity has been known to break down as a result of obesity as observed in obese mice models. The activation of TLR4 further modifies the tight junctions and induces permeability of the intestine, resulting in intestinal inflammation (Li T *et al.* 2018).

In summary, certain factors such as diets or commensal microbiota can alter the relationship of the host–microbiome community. This generates the abnormal signals that influence immune response and barrier function. Disintegration of the gut barrier results in systemic chronic inflammation and organ dysfunction and consequent development of metabolic disease in the host.

17.5.2 Microbial Metabolites

17.5.2.1 Bile Acid

Bile acid facilitates food digestion and dietary lipids and fat-soluble nutrient absorption. Bile acid is also involved in the regulation of several metabolic pathways, including the balance of glucose, lipid and energy. Cholic acid (CA) and chenodeoxycholic acid (CDCA) are the primary bile acids that are synthesized from cholesterol in the liver.

Bile in the gallbladder is secreted into the duodenum after food intake. Almost 95% of primary bile acids are reabsorbed in the ileum and returned to the liver (Chiang 2009). The remaining primary bile acids undergo dehydroxylation, dehydrogenation and deconjugation to form secondary bile acids by the gut microbiota present in the colon (Ajouz *et al.* 2014; Battson *et al.* 2018). The catalyzing enzyme involved in dehydroxylation has been found in various Firmicutes species, particularly *Clostridium scindens* (Ridlon and Hylemon 2012). Thus, the deconjugation and dehydroxylation reactions generate the diversity of bile acids found in the intestine (Sayin *et al.* 2013).

High fat foods induce the secretion of bile acid into the small intestine. An increasing bile acid pool in the small intestine results in a huge increase in specific bile acid within the colon (Ojeda *et al.* 2016). The study of Devkota *et al.* (2012) showed increased taurocholic acid (TCA) when a milkfat-rich diet was consumed. TCA, a sulfur-containing bile acid, promotes the abundance of the pathobiont *Bilophila wadsworthia*, especially in the colon. This pathogenic bacterium is involved in the activation of intestinal inflammation and stimulation of the immune response. This study strengthened the correlation between diet and gut microbiota. Specific types of diet lead to an increase in particular bacterial species that metabolize different bile types. These alterations in gut microbiome and bile acid metabolism may result in disease development in the small intestine (David *et al.* 2014).

Bile acids are also considered as signaling molecules that result in various physiological effects via binding to G protein-coupled bile acid receptor 1 (also known as TGR5) and nuclear receptor (farnesoid X receptor, FXR) (Battson *et al.* 2018). The gut microbiota responds to fat deposition by the regulation of FXR. FXR, a bile acid receptor, regulates the synthesis of bile acid and the accumulation of triglyceride in the liver (Belizário *et al.* 2018).

Recently, the correlation between FXR and metabolic diseases has been extensively researched. FXR may perform differentially in liver and small intestine. Schmitt *et al.* (2015) demonstrated the different impact of FXR on metabolic disorders in an investigation in liver-FXR and intestine-FXR knockout mice. The study showed lipid accumulation with 1% cholesterol intake in the liver-FXR knockout mice, while this effect was not found in intestinal-FXR knockout mice. On the other hand, the intestinal-FXR knockout mice were able to maintain the level of serum cholesterol and bile acids. This finding demonstrates that the activation of liver-FXR can protect fat accumulation due to cholesterol administration, which was not found for intestinal activation. Similarly, Jiang C *et al.* (2015) reported that the antioxidant tempol or antibiotic is able to suppress the expression of FXR in intestinal microbiota. This resulted in the reduction of triglyceride accumulation in the liver and steatosis in a non-alcoholic fatty liver disease model with high-fat diets.

17.5.2.2 Trimethylamine-*N*-oxide (TMAO)

The consumption of dietary choline is necessary for humans to maintain the level of phospholipid synthesis. Certain gut microbiota can produce trimethylamine (TMA), acetate and ethanol through anaerobic choline metabolism. In dysbiosis, abnormal choline metabolism takes place and can potentially contribute to non-alcoholic fatty liver disease. In dysbiosis, the level of TMA is also increased in the circulatory system. This is considered as a risk factor contributing to cardiovascular disease and colon cancer (Krishnan *et al.* 2015). Trimethylamine-*N*-oxide (TMAO) production is a result of secondary ingestion of nutrients consisting of TMA, such as choline, phosphatidylcholine and L-carnitine. These compounds are typically found in animal food sources, such as eggs, red meat, fish, milk, cheese, liver, etc. (Battson *et al.* 2018). These dietary nutrients are converted to TMA by the gut microbial metabolic pathway through the activity of specific enzymes (e.g. lyase) (Vallianou *et al.* 2019). TMA in the circulatory system is transported to the liver and oxidized to TMAO by hepatic flavin monooxygenase 3 (Dannenberg *et al.* 2020). In an animal study, TMAO contributed to a pro-atherogenic state through inhibition of bile acid synthesis and transportation of cholesterol by macrophages in the arterial endothelium. TMAO has also been known to contribute to impaired glucose homeostasis and development of fatty liver (Moran-Ramos *et al.* 2017; Tang and Hazen 2017).

17.6 Gut Microbiome and Metabolic Diseases

17.6.1 Obesity

Obesity is a global public health issue that has been growing rapidly every year. Currently, more than 107.7 million children and 603.7 million adults around the world are obese. Over 60% of deaths are correlated to high body mass index (BMI) (Tseng and Wu 2019). Obesity is related to the imbalance between energy intake and energy expenditure. Higher energy intake and lower energy expenditure lead to excessive fat accumulation, resulting in the enhancement of BMI (obesity is defined as BMI $\geq$30 kg/m^2). Obesity is also one of the factors influencing metabolic syndrome, which significantly increases the incidence of other obesity-related diseases (such as diabetes, cardiovascular diseases, hypertension and liver disorders) and low-grade inflammation (Kho and Lal 2018).

The gut microbiome is a newly identified factor affecting host metabolism regulation and possibly contributing to obesity. There is evidence to show the link between the gut microbiome and obesity. The study of Bäckhed *et al.* (2004) was conducted in bacteria-free or germ-free (GF) mice and mice with normal gut microbiota (N-GM). During fasting, N-GM mice exhibited 40% higher body fat content than GF mice, although N-GM mice were fed with a 30% higher food intake. After the intestinal microflora from N-GM mice was transplanted to GF mice, the researchers found a significant increase (60%) in body fat, a drastic increase in hepatic triglyceride and insulin resistance in the recipients (GF-GM: germ-free mice colonized by gut microbiota). Mainly, two mechanisms have been proposed for these phenomena: (i) the secretion of leptin hormone in GF-GM was related to reduced insulin sensitivity; (ii) the gut microbial colonization in GF-GM is likely to inhibit the expression of fasting-induced adipose factor (FIAF), a lipid metabolism controller. FIAF performs to break down triglyceride in lipoprotein into free fatty acids that are used by muscle and adipose tissue. The inactivation of FIAF thus induces triglyceride accumulation in adipocytes (Bäckhed *et al.* 2004). The mechanism proposed to explain the resistance to diet-induced obesity in GF mice was a release of adenosine monophosphate-activated protein kinase (AMPK). The inhibition of AMPK by gut microbiota suppresses mitochondrial fatty acid oxidation, insulin secretion and ketogenesis, while it promotes lipogenesis and cholesterol and triglyceride synthesis (Boulangé *et al.* 2016).

GF mice inoculated with gut microflora from obese mice exhibited higher body weight and fat tissue than GF mice that received gut microflora from lean mice (Turnbaugh *et al.* 2006). This was due to the gut microbiota received from obese mice harvesting more energy from ingested food. The production of SCFAs seems to be the mechanism that induced gut microbes to increase energy absorption. SCFAs are used as an energy source by gut microbes, and they further have complex metabolic functions. For instance, SCFAs enhance the absorption of monosaccharide, activating the expression of sodium/glucose transporter-1. They also regulate host appetite and food intake by interacting with GPRs of enteroendocrine cells, resulting in stimulation of the secretion of GLP-1 and peptide YY which directly impact satiety of the host (Festi *et al.* 2014). Furthermore, SCFAs trigger lipid metabolism by enhancing lipogenesis and impeding fatty acid oxidation (Bäckhed *et al.* 2004). Ley *et al.* (2005) compared the composition of gut microbiota in genetically obese mice and lean mice. The abundance of Bacteroidetes was reduced by 50% and the proportion of Firmicutes was increased in genetically obese mice. Santacruz *et al.* (2010) also detected the reduction of Bacteroidetes and increase in Firmicutes in overweight humans. However, the alteration in the ratio of Bacteroidetes/Firmicutes composition in obese and lean humans has not been confirmed in all human studies. Duncan *et al.* (2008) exhibited no significant difference in the composition between *Bacteroidetes/Firmicutes* observed in obese and lean individuals.

Consumption of a high-fat diet is likely to increase Gram-negative bacteria in the gut microbiome, resulting in enhanced intestinal permeability to bacterial fragments such as LPS. Elevated LPS level in the circulatory system contributes to metabolic endotoxemia. In an experiment, mice with endotoxemia induced by LPS infusion for 4 weeks exhibited body weight gain, rapid hyperglycemia and hyperinsulinemia; the result was similar in mice fed high-fat diets (Cani *et al.* 2007). The study of De La Serre *et al.* (2010) investigated the role of gut inflammation, intestinal permeability, LPS and gut microbiome on propensity of the obesigenic effected by high fat diet. Sprague Dawley rats could response to a high-fat diet by two different phenotypes in which some individuals are prone (DIO-P) to the obesigenic effects of the high-fat diet, whereas others are resistant (DIO-R). DIO-P only increased the activation of TLR4, gastrointestinal inflammation, LPS, intestinal permeability, but these changes were not observed in rats resistant to obesity (DIO-R). However, changes in gut microbiota were found in rats regardless of phenotype. Thus, consumption of a high-fat diet plays a role in the development of obese phenotype via the activation of TLR4, gut inflammation and LPS.

Fei and Zhao (2013) reported that *Enterobacter cloacae* B29 (obtained from the gut microflora of obese humans) promoted obesity and insulin resistance and increased endotoxin levels in the circulatory system. The authors demonstrated that the presence of endotoxin-producing bacteria is the main cause of obesity and insulin resistance rather than dysbiosis in the host. Thus, it has been suggested that lowering metabolic endotoxemia could be an approach for treatment of metabolic diseases.

17.6.2 Type 2 Diabetes Mellitus

Type 2 diabetes mellitus (T2DM) is a chronic disease associated with metabolic abnormality, mainly determined by elevated blood glucose levels because of insulin resistance and inadequate insulin secretion. This disease develops from the interconnection of genetic and environmental factors and various risk factors such as age, heredity, unhealthy diet, obesity, physical inactivity, smoking, etc. (Mardinoglu *et al.* 2016). The worldwide population with a diagnosis of diabetes is growing. The International Diabetes Federation reported that the number of adults with diabetes increased dramatically from 108 million to 451 million from 1980 to 2017 and is expected to be 693 million in 2045. In 2017, approximately 5 million people globally died as a result of diabetes (Cho *et al.* 2018). Indeed, T2DM is considered one of the most serious health issues in the twenty-first century.

According to gut metagenomic analysis, there is evidence of the association of dysbiosis of the gut microbiota with T2DM (Karlsson *et al.* 2013a; Qin *et al.* 2012). The gut microbiome of T2DM patients showed an increase in opportunistic pathogens and a decrease in SCFA-producing bacteria (Qin *et al.* 2012). Patients with diabetes and glucose intolerance showed a reduction in *Akkermansia muciniphila*, a mucus-colonizing bacterium performing predominantly a gut barrier function (Zhang and Zhang 2013).

LPS-induced metabolic endotoxemia is considered the first step in developing insulin resistance and diabetes (Cani *et al.* 2007). In humans, the level of circulating endotoxin was 20% and 125% higher in obese individuals and T2DM patients, respectively, compared to lean individuals (Harte *et al.* 2012). Shi *et al.* (2013) demonstrated that the gut microbiota potentially links to an inflammatory process in obesity and insulin resistance via LPS. Circulating endotoxin level caused the elevation of pro-inflammatory factors such as TNF-α and IL-6 in adipose cells, in which these factors are associated with the pathway regulating insulin secretion (Ghanim *et al.* 2009).

17.7 Modulation of Gut Microbiome as Target for Prevention of Metabolic Diseases

17.7.1 Role of Dietary Intervention

Diet-induced weight loss is known to be a result of increased diversity of gut bacteria and reduced chronic systemic inflammation. Patients with obesity who consumed low-calorie diets (controlled fat and carbohydrate diets) experienced an enhancement of Bacteroidetes and a reduction in Firmicutes (Bouter *et al.* 2017; Cotillard *et al.* 2013). Different diets contributed to specific gut microbiome communities: animal-based foods were associated with Bacteroidetes while plant-based diets were related to *Prevotella* (Hartstra *et al.* 2015). Among many type of foods, the Mediterranean diet, typically consisting of fish, olive oil, legumes, fruits, vegetables, cereals and nuts, can develop an optimum gut microbial composition (Pascale *et al.* 2018). Olive oil has been proposed to exert anti-inflammatory properties arising from the properties of monounsaturated fatty acid (MUFA) and polyunsaturated fatty acid (PUFA) (Schwingshackl *et al.* 2015). Supplementation with PUFA has beneficial effects on gut microbiota composition, particularly in balancing the ratio of the phyla Bacteroidetes and Firmicutes. PUFA administration also promotes the availability of species *Lachnospiraceae*, *Bifidobacterium* and *Akkermansia* that possess anti-inflammatory effects (Costantini *et al.* 2017). However, the exact mechanisms linking PUFA and the gut microbiota are still poorly understood. Two possible mechanisms have been proposed (Wu W *et al.* 2020). First, the gut microbiome composition could be modulated via PUFA metabolites on bile salt level in the intestine. The other mechanism could be the positive impact of PUFA on intestinal permeability.

Polyphenols (PP) are natural compounds found mostly in plant-based sources such as tea, coffee, wine, fruits, vegetables and cereals. These compounds provide antioxidant and anti-inflammatory properties that reduce the risk of several diseases such as obesity, diabetes and atherosclerosis (Singh *et al.* 2019). PP are poorly absorbed in the small intestine, however the colonic microbiota can break down PP into their absorbable metabolites (Guergoletto *et al.* 2016). A recent study has demonstrated that PP can provide protective effects against obesity-associated diseases via modulation of the gut microbiome (Gowd *et al.* 2019). Administration of a cranberry extract (CE) rich in PP prevented weight gain induced by a high fructose–high sucrose diet and prevented the formation of visceral adiposity in mice. CE administration was also found to decrease triglyceride deposition and suppress hepatic inflammation, resulting in the improvement of insulin sensitivity and the prevention of non-alcoholic fatty liver disease development. The authors further revealed CE consumption's positive effect related to an increased abundance of *Akkermansia* species (Anhê *et al.* 2015). Supplementation of grape polyphenols (GP) to mice fed a high-fat diet significantly modulated the community of gut microbiota, thereby decreasing the Firmicutes to Bacteroidetes ratio. GP administration also supported the growth of *Akkermansia muciniphila*, and these changes prevented the negative effects arising from a high-fat diet (Roopchand *et al.* 2015). In conclusion, PP could prevent metabolic diseases through optimal modulation of the gut microbiome community. PP also promoted the growth of beneficial bacteria and suppressed the growth of harmful microbes.

17.7.2 Role of Probiotics and Prebiotics

Probiotics and prebiotics have been extensively investigated to improve the relationship between the gut microbial and host metabolism, particularly related to metabolic diseases. Probiotics are live microorganisms which, when administered in adequate amounts, have the potential to provide health benefits to the host. Probiotics are able to improve the host's immunity, promote epithelial barrier function and generate antibacterial products. Indeed, probiotics have also been established to prevent metabolic diseases through the modulation of intestinal microbiota (Wang *et al.* 2017). Specific probiotic strains, especially *Lactobacillus*, *Bifidobacterium* and *Akkermansia*, are widely used to diminish obesity and diabetes. They are likely to reduce weight gain, reduce visceral adiposity, improve glucose tolerance and modulate intestinal low-grade inflammation (Festi *et al.* 2014). The potential effect of *Bifidobacterium pseudolongum* on the reduction of triglyceride in induced high-fat diet obese mice was reported in the study of Bo *et al.* (2020). The authors found that treatment of *B. pseudolongum* in obese mice significantly decreased body mass by 12%, plasma triglyceride by 12.4%, total energy intake by 12.8% and visceral fat by 26.5%. *B. pseudolongum* treatment markedly restored the equilibrium of the gut microbiota including the diversity of gut microbia and the Firmicutes to Bacteroidetes ratio. Moreover, the abundance of the strains *Butyricimonas* and *Bifidobacterium* was also observed in the obese mice treated with *B. pseudolongum*. Several reports have shown the potential effects of *Lactobacillus* on the alleviation of overweight and improvement of metabolic disorders such as obesity, T2DM, hypertension and hypercholesterolemia (Park *et al.* 2018; Toral *et al.* 2018; Yan *et al.* 2019). Li *et al.* (2020) reported the preventive effects of *Lactobacillus plantarum* against obesity via the modulation of gut microbiota and their metabolites in high-fat fed mice. High-fat fed mice treated with *L. plantarum* exhibited a decrease in body weight and improved glucose tolerance. *L. plantarum* could lower the level of LPS and inflammatory cytokines in serum while increasing the amount of SCFAs in feces. Indeed, *L. plantarum* could recover the ratio of Firmicutes to Bacteroidetes. Changes in the genera *Akkermansia*, *Lactobacillus* and *Ruminococcus* induced by the high-fat diet were also restored to the level observed in the normal group. Another probiotic strain, *Akkermansia muciniphila*, has been reported to have beneficial effects on host health. Similar reports have been elucidated from Everard *et al.* (2013) and Wu F *et al.* (2020) for the effects of *A. muciniphila* on delaying gain in body weight and helping to control blood glucose. The study of Wu F *et al.* (2020) showed recovery of the adverse changes in gut microbiota induced by a high-fat diet and an increase in the abundance of *Bifidobacterium* for high-fat fed mice treated with *A. muciniphila*. Furthermore, the administration of *A. muciniphila* also restored the reduction of goblet cell production in high-fat fed mice, which provided benefits for maintaining host immunity as well as limiting systemic inflammation.

Prebiotics are non-digestible carbohydrates found in certain plant foods (Choque Delgado and Tamashiro 2018). They are selectively fermented by gut microbiota and promote a desirable growth environment and increase the diversity within the microbiome, supporting host health (Newman and Arshad 2020). The compounds that are recognized as prebiotics include glucose-, fructose-, and xylo-oligosaccharide, inulin and lactulose (Markowiak and Ślizewska 2017). The important fermentative product of prebiotics by commensal organisms is SCFAs, which have beneficial effects on the host (Ahmadi *et al.* 2019). The consumption of prebiotics was reported to promote the growth of specific intestinal microbiota producing SCFAs including *Bifidobacterium* and *Lactobacillus* (Connolly *et al.* 2012). The study of Salazar *et al.* (2015) showed an increase in species *B. longum*, *B. pseudocatenulatum* and *B. adolescentis* in obese women consuming an inulin-type fructan prebiotic. Saccharolytic fermentation by specific microbiota induces the production of SCFAs, which play critical roles in several functions. First, prebiotics have the ability to reduce obesity. Prebiotics contribute to higher production of SCFAs which promotes the secretion of GLP-1 and PYY, resulting in reduced hunger and energy intake (Delzenne *et al.* 2007; O'Connor *et al.* 2017). GLP-1 and PYY serve as satiating hormones regulating food intake. The binding of soluble prebiotics and water in the stomach increases distension, associated with the slowing down of gastric emptying and enhancing the sensation of fullness (Slavin 2013). Second, prebiotics help to reduce inflammation. Low-grade chronic systemic inflammation is indicated by the high level of pro-inflammatory markers in the bloodstream such as TNF-α, IL-6 or C-reactive protein. Low-grade chronic systemic inflammation has been connected to metabolic syndromes and its related components such as obesity, insulin resistance and β-cell dysfunction (Choque Delgado and Tamashiro 2018; Grundy *et al.* 2005). Inflammation induces gut permeability, resulting in the translocation of bacterial toxin into the systemic circulation, a condition known as endotoxemia. Endotoxemia causes an increase in pro-inflammatory components such as LPS in the bloodstream (Shen *et al.* 2013). Prebiotics play a potential role in reducing inflammation by increasing the number of *Bifidobacterium* species producing SCFAs. In particular, butyrate performs beneficial functions in epithelial integrity (O'Connor *et al.* 2017). Indeed, prebiotics can also improve glucose metabolism. The elevation of LPS and pro-inflammatory markers causes the alteration of β-cell function, resulting in fasting hyperglycemia and hyperinsulinemia (Erejuwa *et al.* 2014; Yoo and Kim 2016). The reduction of LPS level and endotoxemia by prebiotics could improve glucose tolerance (Cani and Delzenne 2009). Prebiotic fibers enhance the production of SCFAs, which could also improve the action and sensitivity of insulin (Weickert *et al.* 2006). Slowing down gastric emptying by prebiotics could also decrease the absorption of glucose, thereby regulating the insulin response (Slavin 2013).

17.8 Possible Mechanisms of Gut Microbiome in Prevention of Metabolic Diseases

17.8.1 Roles of Short Chain Fatty Acids

In order to digest complex proteins and polysaccharides, gut microorganisms typically perform their function through enzymatic pathways. SCFAs, 2–6 carbon atoms of organic fatty acids, are synthesized in the colon by the fermentation of non-digestible carbohydrate by gut microbiota. Acetate, propionate and butyrate are the most abundant SCFAs found in the body. SCFAs have been proposed to be microbiome-derived modulators for host metabolism (Warmbrunn *et al.* 2020). Three SCFAs have specific roles in the host. Butyrate acts as the main fuel for colonic epithelial cells. Acetate is involved in fatty acid and cholesterol synthesis (Al-Lahham *et al.* 2010). Butyrate and acetate are further responsible for maintenance of epithelial barrier function; butyrate in particular has been found to enhance mucus secretion and induce tight junction protein expression (Warmbrunn *et al.* 2020). The G protein-coupled receptors (GPRs), which are GPR41 (known as free fatty acid receptor 2) and GPR43 (known as free fatty acid receptor 3), act as receptors for SCFAs (He and Shi 2017). These receptors are present in several tissues including adipose tissue, enteroendocrine cells and inflammatory cells (Belizário *et al.* 2018). SCFAs are able to induce secretion of intestinal hormones such as 5-hydroxytryptamine (5-HT), glucagon-like peptides (GLP-1 and GLP-2) and peptide YY (PYY). 5-HT, a neurotransmitter, regulates the gastrointestinal movement and secretory system. It regulates intestinal permeability and peristalsis and reduces food absorption (He and Shi 2017). GLP-1 stimulates β-cells in the pancreas to secrete insulin and suppress glucagon secretion, gastric emptying and food intake (Dubé and Brubaker 2007). GLP-2 is secreted together with GLP-1 which can increase intestinal epithelial proliferation and reduce gut permeability. Besides, GLP-2 in central neurons increases hepatic insulin sensitivity and is associated with the regulation of glucose homeostasis (Shi *et al.* 2013). PYY decreases the absorption of nutrients in the intestine and modulates the appetite (Belizário *et al.* 2018). Moreover, a number of studies have shown that the presence of SCFAs in the systemic circulation results in a modulatory effect on cardiovascular function (Giles *et al.* 2017).

17.8.2 Role of Bile Salt Hydrolase

The influence of microbial bile salt hydrolase (BSH) on cholesterol lowering in the host has also been revealed. Hypercholesterolemia (high blood cholesterol level) is a risk indicator for coronary heart disease. Although this condition can be treated by pharmacological agents (such as statins or bile acid sequestrants), they often generate undesirable side effects (Begley *et al.* 2006). It was revealed that consumption of probiotics could reduce cholesterol levels by 22–33% in mice fed a high-fat diet. The hypothesis correlated cholesterol-lowering effects with enzymatic deconjugation of bile acids by BSH (He and Shi 2017). Jones *et al.* (2004) reported that *L. plantarum* 80 exhibits lowering of blood serum cholesterol via the activity of BSH. This enzyme has the ability to hydrolyze conjugated glycodeoxycholic acid and taurodeoxycholic acid, resulting in the deconjugation of glycol- and tauro- bile acids. Guo *et al.* (2019) also studied the effect of BSH activity and hypocholesterolemic effect of BSH activity and hypocholesterolemic effect of *Lactobacillus plantarum* KLDS 1.0344. Mice were fed a cholesterol-enriched diet together with administration of the strain *L. plantarum* KLDS 1.0344. The result was that the strain *L. plantarum* KLDS 1.0344 improved lipid profiles in serum and liver and increased fecal total cholesterol and total bile acid level. Besides BSH activity, several possible mechanisms associated with the cholesterol-lowering effects of probiotics include assimilation of cholesterol by the bacteria, binding of cholesterol to the cell wall of bacteria, and physiological actions of the end products of SCFA fermentation (Begley *et al.* 2006). Deconjugated bile acids or free bile acids are less reabsorbed than conjugated bile acids. Thus, huge amounts of free bile acids are excreted in feces. Free bile acids are also poorly effective in the solubilization and absorption of lipids in the intestine. As a consequence, deconjugated bile acids contribute to lowering serum cholesterol either by increasing the demand for cholesterol used for synthesis of bile acids to replace those lost in feces or by reducing cholesterol solubility and thus absorption of cholesterol through the intestinal lumen (He and Shi 2017).

17.8.3 Role on Intestinal Barrier Function

The gut microbiome regulates the host immunity and metabolism via signaling by bioactive molecules. The gut microbiome also plays a vital role in the maintenance of the gut barrier. The epithelial cell connection by tight junctions is a factor indicating the integrity of intestinal epithelium. Levels of the tight junction proteins, such as occludin, claudin and zonulin, in plasma are currently used as indirect markers for the determination of intestinal barrier integrity (Costantini *et al.* 2017). Impairment of the intestinal barrier allows paracellular permeability of bacteria and bacterial products. This situation occurs for example when LPS are transferred from the intestine into the systemic circulation causing chronic inflammation (Wu W *et al.* 2020). Mucosa-associated bacteria respond to the maintenance of the intestinal barrier through TLR and NOD-like receptor (NLR) signaling (reviewed in Ghosh *et al.* 2020). Costantini *et al.* (2017) reviewed the positive impact of polyunsaturated fatty acid administration on gut barrier function as one of the mechanisms mediated by butyrate production by gut microbiota. As a consequence, a healthy gut microbiota and its diversity result in the prevention of chronic inflammation through protection of the gut barrier.

17.9 Conclusion and Future Perspective

The gut microbiome plays a significant role in host metabolism. Host metabolism is regulated by either beneficial or harmful microbial metabolites, such as SCFAs, bile acid, TMAO or gut microbiota composition. Dysbiosis of the gut microbiome arising from some factors, mainly dietary, contributes to the onset of obesity and other related metabolic diseases. However, the manipulation of gut microbial ecology by specific types of diet and the administration of probiotics and prebiotics can be a potential strategy to prevent or act as therapeutic treatment for metabolic diseases. Several studies have been carried out in the animal model but studies in humans are still scarce. Thus, studies in humans are necessary to confirm the interaction and the beneficial effects of gut microbiota on the host.

References

Abid, M.B. and Koh, C.J. (2019). Probiotics in health and disease: fooling Mother Nature? *Journal of Infection*, 47: 911–917.

Ahmadi, S., Nagpal, R., Wang, S., Gagliano, J., Kitzman, D.W., Soleimanian-Zad, S., Sheikh-Zeinoddin, M., Read, R. and Yadav, H. (2019). Prebiotics from acorn and sago prevent high-fat-diet-induced insulin resistance via microbiome–gut–brain axis modulation. *The Journal of Nutritional Biochemistry*, 67: 1–13.

Ajouz, H., Mukherji, D. and Shamseddine, A. (2014). Secondary bile acids: an underrecognized cause of colon cancer. *World Journal of Surgical Oncology*, 12: 164.

Al-Lahham, S.H., Peppelenbosch, M.P., Roelofsen, H., Vonk, R.J. and Venema, K. (2010). Biological effects of propionic acid in humans; metabolism, potential applications and underlying mechanisms. *Biochimica et Biophysica Acta (BBA) - Molecular and Cell Biology of Lipids*, 1801(11): 1175–1183.

Anhê, F.F., Roy, D., Pilon, G., Dudonné, S., Matamoros, S., Varin, T.V., Garofalo, C., Moine, Q., Desjardins, Y., Levy, E. and Marette, A. (2015). A polyphenol-rich cranberry extract protects from diet-induced obesity, insulin resistance and intestinal inflammation in association with increased Akkermansia spp. population in the gut microbiota of mice. *Gut*, 64(6): 872–883.

Asghar, A. and Sheikh, N. (2017). Role of immune cells in obesity induced low grade inflammation and insulin resistance. *Cellular Immunology*, 315: 18–26.

Awadel-Kariem, F.M., Patel, P., Kapoor, J., Brazier, J.S. and Goldstein, E. (2010). First report of Parabacteroides goldsteinii bacteraemia in a patient with complicated intra-abdominal infection. *Journal of Anaeorobe*, 16(3): 223–225.

Bäckhed, F., Ding, H., Wang, T., Hooper, L.V., Gou, Y.K., Nagy, A., Semenkovich, C.F. and Gordon, J.I. (2004). The gut microbiota as an environmental factor that regulates fat storage. *Proceedings of the National Academy of Sciences of the United States of America*, 101(44): 15718–15723.

Bäckhed, F., Ley, R.E., Sonnenburg, J.L., Peterson, D.A. and Gordon, J.I. (2005). Host-bacterial mutualism in the human intestine. *Science*, 307(5717): 1915–1920.

Bárcena, C., Valdés-Mas, R., Mayoral, P., Garabaya, C., Durand, S., Rodríguez, F., Fernández-García, M.T., Salazar, N., Nogacka, A.M. and Garatachea, N. (2019). Healthspan and lifespan extension by fecal microbiota transplantation into progeroid mice. *Nature*, 25(8): 1234–1242.

Barrea, L., Muscogiuri, G., Annunziata, G., Laudisio, D., Pugliese, G., Salzano, C., Colao, A. and Savastano, S. (2019). From gut microbiota dysfunction to obesity: could short-chain fatty acids stop this dangerous course? *Hormones (Athens)*, 18: 245–250.

Battson, M.L., Lee, D.M., Weir, T.L. and Gentile, C.L. (2018). The gut microbiota as a novel regulator of cardiovascular function and disease. *Journal of Nutritional Biochemistry*, 56: 1–15.

Begley, M., Hill, C. and Gahan, C.G.M. (2006). Bile salt hydrolase activity in probiotics. *Applied and Environmental Microbiology*, 72(3): 1729–1738.

Belizário, J.E., Faintuch, J. and Garay-Malpartida, M. (2018). Gut microbiome dysbiosis and immunometabolism: New frontiers for treatment of metabolic diseases. *Mediators of Inflammation*, 2018: 2037838.

Belkaid, Y. and Hand, T.W. (2014). Role of the microbiota in immunity and inflammation. *Journal of Cell*, 157(1): 121–141.

Bo, T., Wen, J., Zhao, Y., Tian, S., Zhang, X. and Wang, D. (2020). Bifidobacterium pseudolongum reduces triglycerides by modulating gut microbiota in mice fed high-fat food. *The Journal of Steroid Biochemistry and Molecular Biology*, 198: 105602.

Bokulich, N.A., Chung, J., Battaglia, T., Henderson, N., Jay, M., Li, H., Lieber, A.D., Wu, F., Perez-Perez, G.I. and Chen, Y. (2016). Antibiotics, birth mode, and diet shape microbiome maturation during early life. *Science Translational Medicine*, 8(343): 343–382.

Bottacini, F., van Sinderen, D. and Ventura, M. (2017). Omics of bifidobacteria: research and insights into their health-promoting activities. *Biochemical Journal*, 474(24): 4137–4152.

Boulangé, C.L., Neves, A.L., Chilloux, J., Nicholson, J.K. and Dumas, M.E. (2016). Impact of the gut microbiota on inflammation, obesity, and metabolic disease. *Genome Medicine*, 8(1), 1–12.

Bouter, K.E., van Raalte, D.H., Groen, A.K. and Nieuwdorp, M. (2017). Role of the gut microbiome in the pathogenesis of obesity and obesity-related metabolic dysfunction. *Gastroenterology*, 152(7): 1671–1678.

Browning, K.N., Verheijden, S. and Boeckxstaens, G. (2017). The vagus nerve in appetite regulation, mood, and intestinal inflammation. *Journal of Gastroenterology*, 152(4): 730–744.

Cabral, C., Kumar, R., Ganguly, R., Gupta, A., Carbone, C., Reis, F. and Pandey, A. (2019) Beneficial effects of dietary polyphenols on gut microbiota and strategies to improve delivery efficiency. *Nutrients*, 11(9): 2216.

Cani, P. and Delzenne, N. (2009). The role of the gut microbiota in energy metabolism and metabolic disease. *Current Pharmaceutical Design*, 15(13): 1546–1558.

Cani, P.D., Amar, J., Iglesias, M.A., Poggi, M., Knauf, C. and Bastelica, D. (2007). Metabolic endotoxemia initiates obesity and insulin resistance. *Diabetes*, 56: 386–389.

Chang, C.J., Lin, T.L., Tsai, Y.L., Wu, T.R., Lai, W.F., Lu, C.C. and Lai, H.C. (2019). Next generation probiotics in disease amelioration. *Journal of Food and Drug Analysis*, 27(3): 615–622.

Chiang, J.Y.L. (2009). Bile acids : regulation of synthesis. *Journal of Lipid Research*, 50: 1955–1966.

Cho, N.H., Shaw, J.E., Karuranga, S., Huang, Y., da Rocha Fernandes, J.D., Ohlrogge, A. W. and Malanda, B. (2018). IDF Diabetes Atlas: Global estimates of diabetes prevalence for 2017 and projections for 2045. *Diabetes Research and Clinical Practice*, 138: 271–281.

Choque Delgado, G.T. and Tamashiro, W.M. da S.C. (2018). Role of prebiotics in regulation of microbiota and prevention of obesity. *Food Research International*, 113: 183–188.

Connolly, M.L., Lovegrove, J.A. and Tuohy, K.M. (2012). In vitro fermentation characteristics of whole grain wheat flakes and the effect of toasting on prebiotic potential. *Journal of Medicinal Food*, 15(1): 33–43.

Costantini, L., Molinari, R., Farinon, B. and Merendino, N. (2017). Impact of omega-3 fatty acids on the gut microbiota. *International Journal of Molecular Sciences*, 18(12): 2645.

Cotillard, A., Kennedy, S.P., Kong, L.C., Prifti, E., Pons, N., Le Chatelier, E., Almeida, M., Quinquis, B., Levenez, F., Galleron, N., Gougis, S., Rizkalla, S., Batto, J. M., Renault, P., Doré, J., Zucker, J. D., Clément, K., Ehrlich, S.D., Blottière, H. and Layec, S. (2013). Dietary intervention impact on gut microbial gene richness. *Nature*, 500(7464): 585–588.

Creely, S.J., McTernan, P.G., Kusminski, C.M., Fisher, F.M., Da Silva, N.F., Khanolkar, M., Evans, M., Harte, A.L. and Kumar, S. (2007). Lipopolysaccharide activates an innate immune system response in human adipose tissue in obesity and type 2 diabetes. *American Journal of Physiology - Endocrinology and Metabolism*, 292(3): 740–747.

Cuervo, A., Hevia, A., López, P., Suárez, A., Diaz, C., Sánchez, B., Margolles, A. and González, S. (2016). Phenolic compounds from red wine and coffee are associated with specific intestinal microorganisms in allergic subjects. *Journal of Food and Function*, 7(1): 104–109.

Daddaoua, A., Puerta, V., Zarzuelo, A., Suárez, M.D., Sánchez de Medina, F., and Martínez-Augustin, O. (2005). Bovine glycomacropeptide is anti-inflammatory in rats with hapten-induced colitis. *Journal of Nutrition*, 135(5): 1164–1170.

Dalile, B., Van Oudenhove, L., Vervliet, B. and Verbeke, K. (2019). The role of short-chain fatty acids in microbiota–gut–brain communication. *Nature Reviews Gastroenterology Hepatology*, 16: 461–478.

Dannenberg, L., Zikeli, D., Benkhoff, M., Ahlbrecht, S., Kelm, M., Levkau, B. and Polzin, A. (2020). Targeting the human microbiome and its metabolite TMAO in cardiovascular prevention and therapy. *Pharmacology & Therapeutics*, 213: 107584

Dash, S., Ng, C.Y. and Maranas, C.D. (2016). Metabolic modeling of clostridia: current developments and applications. *Microbiology Letters*, 363(4).

David, L.A., Maurice, C.F., Carmody, R.N., Gootenberg, D.B., Button, J.E., Wolfe, B.E., Ling, A.V., Devlin, A.S., Varma, Y. and Fischbach, M.A. (2014). Diet rapidly and reproducibly alters the human gut microbiome. *Nature Biotechnology*, 505(7484): 559–563.

De La Serre, C.B., Ellis, C.L., Lee, J., Hartman, A.L., Rutledge, J.C. and Raybould, H.E. (2010). Propensity to high-fat diet-induced obesity in rats is associated with changes in the gut microbiota and gut inflammation. *American Journal of Physiology - Gastrointestinal and Liver Physiology*, 299(2): 440–448.

De Vadder, F., Kovatcheva-Datchary, P., Goncalves, D., Vinera, J., Zitoun, C., Duchampt, A., Bäckhed, F. and Mithieux, G. (2014). Microbiota-generated metabolites promote metabolic benefits via gut-brain neural circuits. *Cell*, 156(1-2): 84–96.

De Vadder, F., Kovatcheva-Datchary, P., Zitoun, C., Duchampt, A., Bäckhed, F. and Mithieux, G. (2016). Microbiota-produced succinate improves glucose homeostasis via intestinal gluconeogenesis. *Cell Metabolism*, 24(1): 151–157.

Delzenne, N.M., Cani, P.D. and Neyrinck, A.M. (2007). Modulation of glucagon-like peptide 1 and energy metabolism by inulin and oligofructose: Experimental data. *Journal of Nutrition*, 137(11): 2547–2551.

Devkota, S., Wang, Y., Musch, M. W., Leone, V., Fehlner-Peach, H., Nadimpalli, A., Antonopoulos, D.A., Jabri, B. and Chang, E.B. (2012). Dietary-fat-induced taurocholic acid promotes pathobiont expansion and colitis in Il10-/- mice. *Nature*, 487(7405): 104–108.

Dhar, D. and Mohanty, A. (2020). Gut microbiota and Covid-19-possible link and implications. *Journal of Virus Research*, 198018.

Dominguez-Bello, M.G., Costello, E.K., Contreras, M., Magris, M., Hidalgo, G., Fierer, N. and Knight, R.J. (2010). Delivery mode shapes the acquisition and structure of the initial microbiota across multiple body habitats in newborns. *Proceedings of the National Academy of Sciences*, 107(26): 11971–11975.

Dominika, Ś., Arjan, N., Karyn, R.P. and Henryk, K. (2011). The study on the impact of glycated pea proteins on human intestinal bacteria. *International Journal of Food Microbiology*, 145(1): 267–272.

Druart, C., Dewulf, E.M., Cani, P.D., Neyrinck, A.M., Thissen, J.-P. and Delzenne, N.M. (2014). Gut microbial metabolites of polyunsaturated fatty acids correlate with specific fecal bacteria and serum markers of metabolic syndrome in obese women. *Journal of Lipids*, 49(4): 397–402.

Dubé, P.E. and Brubaker, P.L. (2007). Frontiers in glucagon-like peptide-2: Multiple actions, multiple mediators. *American Journal of Physiology - Endocrinology and Metabolism*, 293(2).

Dubourg, G., Cornu, F., Edouard, S., Battaini, A., Tsimaratos, M. and Raoult, D. (2017). First isolation of Akkermansia muciniphila in a blood-culture sample. *Clinical Microbiology Infection*, 23(9): 68–683.

Duncan, S.H., Lobley, G.E., Holtrop, G., Ince, J., Johnstone, A.M., Louis, P. and Flint, H.J. (2008). Human colonic microbiota associated with diet, obesity and weight loss. *International Journal of Obesity*, 32(11): 1720–1724.

Eckburg, P.B., Bik, E.M., Bernstein, C.N., Purdom, E., Dethlefsen, L., Sargent, M., Gill, S.R., Nelson, K.E. and Relman, D.A. (2005). Diversity of the human intestinal microbial flora. *Journal of Science*, 308(5728): 1635–1638.

Eid, N., Enani, S., Walton, G., Corona, G., Costabile, A., Gibson, G., Rowland, I. and Spencer, J.P. (2014). The impact of date palm fruits and their component polyphenols, on gut microbial ecology, bacterial metabolites and colon cancer cell proliferation. *Journal of Nutritional Science*, 3.

El Hage, R., Hernandez-Sanabria, E. and Van de Wiele, T. (2017). Emerging trends in "smart probiotics": functional consideration for the development of novel health and industrial applications. *Frontiers in Microbiology*, 8: 1889.

Endo, A., Tanizawa, Y., Tanaka, N., Maeno, S., Kumar, H., Shiwa, Y., Okada, S., Yoshikawa, H., Dicks, L., Nakagawa, J. and Arita, M. (2015). Comparative genomics of Fructobacillus spp. and Leuconostoc spp. reveals niche-specific evolution of Fructobacillus spp. *BMC Genomics*, 16(1): 1117.

Engels, C., Ruscheweyh, H.-J., Beerenwinkel, N., Lacroix, C. and Schwab, C. (2016). The common gut microbe Eubacterium hallii also contributes to intestinal propionate formation. *Frontiers in Microbiology*, 7: 713.

Erejuwa, O.O., Sulaiman, S.A. and Ab Wahab, M.S. (2014). Modulation of gut microbiota in the management of metabolic disorders: The prospects and challenges. *International Journal of Molecular Sciences*, 15(3): 4158–4188.

Everard, A., Belzer, C., Geurts, L., Ouwerkerk, J.P., Druart, C., Bindels, L.B., Guiot, Y., Derrien, M., Muccioli, G.G., Delzenne, N.M., De Vos, W.M. and Cani, P.D. (2013). Cross-talk between Akkermansia muciniphila and intestinal epithelium controls diet-induced obesity. *Proceedings of the National Academy of Sciences of the United States of America*, 110(22): 9066–9071.

Everard, A., Lazarevic, V., Gaïa, N., Johansson, M., Ståhlman, M., Backhed, F., Delzenne, N. M., Schrenzel, J., Francois, P. and Cani, P.D. (2014). Microbiome of prebiotic-treated mice reveals novel targets involved in host response during obesity. *International Society for Microbial Ecology*, 8(10): 2116–2130.

Faith, J.J., Guruge, J.L., Charbonneau, M., Subramanian, S., Seedorf, H., Goodman, A.L., Clemente, J.C., Knight, R., Heath, A.C., Leibel, R.L., Rosenbaum, M. and Gordon, J. I. (2013). The long-term stability of the human gut microbiota. *Science*, 341(6141).

Fava, F., Gitau, R., Griffin, B., Gibson, G., Tuohy, K. and Lovegrove, J. (2013). The type and quantity of dietary fat and carbohydrate alter faecal microbiome and short-chain fatty acid excretion in a metabolic syndrome 'at-risk'population. *International Journal of Obesity*, 37(2): 216–223.

Fei, N. and Zhao, L. (2013). An opportunistic pathogen isolated from the gut of an obese human causes obesity in germfree mice. *ISME Journal*, 7(4): 880–884.

Festi, D., Schiumerini, R., Eusebi, L.H., Marasco, G., Taddia, M. and Colecchia, A. (2014). Gut microbiota and metabolic syndrome. *World Journal of Gastroenterology*, 20(43): 16079–16094.

Flint, H.J., Scott, K.P., Duncan, S.H., Louis, P. and Forano, E. (2012). Microbial degradation of complex carbohydrates in the gut. *Gut Microbes*, 3(4): 289–306.

Foster, J.A. and Neufeld, K.A.M. (2013). Gut–brain axis: how the microbiome influences anxiety and depression. *Trends in Neuroscience*, 36(5): 305–312.

Fraher, M.H., O'toole, P.W., Quigley, E.M. (2012). Techniques used to characterize the gut microbiota: a guide for the clinician. *Nature Reviews Gastroenterology and Hepatology*, 9(6): 312.

Francavilla, R., Calasso, M., Calace, L., Siragusa, S., Ndagijimana, M., Vernocchi, P., Brunetti, L., Mancino, G., Tedeschi, G. and Guerzoni, E. (2012). Effect of lactose on gut microbiota and metabolome of infants with cow's milk allergy. *Pediatric Allergy and Immunology*, 23(5): 420–427.

Geurts, L., Neyrinck, A.M., Delzenne, N.M., Knauf, C. and Cani, P.D. (2014). Gut microbiota controls adipose tissue expansion, gut barrier and glucose metabolism: Novel insights into molecular targets and interventions using prebiotics. *Beneficial Microbes*, 5(1): 3–17.

Ghanim, H., Abuaysheh, S., Sia, C.L., Korzeniewski, K., Chaudhuri, A., Fernandez-Real, J. M. and Dandona, P. (2009). Increase in plasma endotoxin concentrations and the expression of toll-like receptors and suppressor of cytokine signaling-3 in mononuclear cells after a high-fat, high-carbohydrate meal: Implications for insulin resistance. *Diabetes Care*, 32(12): 2281–2287.

Ghosh, S.S., Wang, J., Yannie, P.J. and Ghosh, S. (2020). Intestinal barrier dysfunction, LPS translocation, and disease development. *Journal of the Endocrine Society*, 4(2): 1–15.

Giles, T.D., Cockcroft, J.R., Pitt, B., Jakate, A. and Wright, H.M. (2017). Rationale for nebivolol/valsartan combination for hypertension: review of preclinical and clinical data. *Journal of Hypertension*, 35(9): 1758–1767.

Gomes, J.M.G., Costa, J. de A. and Alfenas, R. de C.G. (2017). Metabolic endotoxemia and diabetes mellitus: A systematic review. *Metabolism: Clinical and Experimental*, 68: 133–144.

Gopalakrishnan, V., Spencer, C.N., Nezi, L., Reuben, A., Andrews, M., Karpinets, T., Prieto, P., Vicente, D., Hoffman, K., and Wei, S. (2018). Gut microbiome modulates response to anti–PD-1 immunotherapy in melanoma patients. *Science*, 359(6371): 97–103.

Gowd, V., Karim, N., Shishir, M.R.I., Xie, L. and Chen, W. (2019). Dietary polyphenols to combat the metabolic diseases via altering gut microbiota. *Trends in Food Science and Technology*, 93: 81–93.

Gregor, M. F. and Hotamisligil, G. S. (2011). Inflammatory Mechanisms in Obesity. *Annual Review of Immunology*, 29(1): 415–445.

Groschwitz, K.R. and Hogan, S.P. (2009). Intestinal barrier function: Molecular regulation and disease pathogenesis. *Journal of Allergy and Clinical Immunology*, 124(1): 3–20.

Grundy, S.M., Cleeman, J.I., Daniels, S.R., Donato, K.A., Eckel, R.H., Franklin, B.A., Gordon, D.J., Krauss, R.M., Savage, P.J., Smith, S.C., Spertus, J.A. and Costa, F. (2005). Diagnosis and management of the metabolic syndrome: An American Heart Association/National Heart, Lung, and Blood Institute scientific statement. *Circulation*, 112(17): 2735–2752.

Guergoletto, K.B., Costabile, A., Flores, G., Garcia, S. and Gibson, G.R. (2016). In vitro fermentation of juçara pulp (*Euterpe edulis*) by human colonic microbiota. *Food Chemistry*, 196: 251–258.

Guerville, M. and Boudry, G. (2016). Gastrointestinal and hepatic mechanisms limiting entry and dissemination of lipopolysaccharide into the systemic circulation. *American Journal of Physiology-Gastrointestinal Boudry, and Liver Physiology*, 311(1): G1–G15.

Guo, L., Wang, L., Liu, F., Li, B., Tang, Y., Yu, S. and Zhang, D. (2019). Effect of bile salt hydrolase-active Lactobacillus plantarum KLDS 1. 0344 on cholesterol metabolism in rats fed a high-cholesterol diet. *Journal of Functional Foods*, 61(600): 103497.

Han, W., Tellez, L.A., Perkins, M.H., Perez, I.O., Qu, T., Ferreira, J., Ferreira, T.L., Quinn, D., Liu, Z.-W. and Gao, X.B. (2018). A neural circuit for gut-induced reward. *Cell* 175(3): 665–678. e623.

Harte, A.L., Varma, M.C., Tripathi, G., Mcgee, K.C., Al-Daghri, N.M., Al-Attas, O.S., Sabico, S., O'Hare, J.P., Ceriello, A., Saravanan, P., Kumar, S. and Mcternan, P.G. (2012). High fat intake leads to acute postprandial exposure to circulating endotoxin in type 2 diabetic subjects. *Diabetes Care*, 35(2): 375–382.

Hartstra, A.V., Bouter, K.E.C., Bäckhed, F. and Nieuwdorp, M. (2015). Insights into the role of the microbiome in obesity and type 2 diabetes. *Diabetes Care*, 38(1): 159–165.

He, M. and Shi, B. (2017). Gut microbiota as a potential target of metabolic syndrome: The role of probiotics and prebiotics. *Cell and Bioscience*, 7(1): 1–14.

Hentges, D.J., Maier, B.R., Burton, G.C., Flynn, M.A. and Tsutakawa, R.K. (1977). Effect of a high-beef diet on the fecal bacterial flora of humans. *Cancer Research* 37(2), 568–571.

Hooper, L.V., Littman, D.R. and Macpherson, A. (2012). Interactions between the microbiota and the immune system. *Science*, 336 (6086): 1268–1273.

Høverstad, T. and Midtvedt, T. (1986). Short-chain fatty acids in germfree mice and rats. *Journal of Nutrition*, 116(9): 1772–1776.

Huttenhower, C., Gevers, D., Knight, R., Abubucker, S., Badger, J.H., Chinwalla, A.T., Creasy, H.H., Earl, A.M., FitzGerald, M.G. and Fulton, R.S. (2012). Structure, function and diversity of the healthy human microbiome. *Nature*, 486(7402): 207.

Ivanov, I.I., Atarashi, K., Manel, N., Brodie, E. L., Shima, T., Karaoz, U., Wei, D., Goldfarb, K.C., Santee, C.A. and Lynch, S. V. (2009). Induction of intestinal Th17 cells by segmented filamentous bacteria. *Cell*, 139(3): 485–498.

Jiang, C., Xie, C., Li, F., Zhang, L., Nichols, R.G., Krausz, K.W., Cai, J., Qi, Y., Fang, Z. Z., Takahashi, S., Tanaka, N., Desai, D., Amin, S.G., Albert, I., Patterson, A.D. and Gonzalez, F.J. (2015). Intestinal farnesoid X receptor signaling promotes nonalcoholic fatty liver disease. *Journal of Clinical Investigation*, 125(1): 386–402.

Jiang, H., Ling, Z., Zhang, Y., Mao, H., Ma, Z., Yin, Y., Wang, W., Tang, W., Tan, Z. and Shi, J. (2015). Altered fecal microbiota composition in patients with major depressive disorder. *Brain, Behavior, and Immunity*, 48:186–194.

Jones, M.L., Chen, H., Ouyang, W., Metz, T. and Prakash, S. (2004). Microencapsulated genetically engineered Lactobacillus plantarum 80 (pCBH1) for bile acid deconjugation and its implication in lowering cholesterol. *Journal of Biomedicine and Biotechnology*, 2004(1): 61–69.

Juge, N. (2012). Microbial adhesins to gastrointestinal mucus. *Trends in Microbiology*, 20(1): 30–39.

Kaklamanos, E.G., Nassar, R., Kalfas, S., Al Halabi, M., Kowash, M., Hannawi, H., Hussein, I., Salami, A., Hassan, A. and Senok, A.C. (2019). A single-centre investigator-blinded randomised parallel group clinical trial to investigate the effect of probiotic strains Streptococcus salivarius M18 and Lactobacillus acidophilus on gingival health of paediatric patients undergoing treatment with fixed orthodontic appliances: study protocol. *BMJ Open*, 9(9): e030638.

Karlsson, F.H., Tremaroli, V., Nookaew, I., Bergström, G., Behre, C.J., Fagerberg, B., Nielsen, J. and Bäckhed, F. (2013a). Gut metagenome in European women with normal, impaired and diabetic glucose control. *Nature*, 498(7452): 99–103.

Karlsson, F., Tremaroli, V., Nielsen, J. and Bäckhed, F. (2013b). Assessing the human gut microbiota in metabolic diseases. *Diabetes*, 62(10): 3341–3349.

Kasubuchi, M., Hasegawa, S., Hiramatsu, T., Ichimura, A. and Kimura, I. (2015). Dietary gut microbial metabolites, short-chain fatty acids, and host metabolic regulation. *Nutrients*, 7(4): 2839–2849.

Kho, Z.Y. and Lal, S.K. (2018). The human gut microbiome – A potential controller of wellness and disease. *Frontiers in Microbiology*, 9.

Kootte, R.S., Levin, E., Salojärvi, J., Smits, L.P., Hartstra, A.V., Udayappan, S.D., Hermes, G., Bouter, K.E., Koopen, A.M. and Holst, J. (2017). Improvement of insulin sensitivity after lean donor feces in metabolic syndrome is driven by baseline intestinal microbiota composition. *Cell Metabolism*, 26(4): 611–619. e616.

Krishnan, S., Alden, N. and Lee, K. (2015). Pathways and functions of gut microbiota metabolism impacting host physiology. *Current Opinion in Biotechnology*, 36:137–145.

Kwon, H.-K., Lee, C.-G., So, J.-S., Chae, C.-S., Hwang, J.-S., Sahoo, A., Nam, J. H., Rhee, J. H., Hwang, K.C. and Im, S.-H. (2010). Generation of regulatory dendritic cells and CD4+ Foxp3+ T cells by probiotics administration suppresses immune disorders. *Proceedings of the National Academy of Sciences*, 107(5): 2159–2164.

Langella, P., Guarner, F. and Martín, R. (2019). Next-generation probiotics: From commensal bacteria to novel drugs and food supplements. *Frontiers in Microbiology* 10: 1973.

Ley, R.E., Bäckhed, F., Turnbaugh, P., Lozupone, C.A., Knight, R.D. and Gordon, J.I. (2005). Obesity alters gut microbial ecology. *Proceedings of the National Academy of Sciences*, 102(31):11070–11075.

Li, C., Chen, X., Kou, L., Hu, B., Zhu, L.P., Fan, Y.R., Wu, Z.W., Wang, J.J. and Xu, G.X. (2010). Selenium-Bifidobacterium longum as a delivery system of endostatin for inhibition of pathogenic bacteria and selective regression of solid tumor. *Experimental and Therapeutic Medicine*, 1(1): 129–135.

Li, T., Gao, J., Du, M. and Mao, X. (2018). Milk fat globule membrane supplementation modulates the gut microbiota and attenuates metabolic endotoxemia in high-fat diet-fed mice. *Journal of Functional Foods*, 47: 56–65.

Li, X., Huang, Y., Song, L., Xiao, Y., Lu, S., Xu, J., Li, J. and Ren, Z. (2020). Lactobacillus plantarum prevents obesity via modulation of gut microbiota and metabolites in high-fat feeding mice. *Journal of Functional Foods*, 73(104103).

Li, Z., Yi, C.-X., Katiraei, S., Kooijman, S., Zhou, E., Chung, C.K., Gao, Y., van den Heuvel, J.K., Meijer, O.C. and Berbée, J.F.J.G. (2018). Butyrate reduces appetite and activates brown adipose tissue via the gut-brain neural circuit. *Gut*, 67(7): 1269–1279.

Lin, T.L., Shu, C.C., Lai, W.F., Tzeng, C.M., Lai, H.C. and Lu, C.C. (2019). Investiture of next generation probiotics on amelioration of diseases–Strains do matter. *Medicine in Microecology*, 1, 100002.

Lukiw, W.J. (2016). Bacteroides fragilis lipopolysaccharide and inflammatory signaling in Alzheimer's disease. *Frontiers in Microbiology*, 7: 1544.

Macfarlane, S. and Macfarlane, G.T. (2003). Regulation of short-chain fatty acid production. *Proceedings of the Nutrition Society*, 62(1): 67–72.

Makki, K., Froguel, P. and Wolowczuk, I. (2013). Adipose tissue in obesity-related inflammation and insulin resistance: cells, cytokines, and chemokines. *International Scholarly Research Notices*, 2013: 139239.

Mangiola, F., Ianiro, G., Franceschi, F., Fagiuoli, S., Gasbarrini, G. and Gasbarrini, A. (2016). Gut microbiota in autism and mood disorders. *World Journal of Gastroenterology*, 22(1): 361.

Manrique, P., Bolduc, B., Walk, S. T., van der Oost, J., de Vos, W.M. and Young, M.J. (2016). Healthy human gut phageome. *Proceedings of the National Academy of Sciences Young*, 113(37): 10400–10405.

Mardinoglu, A., Boren, J. and Smith, U. (2016). Confounding effects of metformin on the human gut microbiome in type 2 diabetes. *Cell Metabolism*, 23(1): 10–12.

Markowiak, P. and Ślizewska, K. (2017). Effects of probiotics, prebiotics, and synbiotics on human health. *Nutrients*, 9(9).

Martin, C.R., Osadchiy, V., Kalani, A. and Mayer, E.A. (2018). The brain-gut-microbiome axis. *Cellular and Molecular Gastroenterology and Hepatology* 6(2): 133–148.

Martín, R., Miquel, S., Benevides, L., Bridonneau, C., Robert, V., Hudault, S., Chain, F., Berteau, O., Azevedo, V. and Chatel, J.M. (2017). Functional characterization of novel Faecalibacterium prausnitzii strains isolated from healthy volunteers: a step forward in the use of F. prausnitzii as a next-generation probiotic. *Frontiers in Microbiology*, 8: 1226.

Martínez, I., Lattimer, J.M., Hubach, K.L., Case, J.A., Yang, J., Weber, C.G., Louk, J.A., Rose, D.J., Kyureghian, G. and Peterson, D.A. (2013). Gut microbiome composition is linked to whole grain-induced immunological improvements. *The ISME Journal*, 7(2): 269–280.

Moran-Ramos, S., López-Contreras, B.E. and Canizales-Quinteros, S. (2017). Gut microbiota in obesity and metabolic abnormalities: A matter of composition or functionality? *Archives of Medical Research*, 48(8): 735–753.

Moreira, A.P.B., Texeira, T.F.S., Ferreira, A.B., Do Carmo Gouveia Peluzio, M. and De Cássia Gonçalves Alfenas, R. (2012). Influence of a high-fat diet on gut microbiota, intestinal permeability and metabolic endotoxaemia. *British Journal of Nutrition*, 108(5): 801–809.

Mowat, A.M. (2003). Anatomical basis of tolerance and immunity to intestinal antigens. *Nature Reviews Immunology*, 3(4): 331–341.

Natividad, J.M., Agus, A., Planchais, J., Lamas, B., Jarry, A.C., Martin, R., Michel, M.L., Chong-Nguyen, C., Roussel, R., Straube, M., Jegou, S., McQuitty, C., Le Gall, M., da Costa, G., Lecornet, E., Michaudel, C., Modoux, M., Glodt, J., Bridonneau, C. and Sokol, H. (2018). Impaired aryl hydrocarbon receptor ligand production by the gut microbiota is a key factor in metabolic syndrome. *Cell Metabolism*, 28(5):737–749.

Newman, A.M. and Arshad, M. (2020). The role of probiotics, prebiotics and synbiotics in combating multidrug-resistant organisms. *Clinical Therapeutics*, 42(9): 1637–1648.

Norman, J.M., Handley, S.A., Baldridge, M.T., Droit, L., Liu, C.Y., Keller, B.C., Kambal, A., Monaco, C.L., Zhao, G. and Fleshner, P. (2015). Disease-specific alterations in the enteric virome in inflammatory bowel disease. *Cell*, 160(3): 447–460.

Noverr, M.C. and Huffnagle, G.B. (2004). Does the microbiota regulate immune responses outside the gut?. *Trends in Microbiology*, 12(12): 562–568.

O'Connor, S., Chouinard-Castonguay, S., Gagnon, C. and Rudkowska, I. (2017). Prebiotics in the management of components of the metabolic syndrome. *Maturitas*, 104: 11–18.

Ojeda, P., Bobe, A., Dolan, K., Leone, V. and Martinez, K. (2016). Nutritional modulation of gut microbiota — the impact on metabolic disease pathophysiology. *The Journal of Nutritional Biochemistry*, 28: 191–200.

Olveira, G. and González-Molero, I. (2016). An update on probiotics, prebiotics and symbiotics in clinical nutrition. *Endocrinología y Nutrición*, 63(9): 482–494.

Park, M.Y., Kim, J., Kim, S. and Whang, K.Y. (2018). Lactobacillus curvatus KFP419 and Leuconostoc mesenteroides subsp. mesenteroides KDK411 isolated from kimchi ameliorate hypercholesterolemia in rats. *Journal of Medicinal Food*, 21(7): 647–653.

Parkar, S.G., Stevenson, D.E. and Skinner, M.A. (2008). The potential influence of fruit polyphenols on colonic microflora and human gut health. *International Journal of Food Microbiology*, 124(3): 295–298.

Parvin, S., Easmin, D., Sheikh, A., Biswas, M., Sharma, S.C.D., Jahan, M.G.S., Islam, M.A., Shovon, M. and Roy, N. (2015). Nutritional analysis of date fruits (Phoenix dactylifera L.) in perspective of Bangladesh. *American Journal of Life Sciences*, 3(4): 274–278.

Pascale, A., Marchesi, N., Marelli, C., Coppola, A., Luzi, L., Govoni, S., Giustina, A. and Gazzaruso, C. (2018). Microbiota and metabolic diseases. *Endocrine*, 61(3): 357–371.

Pérez-Jiménez, J., Neveu, V., Vos, F. and Scalbert, A. (2010). Identification of the 100 richest dietary sources of polyphenols: an application of the Phenol-Explorer database. *European Journal of Clinical Nutrition*, 64(3): S112–S120.

Pistollato, F., Sumalla Cano, S., Elio, I., Masias Vergara, M., Giampieri, F. and Battino, M. (2016). Role of gut microbiota and nutrients in amyloid formation and pathogenesis of Alzheimer disease. *Nutrition Reviews*, 74(10): 624–634.

Plovier, H., Everard, A., Druart, C., Depommier, C., Van Hul, M., Geurts, L., Chilloux, J., Ottman, N., Duparc, T. and Lichtenstein, L. (2017). A purified membrane protein from Akkermansia muciniphila or the pasteurized bacterium improves metabolism in obese and diabetic mice. *Nature Medicine*, 23(1): 107–113.

Puddu, A., Sanguineti, R., Montecucco, F. and Viviani, G. L. (2014). Evidence for the gut microbiota short-chain fatty acids as key pathophysiological molecules improving diabetes. *Mediators of Inflammation*, 2014: 162021.

Qin, J., Li, Y., Cai, Z., Li, S., Zhu, J., Zhang, F., Liang, S., Zhang, W., Guan, Y., Shen, D., Peng, Y., Zhang, D., Jie, Z., Wu, W., Qin, Y., Xue, W., Li, J., Han, L., Lu, D. and Wang, J. (2012). A metagenome-wide association study of gut microbiota in type 2 diabetes. *Nature*, 490(7418): 55–60.

Rajkumar, H., Mahmood, N., Kumar, M., Varikuti, S.R., Challa, H.R. and Myakala, S.P. (2014). Effect of probiotic (VSL#3) and omega-3 on lipid profile, insulin sensitivity, inflammatory markers, and gut colonization in overweight adults: a randomized, controlled trial. *Mediators of Inflammation*, 2014: 348959.

Rajoka, M.S.R., Shi, J., Mehwish, H.M., Zhu, J., Li, Q., Shao, D., Huang, Q., Yang, H. and Wellness, H. (2017). Interaction between diet composition and gut microbiota and its impact on gastrointestinal tract health. *Food Science*, 6(3): 121–130.

Rastelli, M., Knauf, C. and Cani, P.D. (2018). Gut microbes and health: A focus on the mechanisms linking microbes, obesity, and related disorders. *Obesity*, 26(5): 792–800.

Reigstad, C.S., Salmonson, C.E., Rainey, J.F.III, Szurszewski, J.H., Linden, D.R., Sonnenburg, J.L., Farrugia, G. and Kashyap, P.C. (2015). Gut microbes promote colonic serotonin production through an effect of short-chain fatty acids on enterochromaffin cells. *The FASEB Journal*, 29(4): 1395–1403.

Respondek, F., Swanson, K.S., Belsito, K.R., Vester, B.M., Wagner, A., Istasse, L. and Diez, M. (2008). Short-chain fructooligosaccharides influence insulin sensitivity and gene expression of fat tissue in obese dogs. *The Journal of Nutrition*, 138(9): 1712–1718.

Ridlon, J.M. and Hylemon, P.B. (2012). Identification and characterization of two bile acid coenzyme A transferases from Clostridium scindens, a bile acid 7α-dehydroxylating intestinal bacterium. *Journal of Lipid Research*, 53(1): 66–76.

Roopchand, D.E., Carmody, R.N., Kuhn, P., Moskal, K., Rojas-Silva, P., Turnbaugh, P.J. and Raskin, I. (2015). Dietary polyphenols promote growth of the gut bacterium Akkermansia muciniphila and attenuate high fat diet-induced metabolic syndrome. *Diabetes*, 64(8): 2847–2858

Russell, W.R., Gratz, S.W., Duncan, S.H., Holtrop, G., Ince, J., Scobbie, L., Duncan, G., Johnstone, A.M., Lobley, G.E. and Wallace, R.J. (2011). High-protein, reduced-carbohydrate weight-loss diets promote metabolite profiles likely to be detrimental to colonic health. *American Journal of Clinical Nutrition*, 93(5): 1062–1072.

Salazar, N., Dewulf, E.M., Neyrinck, A.M., Bindels, L.B., Cani, P.D., Mahillon, J., de Vos, W.M., Thissen, J.-P., Gueimonde, M., de los Reyes-Gavilán, C.G. and Delzenne, N.M. (2015). Inulin-type fructans modulate intestinal Bifidobacterium species populations and decrease fecal short-chain fatty acids in obese women. *Clinical Nutrition*, 34(3): 501–507.

Sanna, S., van Zuydam, N.R., Mahajan, A., Kurilshikov, A., Vila, A.V., Võsa, U., Mujagic, Z., Masclee, A.A., Jonkers, D.M. and Oosting, M. (2019). Causal relationships among the gut microbiome, short-chain fatty acids and metabolic diseases. *Nature Genetics*, 51(4): 600–605.

Santacruz, A., Collado, M.C., García-Valdés, L., Segura, M.T., Marítn-Lagos, J.A., Anjos, T., Martí-Romero, M., Lopez, R.M., Florido, J., Campoy, C. and Sanz, Y. (2010). Gut microbiota composition is associated with body weight, weight gain and biochemical parameters in pregnant women. *British Journal of Nutrition*, 104(1): 83–92.

Sayin, S.I., Wahlström, A., Felin, J., Jäntti, S., Marschall, H.-U., Bamberg, K., Angelin, B., Hyötyläinen, T., Orešič, M. and Bäckhed, F. (2013). Gut microbiota regulates bile acid metabolism by reducing the levels of tauro-beta-muricholic acid, a naturally occurring fxr antagonist. *Cell Metabolism*, 17(2): 225–235.

Schmitt, J., Kong, B., Stieger, B., Tschopp, O., Schultze, S.M., Rau, M., Weber, A., Müllhaupt, B., Guo, G.L. and Geier, A. (2015). Protective effects of farnesoid X receptor (FXR) on hepatic lipid accumulation are mediated by hepatic FXR and independent of intestinal FGF15 signal. *Liver International*, 35(4): 1133–1144.

Schnorr, S.L., Candela, M., Rampelli, S., Centanni, M., Consolandi, C., Basaglia, G., Turroni, S., Biagi, E., Peano, C. and Severgnini, M. (2014). Gut microbiome of the Hadza hunter-gatherers. *Nature Communications*, 5(1): 1–12.

Schwingshackl, L., Christoph, M. and Hoffmann, G. (2015). Effects of olive oil on markers of inflammation and endothelial function—A systematic review and meta-analysis. *Nutrients*, 7(9): 7651–7675.

Sears, C.L. (2005). A dynamic partnership: celebrating our gut flora. *Anaerobe*, 11(5): 247–251.

Sedwick, C. (2014). A novel regulatory T cell population in the gut. *PLoS Biol*, 12(4): e1001834.

Sekirov, I., Russell, S.L., Antunes, L.C.M. and Finlay, B.B. (2010). Gut microbiota in health and disease. *Physiological Reviews*, 90(3): 859–904.

Selma, M.V., Beltrán, D., Luna, M.C., Romo-Vaquero, M., García-Villalba, R., Mira, A., Espín, J.C. and Tomás-Barberán, F.A. (2017). Isolation of human intestinal bacteria capable of producing the bioactive metabolite isourolithin a from ellagic acid. *Frontiers in Microbiology* 8(1521).

Shang, H., Sun, J. and Chen, Y.Q. (2016). Clostridium butyricum CGMCC0313. 1 modulates lipid profile, insulin resistance and colon homeostasis in obese mice. *PLoS ONE*, 11(4): e0154373.

Sharon, G., Sampson, T.R., Geschwind, D.H. and Mazmanian, S.K. (2016). The central nervous system and the gut microbiome. *Cell*, 167(4): 915–932.

Shen, J., Obin, M.S. and Zhao, L. (2013). The gut microbiota, obesity and insulin resistance. *Molecular Aspects of Medicine*, 34(1): 39–58.

Shen, J., Zuo, Z.-X. and Mao, A.P. (2014). Effect of probiotics on inducing remission and maintaining therapy in ulcerative colitis, Crohn's disease, and pouchitis: meta-analysis of randomized controlled trials. *Inflammatory Bowel Diseases*, 20(1): 21–35.

Sherwin, E., Dinan, T.G. and Cryan, J.F. (2018). Recent developments in understanding the role of the gut microbiota in brain health and disease. *Annals of the New York Academy of Sciences*, 1420(1): 5–25.

Shi, X., Zhou, F., Li, X., Chang, B., Li, D., Wang, Y., Tong, Q., Xu, Y., Fukuda, M., Zhao, J. J., Li, D., Burrin, D.G., Chan, L. and Guan, X. (2013). Central GLP-2 enhances hepatic insulin sensitivity via activating PI3K signaling in POMC neurons. *Cell Metabolism*, 18(1): 86–98.

Silva, Y.P., Bernardi, A. and Frozza, R.L. (2020). The role of short-chain fatty acids from gut microbiota in gut-brain communication. *Frontiers in Endocrinology*, 11: 25.

Singh, A.K., Cabral, C., Kumar, R., Ganguly, R., Rana, H.K., Gupta, A., Lauro, M.R., Carbone, C., Reis, F. and Pandey, A.K. (2019). Beneficial effects of dietary polyphenols on gut microbiota and strategies to improve delivery efficiency. *Nutrients*, 11(9).

Singh, R.K., Chang, H.-W., Yan, D., Lee, K.M., Ucmak, D., Wong, K., Abrouk, M., Farahnik, B., Nakamura, M. and Zhu, T.H. (2017). Influence of diet on the gut microbiome and implications for human health. *Journal of Translational Medicine*, 15(1): 73.

Skelly, A.N., Sato, Y., Kearney, S. and Honda, K. (2019). Mining the microbiota for microbial and metabolite-based immunotherapies. *Nature Reviews Immunology*, 19(5): 305–323.

Slavin, J. (2013). Fiber and prebiotics: Mechanisms and health benefits. *Nutrients*, 5(4): 1417–1435.

Sokol, H., Leducq, V., Aschard, H., Pham, H.-P., Jegou, S., Landman, C., Cohen, D., Liguori, G., Bourrier, A. and Nion-Larmurier, I. (2017). Fungal microbiota dysbiosis in IBD. *Gut*, 66(6): 1039–1048.

Sommer, F. and Bäckhed, F. (2013). The gut microbiota masters of host development and physiology. *Nature Reviews Microbiology*, 11(4): 227–238.

Sprong, R., Schonewille, A. and Van der Meer, R.J. (2010). Dietary cheese whey protein protects rats against mild dextran sulfate sodium–induced colitis: Role of mucin and microbiota. *Journal of Dairy Science*, 93(4): 1364–1371.

Sudo, N. (2012). Role of microbiome in regulating the HPA axis and its relevance to allergy. In: *Allergy and the Nervous System*, Volume 98, 163–175. Karger Publishers.

Sudo, N. (2016). The hypothalamic-pituitary-adrenal axis and gut microbiota: A target for dietary intervention? In: *The Gut-Brain Axis* (ed. N. Hyland and C. Stanton), 293–304. Elsevier.

Sudo, N. (2019). Role of gut microbiota in brain function and stress-related pathology. *Bioscience of Microbiota, Food, and Health*, 38(3): 75–80.

Sudo, N., Chida, Y., Aiba, Y., Sonoda, J., Oyama, N., Yu, X.N., Kubo, C. and Koga, Y. (2004). Postnatal microbial colonization programs the hypothalamic–pituitary–adrenal system for stress response in mice. *The Journal of Physiology*, 558(1): 263–275.

Suez, J., Korem, T., Zeevi, D., Zilberman-Schapira, G., Thaiss, C.A., Maza, O., Israeli, D., Zmora, N., Gilad, S. and Weinberger, A.J.N. (2014). Artificial sweeteners induce glucose intolerance by altering the gut microbiota. *Nature*, 514(7521): 181–186.

Syakila, R.N., Lim, S.M., Agatonovic-Kustrin, S., Lim, F.T. and Ramasamy, K. (2019). In vitro assessment of pediococci-and lactobacilli-induced cholesterol-lowering effect using digitally enhanced high-performance thin-layer chromatography and confocal microscopy. *Analytical*, 411(6): 1181–1192.

Tang, W.H.W. and Hazen, S.L. (2017). Microbiome, trimethylamine N-oxide, and cardiometabolic disease. *Translational Research*, 179: 108–115.

Toral, M., Romero, M., Rodríguez-Nogales, A., Jiménez, R., Robles-Vera, I., Algieri, F., Chueca-Porcuna, N., Sánchez, M., de la Visitación, N., Olivares, M., García, F., Pérez-Vizcaíno, F., Gálvez, J. and Duarte, J. (2018). Lactobacillus fermentum improves tacrolimus-induced hypertension by restoring vascular redox state and improving eNOS coupling. *Molecular Nutrition and Food Research*, 62(14): 1–41.

Torres-Fuentes, C., Golubeva, A.V., Zhdanov, A.V., Wallace, S., Arboleya, S., Papkovsky, D.B., Aidy, S.E., Ross, P., Roy, B.L. and Stanton, C.J.T.F.J. (2019). Short-chain fatty acids and microbiota metabolites attenuate ghrelin receptor signaling. *The FASEB Journal*, 33(12): 13546–13559.

Tseng, C.-H. and Wu, C.-Y. (2019). The gut microbiome in obesity. *Journal of the Formosan Medical Association*, 118: S3–S9.

Tsigos, C. and Chrousos, G.P. (2002). Hypothalamic–pituitary–adrenal axis, neuroendocrine factors and stress. *Journal of Psychosomatic Research*, 53(4): 865–871.

Turnbaugh, P.J., Ley, R.E., Mahowald, M.A., Magrini, V., Mardis, E.R. and Gordon, J.I. (2006). An obesity-associated gut microbiome with increased capacity for energy harvest. *Nature*, 444(7122): 1027–1031.

Urwin, H.J., Miles, E.A., Noakes, P.S., Kremmyda, L.-S., Vlachava, M., Diaper, N.D., Godfrey, K.M., Calder, P.C., Vulevic, J. and Yaqoob, P. (2014). Effect of salmon consumption during pregnancy on maternal and infant faecal microbiota, secretory IgA and calprotectin. *British Journal of Nutrition*, 111(5): 773–784.

Uzal, F.A., Navarro, M.A., Li, J., Freedman, J.C., Shrestha, A. and McClane, B.A. (2018). Comparative pathogenesis of enteric clostridial infections in humans and animals. *Anaerobe*, 53: 11–20.

Vallianou, N., Stratigou, T., Christodoulatos, G.S. and Dalamaga, M. (2019). Understanding the role of the gut microbiome and microbial metabolites in obesity and obesity-associated metabolic disorders: Current evidence and perspectives. *Current Obesity Reports*, 8(3): 317–332.

Wang, P.X., Deng, X.R., Zhang, C.H. and Yuan, H.J. (2020). Gut microbiota and metabolic syndrome. *Chinese Medical Journal*, 133(7): 808–816.

Wang, Y., Wu, Y., Wang, Y., Xu, H., Mei, X., Yu, D., Wang, Y. and Li, W. (2017). Antioxidant properties of probiotic bacteria. *Nutrients*, 9(5).

Warmbrunn, M.V., Herrema, H., Aron-Wisnewsky, J., Soeters, M.R., Van Raalte, D.H. and Nieuwdorp, M. (2020). Gut microbiota: a promising target against cardiometabolic diseases. *Expert Review of Endocrinology and Metabolism*, 15(1): 13–27.

Wei, X., Yang, Z., Rey, F.E., Ridaura, V.K., Davidson, N.O., Gordon, J.I. and Semenkovich, C.F. (2012). Fatty acid synthase modulates intestinal barrier function through palmitoylation of mucin 2. *Cell Host and Microbe*, 11(2): 140–152.

Weickert, M., Möhlig, M., Schöfl, C., Arafat, A., Otto, B., Viehoff, H., Koebnick, C., Kohl, A., Spranger, J. and Pfeiffer, A. (2006). Cereal fiber improves whole-body insulin. *Diabetes Care*, 29(4): 773–780.

Wexler, H.M. (2007). Bacteroides: the good, the bad, and the nitty-gritty. *Clinical Microbiology Reviews*, 20(4): 593–621.

Wostmann, B.S., Larkin, C., Moriarty, A. and Bruckner-Kardoss, E. (1983). Dietary intake, energy metabolism, and excretory losses of adult male germfree Wistar rats. *Laboratory Animal Science*, 33(1): 46–50.

Wrzosek, L., Miquel, S., Noordine, M.-L., Bouet, S., Chevalier-Curt, M.J., Robert, V., Philippe, C., Bridonneau, C., Cherbuy, C. and Robbe-Masselot, C. (2013). Bacteroides thetaiotaomicron and Faecalibacterium prausnitzii influence the production of mucus glycans and the development of goblet cells in the colonic epithelium of a gnotobiotic model rodent. *BMC Biology*, 11(1): 1–13.

Wu, F., Guo, X., Zhang, M., Ou, Z., Wu, D., Deng, L., Lu, Z., Zhang, J., Deng, G., Chen, S., Li, S., Yi, J. and Peng, Y. (2020). An Akkermansia muciniphila subtype alleviates high-fat diet-induced metabolic disorders and inhibits the neurodegenerative process in mice. *Anaerobe*, 61(102138).

Wu, G.D., Chen, J., Hoffmann, C., Bittinger, K., Chen, Y.-Y., Keilbaugh, S.A., Bewtra, M., Knights, D., Walters, W.A. and Knight, R. (2011). Linking long-term dietary patterns with gut microbial enterotypes. *Science*, 334(6052): 105–108.

Wu, T.R., Lin, C.S., Chang, C.J., Lin, T.L., Martel, J., Ko, Y.F., Ojcius, D.M., Lu, C.C., Young, J.D. and Lai, H.C.J.G. (2019). Gut commensal Parabacteroides goldsteinii plays a predominant role in the anti-obesity effects of polysaccharides isolated from Hirsutella sinensis. *Gut*, 68(2): 248–262.

Wu, W.K., Ivanova, E.A. and Orekhov, A.N. (2020). Gut microbiome: A possible common therapeutic target for treatment of atherosclerosis and cancer. *Seminars in Cancer Biology*, 70: 85–97.

Yan, F., Li, N., Shi, J., Li, H., Yue, Y., Jiao, W., Wang, N., Song, Y., Huo, G. and Li, B. (2019). *Lactobacillus acidophilus* alleviates type 2 diabetes by regulating hepatic glucose, lipid metabolism and gut microbiota in mice. *Food and Function*, 10(9): 5804–5815.

Yang, C., Wang, Y., Marty, J.L. and Yang, X.J.B. (2011). Aptamer-based colorimetric biosensing of Ochratoxin A using unmodified gold nanoparticles indicator. *Biosensors*, 26(5): 2724–2727.

Yang, Y.J. and Sheu, B.S. (2012). Probiotics-containing yogurts suppress Helicobacter pylori load and modify immune response and intestinal microbiota in the Helicobacter pylori-infected children. *Helicobacter*, 17(4): 297–304.

Yang, Y., Gu, H., Sun, Q. and Wang, J. (2018). Effects of Christensenella minuta lipopolysaccharide on RAW 264.7 macrophages activation. *Microbial Pathogenesis*, 125: 411–417.

Yelin, I., Flett, K.B., Merakou, C., Mehrotra, P., Stam, J., Snesrud, E., Hinkle, M., Lesho, E., McGann, P. and McAdam, A.J. (2019). Genomic and epidemiological evidence of bacterial transmission from probiotic capsule to blood in ICU patients. *Nature Medicine*, 25(11): 1728–1732.

Yoo, J.Y. and Kim, S.S. (2016). Probiotics and prebiotics: Present status and future perspectives on metabolic disorders. *Nutrients*, 8(3): 1–20.

Zhai, Q., Feng, S., Arjan, N. and Chen, W. (2019). A next generation probiotic, Akkermansia muciniphila. *Critical Reviews in Food Science*, 59(19): 3227–3236.

Zhang, Y. and Zhang, H. (2013). Microbiota associated with type 2 diabetes and its related complications. *Food Science and Human Wellness*, 2(3): 167–172.

18

Overall Safety Considerations and Regulatory Oversight for Probiotics-based Foods and Beverages

Sushil Koirala, Sarina Pradhan Thapa and Anil Kumar Anal

Department of Food, Agriculture, and Bioresources, School of Environment, Resources, and Development, Asian Institute of Technology, Pathumthani, Thailand

18.1 Introduction

The knowledge, attitude and perception of consumers have significantly increased with time on healthier food. Lifestyle-related diseases such as cardiovascular disease, stroke, diabetes and cancers are on the rise and this has prompted consumers to investigate food beyond basic nutrition. Thus, stakeholders in food systems (food scientists, food manufacturers and academia) must produce innovative foods that break away from the conventional approach. One way of doing that can be adding value to the food and making it more functional. Functional foods are superfoods that provide health benefits beyond basic nutrition. One of the first probiotic fermented dairy beverages was Yakult, which contains the probiotic *Lactobacillus casei* Shirota. Yakult trades at an average €4.79 per liter in Europe, while in contrast regular yoghurt can be purchased at as little as €0.75 per liter, confirming what innovations with probiotics in food can do to your business with significantly higher profit margins (Katan 2012). Probiotics also present fewer food safety risks compared to other functional foods (Anal 2019). Common functional foods present in the consumer market domain include probiotics, prebiotics, dietary supplements, vitamins, antioxidants, dietary fiber and other phytochemicals (Anal and Singh 2007; Annunziata and Vecchio 2013; Cencic and Chingwaru 2010; Corbo *et al.* 2014; Granato *et al.* 2020; Koirala and Anal 2021; Kumaree *et al.* 2015).

Among these future foods, probiotic-based functional foods have wider acceptability among consumers due to their long history of safe use, clinical evidence of potential benefits, prevention of foodborne illness, and isolation from healthy gut microbiome (Anal *et al.* 2021; Shi *et al.* 2016). The popularity of probiotics among consumers is reflected in its global market value of USD 42.55 billion in 2017 that is expected to reach USD 74.69 billion by 2024, according to the study by Fortune Business Insights (Figure 18.1). The global paradigm is shifting towards Asia and the Pacific region, which leads when it comes to market

Probiotics, Prebiotics and Synbiotics: Technological Advancements Towards Safety and Industrial Applications, First Edition. Edited by Parmjit Singh Panesar and Anil Kumar Anal.

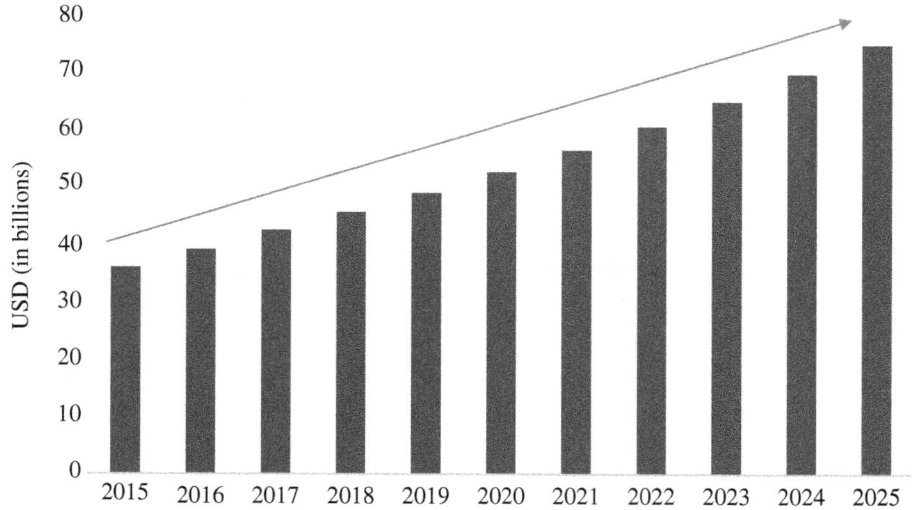

Figure 18.1 Global probiotics market size, 2015–2025. *Source:* Adapted from Fortune Business Insights (2020).

domination of probiotic-based foods, while in Europe regulations with regards to health claims have slowed its growth (Yilmaz-Ersan *et al.* 2020).

Probiotics are live microorganisms that confer health benefits to the host when consumed in an adequate amount. According to the FAO/WHO Expert Consultation (2000), two things can be outlined for probiotics: (i) they are viable microorganisms; and (ii) they exert beneficial effects on host health (Hill *et al.* 2014).

Traditionally fermented foods such as such as yoghurt, fermented milk, chocolate, cereals, dietary supplements and drugs have been known to contain probiotic microorganisms which are available in a wide variety of food products (Araújo *et al.* 2012; Guimarães *et al.* 2020; Kalicka *et al.* 2019; Linares *et al.* 2017; Reid 2015; Roobab *et al.* 2020; Tomar 2019; Zucko *et al.* 2020). Probiotics also offer a legal advantage over other food ingredients with health claims as they are highly patentable, unlike other functional foods. However, the chances of producing new bacterial strains are low with the highly competitive probiotic market. Therefore manufacturers have been stressing the uniqueness of their probiotic strains by giving them different names such as *Lactobacillus immunitas* or *Lactobacillus defensis* (Katan 2012). *Lactobacillus* and *Bifidobacterium* are the most widely found microbial probiotic species in the market (Granato *et al.* 2010; Hekmat and Reid 2006), while next generation probiotics (NGP) that are associated with gut health (Bacteroides, *Faecalibacterium, Clostridium* and *Akkermansia*) are fast entering the global market (Saarela 2019).

Probiotic strains for foods and beverages must be safe for human consumption. Lactic acid bacteria (LAB: *Lactococcus* and *Lactobacillus*) have been classified as generally recognized as safe (GRAS) (Wassenaar and Klein 2008). Having said that, some strains have been found to be opportunistic causing infections (Cannon *et al.* 2005; Gasser 1994). Various factors must be taken into consideration such as origin, nature, pathogenicity, virulome factors, antibiotic resistance genes, infections, and administration process to assure safety of probiotics in food application (Akbar *et al.* 2019; de Simone 2019; Kalhoro *et al.* 2019). While safety is of paramount significance, regulatory frameworks should also be meticulously drafted, updated and regulated considering the intended use of probiotic foods, demographic conditions, consumer behavior and market dynamics (Melchor *et al.* 2019). This chapter focuses on two aspects of probiotics, the first being overall safety, and the second the regulatory framework with some relevant examples.

18.2 Safety Considerations

For a healthy population, probiotics are generally considered to be safe. However, this statement cannot be claimed universally until proper safety and efficacy tests are conducted (Kothari *et al.* 2019). According to a World Health Organization (WHO) report, food poisoning accounts for an estimated 420 000 deaths per year (WHO 2015). This is because food not only acts as a vehicle for nutrients delivery but also for the favorable growth of pathogenic microorganisms. Given the growing interest of consumers in probiotics as the future, research into the genetic components of probiotic strains can have tremendous advantages in eliminating incidences of food poisoning (Terpou *et al.* 2019). It will certainly give insights into how specific probiotic genes can suppress the gene expression and survival of foodborne pathogens, and their toxins, which may give new insights on the propensities and safety of probiotics as future foods (Bian *et al.* 2016; Markowiak and Śliżewska 2017). Overall safety considerations for the selection and application of a probiotic strain in food application are schematically shown in Figure 18.2.

18.2.1 Non-pathogenicity

The probiotic strain used in foods and beverages must be non-pathogenic and should not pose a risk to the host (Khaneghah *et al.* 2020). In the USA, *Lactobacillus* species are commonly classified as Generally Recognized As Safe (GRAS), regulated by the Food and Drug Administration (FDA). In Europe, the conceptual framework of Qualified Presumption of

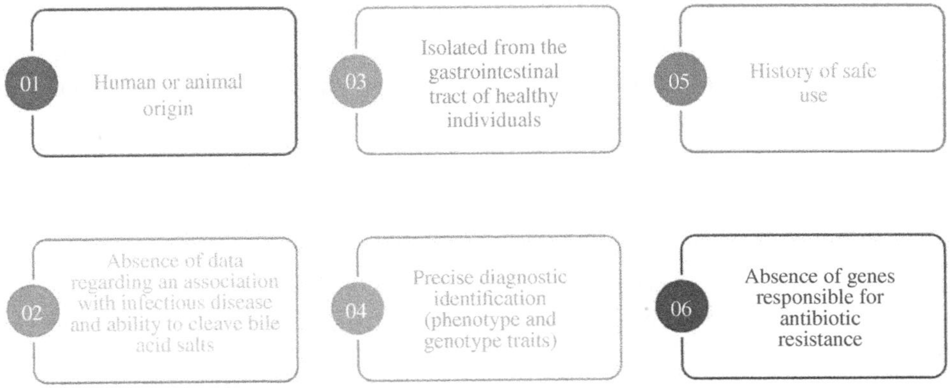

Figure 18.2 Selection criteria for probiotic microorganisms for food application.

Table 18.1 Probiotic microorganisms with long history of safe use.

As a food additive	As a pharmaceutical product
*Lactobacillus acidophilus**	*Lactobacillus amylovorus**
*Lactobacillus casei**	*Lactobacillus casei**
*Lactobacillus gasseri**	*Lactobacillus johnsonii**
*Lactobacillus helveticus**	*Lactobacillus pentosus**
*Lactobacillus reuteri**	*Lactobacillus plantarum**
*Lactobacillus rhamnosus**	*Lactobacillus rhamnosus**
Bifidobacterium adolescentis	*Bifidobacterium breve*
*Bifidobacterium animalis**	*Lactococcus lactis**
Bifidobacterium bifidum	
Bifidobacterium infantis	
*Bifidobacterium longum**	
Enterococcus faecium	
Streptococcus thermophilus	
Bacillus clausii	
Escherichia coli Nissle 1917	
Saccharomyces cerevisiae (boulardii)	

* Qualified Presumption of Safety (QPS) approved.

Safety (QPS) was introduced with additional criteria on transfer of antibiotic resistance genes and history of long use (Markowiak and Śliżewska 2017). More recently, authorities and regulatory bodies have been considerate on history of long use. This makes sense as the safety of these strains is supported by their existence as normal commensals and inhabitants of mammalian flora. The most commonly used probiotics in food application based on the history of safe use are listed in Table 18.1. The FAO/WHO (2002) has theoretically outlined some of the side-effects that may be possible with probiotics in food, which include: (i) systemic infections; (ii) deleterious metabolic activities; (iii) excessive immune stimulation in susceptible individuals; and (iv) gene transfer.

The population most at risk of these infections includes those with weak immune system, dysbiosis and gut–intestinal issues (Peivasteh-Roudsari *et al.* 2019). Hence, it is important to carefully assess the pathogenicity of probiotic strains for food application.

Some studies have been conducted on assessing the pathogenicity of probiotic strains. The study conducted by Cannon *et al.* (2005) with over 200 cases of *Lactobacillus* infections reported cases of bacteremia and endocarditis in the species *casei* and *rhamnosus*. Back in 1990s, Saxelin *et al.* (1996) conducted a 4-year study on the safety assessment of *Lactobacillus* to detect the presence of bacteremia in southern Finland. *Lactobacillus* was identified in eight patients among 3317 blood culture isolates, of which five had a severe bacteremic complication. However, some of the opportunistic infections associated with probiotics are strain-specific and not species-specific. To prove non-pathogenicity, strain-specific evidence is required to establish the claim (Wassenaar and Klein 2008).

In order to prove non-pathogenicity of probiotic bacteria in foods and beverages, the following factors should be taken into consideration (Bernardeau *et al.* 2006).

1) Production of toxin.
2) Survivability in the bloodstream.
3) Host susceptibility.
4) Host resistance.
5) Presence of bacterial virulence factors.
6) Ability of intracellular growth.
7) Replication in the bloodstream.
8) Invasive and translocation attributes.
9) Antibiotic resistance.
10) Ability to acquire foreign DNA.

18.2.2 Virulome Factors

Virulome factors are bacterial associated genes to affect eukaryotic cells by invasion, colonization, immune evasion, suppression of host immune response, and acquisition of nutrition from the host (Wassenaar *et al.* 2015). In order to trace such virulome factors in a given probiotic, whole genome sequencing is essential for safety considerations. Acceptability rests on the complete absence of such genes. However, proving virulence genes in a probiotic strain for food application poses two notable threats. First, the characterization of virulome factors is not yet scientifically understood. For example, the virulence (pathogenicity) of *Campylobacter jejuni* is still unknown (Wassenaar and Blaser 1999). Second, the distinction between colonization and virulence between probiotics and opportunistic pathogens is difficult to distinguish in the gut, which makes it hard to distinguish between probiotic and disease-causing properties (Wassenaar and Klein 2008).

Pieniz *et al.* (2015) evaluated the presence of virulence factors in *Enterococcus durans* LAB18s isolated from frescal cheese. The presence of virulence factors such as adhesion, aggregation and biofilm formation was studied using polymerase chain reaction (PCR) technology. However, the authors reported absence of all tested virulence factors, suggesting the safety of this strain for application in food products. Wassenaar *et al.* (2015) evaluated a probiotic product, Symbioflor2 (DSM 17252) consisting of six different *Escherichia coli,* for virulence factors, only to report several such genes. It is important to note that this virulence did not account to pathogenicity. A 10-year study conducted by Binnewies *et al.* (2006) reported the complete absence of virulence genes is quite common in commensals after complete study of bacterial genomes. Thus, absence of virulence genes is a factor that cannot be overlooked for probiotic-based foods and beverages.

18.2.3 Absence of Antibiotic Resistance

Antibiotic resistance (ABR) is a global health problem due to the indiscriminate use of antibiotics in human and veterinary medicine (Saarela 2019; Saarela *et al.* 2000; Thapa *et al.* 2020). The resistance is due to the ability of bacteria to resist a medication that was once effective against them (D'Costa *et al.* 2011). It is very important to be vigilant that these resistant bacteria are avoided in probiotics for food applications, though the effect on the host is still unclear. Proving the absence of antibiotic resistance in a given bacterial strain is relatively straightforward when compared to the complexities involved with proving absence of virulence factors. The assessment of minimum inhibitory concentration (MIC) is a routine standardized procedure, and evidence for antibiotic resistance genes can be detected by molecular methods.

According to the FAO/WHO (2002) and EFSA (2005) report on guidelines on evaluation of safety of probiotics in food, the following considerations must be taken into account before commercial use of a strain:

1) Screening of the microorganism (strain isolation and identification).
2) Transmissibility of antimicrobial genes.
3) Presence of virulome genes.
4) Toxicological studies.
5) In vitro screening for probiotic potential.
6) In vivo human and animal studies.
7) Product formulation and labeling.

18.3 Regulatory Framework and Labeling Claims Associated with Probiotic-based Foods and Beverages

Probiotic-based foods and beverages can be found in abundance in the market these days due to rising consumer awareness of functional foods that ultimately promote gastrointestinal health and positively affect the whole body. Food products labeled as probiotic can be found on shelves all over the world. However, misuse of the term "probiotic" on foods and beverages has started to take place (Koirala and Anal 2021). This is where regulatory bodies need to step in to ensure that what food manufacturers are selling is authentic and considerate to the consumers.

Generally, probiotics are classified as a "drug" or "dietary supplement" depending on the intended use and claims. Probiotics are classified as a "drug" when a health claim is made for treatment, therapy, prevention or diagnosis, and "drug" regulation may be applied in such conditions (Melchor *et al.* 2019). However, most probiotics in the market do not make specific health claims because of the various complexities associated with the clinical trials it has go through to make such a claim. Hence, most of those probiotics that are added to food directly or in capsules, pills, etc., are all broadly classified as dietary or food supplements (de Simone 2019). This label is very enticing as it is very appealing to the consumer and can immediately boost the market share of a company.

Around the world, countries have enacted laws and frameworks that include labeling requirements, claims permitted, penalties, and closures of business in order to protect consumers from misleading claims. Some of the countries with an assigned regulatory body for the regulation of probiotic-based foods and beverages in the market is presented in Table 18.2. The goal is to maintain the homeostasis in the market in terms of probiotic-based foods and beverages regulation with stringent laws and policies (Arora and Baldi 2015; Venugopalan *et al.* 2010).

Table 18.2 Probiotic food and beverage categorization across the globe.

Serial number	Country	Category	Regulatory authority	References
1.	USA	a) Drugs b) Dietary supplements c) Biological product d) Live therapeutic agent e) Medical food	Food and Drug Administration (FDA) Dietary Supplement Health and Education Act (DSHEA) Biologic License Application (BLA) Food and Drug Administration (FDA) Dietary Supplement Health and Education Act (DSHEA)	FDA (2015) FDA (2006) Maughan *et al.* (2004) Degnan (2008) Arora and Baldi (2015); Degnan (2012)
2.	Europe	a) Functional Food	Functional Food Science in Europe (FUFOSE)	Saxelin (2008)
3.	Japan	a) Probiotics b) Functional foods and nutraceuticals	FAO/WHO Ministry of Health and Welfare (MHLW) Food for Specified Health Use (FOSHU)	Amagase (2008); FAO/WHO, (2002); Nagata and Yamada (2008)
4.	China	a) Functional foods	State Food and Drug Administration (SFDA)	Yang (2016)
5.	Canada	a) Natural health products	Food and Drug Administration (FDA)	Arora and Baldi (2017)
6.	Brazil	a) Functional food	National Health Surveillance Agency Brazil	Frietas (2006)
7.	Thailand	a) Functional food	Thai FDA	FDA (2011)
8.	Malaysia	a) Functional food	Food Safety and Quality Division	Stanton and Emms (2011)
9.	India	a) Functional food b) Drugs	Food Safety and Standards Authority India (FSSAI)	Aggarwal *et al.* (2012); Sharma *et al.* (2013)

Sources: Based on FDA (2015); FDA (2006); Maughan *et al.* (2004); Degnan (2008); Arora and Baldi (2015); Degnan (2012).

The following aspects need to be considered when developing a broad-spectrum framework to develop regulatory policies and labeling claims for probiotic-based foods and beverages:

1) Safety.
2) Efficacy.
3) Market dynamics.
4) International trade and policies.
5) Food laws.
6) Quality control.
7) Health claim regulations.

18.3.1 Key Market Insights

In order to understand the regulatory aspects of probiotic-based foods and beverages, it is necessary to outline the market (Figure 18.3) and distribution channels (Table 18.3) for probiotic-based food products. The global probiotic market share is divided into three sections, with functional foods and beverages covering three-quarters of the total market. The most common probiotic microbes globally are *Lactobacillus* and *Bifidobacterium*.

With more research driving innovation in probiotics, more novel strains are expected in the near future. The major claims for these remain cognitive enhancement and

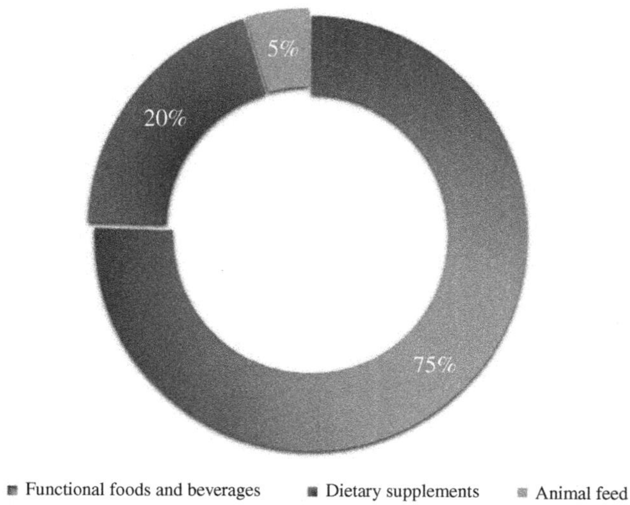

Figure 18.3 Global probiotics market share by application, 2017.

Table 18.3 Global classification of probiotic-based foods and beverages.

Attribute	Details
By microbial genus	*Lactobacillus*
	Bifidobacterium
	Yeast
By application	Functional foods and beverages
	Dietary supplement
	Animal feed
By distribution channel	Pharmacies/health stores
	Supermarkets
	Convenience stores
	Online retail
By geography	North America, Europe, Asia Pacific, South America, Middle East and Africa

strengthening the immune system. In light of this innovation and increasing probiotic research, regulatory frameworks are now becoming more favourable and convenient for sales compared to the past, as consumer preference for healthier foods increases exponentially.

18.3.2 Regional and Country Analysis

Asia Pacific remains the most dominant market for probiotics and probiotic foods and beverages, with market share worth 19 billion USD (Figure 18.4) with China and Japan accounting for half of it, while North America is the most advanced market in terms of consumer space and freedom for manufacturing, sales and consumption of these foods. Consumers are looking for more of these food products with targeted actions and immediate effects.

18.3.2.1 USA

The USA has always been a more liberal and open-minded market when it comes to probiotic-based foods and beverages. This is in part due to the very expensive health care system, dissatisfaction with conventional medical treatments, lack of traditional fermented food products and lower popularity of fermented foods among cosmopolitan societies (Aggarwal *et al.* 2012; Vanderhoof and Young 2008). The major regulatory body for covering probiotic-based foods and beverages in USA is the US Food and Drug Administration (FDA), and the Dietary Supplement Health and Education Act (DSHEA) oversees health and labeling claims for such food products. As per the existing guidelines, probiotic foods are categorized as follows:

1) Dietary supplement: If a probiotic is used as a dietary supplement, then it is considered as "foods" and regulated by the DSHEA/FDA.

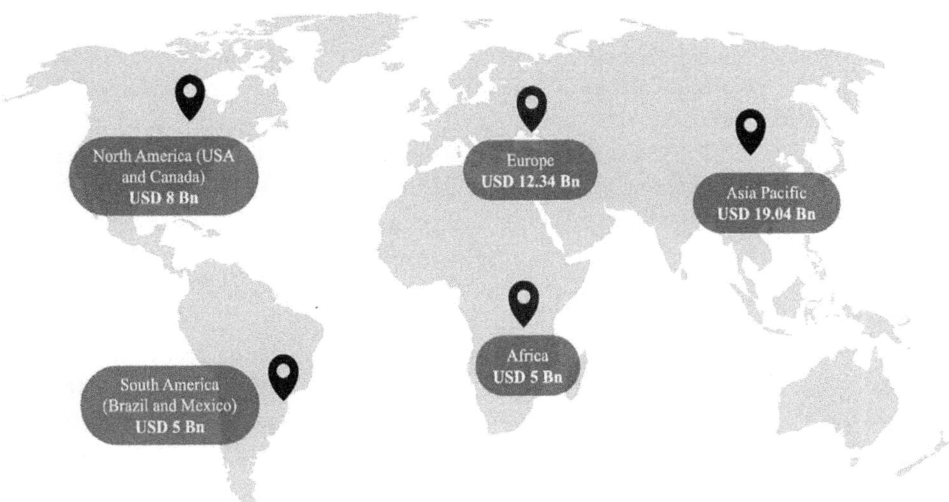

Figure 18.4 World probiotics market share, 2017.

2) Drug: If a probiotic is solely to be used for medical therapeutic purposes, then it is considered as a "drug" and regulated by the FDA.
3) Biological product: For a probiotic to be used as a biological product, approval is necessary via Biologic License Application (BLA) and regulated by the FDA.

The USA does not have a single gold standard or regulation specific to probiotic-based foods and beverages, unlike Europe. As per the definition of a given food product and its intended use, the regulatory body steps in to check the efficacy of specific claims made by the product (Shane *et al.* 2010). The FDA and DSHEA require health claims, nutrient claims and structural claims for probiotics to be used in foods and beverages (Figure 18.5). A petition has to be filed for the health claims that needs a pre-authorization from the FDA (Degnan 2008). Generally, structure and nutrient claims are relatively easier to gain approval from the FDA, as compared to health claims due to the associated test results that need to be submitted to the FDA with clinical trials. Market trail or review among consumers is not necessary for structural and nutrient claims, while it is a must for claims related to health on such food products. Testing, analysis, research, evidence (TARE) is an approach adopted by the FDA based on the recommendation of the Federal Trade Commission (FTC) to produce reliable results while approving these claims. The claims must be substantiated and regulated for any probiotic-based foods and beverages to see the light of the day in the market.

18.3.2.2 Europe

Europe was second to Japan to integrate functional foods and probiotics. Following this, in 1995, Functional Food Science in Europe (FUFOSE) was commissioned by the European Union (EU) to define and regulate functional foods, including probiotics (Stanton *et al.* 2001). Probiotic foods and supplements are regulated under the Food Products Directive and Regulation (regulation 178/2002/EC; directive 2000/13/EU). According to European regulation, all food ingredients including live microbes in probiotics must qualify Qualified Presumption of Safety (QPS) for the safety assessment test (Figure 18.6) (EFSA 2005; Leuschner *et al.* 2010). Also, regulation 1924/2006 from a 2007 guidance document has labeled probiotics under health claim by the European Commission (EC). This means that any probiotic-based food or beverage must prove the health benefits delivered by the probiotic, making it hard for the manufacturers to use the word "probiotic" in the labeling of the food product. Also, probiotics have strain-specific attributes, which is why the health benefits cannot be attributed to an entire genus, hence term "probiotics" cannot per se be used as an object of an authorization as a health claim. Because of these reasons, the term "probiotic" has not been permitted in labeling in the EU since 14 December 2012. It should be noted that some member states have deviated from this interpretation but, in general, this regulation exists all over Europe (Melchor *et al.* 2019). The EC webpage information on the subject of use of the term "probiotic" and nutrition claims states:

> In many Member States, the term 'probiotic' is widely understood as indicating a category of products. This is particularly true of Italy, one of the largest markets in Europe.
>
> After the Regulation (EC) 1924/2006 on nutrition and health claims on foods came into existence, products claiming to be probiotics or to have specific health effects cannot be sold in the EU as use of the term 'probiotic' is considered to be an

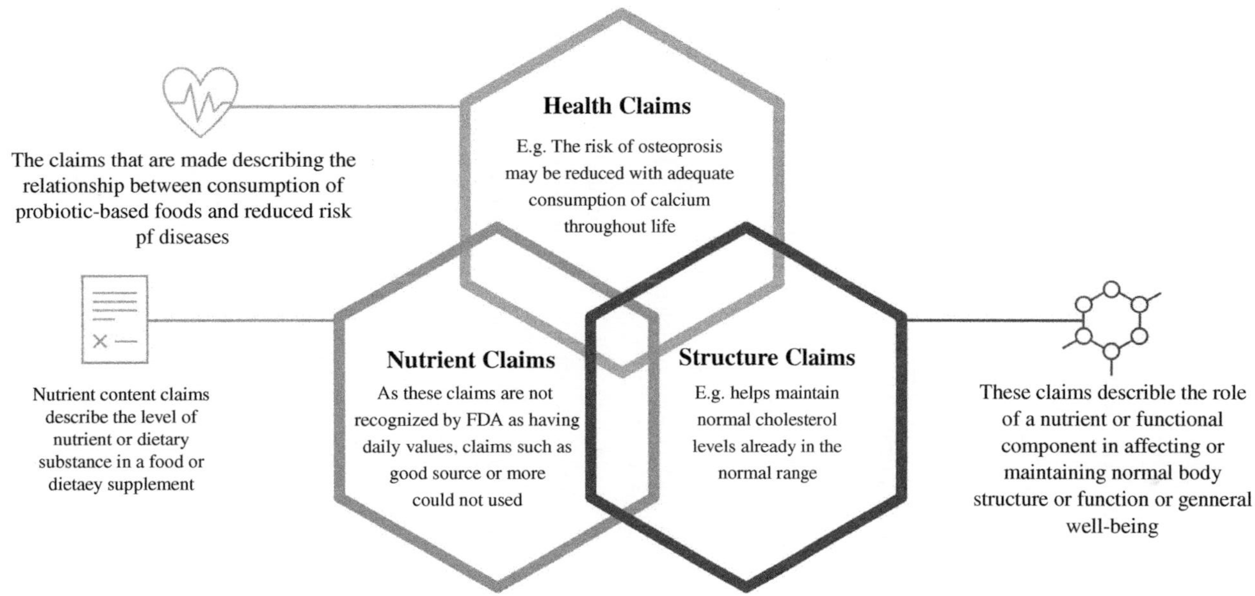

Figure 18.5 Different types of claims regulated by the FDA in the USA for probiotic foods and beverages. *Source:* Based on Koirala and Anal (2021).

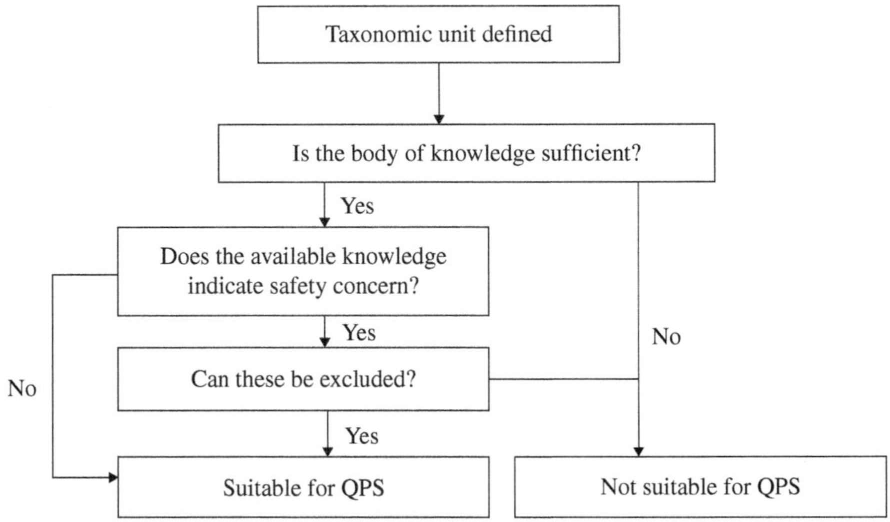

Figure 18.6 Qualified Presumption of Safety (QPS) for safety assessment test. *Source:* Based on EFSA (2005); Leuschner *et al.* (2010).

> unauthorized health claim. According to the Commission, the term implies that a product provides a health benefit, which could be misleading to consumers unless it can be scientifically substantiated (Herman *et al.* 2019).
>
> In spite of many applications having been submitted to the European Food Safety Authority (EFSA), there are no approved health claims for probiotics. As a result, consumers are faced with a label employing the Latin term for a particular strain of bacteria, which is not easily understood and creates confusion rather than clarity" (van Loveren *et al.* 2012).

The European Food Safety Authority (EFSA), as it stands, is the regulatory body along with FUFOSE for functional foods including probiotics in the European market. On 2 December, 2010, EFSA representatives met with food industry stakeholders to discuss health claims made for food that may promote gut health (EFSA-NDA 2011). However, the EFSA rejected all such claims and rather advised negatively to the EC. The EFSA had received almost 3000 health claims by July 2011 and rejected almost 80% of them; even in the 20% of claims approved, none dealt with probiotics (Katan 2012).

18.3.2.3 Japan

Japan is one of the leading countries when it comes to using probiotics as both foods and drugs and became the first to establish regulation on functional foods and nutraceuticals (Japan 1991). The country has established three categories of food that claim health benefits: Foods for Specialized Health Issues (FOSHU), Food with Functional Claims (FFC) and Foods with Nutrient Functional Claims (FNFC) (Figure 18.7).

Foods that fall under the jurisdiction of FOSHU take a minimum of 1 year to be approved which is a scientific review process by a committee. This mandatorily requires statistically

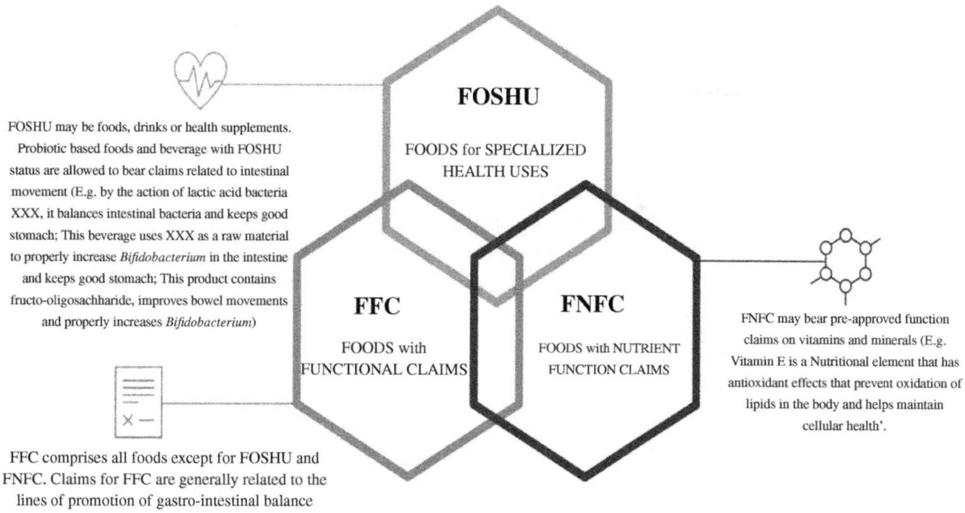

Figure 18.7 Categories of food with health benefit claims in Japan. *Source:* Based on Koirala and Anal (2021).

significant and well-designed epidemiological studies and clinical trials (Japan 2017). Unlike FOSHU, FFC only needs scientific data sourced from clinical trials from human studies and a reputable literature review of the food product (Japan 2013).

18.3.2.4 China

Bifidobacterium animalis and *Bifidus bacterium* are among the list of microorganims that are permitted for food use in the country but there is no law that enacts safety requirements. On the other hand, prebiotic galactooligosaccharides belong to the new food materials category, which has been strictly regulated by the Chinese Ministry of Health.

In general, production of synbiotics is required to adhere to the country's National Food Safety Standards which clearly state that:

1) Conventional foods have the specific ingredient stipulated in the label of the regular foodstuffs.
2) Health foods, on the other hand, are foods that aim to improve bodily functions but not tothe extent of treating a disease.

18.3.2.5 Brazil

As stated in Brazil's Resolution 02 on functional food products, probiotics are classified as food with functional claims, health properties or an isolated probiotic substance. On the other hand, prebiotics can have a claim to have an effect on functional or health properties. On July 2018, a regulation was implemented by the country for both mentioned synbiotics in order to ensure the authenticity and safety of probiotic-based foods and beverages backed by scientific evidence. These are assessed on a case by case basis.

Pre-authorization of application of claims is required to undergo registration with the Brazilian Health Regulatory Agency (ANVISA) through an online petitioning system. The foodstuff registered should follow the guidelines for the analysis and substantiation of functional and health claims in the labeling of foods. The claim is valid as long as there is enough evidence for the safety and efficacy of the food.

The phrase "The (probiotic) (indicated species of the organism) contributes to the balance of the intestinal flora" is the only recently approved standard claim for probiotics in Brazil. In addition, the following species are not considered by ANVISA to have a scientifically proven effect: *Lactobacillus delbrueckii* (subsp. *bulgaricus*), and *Streptococcus salivarius* (subspecies *thermophilus*). Therefore, submitted claims for foodstuffs containing these bacteria are less likely to succeed.

18.3.2.6 Mexico

Mexico does not explicitly regulate and impose safety requirements on the use of probiotics. Mexican general health law categorizes food and food ingredients for health benefits. The Mexican official norm NOM-051-SCFI/SSA1-2010 regulates the usage of food and non-alcoholic drink claims. It allows claims for specific beneficial effects of foods and their constituents in the context of total diet on the normal functions or biological activities of the organism. The claims should relate to a positive correlation for good health. Scientific evidence should support these claims. The claim should represent the nutrient or ingredient and not the product or its brand.

18.3.2.7 India

Probiotics fall into both food and pharmaceutical categories and are regulated depending on their intended use in India. Both food and drugs are currently regulated by the Prevention of Food Adulteration Act (PFA). The Food Safety and Standards Act of 2005 (FSSA) defines foods for particular dietary uses or functional foods, nutraceuticals or health supplements (FSSAI 2016). The FSSAI legally defines functional food categories, such as nutraceuticals or biotherapeutic agent but it is still unclear what these functional foods possess. In addition to this, the PFA regulates labeling and packaging of food products so that necessary information on the food product (ingredients, nutritional information, date of expiry, manufacturer and manufacturing unit details and country of origin and importer) is disclosed to the consumer (Aggarwal *et al.* 2012)

18.3.2.8 Thailand

The use of probiotics in food is documented in notification of the Ministry of Public Health Re: Use of Probiotic Microorganisms in Foods, dated 27 June 2011. The regulatory document defines probiotic microorganisms as viable microbes beneficial to the human body except for biotherapeutic agents, genetically modified microorganisms (GMM), beneficial microorganisms not used in food and others as listed in clause 1.4.1. Clause 2 of the same document states that food that contains probiotic microorganisms must be approved by the Thai Food and Drug Administration (Thai FDA). The Thai FDA has also listed probiotic microorganisms that are permitted to be used in food in the Annex of the same document. The number of viable microbes in such food should be not less than 10^6 CFU/g food at the end of its shelf-life.

Health claims are authorized for probiotic products under the order of the Thai FDA No. 403/2551 (2008) "Consideration for Granting Permission to Make Health Claims for Probiotics in Food Products" if they are backed with scientific evidence sufficient for permission to use these types of claims.

According to the document, health claims mean "a displaying of a picture, photograph, invented mark, mark, trademark, or any statement on the label which is related to the food, food components, or nutrients concerned with health, either directly or indirectly". Based on these, Thailand currently has a stricter approach towards health claims for probiotic-based food products.

18.3.2.9 Malaysia

In the ASEAN region, Malaysia is the only country where nutrition labeling is a requirement. When it comes to health claims, the Malaysian Food Act (1983), enforced by the Food Regulation Act (1983) to implement health and nutrition claims, is the principal legislation covering health and nutrition claims for functional foods. In order to assist with advertisement policies, a guidance document on labeling and claims has also been issued which is in line with Codex Alimentarius guidelines for the same. As in most ASEAN countries, nutrient claims and, more specifically, content claims, comparative claims and nutrient function claims are acceptable.

Functional foods are unofficially defined in Malaysia and still required to follow all of the necessary food regulations. All food and drugs are regulated through a legal system and endorsed by the Food Safety and Quality Division (FSQD), the Drug Control Authority (DCA), the National Pharmaceutical Control Bureau (NPCB) and the Committee for the Classification of Food-Drug Interface Products. All of the laws have been developed referencing the Codex Alimentarius; however, there are no separate guidelines for the probiotic category (Sharma *et al.* 2013). Claims for probiotics are acceptable if they fall into the authorized claims by the Ministry of Health (e.g. "*Bifidobacterium lactis* helps foster a beneficial intestinal environment and may help to reduce the incidence of diarrhea"). The approval of claims involves submission of sufficient scientific evidence (comprised of five clinical trials from recognized countries), while at the same time ensuring that the claims are comprehensible to consumers.

18.3.2.10 Singapore

In Singapore, food regulations are supported by the document "Guide to Food Labelling and Advertisements", which oversees the health claims for foods with probiotic microorganisms. The same regulation, under article 9, states that "Any false or misleading statements, pictures, brands, words or marks purporting to indicate the nature, stability, quantity, strength, purity, composition, weight, origin, age, effects, or proportion of the food or any ingredients are not allowed to be used on food labels and advertisements, unless otherwise specified".

The document permits the claim, "prebiotics promote the growth of good *Bifidus* bacteria to help maintain a healthy digestive system", which is similar to the regulation in Thailand. Companies are also allowed to state that a product "helps to suppress/fight against harmful bacteria in the digestive system, thereby helping to maintain a healthy digestive system".

18.4 Conclusion and Future Expectations

Probiotics are live microorganisms and their application in food has increased over past two decades due to general health benefits and improved immune system of the host. The significance of probiotics is huge and is expected to grow in coming years. As they are live microbes to be ingested into the human body, safety and regulatory frameworks need to be established from the consumer point of view. Probiotic strains should desirably be isolated from human origin with absence of pathogenicity and virulence factors. Another safety concern is transfer of antibiotic resistance genes, which should be absent. Regulatory bodies are necessary to substantiate the claims made by such products in the market. Each country and region has a different set of legislation, policies and government guidance documents as the clinical evidence and human trials are very hard to get approved. The USA and the region (North America) have a diverse and advanced market, while in the EU regulations are strict and limited. Asia and the Pacific account for a significant probiotic foods market share but the regulations are still in the drafting process or not yet framed. One important consideration observed from the experience of various countries is that all stakeholders involved should participate during the process of drafting regulatory guidelines, including government, regulatory bodies and the food industry, so that a harmonized, unanimously accepted framework can be established to regulate the market for the future. Standards and regulations improve continuously, but the rapidly growing market for commercialized probiotic-based foods and beverages requires more intensive efforts to ensure consumer safety.

References

Aggarwal, A., Nagori, B. and Mathur, V. (2012). Regulatory approval of probiotics in US, Japan & India: A comparative study. *International Journal of Pharmaceutical Sciences and Research*, 2: 78–86.

Akbar, A., Sadiq, M.B., Ali, I., Anwar, M., Muhammad, N., Muhammad, J., Shafee, M., Ullah, S., Gul, Z., and Qasim, S. (2019). *Lactococcus lactis* subsp. lactis isolated from fermented milk products and its antimicrobial potential. *CyTA-Journal of Food*, 17(1): 214–220.

Amagase, H. (2008). Current marketplace for probiotics: a Japanese perspective. *Clinical Infectious Diseases*, 46(Suppl_2): S73–S75.

Anal, A.K. (2019). Quality ingredients and safety concerns for traditional fermented foods and beverages from Asia: A review. *Fermentation*, 5(1): 8.

Anal, A.K. and Singh, H. (2007). Recent advances in microencapsulation of probiotics for industrial applications and targeted delivery. *Trends in Food Science & Technology*, 18(5): 240–251.

Anal, A.K., Koirala, S. and Shrestha, S. (2021). Gut microbiome and their possible roles in combating mycotoxins. In: *Mycotoxins in Food and Beverages*, 213–235. CRC Press.

Annunziata, A. and Vecchio, R. (2013). Consumer perception of functional foods: A conjoint analysis with probiotics. *Food Quality and Preference*, 28(1): 348–355.

Araújo, E.A., dos Santos Pires, A.C., Pinto, M.S., Jan, G. and Carvalho, A.F. (2012). Probiotics in dairy fermented products. *Rennes: CC BY*, 3: 129–148.

Arora, M. and Baldi, A. (2015). Regulatory categories of probiotics across the globe: a review representing existing and recommended categorization. *Indian Journal of Medical Microbiology*, 33(5): 2.

Arora, M. and Baldi, A. (2017). Comparative study of regulatory framework for probiotics: current status and future recommendations. *Applied Clinical Research, Clinical Trials and Regulatory Affairs*, 4(2): 140–156.

Bernardeau, M., Guguen, M. and Vernoux, J.P. (2006). Beneficial lactobacilli in food and feed: long-term use, biodiversity and proposals for specific and realistic safety assessments. *FEMS Microbiology Reviews*, 30(4): 487–513.

Bian, X., Muhammad, Z., Evivie, S.E., Luo, G.-W., Xu, M., and Huo, G.-C. (2016). Screening of antifungal potentials of Lactobacillus helveticus KLDS 1.8701 against spoilage microorganism and their effects on physicochemical properties and shelf life of fermented soybean milk during preservation. *Food Control*, 66: 183–189.

Binnewies, T.T., Motro, Y., Hallin, P.F., Lund, O., Dunn, D., La, T., Hampson, D.J., Bellgard, M., Wassenaar, T.M. and Ussery, D.W. (2006). Ten years of bacterial genome sequencing: comparative-genomics-based discoveries. *Functional & Integrative Genomics*, 6(3): 165–185.

Cannon, J., Lee, T., Bolanos, J., and Danziger, L. (2005). Pathogenic relevance of Lactobacillus: a retrospective review of over 200 cases. *European Journal of Clinical Microbiology and Infectious Diseases*, 24(1): 31–40.

Cencic, A. and Chingwaru, W. (2010). The role of functional foods, nutraceuticals, and food supplements in intestinal health. *Nutrients*, 2(6): 611–625.

Corbo, M.R., Bevilacqua, A., Petruzzi, L., Casanova, F.P. and Sinigaglia, M. (2014). Functional beverages: the emerging side of functional foods: commercial trends, research, and health implications. *Comprehensive Reviews in Food Science and Food Safety*, 13(6): 1192–1206.

D'Costa, V.M., King, C.E., Kalan, L., Morar, M., Sung, W.W., Schwarz, C., Froese, D., Zazula, G., Calmels, F., and Debruyne, R. (2011). Antibiotic resistance is ancient. *Nature*, 477(7365): 457–461.

de Simone, C. (2019). The unregulated probiotic market. *Clinical Gastroenterology and Hepatology*, 17(5): 809–817.

Degnan, F.H. (2008). The US Food and Drug Administration and probiotics: regulatory categorization. *Clinical Infectious Diseases*, 46(Suppl_2): S133–S136.

Degnan, F.H. (2012). Clinical studies involving probiotics: when FDA's investigational new drug rubric applies—and when it may not. *Gut Microbes*, 3(6).

EFSA-NDA (2011). Guidance on the scientific requirements for health claims related to gut and immune function. *EFSA Journal*, 9(4): 1984.

EFSA (2005). *Qualified Presumption of Safety of Micro-organisms in Food and Feed* (9291990124).

FAO/WHO (2002). *Guidelines for the Evaluation of Probiotics in Food*. https://www.who.int/foodsafety/fs_management/en/probiotic_guidelines.pdf (accessed 20 January 2020).

FDA (2006). Development & Approval Process of Drugs. http://www.accessdata.fda.gov/scripts/cder/drugsatfda/ (accessed 6 September 2020).

FDA (2011). Re: Use of Probiotic Microorganisms in Foods. http://food.fda.moph.go.th/law/data/announ_moph/V.English/No.%20339%20Use%20of%20Probiotic%20Microorganisms%20in%20Foods.pdf (accessed 20 December 2020).

FDA (2015). Federal Food, Drug, and Cosmetic Act (FD&C Act). http://www.fda.gov/regulatoryinformation/legislation/federalfooddrugandcosmeticactfdcact/default.htm (accessed 28 August 2020).

Fortune Business Insights (2020). Probiotics Market Size, Share and Industry Analysis By Microbial Genus (Lactobacillus, Bifidobacterium, Yeast), By Application (Functional Food and Beverage, Dietary Supplement, Animal Feed), By Distribution Channel (Supermarkets/Hypermarkets, Pharmacies/Health Stores, Convenience Stores, Online Retail), and Regional Forecast 2018-2025. *Fortune Business Insights*. https://www.fortunebusinessinsights.com/industry-reports/probiotics-market-100083 (accessed 29 August 2020).

Frietas, D. (2006). Nutraceuticals in Latin America: Brazil and Beyond at Latin America: Nutraceutical Boom or Bust? https://www.nutraceuticalsworld.com/issues/2006-07/view_features/nutraceuticals-in-latin-america-brazil-and-beyond/ (accessed 20 December 2020).

FSSAI (2016). Food Safety and Standards (Health Supplements, Nutraceuticals, Food for Special Dietary Use, Food for Special Medical Purpose, Functional Food, and Novel Food) Regulations, 2016. https://fssai.gov.in/upload/uploadfiles/files/Nutraceuticals_Regulations.pdf (accessed 22 July 2021).

Gasser, F. (1994). Safety of lactic acid bacteria and their occurrence in human clinical infections. *Bulletin de l'Institut Pasteur*, 92(1): 45–67.

Granato, D., Barba, F.J., Bursać Kovačević, D., Lorenzo, J.M., Cruz, A.G. and Putnik, P. (2020). Functional foods: Product development, technological trends, efficacy testing, and safety. *Annual Review of Food Science and Technology*, 11: 93–118.

Granato, D., Branco, G.F., Nazzaro, F., Cruz, A.G. and Faria, J.A. (2010). Functional foods and nondairy probiotic food development: trends, concepts, and products. *Comprehensive Reviews in Food Science and Food Safety*, 9(3): 292–302.

Guimarães, J.T., Balthazar, C.F., Silva, R., Rocha, R.S., Graça, J.S., Esmerino, E.A., Silva, M.C., Sant'Ana, A.S., Duarte, M.C.K. and Freitas, M. Q. (2020). Impact of probiotics and prebiotics on food texture. *Current Opinion in Food Science*, 33: 38–44.

Hekmat, S., and Reid, G. (2006). Sensory properties of probiotic yogurt is comparable to standard yogurt. *Nutrition Research*, 26(4): 163–166.

Herman, L., Chemaly, M., Cocconcelli, P.S., Fernandez, P., Klein, G., Peixe, L., Prieto, M., Querol, A., Suarez, J.E. and Sundh, I. (2019). The qualified presumption of safety assessment and its role in EFSA risk evaluations: 15 years past. *FEMS Microbiology Letters*, 366(Suppl_1): i17–i23.

Hill, C., Guarner, F., Reid, G., Gibson, G.R., Merenstein, D.J., Pot, B., Morelli, L., Canani, R.B., Flint, H.J. and Salminen, S. (2014). Expert consensus document: The International Scientific Association for Probiotics and Prebiotics consensus statement on the scope and appropriate use of the term probiotic. *Nature Reviews Gastroenterology & Hepatology*, 11(8): 506.

Japan (1991). Food Sanitation Act. http://www.japaneselawtranslation.go.jp/law/detail_main?id=12 (accessed 1 September 2020).

Japan (2013). Overview of FOSHU. https://www.caa.go.jp/policies/policy/food_labeling/health_promotion/pdf/food_labeling_cms206_200122_04.pdf (accessed 1 September 2020).

Japan (2017). Food Labelling and Probiotic Health Claims. https://www.caa.go.jp/policies/policy/food_labeling/health_promotion/pdf/health_promotion_170606_0001.pdf (accessed 1 September 2020).

Kalhoro, M.S., Visessanguan, W., Nguyen, L.T. and Anal, A.K. (2019). Probiotic potential of Lactobacillus paraplantarum BT-11 isolated from raw buffalo (Bubalus bubalis) milk and characterization of bacteriocin-like inhibitory substance produced. *Journal of Food Processing and Preservation*, 43(8): e14015.

Kalicka, D., Znamirowska, A., Pawlos, M., Buniowska, M. and Szajnar, K. (2019). Physical and sensory characteristics and probiotic survival in ice cream sweetened with various polyols. *International Journal of Dairy Technology*, 72(3): 456–465.

Katan, M. (2012). Why the European Food Safety Authority was right to reject health claims for probiotics. *Beneficial Microbes*, 3(2): 85–89.

Khaneghah, A.M., Abhari, K., Eş, I., Soares, M.B., Oliveira, R.B., Hosseini, H., Rezaei, M., Balthazar, C.F., Silva, R. and Cruz, A.G. (2020). Interactions between probiotics and pathogenic microorganisms in hosts and foods: A review. *Trends in Food Science & Technology*, 95: 205–218.

Koirala, S. and Anal, A.K. (2021). Probiotics-based foods and beverages as future foods and their overall safety and regulatory claims. *Future Foods*: 100013.

Kothari, D., Patel, S. and Kim, S.-K. (2019). Probiotic supplements might not be universally-effective and safe: A review. *Biomedicine & Pharmacotherapy*, 111: 537–547.

Kumaree, K.K., Akbar, A. and Anal, A.K. (2015). Bioencapsulation and application of Lactobacillus plantarum isolated from catfish gut as an antimicrobial agent and additive in fish feed pellets. *Annals of Microbiology*, 65(3): 1439–1445.

Leuschner, R.G., Robinson, T.P., Hugas, M., Cocconcelli, P.S., Richard-Forget, F., Klein, G., Licht, T.R., Nguyen-The, C., Querol, A. and Richardson, M. (2010). Qualified presumption of safety (QPS): a generic risk assessment approach for biological agents notified to the European Food Safety Authority (EFSA). *Trends in Food Science & Technology*, 21(9): 425–435.

Linares, D.M., Gomez, C., Renes, E., Fresno, J.M., Tornadijo, M.E., Ross, R.P., and Stanton, C. (2017). Lactic acid bacteria and bifidobacteria with potential to design natural biofunctional health-promoting dairy foods. *Frontiers in Microbiology*, 8: 846.

Markowiak, P. and Śliżewska, K. (2017). Effects of probiotics, prebiotics, and synbiotics on human health. *Nutrients*, 9(9): 1021.

Maughan, R.J., King, D.S. and Lea, T. (2004). Dietary supplements. *Journal of Sports Sciences*, 22(1): 95–113.

Melchor, S.R., Skoblikov, L. and Schütte, B. (2019). The regulatory framework for the use of probiotics claims in food and food supplements around the world: a comparative analysis. In: *The Functional Field Of Food Law: Reconciling the Market and Human Rights*, 155–169. Wageningen Academic Publishers.

Nagata, J. and Yamada, K. (2008). Foods with health claims in Japan. *Food Science and Technology Research*, 14(6): 519.

Peivasteh-Roudsari, L., Pirhadi, M., Karami, H., Tajdar-oranj, B., Molaee-Aghaee, E. and Sadighara, P. (2019). Probiotics and food safety: an evidence-based review. *Journal of Food Safety and Hygiene*, 5(1).

Pieniz, S., de Moura, T.M., Cassenego, A.P.V., Andreazza, R., Frazzon, A.P.G., de Oliveira Camargo, F.A., and Brandelli, A. (2015). Evaluation of resistance genes and virulence factors in a food isolated Enterococcus durans with potential probiotic effect. *Food Control*, 51: 49–54.

Reid, G. (2015). The growth potential for dairy probiotics. *International Dairy Journal*, 49: 16–22.

Roobab, U., Batool, Z., Manzoor, M.F., Shabbir, M.A., Khan, M.R. and Aadil, R.M. (2020). Sources, formulations, advanced delivery and health benefits of probiotics. *Current Opinion in Food Science*, 32: 17–28.

Saarela, M., Mogensen, G., Fonden, R., Mättö, J. and Mattila-Sandholm, T. (2000). Probiotic bacteria: safety, functional and technological properties. *Journal of Biotechnology*, 84(3): 197–215.

Saarela, M.H. (2019). Safety aspects of next generation probiotics. *Current Opinion in Food Science*, 30: 8–13.

Saxelin, M. (2008). Probiotic formulations and applications, the current probiotics market, and changes in the marketplace: a European perspective. *Clinical Infectious Diseases*, 46(Suppl_2): S76–S79.

Saxelin, M., Chuang, N.-H., Chassy, B., Rautelin, H., Mäkelä, P.H., Salminen, S. and Gorbach, S.L. (1996). Lactobacilli and bacteremia in southern Finland, 1989–1992. *Clinical Infectious Diseases*, 22(3): 564–566.

Shane, A.L., Cabana, M.D., Ellis, C.L., Heimbach, J.T., Hempel, S., Hummelen, R., Lynch, S., Merenstein, D.J., Sanders, M.E. and Tancredi, D.J. (2010). Guide to designing, conducting, publishing, and communicating results of clinical studies involving probiotic applications in human participants. *Gut Microbes*, 1(4): 243–253.

Sharma, S., Arora, M. and Baldi, A. (2013). Probiotics in India: Current status and future prospects. *Pharm Aspire*, 1: 1–12.

Shi, L.H., Balakrishnan, K., Thiagarajah, K., Ismail, N.I.M. and Yin, O.S. (2016). Beneficial properties of probiotics. *Tropical Life Sciences Research*, 27(2): 73.

Stanton, C., Gardiner, G., Meehan, H., Collins, K., Fitzgerald, G., Lynch, P.B., and Ross, R.P. (2001). Market potential for probiotics. *The American Journal of Clinical Nutrition*, 73(2): 476s–483s.

Stanton, E. and Emms, S. (2011). Malaysia's markets for functional foods, nutraceuticals and organic foods: An introduction for Canadian producers and exporters. The Counsellor and Regional Agri-Food Trade Commissioner, Southeast Asia, and the High Commission of Canada in Malaysia.

Terpou, A., Papadaki, A., Lappa, I.K., Kachrimanidou, V., Bosnea, L.A. and Kopsahelis, N. (2019). Probiotics in food systems: Significance and emerging strategies towards improved viability and delivery of enhanced beneficial value. *Nutrients*, 11(7): 1591.

Thapa, S.P., Shrestha, S. and Anal, A.K. (2020). Addressing the antibiotic resistance and improving the food safety in food supply chain (farm-to-fork) in Southeast Asia. *Food Control*, 108: 106809.

Tomar, O. (2019). The effects of probiotic cultures on the organic acid content, texture profile and sensory attributes of Tulum cheese. *International Journal of Dairy Technology*, 72(2): 218–228.

van Loveren, H., Sanz, Y. and Salminen, S. (2012). Health claims in Europe: probiotics and prebiotics as case examples. *Annual Review of Food Science and Technology*, 3: 247–261.

Vanderhoof, J.A. and Young, R. (2008). Probiotics in the United States. *Clinical Infectious Diseases*, 46(Suppl_2): S67–S72.

Venugopalan, V., Shriner, K.A. and Wong-Beringer, A. (2010). Regulatory oversight and safety of probiotic use. *Emerging Infectious Diseases*, 16(11): 1661.

Wassenaar, T.M. and Blaser, M.J. (1999). Pathophysiology of Campylobacter jejuni infections of humans. *Microbes and Infection*, 1(12): 1023–1033.

Wassenaar, T.M. and Klein, G. (2008). Safety aspects and implications of regulation of probiotic bacteria in food and food supplements. *Journal of Food Protection*, 71(8): 1734–1741.

Wassenaar, T., Zschüttig, A., Beimfohr, C., Geske, T., Auerbach, C., Cook, H., Zimmermann, K. and Gunzer, F. (2015). Virulence genes in a probiotic E. coli product with a recorded long history of safe use. *European Journal of Microbiology and Immunology*, 5(1): 81–93.

WHO (2015). WHO's first ever global estimates of foodborne diseases find children under 5 account for almost one third of deaths. https://www.who.int/news/item/03-12-2015-who-s-first-ever-global-estimates-of-foodborne-diseases-find-children-under-5-account-for-almost-one-third-of-deaths (accessed 10 July 2021).

Yang, M.S. (2016). Regulatory aspects of nutraceuticals: Chinese perspective. In: *Nutraceuticals*, 947–957). Elsevier.

Yilmaz-Ersan, L., Ozcan, T. and Akpinar-Bayizit, A. (2020). Assessment of socio-demographic factors, health status and the knowledge on probiotic dairy products. *Food Science and Human Wellness*, 9(3): 272–279.

Zucko, J., Starcevic, A., Diminic, J., Oros, D., Mortazavian, A.M. and Putnik, P. (2020). Probiotic–friend or foe? *Current Opinion in Food Science*, 32: 45–49.

Index

Page numbers in **bold** refer to Tables
Page numbers in *italics* refer to Figures

Probiotics, Prebiotics and Synbiotics: Technological Advancements Towards Safety and Industrial Applications, First Edition. Edited by Parmjit Singh Panesar and Anil Kumar Anal.

b

d

g

h

m

q

r

Recent Advances in Micro- and Macroalgal Processing

Recent Advances in Micro- and Macroalgal Processing

Food and Health Perspectives

Edited by

Gaurav Rajauria
University College Dublin, Ireland

Yvonne V. Yuan
Ryerson University, Canada

WILEY Blackwell

This edition first published 2021

Registered Office(s)
John Wiley & Sons, Inc., 111 River Street, Hoboken, NJ 07030, USA
John Wiley & Sons Ltd, The Atrium, Southern Gate, Chichester, West Sussex, PO19 8SQ, UK

Editorial Office
The Atrium, Southern Gate, Chichester, West Sussex, PO19 8SQ, UK

For details of our global editorial offices, customer services, and more information about Wiley products visit us at www.wiley.com.

Wiley also publishes its books in a variety of electronic formats and by print-on-demand. Some content that appears in standard print versions of this book may not be available in other formats.

Library of Congress Cataloging-in-Publication Data

Names: Rajauria, Gaurav, editor. | Yuan, Yvonne V., editor.
Title: Recent advances in micro and macroalgal processing : food and health perspectives / edited by Gaurav Rajauria, University College Dublin, Ireland, Yvonne V. Yuan, Ryerson University, Canada.
Description: First edition. | Hoboken, NJ, USA : Wiley-Blackwell, 2021. | Series: IFST advances in food science book series | Includes bibliographical references and index.
Identifiers: LCCN 2020048355 (print) | LCCN 2020048356 (ebook) | ISBN 9781119542582 (hardback) | ISBN 9781119542629 (adobe pdf) | ISBN 9781119542612 (epub)
Subjects: LCSH: Algae–Biotechnology. | Algae as food. | Microalgae–Industrial applications.
Classification: LCC TP248.27.A46 R43 2021 (print) | LCC TP248.27.A46 (ebook) | DDC 660.6–dc23
LC record available at https://lccn.loc.gov/2020048355
LC ebook record available at https://lccn.loc.gov/2020048356

Cover Design: Wiley
Cover Images: Lab & Science Vector Icon Set, © fleaz / iStockphoto, Beautiful tropical seascape. Sky and sea © Efired / Shutterstock, farming icons © bioraven / Shutterstock, Coal industry icons black set with train truck factory isolated vector illustration © Macrovector / Shutterstock, Green Seaweed © divedog / Shutterstock, Single-cell algae with lipid droplets. Biofuel production. Illustration of microalgae under the microscope, isolated on white © Perception7 / Shutterstock

Set in 9.5/11.5pt, TimesLTStd by SPi Global, Chennai, India.

C9781119542582_290321
Printed and bound by CPI Group (UK) Ltd, Croydon CR0 4YY

Acknowledgments

In our preparation and editing of this book we have had the assistance of numerous colleagues and support from friends and family for which we are both greatly appreciative.

When we first started this project, we never dreamed that the global community would be challenged by the COVID-19 pandemic, which is now a reality as we finalize this volume for publication. We are extremely grateful to our contributors from across the globe who have been diligently laboring from their homes during these difficult times and continued to successfully complete the chapters with revisions provided by the editors.

In addition, we are deeply humbled and want to thank our passionate managing editor, project editor, copy editor, and our fabulous commissioning team, production team, administrative, IT, and support staff at Wiley.

Finally, we would like to dedicate this work with a huge thank you to the array of frontline workers across the world who are courageously and valiantly working every day to support us all in the fight against the deadly COVID-19 virus. There are no words that can adequately express our gratitude for all that you are doing during this difficult time. We wish you and your families safety and health as you forge ahead to get us to the other side of this pandemic. Your contributions are appreciated, and we thank you in our prayers, hearts, and minds every day. WE SALUTE YOU!

Contents

About the IFST Advances in Food Science Book Series

The Institute of Food Science and Technology (IFST) is the leading qualifying body for food professionals in Europe and the only professional organization in the UK concerned with all aspects of food science and technology. Its qualifications are internationally recognized as a sign of proficiency and integrity in the industry. Competence, integrity, and serving the public benefit lie at the heart of the IFST philosophy. IFST values the many elements that contribute to the efficient and responsible supply, manufacture, and distribution of safe, wholesome, nutritious, and affordable foods, with due regard for the environment, animal welfare, and the rights of consumers. **IFST Advances in Food Science** is a series of books dedicated to the most important and popular topics in food science and technology, highlighting major developments across all sectors of the global food industry. Each volume is a detailed and in-depth edited work, featuring contributions by recognized international experts, and which focuses on new developments in the field. Taken together, the series forms a comprehensive library of the latest food science research and practice, and provides valuable insights into the food processing techniques that are essential to the understanding and development of this rapidly evolving industry. The IFST Advances series is edited by Dr. Brijesh Tiwari, who is Senior Research Officer at Teagasc Food Research Centre in Ireland.

List of Contributors

Ahmad Adnan, Department of Chemistry, GC University, Lahore, Pakistan

Sumia Akram, Division of Science and Technology, University of Education, Lahore, Pakistan

Sara Amiri Samani, Department of Food Science and Technology, Shahrekord Branch, Islamic Azad University, Shahrekord, Iran

Lucie Beaulieu, Institut sur la nutrition et les aliments fonctionnels (INAF), Département des Sciences des aliments, Université Laval, Québec, Canada

Gilles Bedoux, Laboratoire de Biotechnologie et Chimie Marines EA 3884, Université Bretagne Sud, IUEM, Vannes, France

Rajeev Bhat, RA-Chair in VALORTECH, Estonian University of Life Sciences, Tartu, Estonia

Nathalie Bourgougnon, Laboratoire de Biotechnologie et Chimie Marines EA 3884, Université Bretagne Sud, IUEM, Vannes, France

Benoît Chénais, Mer Molécules Santé EA2160, Le Mans Université, Le Mans, France

Kit-Leong Cheong, Guangdong Provincial Key Laboratory of Marine Biotechnology, STU-UNIVPM Joint Algal Research Center, Department of Biology, College of Science, Shantou University, Shantou, China

Solène Connan, Univ Brest, CNRS, IRD, Ifremer, LEMAR, F-29280, Plouzane, France

Hong Du, Guangdong Provincial Key Laboratory of Marine Biotechnology, STU-UNIVPM Joint Algal Research Center, Department of Biology, College of Science, Shantou University, Shantou, China

Sidra Ehsan, Department of Chemistry, GC University, Lahore, Pakistan

Froylán Mario Espinoza Escalante, Department of Chemistry, Autonomous University of Guadalajara, Zapopan, Mexico

Mathilde Fournière, Laboratoire de Biotechnologie et Chimie Marines EA 3884, Université Bretagne Sud, IUEM, Vannes, France

Leslie Gager, Univ Brest, CNRS, IRD, Ifremer, LEMAR, F-29280, Plouzane, France

Abirami Ramu Ganesan, Department of Food Science and Home Economics, School of Applied Sciences, College of Engineering, Science and Technology, Fiji National University, Nasinu, Fiji Islands

Marco Garcia-Vaquero, Section of Food and Nutrition, School of Agriculture and Food Science, University College Dublin, Dublin, Ireland

Francesco Gentili, Department of Forest Biomaterials and Technology, Swedish University of Agricultural Sciences, Umeå, Sweden

Carmen P. Gómez, Applied Physics Department, Faculty of Sea Sciences, University of Vigo, Vigo, Spain

Maryam Jafari, Research Center of Nutrition and Organic Products, Shahrekord Branch, Islamic Azad University, Shahrekord, Iran

Valentina Jesumani, Guangdong Provincial Key Laboratory of Marine Biotechnology, STU-UNIVPM Joint Algal Research Center, Department of Biology, College of Science, Shantou University, Shantou, China

Bilal Muhammad Khan, Guangdong Provincial Key Laboratory of Marine Biotechnology, STU-UNIVPM Joint Algal Research Center, Department of Biology, College of Science, Shantou University, Shantou, China

K. Suresh Kumar, Department of Botany, University of Allahabad, Prayagraj, India

Sushma Kumari, Department of Botany, University of Allahabad, Prayagraj, India

Pratibha Kushwaha, Department of Botany, University of Allahabad, Prayagraj, India

Fanny Lalegerie, Univ Brest, CNRS, IRD, Ifremer, LEMAR, F-29280, Plouzane, France

Duu-Jong Lee, Department of Chemical Engineering, National Taiwan University, Taipei, Taiwan

José L. Legido, Applied Physics Department, Faculty of Sea Sciences, University of Vigo, Vigo, Spain

Yang Liu, Guangdong Provincial Key Laboratory of Marine Biotechnology, STU-UNIVPM Joint Algal Research Center, Department of Biology, College of Science, Shantou University, Shantou, China

Shingo Matsukawa, Department of Food Science and Technology, Tokyo University of Marine Science and Technology, Tokyo, Japan

Kannan Mohan, Postgraduate and Research Department of Zoology, Sri Vasavi College, Erode, India

María Lourdes Mourelle, Applied Physics Department, Faculty of Sea Sciences, University of Vigo, Vigo, Spain

Shanmugam Munisamy, Research and Development Division (DSIR-Lab), Aquagri Processing Private Limited, Manamadurai, India

S. Murugesan, Unit of Algal Biotechnology Bio-nanotechnology, Postgraduate and Research Department of Botany, Pachaiyappa's College, Chennai, India

Muhammad Mushtaq, Department of Chemistry, GC University, Lahore, Pakistan

Calle Niemi, Department of Forest Biomaterials and Technology, Swedish University of Agricultural Sciences, Umeå, Sweden

John O'Doherty, School of Agriculture and Food Science, University College Dublin, Lyons Research Farm, Celbridge, Ireland

Daniel A. Pérez-Rico, Department of Chemistry, Autonomous University of Guadalajara, Zapopan, Mexico

Muhammad Pervaiz, Department of Chemistry, GC University, Lahore, Pakistan

Akanksha Priyadarshini, UCD Michael Smurfit Graduate Business School, University College Dublin, Blackrock, Ireland

Anushree Priyadarshini, College of Business, Technological University Dublin, Dublin, Ireland

Rashida Qari, Department of Maritime Sciences, Bahria University, Karachi, Pakistan

D. Radhika, Postgraduate and Research Department of Zoology, V.O.Chidambaram College, Tuticorin, India

Gaurav Rajauria, School of Agriculture and Food Science, University College Dublin, Belfield, Dublin, Ireland

Shakeel Ramzan, Department of Chemistry, GC University, Lahore, Pakistan

Rajeev Ravindran, School of Agriculture and Food Science, University College Dublin, Belfield, Dublin, Ireland

Shahin Roohinejad, Burn and Wound Healing Research Center, Division of Food and Nutrition, Shiraz University of Medical Sciences, Shiraz, Iran

Zohaib Saeed, Department of Chemistry, GC University, Lahore, Pakistan

Sayed Mohammad Sahafi, Department of Food Science and Technology, Isfahan University of Technology, Isfahan, Iran

Palaniappan Seedevi, Department of Enviromental Science, Periyar University, Salem, India

K.Y. Show, Puritek Research Institute, Puritek Co. Ltd., Nanjing, China

Kamleshwar Singh, Department of Botany, University of Allahabad, Prayagraj, India

V. Sivamurugan, Postgraduate and Research Department of Chemistry, Pachaiyappa's College, Chennai, India

Valerie Stiger-Pouvreau, Univ Brest, CNRS, IRD, Ifremer, LEMAR, F-29280, Plouzane, France

Torres Sweeney, School of Veterinary Medicine, Veterinary Sciences Centre, University College Dublin, Belfield, Dublin, Ireland

Nolwenn Terme, Laboratoire de Biotechnologie et Chimie Marines EA 3884, Université Bretagne Sud, IUEM, Vannes, France

Ariane Tremblay, Institut sur la nutrition et les aliments fonctionnels (INAF), Département des Sciences des aliments, Université Laval, Québec, Canada

Y.G. Yan, Puritek Research Institute, Puritek Co. Ltd., Nanjing, China

Yvonne V. Yuan, School of Nutrition, Ryerson University, Toronto, Ontario, Canada

Preface

Micro- and macroalgae are among the most ancient functional foods or "superfoods" known to mankind given the origin of cyanobacteria on Earth approx. 3 billion years ago. For example, consumption of marine macroalgae was identified at the Monte Verde II archeological site dating approx. 14 000 years ago; the Aztecs were known to consume the microalga *Spirulina platensis*; and micro- and macroalgae have long been consumed by coastal communities across the globe. Not only are micro- and macroalgae valorized for their macronutrient contents (proteins, soluble and insoluble carbohydrates, long-chain marine polyunsaturated fatty acids), and micronutrients (minerals, vitamins), but also for a plethora of non-nutritive secondary metabolites or phytochemicals (mycosporine-like amino acids, fucoidans, carotenes, tocols, polyphenols, phenolic acids, phlorotannins, lignans, pterins, scytonemins, etc.). The valorization of edible micro- and macroalgae includes intact dehydrated or rehydrated plant material consumed in macrobiotic diets, as well as salads, soups, stews, sushi wraps, and condiments. Aqueous extracts from algae are often used in gelled desserts and beverages, and more widely as hydrocolloids; as well, crude and purified isolates of potentially biologically active phytochemicals have been used to develop nutraceuticals. It is this latter group of phytochemicals, identified above, with the potential to reduce chronic disease risk factors, which has resulted in micro- and macroalgae being described as functional foods or "superfoods." Coincident with the term superfood being a part of the marketing and broader vernacular since 2004 (referring to foodstuffs with *in vitro* antioxidant capacity and potential positive effects to reduce diet-related chronic disease risk factors), consumer and lay press interest in adding micro- and macroalgae to the diet has been steadily growing as evidenced by magazine articles and the addition of seaweeds to restaurant menus and grocery store shelves.

As photosynthetic organisms, whether prokaryotes or eukaryotes, the composition of micro- and macroalgae is highly variable as a function of tidal zone habitat, nutrient availability, light irradiance, latitude, temperature, and seasonality, and thereby is susceptible to oxidative stress. Thus, despite the fact that 71% of the Earth's surface is covered by oceans, in addition to less than 1% as freshwater for potentially wild-harvesting many algal species, there is a burgeoning mariculture industry for the cultivation of many micro- and macroalgal species of commercial interest. Cultivation of micro- and macroalgae allows for biomass to be sustainably produced with consistent morphology and composition by controlling seed stock, nutrients, light irradiance, temperature, and agitation. Thus, the scientific literature has been greatly enriched by basic and applied research focused on the nutritional, functional food, and nutraceutical benefits of micro- and macroalgae. As well, the potential biological activities of micro- and macroalgal extractables *in vitro*, *in situ*, and *in vivo* from animal model studies, case-control, and epidemiological studies are being extensively explored. Moreover, applied phycological research has been expanded by studies focused on micro- and macroalgal growth and metabolism, mariculture cultivation, and processing for extraction and isolation of biologically active constituents.

It is noteworthy that capturing this diversity and controlling variability in algal chemical composition and linked bioactivities are key challenges for future commercial applications, particularly in the mariculture industries. Additionally, processing and extraction of active fractions that are bioavailable upon consumption, and further understanding the biological activity of these extracts, their potential roles in chronic disease risk reduction, and potential applications in the functional food and nutraceutical sectors are critical. Superimposed upon these considerations are the effects of harvesting, storage, and novel processing techniques that can dramatically influence the potential nutritive value and bioactivity of algal derived foods. There are many emerging technologies available to process algae, but optimization and greater efficiency of processing techniques are still required. Therefore, a sustainable supply (without impacting the environment) along with an increasing requirement for novel processing and extraction techniques to explore and harness the immense potential of algae form the premise of this book. There is a need to document not only the conventional methods to extract algal bioactives, but also to know how novel processes can be exploited industrially. The challenge to find all of this information in one expert monograph has been unmet to date, which explains why hitherto there has been limited availability of a comprehensive book that covers the health and nutraceutical aspects of micro- and macroalgae.

This volume offers readers a broad review of the applications of conventional and new processing/extraction techniques for algal bioactive compounds and their potential health impacts. With book chapter contributions authored and co-authored by researchers from India, Taiwan, Ireland, Sweden, Canada, Fiji, Pakistan, China, France, Estonia, Japan, Iran, Mexico, and Spain, the present volume focuses on *Recent Advances in Micro- and Macroalgal Processing* in a truly international collaboration. What makes this work of particular note is its intentional discussion of not only well-known and lesser-known microalgal species, but also macroalgal species of economic and nutritional importance across the globe. Our sincere hope is that this volume will be a valuable and comprehensive resource for students, teachers and researchers across academia and industry. We owe a deep debt of gratitude to all the authors and co-authors who have contributed their works in a comprehensive and timely manner for publication, as well as the editorial staff of Wiley.

Yvonne V. Yuan and Gaurav Rajauria
June 2020

Section I
Composition and Extraction Technologies for Algal Bioactives

1
Algae: A Functional Food with a Rich History and Future Superfood

Gaurav Rajauria[1] and Yvonne V. Yuan[2]
[1]*School of Agriculture and Food Science, University College Dublin, Lyons Research Farm, Celbridge, Ireland*
[2]*School of Nutrition, Ryerson University, Toronto, Ontario, Canada*

1.1 Introduction

With increased consumer interest in simple, clean, minimally processed, and additive- or preservative-free food products and ingredients, it is only natural that interest in macro- and microalgae as foodstuffs has grown exponentially in recent years. This consumer interest in macro- and microalgae-based foods is supported by lay press sources including fashion and beauty industry magazines such as *Elle Magazine* (Davidson 2019); television and media personality websites such as that of Dr. Mehmet Oz (Ni 2018); daily newspapers (Liu 2020); as well as food and beverage industry trade publications (Hein 2016). Specific examples of this burgeoning consumer demand and interest include seaweed salads appearing on menus of mainstream seafood (non-Asian) restaurants; roasted seaweed snacks being sold in many mainstream supermarkets (Sloan 2018); dried seaweed flakes being offered as condiments in restaurants; dehydrated seaweeds and seaweed salad kits being sold in mainstream and specialty grocery stores; and nutritional supplement products such as GREENS+™, which include microalgae such as *Spirulina* sp., *Chlorella* sp., *Dunaliella salina*, the macroalga dulse (*Palmaria palmata*) (https://www.greensplus.com/superfood-powders), and numerous microalgae powders containing *Spirulina* sp. and *Chlorella* sp.

Moreover, there is a steadily increasing body of knowledge in the scientific literature about the potential nutritional, functional food, and nutraceutical benefits of

Recent Advances in Micro- and Macroalgal Processing: Food and Health Perspectives, First Edition.
Edited by Gaurav Rajauria and Yvonne V. Yuan.

whole micro- and macroalgae consumption as well as the potential biological activities of micro- and macroalgal extracts and extractable constituents *in vitro*, *in situ*, and *in vivo* from animal model studies, case-control, and epidemiological studies in reducing chronic disease risk factors, as well as inflammation. Key areas of investigation continue to be the chemical characterization of unique micro- and macroalgal specimens collected and isolated from terrestrial as well as fresh-, brackish, and marine environments due to the influence of oxidative stress on these algae from exposure to varying nutrient levels, temperatures, tides and/or desiccation, and UV irradiation. Oxidative stress experienced by these photosynthetic organisms can ultimately influence growth rates, metabolism, and synthesis of secondary metabolites, with many of the latter compounds of interest as potential nutraceuticals, cosmeceuticals, or in pharmacognosis. While bench-top and *in vitro* cell culture studies are key to understanding the mechanisms of action of extracts and/or their constituent purified compounds, the *in vivo* bioaccessibility and ultimately bioavailability and metabolism of these molecules are key to determining their potential to influence and protect human health. A particularly intriguing avenue of investigation is evaluating the efficacy of UV-absorbing compounds from micro- and macroalgae as potential nutraceuticals, antioxidants, and sunscreen molecules in cosmeceuticals.

1.2 History of Macro- and Microalgae Consumption

Edible marine macroalgae, often referred to as seaweeds or sea vegetables, as well as marine and freshwater microalgae have a long history in the diets of ancient cultures and increasingly in modern, health-conscious, and environmentally sustainable cuisines as recently reviewed (Pérez-Lloréns et al. 2020; Tou et al. 2020; Gomez-Zavaglia et al. 2019; Mac Monagail et al. 2017; Talero et al. 2015; Athukorala and Yuan 2013; Yuan and Athukorala 2012; Christaki et al. 2011; Lordan et al. 2011). For example, the importance of edible seaweeds in East and Southeast Asian (e.g. China, Japan, Korea, Vietnam, Indonesia, Philippines) cultures is commonly known, as well as in Pacific (e.g. Hawai'i, Maori of New Zealand), Caribbean (e.g. Jamaica, Saint Lucia, Grenadines), Central (e.g. Belize, Honduras, Panama) and South American cultures (e.g. Chile, Argentina, Brazil, Peru, Venezuela) (Figure 1.1). Conversely, seaweeds are not as common in Northern American or European cultures with some local exceptions such as Atlantic Canada and the USA, Mexico as well as Iceland, Ireland, Norway, Wales, Spain, and more recently France. Many of these cultures have incorporated macro- and microalgae as well as seaweed extracts throughout the diet in salads, soups, stews, sushi wraps, condiments, gelled desserts, and beverages (Tou et al. 2020; Yuan 2008; Robledo and Freile Pelegrín 1997).

The edible marine macroalgae comprise the Ochrophyta (containing those of the Phaeophyceae class [brown (B)]), Chlorophyta (the Chlorophyceae class [green (G)]), and Rhodophyta (the Rhodophyceae class [red (R)]) phyla or divisions, with species valued, and therefore, wild-harvested or cultivated as sources of hydrocolloids (e.g. agar agar, alginates, carrageenans), other soluble (e.g. Floridean starch, fucoidans) and insoluble dietary fibers (e.g. cellulose, mannans, xylans), proteins,

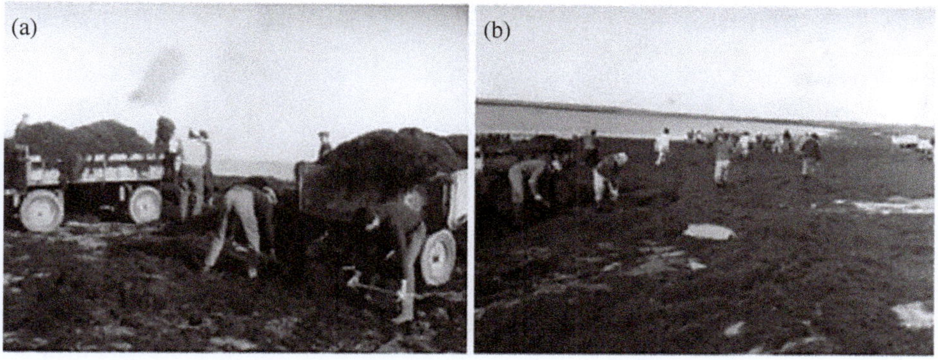

Figure 1.1 "Seaweed Gatherers" (a) Loading trailers on the shore; (b) Beach collection of Gracilaria after wash up, Bahia Bustamante, Argentina, (1960). Source: Adopted from (with permission) Mac Monagail et al. (2017).

minerals, vitamins, small amounts of long-chain n-3 polyunsaturated fatty acids (PUFAs), as well as a host of nutraceutical compounds including mycosporine-like amino acids, fucoidans, carotenoids, tocols, polyphenols, phenolic acids, phlorotannins, and lignans with potential biological activities (Tou et al. 2020; Athukorala and Yuan 2013; Plaza et al. 2008; Yuan 2008). It is noteworthy that the medicinal or functional food properties of edible macroalgae in the treatment or prevention of chronic disease risks such as breast cancer were noted as far back as approx. 1534 BCE in the Egyptian "Ebers Papyrus." Moreover, nine species of marine algae were recovered from the hearths of homes in the archeological site of Monte Verde II in southern Chile dating from approx. 14 000 years ago, indicating the use of seaweeds from coastal and estuarine environments for food and medicine by these peoples.

Unicellular microalgae are similarly diverse including Dinoflagellata (eukaryotic, photosynthetic, marine and freshwater dinoflagellates or plankton), Cryptophyta (eukaryotic, freshwater algae, but also in marine and brackish waters), Raphidophyta (eukaryotic, marine and freshwater algae), and Cyanophyta (prokaryotic, photosynthetic blue-green algae, e.g. Cyanophyceae) phyla or divisions (Tou et al. 2020; Garcia et al. 2017). Microalgae, wild-harvested worldwide or even grown in culture, have been valued as part of macrobiotic diets and dietary supplements for nutritional (e.g. protein, PUFAs, carotenoids, carbohydrates) or nutraceutical benefits in modern times (Garcia et al. 2017), but also have an ancient history, such as with the Aztecs harvesting *Spirulina platensis* (or *Arthrospira platensis*) (Cyanophyceae) from Lake Texcoco as tecuitlatl, which was eaten with roasted corn or tortillas; or the consumption *of S. platensis in* Chad from Lake Kossorom, where it is known as dihé; or the consumption of *Nostoc commune* (Cyanophyceae) in China, where it is known as fah-tsai or dacai; or *Spirogyra varians* (eukaryotic, Charophyta division, Zygnematophyceae class) known as Tao or water silk, pond silk or mermaid's tree in Thailand (Tou et al. 2020; Garcia et al. 2017).

1.3 Economic Relevance of Macro- and Microalgae

With 71% of the Earth's surface covered by oceans, comprising 97% of the Earth's water, and with less than 1% of the Earth's water as freshwater with the remaining 2–3% contained in glaciers and ice caps, it is no surprise that wild harvesting of macroalgae for food, animal feed, fertilizer, and even fuel has been instrumental in the establishment of coastal communities across the globe. Countries including Chile, Norway, France, Ireland, Iceland, the Russian Federation, Spain, Italy, Denmark, Portugal, Indonesia, Korea, South Africa, Japan, China, the UK, Canada, and the USA are among those playing a role in wild-harvesting of macroalgae historically and today. Statistics from 2014 indicate that global macroalgal harvests have increased approx. 5.7% annually with Europe, Asia, Africa, North and South America, and Oceania accounting for 1.3, 1.9, 0.10, 2.4, and 0.015 million t, respectively (Mac Monagail et al. 2017). Approximately 20 countries are harvesters of brown macroalgae, including Norway, Chile, and Ireland, with 0.6 million t of kelps harvested for alginates annually. On the other hand, 32 countries are harvesters of Rhodophyceae with 0.22 million t harvested annually, dominated by Chile and Indonesia representing 76% of the harvest, while 11 countries harvest Chlorophyceae with 1661 t collected annually, mostly by Korea (Mac Monagail et al. 2017). Interestingly, while there are more than 10 000 species of macroalgae that have been reported to exist, of these, only approx. 200 species are consumed across the globe as discussed above. However, today, wild harvesting of macroalgae comprises only approx. 4% of the total annual global production in 2014 of 28.5 million t, with 96% of production from mariculture cultivation. Current global macroalgae production for all uses is worth approx. US$11.7 billion.

Because the composition of macroalgae within the same species may be highly variable when wild-harvested as a function of growth conditions, UV- and photosynthetically active radiation (PAR) exposure and desiccation, it is noteworthy that mariculture researchers and producers are cultivating macroalgae from uniform seed stocks in tanks with filtered seawater and fertilizer and/or other essential nutrients as well as controlled exposure to light (Athukorala et al. 2016; Ceccoli et al. 2008; Shacklock and Craigie 1986). These management techniques thereby ensure a reliable, year-round supply of biomass with the desired attributes, but also generate genetic variants of target species. A prime example of the innovation of mariculture industries such as these is Acadian Seaplants Limited (Nova Scotia, Canada), which generates approx. US$133 million in annual revenue from products including Hana Tsunomata™, a cultivated Irish moss (*Chondrus crispus* [R]) sold to the Japanese market. Cultivation of macroalgae contributes to the profitability and sustainability of the industry given that historically wild harvesting of macroalgae has involved labor-intensive hand-harvesting using sickles to selectively cut plants, or gathering "storm-cast" fronds on beaches, or on a larger scale using nets, horse-drawn rakes, bulldozers, tractors, diving, or mechanical methods including suction harvesters. However, this latter technology was discontinued in the Canadian Maritimes in 1994 due to overexploitation of natural stocks of Irish moss (*Ascophyllum nodosum*) and kelps in favor of a return to manual or rake harvesting (Mac Monagail et al. 2017). Indeed, the overexploitation of Irish moss in Prince Edward Island and Nova Scotia (Canada) resulted in the *C. crispus* beds being dominated and overtaken by *Furcellaria lumbricalis* (R). Other consequences of overexploitation include effects on the food, habitat, and shelter of intertidal species such as sea urchins and fish, or even effects on tidal surges and wave action and thereby erosion of coastlines, cliffs, and sedimentation.

One recent estimate suggested that approx. 5000 metric t of dry microalgal biomass processed for bioproducts including food, functional foods and nutraceuticals, nutritional supplements, and animal feed could be valued at approx. US$1.25 billion (Khan et al. 2018). As mentioned above, microalgae represent a locally available, renewable, sustainable, reliable source of nutrition, functional foods and nutraceuticals, bioactives, and food ingredients. For example, under optimal conditions, microalgae are theoretically capable of transforming approx. 9% of solar irradiance into 77 g biomass m^{-2} day^{-1} equivalent to 280 t ha^{-1} $year^{-1}$; this yield would be reduced in culture conditions due to loss of absorbed radiation (Khan et al. 2018). The environmental sustainability of culturing microalgae is supported by the technology's CO_2 utilization, in that 1 kg of algal biomass can fix approx. 1.83 kg CO_2. Large-scale cultivation of microalgae requires light (200–400 μM photons m^{-2} $second^{-1}$); major nutrients including carbon, nitrogen, and phosphorus; macronutrient minerals such as Na, Mg, Ca, and K; micronutrient minerals including Mo, Mn, B, Co, Fe, and Zn; as well as temperature control, typically in the range of 20–30 °C. Conditions can be optimized, including the mixing of the culture in the photobioreactor to ensure uniform exposure to the light source for photosynthesis. It has been estimated that a feasible operation should have a production output in the range of greater than 30 g biomass m^{-2} day^{-1}.

Another way of valuing the microalgal cultivation industry is to look at the value of microalgal products, such as the carotenoids: the global carotenoid market was valued at US$1.24 billion in 2016 and is projected to reach $1.53 billion by 2021 (Novoveská et al. 2019). Similarly, microalgal derived long-chain marine PUFAs, including eicosapentaenoic acid (EPA) and docosahexaenoic acid (DHA), are valued at US$10 billion annually. Thus, it is of vital importance to carefully choose the microalgal species of interest and culture conditions to optimize the production of the primary or secondary metabolites of interest.

1.4 Book Objectives

The overarching objective of *Recent Advancements in Micro- and Macroalgal Processing: Food and Health Perspectives* is to provide a bird's eye view of algal biomolecules, the role of emerging processing techniques, biological and health benefits and their applications in food, pharmaceuticals, and cosmetic products. A key objective of the book is to critically evaluate the role of emerging technologies in algal processing. Recent developments in drying and milling technologies are discussed along with advances in greener techniques in the extraction of bioactives from algae, which is critical for the industry. Determination of recent applications of algae for food, feed, pharmaceutical, and cosmetic products as well as economic feasibility, market trends and considerations, and health hazards associated with algae for its commercial applications, can provide a holistic picture to the industrial community. Compiling all this information in one expert monograph, this comprehensive book covers almost all aspects of algae and will establish itself as a standard reference book on the advancements in algal processing for food and health.

1.5 Book Structure

The book contains 20 chapters, which are divided into three sections. Section I explores the composition and conventional and emerging extraction technologies for algal bioactives; Section II focuses on potential biological properties and the role of algal derived compounds in promoting health; while Section III covers the advancements of algae and algal components in pharmaceutical and cosmetics products as well as application in functional foods or as nutraceuticals.

Section I, which has a stress on *relevance and processing* of algae, comprises eight chapters, wherein **Chapter 2** aims to offer insights on the influence of seasonality on the chemical composition and nutritional profile of micro- and macroalgae for their better utilization. Apart from being influenced by species and geography, the biochemistry of algae, and their nutritive and bioactive profiles, is influenced by factors such as seasons and the changing physical and chemical parameters (wave exposure, depth, temperature, irradiation, salinity, pH, etc.). Understanding seasonal differences in biochemical constituents of algae would help determine the optimal algal-harvesting time to obtain a specific composition. **Chapter 3** gives a brief overview on recent advancements in algal cell drying and milling technologies. Production of value-added products requires algal cultivation and harvesting, drying, and disruption of the algal cells for subsequent extraction and processing of the intended products. A major hurdle to the utilization of algal biomass for large-scale commercial applications is the high processing costs. Increasing the recovery of intracellular substances from algal cells could result in greater product yields and lower production costs. Drying and milling are two integral processes for effective production of value-added products from algae. Technology development, energy requirements, and comparisons in the processing methods along with challenges and prospects of algae drying and milling for sustainable and viable algal biorefineries are outlined in this chapter. After the drying and milling, the recovery or extraction of valuable bioactive compounds is the next key step. These interesting compounds are often tightly entrapped inside the algal cells; hence they need to be extracted and collected, which is covered in **Chapter 4**. This chapter focuses on recent advances in the use of greener extraction technologies for the recovery of valuable bioactive compounds from algae. Algae synthesize a range of bioactive compounds including polysaccharides, proteins and peptides, lipids, polyphenols, and carotenoids with potent biological activities. The exploitation of these molecules requires the development of extraction protocols that should ideally be food-safe/nontoxic, selective, achieve high yields of compounds, minimize the generation of waste, and reduce the use of solvents and energy during the process. This chapter summarizes the main innovative technologies (pulsed electric fields, supercritical fluid extraction, pressurized liquid extraction, microwave assisted extraction, and ultrasound assisted extraction) used to extract high-value compounds from algae. The concepts of green chemistry and biorefinery together with the principles, advantages, applications, future trends, and challenges of novel green extraction technologies are discussed in detail. Extraction methods can be divided into conventional and nonconventional or advanced extraction methods. Conventional methods are based on traditional organic solvents, while novel methods include new greener and environmentally friendly solvents such as ionic liquid and/or method. **Chapters 5–8** together explore the roles and applications of conventional and advanced extraction technologies for the recovery of individual compounds such as lipids, proteins and peptides, polyphenols, and polysaccharides from algae. Conventional extraction technologies can lead to longer processing, high energy consumption, slow extraction rate, can be time-consuming, and may cause degradation or lower yields of algal extractives. To overcome those disadvantages, extraction technologies with relatively lower energy inputs, rapid treatment times, and avoidance of hazardous solvents, increasing yields and purity levels have been developed. The future outlook, including challenges and recommendations for further development and optimization of extraction technologies for individual compounds needed to extend industrial applications, is widely discussed in these chapters.

There are ancient histories of macro- and microalgae consumption, while dietary patterns between populations are coincident with differences in diet-related chronic disease risks in populations. Marine algae have attracted a great deal of interest as excellent sources of nutrients. There is a growing global interest in the idea that algal derived bioactive compounds can play a major therapeutic role in disease prevention in humans. The fact that most of these bioactives are known to exhibit antioxidant, antimicrobial, antiviral, anti-inflammatory, anticancer, anti-proliferative, antidiabetic, antitumor, anticoagulant, and apoptosis-inducing effects demonstrates their potential use in nutraceuticals, functional foods, pharmaceuticals, and cosmetics. Therefore, **Section II** of the book, which contains seven chapters emphasizing *bioactivities*, largely focuses on the potential biological properties of algal derived compounds and their role in promoting health and disease prevention. This section is focused on individual groups of compounds such as polysaccharides, proteins, polyphenols, carotenoids, lipids, and fiber from algae and has covered purification and characterization strategies along with their biological properties and possible health effects. **Chapter 9** critically examines the existing scientific knowledge on secondary metabolites and their biological activities ascribed to macro- and microalgae including anticarcinogenic, antiobesogenic, modulation of blood glucose, lipids, and antioxidant capacities. The chapter reviews the evidence underlying the biological activities of macro- and microalgal constituents and the proposed mechanisms of action. **Chapter 10** is primarily focused on polysaccharides, the main constituents in marine algae, which have numerous beneficial health effects on human health. The biological activities including antioxidant, immunomodulatory, anticancer, antiviral, hypolipidemic, anticoagulant, and antimicrobial effects are discussed. This contribution is an overview of the biological activities and potential health benefits, along with the chemical structure, extraction, and purification approaches used for marine algal polysaccharides. **Chapter 11** investigates the phenolic compounds encountered in micro- and macroalgae, their chemical structures together with their biological activities and potential valorization for medical and cosmetic industries. For example, phenolic compounds in marine algae are known to be synthesized in response to different environmental conditions. Polyphenols protect these organisms against herbivores or epiphytes, bacterial infection, or UV radiation. Once consumed, they may be beneficial to human health and assist with chronic disease risk prevention since they have a wide range of bioactivities. They can exhibit antioxidant, antimicrobial, anti-inflammatory, antitumor, antiaging, pro-mineralogenic activities or can act as modulators of cardiovascular disease risk. **Chapter 12** delineates the commercial and nutraceutical importance of carotenoids, an important bioactive compound from algal biomasses. The growing importance of carotenoids has an immense impact on the cosmetics and nutraceuticals markets. Hence, the chemical structure, isolation, and biological applications and commercialization of different types of carotenoids and xanthophylls are described herein. The biological importance of algal carotenoids in relation to chronic disease risk reduction, such as in various cancers, diabetes mellitus, antiaging, skin diseases, and other ailments, along with their marketable production, commercial aspects, and future prospects are elaborated on in this chapter. **Chapter 13** presents information about the structure and distribution of fatty acids in micro- and macroalgae, and various parameters affecting lipid and fatty acid contents as well as their distribution. Algal fatty acids are known as sources of bioactive compounds for health promotion and wellness. Lipid fractions and fatty acids act as bioactive ingredients or additives for cosmeceutical applications. Algae are organisms with enormous biodiversity and contain manifold fatty acid molecular structures and ratios. Methods for isolation and purification of fatty acids from algae, in order to obtain highly pure fatty acid or fatty acid fractions with good overall yields as well as preventive effects of n-3 PUFAs on cardiovascular disease, metabolic syndrome, and cancer are discussed therein. Furthermore, the potential role of n-3 fatty acids in cancer risk reduction therapies and antiviral activities of lipids for health promotion and potential commercial application are reviewed in this chapter. **Chapter 14** provides an overview of algal peptides investigated for their potential health benefits and functionality, and also outlines research challenges in their extraction, as well as their global market position. Proteins are the fundamental growth factors of living organisms while various algae are known to be rich sources of protein. Algal proteins have distinctive structures and their peptides have various functionalities that are not seen in higher plants. With the increasing number of metabolic disorders in aging populations, algal peptides have gained more attention in recent times. Lastly, for Section II, **Chapter 15** is focused on the physicochemical characteristics and potential health impacts of algal dietary fiber. It is commonly known that dietary fiber is the nondigestible food component present in the human diet. Epidemiological research suggests that fiber and polysaccharides, particularly sulfated polysaccharides, are effective in modulating immunity, mutagens, coagulants, cholesterol, and blood glucose levels. It is interesting to note that algal biomass comprises about 30–70% of fiber on a dry weight basis and that the majority of this fiber is water-soluble or water-dispersable as hydrocolloids. The chemical, physical, and rheological properties of algal dietary fiber are most suitable for dietary purposes. In particular, the viscosity, dispersibility, water-holding capacity, fermentability, and fecal bulking capacity of algal fiber renders it a potential candidate for the food, feed, and pharmaceutical industries.

The multiple benefits of algal derived functional ingredients with their unique structures and nutritional and therapeutic activities provide many opportunities for the development of healthier foods, pharmaceutical and even cosmeceutical products. Despite the prominence of both microalgae and seaweeds in the human diet for thousands of years, only in recent years with the new technological outcomes has the functional food and nutraceutical potential of algae been explored and reported. Some epidemiological studies indicate that consumption of algae can reduce the risk of certain chronic diseases such as allergies, cardiovascular diseases, cancer, obesity, diabetes, high blood pressure, atopic dermatitis, or Alzheimer's disease, and this has led to *in vitro* and *in vivo* studies to elucidate their possible mechanisms of action. Even though clinical trials are scarce, the pharmaceutical industry is keen on developing drugs of natural origin from marine organisms (e.g. Adcetris®), with fewer side effects and reduced toxicity to humans.

Thus, considering the above, **Section III** of the book, which contains five chapters, is entirely focused on the *application* of this subject matter by addressing the utilization of whole algae or algal compounds in food, cosmetics, and pharmaceuticals with an overview of their impact on health. **Chapter 16** explores the feasibility of using whole algae in animal feed and as an ingredient in various human food products (e.g. muscle-based foods, cereal-based foods, dairy products, and beverages) along with their functional and nutritional impacts. **Chapters 17–19** explore the potential of algae to benefit human health and highlight the potential use of functional ingredients in the food and pharmaceutical industries. These chapters present an overview of the main molecules that have been recovered from microalgae and macroalgae and review their nutraceutical benefits and applications. They also summarize current knowledge on algal compounds of interest for the formulation of nutraceutical, pharmaceutical, and cosmeceutical preparations. The final chapter (**Chapter 20**) of the book is focused on the commercial cultivation and exploitation of seaweeds. Commercial exploitation of seaweeds is primarily focused on farming the edible species for production of hydrocolloids. However, due to advances in algal research, opportunities for commercial exploitation of seaweed have included processing for functional ingredients, nutraceuticals, pharmaceuticals and dentistry, health and beauty industries, animal stock feeds, soil conditioners, fertilizers, biofuels, water filtration, and livestock and fishery diets as discussed above. Global seaweed production has been experiencing steady growth in recent years and the statistics on production have been widely captured in the Food and Agriculture Organization's (FAO) annual publications, which are the primary source of production data. This final chapter reviews the recently published literature on commercial aspects of seaweed, including its production statistics and usage details, and presents a comprehensive business overview of this unique resource. Finally, in order to provide a holistic picture to the industry community, this chapter will finish by looking at the economic feasibility, market trends and considerations, and health hazards associated with the industrial applications of algae.

To conclude, we hope that this book will be a valuable resource for information relating to algal processing. This volume includes contributions from leading international experts from world-renowned universities and institutions, and we are confident that the chapters are informative and concise, and will provide meaningful perspectives on a subject of growing interest and importance to researchers and industry. This book will offer the reader a broad review of conventional techniques and application of novel processing/extraction techniques for algal bioactive compounds. Thus, it is hoped that this text will serve as a comprehensive reference book for students, educators, researchers, food ingredients specialists, and product developers providing up-to-date insights into algal processing. The range of processes covered will provide food technologists, professionals, engineers, and scientists working in the food and nutraceutical industry with a valuable resource for their work. Thus, it is particularly timely to be able to contribute a volume focused on *Recent Advances in Micro- and Macroalgal Processing: Food and Health Perspectives* to the teaching, research, and industrial communities including students at all levels, faculty members, researchers, and allied professionals.

References

Athukorala, Y. and Yuan, Y.V. (2013). Fucoidans from marine brown macroalgae: isolation, identification and potential biological activities. Ch. 24. In: *Marine Nutraceuticals: Prospects and Perspectives* (ed. S.-K. Kim), 393–435. Boca Raton, FL: CRC Taylor & Francis Press Inc.

Athukorala, Y., Trang, S., Kwok, C., and Yuan, Y.V. (2016). Antiproliferative and antioxidant activities and mycosporine-like amino acid profiles of wild-harvested and cultivated edible Canadian marine red macroalgae. *Molecules* **21** (1): 119. https://doi.org/10.3390/molecules21010119.

Ceccoli, J., Costello, B., and Pillai, S. (2008). Marine extracts and biofermentations for use in cosmetics. US Patent 8,202,519 B2.

Christaki, E., Florou-Paneri, P., and Bonos, E. (2011). Microalgae: a novel ingredient in nutrition. *International Journal of Food Sciences and Nutrition* **62** (8): 794–799.

Davidson, K. (2019). 7 Reasons seaweed belongs in your diet and beauty routine. *Elle Magazine* (March 25). https://www.elle.com/beauty/health-fitness/news/a26568/seaweed-snacks-healthy (accessed August 28, 2020).

Garcia, J.L., de Vicente, M., and Galán, B. (2017). Microalgae, old sustainable food and fashion nutraceuticals. *Microbial Biotechnology* **10** (5): 1017–1024.

Gomez-Zavaglia, A., Prieto Lage, M., Jiminez-Lopez, C. et al. (2019). The potential of seaweeds as a source of functional ingredients of prebiotic and antioxidant value. *Antioxidants* **8**: 406. https://doi.org/10.3390/antiox8090406.

Hein, T. (2016). Sea superfood. Canada and other Western countries have been slow to realize the benefits of seaweed – but that's now changing. *Food in Canada*. https://www.foodincanada.com/features/sea-superfood (accessed August 28, 2020).

Khan, M.I., Shin, J.H., and Kim, J.D. (2018). The promising future of microalgae: current status, challenges, and optimization of a sustainable and renewable industry for biofuels, feed, and other products. *Microbial Cell Factories* **17** (1): 36. https://doi.org/10.1186/s12934-018-0879-x.

Liu, K. (2020). It's been banned in China for 20 years. But it's still a popular Chinese New Year ingredient in Toronto. *The Star* (January 22). https://www.thestar.com/life/food_wine/2020/01/22/fat-choy-the-lucky-but-not-so-environmentally-friendly-lunar-new-year-ingredient.html (accessed August 28, 2020).

Lordan, S., Ross, R.P., and Stanton, C. (2011). Marine bioactives as functional food ingredients: potential to reduce the incidence of chronic diseases. *Marine Drugs* **9**: 1056–1100.

Mac Monagail, M., Cornish, L., Morrison, L. et al. (2017). Sustainable harvesting of wild seaweed resources. *European Journal of Phycology* **52** (4): 371–390. https://doi.org/10.1080/09670262.2017.1365273.

Ni, M. (2018). seaweed: miracle vegetable from the sea. doctoroz.com. https://www.doctoroz.com/blog/mao-shing-ni-lac-dom-phd/seaweed-miracle-vegetable-sea (accessed August 28, 2020).

Novoveská, L., Ross, M.E., Stanley, M.S. et al. (2019). Microalgal carotenoids: a review of production, current markets, regulations, and future direction. *Marine Drugs* **17** (11): 640. https://doi.org/10.3390/md17110640.

Pérez-Lloréns, J.L., Mouritsen, O.G., Rhatigan, P. et al. (2020). Seaweeds in mythology, folklore, poetry, and life. *Journal of Applied Phycology* https://doi.org/10.1007/s10811-020-02133-0.

Plaza, M., Cifuentes, A., and Ibáñez, E. (2008). In the search of new functional food ingredients from algae. *Trends in Food Science and Technology* **19**: 31–39.

Robledo, D. and Freile Pelegrín, Y. (1997). Chemical and mineral composition of six potentially edible seaweed species of Yucatán. *Botanica Marina* **40**: 301–306.

Shacklock, P.F. and Craigie, J.S. (1986). Winter survival and growth of *Chondrus crispus* in onshore culture tanks. *Canadian Journal of Fisheries and Aquatic Sciences* **43**: 263–268.

Sloan, A.E. (2018). Top 10 functional food trends. *Food Technology* **72** (4): 26–28, 31–32, 35–43.

Talero, E., García-Mauriño, S., Ávila-Román, J. et al. (2015). Bioactive compounds isolated from microalgae in chronic inflammation and cancer. *Marine Drugs* **13**: 6152–6209.

Tou, J., Oldaker, C., and Yuan, Y.V. (2020). Novel marine sources of nutraceuticals and functional foods: the marine crustacean krill, macro- and microalgae. In: *Encyclopedia of Marine Biotechnology* (ed. S.-K. Kim). Chichester: Wiley in press.

Yuan, Y.V. (2008). Marine algal constituents. In: *Marine Nutraceuticals and Functional Foods* (eds. C. Barrow and F. Shahidi), 259–296. Boca Raton, FL: CRC Taylor & Francis Press Inc.

Yuan, Y.V. and Athukorala, Y. (2012). Red algal mycosporine-like amino acids (MAAs) as potential cosmeceuticals. In: *Marine Cosmeceuticals: Trends and Prospects* (ed. S.-K. Kim), 143–167. Boca Raton, FL: CRC Taylor & Francis Press Inc.

2

Influence of Seasonal Variation on Chemical Composition and Nutritional Profiles of Macro- and Microalgae

K. Suresh Kumar, Sushma Kumari, Kamleshwar Singh, and Pratibha Kushwaha
Department of Botany, University of Allahabad, Prayagraj, India

2.1 Introduction

Escalation in the human population has accelerated the desire to find new resources to meet the growing demand for food, medicine, fuel, etc. The aquatic environment, containing a variety of unique organisms, comprises one of the most underutilized biological resources. Having explored colossal terrestrial alternatives, utilization of aquatic (marine and freshwater) resources has now emerged as a feasible unconventional alternative to fulfill human necessities.

Algae are a complex and heterogeneous group of organisms characterized by their photosynthetic nature and their simple reproductive structures (Ibañez et al. 2012; Balakrishnan et al. 2014). They are often found in aquatic (freshwater and marine) as well as certain terrestrial habitats; they can survive extreme environments (light, salinity, and temperature). Having a paramount role as primary producers in the ocean and the food web, they perform significant ecological functions (capturing carbon, providing habitat, being a part of the food web, etc.). Based on their size, algae are divided into unicellular organisms, known as microalgae (including blue-green algae and phytoplanktons), and multicellular organisms, referred to as macroalgae (seaweeds) (Anbuchezhian et al. 2015). The vast diversity of species of macro- and microalgae, their prevalence in the aquatic ecosystems, and tolerance to hostile environments, coupled with their versatility, make these organisms key targets for screening projects for food, functional food ingredients, minerals, medicine,

Recent Advances in Micro- and Macroalgal Processing: Food and Health Perspectives, First Edition.
Edited by Gaurav Rajauria and Yvonne V. Yuan.

insulation, fertilizer, fodder, bioactive compounds, etc. (Balakrishnan et al. 2014; Ibañez et al. 2012). With high species diversity and myriad forms and sizes, freshwater algae are universal (Sheath and Wehr 2015). However, Anbuchezhian et al. (2015) describe the marine environment as home to the majority of algal classes (including micro- and macroalgae). Macroalgae comprise a taxonomically diverse group of organisms that often have a plant-like appearance; however, they do not have roots, stems, leaves, and well-defined vascular tissues (Barsanti and Gualtieri 2006). Forming an important food or a breeding ground for several marine organisms, they also serve as a sink for additional carbon dioxide and nutrients. Algae have turned into a multibillion dollar industry due to high productivity, unequaled species diversity, and the plethora of industrially important chemicals that they produce (Stengel and Connan 2015). They hold the potential for tremendous applicability in various sectors such as food (and food ingredients), feed (animal feed and plant stimulants), bioremediation, biofuel, as well as the pharmaceutical, nutraceutical, and cosmeceutical industries.

Macroalgae are a rich natural resource of valuable biochemicals such as high-quality proteins, bioactive peptides, dietary fiber, polysaccharides, lipids, fatty acids (FAs), minerals, vitamins, pigments, and phytochemicals such as polyphenols, and also have protective effects (against allergy, cancers, degenerative disorders, diabetes, digestive disorders, heart disease, hypertension, inflammation, lipidemia, obesity, and oxidative stress; Paiva et al. 2018). They are reported to produce industrially important polysaccharides and sugars (agar, carrageenan, alginates, ulvan, furcellaran, hypnean, funoran, iridophycan, phyllophoran, laminaran, fucoidan, and mannitol) and fascinating natural metabolites with novel structures and biological activities (carotenoids, polyketides, polyphenols, peptides, halogenated compounds, FAs, steroids, lectins, etc.; Anbuchezhian et al. 2015). The chemical compositions of various types of algae can be viewed in Table 2.1. On the other hand, microalgae (including diatoms, dinoflagellates, green algae, and blue-green algae) are distributed throughout the ocean, and occupy the bottom of the food chain; they are one of the important sources of food for various organisms in the marine environment (Anbuchezhian et al. 2015). Microalgae provide a variety of high-value products such as polyunsaturated fatty acids (PUFAs), pigments (carotenoids and phycobiliproteins), and, bioactive compounds, which are useful as nutraceuticals and pharmaceuticals and in industrial applications. *Spirulina* and *Chlorella* have high nutritional value and are mass cultured for health food. Microalgae are used for bioremediation and biomonitoring of environmental toxicants, and as feedstock for several different types of renewable fuels (biodiesel, methane, hydrogen, and ethanol) (Chu 2012). Nowadays, there is a growing demand for algae, but this rise in demand for algae is no longer met by the natural availability, which has promoted technical developments in cultivation of algae (aquaculture). The supply of a sufficient quantity of algae that meets the quality mark has always been a matter of concern with the conflicting environmental pressures.

Environmental and physical conditions (habitat, light, substrate, topography, temperature, salinity, humidity, tides, waves, wind, currents, and pollutants) prevailing in the aquatic body determine the occurrence, distribution, growth, abundance, and chemical constitution of algae. For example, certain algae endure strong waves, others prefer calm water or sea bays; some algae tolerate drier conditions and grow in the supralittoral fringe, while others survive extra ordinal environmental changes (dry or wet) in the littoral zone (which occurs at low tide twice daily). Growth of algae also

Table 2.1 Chemical composition of various algae (% dry weight).

Algae	Protein	Carbo-hydrate	Fiber	Lipid	Ash	References
Microalgae						
Anabaena cylindrica	43–56	25–30		4–7		Becker (2007)
Anabaena cylindrica	43–56	25–30		4–7		Becker (2007)
Anabaena cylindrica	43–56	25–30		4–7		Spolaore et al. (2006)
Aphanizomenon sp.	1.0	23.0				Bishop and Zubeck (2012)
Aphanizomenon flos-aquae	62	23		3		Becker (2007)
Arthrospira maxima	60–71	13–16		6–7		Becker (2007)
Catenella repens	8.42	28.96		5.29		Chakraborty and Santra (2008)
Chlamydomonas rheinhardii	48	17		21		Becker (2007)
Chlamydomonas rheinhardii	48	17		21		Spolaore et al. (2006)
Chlorella	64.5	15.0				Bishop and Zubeck (2012)
Chlorella pyrenoidosa	57	26		2		Becker (2007)
Chlorella pyrenoidosa	57	26		2		Becker (2007)
Chlorella pyrenoidosa			1.97			Mišurcová et al. (2010)
Chlorella vulgaris	51–58	12–17		14–22		Becker (2007)
Chlorella vulgaris	51–58	12–17		14–22		Becker (2007)
Chlorella vulgaris	51–58	12–17		14–22		Spolaore et al. (2006)
Dunaliella	7.4	29.7				Bishop and Zubeck (2012)
Dunaliella salina	57	32		6		Becker (2007)
Dunaliella salina	57	32		6		Spolaore et al. (2006)
Dunaliella tertiolecta	43			17	8	Diprat et al. (2017)
Enteromorpha intestinalis	6.15	30.58		7.13		Chakraborty and Santra (2008)
Euglena gracilis	39–61	14–18		14–20		Becker (2007)
Haematococcus	23.6	38.0				Bishop and Zubeck (2012)
Heterochlorella luteoviridis	29			11	14	Diprat et al. (2017)

(*continued overleaf*)

Table 2.1 (*continued*)

Algae	Protein	Carbo-hydrate	Fiber	Lipid	Ash	References
Lola capillaris	40.87	22.32		4.05		Chakraborty and Santra (2008)
Polysiphonia mollis	16.59	25.81		5.79		Chakraborty and Santra (2008)
Porphyridium cruentum	28–39	40–57		9–14		Becker (2007)
Porphyridium cruentum	28–39	40–57		9–14		Becker (2007)
Porphyridium cruentum	28–39	40–57		9–14		Spolaore et al. (2006)
Prymnesium sp.	28–45	25–33		22–38		Ricketts (1966)
Rhizoclonium riparium	21.09	15.34		3.37		Chakraborty and Santra (2008)
Scenedesmus obliquus	50–56	10–17		12–14		Becker (2007)
Scenedesmus obliquus	50–56	10–17		12–14		Spolaore et al. (2006)
Spirogyra	6–20	33–64		11–21		Becker (1994)
Spirogyra sp.	6–20	33–64		11–21		Becker (2007)
Spirulina maxima	60–71	13–16		6–7		Spolaore et al. (2006)
Spirulina platensis	46–63	8–14		4–9		Becker (2007)
Spirulina platensis	65.6	10.7		14.2	9.5	Yucetepe et al. (2018)
Spirulina platensis	46–63	8–14		4–9		Becker (2007)
Spirulina pacifica			0.18			Mišurcová et al. (2010)
Spirulina platensis			0.10			Mišurcová et al. (2010)
Synechococcus sp.	63	15		11		Becker (2007)
Synechococcus sp.	63	15		11		Spolaore et al. (2006)
Macroalgae/seaweed						
Chlorophyta						
Ascophyllum nodosum	8.70			3.62	30.89	Lorenzo et al. (2017)
Alaria esculenta	9–20	46–51		1–2		Pereira (2011)
Ascophyllum nodosum	1.2–17			0.5–4.8	18–30	Turan and Cırık (2018)
Ascophyllum nodosum	4.8–9.8			1.9–4.8	18–24	Ghadiryanfara et al. (2016)
Ascophyllum nodosum		13.1	8.8			MacArtain et al. (2007)

(*continued overleaf*)

Table 2.1 (*continued*)

Algae	Protein	Carbo-hydrate	Fiber	Lipid	Ash	References
Bifurcaria bifurcata	8.92			6.54	31.68	Lorenzo et al. (2017)
Caulerpa racemosa	17.8–18.4	33.41	64.9	9.8	7–19	Pereira (2011)
Caulerpa lentillifera	10–13	38–59	33	0.86–1.11	24–37	Pereira (2011)
Caulerpa racemosa				2.64		Kumari et al. (2010)
Caulerpa sp.	10–18.40					Pereira (2011)
Caulerpa veravalnensis				2.83		Kumari et al. (2010)
Codium fragile	8–11	39–67	5.1	0.5–1.5	21–39	Pereira (2011)
Cystoseira indica				1.23		Kumari et al. (2010)
Cystoseira abies-marina	6.81		56.34			Patarra et al. (2011)
Enteromorpha linza	12.5		7.14	4.10	28.33	Ganesan et al. (2014)
Enteromorpha tubulosa	19.09		6.28	5.56	17.01	Ganesan et al. (2014)
Eisenia bicyclis	7.5	60.6		0.1	9.72	Pereira (2011)
Enteromorpha compressa	17.48		2.93	3.56	31.21	Ganesan et al. (2014)
Enteromorpha sp.		7.8	4.9			MacArtain et al. (2007)
Fucus vesiculosus	12.99			3.75	20.71	Lorenzo et al. (2017)
Fucus sp.	3.00–14.00					Pereira (2011)
Fucus spiralis	10.77		63.88			Pereira (2011)
Fucus vesiculosus	3–14	46.8	45–59	1.9	14–30	Pereira (2011)
Himanthalia elongata	5–15	44–61	33–37	0.5–1.1	27–36	Pereira (2011)
Himanthalia elongata	6–13	65				Arumugam et al. (2018)
Himanthalia elongata		15.0	9.8			MacArtain et al. (2007)
Macrocystis	17.3				41.1	Ghadiryanfara et al. (2016)
Ulva lactuca (autumn)	16.78	42.09		3.14	23.19	Khairy and El-Shafay (2013)
Ulva lactuca (spring)	20.12	44.81		4.09	22.08	Khairy and El-Shafay (2013)

(*continued overleaf*)

Table 2.1 (*continued*)

Algae	Protein	Carbo-hydrate	Fiber	Lipid	Ash	References
Ulva lactuca (summer)	17.88	46.42		3.57	17.56	Khairy and El-Shafay (2013)
Ulva lactuca	10–25	36–43	29–55	0.6–1.6	12.9	Pereira (2011)
Ulva pertusa	20–26	47.0				Pereira (2011)
Ulva reticulata	17–20	50–58	65.7	1.7–2.3		Pereira (2011)
Ulva rigida	18–19	43–56	38–41	0.9–2.0	28.6	Pereira (2011)
Ulva compressa	21–32	48.2	29–45	0.3–4.2	17–19	Pereira (2011)
Ulva compressa	26.62		41.16			Patarra et al. (2011)
Ulva fasciata				1.83		Kumari et al. (2010)
Ulva lactuca	8.44	35.27		4.36		Chakraborty and Santra (2008)
Ulva sp.		4.1	3.8			MacArtain et al. (2007)
Ulva sp.	10–32					Pereira (2011)
Ulva sp.	13.6			2.7	30.2	Ghadiryanfara et al. (2016)
Ulva lactuca	13.84	43.19	53.62		12.41	Debbarma et al. (2016)
Ulva reticulata				2.00		Kumari et al. (2010)
Ulva sp.	4–44			0.3–1.6	26; 52–55	Turan and Cırık (2018)
Ulva tubulosa				2.13		Kumari et al. (2010)
Phaeophyta						
Saccharina japonica	7–8	51.9	10–41	1–1.9	27–33	Pereira (2011)
Hizikia fusiformis			12.55			Mišurcová et al. (2010)
Laminaria japonica			5.45			Mišurcová et al. (2010)
Undaria pinnatifida			2.94			Mišurcová et al. (2010)
Saccharina sp.	5–26					Pereira (2011)
Saccharina latissima	6–26	52–61	30	0.5–1.1	34.78	Pereira (2011)
Sargassum sp.	18.21	30.32	58.25		12.95	Debbarma et al. (2016)
Sargassum fusiforme	11.6	30.6	17–69	1.4	19.77	Pereira (2011)
Sargassum sp.	9–20			0.5–3.9	44	Turan and Cırık (2018)
Sargassum tenerrimum				2.03		Kumari et al. (2010)

(*continued overleaf*)

Table 2.1 (*continued*)

Algae	Protein	Carbo-hydrate	Fiber	Lipid	Ash	References
Sargassum vulgare	9.19–19.94	52.62–68.54	4.8–10.51	0.15–0.79	13.07–3.19	Marinho-Soriano et al. (2006)
Jania rubens (spring)	12.93	42.18		2.39	39.25	Khairy and El-Shafay (2013)
Jania rubens (summer)	11.14	39.20		2.30	42.3	Khairy and El-Shafay (2013)
Jania rubens (autumn)	9.76	34.57		1.47	50.54	Khairy and El-Shafay (2013)
Pterocladiella capillacea (spring)	23.72	50.49		2.71	13.02	Khairy and El-Shafay (2013)
Pterocladiella capillacea (summer)	20.95	50.96		2.09	15.81	Khairy and El-Shafay (2013)
Pterocladiella capillacea (autumn)	17.35	47.98		1.76	23.68	Khairy and El-Shafay (2013)
Laminaria digitata	4.63			0.53	26.5	Ghadiryanfara et al. (2016)
Laminaria digitata	8–15	48	36–37	1.0	38	Pereira (2011)
Laminaria digitata	8–14	48				Arumugam et al. (2018)
Laminaria digitata		9.9	6.2			MacArtain et al. (2007)
Laminaria longicruris	3–21			0.3–2.9	15–45	Turan and Cırık (2018)
Laminaria ochroleuca	7.49			0.92	29.47	Pereira (2011)
Laminaria sp.	7.49–15.00					Pereira (2011)
Laminaria sp.	12			2	26	Ghadiryanfara et al. (2016)
Undaria pinnatifida	12–23	45–51	16–51	1.05–4.5	26–40	Pereira (2011)
Undaria pinnatifida	11–24			1–4.5	27–40	Turan and Cırık (2018)
Undaria pinnatifida		4.6	3.4			MacArtain et al. (2007)
Rhodophyta						
Gracilaria edulis	14.26		63.17		7.63	Debbarma et al. (2016)
Chondrus crispus	11–21	55–68	10–34	1.0–3.0	21	Pereira (2011)
Chondrus crispus	6–29			0.7–3	21	Turan and Cırık (2018)

(*continued overleaf*)

Table 2.1 (*continued*)

Algae	Protein	Carbo-hydrate	Fiber	Lipid	Ash	References
Chondrus crispus	11.00–21.00					Pereira (2011)
Chondrus crispus	11–18	55–66				Arumugam et al. (2018)
Gelidium microdon	15.18		57.37			Patarra et al. (2011)
Gracilaria sp.	6.90–13.70					Pereira (2011)
Gracilaria sp.	11.4				37.7	Ghadiryanfara et al. (2016)
Gracilaria cervicornis	14.29–22.71	57.72–68.29	4.87–7.67	0.33–0.52	8.07–13.11	Marinho-Soriano et al. (2006)
Gracilaria changii	6.9		24.7	3.3	22.7	Pereira (2011)
Gracilaria chilensis	13.7	66.1		1.3	18.9	Pereira (2011)
Gracilaria debilis				1.23		Kumari et al. (2010)
Gracilaria dura				1.10		Kumari et al. (2010)
Gracilaria furgosonii				0.57		Kumari et al. (2010)
Gracilaria sp.	5–23			0.4–2.6	8–29	Turan and Cırık (2018)
Hypnea esperi				1.00		Kumari et al. (2010)
Hypnea musciformis				1.07		Kumari et al. (2010)
Kappaphycus alvarezii				1.50		Kumari et al. (2010)
Laurencia cruciata				1.53		Kumari et al. (2010)
Laurencia papillosa				1.73		Kumari et al. (2010)
Osmundea pinnatifida	20.64		33.82			Patarra et al. (2011)
Palmaria palmata	8–35					Pereira (2011)
Palmaria palmata	8–35	46–56	29–46	0.7–3	12–37	Pereira (2011)
Palmaria palmata		10.6	5.4			MacArtain et al. (2007)
Palmaria palmata	12–21	46–50				Arumugam et al. (2018)
Palmaria palmata	8–35			0.2–3.8	12–37	Turan and Cırık (2018)
Porphyra sp.	25.80		40.98			Patarra et al. (2011)

(*continued overleaf*)

Table 2.1 (*continued*)

Algae	Protein	Carbo-hydrate	Fiber	Lipid	Ash	References
Porphyra columbina	24.61		48.02	0.25	6.46	Cian et al. (2014)
Porphyra sp.	7–50			0.12–2.8	7–21	Turan and Cırık (2018)
Porphyra tenera	28–47	44.3	12–35	0.7–1.3	8–21	Pereira (2011)
Porphyra umbilicalis	29–39	43	29–35	0.3	12	Pereira (2011)
Porphyra yezoensis	31–44	44.4	30–59	2.1	7.8	Pereira (2011)
Porphyra yezoensis	29–44					Pereira (2011)
Pterocladiella capillacea	20.52		52.08			Patarra et al. (2011)
Pyropia tenera	28–47					Pereira (2011)
Sarconerna filiforme				1.47		Kumari et al. (2010)
Sphaerococcus coronopifolius	19.56		41.25			Patarra et al. (2011)

varies depending on the substrate (lithoherm, coral reefs, stone blocks, shells, and mud); generally, they tend to grow on lithoherm or coral reefs in the coastal regions, especially in tidal pools or reef grooves (National Taiwan Museum 2006).

Algal flora undergo seasonal changes in occurrence as well as biochemical constituents. Osman et al. (2011) point out that seasonal changes in lipid, carbohydrate, and protein quantities are possible indicators of the physiological state of the algae. For example, certain algae could flourish in winter and spring, but decrease significantly in richness and species during summer and autumn. In summer, the prevalent strong sunlight and high temperature make it difficult for algae to survive, therefore algae are often absent in certain habitats; this could be due to changes in light intensity, light duration, temperature, water composition, wave motion, etc. (Paiva et al. 2018) particularly state that the biochemical composition of seaweeds, and their nutritional and commercial value, depends on factors such as species, its developmental stage, spatial and temporal changes in environmental parameters (including light, temperature, nutrients, and salinity), and biotic interactions. This chapter discusses the chemical composition of algae and its seasonal variability.

2.2 Influence of Seasonal Variation on Biochemical Composition of Micro- and Macroalgae

The biochemical composition of algae displays considerable diversity between and within taxa, i.e. the biochemistry of closely related algal species is usually more similar than that of unrelated species. Nonetheless, the biochemical composition of every member within a single species, or an individual organism, is distinct (Table 2.1). The growth, occurrence, abundance (availability), the biochemical composition of algae, and, consequently their nutritional and medicinal value, depend on several variable including: species and its developmental stage, spatial and temporal changes inenvironmental parameters (light, temperature, nutrient, salinity, wave motion, etc.) as well as biotic interactions (Marinho-Soriano et al. 2006).

Most environmental parameters vary with season and with changes in ecological conditions; this in turn could stimulate or inhibit the biosynthesis of several nutrients. This makes it nearly impossible to review the vast chemical diversity that exists for the whole range of algae as a group or its compounds (Stengel et al. 2011). It is important to understand and quantify existing chemical diversity and variability of these compounds in algae in order to better utilize them.

Seasonal evaluations and comparisons of the chemical composition (protein, carbohydrate, lipids, fiber, ash, and nitrogen) of various algae species provide an insight into their commercial value and the best period of harvest from an economic perspective. Compounds of particular commercial interest include pigments, lipids and FAs, proteins, polysaccharides, and phenolics. Even though it has been known that ecological conditions could stimulate or inhibit the biosynthesis of several nutrients (Marinho-Soriano et al. 2006), less emphasis has been placed on the nutritional properties of algae in context to facilitate their better utilization. The few reports evaluating the chemical composition of algae also highlight the challenge put forward by seasonality in terms of fluctuations in chemical composition (Mabeau and Fleurence 1993; van Hal Jaap et al. 2014).

Seasonal variations in chemical composition and nutritive value have been reported in common seaweeds from different parts of the world; for example, north-east Brazil (*Gracilaria cervicornis* and *Sargassum vulgare*; Marinho-Soriano et al. 2006), Hong Kong (Kaehler and Kennish 1996), coastal India (Kumar 1993), and Ireland (Mercer et al. 1993). Stengel et al. (2011) reviewed temporal (seasonal and diurnal) changes and reproductive development in algae, stating that the seasonality of chemical composition mainly results from two distinct yet complementary factors: (i) physiological changes in response to ambient environmental conditions, and (ii) seasonal vegetative and reproductive development. They reported comprehensive changes in levels and composition of minerals, vitamins, amino acids, carbohydrates, FAs, and proteins of algae with considerable seasonal differences, e.g. Pacific kelp *Eisenia arborea*, *Fucales*, and *Laminariales* (Stengel et al. 2011). Contrarily, in certain species with distinct seasonal phenologies (kelps) and the bi-annual *Himanthalia elongata*, seasonal changes in carbohydrates and nitrogen-containing substances are attributed to various growth phases like the annual cycle of receptacle development, where the mature alga consists predominantly of reproductive structures (*H. elongata*). In other perennial algae like *Ascophyllum nodosum*, apart from seasonal occurrence of reproductive structures (which varies according to geographic location and shore level; Stengel et al. 2011), the seasonal variability in chemical composition is also influenced by physiological changes within vegetative thalli (Stengel et al. 2011).

Seasonality (accompanied by varying light density and quality, photoperiod, light, temperature, salinity, currents, nutrients, etc.) also influences the composition, occurrence, abundance, community dynamics, and biochemistry of microalgae. Al-Harbi (2017) observed seasonal and regional fluctuations in algae and stated that the convergence zone of the Red Sea was poorer in microalgal species; the diatoms were the major group of epilithic microalgae (and showed high abundance in summer at the north-west coast of Jeddah of the Red Sea), where the dominant species was *Spirulina subsalsa* among the epilithic microalgal community.

It is absolutely essential for researchers and industrialists interested in production of a particular algal constituent to first understand the potent role of seasonality, and thereafter determine the period of harvest for optimal production of a desired composition. The role of seasonality in the composition of algae, highlighting major biochemical moieties with certain examples, is discussed herein.

2.3 Pigments

Photosynthetic pigments utilize sunlight for the production of carbohydrates through the process of photosynthesis and further supply this energy to herbivores and carnivores in an ecosystem, thereby playing a vital role in the growth and development of photosynthetic organisms. Pigments are broadly classified into photosynthetic pigments (chlorophyll, chl) and other accessory pigments (carotenoids [Car], phycoerythrin [PE], and phycocyanin [PC]). Car, phycobilins (PBs), PE, and PC help in capturing light energy for chl. Car also play an important role in antioxidant activities of plants to enable them to cope with biotic and abiotic stress. Algae are known to possess photosynthetic pigments such as chl, Car (carotenes and xanthophylls), and PBs. The light-harvesting processes of photoautotrophic algae suggest involvement of chl (i.e. all groups possess chl *a*) and various groups of accessory pigments; these are specific to a particular algal group, with major groups delimited by the presence of PBs and Car. The diversity of the pigments that exists within algal divisions has been emphasized in several reports (e.g. Prasanna et al. 2007; Prasanna and Kaushik 2010); a summary of algal pigments based on various groups has been provided in Table 2.2. Takaichi (2011) evaluated several algal Car, observing that approximately 30 types have photosynthetic functions, while others could be intermediates of carotenogenesis or accumulated Car. They suggested the use of Car and chl as chemotaxonomic markers (due to their distribution in algae). They state that Car contain a unique allene (C=C=C); nevertheless, some classes contain additional Car, such as loroxanthin, siphonaxanthin, and prasinoxanthin, which are derivatives of lutein, and are class-specific acetylenic Car (acetylene C≡C) found only in algae (Takaichi 2011).

In the applicability context, Stengel and Connan (2015) describe commercial utilization of pigments such as β-carotene (*Dunaliella salina*, *Haematococcus pluvialis*) and astaxanthin (*H. pluvialis*, *Chlorella* sp.) in animal feed, human food, pharmaceuticals, and nutraceuticals. Canthaxanthin (*Chlorella* sp., *H. pluvialis*) is used in as a colorant in animal feed (aquaculture, poultry, food), while echineone (*Botryococcus braunii*, Cyanobacteria) and zeaxanthin (*Chlorella ellipsoidea*, *D. salina* [mutant]) work as colorants cum antioxidants in animal feed. Fucoxanthin (*Phaeodactylum tricornutum*) and lutein (*Scenedesmus* sp., *Muriellopsis* sp.) have nutraceutical and pharmaceutical uses. The phycobiliproteins (PC, PE, allophycocyanin [APC]) obtained from *Spirulina*/*Arthrospira* sp., *Pophyridium* sp., *Rhodella* sp., *Galdieria* sp., Cyanobacteria, Rhodophyta, Cryptophyta, and Glaucophyta are used in human food (colorant), cosmetics (colorant + antioxidant), histochemistry, fluorescence microscopy, flow cytometry (fluorescent conjugates/probes; prozyme), the nutraceutical industry, and medical applications (photodynamic therapy in cancer) (Stengel and Connan 2015).

To give an idea of the quantities involved, microalgae are reported to contain pigments like chl (0.5–1% of dry weight), Car (0.1–0.2% of dry weight on average and up to 14% of dry weight for β-carotene of *Dunaliella*), and phycobiliproteins (Spolaore et al. 2006). Seaweeds *Enteromorpha intestinalis*, *Rhizoclonium riparium*, *Lola capillaris*, *Ulva lactuca*, *Dictyota ceylinica*, *Catenella repens*, *Polysiphonia mollis*, and *Gelidiella acerosa* have 1.70, 2.45, 1.76, 2.06, 2.15, 0.37, 1.17, and 0.62 Chl *a* (mg g^{-1} DW) (respectively); 1.04, 1.77, 1.21, 1.35, 0.58, 0.09, 0.24, and 0.09 Chl *b* (mg g^{-1} DW), and

Table 2.2 A summary of algal pigments.

Highlights	Group of algae: their pigment(s)	References
Evaluated several algal carotenoids, observing that approx. 30 types of them have photosynthetic functions, while others could be intermediates of carotenogenesis or accumulated carotenoids; they also suggest use of carotenoids and chlorophyll (chl) as chemotaxonomic markers (due to their distribution in algae). They described carotenoids that contain a unique allene (C=C=C). Acetylenic carotenoids (acetylene C≡C) are found only in algae Some classes contain additional carotenoids, such as loroxanthin, siphonaxanthin, and prasinoxanthin, which are derivatives of lutein, and are class-specific	• Brown algae and diatoms: fucoxanthin • Haptophyta and Dinophyta: 19′-acyloxyfucoxanthin • Dinoflagellates: peridinin • Green algae and land plants: 9′-cis neoxanthin • Cryptophyta: diadinoxanthin alloxanthin, crocoxanthin, and monadoxanthin • Heterokontophyta, Haptophyta, Dinophyta, and Euglenophyta: have diatoxanthin • Heterokontophyta, Haptophyta, and Dinophyta: have acetylated carotenoids (-O-CO-CH_3), such as fucoxanthin, peridinin, and dinoxanthin • Many Cyanobacteria: contain β-carotene, zeaxanthin, echinenone, and myxol pentosides (myxoxanthophyll), while some species lack part of these and some contain additional carotenoids, such as nostoxanthin, canthaxanthin, and oscillol dipentoside. Essentially, the carotenoid compositions of Cyanobacteria are different from those of chloroplasts in algae; consequently, during symbiosis of Cyanobacteria to eukaryotic cells, carotenoids might be considerably restructured. Since the name of myxoxanthophyll cannot specify the glycoside moieties, Takaichi (2011) proposed the name of myxol glycosides to specify the glycosides, such as myxol 2′-α-L-fucoside, 4-ketomyxol 2′-rhamnoside, and oscillol dichinovoside • Rhodophyta (red algae): the unicellular type (containing only β-carotene and zeaxanthin), and the macrophytic type (containing additional α-carotene and lutein). Nevertheless, the relationship between phylogenetics of red algae and carotenoid composition is not clear • Cryptophyta: α-carotene and its acetylenic derivatives, crocoxanthin, and monadoxanthin, which are only found in this division	Takaichi (2011)

(*continued overleaf*)

Table 2.2 *(continued)*

Highlights	Group of algae: their pigment(s)	References
	• Heterokontophyta, Haptophyta, and Dinophyta: β-carotene and its derivatives as well as chl *c*. Fucoxanthin and peridinin have unique structures and are class-specific carotenoids. Fucoxanthin and its derivatives are found in only four classes of Heterokontophyta (Chrysophyceae, Raphidophyceae, Bacillariophyceae, and Phaeophyceae), Haptophyta, and Dinophyta. Peridinin and its derivatives are found only in Dinophyta • Euglenophyta, Chlorarachniophyta, and Chlorophyta: the same carotenoids as land plants, namely β-carotene, violaxanthin, 9′-cis neoxanthin, and lutein, as well as chl *a* and *b*	
Pigments are characteristic of particular algal groups Compiling algal pigments, they mention the main accessory pigments, and minor pigments (or pigments with limited distribution within groups) in algae	• Cyanobacteria (including Prochlorophyta): chl *a*, β-carotene, c-phycoerythrin (c-PE), allophycocyanin, c-phycocyanin (c-PC), zeaxanthin, cryptoxanthin; some of them also have minor pigments such as β-cryptoxanthin, caloxanthin, canthaxanthin, echinenone, myxoxanthophylls, nostoxanthin, and oscillaxanthin distributed within groups • Rhodophyta: chl *a* or *d*, r-phycocyanin (r-PC), allophycocyanin, α- and β-carotene, as well as, b-, c-, and r-phycoerythrin; some contain antheraxanthin, cryptoxanthin, lutein, violaxanthin, zeaxanthin • Chrysophyceae: fucoxanthin, violaxanthin, zeaxanthin, β-carotene, and minor pigments as diadinoxanthin or diatoxanthin. Both Prymnesiophyceae (Haptophyta) and Bacillariophyta contain chlorophyll a (chl *a*), chlorophyll c1 (chl *c*1), and chlorophyll *c*2 (chl *c*2); they differ in their other major and minor pigments. Prymnesiophyceae have β-carotene, diadinoxanthin, diatoxanthin, and fucoxanthin. Bacillariophyta comprise β-carotene, fucoxanthin, diatoxanthin, diadinoxanthin, and could also have canthaxanthin, echinonene, fucoxanthinol	Stengel et al. (2011)

(continued overleaf)

Table 2.2 (*continued*)

Highlights	Group of algae: their pigment(s)	References
	• Phaeophyceae: chl *a*, *c*1, and *c*2; they also have major pigments such as β-carotene, fucoxanthin, zeaxanthin, violaxanthin, and minor pigments such as antheraxanthin-like, cryptoxanthin-like, cryptoxanthin-5,6-epoxide-like, latoxanthin-like, and mactraxanthin-like carotenoids, and neoxanthin • Raphidophyceae: chl *a* and *c*2 along with diatoxanthin, diadinoxanthin, heteroxanthin, and fucoxanthin, and minor pigments could include dinoxanthin, heteroxanthin, neoxanthin, and vaucheriaxanthin • Both Xanthophyceae and Eustigmatophyceae: chl *a*, *c*, and β-carotene, and minor pigments like violaxanthin and vaucheriaxanthin, but the former have diatoxanthin, diadinoxanthin, heteroxanthin, vaucheriaxanthin ester, and antheraxanthin • Eustigmatophyceae have neoxanthin and zeaxanthin • Cryptophyceae: chl *a* and *c*; they have major pigments such as α-carotene, diatoxanthin, phycoerythrin, phycocyanin, and minor pigments like alloxanthin, crocoxanthin, and monadoxanthin • Chlorophyta (green algae), Charophyta (Charophytes), and Euglenophyta (Euglenoids): chl *b* as the major pigment • In Chlorophyta: Chlorophyceae, Charophyceae, and Prasinophyceae: chl *a* and *b*. Chlorophyceae consist of α-, β-, and γ-carotenes, lutein, siphonaxanthin, siphonein. Antheraxanthin, astaxanthin, canthaxanthin, echinone, neoxanthin, violaxanthin, zeaxanthin. Charophyceae have α-, β-, and γ-carotenes, and could also have antheraxanthin, loroxanthini, lutein, neoxanthin, violaxanthin, zeaxanthin. Prasinophyceae have major pigments such as β-carotene, siphonoxanthin, siphonein and minor pigments like anhydromicromonal, anhydroprasinoxanthin, anhydrouriolide, antheraxanthin, deepoxyuriolide, dehydrouriolide, dihydrolutein, lutein, micromonol, neoxanthin, prasinoxanthin, preprasinoxanthin, violaxanthin, and zeaxanthin	

(*continued overleaf*)

Table 2.2 *(continued)*

Highlights	Group of algae: their pigment(s)	References
	• Phaeophyta (brown algae) and Chrysophyta (yellow-brown or golden-brown algae): chl $c1 + c2$ along with fucoxanthin (Dring 1982) • Dinoflagellates (Pyrrhophyta) and Cryptophyta (Cryptomonads): chl $c2$ and peridinin • Rhodophyta and Cyanophyta: PC and PE (Robertson 2019)	

18.85, 19.16, 20.19, 19.55, 29.02, 21.08, 25.09, and 22.53 Car (μg g^{-1} DW), respectively (Chakraborty and Santra 2008). Further, *Cheatomorpha antennina*, *E. intestinalis*, *Ulva fasciata*, *Padina gymnospora*, *Grateloupia lithophila* and *Hypnea valentiae* are said to contain 0.68, 0.54, 0.60, 0.66, 0.51, and 0.63 mg g^{-1} total chl (*a* and *b*) along with 0.26, 0.38, 0.37, 0.63, 0.6, and 0.49 (mg g^{-1}) Car, respectively (Chinnadurai et al. 2013).

Seasonality influences the temperature, light exposure, light intensity, and nutrient composition of a water body (e.g. winters could be accompanied by lower irradiance levels and higher nutrient contents), and it also impacts the aquatic dwellers, e.g. aquatic plants and algae. Ansari and Ghanem (2017) affirm that changing climatic conditions such as nutrient availability, pH, temperature, light, and precipitation affect vital plant processes. Seasonal variations in chemical composition and nutritive value have been reported in macroalgae across the world (Banerjee et al. 2009; Kaehler and Kennish 1996; Kumar 1993; Mercer et al. 1993). Dere et al. (2003) studied the role of environmental factors in quantity of algal pigment, stating that salinity, temperature, nutrients, and intense irradiance could cause a high rate of pigment production. Nutrients are also known to affect macroalgal pigmentation, thereby affirming the role of rainfall/monsoon in pigmentation. The concentration and distribution of photoprotective plant pigments are reported to vary with season in micro- and macroalgae and with tissue type in macroalgal species (Sarojini and Sujata 2015; Paerl 1984). Stengel et al. (2011) highlighted the influence of seasonal changes in brown macroalgal pigments including commercially important Car, also mentioning that acclimations may result in conspicuous color changes and bleaching events. In addition to the seasonal changes over several months, short-term fluctuations in pigment levels may occur within a daily cycle (e.g. López-Figueroa 1992).

Parameters such as sun exposure and tide are known to vary on a day-to-day basis as well as seasonally in any marine system. Sampath-Wiley et al. (2008) undertook studies on seasonal effects of sun exposure and emersion on intertidal seaweed physiology, particularly *Porphyra umbilicalis*, and stated that prolonged exposure to high light intensities can damage the photosynthetic system and contribute to decreases in both quantum efficiency and maximum photosynthetic rates. This damage could be further escalated when coupled with stress such as desiccation and/or temperature (Davison and Pearson 1996). Several intertidal seaweeds have developed mechanisms to cope with the lethal physiological damages incurred; they maintain physiological integrity even in response to high irradiance levels suggesting that there are certain repair mechanisms. However, at low light levels photosynthetic efficiency is heightened and greater amounts of pigments are required to drive photosynthetic electron transport, while under high irradiance levels, photosynthetic efficiency declines and photosynthetic pigment contents decrease to protect sensitive

PSII machinery against irreversible photodamage and/or photoinhibition (Lüning et al. 1990). Certain green and brown seaweed also demonstrate adjustments in pigment ratios and thallus absorbance properties (Sampath-Wiley et al. 2008). Neish et al. (1977) reported red algae to demonstrate a characteristic summer discoloration, which is regarded as a loss of pigment related to environmental conditions.

Ismail and Osman (2016) investigated red algae *Corallina elongata*, *Corallina officinalis*, *Jania rubens*, *Polysiphonia elongata*, and *Pterocladia* sp. for their photosynthetic pigment production during different seasons; they observed maximum quantities of chl *a* in winter and minimum values in the summer. The total chl content of *P. elongata* was 5.63 mg g^{-1} FW in winter and 3.82 mg g^{-1} FW in summer, while *J. rubens* had 2.73 mg g^{-1} FW total chl content in winter. On the other hand, *C. elongata* had a total chl content of 1.75 and 1.55 mg g^{-1} FW in spring and autumn, respectively, while *C. officinalis* had a total chl content of 1.69 mg g^{-1} FW in summer. Ismail and Osman (2016) observed that Car showed a similar pattern to total chl in the tested seaweeds, i.e. *P. elongata* exhibited a higher content of 0.609 mg g^{-1} FW, whereas a lower content (0.28 mg g^{-1} FW) was recorded in *J. rubens* in winter seasons. Their study showed that *P. elongata* also showed the highest concentration of PC, APC, and PE (2.38, 6.23, and 3.70 mg g^{-1} FW, respectively), whereas *J. rubens* had the lowest quantities of PC, APC, and PE (0.51, 2.05, and 0.91 mg g^{-1} FW) in winter. Additionally, they observed that the changes in the Car/Chl *a* ratio of all tested seaweeds during the four seasons showed highly significant differences between species and seasons (Ismail and Osman 2016). In another study, Ansari and Ghanem (2017) showed significant variation in the photosynthetic and accessory pigments of chlorophytic algae of the Red Sea in different seasons. According to this study, chl contents in *U. lactuca* and *Caulerpa prolifera* showed a significant increase in July, whereas in *Enteromorpha flexuoca* and *Chaetomorpha linum* high chl content was observed in April and October, respectively; a significantly higher accumulation of PE in *E. flexuoca*, *C. prolifera*, and *C. linum* was recorded in October, whereas in *U. lactuca* they were higher in July. Ansari and Ghanem (2017) also observed a significant increase in the PC and Car content of selected species of green algae during July; they noticed in particular that chl, PE, PC, and Car pigments significantly decreased in January. Seasonal variation in PE content (major water-soluble pigments; high in autumn and winter with a maximum of 2.85 mg g^{-1} of fresh matter noticed in November and low at the end of spring and at the beginning of summer with a minimum of 0.46 mg g^{-1} of fresh matter recorded in June) has been reported by Aziza et al. (2008). The PC content varied between 0.07 and 0.75 mg g^{-1} fresh weight, while chl *a* did not show marked seasonal variations (with the highest value in November 0.88 mg g^{-1} of fresh matter). Sarojini and Sujata (2015) reported seasonal variations in pigment content of *Padina tetrastromatica*. They observed high chl *a* values in February to April 2012, chl *c* in December 2012, fucoxanthin in August to September 2012, and high Car in August and October 2012. They also reported seasonal variations in distribution of photosynthetic pigments of *S. vulgare* wherein high values of chl *a*, chl *c* and fucoxanthin were recorded in August 2012, while the Car values were high in May 2012, August 2012, and January 2013. According to Sarojini and Sujata (2015) the variation in pigment composition was species-specific, as no similar trend in variation between seasons was evidenced. Schreiber (1979) reported that PB content varied seasonally in different seaweeds.

Light intensity plays an important role in controlling the pigment accumulation in microalgal cells. Apart from season and geography, the light quality and intensity varies. According to Wang et al. (2003) irradiance influences the culture density, cell maturity, medium nutrient profile, and light path; however, there is a relationship between the light color and pigment production in different microalgal species. Essentially, the light quality that is known to vary with season could also influence the pigment of algae; for example, Rodriguez et al. (1991) reported that a decrease in irradiance led to an increase in phycobiliprotein production in nitrogen-fixing Cyanobacteria. Green light induced an increase in the C-PE content, whereas red light enhanced C-PC content (Begum et al. 2016). The light intensity varies with the season; as per the report of Imamoglu et al. (2009) high light intensity (546 μmol photons m^{-2} s^{-1}) is known to cause high (30 mg g^{-1}) astaxanthin accumulation in green microalgae (*H. pluvialis*). This could be explained by the fact that intense illumination induced oxidative stress resulting in an increase of astaxanthin synthesis; active oxygen molecules are produced by excess photo oxidation.

Begum et al. (2016) elaborately describe the role of various proportions of light spectra (such as red:far red, blue:red, green:red, and blue:green) in influencing the relative pigment composition in microalgae; they suggest that the proportions of light spectra act as photomorphogenic signals. While the productivity of microalgae is affected by the individual light regimen, variations in chl and PB levels are subject to an adaptive response that allows proficient light-harvesting. Cyanobacteria favor low light intensities, which stimulate phycobiliprotein production; they are reported to prefer low light intensity because of their low specific maintenance energy rate and pigment composition. Low irradiance favors more accessory pigment synthesis; Begum et al. (2016) mention that 25 μmol photons m^{-2} s^{-1} is the best intensity for PB production in the case of blue-green microalgae such as *Spirulina maxima*, *Anabaena* NCCU-9, and *Synechococcus* NKBG, whereas 60 μmol photons m^{-2} s^{-1} was suitable for blue-green microalgae *Nostoc* UAM 206. However, Madhyastha and Vatsala (2007) observed that the production of PC and PE in *Spirulina* was enhanced by higher light intensity (135 μmol photons m^{-2} s^{-1}). While an inverse relationship was found in chl content per cell (i.e. high irradiance/intensity caused a decrease in chl content of *D. salina* and *Spirulina platensis*), β-carotene content per cell sharply increased with light intensity in *D. salina* (Pisal and Lele 2005). Nonetheless, seasonality also influences the occurrence of other algal canopies and organisms that could change the light intensity in any water body and indirectly influence the occurrence of certain microalgae.

In addition to light, seasonal changes in temperature are also known to occur in the open environment. Temperature comprises one of the most elementary factors that affects metabolic processes and biochemical composition of all living organisms. While optimal growth temperature and tolerance of extreme values generally differ for different microalgae strains, seasonal changes in temperature could cause fluctuation in the pigment content of algae. Hemlata and Fatma (2009) observed that the optimum temperature for production of phycobiliproteins was 30 °C for *Anabaena* sp., while a temperature of 25, 35, and 36 °C was optimum for *S. platensis*, *Anaebaena* sp., *Nostoc* sp., and *Spirulina* sp., respectively. Likewise, the optimum temperature for production of astaxanthin was 25 and 28 °C for green microalgae *H. pluvialis* and *Chlorella zofingiensis*, respectively. Furthermore, according to the study by Hemlata and Fatma (2009) 25 and 30 °C are regarded as optimum for β-carotene production in blue-green microalgae *D. salina*, while the optimum temperature for production of Car (lutein) is 28 °C for *Muriellopsis* sp., *Chlorella protothecoides*, *C. zofingiensis*, and *Neospongiococcus gelatinosum*. Essentially, for temperatures above optimum, heat stress causes inactivation or denaturation of enzymes, or modification of proteins involved in photosynthetic processes, which in turn could influence growth (Ras et al. 2013).

2.4 Carbohydrates/Polysaccharides

Carbohydrate is the most important component for metabolism (Khairy and El-Shafay 2013). Production of carbohydrates serves two main functions in algae: they act as structural components in the cell walls, and as storage components inside the cell. As storage compounds, carbohydrate provides the energy needed for the metabolic processes of the organisms and allows temporary survival in dark conditions (Markou et al. 2012). Polysaccharides are polymers of simple sugars (monosaccharides) linked together by glycosidic bonds. The most representative polysaccharides in the marine environment are cellulose and chitin, which are the most abundant biopolymers, followed by agar, alginates, and carrageenans. Algae contain large amounts of polysaccharides (a type of bio-macromolecule) that can either be a part of cell wall structure (cellulose, hemicellulose), or occur as mycopolysaccharides and storage polysaccharides (e.g. sulfuric acid polysaccharides, galactans, xylans, fudoidan, laminarin etc.; Xu et al. 2017; Kraan 2012). In general, green algae contain sulfated galactans and xylans, while brown algae have alginic acid, fucoidan (sulfated fucose), laminarin (β-1,3 glucan), and sargassan. Red algae contain agars, carrageenans, xylans, Floridean starch (amylopectin like glucan), water-soluble sulfated galactan, as well as porphyran, as mucopolysaccharides, located in the intercellular spaces (Kumar et al. 2008). According to Stengel et al. (2011), the main storage carbohydrate in Cyanobacteria is glycogen, but they also contain other complex mucilages (rich in Glc-, Xyl-, and GlcA), glucans, lipopolysaccharides, peptidoglycan (murein), and xylans.

Algae polysaccharides have multiple end uses based on their physico-chemical properties and biological activities (e.g. molecular sizes, types, ratios of constituent monosaccharides, and features of glycosidic linkages). Stengel and Connan (2015) describe various uses of hydrocolloid agar from *Gelidium* sp. and *Gracilaria* sp. in biotechnology (bacteriological agar), human food (agar-agar), health and horticulture; alginate from *A. nodosum*, *Durvillaea potatorum*, *Ecklonia maxima*, *Laminaria/Saccharina* sp., *Lessonia nigrescens*, and *Macrocystis pyrifera* in the pharmaceutical and medical industries, cosmetics, human food, immobilized biocatalysts, the paper industry, animal feed, and textile printing; carrageenan from *Eucheuma denticulatum*, *Kappaphycus alvarezii*, *Gigartina skottsbergii*, *Sarcothalia crispata*, and *Chondrus crispus* in human food, the pharmaceutical and medical industries (vaginal suppositories), immobilized biocatalysts, and home care; ulvans (from *Ulva* sp.) for animal feed; laminarin (from Laminarales) in horticulture; fucanes (or fucoidan; from *A. nodosum*) in cosmetics, human food, nutraceutical and animal feed; and cyanobacterial polysaccharides from *Mastocarpus stellatus*, *Porphyridium cruentum*, and *Rhodella* sp. in cosmetics. According to Offei et al. (2018) nearly 50–70% of the seaweed carbohydrates can be converted to fermentable sugars; further, red (*Kappaphycus* sp., *Gelidium* sp., and *Gracilaria* sp.), brown (*Laminaria* sp. and *Sargassum* sp.), and green (*Ulva* sp., *Chaetomorpha* sp., and *Rhizoclonium* sp.) seaweed could be used as a good raw material for bioethanol production. Chen et al. (2013) have listed a few groups of algae with their cell wall and storage products with a biofuel perspective; these include: Cyanophyta (lipopolysaccharides, peptidoglycan; cyanophycean starch), Chlorophyta (cellulose, hemicellulose; starch/lipid), Dinophyta (contain little cellulose; starch), Cryptophyta (periplast; starch), Euglenophyta (paramylum/lipid), and Rhodophyta (agar, carrageenan, cellulose, calcium carbonate; Floridean starch). Polysaccharides of *P. cruentum*, *Chlorella pyrenoidosa*, and *Chlorella stigmatophora* are reported to be used as viscosifiers, lubricants, and flocculants for industrial applications; to work as antiviral agents; to have immunostimulatory effects; antitumor activities; and anti-inflammatory and immunosuppressive properties (Sathasivam et al. 2019). Sulfonated polysaccharides of *Chlorella vulgaris* and *Scenedesmus quadricauda* have anticoagulant, antiviral, antioxidative, and anticancer activities (Sathasivam et al. 2019).

The quantity of polysaccharides as well as the type and quantity of individual sugar content vary with the algal species. From the quantitative perspective, Holdt and Kraan (2011) reported the total polysaccharide content of macroalgae to vary from 4 to 76% DW; *Ulva* sp. had a high content, up to 65% of DW. They observed the highest polysaccharide content in *Ascophyllum*, *Porphyra*, and *Palmaria*.

Some microalgae may contain a large amount of carbohydrates in the cell wall (mainly in the form of cellulose and soluble polysaccharides) and plastids (mainly in the form of starch), which can potentially be used as carbon sources for fermentation (Chen et al. 2013). Julius (2018) detailed carbohydrate diversity in microalgae from a phylogenetically arranged perspective. Several microalgal species, such as *P. cruentum* (40–57%) and *Spirogyra* sp. (33–64%) have high innate carbohydrate content (Harun et al. 2010). Schulze et al. (2017) evaluated 46 tested algae species and revealed total carbohydrate contents in a range from 16.5% (*Mychonastes* sp.) to 71.6% (*Porphyridium purpureum*); they performed thin layer chromatography (TLC) and observed the presence of glucose in every screened alga, but the presence of galactose, mannose, rhamnose, arabinose, xylose, ribose, and fucose depended on the species. Their liquid chromatography-mass spectrometry (LC-MS) analysis also revealed glucose as the main monosaccharide, and its quantity varied with species (5.6–66.8%). Mannose, galactose, rhamnose, and xylose were detected in most algae species in higher amounts (up to 15, 7, 3, and 17%, respectively), but arabinose, ribose, and fucose were only present in lower concentrations (<5%).

Seasonality apart from influencing the biomass also influences carbohydrate content of several algae. The carbohydrate content of *U. lactuca*, *J. rubens*, and *Pterocladia capillacea* is known to show seasonal fluctuations in spring, summer, and autumn (44.81, 46.42, 42.09; 42.18, 39.20, 34.75; 50.49, 50.96, 47.98% DW, respectively; Khairy and El-Shafay 2013). Ansari and Ghanem (2017) observed that the total carbohydrates in *U. lactuca* and *E. flexuoca* were significantly higher in July; however, in the case of *C. prolifera* and *C. linum*, maximum accumulation was observed in October. Renaud and Luong-Van (2006) evaluated 30 common species of tropical Australian marine macroalgae from Darwin Harbour, reporting that they comprised mainly soluble carbohydrate (chlorophytes range 2.5–25.8% DW, phaeophytes range 8.4–22.2% DW, rhodophytes range 18.7–39.2% DW), with significantly higher percentages only in winter-season rhodophytes. Paiva et al. (2018) obtained a contrasting pattern in the case of *Fucus spiralis*, wherein higher carbohydrate and protein contents were recorded in winter, rather than summer; they acknowledge the influence of increased values of seawater temperature, salinity, and sunlight intensity on carbohydrate synthesis of *F. spiralis*, which caused an inverse relationship between carbohydrates (higher in summer) and protein (higher in winter). Highest carbohydrate contents have been reported in *U. lactuca* and *P. capillacea* (46.42 and

50.96% of DW, respectively) during summer, and in *J. rubens* (42.18% of DW) during spring (Khairy and El-Shafay 2013).

Commercially important phycocolloids are also known to vary seasonally; for example, in *Myagropsis* and *Sargassum* the alginic acid levels and composition (i.e. M/G ratios) vary resulting in different chemical properties of extracts (Stengel et al. 2011). Agar levels and quality, and thus economic value of the harvested biomass, are also known to fluctuate seasonally (Stengel et al. 2011); in the case of *Gracilaria confervoides* high agar yields were reported by Whyte et al. (1981) in August, while peak biomass occurred in October. However, Humm (1951) reported that agar content of *Gracilaria foliifera* declined in autumn as the alga reached maximum abundance. John and Asare (1975), as well as Rao (1969), observed that the abundance and agar content peaked simultaneously in *Gracilaria dentata* (from Ghana) and *Gracilaria corticata* (India), respectively. Particularly, John and Asare (1975) reported that reduced salinity, high turbidity, and sedimentation led to lowered phycocolloid yields and reduced abundance of plants during the wet season.

Hoyle (1978) too observed low agar yield from *Gracilaria bursa-pastoris* and *Gracilaria coronopifolia* in January and February, which indicated a winter reduction in phycocolloid production; occurrence of low biomasses in winter was coincident with low agar yield in these two species. However, the relationship was less clear with *G. bursa-pastoris* in which maximum biomass in autumn seems to be accompanied by a decrease in agar yield. Essentially, the important factor governing agar seasonality is the same as that in carrageenan-producing algae, i.e. the nitrogen concentration in the ambient seawater. In the case of Hoyle (1978), an increase in the seawater reactive NO_3-N concentration occurred during late autumn and early winter, which led to a concomitant seasonality in the total nitrogen content within two *Gracilaria* species, thereby indicating that protein synthesis was favored over carbohydrate synthesis at the time of greater nitrogen availability. Here, the seasonality expressed as low gel strength in agar from August through November in *G. coronopifolia* while the period of low gel strength in *G. bursa-pastoris* was from April through June. Looking into the two different periods of low gel strength in two different *Gracilaria* species from the same environment, it could be said that gel strength of polysaccharides is seasonality as well as species dependent. In yet another study, Yenigil (1993) observed that the 3,6-anhydrogalactose and sulfate contents of *Gracilaria* were the highest between June and November and January and July; they state that long summers probably caused the gel strength to increase up to 1250 $N\,m^{-2}$ in November, which results from the increase in 3,6-anhydrogalactose determined in agar extracted from *Gracilaria* throughout the year. Similarly, Lahaye and Yaphe (1988) investigated *G. bursa-pastoris* and observed that the agar fractions from the summer-collected sample had higher gel strength than those of the winter ones; the algae collected in winter contained agar molecules richer in alkali-stable sulfate groups attributed in part to D-galactose-4-sulfate. Kumar et al. (2015) also report the influence of seasonality on the chemical composition (carbohydrate, protein, fiber, lipid content) of *K. alvarezii*, stating that the gel strength of the semi-refined carrageenan (SRC) (ranging from 348.33 to 783.33 $g\,cm^{-2}$) was also influenced by seasonality. As per the report of Lahaye and Yaphe (1988), the chemical and rheological variations (due to seasonal changes) reflect the ratio of actively growing (young) to resting (old) tissue in the alga and are proposed to represent a type of "secondarization" of the algal cell wall. In their study, a similar total concentration of 6-O-methylated agarobiose repeat units was present in the agar from both algal samples but the distribution of the methylated disaccharide varied in the fractions. Christiaen et al. (1987) also found an inverse relationship between gel strength and seawater temperature (which varies seasonally).

Successful and sustainable algal exploitation and domestication require excellent control of factors controlling growth and reproduction; further, photoperiodism, temperature, and nutrients influence the thresholds for life stage transitions in algae (Liu et al. 2017). Seasonal periodicities of life cycles of algae (that depend on environmental factors and vary seasonally) also influence the carbohydrate content. Different phases of algae could influence occurrence of the type of carbohydrate that occurs in macroalgae, for example the gametophytic and sporophytic phases of members of the family Gigartinaceae (*Chondrus*, *Gigartitia*, *Iridaea*, and *Rhodoglossum*) have been known to produce predominantly kappa and lambda carrageenans, respectively (Whyte et al. 1981). Although this phenomenon of reproductive condition dictating the type of polysaccharide has been sparsely elaborated in the agarophytes, Whyte et al. (1981) observed a general increase in the anhydrogalactose content in certain macroalgae with season, which was evident with maximum inclusions for the tetrasporic, cystocarpic, and vegetative forms occurring in July and for the male gametophytic samples of *Gracilaria verrucosa* in the following month. They observed that inclusion of sulfate ester in the agars was lowest in June samples of the male gametophytic and vegetative plants and in July samples of the cystocarpic and tetrasporic alga. They also found evidence that the percentage of 6-O-methylgalactose in the total content of galactose in the agars was seasonally greater in the vegetative and male plants, averaging 35.2 and 32.7%, respectively, than in the cystocarpic and tetrasporic plants with seasonal averages of 26.2 and 20.8%, respectively. Whyte et al. (1981) compared several data stating that July to August would be the optimum period for harvesting *G. verrucosa*; they reported that the production and quality of the agar depended on the following reproductive categories of the *Gracilaria* in decreasing order of merit: cystocarpic, tetrasporic, vegetative, and male gametophytic plants. Monosaccharide composition of fucoidan in *Undaria pinnatifida* is reported to have fluctuated monthly according to blade age; in addition, total fucoidan content, and the proportion of galactose residues present, is reported to be positively correlated with sori development (Skriptsova et al. 2010). Similarly, monthly variation was observed in cultivated *Saccharina* (*Laminaria*) *japonica* where fucan levels peaked in summer, and composition and levels of laminaran, alginate, mannose, glucuronic acid, fucose, and sulfate were related to reproductive development and plant maturity (Honya et al. 1999).

Kraan (2012) report that the laminaran content showed extreme variations during the year with very small amounts or none at all in February to June and maximum amounts from September to November. Furthermore, they stated that in the fronds of *Saccharina* and *Laminaria* maximum alginic acid content occurred from March to June, while the minimum occurred from September to October. Jensen and Haug (1956) also observed the highest contents of alginic acid during winter for *Laminaria* species from Norway. Alginate and fucoidan as matrix substances can be found at any time in the seaweeds of the Laminariaceae, but Manns et al. (2014) report that their relative amounts vary with the season; for alginate the levels vary from 17 to 45%, while for fucoidan they vary between 3 and 10% (w/w).

Seasonal variation in the amount of particular sugars in seaweeds has also been reported; for example, rhamnose in *Ulva* sp. was reported to vary from 17 to 23% over a period from June to September, and mannitol in *Laminaria digitata* varies from

5 to 32% over a year (van Hal Jaap et al. 2014). Kraan (2012) also reported that contents of both total and species-specific polysaccharides show seasonal variations; he observed that the mannitol content varied markedly in the fronds of *Saccharina* and *Laminaria* species with maximum amounts found during summer and autumn, from June to November. The amounts of laminarin and mannitol found in the most studied brown seaweed species *L. digitata* and *Saccharina latissima*, both belonging to the Laminariaceae family, are reported to differ widely due to large seasonal variations (depending on the harvest month 0–33% w/w of the total dry matter for laminarin and 2–20% w/w for mannitol) (Manns et al. 2014). Adams et al. (2011) talk about utilization of *L. digitata* for both methane and ethanol production, wherein they observed that minimum yields were seen in material harvested in March when the carbohydrates laminarin and mannitol were lowest. Adams et al. (2011) observed a seasonal variation of the mannitol content of *L. digitata* (minimum 5% w/w in the beginning of the year to a peak in June before the mannitol levels determined remained constant between 15 and 20% w/w). This highlights the necessity for seasonal harvesting and the development of storage technologies for better end utilization.

For microalgae, light intensity and duration is one of the major factors impacting growth; light not only affects photosynthesis but also influences the biochemical composition of microalgae and biomass yield. Therefore, optimal light intensity is needed to maximize CO_2 assimilation with a minimum rate of photorespiration and as little photoinhibition as possible; additionally, a specific duration of light/dark periods is required for algal photosynthesis (Khan et al. 2018). Higher light intensities will increase the photosynthetic rate to some maximum point, after which it levels off until the photosynthetic rate is balanced by photorespiration and photoinhibition. The growth rate and biomass productivity decrease with decreasing light duration. Most studies have shown that 16 hours' light/8 hours' dark is most suitable for algae growth; however, this is not the case in every season in the open environment. *Microcystis aeruginosa* is reported to yield maximum biomass and carbohydrate productivity at red LED light of about 5000 lx (Khan et al. 2017). While light directly affects the final yield of biomass and synthesis and accumulation of carbohydrates in the algal cells, temperature is another important factor in the growth of microalgae and directly influences the biochemical processes, including photosynthesis, in the algal cell factory (Khan et al. 2018).

An increase or decrease in the temperature beyond the optimal point retards or even stops algae growth and activity. Low temperatures affect photosynthesis by reducing carbon assimilation activity, whereas too-high temperatures reduce photosynthesis by inactivating the photosynthetic proteins and disturbing the balance of energy in the cell (Khan et al. 2018). High temperature reduces cell size and respiration; a decline in photosynthesis results in a decreased growth rate, and this in turn impacts the cellular composition. Converti et al. (2009) found that a culture of *C. vulgaris* produced more carbohydrates and lipids if grown at 25 °C than at 30 °C. Each season has a different temperature and light duration and intensity; it becomes essential to view the impact of these two factors on polysaccharide content of microalgae. Essentially, with the growing concern regarding global warming, there has been a continuous hike in the ocean and atmospheric temperatures, which thereby need to be researched in the algal context seasonally. In the context of microalgae, Pierre et al. (2014) mention that variations in sediment dynamics and compositions could result from seasonal fluctuations, particularly in extracellular polymeric substances (EPS) composing benthic biofilms. They reported that more colloidal carbohydrates were extracted from the sediment in winter (5.28 µg.µg chl a^{-1}) than summer (2.04 µg.µg chl a^{-1}), similarly 2.5 times more bound and residual carbohydrates were found in the winter samples. Although the neutral sugars were the main component of the fractions in both summer and winter, their ratios varied during these two periods (Pierre et al. 2014).

Today, both micro- and macroalgal polysaccharides have gained in popularity owing to their multifaceted applications, in terms of edibility, medicine and medicinal foods (anticoagulant sulfated galactans), pharmaceuticals, cosmeceuticals, nutraceuticals, functional food molecules, etc. In fact, microalgal biomass rich in carbohydrates is used directly for animal feed. This makes it all the more essential to understand the effect of seasonality on their production.

2.5 Fiber Content

Humans lack the ability to digest β (1→4) linkages in glucan polysaccharides, as in cellulose and hemicelluloses such as xyloglucan; this indigestible material or the resistant polysaccharides are referred to as dietary fiber. Dietary fiber means the edible parts of plants or analogous carbohydrates that are resistant to digestion and absorption in the human small intestine with complete or partial fermentation in the large intestine. Dietary fiber includes polysaccharides, oligosaccharides, lignin, and associated plant substances. Dietary fiber promotes beneficial physiological effects including laxation and blood cholesterol or glucose attenutation (Mišurcová et al. 1982). Dietary fiber from different sources is known to decrease the risk of coronary heart disease, mainly owing to its characteristics of dispersibility in water (water-holding capacity), viscosity, binding ability, absorptive capacity, fecal-bulking capacity, and fermentability in the alimentary canal. Furthermore, dietary fiber can be classified as either soluble or insoluble, based on whether it forms a dispersion when mixed with water (soluble fiber), or not (insoluble fiber) (Jiménez-Escrig and Sánchez-Muniz 2000). While soluble and insoluble fractions share many of the same physical properties, soluble fiber can be distinguished by its ability to form viscous gels in the intestinal tract. Insoluble fiber does not exhibit viscosity but can instead be characterized by its fecal-bulking capacity. Soluble and insoluble dietary fibers are recognized to have different physiological responses (Wang et al. 2001). Both these forms of fiber share the ability to bind water or mineral cations; further, they may be used by colonic microflora as fermentable substrate.

The fiber contents of a few algae species are detailed in Table 2.1. Kılınç et al. (2013) observed that the fiber content of seaweed varieties is higher than those found in most fruits and vegetables. The typical algae carbohydrates are indigestible by the human gastrointestinal tract and therefore Dawczynski et al. (2007) consider them as dietary fibers. Consumption of algal fiber has been proven to be health-promoting for human in the following ways: (i) it promotes the growth and protection of the beneficial intestinal flora; (ii) its consumption, in combination with high glycemic load foods, reduces the overall glycemic response, and macroalgae fiber acts as a hypoglycemic; (iii) it increases stool volume; and (iv) it reduces the risk of colon cancer (Kılınç et al. 2013).

Wong and Cheung (2000), investigated the chemical compositions of *Hypnea charoides*, *Hypnea japonica*, and *U. lactuca*, and found relatively high fiber (50.3–55.4%) and ash (21.3–22.8%) levels, while its lipid levels were low (1.42–1.64%).

According to McDermid et al. (2005), a cup of fresh *Gracilaria*, *Grateloupia*, *Dictyopteris*, or *Codium* (equivalent to about 20 g DW) with a meal could provide approximately 5–10 g of total dietary fiber (TDF) depending on the species. The soluble fiber fraction accounts for 51–56% of total fibers in green (ulvans) and red algae (agars, carrageenans, and xylans), and for 67–87% in brown algae (*Laminaria* and *Fucus*). Arame (*Eisenia bicyclis*), with 74.6% of TDF and 59.7% in the soluble form, is markedly richer in fibers than conventional vegetables (Lahaye 1991).

Marine algae, rich in polysaccharides that are indigestible by humans, appear to be good sources of soluble dietary fiber; the dietary fiber, which constitutes 2.57% of the dry weight of marine algae and represents their major component, is primarily soluble fiber. Soluble dietary fiber could include xyloglucans and galactomannan hemicelluloses, glucans and pectic substances, gums and mucilages, while celluloses, lignin arabinoxylan hemicelluloses, and resistant starch comprise the insoluble fraction. Jiménez-Escrig and Sánchez-Muniz (2000) provide the insoluble, soluble, and total fiber content of nori (16.8, 17.9, 34.7%, respectively), hijiki (16.3, 32.9, 49.2%), wakame (5.3, 30.0, 35.3%, respectively), *U. lactuca* (16.8, 21.3, 38.1%, respectively), *Enteromorpha* sp. (16.2, 17.2, 33.4%, respectively), *H. elongata* (7.0, 25.7, 32.7%, respectively), and *E. bicyclis* (14.9, 59.7, 74.6%, respectively). Total fiber content of *A. nodosum*, *L. digitata*, *H. elongata*, *U. pinnatifida*, *P. umbilicalis*, *Palmaria palmata*, *Ulva* sp., and *Enteromorpha* sp. was 8.8, 6.2, 9.8, 3.4, 3.8, 5.4, 3.8, and 4.9 g $100\,g^{-1}$ wet weight seaweed; here, the soluble fiber content was 7.5, 5.4, 7.7, 2.9, 3.0, 3.0, 2.1, and 2.9 g $100\,g^{-1}$ wet weight, while the insoluble fiber content was 1.3, 0.8, 2.1, 0.5, 1.0, 2.3, 1.7, and 2.1 g $100\,g^{-1}$ wet weight, respectively (MacArtain et al. 2007). The percentages of soluble, insoluble, and total fiber content of wakame *U. pinnatifida* (30.0, 5.3, 35.3%), *Hizikia fusiformis* (32.9, 16.3, 49.2%), sea spaghetti *H. elongata* (25.7, 7.0, 32.7%), arame *E. bicyclis* (59.7, 14.9, 74.6%), sea lettuce *U. lactuca* (21.3, 16.8, 38.1%), aonori *Enteromorpha* sp. (17.2, 16.2, 33.4%), and nori *Porphyra tenera* (17.9, 16.8, 34.7%) have also been reported by Lahaye (1991).

Dietary fiber from edible seaweeds show physico-chemical properties (water retention capacity, binding capacity, cation exchange capacity, fermentability, etc.) that show beneficial effects on body weight, cholesterol metabolism, and blood lipid levels (McDermid et al. 2005). Fiber content also influences palatability, digestibility, and nutritional quality of seaweeds in the diets of other organisms, such as green sea turtles, reef fish, shore crabs, invertebrates, etc. Apart from the food industry algal fibers have also been used for other purposes; for example, Pauli (2010) mention a team of Chinese researchers who were inspired by the fact that each year in June and July green algae appear along the Qingdao coastline, and decided to utilize them as a source of fiber. They initially obtained fragile fibers that only served for medical textiles (bandages and surgical dressing); thereafter the team extracted fibers from kelp that were stronger and more durable than cotton. They also tested high-strength alginate fibers from a wide variety of brown, green, and red algae, and found that they were resistant to fire and electromagnetic waves and could provide a unique raw material to manufacture special clothing, such as fireproof gear, medical uniforms, and protective clothing with military applications.

On the other hand, TDF of microalgae *Arthrospira platensis*, *Scenedesmus almeriensis*, *C. vulgaris*, *H. pluvialis* (green phase), *H. pluvialis* (red phase), *D. salina*, and *Nannochloropsis* sp. is reported to be 42.82, 22.60, 35.04, 34.56, 58.52, 8.97, and 17.67% DW, respectively (Molino et al. 2018). The high percentage of fiber in the microalgae *H. pluvialis* in the red phase 58.52% DW is due to the structural characteristics of the cell wall of the cyst, which is mainly made up of sporopollenin, a complex and very resistant polysaccharide. PC extracts and whole *A. platensis* are reported to have added health benefits and to enhance protein and fiber content when used in cookie production (Singh et al. 2015).

The fiber content of algae varies not only with species (e.g. Dawczynski et al. 2007 studied 34 edible seaweeds, stating that the highest fiber content was in *H. fusiformis* [62 g 100 g^{-1} s.w.], and the lowest in *Laminaria* sp.), but varies with season. Kumar et al. (2015) reported seasonal variation in fiber content (9.68–18.57 g 100 g^{-1} DW) of *K. alvarezii* from the west coast of India. The soluble dietary fiber of *H. fusiformis* is reported to fluctuate from 9.3 g 100 g^{-1} DW in April to 13.4 g in February (Suzuki et al. 1993). Similarly, Indergaard and Knutsen (1990) found the fiber content of *Furcellaria lumbricalis* to vary from 4.9% in February to 3.4% in September 1983. Suzuki et al. (1993) recognized seasonal variation in fiber content in *H. fusiformis* (Harvey) Okamura in Japan (36–54%).

In fact, Marinho-Soriano et al. (2006) reported seasonal variation in the fiber content of *G. cervicornis* (48.70–76.67 mg g^{-1}) and *S. vulgare* (48.00–105.10 mg g^{-1}); they specified a negative correlation between the solar radiation and fiber content. Paiva et al. (2018) also observed a difference in the values of the TDF, soluble dietary fiber, and insoluble dietary fiber of *F. spiralis* collected from Santa Maria Island (Azores) and Santa Maria Island (Azores) in summer (52.27, 24.77, 27.50 and 50.24, 24.71, 25.53% DW, respectively) and winter (40.47, 17.77, 22.7 and 40.44, 18.75, 21.69% DW, respectively).

Murakami et al. (2016) observed that ocean depth and seasonality influenced the TDF content of *Sargassum horneri*; in the case of samples collected from 1 m ocean depth the TDF increased gradually until June (74.2 mg g^{-1} and 69.0 mg g^{-1} for females and males, respectively) and this increase in fiber content from to June corresponded to plant maturity. They mention that the mean TDF content was higher in the case of plants harvested at a 5-m ocean depth (477 mg g^{-1}) than for those harvested at a 1–2-m ocean depth (409 mg g^{-1}).

2.6 Proteins

Both macro- and microalgae have adapted to survive in highly complex and competitive environments (extreme salinity levels, temperature variations, low light intensities, and nutrient-deficient habitats; Plaza et al. 2008); bearing this in mind, it is logical to consider that they could be a rich source of secondary metabolites, including functional nutrients and associated bioactive peptides (Samarakoon and Jeon 2012). Proteins, in algae, are present in a diverse range of forms and cellular locations (as a component of the cell wall, as enzymes, and bound to pigments and carbohydrates), but data regarding their occurrence (that enable elucidation of their taxonomic distribution) are sparse, with exceptions for the light-harvesting proteins of eukaryotic algae and the green algal cell wall glycoproteins (Stengel et al. 2011). Algal proteins have a high nutritional value in terms of protein content, amino acid quality, and nutritional acceptability; in addition, algal proteins have functional properties (such as gelation, water and fat absorption capacity, emulsification capacity, foaming capacity, etc.) comparable with terrestrial plants (Chronakis and Madsen 2011). Algae are considered a viable source of protein; algal proteins are of importance as a source of dietary protein and essential amino acids (EAAs) (Bleakley and Hayes 2017), as well as for the bioactive potentials of specific lectins, enzymes, and protein derivatives such as peptides. In fact, some species of seaweed and microalgae are known to contain protein levels similar to those of traditional protein sources, such as meat, egg, soybean, and milk (Bleakley and Hayes 2017; Koyande et al. 2019). Besides being easy cultivatable, their capability for rapid growth and controlled production (by manipulating cultivation conditions) contributes to their great economic potential for utilization in functional, processed foods and health foods. Moreover, they do not compete with traditional terrestrial crops in terms of space.

Protein content is a major factor determining the nutritional value of microalgae; Chronakis and Madsen (2011) stated that algae, particularly blue-green and green algae, contain very high levels of protein, typically 40–60% DW, which can be used as functional food ingredients. Green algal cell walls are rich in hydroxyproline-glycoproteins, one of the few protein groups to contain high levels of hydroxyproline. *Arthrospira* is used in human nutrition because of its high protein content and has excellent nutritive value (Spolaore et al. 2006). Bleakley and Hayes (2017) report that *A. platensis* (a filamentous Cyanobacterium originally referred to as *Spirulina* sp.) has the highest recorded protein content of any whole food, while *C. vulgaris* is the most commonly exploited industry species due to its high protein content (51–58% DW) and favorable EAA composition. *Spirulina platensis*, *Chlorella* sp., *D. salina*, and *Aphanizome nonflosaquae* are also widely used in food owing to their high protein content and nutritional value. Large-scale production of the Chlorophyceae *Chlorella* sp. and *Scenedesmus obliquus*, as well as the Cyanobacteria *Spirulina* sp. and *Athrospira* sp. is popular. *Spirulina* sp., also known as a "superfood," with protein content reaching up to 70%, also contains vitamins A, B_1, B_2, and B_{12} along with essential FAs and useful pigments like xanthophyll and Car (Koyande et al. 2019). *Spirulina* is reported to contain protein levels as high as 670% compared with tofu (Capelli and Cysewski 2010). In addition, the protein derivatives from Cyanobacteria also have the potential for bioactivity such as the inhibition of microtubule assembly, and anticancer, and anti-fungal activities, which are associated with cyclic peptides (Stengel et al. 2011).

The protein content of red macroalgae commonly reaches up to 47% DW, while green and brown macroalgae typically contain lower levels (i.e. 9–26 and 3–15% DW, respectively) of protein (Stengel et al. 2011). Proteins extracted from seaweeds have a high degree of *in vitro* digestibility; thus, apart from being used as food dyes, e.g. phycobiliproteins from red macroalgae, they have nutritive value. In context to the amino acid content, most macroalgae are rich in aspartic and glutamic acids (Fleurence 1999), but their protein content and composition vary with season and species; for example, glutamic acid, serine, and alanine were present in high concentrations in *P. palmata* harvested in late winter/early spring but absent at other times of year (Galland-Irmouli et al. 1999).

MacArtain et al. (2007) and Stengel et al. (2011) ascertained the relatively high protein content of algae, stating that the protein content could be as high as 47% DW, but they observed variation with season, source, species, and nutrient supply. Protein contents of various macroalgae are provided in Table 2.1.

Proteins are composed of different amino acids and hence the nutritional quality of a protein is determined basically by the content, proportion, and availability of its amino acids. Selected amino acid profiles of various algae have been compiled in Table 2.3. The algal cells are capable of synthesizing all amino acids; having an EAA composition that meets Food and Agriculture Organization (FAO) requirements and

Table 2.3 Amino acid content of algae compared with egg and soybean (mg g^{-1} protein).

Source	Ile	Leu	Val	Lys	Phe	Tyr	Met	Cys	Try	Thr	Ala	Arg	Asp	Glu	Gly	His	Pro	Ser	References
World Health Organization/ United Nations Food and Agriculture Organization	4.0	7.0	5.0	5.5	6.0	3.5	1.0												Becker (2007)
Egg	6.6	8.8	7.2	5.3	5.8	4.2	3.2	2.3	1.7	5.0		6.2	11.0	12.6	4.2	2.4	4.2	6.9	Becker (2007)
Soybean	5.3	7.7	5.3	6.4	5.0	3.7	1.3	1.9	1.4	4.0	5.0	7.4	1.3	19.0	4.5	2.6	5.3	5.8	Becker (2007)
Chlorella vulgaris	3.8	8.8	5.5	8.4	5.0	3.4	2.2	1.4	2.1	4.8	7.9	6.4	9.0	11.6	5.8	2.0	4.8	4.1	Becker (2007)
Dunaliella bardawil	4.2	11.0	5.8	7.0	5.8	3.7	2.3	1.2	0.7	5.4	7.3	7.3	10.4	12.7	5.5	1.8	3.3	4.6	Becker (2007)
Scenedes musobliquus	3.6	7.3	6.0	5.6	4.8	3.2	1.5	0.6	0.3	5.1	9.0	7.1	8.4	10.7	7.1	2.1	3.9	3.8	Becker (2007)
Arthrospira maxima	6.0	8.0	6.5	4.6	4.9	3.9	1.4	0.4	1.4	4.6	6.8	6.5	8.6	12.6	4.8	1.8	3.9	4.2	Becker (2007)
Spirulina platensis	6.7	9.8	7.1	4.8	5.3	5.3	2.5	0.9	0.3	6.2	9.5	7.3	11.8	10.3	5.7	2.2	4.2	5.1	Becker (2007)
Aphanizomenon sp.	2.9	5.2	3.2	3.5	2.5		0.7	0.2	0.7	3.3	4.7	3.8	4.7	7.8	2.9	0.9	2.9	2.9	Becker (2007)
Heterosiphonia japonica	44.8	97.9	56.3	66.3	37.2	27.9	18.5	29.1		45.9	57.4	66.8	98.4	110	54.2	6.89	45.4	47.5	Wong and Cheung (2000)
Hypnea charoides	48.5	72.3	61.4	64.9	56.0	26.0	16.8	28.1		51.3	52.3	63.6	88.6	98.4	50.6	6.58	47.9	44.9	Wong and Cheung (2000)
Ulva lactuca	38.2	67.1	55.0	65.8	35.0	35.0	15.7	13.3		50.6	73.9	84.4	98.7	87.3	67.4	4.82	44.6	55.4	Wong and Cheung (2000)
Sargassum wightii	0.55	0.55	0.5	0.5	0.63	0.49	0.37	0.25		0.71	0.44	0.6	1.8	1.15	0.45	0.45	0.38		Kumar and Kaladharan (2007)
Ulva lactuca	0.38	0.72	0.66	0.46	0.6	0.39	0.19	0.1		0.99	0.85	0.89	1.59	1.4	0.71	0.31	0.41		Kumar and Kaladharan (2007)
Kappaphycus alvarezii	0.21	0.33	0.31	0.2	0.24	0.13	0.19	0.06		0.39	0.25	0.46	0.66	0.73	0.28	0.08	0.17		Kumar and Kaladharan (2007)
Hypnea musciformis	0.9	1.33	1.07	1.13	0.91	0.46	0.43	0.21		1.78	0.97	1.04	2.46	2.67	0.95	0.4	0.82		Kumar and Kaladharan (2007)
Gracilaria corticata	0.63	1.06	0.9	0.68	0.76	0.44	0.15	0.12		1.23	0.81	0.89	1.99	1.85	0.85	0.33	0.58		Kumar and Kaladharan (2007)
Acanthophora spicifera	0.37	0.49	0.44	0.43	0.54	0.62	0.32	0.13		0.5	0.34	0.51	1.42	1.21	0.33	0.38	0.31		Kumar and Kaladharan (2007)

Table 2.4 Macro (g.100 g^{-1} DW), micro and trace elements (mg.100 g^{-1} DW) of various algae.

Seaweed	Calcium	Potassium	Magnesium	Sodium	Copper	Iron	Iodine	Zinc	References
Ascophyllum nodosum	575.0	765.0	225.0	1173.8	0.8	14.9	18.2	NA	Sundaramurthy and Shantaram (2016)
Caulerpa racemosa	1852	318	384–1610	2574	0.6–0.8	30–81		1–7	Pereira (2011)
Caulerpa stigmatophora	1510	1120	0.78 ppm	980	108.00 ppm	180		30	Fábregas and Herrero (1986)
Caulerpa lentillifera	780–1874	700–1142	630–1650	8917	0.11–2.2	9.3–21.4		2.6–3.5	Pereira (2011)
Chaetomorpha linum	7.30	15.44	2.50	3.09	0.76	105.97		1.87	Panayotova and Stancheva (2013)
Chondrus crispus	373.8	827.5	573.8	1572.5	0.1	6.6	6.1	NA	Sundaramurthy and Shantaram (2016)
Chondrus crispus	420–1120	1350–3184	600–732	1200–4270	<0.5	4–17	24.5	7.14	Pereira (2011)
Cystoseira barbata	21.40	11.93	4.14	1.92	0.77	33.43		1.43	Panayotova and Stancheva (2013)
Cystoseira crinita	19.93	17.95	4.22	5.16	0.24	6.10		1.63	Panayotova and Stancheva (2013)
Dunaliella tertiolecta	2090	740	0.63 ppm	920	65.00 ppm	200		30	Fábregas and Herrero (1986)
Enteromorpha sp.	104.0	351.1	455.1	52.0	0.1	22.2	97.9	1.2	Sundaramurthy and Shantaram (2016)
Fucus vesiculosus	725–938	2500–4322	670–994	2450–5469	<0.5	4–11	14.5	3.71	Pereira (2011)
Gelidium crinale	8.68	5.57	2.31	5.32	0.91	89.27		3.80	Panayotova and Stancheva (2013)
Gracilaria sp.	402	3417	565	5465		3.65		4.35	Pereira (2011)
Himanthalia elongata	30.0	1351.4	90.1	600.6	0.1	5.0	10.7	1.7	Sundaramurthy and Shantaram (2016)
Himanthalia elongata	720	8250	435	4100		59	14.7		Pereira (2011)
Isochrysis galbana	1620	560	1.15 ppm	720	204.00 ppm	360		60	Fábregas and Herrero (1986)

(continued overleaf)

Table 2.4 (*continued*)

Seaweed	Calcium	Potassium	Magnesium	Sodium	Copper	Iron	Iodine	Zinc	References
Laminaria digitata	364.7	2013.2	403.5	624.6	0.3	45.6	70.0	1.6	Sundaramurthy and Shantaram (2016)
Laminaria digitata	1005	11 579	659	3818	<0.5	3.29		1.77	Pereira (2011)
Porphyra umbilicalis	330	2030	370	940		23	17.3		Pereira (2011)
Porphyra yezoensis	440	2400	650	570	1.47	13		10	Pereira (2011)
Palmaria palmata	148.8	1169.6	97.6	255.2	0.4	12.8	10.2	0.3	Sundaramurthy and Shantaram (2016)
Palmaria palmata	560–1200	7000–9000	170–610	1600–2500	0.3–76	50	10–100	2.86	Pereira (2011)
Porphyra tenera	390	3500	565	3627	<0.63	10–11	1.7	2–3	Pereira (2011)
Porphyra umbilicalis	34.2	302.2	108.3	119.7	0.1	5.2	1.3	0.7	Sundaramurthy and Shantaram (2016)
Saccharina latissima	810	4330	715	2620			15.9		Pereira (2011)
Saccharina japonica	225–910	4350–5951	550–757	2532–3260	0.25–0.4	1.19–43	130–690	0.89–1.63	Pereira (2011)
Sargassum fusiforme	1860		687			88.6	43.6	1.35	Pereira (2011)
Tetraselmis suecica	2080	1200	0.78 ppm	1040	652.00 ppm	100		150	Fábregas and Herrero (1986)
Ulva rigida	524	1561	2094	1595	0.5	283		0.6	Pereira (2011)
Ulva lactuca	840					66			Pereira (2011)
Ulva rigida	5.52	4.60	7.85	5.90	0.82	24.53		1.30	Panayotova and Stancheva (2013)
Ulva sp.	325.0	245.0	465.0	340.0	0.3	15.3	1.6	0.9	Sundaramurthy and Shantaram (2016)
Undaria pinnatifida	112.3	62.4	78.7	448.7	0.2	3.9	3.9	0.3	Sundaramurthy and Shantaram (2016)
Undaria pinnatifida	680–1380	5500–6810	405–680	1600–7000	0.1–85	1.54–30	22–30	0.944	Pereira (2011)

often being on a par with other protein sources, algae are generally considered viable protein sources. Becker (2007) suggests that based on the amino acid pattern of algae they could be utilized as food proteins. Spolaore et al. (2006) also confirm that amino acid patterns of almost all algae are comparable with other food proteins, thereby making them favorable for consumption in food and feed. The high arginine contents of *Tetraselmis suecica*, *Tetraselmis chuii*, and *Pavlova lutheri* make them nutritionally superior (Webb and Chu 1983). The amino acid profile of *S. platensis* is reported to be similar to that of egg. Chakraborty and Santra (2008) analysed the free amino acid content of eight benthic algae. EAAs such as histidine, leucine, isoleucine, and valine are present in many seaweeds such as *P. palmata* (dillisk/dulse) and *Ulva* sp. (sea lettuce). Being a good source of EAAs, *Ulva pertusa* contains histidine at similar levels to legume and egg proteins, while taurine (identified as having antihypertensive, antichloesterolemic, and antioxidant properties) occurs in brown macroalgae *Undaria*, *Laminaria*, and *Hizikia* sp. The levels of isoleucine and threonine in *P. palmata* are equivalent to those found in legumes, while histidine in *U. pertusa* is on a par with egg proteins (MacArtain et al. 2007). Although, there is limited comparison made between the algal protein content and quality based on different algae species and season, most species have aspartic and glutamic acids as a large part of their amino acid make-up. Aspartic and glutamic acids exhibit interesting properties in flavor development, and glutamic acid is a main component in the taste sensation of "umami" (MacArtain et al. 2007; Bleakley and Hayes 2017). The seaweed *Laminaria japonica* (kombu) is considered as the original source of the flavor enhancer monosodium glutamate, which was discovered through its use in Asian cooking; the levels are highest in brown seaweeds, with red seaweeds having lower amounts of these two amino acids. Aspartic acid and glutamic acid are present as approximately 22–44% of total amino acids in *Fucus* sp. and 26–32% in *Ulva* sp. – apart from this, the amino acid pattern of almost all algae is comparable with other food proteins. Reports (Becker 2004; Roy and Pal 2014) also state that there are minor deficiencies in sulfur-containing amino acids methionine and cysteine. Bleakley and Hayes (2017) point out that tryptophan and lysine are often limiting amino acids in most algae species, while leucine and isoleucine are commonly found in low concentrations in red species of algae. Methionine, cysteine, and lysine are often limiting in brown algae species, and cysteine typically occurs at low levels in many seaweed species, and is often not detectable. MacArtain et al. (2007) particularly reported that seaweed proteins are very low in cysteine. Other amino acids like laminine and kainoids found in macroalgae have been investigated for their potential to treat neurophysiological disorders such as epilepsy, Alzheimer's, and Parkinson's disease (Stengel et al. 2011).

The protein content of algae varies based on species, seasonal period (Khairy and El-Shafay 2013), and geography. Seaweeds are exposed to abiotic factors that influence their metabolic responses (photosynthesis and growth rates) and levels of proximate constituents, which are demonstrated as seasonal variations (Banerjee et al. 2009). For example, in the case of subtropical species, the seawater temperature, light, and nutrients are the primary factors that modify the seasonal photosynthesis in *Hypnea musciformis* (Wulfen) Lamouroux (Durako and Dawes 1980) and *Gracilaria tikvahiae* McLachlan (Banerjee et al. 2009). Marinho-Soriano et al. (2006), in their study on the chemical composition of red algae *G. cervicornis* (Turner) J. Agardh and brown algae *S. vulgare* C. Agardh takson, reported protein contents ranging from 15.97–23.05%, with the highest protein content found in *G. cervicornis* takson. Khairy and El-Shafay (2013) report the protein content of *U. lactuca* to be 20.12, 17.88, and

16.78% in spring, summer, and autumn, respectively; they also report protein contents of *J. rubens* (12.93, 11.14, and 9.76% in spring, summer, and autumn) and *P. capillacea* (23.72, 20.95, 17.35% in spring, summer, and autumn) to vary seasonally. Protein levels of *P. palmata* (dulse) from the French Atlantic coast seasonally varied from 9 to 25% DW (Fleurence 2004). In research on seasonal and geographic changes, Rodde et al. (2004) evaluated the chemical composition of red algae *P. palmata*, stating protein and carbohydrate contents ranging between 14 and 30%, and 3.3–25% of DW, respectively. Further, Banerjee et al. (2009) observed that protein levels were positively correlated with dissolved nitrate content and negatively correlated with water temperature and salinity; they reported protein content of *C. repens* varied from 2.78 to 16.03% DW at station 3 and 1 of their study, respectively, with the highest values during monsoon. Ansari and Ghanem (2017) reported a significant increase in total protein contents of *U. lactuca*, *E. flexuoca*, and *C. prolifera* during July, while *C. linum* accumulated higher protein levels during October. Kumar et al. (2015) reported seasonal variation in the protein content of *K. alvarezii* (12.69–23.61 g $100\,g^{-1}$ DW). Rodde et al. (2004), in their research on the seasonal and geographic changes of the chemical composition of red algae *P. palmata* found that protein contents were between 14 and 30% DW.

A few reports on protein content of marine algae, stating its dependence on species and season, mention that higher protein levels occur at the end of the winter and spring, while less protein is recorded in summer (Fleurence 1999; Augier and Santimoine 1978; Abdel-Fattah and Sary 1987). However, Stengel et al. (2011) vividly narrate that temporal changes in algal protein levels are directly related to nitrogen levels in surrounding waters; for example, total protein levels in *Sargassum muticum* were highest in winter and early spring (Gorham and Lewey 1984); in red (*Gracilaria* sp.) and brown algae (*Sargassum* sp.) too protein levels positively correlate with water nitrogen level (Marinho-Soriano et al. 2006). Marinho-Soriano et al. (2006) in their study on chemical composition of *G. cervicornis* and *S. vulgare* from Brazil establish the relationship between the nutritive components of each species and the environment (reporting variation in protein content from 23.05 to 15.97%); according to them, the protein levels were positively correlated with nitrogen content and negatively with water temperature and salinity. According to Stengel et al. (2011), light-harvesting proteins additionally respond to season and even diurnally to light. Observed levels of phycobiliproteins, which constitute a significant proportion of proteins in red algae, were lowest during summer (e.g. *Gelidium*; Rico and Fernandez 1996). Hoyle (1978) studied seasonality in agar and nitrogen content of *Gracilaria* sp. in Hawaii, stating that, unlike agar, the crude protein was lower in summer and higher in winter. Zavodnik (1973) also reported a maximum protein in winter (12.3% DW) and a minimum in summer (5.1% DW) for *Fucus virsoides*. Rupérez and Saura-Calixto (2001) and Rodrigues (2013) too describe high protein content for *Fucus vesiculosus* collected in Pontevedra (Spain) (6.19% DW) and Aveiro (Portugal) (13.2% DW), respectively, during winter. Paiva et al. (2018) observed the protein composition of *F. spiralis* during the winter season and stated that the lower seawater temperature and salinity in winter could be responsible for this. The protein content of *Polysiphonia morrowii* is reported to vary from winter (11.71–34.49% in various locations in Canakkale Strait) to spring (16.74–29.13% in various locations). Short-term and small-scale changes in phycobiliproteins are reported by López-Figueroa (1992) as well as Sampath-Wiley et al. (2008).

Contrarily, Renaud and Luong-Van (2006) obtained the highest percentages of protein in rhodophytes collected in the summer (range 4.8–12.8% DW), with significantly lower percentages during winter. They further provide substantial evidence that protein synthesis dominates polysaccharide synthesis in winter along with seasonally high total nitrogen content in the *Gracilaria* thalli in winter (which correlates well with the level of nitrate in the seawater). Irkin and Erdugan (2014) too obtained relatively higher protein levels for red algae (4.8–12.8%), reporting higher energy levels and inorganic materials in the case of winter samples as compared with those collected during summer.

Historic harvesting times and current harvesting regimes differ with changing times. However, apart from the quantity of protein, the amino acid content of algae is also known to fluctuate seasonally (Stengel et al. 2011). There is remarkably poor documentation of seasonal changes in protein content and amino acid profiles (Wells et al. 2017). Especially in the food context, it is essential to determine the seasonal optima for harvesting algae based on the variation in their amino acid content. A comparison of amino acid compositions of algae (especially seaweeds) with the FAO reference pattern (FAO 1981) and those of other food proteins (Orr and Watt 1968) indicates that the total required amount of EAAs plays an important role is establishing the high nutritional value of seaweed proteins as food. Fluctuation in the amino acid content is often linked to the types of proteins or enzymes present at specific times of year.

In the case of macroalgae, the amounts of amino acids seem to vary in different algal species. For example, glutamic acid, serine, and alanine were present at high concentrations in *P. palmata* harvested in late winter/early spring but were absent at other times of year (Galland-Irmouli et al. 1999).

It was Mohsen et al. (1975) who first evaluated amino acid patterns, either free or combined (in the peptide form), during the different seasons of the year in *Laurencia papillosa*, *Cystoseira barbata*, and *E. intestinalis* (representing the three major classes Rhodophyceae, Phaeophyceae, and Chlorophyceae, respectively); they stated that since the amino acid metabolism depends on the individual alga, so the algal classes may differ from each other in their amino acid patterns constituting the individual proteins. As per their study, the free amino acids were more abundant in autumn and winter than in spring and summer; this could be due to incorporation of such amino acids into higher building units. They also suggest that some of the conjugated amino acids might have been utilized in the formation of the reproductive cells that ultimately become freed into the surrounding medium, which could be true owing to the fact that, during winter, reproduction (especially sexual) is intensive for most algae. During this period, a drop in protein content of these algae was recorded, following the formation of countless numbers of gametes (Mohsen et al. 1975). Several studies examining the amino acid content of seaweeds have been undertaken. Khairy and El-Shafay (2013) reported that EAAs made up over 30% of the total amino acids in different seaweeds, while other studies recorded 37% in *P. tenera*, *Grateloupia turuturu*, *U. pertusa*, and *Codium fragile* (Fujiwara-Arasaki et al. 1984); 37–42% in *U. lactuca* and *Gelidium amansii* (Ochiai et al. 1987); 36.56% in *Ulva rigida* and *Ulva rotundata* (Fleurence et al. 1995); and 45.49% in *K. alvarezii*, and *H. musciformis* (Kumar and Kaladharan 2007).

Khairy and El-Shafay (2013) detailed the seasonal profiles of amino acids in the three seaweed species, stating that proline was the major amino acid in *U. lactuca*, accounting for 34.8, 23.3, and 37.6% of the total amino acids during spring, summer, and autumn, respectively. Proline is known to accumulate in large quantities in higher plants in response to environmental stresses, and many plants accumulate proline as a nontoxic and protective osmolyte under saline conditions. Khairy and El-Shafay (2013) reported *U. lactuca* and *P. capillacea* contained distinctly higher concentrations of valine than *J. rubens*, especially during spring. Their results coincide with the findings of Ratana-arporn and Chirapart (2006), who reported that EAAs made up almost 40% of the total amino acids in *Caulerpa lentillifera* and *U. reticulata*.

Microalgae are considered as an unconventional source of amino acids; therefore microalgal proteins hold great potential as an alternative protein source as they contain all EAAs, and it is important to monitor their amino acid composition (Waghmare et al. 2016). Uslu et al. (2009) observed that the protein content (72.9%) and the amino acid concentrations of *S. platensis* grown in summer were higher than in winter (summer 33.09 mg 100 g^{-1} wet biomass, and, winter 20.88 mg 100 g^{-1} wet biomass); some of the amino acids, namely proline, cystine, and arginine, were observed only in winter.

2.6.1 Mycosporine-Like Amino Acids (MAAs)

MAAs are water-soluble molecules; they are potent and stable absorbers of ultraviolet light (MacArtain et al. 2007). MAAs, known for their UV-absorbing properties (λ_{max} = 310–362 nm), are either biosynthesized and/or accumulated by both marine and freshwater primary producers and consumers. Algae biosynthesize MAAs while other marine organisms acquire MAAs by diet transfer and symbiotic or bacterial associations; apart from their role as sunscreens in aquatic organisms, some MAAs act as antioxidants, providing some protection against photo-oxidative stress induced by reactive oxygen species (ROS). Although they are most commonly produced and best characterized in Cyanobacteria and Rhodophyta, they are detected in (green algal) *Prasiola* sp. as well as several groups of microalgae. MAAs are also present in macroalgae belonging to other Chlorophyta and Phaeophyceae (Stengel et al. 2011; Sinha et al. 2007), and red seaweeds such as *C. crispus* (MacArtain et al. 2007). Helioguard®365, which contains MAAs, is obtained from the red alga *P. umbilicalis* (Cardozo et al. 2007). MAAs from *P. umbilicalis* (Porphyra-334 + shinorine), Cyanobacteria and organohalogenated compounds (from *Asparagopsis armata*), phytoene and phytofluene (*Dunaliella* sp.), and squalene (*Aurantiochytrium* sp.) are used in cosmetics (Stengel and Connan 2015).

Nevertheless, seasonal changes in UV radiation have been reported to influence the quantity and production of MAAs (Ha et al. 2015). Carreto and Carignan (2011) highlight the synergistic effect of increased temperature (occurring seasonally) with high levels of solar radiation; they showed that a complex set of interactions between environmental factors can lead to differential responses to a stress. Evaluation of MAAs from three commercially important red macroalgae (*P. palmata*, *C. crispus*, and *Porphyra dioica*), with respect to seasonal changes at three locations in Galway Bay (western Ireland), carried out by Guihéneuf et al. (2018), revealed an increase in total MAA contents was induced by increasing daily light doses and irradiance levels, from winter to spring, but without clear significant correlations with light and/or temperature. They explained that low nutrient concentrations observed in summer months limited the synthesis and accumulation of MAAs, even when exposed to high irradiance levels. Further, nutrient availability, in particular nitrate, appears to be a limiting factor for the red algal species that they investigated, to synthetize MAA compounds when exposed to extreme light/irradiance stress. These reports ascertain the influence of seasonality on the production of MAAs in algae.

2.6.2 Phycobiliproteins and Lectins

The algal proteins, lectins and phycobiliproteins, exhibit the greatest bioactive potential. Lectins can recognize and bind to specific carbohydrate structures. Only a few algal lectins have been characterized; however, most appear to be low molecular weight, thermostable proteins that exhibit affinity for oligosaccharides or glycoproteins; nevertheless, those isolated to date have novel amino acid sequences (Stengel et al. 2011). Several bioactivities have been attributed to macroalgal lectins including antibiotic, mitogenic, cytotoxic, anti-inflammatory, antiadhesion, anti-HIV, reduction to pain sensitivity, and human platelet aggregation inhibition (Stengel et al. 2011). Sometimes, multiple lectins with a variety of activities are found in the same species (e.g. lectins from *Eucheuma serra* have mitogenic, cytotoxic, and antibacterial activities). On the other hand, endogenous peptides at times exhibit similar activities to lectins; for example, a hexapeptide isolated from *Ulva* sp. has mitogenic activity. According to Wang et al. (2004), marine alga lectins have a proteinaceous nature similar to those from land plants, but are different in some of their properties. They have generally lower molecular masses than most land plant lectins and are more specific for complex oligosaccharides or glycoproteins. In general, most marine algal lectins do not require divalent cations for their biological activity (Wang et al. 2004); further, they occur mainly in monomeric forms and have a high content of acidic amino acids, with isoelectric points from 4 to 6. Even though several studies on lectins from marine algae have been reported, only a few lectins from algae have been characterized in detail (Wang et al. 2004). The full amino acid sequence of the lectins from the marine red algae *Bryothamnion triquetrum* and *H. japonica* have been detailed (Hori et al. 2000; Calvete et al. 2000).

Macroalgal peptides could also have bioactivities such as anticancer, antimicrobial, antiviral, and antihypertensive angiotensin I-converting enzyme (ACE) inhibitory, antioxidant, antimicrobial, antithrombotic, immune-modulatory, and mineral binding (Harnedy and FitzGerald 2011).

Further, seaweeds also contain a group of proteins called biliproteins, some of which are extracted for their valuable use as fluorescent markers. While phycoerythrin (a major light-harvesting pigment in red algae) is used as a fluorescent probe in scientific experiments, other members of this phycobiliprotein group include PCs and APCs. These proteins are assembled into a structure in the cell that absorbs light where chl absorbs poorly (wavelength 450–650 nm). This facilitates certain red seaweeds to survive in relatively deep water, depending on opacity and other conditions.

Just like the other biochemical constituents, seasonal variations in PBs and lectins have also been reported. For example, Asai et al. (2001) detected seasonal changes in PBs of the water bloom phytoplankton *M. aeruginosa* in Lake Kasumiguara. Sampaio et al. (1996) reported seasonal variation in production of lectins by *U. lactuca*, while Hung et al. (2009) witnessed seasonal changes in lectin content in the red alga *K. alvarezii* cultivated in Camranh Bay, Vietnam.

2.7 Lipids and PUFAs

Algal lipids comprise phospholipids, glycolipids (glycosylglycerides), and nonpolar glycerolipids (neutral lipids) analogous to higher plants, along with betaine and some unusual lipids that may be characteristic of a particular genus or species (Kumari et al. 2013). Phospholipids (PL) represent 10–20% of total lipids (TL) in algae except dinophytes such as *Kraenia*, *Karlodinium*, and *Takayama* species (Mooney et al. 2007), and *Polarella glacialis*, where its content is 78–95% (Aakanksha et al. 2010). Microalgae are a promising source of lipid; the lipid classes usually present in all the algal species include C16:0, C16:1ω7, C18:1ω9, C18:3ω3, and C18:3ω6 (Aakanksha et al. 2010). Species with high lipid productivity are desirable for biofuel production. With a lipid content of 50–60% DW, the proportions of the various lipid classes (particularly triglycerides) vary with environmental conditions (nutrient deficiency, light intensity, temperature, growth phase, etc.); this could lead to triacylglycerol (TAG) accumulation. Certain microalgae produce substantial amounts (e.g. 20–50% dry cell weight) of TAG as a storage lipid under photo-oxidative stress or other adverse environmental conditions. There are two main types of lipids found in algal cells: polar lipids and nonpolar lipids. In the algal cell, the polar lipids form the part of structural lipids, while the nonpolar or neutral lipids are storage. FAs are the building blocks of lipids; they can be either saturated or unsaturated. Storage lipids are basically made up of saturated and monosaturated FAs. The PUFAs, which are generally part of the membrane lipids, act as essential FAs. Especially ω3 and ω6 unsaturated FAs are essential FAs. While storage lipids are used for the production of the biofuels, the essential FAs like eicosapentaenoic acid (EPA) and docosahexaenoic acid (DHA) could be utilized as a nutrient supplement. Stengel and Connan (2015) explained the commercial importance of algal FAs, e.g. FAs from *Chlorella* sp., *Synechocystis* sp., *Chlamydomonas* sp., and, *Isochrysis* sp., in biofuel, while DHA and EPA from *Crypthecodinium cohnii*, *Schizochytrium* sp., *Nannochloropsis* sp., *Spirulina/Arthrospira* sp., and *Ulkenia* sp. could be used for culture, genetic engineering, nutraceuticals, bioceuticals, pharmaceuticals, and animal feed.

Kumari et al. (2013) elaborate the distribution of algal lipids, according to which the Euglenophyta, Rhodophyta, and diatoms have unusual sulfur-containing PL, phosphatidylsulfocholine (PSC). Brown algae have phosphatidyl O-[N-(2-hydroxyethyl) glycine] (PHEG) containing a glycine head group (3–25% of PL) and are rich in arachidonic acid (AA 80%) and EPA (10%). While the brown algae have amino acids containing PL, *Ochromonas danica* and *P. lutheri* contain carboxylated glycoglycerolipid, diacylglyceryl glucuronide (DGGA) containing AA, and docosapentaenoic acid (DPA). Furthermore, *P. lutheri*, *Scytonema* sp., and *Oscillatoria raoi* have acylated and diacylated sulfoquinovosyldiacylglycerol (SQDG), and *Chondria armata* contains sulfonoglycolipid crassiculisine with α-O-(6-sulfo-α-D-quinovopyranosyl)-glycerol as a sugar moiety and methyl myristate and palmitate as acyl chains. The freshwater and marine algae both have chlorosulfolipids. *Botryococcus braunii* possesses unusual hydrocarbons (C23–C40) and ether lipids accounting for 80% of cell dry weight. *Emiliania huxleyi* and *Isochrysis galbana* are reported to contain long-chain (C35–C40) alkenes, alkenones, and alkenoates, while *Arainvillea nigricans* has arainvilloside containing a 6-deoxy-6-aminoglucose moiety. *A. nigricans* contains antimitotic ether-linked glycoglycerolipids nigricanosides A and B, while *Sargassum thunbergii* contains (2S) -1-O-(5Z,8Z,11Z,14Z,17Z-eicosapentaenoyl)-2-O-(9Z,12Z,15Z-octadecatrienoyl)-3-O-b-D-galactopyranosyl-sn-glycerol (1) and (2S)-1-O-(9Z,12Z,15Z-octadecatrienoyl) -2-O-(6Z,9Z,12Z,15Z-octadecatetraenoyl)-3-O-b-D-galactopyranosyl-sn-glycerol(Kim et al. 2007). *Chondria armata* has six minor new glycolipids in crude methanolic extracts that include 1,2-diO-acyl-3-O-(acyl-6′-galactosyl)-glycerol (GL 1a) and sulfonoglycolipids 2-O-palmitoyl-3-O-(6'sulfoquinovopyranosyl)-glycerol and its ethyl ether derivative according to Al-Fadhli et al. (2006). Kumari et al. 2013 found that *Gymnodinium* sp. have a trigalactosyl diacylglycerol containing 18:1/14:0, 18:1/16:0, and 18:1/18:1 at sn-1 and sn-2 positions, while *P. tricornutum* has SQDG and acylated SQDG containing sn-1: C16:0/sn-2: C16:0/2' C20:5, and sn-1: C20:5/sn-2: C16:0/2' C20:5.

However, in a discrete study on seasonality, Henderson et al. (1998) investigated ice algae sampled from the Barents Sea, finding that during spring, *Nitzschia frigida* was the most common species, while resting stages of *Thalassiosira bioculata* and *Actinocyclus cf. curvatulus* predominated in autumn. In their study, the neutral lipids predominated over glycolipids and phospholipids in all algal samples; in the spring samples the major FAs of the neutral lipid fraction were 16:0, 16:1(n-7), and 20:5(n-3), while the glycolipid fraction was characterized by higher levels of 20:5(n-3) and C16 PUFAs, particularly 16:4(n-1). Phospholipids contained higher levels of 22:6(n-3) than the other two lipid fractions, but 20:5(n-3) was still the major polyunsaturated FA. In the autumn samples of Henderson et al. (1998), the neutral lipid fraction contained higher proportions of saturated FAs and 16:1(n-7) than the two polar lipid fractions and 22:6(n-3) was most abundant in phospholipids. Just as in the spring samples, 20:5(n-3) was the major polyunsaturated FA in all lipid fractions of the autumn algae. Nevertheless, Henderson et al. (1998) reported some species-specific differences in lipid production as the neutral lipid content of autumn samples containing mainly *Actinocyclus curvatulus* was substantially higher than those in which *T. bioculata* predominated.

Olofsson et al. (2012) reported seasonal variation of TL content of *Nannochloropsis oculata* grown outdoors (winter and spring [11–24%] and [13–22%]; summer and autumn [20–30%]), and underlined the important role of light and temperature in algal lipid synthesis and accumulation. High lipid contents related to high light, measured as total global radiation (TGR), and high temperature are reported, and vice versa. The highest lipid content was recorded during autumn indicating an optimal, nonlinear response to light and temperature that enhanced thylakoid stacking under reduced light conditions resulting in more structural lipids, concomitantly with the increase in glycerides due to released photo-oxidative stress. High lipid accumulation has also been reported in *Dunaliella* cells grown at low (12 °C) temperature as compared with high (30 °C) temperature, and even more lipid accumulation was reported when cells responded to a sudden shift from 30 to 12 °C (Lynch and Thompson 1982); here, lower temperature could lead to enhancement of structural lipids to facilitate cell membrane fluidity. For *N. oculata* grown outdoors, Olofsson et al. (2012) report that the total glycerides increased during late summer–autumn in relation to free fatty acids (FFAs), concomitant with the rise in TL, indicating a significant glyceride synthesis. TAGs are storage lipids usually synthesized under adverse environmental conditions (low light and temperature) or photo-oxidative stress; they serve as electron sinks during photo-oxidative stress preventing ROS damage to membrane lipids and proteins. During summer, clouds do not reflect sunlight and shortwave radiations (UV) increase, possibly triggering photoinhibition. While the overall PUFA levels in Olofsson et al. (2012) study increased in winter, when light intensity was low, the monounsaturated fatty acids (MUFAs) were high in the autumn possibly as a result of more C16:1 allocated to TAGs, and PUFAs (mainly C16:3ω4 and C18:3ω3) decreased, potentially converted into C16:1 and C18:1. They point out that while temperature affects the FA composition of microalgae, the degree of unsaturation in FAs usually has a negative relationship with temperature. At higher temperatures, PUFAs in various microalgae decreased, while saturated fatty acids (SAFAs) increased probably due to the fluidity of cell membranes. Although many reports suggest microalgae form a larger amount of PUFAs in response to low temperature, this is species-specific. Olofsson et al. (2012) determined that there was seasonal variation in the saturated to unsaturated ratio of FAs in *N. oculata*; together with temperature, the TGR played a role in the elevated TL, TAGs, SAFAs, and MUFAs. Since the proposed most suitable FA for algal biofuel production consisted of SAFAs and MUFAs, autumn conditions seemed to favor optimal lipid accumulation in *N. oculata*. They suggested an appealing concept for utilization of PUFAs as high-value FAs for food and feed in the summer season perhaps, which probably is necessary for making microalgal fuel production environmentally and economically sustainable (Olofsson et al. 2012). Sushchik et al. (2009) observed the FA composition in the microalgae of the Yenisei River, reporting seasonal changes to be caused by seasonal succession of species composition of the community; they found that populations of both diatoms and green algae grown in summer at a higher water temperature were lower in PUFAs than those in spring, at a lower temperature.

Seaweeds, on the other hand, could contain up to 1–5% TL on DW basis; although seaweeds have significantly lower lipid contents than marine fish, they are still a potential source of functional lipids due to their large stock in coastal waters (Miyashita et al. 2013). A study of 34 edible seaweed products of the *Laminaria* sp., *U. pinnatifida*, *H. fusiformis*, and *Porphyra* sp., revealed the presence of approximately 2 g lipid 100 g^{-1} semi-dry sample weight (s.w.); geography and species influenced the lipid content, i.e. the low lipid contents of *Porphyra* sp., *Laminaria* sp., and *H. fusiformis* from China differed significantly from the lipid content of *U. pinnatifida* and *Porphyra* sp. from Japan and Korea.

Khairy and El-Shafay (2013) stated that the environmental factors that influenced the growth of the seaweed also influenced the lipid content; essentially, seasonal changes in temperature have a major effect on the FA composition of cell membranes (Phleger 1991). Ahmed and Ahmed (2016) report that contents of TL and omega-3 PUFAs of seaweeds vary seasonally, indicating that the TL of some Sargassaceae brown seaweeds could reach 15 wt.% TL per DW and could contain over 40 wt.% omega-3 PUFAs per total FAs. Brown seaweed lipids contain many types of bioactive compounds, such as omega-3 PUFAs, omega-6 AA, fucoxanthin, fucosterol, and some polyphenols. Kendel et al. (2015) mention that lipid composition in marine algae (seaweed) has been of considerable interest due to its high PUFA content, specifically α-linolenic (18:3 n-3), octadecatetraenoic (18:4 n-3), arachidonic (20:4 n-6), and EPAs (20:5 n-3). This class of acids is nutritionally essential for humans and animals; they help in preventing cardiovascular diseases, osteoarthritis, diabetes, and possess antimicrobial, antiviral, anti-inflammatory, and antitumoral properties. The total FA content of *H. elongata*, *Laminaria ochroleuca*, *U. pinnatifida*, *Palmaria* sp., and *Porphyra* sp. is reported to comprise saturated FAs (39.06, 33.82, 20.39, 60.48, 64.95%), monounsaturated FAs (22.75, 19.23, 10.5, 10.67, 18.91%), PUFAs (38.16, 46.94, 69.11, 28.86, 16.1%), ω6 PUFAs (15.08, 20.99, 22.1, 2.14, 7.97%), and ω3 PUFAs (18.7, 25.08, 44.7, 25.52, 7.2%) (MacArtain et al. 2007). *U. fasciata* and *Dilophys fasciola* have mannose- and rhamnose-containing glycolipids.

Evaluating Egyptian seaweeds *U. lactuca*, *J. rubens*, and *P. capillacea*, Khairy and El-Shafay (2013) report seasonal differences between the lipid content (with *J. rubens* being an exception); they observed a decrease in lipid contents from spring till autumn. During spring, summer, and autumn, they observed varying lipid content in *U. lactuca* (4.09, 3.57, and 3.14, respectively), *J. rubens* (2.39, 2.30, and 1.47, respectively), and *P. capillacea* (2.71, 2.09, and 1.76, respectively). Renaud and Luong-Van (2006) evaluated 30 common Australian macroalgae, observing the highest lipid content in phaeophytes in summer. Paiva et al. (2018) too reported high crude lipid content (DW) in *F. spiralis* in summer as compared with winter samples. Similarly, *Fucus serratus*, *F. virsoides*, and *Fucaceae* sp. have been reported to show high lipid content in summer (Kim et al. 1996; Zavodnik 1973; Schmid et al. 2017). Sanchez-Machado et al. (2004) observed that as the temperature increased, the lipid level decreased and remained almost stable until the end of the growing season; even Kumari et al. (2013) cite examples of high lipid content in winter and autumn as compared with summer in the case of *U. pinnatifida*, *L. japonica*, *F. serratus*, *Egregia menziesii*, *Condrocanthus canaliculatus*, and *Ulva lobata*. According to them, changes in other abiotic factors (light, salinity, and nutrients/nutrient availability), physiological state of the algae, and interactions between factors could also contribute to variations in lipid content (Kumari et al. 2013; Paiva et al. 2018). Kumari et al. (2013) mention that polar lipids depend on the algal development stages throughout the year while high TAG contents are observed in summer. The higher lipid content in summer (during high temperatures) could be caused by an accumulation of TAGs as storage compounds (Paiva et al. 2018).

In contrast, Kendel et al. (2012) studied *G. turuturu* and observed the highest neutral lipids in winter (42% of TL) and the lowest in summer (20%), while they reported a vice versa trend in the case of phospholipid content, stating that this could be due to the use of lipid reserves for the growth of the thalli during the summer.

PUFAs are also responsive to species, environmental changes (Nichols et al. 1998), or a combination of both. The higher percentage of PUFAs during winter benefits low-temperature acclimatization and protects photosynthetic machinery from low-temperature photoinhibition (Gombos et al. 1994). Khairy and El-Shafay (2013) particularly reported the highest monounsaturated FAs in the three algae during autumn; further, *J. rubens* had the highest amount of PUFAs among the three, and DHA was the predominant component in autumn. Paiva et al. (2018) found high MUFAs in summer samples, with oleic acid (C18:1n9) being the dominant one (20.36–38.04%), and high PUFAs in winter (28.17–40.59%); similarly, Schmid et al. (2014, 2017) reported seasonal variation in Fucaceae species from upper to mid-shore (*A. nodosum*, *F. serratus*, and *F. vesiculosus*). According to Paiva et al. (2018), an increase in PUFAs in winter facilitates greater cell membrane fluidity at low temperatures; among the PUFA group, they observed that dihomo-γ-linolenic (DHGLA, C20:3n6) and eicosatrienoic (C20:3n3) acids were found in appreciable quantities (9.40–13.83 and 4.33–11.31%, respectively). Gerasimenko et al. (2010) also report higher TAG content for *Costaria costata* in May at the time of sporulation; they state that lipid changes were often accompanied by high PUFAs, high unsaturation index (UI), and n-3 > n-6 PUFAs in winter versus summer season, citing examples of *Ahnfeltia touchiensis*, *L. japonica*, *Ulva fenestrata*, *Sargassum pallidum*, *U. pinnatifida*, and *Caulerpa taxifolia*.

2.8 Inorganic Elements and Minerals

Evaluating the inorganic element composition of algae is imperative in the algal physiology and applicability (industrial, agricultural, nutritional, and pharmaceutical areas) context. Certain algae, especially seaweeds, are known to be rich in nutritional supplements such as minerals and essential metals (e.g. Kumar et al. 2008). Although more than 30% of the dry weight of marine algae is ash, which contains various kinds of minerals, there is inadequate literature documentation (Table 2.4) describing the mineral contents of macroalgal and microalgal foods (Wells et al. 2017; Cabrita et al. 2016). Macroalgae are rich in several essential minerals and trace elements required for human nutrition; reports suggest that their mineral content could be higher than that of edible land plants (Kumar et al. 2015). On the other hand, several species of microalgae being used as animal or aquacultural feeds could also be useful sources of minerals and single cell protein (SCP). Fábregas and Herrero (1986) highlight the mineral composition, in terms of major and trace elements, suggesting the utilization of marine microalgae *T. suecica*, *I. galbana*, *Dunaliella tertiolecta*, and *C. stigmatophora* in marine aquaculture and as a new SCP source.

Nevertheless, changes in environmental and physiological conditions influence occurrence and quantity of minerals in any water body, and thereby govern seasonal, geographic, and taxonomic variations in mineral contents of marine algae. According to Jensen (1993), algal mineral contents are subjected to seasonal, geographic, and taxonomic variations, which make their nutritional generalization somewhat difficult. For example, in terms of geographic variation, Wells et al. (2017) reported macroalgal harvests from warm equatorial areas to have lower mineral nutritional value than those from higher latitude regions. Indonesian green, brown, and red algae contain high levels of potassium, calcium, and sodium, but significantly lower levels of iron and zinc than reported for Japanese pyropia (as *Porphyra*) *yezoensis*, *E. intestinalis*, and *H. fusiformis*.

Most macroalgae have high calcium, magnesium, phosphorus, potassium, sodium, and iron (i.e. Ca, Mg, P, K, Na, and Fe, respectively) contents (Table 2.3); they also have other minerals such as chloride, manganese, magnesium, zinc, copper, cobalt, selenium, fluoride, and vanadium (i.e. Cl, Mn, Mg, Zn, Cu, Co, Se, Fl, and V, respectively). Essentially, all seaweeds offer an extraordinary level of K that is very similar to our natural plasma level. On the other hand, certain minerals have biological functions, either in elemental form or when incorporated into specific compounds, including Ca, P, Mg, Na, P, Cl, Fe, Co, Cu, Mn, Zn, and also, sulfur (S), iodine (I), molybdenum (Mo), selenium (Se), and fluorine (F). Panayotova and Stancheva (2013) analyzed various seaweeds belonging to the Chlorophyceae (*U. rigida* and *C. linum*), Phaeophyceae (*C. barbata* and *Cystoseira crinita*), and Rhodophyceae (*Gelidium crinale*) groups, and observed that they were rich in minerals such as Na, K, Ca, Mg, Sr (2.59–5.90; 0.28–10.9, 5.52–21.4; 2.31–4.22; 0.05–1.18 mg g^{-1} DW, respectively), and contained Pb, Cr, Co, Fe, Zn, Mn, Cu, As, Ni, Ba, Se (0.02–0.12; 0.02–0.33; 0.02–0.15; 6.1–105; 1.30–3.80; 1.60–29.4; 0.24–0.91; 0.18–1.54; 0.04–0.11; 0.01–1.95; 0.004–0.12 mg 100 g^{-1} DW, respectively), as well as Hg and Cd (0.01–0.03, 0.03–0.34 μg g^{-1} DW). According to them, the green algae *C. linum* and *U. rigida* were rich in mineral elements such as Mg, Na, Cr, Co, Fe, Mn, As, Pb, and Hg, while the red alga *G. crinale* had good Cu, Zn, and Se levels ; the brown algae *C. barbata* and *C. crinita* were rich in Ni, Cd, Ca, K, Sr, and Ba. The mineral composition of different Black Sea macroalgae species was found to be relatively higher than land vegetables as well as than other edible seaweeds; thereby proving their applicability as a food supplement or as a spice to improve the nutritive value in animal or human diet.

However, Kumar et al. (2015) reported seasonal variation in the mineral composition of *K. alvarezii*; they recorded the highest mineral content in *K. alvarezii* (29 939.61 mg 100 g^{-1} DW) during April 2005, and the lowest values (10 997.62 mg 100 g^{-1} DW) in January 2006. They observed that accumulation of Na and K salts generally depended upon the physiology and season; Na:K ratio of *K. alvarezii* varied from 0.34 to 0.87. Schiener et al. (2015) found the levels of the major metal salts of Ca and K and the trace element Fe more than doubled during spring and summer months in the brown algae *L. digitata*, *Laminaria hyperborea*, and *S. latissima*. Evaluation of several macronutrients (C, N, P, Na, K, Ca, Mg, and S) and micronutrients (Fe, Mn, Cu, and Zn) in the brown seaweeds *A. nodosum*, *F. vesiculosus*, and *F. spiralis* in Spain, conducted by Villares et al. (2013), revealed seasonal variability in N and K in the three seaweeds (minimum values in summer). They observed minimum N values in summer in all three species, which, together with high C:N and low N:P ratios may indicate nutrient limitation by this element. Among the other elements considered, only K displayed a seasonal trend in all species they evaluated (most evident in *F. vesiculosus*); minimum K was observed in summer. They stated that seasonal variation in nutrients that usually limit the growth of macroalgae (N or P) is often observed, with minimum concentrations in summer due to a dilution effect by growth in a favorable season and the fact that at this time of year, nutrient concentrations in water are usually minimal. The highest concentrations of P and Zn were observed in *F. vesiculosus* during spring and no seasonal trends were observed in the remaining minerals. In *F. vesiculosus* and *F. spiralis*, the concentrations of C followed the reverse pattern to that observed for N and K, as peaks occurred in summer, possibly as a result of the accumulation of carbohydrates as an energy reserve.

It has been known that seasonality and environment influence growth of seaweeds; however, Hou and Yan (1998) evaluated the influence of growth stage on the variations in the elemental profile of *Sargassum kjellmanianum*; remarkably, they observed no significant variations in major elements (namely Na, Ca, and Mg) during the full growth period; however, Cl and K were slightly higher in the later growth stage. The trace elements scandium (Sc), cesium (Cs), vanadium (V), Cr, thorium (Th), aluminum (Al), and Fe, and the rare earth elements, were at lower concentrations in the initial and later growth stages, while the highest concentrations were recorded in February (the mid-growth stage). Highest I concentrations were recorded during March. The Mn concentration was lowest in February, and the highest in the later growth stage. Hou and Yan (1998) demonstrated no significant seasonal variations in Br, Rb, and Zn; they also studied seasonal variations in the water-soluble states of inorganic elements for *S. kjellmanianum* and stated that three times leaching with de-ionized water (with stirring), successfully leached out the water-soluble part of elements; water leaching ratios of various elements showed seasonal variations based on the chemical species. Cl, Na, and K exhibited no significant seasonal variations in leaching ratio, while Mg leaching was the lowest in the initial growth stage, and gradually increased, reaching the highest value in March, followed by a decrease. Similarly seasonal variations in leaching ratios of Sb, Sc, Cs, Co, Zn, Ba, Fe, and Sr were also found (highest in January and low in February and December). The seasonal variation of the I leaching ratio was the same as its total content variation.

Marine macroalgae are particularly rich in I and Fe. I deficiency has been known to cause hypothyroidism while excess I uptake can induce either hyper- or hypothyroidism (Wells et al. 2017). Marine algae can hyperaccumulate I (which also has associated health risks), but I content and bioavailability depend on species, with generally higher levels in kelps, and also vary seasonally and geographically (Stengel and Connan 2015). Macroalgae such as kelps (*Laminaria* sp. and *Saccharina* sp.) have high I level and salts. Kelps such as *Undaria* (wakame) and *Alaria* (Atlantic wakame) too have I but at a lower concentration than *P. palmata* (dulse, a Red Sea vegetable). The method of extraction (many iodine compounds are water-soluble) and the duration of storage (I may vaporize under humid conditions) are other influential factors. Processing of macroalgae, i.e. washing and drying for storage, followed by rehydration (of *Alaria esculenta*, *P. palmata*, and *E. intestinalis*) could decrease the I content from 14 to 75% (Nitschke and Stengel 2016). Young and Langille (1958) reported seasonal variation in I for *C. crispus* (from 180 ppm [in April] to 310 ppm [July and December]); further, total ash and potassium are highest in the winter months and lowest in summer. On the other hand, macroalgae are also a potentially rich source of Fe for human diets. The Fe content of naturally occurring wild algae has also been known to vary seasonally and geographically depending on the metal content of coastal waters, in addition to being species-specific. Cabrita et al. (2016) established that Fe content (and other metal) varied, in some cases substantially, among macroalgal species collected at the same sites and time, and this was presumably linked with the differences in metabolic requirements. Wells et al. (2017) have detailed seasonal differences in the Fe content of four seaweed species (*Ulva* sp., *Sargassum* sp., *Porphyra* sp., and *Gracilariopsis* sp.). Garcia-Casal et al. (2009) established that apart from enhancing total dietary Fe content, seaweeds synergistically facilitated Fe uptake from wheat and maize, which could possibly be related to high levels of ascorbic acid (vitamin C), which converts Fe to the more readily absorbed ferrous form. Wells et al. (2017) looked at Fe levels in *Ulva* sp., *Sargassum* sp., *Porphyra* sp., and *Gracilariopsis* sp., and found that *Gracilariopsis* sp. and *Sargassum* sp. had substantially higher Fe content compared with *Porphyra* sp.; however, they found a distinct seasonal cycle whereby Fe content was highest in spring and summer and lowest in autumn and winter. *Gracilariopsis* sp. and *Sargassum* sp. have been reported to contain substantially higher Fe content as compared with *Porphyra* sp. from Venezuelan waters; nevertheless, Garcia-Casal et al. (2007) and (2009) revealed seasonal differences in the Fe content of *Ulva* sp., *Sargassum* sp., *Porphyra* sp., and *Gracilariopsis* sp., stating that the Fe content was highest in spring and summer, and lowest in autumn and winter. *Sargassum*, *Ulva*, and *Porphyra* sp. have high iron content, and 15 g day^{-1} of *Sargassum* provided substantially higher amounts than daily recommended intakes ($\leq$18 mg Fe day^{-1}, Institute-of-Medicine 2001).

Nowadays researchers tend to evaluate seasonal variations in elements that are considered toxic at low concentrations owing to their significance in marine pollution. For example, Perez et al. (2007) evaluated *Porphyra columbina* and *Ulva* sp., noticing significant seasonal variations in metal loading, with *Pyropia columbina* having maximum Cd concentrations during winter; however, *Ulva* sp. showed highest Pb concentrations during summer. Riosmena-Rodríguez et al. (2010) found elevated concentrations of Cd in several algal species during April that appeared to be related to local upwelling events. This seasonality in metal concentrations of algae may result not only from metabolic controls but also oceanographic influences (Wells et al. 2017). Similarly, monthly variations in metal contents in *U. lactuca* from El Jadida city (Morocco) were reported by Kaimoussi et al. (2004); Fe contents of *U. lactuca* showed large variations, with low levels during summer. Cu exhibited fluctuations during the season, while less marked seasonal variations of Zn were observed. Cd value for the S4 station was highest in June 1998 (2.15 $\mu g\ g^{-1}$ DW). Although a less significant seasonal variation of Mn in *U. lactuca* was evidenced in their study, maximum values were recorded in June 1998 for station S1, in April 1998 for station S2, in November 1998 for station S3, and in May 1998 for station S4. Kaimoussi et al. (2004) suggest intensification of urbanization and socio-economic activities were also responsible for some of the variations.

In contrast, in a study on natural seasonal variations of certain metals, Riget et al. (1995) studied growing tips of *F. vesiculosus*, reporting variation in cadmium (Cd) and Zn metal levels between samples taken at different times of the year. In their study, seasonal variations in Cu and Pb concentrations were less clear. Fuge and James (1973) reported that seasonal variation in metal content could be a function of seaweed growth; according to their theory, the concentration would rise in slow-growing wintering plants, until the spring, when growth resumes; thereafter, concentrations would fall until the beginning of winter, as a result of continuing growth. Thus, Riget et al. (1995) affirm that seasonal pattern of metal concentrations found in their study fits this theory of Fuge and James (1973). Miramand and Bentley (1992) also reported no seasonal variation of Pb levels in the brown alga *F. serratus*, but a pronounced seasonal pattern of Zn and Cd.

Remarkably, seasonal variations of seaweed chemical composition are linked with the particular life stage. Mišurcová et al. (2011) confirmed this by reporting that in periods of maximum growth, photosynthetic activity increased, which resulted in higher content of carbohydrates with many binding sites for metals. They observed maximum and minimum concentrations of Cd, Cu, and Pb in February (middle growth stage) and August (initial and latter growth stage), respectively; for Zn, maximum and minimum concentrations occurred in March and September, respectively (similar to Lares et al. 2002). However, they recorded the highest Cd content in June and the lowest in October in brown seaweed *M. pyrifera*. Eide et al. (1980) too reported marked differences in the rates of uptake of Cd and Zn between seasons in the seaweed *A. nodosum*; they proposed that the uptake of these metals was linked with metabolic processes. They found less difference in bioaccumulation of lead between seasons, suggesting that an ion-exchange process could be involved in Pb uptake. Nevertheless, growth activities alone do not completely explain the difference in seasonal variability between metals. According to Villares et al. (2002), seasonal changes in levels of different metals followed a similar pattern in both *Ulva* and *Enteromorpha*, with minimum values being found in summer and maximum values in autumn/winter. This is apparently caused by a dilution effect due to growth during favorable periods and in winter to a large decrease in metabolic rates. This pattern was probably accentuated in the levels of Al, Fe, and Mn in autumn and winter because of fluvial inputs.

Villares et al. (2002) suggest that the temporal variability in these elements could be related to environmental factors (e.g. the increased river inputs of metals during rainy seasons could lead to greater accumulation by seaweeds); in addition, salinity may cause physico-chemical changes in the water and physiological changes in the macroalgae (e.g. reduced salinity can reduce the production of metal-binding phenols in brown seaweeds).

2.9 Vitamins

Vitamins are essential organic micronutrients that cannot be synthesized by an organism directly in sufficient quantities, thus they should be obtained from the diet. They serve as precursors for essential enzyme cofactors and are needed for essential metabolic functions. Vitamin-deficiency diseases include beriberi (deficiency in thiamine, vitamin B_1), pellagra (niacin), pernicious anemia (cobalamin, vitamin B_{12}), and scurvy (ascorbic acid, vitamin C) (Wells et al. 2017). The vitamin content of several species of algae has been provided by Wells et al. (2017); *T. suecica*, *I. galbana*, *D. tertiolecta*, and *C. stigmatophora* are rich in lipid-soluble (A and E) and B-group vitamins (including vitamins B_1, B_2 [riboflavin], B_6 [pyridoxal], and B_{12}). *Cyanobacterium Arthrospira* sp. (*Spirulina*) contains pseudovitamin B_{12}. Lordan et al. (2011) reported *D. tertiolecta* to contain 200–500 $\mu g\, g^{-1}$ DW vitamin E. On the other hand, as seaweed species are rich in beneficial nutrients and are rich sources of vitamin C, vitamin B-complex, e.g. folic acid and B_{12}, and vitamin A precursors, such as β-carotene, they have been consumed in several countries (Chapman and Chapman 1980); they could an provide an important amount of the daily requirement levels for vitamins. Algal foods are one of the vegetarian alternatives for cobalamin (vitamin B_{12}) in the diet; for example, kelps (including wakame), hijiki, "green" (*Ulva* [formerly *Enteromorpha* sp.]), and "purple" (*Pyropia* [formerly *Porphyra*] sp.) laver, as well as nori. Several sea vegetables (laver [*P. umbilicalis*], sea spaghetti [*H. elongata*], and *Gracilaria changii*) contain levels of vitamin C comparable with common vegetables such as tomatoes and lettuce, while brown seaweed *E. arborea* (34.4 mg 100 g^{-1} DW) has vitamin C levels close to those found in mandarin oranges (Hernandez-Carmona et al. 2009). *Ulva rigida*, *A. nodosum*, *U. pinnatifida*, *L. digitata*, *P. umbilicalis*, and *P. palmata* contain 19.70, 3.63, 145–174, 34.38, 14.25, and 162 $\mu g\, g^{-1}$ DW vitamin E, respectively (Lordan et al. 2011). The kelp *M. pyrifera* contains α-tocopherol (the most biologically active form of vitamin E) on a par with plant oils rich in this vitamin, such as palm, sunflower seed, and soybean oil; further, β-carotene (provitamin A) values of *C. fragile* and *Gracilaria chilensis* are greater than carrots (Ortiz et al. 2009). Vitamin B_1, B_2, B_3, B_6, B_8, B_9, C, E, B_{12} content (mg 8 g^{-1} dry portion) values of *A. nodosum* (0.216, 0.058, 0.000, 0.001, 0.001, 3.648, 0.654, 0.029, 0.131), *L. digitata* (0.011, 0.011, 4.896, 0.513, 0.513, 0.000, 2.842, 0.275, 0.495), *U. pinnatifida* (0.403, 0.936, 7.198, 0.259, 0.015, 0.528, 14.779, 1.392, 0.345), *P. umbilicalis* (0.077, 0.274, 0.761, 0.119, 1.003, 12.885, 0.114, 0.769), *P. palmata* (0.024, 0.080, 0.800,0. 002, 0.002, 0.021, 5.520, 1.296, 1.840), and *Ulva* sp. (0.060,0.030, .000, 0.012, 1.000, 6.300) have been provided by Fábregas and Herrero (1990). Thus algal foods can be an excellent source for a wide range of these essential micronutrients.

Although macro- and microalgae are an incredible source of vitamins, variability between samples can make direct comparisons difficult; differences can also occur owing to environmental and seasonal factors. Seasonal variation in vitamin content of algae has been sparsely deliberated, for example Hernandez-Carmona et al. (2009) carried out monthly quantitation of vitamins C, B_2, B_1, and A in *E. arborea* over a 12-month period, revealing low levels in the summer (June, July, August); the highest vitamins C, B_2, B_1 concentrations were reported in April/September, while provitamin A peaked in January. Evaluation of vitamin C in several macroalgae by Sarojini and Sarma (1999) revealed seasonal variability based on the species investigated; most of the species showed two peaks with one corresponding to the vegetative part of the early growth phase, and the other to the reproductive phase of the thalli. Such phases observed in *U. fasciata* are one in August and another in March; *Chaetomorpha antenina* in September and November; *Chaetomorpha brachygona* in August and February; *Caulerapa racemosa* in September and February; *Caulerpa sertularioides* in August and December; *Spongomorpha indica* in September and December; while *Enteromorpha compressa* shows high vitamin C levels in February. Among the Phaeophyceae, *P. tetrastromatica* showed two peaks for high vitamin C in May and January, and *Sargassum tenerrimum* showed high vitamin C in June and December. According to them, among the Rhodophyceae, *G. corticata* showed two peaks, one in September and another in February–March. High vitamin C was observed in June and January in *Pterocladia heteroplatos*, while in *Amphiroa fragilissima* vitamin C reportedly peaked in June and October (Sarojini and Sarma 1999).

2.10 Phenolic Compounds

Phenolic compounds are secondary metabolites; they are not directly involved in algal primary processes such as photosynthesis, cell division, and reproduction. Usually characterized as stress compounds, phenolics are involved in chemical protective mechanisms against biotic factors such as grazing, settlement of bacteria or other fouling organisms, and against abiotic stressors such as UV radiation and metal contamination (Stengel et al. 2011). Phenolic compounds contain one or more phenolic rings, which may be halogenated conferring different and often stronger biological activities; they are present in many algal groups. Stengel et al. (2011) provided a discrete description of the various algal phenolic compounds; according to them bromophenols are common to all major algal groups. Bromophenols are found in red seaweeds, mainly in Ceramiales (*Laurencia* sp.) as well as Gelidiales and Corallinales; they also occur in brown and green seaweed. Certain phenolic compounds, such as phlorotannins in brown seaweeds, exhibit primary functions, e.g. in growth and the development of the cell wall in Fucales. Further, phenolic terpenoids occur in brown and red algae; for example, Sargassaceae exclusively have meroditerpenoids (plastoquinones, chromanols, chromenes), while red algae contain mainly diterpenes, with sesquiterpenes present in Rhodomelaceae (*Laurencia* sp.), and the secondary cyclization forming a macrolide in *Callophycus serratus* (bromophycolides). In the Phaeophyceae, the majority of the described phenolic compounds are phlorotannins: polymers of phloroglucinol such as fucols, fuhalols, phlorethols, eckols, and carmalols. They are only present in brown seaweeds but are widespread among them, occurring in greatest abundance in the Fucales (approx. 20% DW) (Stengel et al. 2011). *Fucus* sp., *Laminaria* sp., *Porphyra* sp., *Spongiochloris spongiosa*, and *Undaria* sp. are known to contain 41 400, 7300, 5700, 5.65, and 6600 $\mu g\,g^{-1}$ DW polyphenol, respectively (Lordan et al. 2011). Other nontypical phenolic compounds in algae include: colpol (in the brown seaweed *Colpomenia sinuosa*), tichocarpols (phenylpropanoid derivatives; in the red macroalga *Tichocarpus crinitus*), coumarins (in green seaweeds such as *Dasycladus vermicularis*), vanillic acid derivatives (in the green macroalga *Cladophora socialis*), and a polyphenolic pigment marennine in the diatom *Haslea ostrearia* responsible for oyster greening; furthermore, another polyphenolic pigment, scytonemin, and phenolic toxins such as microcystin are produced in certain Cyanobacteria. Lignin (polymerized hydroxycinnamyl alcohols), which commonly occurs in vascular land plants, also occurs in calcified intertidal red seaweed *Calliarthron cheilosporioides* (Stengel et al. 2011).

From the applicability perspective, phenolic compounds are known to have a wide range of applications; for example, purified phenolic compounds exhibit antioxidant, antiradical, UV-protective, metal-chelation, and antifouling activity, whereas the activity of phlorotannins varies according to concentration and molecular-size profile (Stengel et al. 2011). Phlorotannins (phenolics) from Fucales have pharmaceutical uses (Stengel and Connan 2015). Eckols exhibit antiviral (anti-HIV) and antiallergic activities; having antiadipogenic and neuroprotective effects, they have potential application in the treatment of Alzheimer's disease, and are inhibitors of melanin formation. Further, bromophenols are used as marine flavor agents in farmed fish and prawns, while certain meroditerpenoids from *Sargassum fallax* exhibit antitumor activities. Elatol, a sesquiterpene found in *Laurencia obtusa* var. *dendroidea*, is an antiparasitic agent. Some specific terpenoids of *C. serratus*, bromophycolides, have antimalaria properties due to their macrolide structure (Stengel et al. 2011). Polyhydroxyalkanoates (P3HB; PHA) from *Synechocystis* sp., *Nostoc* sp., and Cyanobacteria are utilized as bioplastic.

Stengel et al. (2011) studied *S. muticum* and its annual growth cycle, and observed that the phenolic compounds and mannitol levels peak in fully mature plants, while protein levels are lower in young plants but no significant laminaran variability in alginate content has been observed. Stengel et al. (2011) attributed the temporal variation in phenolics in fucoids to developmental stage and light environment. Diurnal (in addition to seasonal) changes in phenolic compound levels in response to irradiance levels have been observed in *Cystoseira tamariscifolia*, but short-term changes depended on season and plant part, suggesting rapid cycling of phenolic compounds in response to short-term environmental fluctuations (Abdala-Diaz et al. 2006). According to Geider and Osborne (1992), the photosynthetic apparatus of most algae acclimatizes to seasonal and microhabitat light climate by optimizing pigment levels and composition, but the ability of macroalgae to respond to short-term changes in light climate depends on their natural sensitivity. Fellah et al. (2017) reported seasonal variations in the total phenolic contents and potential antioxidant activities of three seaweed species (*Halopteris scoparia*, *Zonaria tournefortii*, and *Sphaerococcus coronopifolius*), where the highest total phenolic content was recorded during autumn in *S. coronopifolius* (144.33 mg gallic acid equivalent [GAE] $100\,g^{-1}$) and *H. scoparia* (105.40 mg GAE $100\,g^{-1}$), and the highest ascorbic acid content was observed in *H. scoparia* (125.52 mg ascorbic acid equivalents [AAE] $100\,g^{-1}$) in spring.

On the other hand, Connan et al. (2004) reported seasonal variation in phlorotannins in several brown algal families; *L. digitata* had the lowest phlorotannin concentrations in summer (0.09 DW), while in *F. vesiculosus* the highest levels occurred in spring (7.84% DW). *H. elongata* showed an exceptional seasonal variation in mean phenolic content, with 0.49% DW in winter and 4.84% DW in summer; according to them, this 10-fold variation may be related to reproductive strap elongation, since the lowest phenolic content was recorded in spring, when receptacles were still short. Phenolic levels increased with strap length, and decreased when aging straps started to degenerate. More generally, members of the Fucales exhibited maximal phenolic levels in summer (3.72% DW in *Pelvetia canaliculata* to 7.18% DW in *A. nodosum*) as opposed to *L. digitata*, which showed the highest phenolic content in winter (0.19% DW). Among the eight species studied in fucaleans, the highest levels of phlorotannins were recorded in summer, again supporting the idea of a photoprotective role for phenolic accumulation. According to their report, in spring, nonfertile receptacles proved to be poor in phenolics, whereas during summer, when receptacles were fertile, phenolic contents were higher. An increase has been reported in *S. muticum* (Yendo) Fensholt just after the period of highest fertility (Gorham and Lewey 1984), but in members of the Fucaceae phenolic contents are generally reported as higher in nonfertile plants (Ragan and Jensen 1978; Rönnberg and Ruokolahti 1986). Other reports (Rönnberg and Ruokolahti 1986; Steinberg and Van Altena 1992) also state maximal phlorotannin content in spring or summer, especially in phenol-rich species. In contrast, Ragan and Jensen (1978) report maximum levels for *Fucales* sp. in winter, while Ragan and Glombitza (1986) obtained high levels from late summer to the middle of winter, depending on the species.

Paiva et al. (2018) observed seasonality in the total phenol content of an *F. spiralis* sample at two sites SMA and SMG (172, 187 mg g^{-1} of DW summer, and 113, 153 mg g^{-1} of DW winter) in the methanolic extracts; he also observed seasonality in acetone:water extracts. The polyphenol contents of *L. digitata*, *Laminaria hyperborea*, *A. esculenta*, and *S. latissima* are known to have seasonal and species-related differences; Schiener et al. (2015) report accumulation of polyphenols that began with the onset of the growth phase and declined toward the autumn months. The highest polyphenol levels in the aforesaid seaweeds were observed between May and July; however, *Laminaria* sp. had the lowest polyphenol content in October, while *A. esculenta* and *S. latissima* had low polyphenol levels in March (Schiener et al. 2015).

2.11 Other Compounds

The chemical composition of algae has been researched and several components have been identified; however, there are several other components that need to be uncovered, focused on, or deliberated. For example, an invasive alga, *C. fragile* ssp. *tomentosoides*, is chemically defended against grazing by a wound-activated chemical defense mechanism (involving dimethylsulfoniopropionate [DMSP] and the products of its cleavage, dimethylsulfide [DMS], and acrylic acid). DMSP not only acts as a feeding deterrent, but functions as an antioxidant, a compatible solute, a cryoprotectant, and a waste molecule used to expel excess sulfur and energy; in terms of seasonality, Lyons et al. (2007) suggest that DMSP concentration in *C. fragile* ssp. *tomentosoides* correlates strongly with water temperature (which depends on season). Elevated DMSP concentration in winter may be a physiological response to increased antioxidant or cryoprotection requirements during periods of senescence and cold temperature. DMSP concentrations in several Antarctic and temperate algae are reported to change in response to changes in irradiance and salinity, which can be interpreted to vary with season (Karsten et al. 1992).

2.12 Conclusion

Algae comprise one of the most valuable yet underutilized resources that hold great potential. Appreciation with regard to their nutritional and health benefits has escalated over time leading to their utilization as high-value food sources; they also have multifaceted applications in several industries (phycocolloids, pigments, bioactives, pharmaceuticals, and cosmeceuticals). The biochemical composition of algae (which determines its applicability) varies with species, other physical and chemical parameters (wave exposure, seawater temperature, light, salinity, pH, oxidation state of minerals, etc.), geography, and season. Seasonality-dependent chemical composition of macroalgae is definitely of interest for the production of specific compounds (e.g. polysaccharide) especially on an industrial scale. In today's scenario where man is combating climate change and population rise, algae hold great potential as an income source. It is essential to create an awareness regarding the impact of biotic pressures on natural algae, harvesting of natural algae, various aquaculture techniques, and microalgal cultivation. This study summarizes the tremendous role of seasonality on the biochemical components of algae; understanding this aspect would benefit researchers and industrialists seeking to utilize particular algae or algal products.

References

Aakanksha, Samantray, S., Guruprasad, S., and Ramachandra, T.V. (2010). Diversity of lipids in algae. Lake 2010: Wetlands, Biodiversity and Climate Change 22nd–24th December 2010. http://wgbis.ces.iisc.ernet.in/energy/lake2010/Theme%201/T1_Poster_27.pdf (accessed on September 16, 2020).

Abdala-Diaz, R.T.A., Cabello-Pasini, A., Pérez-Rodríguez, E. et al. (2006). Daily and seasonal variations of optimum quantum yield and phenolic compounds in *Cystoseira tamariscifolia* (Phaeophyta). *Marine Biology* **148**: 459–465.

Abdel-Fattah, A.F. and Sary, H.H. (1987). Selective isolation of glycoprotein materials from the green seaweed *Ulva lactuca. Pakistan Journal of Biochemistry* **20**: 61–65.

Adams, J.M.M., Toop, T.A., Donnison, I.S., and Gallagher, J.A. (2011). Seasonal variation in *Laminaria digitata* and its impact on biochemical conversion routes to biofuels. *Bioresource Technology* **102** (21): 9976–9984.

Ahmed, N. and Ahmed, K. (2016). Chemical and different nutritional characteristics of brown seaweed lipids. *Advances in Science, Technology and Engineering Systems Journal* **1** (1): 23–22.

Al-Harbi, S.M. (2017). Seasonal dynamics and community composition of epilithic microalgae in relation with environmental factors at northwest coast of Jeddah: the Red Sea. *Journal of Oceanography and Marine Research* **5** (152): 1–8. https://doi.org/10.4172/2572-3103.1000152.

Al-Fadhli, A., Wahidulla, S., and D'Souza, L. (2006). Glycolipids from the red alga *Chondria armata* (Kütz.) Okamura. *Glycobiology* **16** (10): 902–915.

Anbuchezhian, R., Karuppiah, V., and Li, Z. (2015). Prospect of marine algae for production of industrially important chemicals. In: *Algal Biorefinery: An Integrated Approach* (ed. D. Das), 195–217. New York: Capital Publishing Company.

Ansari, A.A. and Ghanem, S.M. (2017). Seasonal variation in the growth responses of some chlorophytic algal flora of the Red Sea. *The Egyptian Journal of Aquatic Research* **43** (2): 129–134.

Arumugam, A., Uthra, S., and Muthuvel, A. (2018). Nutritional value of seaweeds and their potential pharmacological role of polyphenolics substances: a review. https://www.researchgate.net/publication/327363984_NUTRITIONAL_VALUE_OF_SEAWEEDS_AND_THEIR_POTENTIAL_PHARMACOLOGICAL_ROLE_OF_POLYPHENOLICS_SUBSTANCES_A_REVIEW (accessed September 2, 2020).

Asai, R., Horiguchi, Y., Yoshida, A. et al. (2001). Detection of phycobilin pigments and their seasonal change in Lake Kasumigaura using a sensitive in situ fluorometric sensor. *Analytical Letters* **34** (14): 2521–2533.

Augier, H. and Santimoine, M. (1978). Contribution á l'étude de la composition en azote total, en protéines et en acides aminés protéiniques des différentes parties du thalle de *Laminaria digitata* (Huds.) Lamour. dans le cadre de son exploitation industrielle et agricole. *Bulletin de la Société Mathématique de France* **23**: 19–28.

Aziza, M., Givernaud, T., Chikhaoui-Khay, M., and Bennasser, L. (2008). Seasonal variation of the growth, chemical composition and carrageenan extracted from *Hypnea musciformis* (Wulfen) Lamouroux harvested along the Atlantic coast of Morocco. *Scientific Research and Essay* **2**: 509–514.

Balakrishnan, D., Kandasamy, D., and Nithyanand, P. (2014). A review on antioxidant activity of marine organisms. *International Journal of ChemTech Research* **6** (7): 3431–3436.

Banerjee, K., Ghosh, R., Homechaudhuri, S., and Mitra, A. (2009). Seasonal variation in the biochemical composition of red seaweed (*Catenella repens*) from Gangetic delta, northeast coast of India. *Journal of Earth System Science* **118** (5): 497–505.

Barsanti, L. and Gualtieri, P. (2006). General overview. In: *Algae: Anatomy, Biochemistry, and Biotechnology* (eds. L. Barsanti and P. Gualtieri), 1–48. Boca Raton, FL: CRC Press/Taylor & Francis Group.

Becker, E.W. (1994). *Microalgae – Biotechnology and Microbiology*. Cambridge: Cambridge University Press.

Becker, E.W. (2004). Microalgae in human and animal nutrition. In: *Handbook of Microalgal Culture. Biotechnology and Applied Phycology* (ed. A. Richmond), 312–351. Oxford: Blackwell Science.

Becker, E.W. (2007). Micro-algae as a source of protein. *Biotechnology Advances* **25**: 207–210.

Begum, H., Yusoff, F.M., Banerjee, S. et al. (2016). Availability and utilization of pigments from microalgae. *Critical Reviews in Food Science and Nutrition* **5**: 2209–2222.

Bishop, W.M. and Zubeck, H.M. (2012). Evaluation of microalgae for use as nutraceuticals and nutritional supplements. *Journal of Nutrition & Food Sciences* **2**: 147–152.

Bleakley, S. and Hayes, M. (2017). Algal proteins: extraction, application, and challenges concerning production. *Food* **6** (5): 1–33.

Cabrita, A.R.J., Maia, M.R.G., Oliveira, H.M. et al. (2016). Tracing seaweeds as mineral sources for farm-animals. *Journal of Applied Phycology* **28**: 3135–3150.

Calvete, J.J., Costa, F.H.F., Saker-Sampaio, S. et al. (2000). The amino acid sequence of the agglutinin isolated from the red marine alga *Bryothamnion triquetrum* defines a novel lectin structure. *Cellular and Molecular Life Sciences* **57**: 343–350.

Capelli, B. and Cysewski, G.R. (2010). Potential health benefits of *Spirulina* microalgae. *Nutrafoods* **9**: 19–26.

Cardozo, K.H.M., Guaratini, T., Barros, M.P. et al. (2007). Metabolites from algae with economical impact. *Comparative Biochemistry and Physiology Part C: Toxicology & Pharmacology* **146**: 60–78.

Carreto, J.I. and Carignan, M.O. (2011). Mycosporine-like amino acids: relevant secondary metabolites. Chemical and ecological aspects. *Marine Drugs* **9** (3): 387–446.

Chakraborty, S. and Santra, S.C. (2008). Biochemical composition of eight benthic algae collected from Sunderban. *Indian Journal of Marine Sciences* **37** (3): 329–332.

Chapman, V.J. and Chapman, D.J. (1980). *Seaweeds and Their Uses*, 3e, 334. New York: Chapman and Hall.

Chen, C.Y., Zhao, X.Q., Yen, H.W. et al. (2013). Microalgae-based carbohydrates for biofuel production. *Biochemical Engineering Journal* **78**: 1–10.

Chinnadurai, S., Girija, K., Parthiban, C. et al. (2013). Eestimation of major pigment content in seaweeds collected from Pondicherry coast. *International Journal of Science and Technology* **9**: 522–525.

Christiaen, D., Stadler, T., Ondarza, M., and Verdus, M.C. (1987). Structures and functions of the polysaccharides from the cell wall of *Gracilaria verrucosa* (Rhodophyceae, Gigartinales). *Hydrobiologia* **151** (152): 139–146.

Chronakis, I.S. and Madsen, M. (2011). Algal proteins. In: *Handbook of Food Proteins* (eds. G.O. Phillips and P.A. Williams), 353–394. Cambridge: Woodhead Publishing.

Chu, W.L. (2012). Biotechnological applications of microalgae. *International e-Journal of Science, Medicine & Education* **6**: S24–S37.

Cian, R.E., Fajardo, M.A., Alaiz, M. et al. (2014). Chemical composition, nutritional and antioxidant properties of the red edible seaweed *Porphyra columbina. International Journal of Food Sciences and Nutrition* **65**: 299–305.

Connan, S., Goulard, F., Stiger, V. et al. (2004). Interspecific and temporal variation in phlorotannin levels in an assemblage of brown algae. *Botanica Marina* **47**: 410–416.

Converti, A., Casazza, A.A., Ortiz, E.Y. et al. (2009). Effect of temperature and nitrogen concentration on the growth and lipid content of *Nannochloropsis oculata* and *Chlorella vulgaris* for biodiesel production. *Chemical Engineering and Processing* **48**: 1146–1151.

Davison, I.R. and Pearson, G.A. (1996). Stress tolerance in intertidal seaweeds. *Journal of Phycology* **32**: 197–211.

Dawczynski, C., Schubert, R., and Jahreis, G. (2007). Amino acids, fatty acids, and dietary fibre in edible seaweed products. *Food Chemistry* **103**: 891–899.

Debbarma, J., Rao, B.M., Murthy, L.N. et al. (2016). Nutritional profiling of the edible seaweeds *Gracilaria edulis*, *Ulva lactuca* and *Sargassum* sp. *Indian Journal of Fisheries* **63**: 81–87.

Dere, Ş., Dalkiran, N., Karacaoğlu, D. et al. (2003). The determination of total protein, total soluble carbohydrate and pigment contents of some macroalgae collected from GemlikKaracaali (Bursa) and Erdek–Ormanlı (Balikesir) in the Sea of Marmara, Turkey. *Oceanologia* **45**: 453–471.

Diprat, A.B., Menegol, T., Boelter, J.F. et al. (2017). Chemical composition of microalgae *Heterochlorella luteoviridis* and *Dunaliella tertiolecta* with emphasis on carotenoids. *Journal of the Science of Food and Agriculture* **97**: 3463–3468.

Dring, M.J. (1982). *The Biology of Marine Plants*. Edward Arnold.

Durako, M.J. and Dawes, C.J. (1980). A comparative seasonal study of two populations of *Hypnea musciformis* from the east and west coasts of Florida, USA. I. Growth and chemistry. *Marine Biology* **59**: 151–156.

Eide, I., Adjers, K., Ruokolahti, C., and Bondestam, M. (1980). Longterm uptake and release of heavy metals by *Ascophyllum nodosum* (L) Le Jol. (Phaeophyceae) in situ. *Environmental Pollution* **23**: 19–28.

Fábregas, J. and Herrero, C. (1986). Marine microalgae as a potential source of mínerals in fish diets. *Aquaculture* **51** (3–4): 237–243.

Fabregas, J. and Herrero, C. (1990). Vitamin content of four marine microalgae. Potential use as source of vitamins in nutrition. *Journal of Industrial Microbiology and Biotechnology* **5**: 259–263. https://doi.org/10.1007/BF01569683.

FAO. (1981). Amino acid scoring patterns. FAO/WHO/UNUEPR/81/31. www.fao.org/3/M3013E/M3013E00.htm (accessed September 2, 2020).

Fellah, F., Louaileche, H., Dehbi-Zebboudj, A., and Touati, N. (2017). Seasonal variations in the phenolic compound content and antioxidant activities of three selected species of seaweeds from Tiskerth islet, Bejaia, Algeria. *Journal of Materials and Environmental Science* **8** (12): 4451–4456.

Fleurence, J. (1999). Seaweed proteins: biochemical, nutritional aspects and potential uses. *Trends in Food Science and Technology* **10**: 25–28.

Fleurence, J. (2004). Seaweed proteins. In: *Proteins in Food Processing* (ed. R.Y. Yada), 197–213. Cambridge: Woodhead Publishing.

Fleurence, J., Le Coeur, C., Mabeau, S. et al. (1995). Comparison of different extractive procedures from the edible seaweeds *Ulva rigida* and *Ulva rotundata*. *Journal of Applied Phycology* **7** (6): 577–582.

Fuge, R. and James, K.H. (1973). Trace metal concentrations in brown seaweeds, Cardigan Bay, Wales. *Marine Chemistry* **1**: 281–293.

Fujiwara-Arasaki, T., Mino, N., and Kuroda, M. (1984). The protein value in human nutrition of edible marine algae in Japan. *Hydrobiologia* **116–117** (1): 513–516.

Galland-Irmouli, A.V., Fleurence, J., Lamghari, R. et al. (1999). Nutritional value of proteins from edible seaweed *Palmaria palmata* (dulse). *The Journal of Nutritional Biochemistry* **10**: 353–359.

Ganesan, K., Suresh Kumar, K., Subba Rao, P.V. et al. (2014). Studies on chemical composition of three species of *Enteromorpha*. *Biomedicine & Preventive Nutrition* **4** (3): 365–369.

Garcia-Casal, M.N., Pereira, A.C., Leets, I. et al. (2007). High iron content and bioavailability in humans from four species of marine algae. *The Journal of Nutrition* **137**: 2691–2695.

Garcia-Casal, M.N., Ramirez, J., Leets, I. et al. (2009). Antioxidant capacity, polyphenol content and iron bioavailability from algae (*Ulva* sp., *Sargassum* sp., and *Porphyra* sp.,) in human subjects. *British Journal of Nutrition* **101**: 79–85.

Geider, R.J. and Osborne, B.A. (1992). *Algal Photosynthesis*. Dordrecht: Springer Science+Business Media.

Gerasimenko, N.I., Busarova, N.G., and Moiseenko, O.P. (2010). Seasonal changes in the content of lipids, fatty acids, and pigments in brown alga *Costaria costata*. *Russian Journal of Plant Physiology* **57** (2): 205–211.

Ghadiryanfara, M., Rosentraterb, A.K., Keyhanic, A., and Omidc, M. (2016). A review–macroalgae production, with potential applications in biofuels and bioenergy. *Renewable & Sustainable Energy Reviews* **54**: 473–481.

Gombos, Z., Wada, H., and Murata, N. (1994). The recovery of photosynthesis from low temperature photoinhibition is accelerated by the unsaturation of membrane lipids: a mechanism of chilling tolerance. *Proceedings of the National Academy of Sciences of the United States of America* **91**: 8787–8791.

Gorham, J. and Lewey, S.A. (1984). Seasonal changes in the chemical composition of *Sargassum muticum*. *Marine Biology* **80**: 103–107.

Guihéneuf, F., Gietl, A., and Stengel, D.B. (2018). Temporal and spatial variability of mycosporine-like amino acids and pigments in three edible red seaweeds from western Ireland. *Journal of Applied Phycology* **30**: 2573–2586.

Ha, S.J., Lee, Y., Kim, M.S. et al. (2015). Seasonal changes in mycosporine like amino acids production rate with respect to natural phytoplankton species. *Marine Drugs* **13**: 6740–6758.

van Hal Jaap, W., Huijgen, W.J.J., and López-Contreras, A.M. (2014). Opportunities and challenges for seaweed in the biobased economy. *Trends in Biotechnology* **32** (5): 231–233.

Harnedy, P. and FitzGerald, R.J. (2011). Review of bioactive protein, peptides and amino acids from macroalgae. *Journal of Phycology* **47**: 218–232.

Harun, R., Danquah, M.K., and Forde, G.M. (2010). Microalgal biomass as a fermentation feedstock for bioethanol production. *Journal of Chemical Technology and Biotechnology* **85**: 199–203.

Hemlata, A.E. and Fatma, T. (2009). Screening of cyanobacteria for phycobiliproteins and effect of different environmental stress on its yield. *Bulletin of Environmental Contamination and Toxicology* **83** (4): 509–515.

Henderson, R.J., Hegseth, E.N., and Park, M.T. (1998). Seasonal variation in lipid and fatty acid composition of ice algae from the Barents Sea. *Polar Biology* **20**: 48–55.

Hernandez-Carmona, G., Carrillo-Dominguez, S., Arvizu-Higuera, D.L. et al. (2009). Monthly variation in the chemical composition of *Eisenia arborea* JE Areschoug. *Journal of Appled Phycology* **21**: 607–616.

Holdt, S. and Kraan, S. (2011). Bioactive compounds in seaweed: functional food applications and legislation. *Journal of Applied Phycology* **23**: 543–597.

Honya, M.H., Mori, M., Anzai, M. et al. (1999). Monthly changes in the content of fucans, their constituent sugars and sulphate in cultured *Laminaria japonica*. *Hydrobiologia* **398/399**: 411–416.

Hori, K., Matsubara, K., and Miyazawa, K. (2000). Primary structures of two hemagglutinins from the marine red alga, *Hypnea japonica*. *Biochimica et Biophysica Acta* **1474** (2): 226–236.

Hou, X. and Yan, X. (1998). Study on the concentration and seasonal variation of inorganic elements in 35 species of marine algae. *Science of the Total Environment* **222** (3): 141–156.

Hoyle, M.D. (1978). Agar studies in two *Gracilaria* species (*G. bursapastoris* (Gmelin) Silva and *G. coronopifolia* J. Ag.) from Hawaii. H. Seasonal Aspects1 M. *Botanica Marina* **21**: 347–352.

Humm, H.J. (1951). The seaweed resources of North Carolina. In: *Survey of Marine Fisheries of North Carolina* (ed. H.F. Taylor), 231–250. Chapel Hill, NC: University of North Carolina Press.

Hung, L.D., Hori, K., Nang, H.Q. et al. (2009). Seasonal changes in growth rate, carrageenan yield and lectin content in the red alga *Kappaphycus alvarezii* cultivated in Camranh Bay, Vietnam. *Journal of Applied Phycology* **21** (3): 265–272.

Ibañez, E., Herrero, M., Mendiola, J.A., and Castro-Puyana, M. (2012). Extraction and characterization of bioactive compounds with health benefits from marine resources: macro and micro algae, cyanobacteria, and invertebrates. In: *Marine Bioactive Compounds: Sources, Characterization and Applications* (ed. M. Hayes), 55–98. Boston, MA: Springer.

Imamoglu, E., Dalay, M.C., and Sukan, F.V. (2009). Influences of different stress media and high light intensities on accumulation of astaxanthin in the green alga *Haematococcus pluvialis*. *New Biotechnology* **26**: 199–204.

Indergaard, M. and Knutsen, S.H. (1990). Seasonal differences in ash, carbon, fibre and nitrogen components of *Furcellaria lumbricalis* (Gigartinales, Rhodophyceae), Norway. *Botanica Marina* **33**: 327–334.

Institute-of-Medicine (2001). Iron. In: *Dietary Reference Intakes for Vitamin a, Vitamin K, Arsenic, Boron, Chromium, Copper, Iodine, Iron, Manganese, Molybdenum, Nickel, Silicon, Vanadium, and Zinc*. A Report of the Panel on Micronutrients, Subcommittees on Upper Reference Levels of Nutrients and of Interpretation and Uses of Dietary Reference Intakes, and the Standing Committee on the Scientific Evaluation of Dietary Reference Intakes, 290–378. Washington, DC: National Academy Press.

Irkin, L.C. and Erdugan, H. (2014). Investigation of seasonal variations in biochemical composition of *Polysiphonia morrowii* (Harvey) from different locations in the strait of Canakkale. *Marine Science and Technology Bulletin* **3** (1): 11–13.

Ismail, M.M. and Osman, M.E.H. (2016). Seasonal fluctuation of photosynthetic pigments of most common red seaweeds species collected from Abu Qir, Alexandria, Egypt. *Revista de Biología Marina y Oceanografía* **51** (3): 515–525.

Jensen, A. (1993). Present and future needs for algae and algal products. *Hydrobiologia* **261**: 15–23.

Jensen, A. and Haug, A. (1956). Geographical and seasonal variation in the chemical composition of *Laminaria hyperborea* and *Laminaria digitata* from the Norwegian Coast. Norsk Institutt for Tang- og Tareforskning, report 14. Oslo: Akademisk trykningssentral.

Jiménez-Escrig, A. and Sánchez-Muniz, F.J. (2000). Dietary fibre from edible seaweeds: chemical structure, physicochemical properties and effects on cholesterol metabolism. *Nutrition Research* **20**: 585–598.

John, D.M. and Asare, S.O. (1975). A preliminary study of the variations and properties of phycocolloids from Ghanaian seaweeds. *Marine Biology* **30**: 325–330.

Julius, M.L. (2018). Microalgae in health and disease prevention. In: *Carbohydrate Diversity in Microalgae: A Phylogenetically Arranged Presentation* (eds. I.A. Levine and J. Fleurence), 133–144. San Diego, CA: Academic Press.

Kaehler, S. and Kennish, R. (1996). Summer and winter comparisons in the nutritional value of marine macroalgae from Hong Kong. *Botanica Marina* **39**: 11–17.

Kaimoussi, A., Mouzdahir, A., and Saih, A. (2004). Variations saisonnières des teneurs en métaux (Cd, Cu, Fe, Mn et Zn) chez l'algue *Ulva lactuca* prélevée au niveau du littoral de la ville d'El Jadida (Maroc). *Comptes Rendus Biologies* **327** (4): 361–369.

Karsten, U.C., Wiencke, C., and Kirst, G.O. (1992). Dimethylsulphoniumpropionate (DMSP) accumulation in green macroalgae from polar to temperate re-gions: interactive effects of light versus salinity and light versus temperature. *Polar Biology* **12**: 603–607.

Kendel, M., Couzinet-Mossion, A., Viau, M. et al. (2012). Seasonal composition of lipids, fatty acids, and sterols in the edible red alga *Grateloupia turuturu*. *Journal of Applied Phycology* **25** (2): 425–432.

Kendel, M., Wielgosz-Collin, G., Bertrand, S. et al. (2015). Lipid composition, fatty acids and sterols in the seaweeds *Ulva armoricana*, and *Solieria chordalis* from Brittany (France): an analysis from nutritional, chemotaxonomic, and antiproliferative activity perspectives. *Marine Drugs* **13**: 5606–5628.

Khairy, H.M. and El-Shafay, S.M. (2013). Seasonal variations in the biochemical composition of some common seaweed species from the coast of Abu Qir Bay, Alexandria, Egypt. *Oceanologia* **55** (2): 435–452.

Khan, M.I., Lee, M.G., Shin, J.H., and Kim, J.D. (2017). Pretreatment optimization of the biomass of *Microcystis aeruginosa* for efficient bioethanol production. *AMB Express* **7**: 19. https://doi.org/10.1186/s13568-016-0320-y.

Khan, M.I., Shin, J.H., and Kim, J.D. (2018). The promising future of microalgae: current status, challenges, and optimization of a sustainable and renewable industry for biofuels, feed, and other products. *Microbial Cell Factories* **17**: 1–21.

Kılınç, B., Cirik, S., Turan, G. et al. (2013). Seaweeds for food and industrial applications. In: *Food Industry* (ed. I. Muzzalupo), 735–748. Croatia: InTech.

Kim, M.-K., Dubacq, J.-P., Thomas, J.-C., and Giraud, G. (1996). Seasonal variations of triacylglycerols and fatty acids in *Fucus serratus*. *Phytochemistry* **43**: 49–55.

Kim, Y.H., Kim, E.H., Lee, C. et al. (2007). Two new monogalactosyl diacylglycerols from brown alga *Sargassum thunbergii*. *Lipids* **42**: 395–399.

Koyande, A.K., Chew, K.W., Rambabu, K. et al. (2019). Microalgae: a potential alternative to health supplementation for humans. *Food Science and Human Wellness* **8** (1): 16–24.

Kraan, S. (2012). Algal polysaccharides, novel applications and outlook. In: *Carbohydrates – Comprehensive Studies on Glycobiology and Glycotechnology* (ed. C.-F. Chang), 489–532. Croatia: InTech.

Kumar, V. (1993). Biochemical constituents of marine algae from Tuticorin coast. *Indian Journal of Marine Science* **22**: 138–140.

Kumar, V.V. and Kaladharan, P. (2007). Amino acids in the seaweeds as an alternate source of protein for animal feed. *Journal of the Marine Biological Association of India* **49** (1): 35–40.

Kumar, C.S., Ganesan, P., and Bhaskar, N. (2008). In vitro antioxidant activities of three selected brown seaweeds of India. *Food Chemistry* **107** (2): 707–713.

Kumar, K.S., Ganesan, K., and Rao, P.S. (2015). Seasonal variation in nutritional composition of *Kappaphycus alvarezii* (Doty) Doty – an edible seaweed. *Journal of Food Science and Technology* **52**: 2751–2760.

Kumari, P., Kumar, M., Gupta, V. et al. (2010). Tropical marine macroalgae as potential sources of nutritionally important PUFAs. *Food Chemistry* **120**: 749–757.

Kumari, P., Kumar, M., Reddy, C.R.K., and Jha, B. (2013). Algal lipids, fatty acids and sterols. In: *Functional Ingredients from Algae for Foods and Nutraceuticals* (ed. H. Dominguez), 87–134. Cambridge: Woodhead Publishing.

Lahaye, M. (1991). Marine algae as sources of fibres: determination of soluble and insoluble dietary fibre contents in some "sea vegetables". *Journal of the Science of Food and Agriculture* **54** (4): 587–594.

Lahaye, M. and Yaphe, W. (1988). Effects of seasons on the chemical structure and gel strength of *Gracilaria* pseudoverrucosa agar (*Gracilariaceae*, rhodophyta). *Carbohydrate Polymers* **8** (4): 285–301.

Lares, M.L., Flores-Munŏz, G., and Lara-Lara, R. (2002). Temporal variability of bioavailable Cd, Hg, Zn, Mn and Al in an upwelling regime. *Environmental Pollution* **120**: 595–608.

Liu, X., Bogaert, K., Engelen, A.H. et al. (2017). Seaweed reproductive biology: environmental and genetic controls. *Botanica Marina* **60**: 89–108.

López-Figueroa, F. (1992). Diurnal variations in pigment contents in *Porphyra laciniata* and in *Chondrus crispus* and its relation to the diurnal changes of underwater light quality and quantity. *Marine Ecology* **13**: 285–305.

Lordan, S., Ross, R.P., and Stanton, C. (2011). Marine bioactives as functional food ingredients: potential to reduce the incidence of chronic diseases. *Marine Drugs* **9** (6): 1056–1100. https://doi.org/10.3390/md9061056.

Lorenzo, J.M., Agregán, R., Munekata, P.E. et al. (2017). Proximate composition and nutritional value of three macroalgae: *Ascophyllum nodosum, Fucus vesiculosus* and *Bifurcaria bifurcata. Marine Drugs* **15** (360): 1–11.

Lüning, K., Yarish, C., and Kirkman, H. (1990). *Seaweeds – Their Environment, Biogeography and Ecophysiology*. New York: Wiley.

Lynch, D.V. and Thompson, G.A. (1982). Low temperature-induced alterations in the chloroplast and microsomal-membranes of *Dunaliella salina. Plant Physiology* **69**: 1369–1375.

Lyons, D.A., Van Alstyne, K.L., and Scheibling, R.E. (2007). Anti-grazing activity and seasonal variation of dimethylsulfoniopropionate-associated compounds in the invasive alga *Codium fragile* ssp. Tomentosoides. *Marine Biology* **153**: 179–188.

Mabeau, S. and Fleurence, J. (1993). Seaweed in food products: biochemical and nutritional aspects. *Trends in Food Science and Technology* **4**: 103–107.

MacArtain, P., Gill, C.I.R., Brooks, M. et al. (2007). Nutritional value of edible seaweeds. *Nutrition Reviews* **65**: 535–543.

Madhyastha, H.K. and Vatsala, T.M. (2007). Pigment production in *Spirulina fussiformis* in different photophysical conditions. *Biomolecular Engineering* **24**: 301–305.

Manns, D., Deutschle, A.L., Saake, B., and Meyer, A.S. (2014). Methodology for quantitative determination of the carbohydrate composition of brown seaweeds (*Laminaria*ceae). *RSC Advances* **4**: 25736–25746.

Marinho-Soriano, E., Fonseca, P.C., Carneiro, M.A.A., and Moreira, W.S.C. (2006). Seasonal variation in the chemical composition of two tropical seaweeds. *Bioresource Technology* **97** (18): 2402–2406.

Markou, G., Angelidaki, I., and Georgakakis, D. (2012). Microalgal carbohydrates: an overview of the factors influencing carbohydrates production, and of main bioconversion technologies for production of biofuels. *Applied Microbiology and Biotechnology* **96**: 631–645.

McDermid, K.J., Stuercke, B., and Haleakala, O.J. (2005). Total dietary fiber content in Hawaiian marine algae. *Botanica Marina* **48**: 437–440.

Mercer, J.P., Mai, K.S., and Donlon, J. (1993). Comparative studies on the nutrition of two species of abalone, *Haliotis tuberculata coccinea* Linneaeus and *Haliotis discus hannai* Ino: 1 Effects of algal diets on growth and biochemical composition. *Invertebrate Reproduction & Development* **23**: 75–88.

Miramand, E. and Bentley, D. (1992). Heavy metal concentrations in two biological indicators (*Patella vulgata* and *Fucus* serratus) collected near the French nuclear fuel reprocessing plant of La Hague. *Science of the Total Environment* **111**: 135–149.

Mišurcová, L., Kračmar, S., Klejdus, B., and Vacek, J. (2010). Nitrogen content, dietary fiber, and digestibility in algal food products. *Czech Journal of Food Sciences* **28**: 27–35.

Mišurcová, L., Machů, L., and Orsavová, J. (2011). Seaweed minerals as nutraceuticals. In: *Advances in Food and Nutrition Research*, vol. **64** (ed. S.-K. Kim), 371–390. Burlington, VA: Academic Press.

Miyashita, K., Mikami, N., and Hosokawa, M. (2013). Chemical and nutritional characteristics of brown seaweed lipids: a review. *Journal of Functional Foods* **5** (4): 1507–1517.

Mohsen, A.F., Kharboush, A.M., Khaleafa, A.F. et al. (1975). Amino acid pattern and seasonal variation in some marine algae from Alexandria. *Botanica Marina* **18**: 167–178.

Molino, A., Iovine, A., Casella, P. et al. (2018). Microalgae characterization for consolidated and new application in human food, animal feed and nutraceuticals. *International Journal of Environmental Research and Public Health* **15**: 2436.

Mooney, B.D., Nicholas, P.D., De Salas, M.F., and Halleggraeff, G.M. (2007). Lipid, fatty acid, and sterol composition of eight species of Kareniaceae (Dinophyta): chemotaxonomy and putative lipid phycotoxins. *Journal of Phycology* **43**: 101–111.

Murakami, K., Yamaguchi, Y., Sugawa-Katayama, Y., and Katayama, M. (2016). Effect of water depth on seasonal variation in the chemical composition of Akamoku, *Sargassum horneri* (turner) C. Agardh. *Natural Resources* **7**: 147–156. http://dx.doi.org/10.4236/nr.2016.74015.

National Taiwan Museum (2006). Introduction. http://formosa.ntm.gov.tw/seaweeds/english/d/d1_01.asp (accessed July 11, 2019).

Neish, A.C., Shacklock, P.F., Fox, C.H., and Simpson, F.J. (1977). The cultivation of *Chondrus crispus*. Factors affecting growth under greenhouse conditions. *Canadian Journal of Botany* **55**: 2263–2271.

Nichols, P.D., Virtue, P., Mooney, B.D. et al. (1998). *Seafood the Good Food: The Oil (Fat) Content and Composition of Australian Commercial Fishes, Shellfishes and Crustaceans*. Hobart: CSIRO, 100 pp.

Nitschke, U. and Stengel, D.B. (2016). Quantification of iodine loss in edible Irish seaweeds during processing. *Journal of Applied Phycology* **28**: 3527–3533.

Ochiai, Y., Katsuragi, T., and Hashimoto, K. (1987). Proteins in three seaweeds: 'Aosa' *U. lactuca*, 'Arame' *Eisenia bicyclis*, and 'Makusa' *Gelidium amansii*. *Bulletin of the Japanese Society for the Science of Fish* **53** (6): 1051–1055.

Offei, F., Mensah, M., and Thygesen, A. (2018). Seaweed bioethanol production: a process selection review on hydrolysis and fermentation. *Fermentation* **4**: 1–18.

Olofsson, M., Lamela, T., Nilsson, E. et al. (2012). Seasonal variation of lipids and fatty acids of the microalgae *Nannochloropsis oculata* grown in outdoor large-scale photobioreactors. *Energies* **5**: 1577–1592.

Orr, M.L. and Watt, B.K. (1968). Amino acid content of foods. Home Economics Research Report No. 4. Washington, DC: ARS-USDA.

Ortiz, J., Uquiche, E., Robert, P. et al. (2009). Functional and nutritional value of the Chilean seaweeds *Codium fragile*, *Gracilaria chilensis* and *Macrocystis pyrifera*. *European Journal of Lipid Science and Technology* **111**: 320–327.

Osman, N.A., El-Manawy, I.M., and Amin, A.S. (2011). Nutritional composition and mineral content of five macroalgae from Red Sea. *Egyptian Journal of Phycology* **12** (1): 89–102.

Paerl, H. (1984). Cyanobacterial carotenoids: their roles in maintaining optimal photosynthetic production among aquatic bloom forming genera. *Oecologia* **61**: 143–149.

Paiva, L., Lima, E., Neto, A., and Baptista, J. (2018). Seasonal variability of the biochemical composition and antioxidant properties of *Fucus spiralis* at two Azorean Islands. *Marine Drugs* **16** (8): 248.

Panayotova, V. and Stancheva, M. (2013). Mineral composition of marine macroalgae from the Bulgarian Black Sea coast. *Scripta Scientifica Medica* **45** (6): 42–45.

Patarra, R.F., Paiva, L., Neto, A.I. et al. (2011). Nutritional value of selected macroalgae. *Journal of Applied Phycology* **23**: 205–208.

Pauli, G. (2010). Fibers from algae. https://www.theblueeconomy.org/uploads/7/1/4/9/71490689/case_77_fibers_from_algae.pdf (accessed July 10, 2019).

Pereira, L. (2011). A review of the nutrient composition of selected edible seaweeds. In: *Seaweed* (ed. V.H. Pomin), 15–47. Hauppauge, NY: Nova Science Publishers, Inc.

Perez, A.A., Farias, S.S., Strobl, A.M. et al. (2007). Levels of essential and toxic elements in *Porphyra columbina* and *Ulva* sp from San Jorge Gulf, Patagonia Argentina. *Science of the Total Environment* **376**: 51–59.

Phleger, C.F. (1991). Biochemical aspects of buoyancy in fishes. In: *Biochemistry and Molecular Biology of Fishes*, Phylogenetic and Biochemical Perspectives, vol. **I** (eds. P.W. Hochachka and T.P. Mommsen), 209–247. Amsterdam: Elsevier.

Pierre, G., Zhao, J.M., Orvain, F. et al. (2014). Seasonal dynamics of extracellular polymeric substances (EPS) in surface sediments of a diatom-dominated intertidal mudflat (Marennes–Oléron, France). *Journal of Sea Research* **92**: 26–35.

Pisal, D.S. and Lele, S.S. (2005). Carotenoid production from microalgae, *Dunaliella salina*. *Indian Journal of Biotechnology* **4**: 476–483.

Plaza, M., Cifuentes, A., and Ibanez, E. (2008). In the search of new functional food ingredients from algae. *Trends in Food Science & Technology* **19**: 31–39.

Prasanna, R. and Kaushik, B.D. (2010). Evolutionary relationships among cyanobacteria, algae and plants: revisited in the light of Darwinism. In: *Nature at Work-Ongoing Saga of Evolution* (ed. V.P. Sharma), 119–140. New Delhi: The National Academy of Sciences, Springer.

Prasanna, R.A., Sood, A., Suresh, S. et al. (2007). Potentials and applications of algal pigments in biology and industry. *Acta Botanica Hungarica* **49**: 131–156.

Ragan, M.A. and Glombitza, K.W. (1986). Phlorotannins, brown algal polyphenols. *Progress in Phycological Research* **4**: 129–241.

Ragan, M.A. and Jensen, A. (1978). Quantitative studies on brown algal phenols. II. Seasonal variation in polyphenol content of *Ascophyllum nodosum* (L.) Le Jol. and *Fucus vesiculosus* (L.). *Journal of Experimental Marine Biology and Ecology* **34**: 245–258.

Rao, U.M. (1969). Agar and algin-yielding seaweeds of India! In: *Proceedings of the International Seaweed Symposium*, vol. **6**, 715–721.

Ras, M., Steyer, J.P., and Bernard, O. (2013). Temperature effect on microalgae: a crucial factor for outdoor production. *Reviews in Environmental Science and Bio/Technology* **12**: 153–164.

Ratana-arporn, P. and Chirapart, A. (2006). Nutritional evaluation of tropical green seaweeds *Caulerpa lentillifera* and *Ulva reticulata*. *Kasetsart Journal (Natural Science)* **40S**: 75–83.

Renaud, M.S. and Luong-Van, T.J. (2006). Sesonal variation in the chemical composition of tropical Australian marine macroalgae. *Journal of Applied Phycology* **18**: 381–387.

Ricketts, T.R. (1966). On the chemical composition of some unicellular algae. *Phytochemistry* **5**: 67–76. 120.

Rico, J.M. and Fernandez, C. (1996). Seasonal nitrogen metabolism in an intertidal population of *Gelidium latifolium* (Gelidiaceae). *European Journal of Phycology* **31**: 149–155.

Riget, F., Johansen, P., and Asmund, G. (1995). Natural seasonal variation of cadmium, copper, lead and zinc in brown seaweed (*Fucus vesiculosus*). *Marine Pollution Bulletin* **30** (6): 409–413.

Riosmena-Rodríguez, R., Talavera-Sáenz, A., Acosta-Vargas, B., and Gardner, S.C. (2010). Heavy metals dynamics in seaweeds and seagrasses in Bahía Magdalena, B.C.S., México. *Journal of Applied Phycology* **22**: 283–291.

Robertson, D. (2019). Algal pigments (protocols). https://wordpress.clarku.edu/debrobertson/laboratory-protocols/algal-pigments (accessed July 10, 2019).

Rodde, R., Varum, K., Larsen, B., and Myklestad, S. (2004). Seasonal and geographical variation in the chemical composition of the red alga *Palmaria palmata* (L.) Kuntze. *Botanica Marina* **47**: 125–133.

Rodrigues, J.M. (2013). Avaliação do valor Nutricional e de Propriedades Antioxidantes das Macroalgas *Chaetomorpha* linum, *Ulva lactuca*, *Gracilaria vermiculophylla* e *Fucus vesiculosus*. Master's Thesis, Escola Superior Agrária, Instituto Politécnico de Coimbra, Coimbra, Portugal.

Rodriguez, H., Rivas, J., Guerrero, M.G., and Losada, M. (1991). Enhancement of phycobiliprotein production in nitrogen-fixing cyanobacteria. *Journal of Biotechnology* **20**: 263–270.

Rönnberg, O. and Ruokolahti, C. (1986). Seasonal variation of algal epiphytes and phenolic content of *Fucus vesiculosus* in a northern Baltic archipelago. *Annales Botanici Fennici* **23**: 317–323.

Roy, S.S. and Pal, R. (2014). Microalgae in aquaculture: a review with special references to nutritional value and fish dietetics. *Proceedings of the Zoological Society* **68**: 1–8.

Rupérez, P. and Saura-Calixto, F. (2001). Dietary fibre and physicochemical properties of edible Spanish seaweeds. *European Food Research and Technology* **212**: 349–354.

Samarakoon, K. and Jeon, Y.J. (2012). Bio-functionalities of proteins derived from marine algae–a review. *Food Research International* **48**: 948–960.

Sampaio, A.H., Rogers, D.J., Barwell, C.J., and Farnham, W.F. (1996). Seasonal variation in production of lectins by *Ulva lactuca*. *Lectins: Biology, Biochemistry, Clinical Biochemistry* **11**: 101–106.

Sampath-Wiley, P., Neefus, C.D., and Jahnke, L.S. (2008). Seasonal effects of sun exposure and emersion on intertidal seaweed physiology: fluctuations in antioxidant contents, photosynthetic pigments and photosynthetic efficiency in the red alga *Porphyra umbilicalis* Kützing (Rhodophyta, Bangiales). *Journal of Experimental Marine Biology and Ecology* **361** (2): 83–91.

Sanchez-Machado, D.I., Lopez-Cervantes, J., Lopez-Hernandez, J., and Paseiro-Losada, P. (2004). Fatty acids, total lipid, protein and ash contents of processed edible seaweeds. *Food Chemistry* **85**: 439–444.

Sarojini, Y. and Nittala, S.S. (1999). Vitamin C content of some macroalgae of Visakhapatnam, east coast of India. *Indian Journal of Marine Sciences* **28**: 408–412.

Sarojini, Y. and Sujata, B. (2015). The seasonal variations in distribution of photosynthetic pigments in two species of Phaeophyceae and the effect of light, dissolved oxygen and nutrients on their distribution. *Der Pharmacia Lettre* **7** (5): 140–145.

Sathasivam, R., Radhakrishnan, R., Hashem, A., and Abd-Allah, E.F. (2019). Microalgae metabolites: a rich source for food and medicine. *Saudi Journal of Biological Sciences* **26** (4): 709–722.

Schiener, P., Black, K.D., Stanley, M.S., and Green, D.H. (2015). The seasonal variation in the chemical composition of the kelp species *Laminaria digitata*, *Laminaria hyperborea*, *Saccharina latissima* and *Alaria esculenta*. *Journal of Applied Phycology* **27**: 363–373.

Schmid, M., Guihéneuf, F., and Stengel, D.B. (2014). Fatty acid contents and profiles of 16 macroalgae collected from the Irish Coast at two seasons. *Journal of Applied Phycology* **26**: 451–463.

Schmid, M., Guihéneuf, F., and Stengel, D.B. (2017). Ecological and commercial implications of temporal and spatial variability in the composition of pigments and fatty acids in five Irish macroalgae. *Marine Biology* **164**: 158.

Schreiber, U. (1979). Cold-induced uncoupling of energy transfer between phycobilins and chlorophyll in Anacytisnidulans. *FEBS Letters* **107** (1): 4–9.

Schulze, C., Strehle, A., Merdivan, S., and Mundt, S. (2017). Carbohydrates in microalgae: comparative determination by TLC, LC-MS without derivatization, and the photometric thymol-sulfuric acid method. *Algal Research* **25**: 372–380.

Sheath, R.G. and Wehr, J.D. (2015). Introduction to the freshwater. Algae. In: *Aquatic Ecology, Freshwater Algae of North America*, 2e (eds. J.D. Wehr, R.G. Sheath and J.P. Kociolek), 1–11. New York: Academic Press.

Singh, P., Singh, R., Jha, A. et al. (2015). Optimization of a process for high fibre and high protein biscuit. *Journal of Food Science and Technology* **52**: 1394–1403.

Sinha, R.P., Singh, S.P., and Häder, D.P. (2007). Database on mycosporines and mycosporine-like amino acids (MAAs) in fungi, cyanobacteria, macroalgae, phytoplankton and animals. *Journal of Photochemistry and Photobiology B* **89**: 29–35.

Skriptsova, A.V., Shevchenko, N.M., Zvyagintseva, T.N., and Imbs, T.I. (2010). Monthly changes in the content and monosaccharide composition of fucoidan from *Undaria pinnatifida* (*Laminaria*les, Phaeophyta). *Journal of Applied Phycology* **22**: 79–86.

Spolaore, P., Joannis-Cassan, C., Duran, E., and Isambert, A. (2006). Commercial applications of microalgae. *Journal of Bioscience and Bioengineering* **101** (2): 87–96.

Steinberg, P.D. and Van Altena, I. (1992). Tolerance of marine invertebrate herbivores to brown algal phlorotannins in temperate Australasia. *Ecological Monographs* **62**: 189–222.

Stengel, D.B. and Connan, S. (2015). Marine algae: a source of biomass for biotechnological applications. *Methods in Molecular Biology* **1308**: 1–37.

Stengel, D.B., Connan, S., and Popper, Z.A. (2011). Algal chemodiversity and bioactivity: sources of natural variability and implications for commercial application. *Biotechnology Advances* **29** (5): 483–501.

Sundaramurthy, A. and Shantaram, M. (2016). Biochemical composition of seaweeds and their anti–cancer properties against human papillomavirus (HPV) – a review. *International Journal of Pharmaceutical, Chemical, and Biological Sciences* **6**: 271–279.

Sushchik, N.N., Gladyshev, M.I., Ivanova, E.A., and Kravchuk, E.S. (2009). Seasonal distribution and fatty acid composition of littoral microalgae in the Yenisei River. *Journal of Applied Phycology* **22** (1): 11–24.

Suzuki, T., Nakai, K., Toshie, Y. et al. (1993). Seasonal variation in the dietary fiber content and molecular weight of soluble dietary fiber in brown algae, Hijiki. *Nippon Suisan Gakkaishi* **59**: 1633.

Takaichi, S. (2011). Carotenoids in algae: distributions, biosyntheses and functions. *Marine Drugs* **9** (1119): 1101–1118.

Turan, G. and Cırık, S.. (2018). Sea vegetables. https://www.intechopen.com/books/vegetables-importance-of-quality-vegetables-to-human-health/sea-vegetables (accessed September 2, 2020).

Uslu, L.H., Işık, O., Sayın, S. et al. (2009). The effect of temperature on protein and amino acid composition of *Spirulina platensis*. *E.U. Journal of Fisheries & Aquatic Sciences* **26**: 139–142.

Villares, R., Puentecarballeir, X., and Acarballeira, A. (2002). Seasonal variation and background levels of heavy metals in two green seaweeds. *Environmental Pollution* **119** (1): 79–90.

Villares, R., Fernández-Lema, E., and López-Mosquera, M.E. (2013). Seasonal variations in concentrations of macro- and micronutrients in three species of brown seaweed. *Botanica Marina* **56** (1): 49–61.

Waghmare, A.G., Salve, M.K., LeBlanc, J.G., and Arya, S.S. (2016). Concentration and characterization of microalgae proteins from *Chlorella pyrenoidosa*. *Bioresources and Bioprocessing* **3**: 1–11.

Wang, W., Onnagawa, M., Yoshie, Y., and Suzuki, T. (2001). Binding of bile salts to soluble and insoluble dietary fibers of seaweeds. *Fisheries Science* **67** (6): 1169–1173.

Wang, B., Zarka, A., Trebst, A., and Boussiba, S. (2003). Astaxanthin accumulation in *Haematococcus pluvialis* (Chlorophyceae) as an active photoprotective process under high irradiance. *Journal of Phycology* **39**: 1116–1124.

Wang, S., Zhong, F.D., Zhang, Y.J. et al. (2004). Molecular characterization of a new lectin from the marine alga *Ulva pertusa*. *Acta Biochimica et Biophysica Sinica* **36**: 111–117.

Webb, K.L. and Chu, F.L.E. (1983). Phytoplankton as a food source for bivalve larvae. In: *Proceedings of the Second International Conference on Aquaculture Nutrition: Biochemical and Physiological Approaches to Shellfish Nutrition* (eds. G.D. Pruder, C. Langdon and D. Conklin), 272–291. Baton Rouge, LA: Louisiana State University.

Wells, M.L., Potin, P., Craigie, J.S. et al. (2017). Algae as nutritional and functional food sources: revisiting our understanding. *Journal of Applied Phycology* **29** (2): 949–982.

Whyte, J.N.C., Englar, J.R., Saunders, R.G., and Lindsay, J.C. (1981). Seasonal variations in the biomass, quantity and quality of agar, from the reproductive and vegetative stages of *Gracilaria* (*verrucosa* type). *Botanica Marina* **24**: 493–501.

Wong, K.H. and Cheung, P.C.K. (2000). Nutritional evaluation of some subtropical red and green seaweeds Part I – proximate composition, amino acid profiles and some physico-chemical properties. *Food Chemistry* **71**: 475–482.

Xu, S.Y., Huang, X., and Cheong, K.L. (2017). Recent advances in marine algae polysaccharides: isolation, structure, and activities. *Marine Drugs* **15** (12): 388.

Yenigil, M. (1993). Seasonal changes in the chemical and gelling characteristics of agar from *Gracilaria verrucosa* collected in Turkey. *Hydrobiologia* **260/261**: 627–631.

Young, E.G. and Langille, W.M. (1958). The occurrence of inorganic elements in marine algae of the Atlantic provinces of Canada. *Canadian Journal of Botany* **36** (3): 301–310.

Yucetepe, A., Saroglu, O., Bildik, F. et al. (2018). Optimisation of ultrasound-assisted extraction of protein from *Spirulina platensis* using RSM. *Czech Journal of Food Sciences* **36** (1): 98–108.

Zavodnik, N. (1973). Seasonal variations in rate of photosynthetic activity and chemical composition of the littoral seaweeds common to the north Adriatic. Part I. *Fucus virsoides* (Don) J. AG. *Botanica Marina* **16**: 155–165.

3
Advances in Drying and Milling Technologies for Algae

K.Y. Show[1], Y.G. Yan[1], and Duu-Jong Lee[2]
[1]*Puritek Research Institute, Puritek Co. Ltd., Nanjing, China*
[2]*Department of Chemical Engineering, National Taiwan University, Taipei, Taiwan*

3.1 Introduction

Algae are versatile crops and their cultivation has attracted extensive global interest in the past two decades or so. Other than biofuel, cultivated microalgae can be processed for bulk value-added commodities such as animal feeds, pharmaceuticals, cosmetics, nutraceuticals, and nutritional and health supplements (Mata et al. 2010; Barros et al. 2015). Production of algal products entails numerous levels of processing commencing with algal cultivation, harvesting, drying, cell disruption, oil extraction, and fractionation (Figure 3.1).

Conversion of algal biomass into biofuels and value-added products through gasification, pyrolysis, combustion, fermentation, and transesterification necessitates a further removal of water from dewatered algal slurry via drying (Bennion et al. 2015; Azizi et al. 2018). Upon harvesting and dewatering, algal slurry is dried for material preservation, convenience of storage, prolonged product shelf-life, cell disintegration, extraction, and other processing (Mujumdar and Law 2010; Guine et al. 2012). The algae must be completely dried, for instance, before press extraction of lipids, which could then be converted into biodiesel. In general, algae are regarded as dried with water content below 10% (Villagracia et al. 2016). Drying of algae is a complex process involving simultaneous heat and mass transfer with different rate processes. The drying rate is dictated by the water content and temperature of algal slurry, the humidity, and the speed of air in contact with the slurry.

A life cycle assessment (LCA) revealed that, besides harvesting, drying of algae contributed predominantly to the energy requirements and hence the total cost of biofuel production (Maity 2015). It has been reported that about 69% of the overall energy demand for biodiesel production was contributed by gas drying of algal slurry (Sander and Murthy 2010). Other studies indicated that the energy requirements for drying were more than that needed for dewatering (Singh and Gu 2010; Bennion et al. 2015; Hognon et al. 2015). In fact, it was found that drying of *Laminaria digitata* removed

Recent Advances in Micro- and Macroalgal Processing: Food and Health Perspectives, First Edition.
Edited by Gaurav Rajauria and Yvonne V. Yuan.

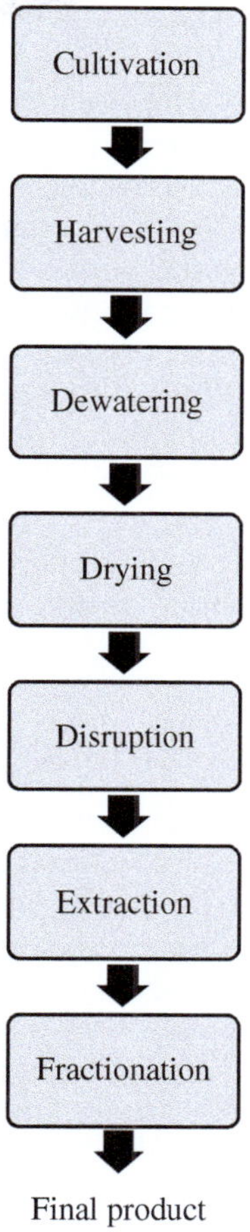

Figure 3.1 Schematic processes for algal products.

not only the free water but also the water trapped between particles and molecularly bound water (Adams et al. 2011). Drying appears to be the largest challenge for algae conversion into biofuel considering the high energy cost. Thus, viable production of algal biofuels calls for the development of an efficient drying technique.

Upon drying, the cells should be disrupted for extraction of intracellular substances. The main components of cell walls in algae are cellulose fibrils and crystalline polymers, which are sturdy in nature (Aarthy et al. 2018). The fibrillar and polymeric materials of cell walls have varying compositions, so different species of algae require different cell disruption methods to break them up. A wide range of disruption methods engaging mechanical and liquid shear forces, ultrasonication, thermal disintegration, electromagnetic radiation, and enzymatic hydrolysis have been developed (Al Hattab and Ghaly 2015). Selection of disruption method depends upon the algae species, cellular wall nature, and constitution. For instance, disrupting the cell wall of *Chlorella vulgaris* (which consists mainly of hemicellulose and saccharides) with liquid nitrogen exhibited improved disruption (Zheng et al. 2011).

A common approach to algal cell disruption is bead milling, which engages agitated beads in disrupting cell walls. The method has been frequently employed in the chemical manufacturing of minerals and paints/lacquers (Kula and Schütte 1987). It has been effectively used for disruption of yeast (Bunge et al. 1992), cyanobacteria (Balasundaram et al. 2012), and microalgae (Postma et al. 2015; Günerken et al. 2016), in extraction of intracellular compounds with low energy requirements and mild disintegration. The efficacy of cell disruption relies on numerous factors such as chamber size, agitator configuration and speed, algae concentration, slurry feed rate, bead material and size, and bead to cell ratio (Postma et al. 2017).

Drying and milling are two primary processes for effective production of value-added products from algae (Guldhe et al. 2014). This chapter focuses on recent advancements in algal cell drying and milling technologies along with a brief discussion of technology development, energy requirements, and comparisons of the processing methods. Challenges and prospects of algae drying and milling for sustainable and viable algal biorefineries are also outlined.

3.2 Algal Cell Drying Technologies

In selecting the drying technology, the key selection criterion depends on the scale of production and the intended algal product (Show et al. 2013, 2015). The main purpose of the selection is to achieve production with practical cost and simple operation. The selected drying method should also avoid deterioration of algal quality resulting from the drying process. Drying engages concurrent mass transfer and coupled heat (Diamante et al. 2010). Thus, heat and mass transfer characteristics of algae like water diffusivity, activation energy, and energy demand are important considerations for dryer design. Various algal drying options, from the simplest solar drying to the advanced refractance window drying as depicted in Figure 3.2, are delineated in the following sections.

3.2.1 Solar Drying

In distant areas where grid energy supply is deficient, natural drying methods such as solar drying emerge as the most practical method of drying. Algal drying by sunlight could be accomplished either through natural convection caused by direct solar radiation, or through solar water heating. While solar drying appears to be the most cost-effective and environmentally friendly, solar radiation is weather-dependent and hence unreliable. Uncontrollable sun radiation also causes erratic texture and color thereby affecting the final product quality.

Irregular heating can be evaded in a solar water heating system, in which solar thermal energy is derived by glass tubes used to heat up the water. Some proprietary solar water heating systems provide regulated and higher algal drying rates. In comparison with direct solar radiation, solar water heating is less feasible due to higher capital investment (Show et al. 2013).

Long-period solar drying of cyanobacterium *Microcystis aeruginosa* stretching over a year was investigated (Brink and Marx 2013). Assuming 300 effective drying days a year and a mean day-time temperature of 24.0 °C, an annual renewable energy of 9938 GJ ha^{-1} with an algal calorific value of 21 MJ kg^{-1} can be generated. Solar drying

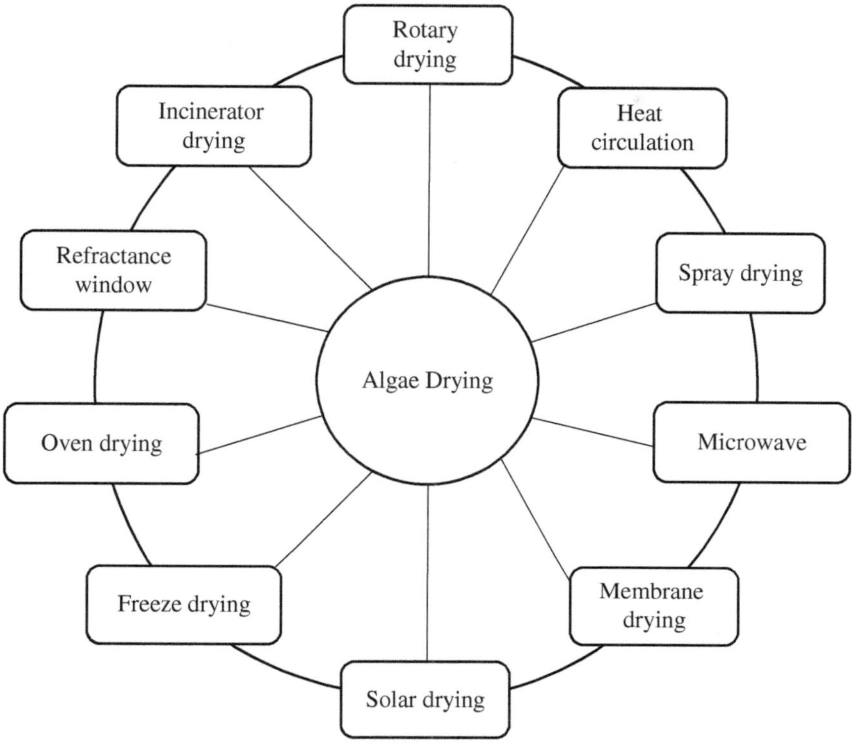

Figure 3.2 Process options for algae drying.

recorded the lowest energy consumption but required a longer drying time at 72 hours, in comparison with freeze drying (24 hours) and oven drying (12 hours) (Guldhe et al. 2014). However, more sophisticated equipment and energy were required for oven drying (6 kW) and freeze drying (22 kW). In another study, sun drying was reportedly the best drying option among the methods of drum drying, freeze drying, and spray drying (Tan et al. 2016).

Use of a solar dryer made of a wooden compartment with the top veiled by a glass panel and painted black internally for drying *Spirulina* algae was reported by Becker and Venkataraman (1982). Drying for about 5.5 hours at 60–65 °C, the solar dryer achieved an algal product of below 8% moisture content (Gupta et al. 2011). Similar to solar radiation drying, the solar dryer method appears to be low-tech, simple, and low-cost but is highly unreliable. A solar dryer made of concrete base, a wooden back wall, polycarbonate lateral and front walls, and a glass roof achieving 85% light transmittance and 0.8 $W\,m^{-1}\,°C^{-1}$ thermal conductivity transmittance was investigated (Poblete et al. 2018). A closed solar dryer unit was found to be more efficient than its open-air counterpart in terms of water evaporation rate (86.1% versus 67.6%). Hybrid solar dryers are devices that integrate solar energy with other energy sources like fossil fuel or biomass. Although the rates of drying are higher, their operation is costly particularly where fuel prices are high (El Hage et al. 2018).

In areas with scarce electricity supply, a greenhouse dryer constructed with glass or polycarbonate sheets may be suitable (Singh et al. 2018). It was found that a dome-structured greenhouse dryer was superior in harnessing solar radiation, while the effect of mixing by air in an even-roof greenhouse was better (Prakash and Kumar 2014). A productivity and economic assessment on combined production of algae and tomato in a greenhouse dryer was studied (Slager et al. 2014). It was deduced that the dry mass (DM) cost at €11 kg^{-1} algae DM of the combined production was lower than that of the individual production. The production cost at €70 kg^{-1}, however, was higher than the assumed price of €50 kg^{-1}.

A cabinet solar dryer was constructed of a large metal or wood box, in which shelves were installed between the walls. A heat storage system can also be installed within the box (El Hage et al. 2018). A hybrid solar tunnel dryer was designed and constructed using a photovoltaic (PV) system and a flat-plate solar energy collector (Eltawil et al. 2018). The PV system was installed to transfer hot air from the solar collector to the dryer via an insulated tube.

Heat pump technology using renewable energy for heat generation was recommended for reasons of economic viability and superior thermodynamic performance (Ommen et al. 2014). To enhance drying efficiency and reduce operational problems of heat pumps combined systems integrating heat pumps and solar energy utilizing direct and indirect solar irradiation can be adopted (Dott et al. 2012).

In summary, solar drying is more economical and suitable in places with consistent solar radiation throughout the year (Zhang et al. 2014). If land cost is taken into account, sun drying may not be viable as it entails use of a large land area. Solar drying is not recommended for algal products for human consumption, as algal biomass is open to contamination with dust, insects, and other contaminants. The low rates and uncontrolled drying generate repulsive odor and inferior texture of the final product. Solar drying, however, may be a feasible solution for production of algal animal feed.

3.2.2 Oven Drying

Oven drying is a common and easy-to-operate drying method for algae (Balasubramanian et al. 2011). Drying of *Scenedesmus obliquus* using an oven operated at different temperature settings was investigated (Abomohra et al. 2014). The content of extracted esterified fatty acids was correlated to the drying temperature, which increased by 6% and 12% when dried at 75 °C and 100 °C, respectively. The time taken for drying at 100 °C was reduced but the fatty acid composition remained consistent. Conversely, it was observed that operating conditions affected the algal chemical characteristics (Syed et al. 2016). The physical characteristics such as cell size, thickness, density, and strength, however, were dependent on drying methods.

Energy requirements for drying of microalgae in a laboratory-scale hot air oven dryer at 30–60 °C were investigated (Agbede et al. 2018). Drying rate and moisture diffusivity (4.13×10^{-10} to 1.18×10^{-9} m^2 $second^{-1}$) increased with the working temperature. It was concluded that elevated temperatures lead to higher moisture diffusivities, which boosts the diffusion controlled rate of drying in a hot air oven dryer. An activation energy of 30.6 kJ per mol algal mass was required based on an Arrhenius-type model. Total energy of 1.39–3.16 kWh and specific energy of 278–631 kWh per kg algal mass derived from the study are shown in Figure 3.3. The authors deduced that the energy requirements can be abated by drying at elevated temperatures. An increase in temperature leads to higher drying rate, thus shortening the drying time and thus lowering the energy requirement. Similar findings have also been documented in other studies (Aghbashlo et al. 2008; Tunde-Akintunde and Ogunlakin 2011; Motevali et al. 2011).

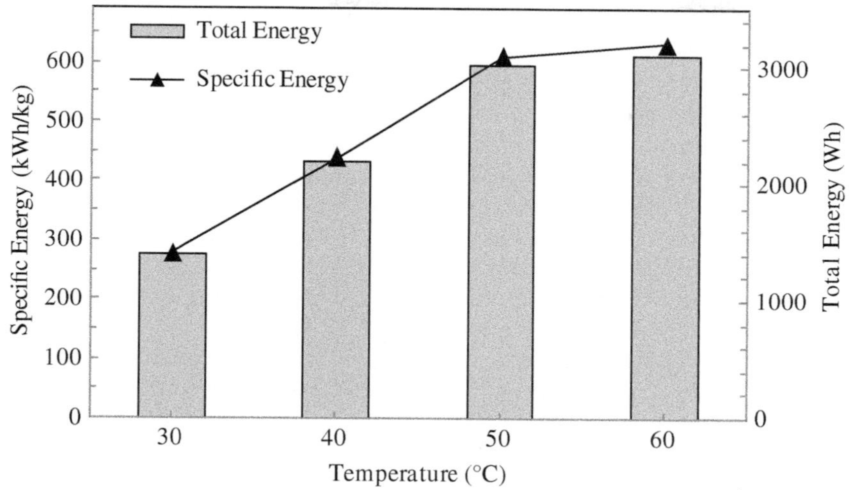

Figure 3.3 Total and specific energy demands by oven drying.

It appears that large-scale industrial applications of oven drying may not be feasible because of high energy demands. From an economic point of view, it may be more cost-effective to carry out oven drying with shorter heating times and higher temperatures.

3.2.3 Freeze Drying

In the freeze drying technique, wet algae is vacuum-frozen at −84 °C to crystallize the intracellular fluid (Guldhe et al. 2014). Subsequent to freezing, the ice crystals are subject to thawing, resulting in expansion of the cellular structure, which leads to cell lysis. Freeze drying enables easy lipid extraction from thawed and disintegrated algal biomass (Munir et al. 2013). Loss of lipids that are volatile upon heating is minimized (Pourmortazavi and Hajimirsadeghi 2007). Freeze drying can be incorporated into other disruption methods such as bead milling, microwave, or ultrasound to increase extraction yield (Prakash and Raja 2014). It has been reported that lipid extraction was enhanced by incorporating freeze drying prior to bead milling (Halim et al. 2013). The yield enhancement is due to increased specific cell area and lower diffusion gradient. A comparative study indicated that the differences in lipid yields of *Scenedesmus* sp. among freeze drying, sun drying, and oven drying were insignificant (Guldhe et al. 2014). While freeze drying process is effective in algal cell disintegration and recovery of high product quality, it is very costly in terms of energy input (Liapis and Roberto 2014).

3.2.4 Rotary Drum Drying

Rotary drum drying engages an inclined rotating vessel (also called a rotary dryer) to dry and move the algae from a feed inlet to the discharge outlet by gravity. With a drum surface area of 2.5 m^2, an algal suspension was dried in a rotary dryer to reach solids content of 25% (Mohn and Soeder 1978). Energy up to 15.7 Mcal was required for drying algal slurry with 4% water content, achieving water removal by 18.2 kg kg^{-1} dry algal mass (Soeder and Pabst 1975). Besides, an additional electric power input of 1.4 kWh was required to drive the dryer. Drying a slurry composed of 30% *Scenedesmus* sp. by weight at 120 °C for 10 seconds using a pilot-scale rotary drum consumed 52 kWh of energy (Becker and Venkataraman 1982). Replacing the electric drying with steam heating, the operating cost was markedly reduced by 6.8-fold. Up to 50 kg m^{-2} of water was evaporated in a steam heated rotary dryer working at a steam pressure of 0.8 MPa (Mohn and Soeder 1978). The energy expenditure can certainly be drastically reduced if waste steam can be used for heating.

Rotary drum drying of *Scenedesmus* sp. blended with terrestrial biomass such as ground pine, sorghum, corn stover, and dried algae was examined (Wahlen et al. 2017). Operating at an internal temperature of 50 °C, the experimental results showed that the drying rate of algae alone was markedly influenced by moisture and lignocellulosic contents. Blending other biomass at an optimal mix would increase the drying rate significantly. Blended algae may be applicable in situations such as if a certain rotary dryer throughput needs to be maintained when drying of algae alone is not feasible, for example, in low-demand season. Another advantage of blended algae is a lower drying cost. It was reported that drum drying exhibited superior digestibility, lower energy consumption, and smaller required investment than spray drying (Mohn and Soeder 1978; Show et al. 2015).

3.2.5 Incinerator Drying

An incinerator incorporating a cylindrical steel vessel containing multiple vertical hearths is often used for drying and firing wastewater sludge. The multiple-hearths incinerator can be improvised with lower heat inputs for use as an algae dryer. With a supply of hot gas, both the hot drying gas and wet algal slurry flow downward in parallel through the incinerator (Shelef et al. 1984). Such a parallel flow pattern is a technique frequently used in drying to avoid scorching or igniting a heat-sensitive material like algae. A fluidized bed incinerator is another sludge incinerator that could be improvised for algae drying. This incinerator uses a fluidized sand bed as a heat source to support uniform drying of algal biomass. Upon drying, dried algae can be separated from sand particles using a cyclone separator (Shelef et al. 1984). As the fluidized bed has to be preheated using auxiliary fuel before the algal slurry is fed, the energy demand and operating cost are high.

3.2.6 Spray Drying

Spray drying is a technique of generating a dry algal product from a suspension or slurry by rapid hot gas drying. A spray nozzle or atomizer is used to disperse the liquid/slurry into a controlled droplet-sized spray (Shelef et al. 1984). The atomized droplets are sprayed downward into a drying chamber through which hot drying gas flows downward. Drying is achieved rapidly in just a few seconds. The dried product in powder form is collected at the bottom of a cyclone, where the waste gas is exhausted through a vent on top.

Spray drying is an appropriate drying method for production of algae for human consumption and many other heat-sensitive and high-value nutritious products and pharmaceuticals (Soeder 1980). In spray drying of *Dunaliellasalina*, β-carotene-rich powder was retained in the dried product. For economical processing, the salt content in algae was reduced to below 2% by centrifugation without disintegrating the cells (Leach et al. 1998). It was cautioned that the heating temperature affected the structure of the algal polymer. As temperature rises during the drying process, pressure is built up causing the release of water vapor, which leads to a porous matrix. During storage, oxygen permeates into the porous matrix and degrades the product quality over time. To curtail product degradation, it was suggested that the algal dried powder be kept in capsules. Nevertheless, deterioration of some algae pigments was still reported (Desmorieux and Decaen 2005).

In spite of the fact that spray drying is very efficient, it could disrupt cellular cells from the pressurized atomization, and give rise to undesirable product degradation. Another drawback of spray drying is its high operating expenditure and poor digestibility of the dried product. In a comparative study involving algal spray drying and drum drying, the latter was recommended by virtue of enhanced digestibility, lower energy demands, and lower required investments (Mohn and Soeder 1978; Syed et al. 2016). An energy assessment of various drying methods found that spray drying required the highest energy input among the methods examined as depicted in Figure 3.4 (Xu et al. 2011; Bennion et al. 2015; Villagracia et al. 2016).

3.2.7 Heat Circulation Drying

Heat circulation drying is based upon the principles of exergy elevation and heat coupling for latent and sensible heat alike (Aziz et al. 2013). There is a major energy reduction of up to 90% when drying the brown seaweed *Laminaria japonica* using this method compared with the energy consumed in the conventional heat cascade drying technology. Interestingly, the temperature–enthalpy analysis revealed the hot air stream plot corresponded well with the cold air curve, indicating minimization of exergy losses.

Consequently, an integrated scheme incorporating a drying–gasification combined cycle embracing principles of exergy recovery and process integration was developed (Aziz et al. 2015). The heating elements of this system consisted of a preheater, main dryer, and super heater. A steam rotary tube dryer with an internal heat exchanger was used for drying. The rotary dryer was revolved at a regular speed to accomplish drying and conveying of the algae by gravity. Gasification was realized by a fluidized bed gasifier, which is well regarded with the merits of high algal mass processing, better heat transfer, and high efficiency. It was observed that the initial exergy elevation took place while purged steam was compressed, and this resulted in a high exergy rate of the hot air stream. Electrical and heat energy were combined in the process, which elevated the exergy rate of heat energy. Subsequent exergy elevation developed during the gasification when the steam was superheated by hot gas. Apparently, the elevation of the lower exergy rate was derived from coupling of different forms of energy. Approx. 40% of energy could be harvested from this system leading to high energy efficiency.

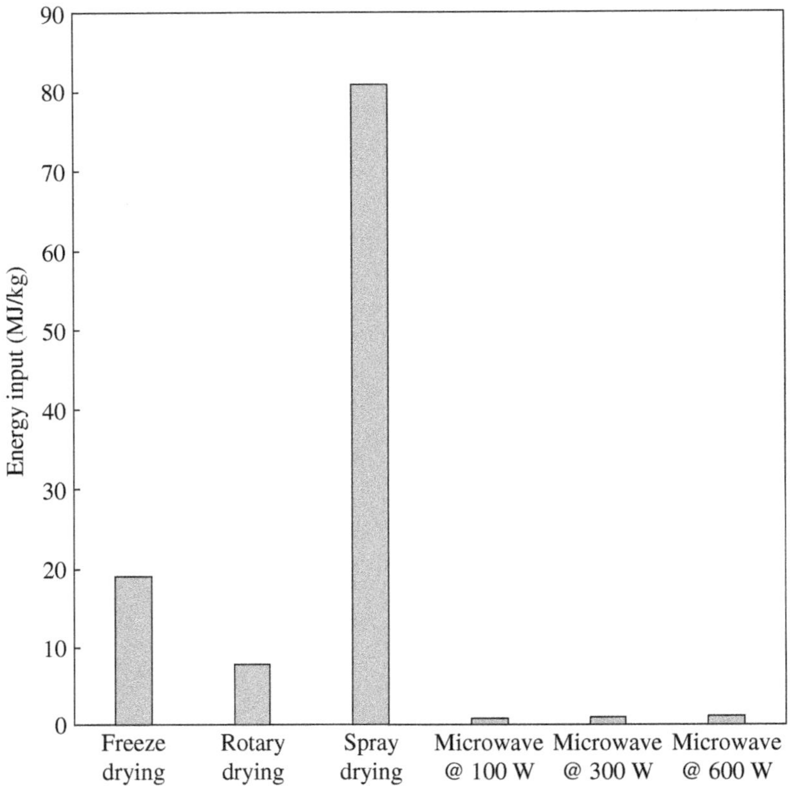

Figure 3.4 Specific energy demand of different algae drying methods. Source: adapted from (Xu et al. 2011; Bennion et al. 2015; Villagracia et al. 2016).

3.2.8 Microwave Drying

Microwave is a novel initiative for rapid drying of algae while keeping the cell matrix intact. Different microwave intensities (300, 600, and 900 W) at a fixed frequency of 2450 MHz were examined in drying *C. vulgaris* (Villagracia et al. 2016). The results demonstrated that lower specific energy demand corresponded to a specific microwave intensity of 20 W g^{-1}. The microwave drying also preserved the rich lipids content of the algae. As illustrated in Figure 3.4, microwave drying consumed the lowest energy (<1.03 MJ kg^{-1}) among the drying methods evaluated (Xu et al. 2011; Bennion et al. 2015; Villagracia et al. 2016). The microwave power tested (100, 300, and 600 W) did not indicate much difference in the energy demand. Spray drying, on the other hand, required exceptionally high energy (80.9 MJ kg^{-1}) among the drying methods examined.

3.2.9 Polypropylene Nonwoven Membrane Drying

Use of polypropylene nonwoven fabric membrane (PNFM) for dewatering and drying of *Scenedesmus* sp. and *Chlorella sorokiniana* was studied (Sahoo et al. 2017). Algal moisture content was lowered to 10.5 and 7.2% in 2 and 24 hours, respectively, upon drying on a PNFM propped with wire gauge stand and then on a sand bed. The calculated cost of pilot dewatering–drying was US$0.048 per kilogram of dry algal biomass. Dehydration using PNFM followed by natural drying was found to be energy-efficient and very cost-effective for pilot-scale harvesting (Sahoo et al. 2017). While drying by PNFM technique is novel, literature on this method is somewhat limited.

3.2.10 Refractance Window® Drying

Refractance Window® system is a proprietary drying technique employed for food products (Nindo and Tang 2007). The technique involves placing purées and liquids over a thin infrared translucent film that basically becomes a 'window' through which drying takes place (Raghavi et al. 2018). Other than the food industries, Refractance Window® drying has been used in numerous applications such as the cosmetic, nutraceutical, pharmaceutical, and pigment handling industries. Product temperatures are kept low and rapid drying transpires as all modes of heat transfer, namely conduction, convection, and radiation, are involved. For commercial production of algal products, this technique is used to dry high carotenoid-containing algae. Thermal energy is transmitted from hot water to the algal biomass spread thinly on a conveyor belt. The rapid drying process (3–5 minutes) converts the materials into powders, sheets, or flakes while retaining algal characteristics. Operating at atmospheric pressure, this patented drying system is considered inexpensive comparing with freeze drying.

3.3 Algal Cell Milling Technologies

A major barrier for applying algae on commercial scales is the high processing costs. One of the major costs of processing is associated with cell disruption for lipid extraction. Disruption of algal cellular wall facilitates the release of intracellular components for subsequent extraction, and enhancing lipid extraction from algal biomass could result in greater product yields and a cost-effective extraction. For this purpose, appropriate disruption technology for algal cells should be carefully selected and incorporated into the processing. Various cell disruption methods involving mechanical and liquid shear forces, ultrasound techniques, thermal treatment, electromagnetic radiation, and enzymatic hydrolysis have been reported (Al Hattab and Ghaly 2015). This section reviews the development and advancement in algal cell milling technologies.

3.3.1 Vortex-Bead Milling

In vortex-bead milling, fine beads and algal suspension are mixed and agitated in the vessels (Lee et al. 2017). The high-speed spinning beads produce sudden compression and vigorous shear forces leading to efficient rupture of the algal cell walls (Munir et al. 2013; Günerken et al. 2015). The rapid rotating agitator produces heat arising from the mechanical work; hence the vortex-bead mill is usually installed with cooling jackets for milling heat-sensitive cells. This milling method accomplishes simultaneous agitation–collision–grinding of the algal cells, resulting in efficient cell disruption (Lee et al. 2012).

It has been reported that 17.5% of microalgae *Chlorococcum* sp. cells were disrupted (Halim et al. 2012), 20.5% oil recovery from *Chlorella protothecoides* (Shen et al. 2009), 33% oil extraction from *Nannochloropsis* sp. (Gouveia et al. 2012), and 100% increase in lipid yield from *Scenedesmus* sp. disruption (Baldev et al. 2014) using vortex-bead milling. Oil yields ranging from 7.9 to 8.1 g l^{-1} from *Botryococcus* sp., *C. vulgaris*, and *Scenedesmus* sp. had been achieved (Lee et al. 2010). With a laboratory-scale vortex-bead mill made of glass tube, 50 mg of *Thraustochytrid* cells was suspended in a vessel filled with 3 ml of extraction organic solvent and 1 ml of zirconia beads (diameter 0.4–0.6 mm). The mixture was agitated using a vortex in 30-second bursts for 20 minutes, and 22.8% lipid was extracted from the algal cells (Avinesh et al. 2015).

Over 97% of the cells were disrupted in all the experiments conducted by Postma et al. (2015). The water-soluble proteins could be released with an 85% lower energy requirement than for cell disruption, giving rise to specific energy demands well below 2.5 kWh for every kilogram of dry algal mass. The extracellular wall fragility of *Nannochloropsis oculata* was measured through a high-pressure vortex-bead mill (Taleb et al. 2016). As much as 98% cell disruption was accomplished at a pressure of 175 MPa for triacylglycerol extraction in wet slurry.

The efficiency of cell disruption is dictated by the toughness of the cellular walls, collision between the beads and the cells, and the size, shape, and amount of the beads (Doucha and Livansky 2008; Greenwell et al. 2010). Work on disintegration of *C. vulgaris, Neochloris oleoabundans, and Tetraselmis suecica* in a laboratory-scale bead mill was carried out using different bead sizes (0.3–1 mm). The experiments showed that liberation rates of intracellular protein and carbohydrates were faster with the lowest energy requirement for finer beads (Postma et al. 2015). Finer beads produced higher kinetic rates, with the lowest specific energy demand of 60.47 kWh per kg of dried cells for 0.3 mm beads (Postma et al. 2017). Further analysis by the same authors (Postma et al. 2017) indicated that optimal cell disruption and energy needs for all algal strains tested occurred in the 0.3–0.4 mm bead size range. In other separate studies, the optimal bead diameter for effective cellular wall rupture was 0.3–0.5 mm (Hopkins 1991; Doucha and Livansky 2008).

On the other hand, algal concentration, bead retention time, and agitator speed have been found to be most critical for cell disruption efficiency, processing time, and energy requirement (Doucha and Livansky 2008; Postma et al. 2015; Greenwell et al. 2010). Microalgae *C. vulgaris* cells were successfully disrupted at different dried algal concentrations in the range of 25–145 g kg^{-1} agitated at speeds varying between 6 and 12 m $second^{-1}$ (Postma et al. 2015). Bead milling is effective with energy use when algal cell concentrations of 100–200 g l^{-1} were disrupted (Northcote et al. 1958; Scott et al. 2010). At an agitator speed of 9–10 m $second^{-1}$, a distinct optimum cell disruption rate and soluble protein release was observed irrespective of the biomass content.

Disruption of cellular walls improved from 67 to 95% as the bead milling time extended from 30 to 90 minutes (Doucha and Livansky 2008). It was reported that bead milling for 500 seconds of *C. vulgaris* gave rise to 99% cell disruption (Postma et al. 2015). However, 90–95% of the cell disintegration occurred between 200 and 250 seconds. Conversely, it was reported that extending the disintegration up to the longest milling time of 40 minutes on *C. vulgaris* enhanced the cell wall disruption, leading to higher pigment and protein recoveries (Safi et al. 2015). In another work,

87% of *Scenedesmus quadricauda* cells were disintegrated in the first 5 minutes of milling (Hedenskog et al. 1969).

3.3.2 Shake-Bead Milling

Shake-bead milling is a type of bead milling for disruption of the extracellular walls through shaking the vessel containing the beads and algal culture (Kumar et al. 2015). Algal extracellular walls are disintegrated by grinding the cells on the surfaces of glass beads (Mercer and Armenta 2011). Beads are normally made of strong materials such as zirconia-silica, zirconium oxide, or titanium carbide (Hopkins 1991). Single or multiple vessels are mechanized to vibrate, causing the beads to collide and grind against the cells.

Lipid recovery of 11% from *C. vulgaris* using bead milling was reported (Zheng et al. 2011). The highest lipid recovery of 18.8% from *C. protothecoides* was achieved by shake-bead milling among the extraction methods tested (Shen et al. 2009). Higher rates of lipid recovery were noted from other studies on shake-bead mills. These include 28% recovery from *Botryococcus* sp. cells (Lee et al. 2010), 25–30% from *Chlorella* sp., *Nostoc* sp., and *Tolypothrix* sp. cells (Prabakaran and Ravindran 2011), 30.5% from Thraustochytrid strains (Avinesh et al. 2015), and 40% from *P. tricronutum* (Ryckebosch et al. 2011). In the study by Avinesh and his coworkers (2015), the Thraustochytrid cells were disrupted in a shake-bead mill based on a biomass/bead ratio of 3 : 1. Zirconia beads of sizes in the range of 0.4–0.6 mm were shaken at the maximum speed of 1060 cycle minutes^{-1} for duration of 5 minutes. Use of shake-bead milling, however, is limited to laboratory research. Compared with the vortex-bead mills method, shake-bead milling is relatively less effective in disrupting algal cell walls (Zheng et al. 2011; Kumar et al. 2015).

Cellular wall disintegration by shake-bead milling consumed a specific energy of 35–810 Wh kg^{-1} (Greenwell et al. 2010; Doucha and Livansky 2008; Postma et al. 2015) and 300–400 Wh kg^{-1} (Greenwell et al. 2010). This energy consumption disparity was due to the diverse microalgae species and operation parameters tested. Conversely, a lower energy range of 35–250 Wh kg^{-1} was reported in disintegrating *Chlorella* using an agitated bead mill (Doucha and Livansky 2008). Also using an agitated bead mill, disruption of microalgae *Botryococcus*, *Chlorella*, and *Scenedesmus* required an energy input of 140 Wh kg^{-1} (Lee et al. 2010). It appears from these studies that agitated shake-bead milling requires higher energy consumption than bead–bead milling.

Comparative energy consumptions, lipid yields, and processing times of laboratory-scale vortex-bead milling, shake milling, and liquid nitrogen grinding of Thraustochytrids are presented in Table 3.1 (Avinesh et al. 2015). Shake-bead milling resulted in the highest energy consumption of 690 MJ kg^{-1} DM corresponding to a lipid recovery of 30.5%. Vortex-bead milling consumed a modest amount of energy (48 MJ kg^{-1}) associated with the lowest lipid recovery (22.8%). The liquid nitrogen grinding extracted 44.6% of lipids, but the energy consumption was not determined because the physical grinding work cannot be quantified. No energy was consumed in the case of control sample without milling.

In summary, shake-bead milling appears to have a good potential for commercial applications due to its high disintegration efficiency in batch operations, simple scale-up, and low labor requirement (Jahanshahi et al. 2002). Vortex-bead milling is

Table 3.1 Comparison of energy consumptions, lipid yield, and processing time.

Milling method	Lipid yield (%)	Energy consumption MJ $kg_{Dry\ mass}^{-1}$	Processing time (minutes)
Control	22.04	0	0
Liquid nitrogen grinding	44.6	ND	2
Vortex-bead	22.8	48	20
Shake-mill	30.5	690	5

Source: Adapted from Avinesh et al. 2015.

generally more efficient in cell disruption. In a laboratory-scale set-up, the product could be readily extracted by pipetting once the beads settle to the vessel bottom by gravity after vortex-bead milling (Miranda et al. 2012). For large-scale applications, relatively high energy demand and elaborate product extraction of vortex-bead milling may hinder large-scale implementation. Another drawback is that upscaling the process requires an extensive cooling system to prevent overheating from the heat generated in order to prevent deterioration of the product quality (Kim et al. 2013).

3.3.3 High-Pressure Homogenization

High-pressure homogenization (HPH) is a fairly simple cell disruption method whereby the cell slurry is pumped under high pressure through a fine orifice producing an accelerated jet. The suspension is impinged on the stationary valve surface creating powerful mechanical forces such as hydraulic turbulence, shear stress, and cavitation, which give rise to effective cell rupture (Lee et al. 2017). Basically, cell disruption is caused by the release of large amounts of energy per unit suspension volume (Petrier et al. 1998).

Loading pressure applied at the valve is a major operating parameter in HPH cell disruption. Other key parameters dictating the disruption efficiency are associated with the suspension attributes, which include viscosity, size, and concentration of cells (Lee et al. 2012). Increasing the loading pressure raises the impact force deriving from cell collision within the valve seat. The cells spread across the valve seat surface upon collision, followed by further collision with the impact ring. Such immense impact brings about efficient cell disintegration and release of intracellular substances. It has been reported that high loading pressure along with the quantity of cycles directly affects the cell disruption (Günerken et al. 2015). The extent of cell disruption depends on the working pressure and the resilience of the cell walls (Greenwell et al. 2010).

A study found that loading pressures between 40 and 80 MPa largely effected cell disruption (Wang et al. 2015). The highest disintegration efficiency of 35.2% corresponded to the pressure increase from 40 to 60 MPa. Further increase in the pressure up to 70 MPa and then 80 MPa resulted in only marginal improvement in the disintegration (4.6 and 2.0%, respectively). The optimum loading pressure of the HPH was recommended as 60 MPa. Another study showed that effective disintegration of *Chlorococcum* was achieved at a working pressure of 85 MPa (Halim et al. 2011).

The requirement for high pressure in HPH disruption leads to a conflict between high energy demand and favorable energy efficiency. An algal biomass concentration of 20 g l^{-1} disrupted by a 4 kW HPH for 4 minutes pressurized at 80 MPa achieved a disruption efficiency of 83.07% with an energy input of 48 kJ per g of DM (Wang et al. 2015). This energy demand, however, was lower than those reported in other similar studies (Spiden et al. 2013; Halim et al. 2012). One possible explanation for the lower energy demand is that the high algal mass content (20 g l^{-1}) gave rise to lower energy input calculated on the basis of per gram of mass.

Just like other cell disruption methods, the lipid yield through HPH is dependent on the extraction method. Using petroleum ether as an extraction solvent, lipid yields from *N. oculata* of 8.2–16.2% were achieved under a Soxhlet extraction environment (Shene et al. 2016). A much higher yield of 34% was achieved from the combined petroleum ether and HPH disruption (230 MPa with six passes) relative to the Soxhlet method. An investigation using HPH for lipid recovery from *Chlorella saccharophila* found that at an optimal pressure of 80 MPa/ten passes, close to 90% of the lipid can be extracted using organic solvent tert-butanol (Mulchandani et al. 2015).

A study investigating the influence of alga biomass concentration on HPH disruption was carried out (Wang et al. 2015). It was reported that cell concentrations ranging from 4 to 20 g l^{-1} dry weight did not show significant impact on the disruption efficiency. Olmstead et al. (2013a) reported that HPH can be applied for microalgae with high slurry concentrations (20–25% w/w).

Comparisons of cell disruption by bead mill and high-pressure homogenizer and their effects on algae separation were examined (Agerkvist and Enfors 1990). Both disruption methods produced almost the same enzyme and protein yields, but produced disintegrated cells with different physical characteristics. The varying characteristics of the disrupted cells resulted in different impacts on subsequent separation. The separation through centrifugation was only marginally influenced by the extent of bead milling, but the increase in HPH disruption hampered the separation efficiency of centrifugation. Nonetheless, increase in disruption extent by bead milling and HPH alike shortened the filtration time. It was also found that cell concentration did not show any major influence on protein releases in the HPH, but increasing the algal concentration would diminish the separation efficiencies of the filtration and centrifugation alike. This finding corresponds well with those reported by Wang et al. (2015).

In summary, HPH confers various merits such as lower cooling expenditure, lower heat generation, simple upscaling, and low potential of thermal deterioration (Aarthy et al. 2018). Cell disintegration can be maximized as there is a variety of valve seat designs. This technique can be applied for algae with sturdy cell walls (Olmstead et al. 2013a), even for the most tough-walled algae such as *Nannochloropsis* (Spiden et al. 2013). In addition, it can be used for suspensions with high biomass concentrations, for example, pretreated concentrated pastes (Olmstead et al. 2013b). A study examining energy efficiency concluded that thermal pretreatments up to 123 °C resulted in effective disruption of *Chlorella* cells by HPH (Spiden et al. 2015). The thermal pretreatments also brought about solidification of the extracted cellular protoplasts.

While HPH offers many advantages and seems to be a feasible option for commercial applications judging from its high disruption efficiency and ease of upscale, it remains unfit for large-scale installations due to its high energy demand and relatively expensive equipment (Kim et al. 2013). System scale-up also reduces processing capability because of the elevated homogenizing pressure (Yap et al. 2014). Particular care needs to be taken to reduce the product deterioration that might result from the cavitation.

3.3.4 High-Speed Homogenization

High-speed homogenization comprises a stainless steel stator and a rotor assembly operating at high rotation per minute. A hydrodynamic cavitation is created in the suspension due to the vigorous mixing and formation of shear forces at the liquid–solid interphase (Aarthy et al. 2018). When the critical speed is attained by the impeller, cavitation is created, which reduces the ambient pressure to the point of vapor pressure of the fluid. This drives the fluid away from the impeller. The pressure balance is then reinstalled, which moves the fluid back to the impeller. The pressure reestablishment creates rarefaction (negative pressures) and compressions (positive pressures). It is these alternating cycles of compression and rarefaction that create the cavitation, a phenomenon describing the formation, growth, and collapse through implosion of microbubbles (Kuttruff 1991). At implosion of the bubbles, dramatic conditions exist in the gaseous phase: extreme temperatures (5000 K) and high pressures (50 MPa) (Neis 2000). The bubble implosions produce short-lived (micro-seconds) "hot spots" in the liquid, which release huge energy to drive a variety of chemical reactions (Clark and Nujjoo 2000; Chemat et al. 2011).

High-speed homogenization is a simple, efficient, and vigorous cell disruption method. The homogenization is able to handle suspensions with relatively dense cell concentrations (2–6% w/w) with short processing time, thus lowering the vessel footprint and the expenditure of downstream processing. Respective lipid yields of up to 38 and 76% from *Nannochloropsis* sp. using high-speed homogenization have been reported (Balasubramanian et al. 2013; Wang and Wang 2012).

3.3.5 Liquid Nitrogen Grinding

Liquid nitrogen grinding is not a common disruption technique for algal cell disruption. It remains confined to laboratory research, and literature reporting this technique is somewhat limited. In a laboratory-scale study, liquid nitrogen was added as a cryogenic agent in freezing Thraustochytrid cells in the grinding vessel (Avinesh et al. 2015). The mixture was left to thaw and then ground manually with a pestle. Lipid was extracted by organic solvents after grinding. About 44.6% of the lipids were extracted from the Thraustochytrids by the liquid nitrogen grinding. Further analysis of the research found that, in *Schizochytrium* sp. S31, the prominent fatty acid of the lipids extracted consisted of saturated (49–57%), monounsaturated (31–35%), and polyunsaturated fatty acids (2–18%), making it a potential feedstock for biodiesel production. Notably, saturated and monounsaturated fatty acids are key constituents for algal biodiesel because of their comparatively high oxidative consistency (Cao et al. 2014). In *Thraustochytrium* sp. AMCQS5-5, the highest percentage of polyunsaturated fatty acid (67%) was extracted among the extraction methods tested. In another study, grinding with liquid nitrogen promoted higher efficiencies of lipid recovery from *C. vulgaris* (Zheng et al. 2011).

3.4 Challenges and Prospects

Applications of algae for biofuel and value-added products are a hot-spot issue in terms of sustainability and environmental impact (Show et al. 2013, 2015; Vassilev and Vassileva 2016). There are no major restrictions to large-scale production other than the high capital investment and excessive energy consumption required for algae processing. Algae must be dried and milled in an economic way prior to extraction. For large-scale commercial or industrial applications, cost-effective production remains an important consideration (Chen et al. 2015). Challenges and prospects associated with practical production such as processing technology, product quality, energy requirement, and environmental impacts are discussed in the following sections.

3.4.1 Processing Technology

Several advanced drying and milling technologies developed from laboratory- or pilot-scale studies are hitherto to be proven viable in terms of upscaling feasibility, energy efficiency, costs, and product quality. For practical applications, technology innovations or modifications could be adopted. The implementation of a layered drying technique via hot air/heat circulation or insulation in a vessel may be viable for places where land space is restricted. Moreover, the heating system should be designed with a controllable device in order to achieve optimum drying leading to desirable yield and product quality in subsequent processing. In addition, the design can consider gravitational force for transporting or collecting the dried materials. This can lower the operating cost that would be required for an electrical and mechanical conveyor and collector. Most of the algae drying methods were developed from conventional dewatering of sewage sludge (Show et al. 2015). As sludge and algae differ greatly in their characteristics, innovative modifications or improvised designs on the dryers may be considered. A belt dryer, for instance, could be improved to further reduce its energy requirement. A conventional belt could efficiently dry up to 90% solids, but with a relatively high electricity input of 400 Wh and 13.8 MJ of heat for every kilogram of dry biomass processed (Lardon et al. 2009; Hassebrauck and Ermel 1996).

For multi-criteria technology evaluation, systematic methodology such as a fuzzy analytic hierarchy process approach can be used, for example, in comparing feasibilities of two drying methods (Tan et al. 2016). The effects of different bead mill operating parameters for grinding *Nannochloropsis* sp. were assessed (Fernando et al. 2016). MATLAB Artificial Neural Network was used as an optimization tool to ascertain the best process configuration for the pilot set-up. Based on input parameters like milling speed and duration, bead material and diameter, chamber diameter, loading percentage, and bead : algae ratio, the neural network approach was reportedly effective in optimizing and improving the configuration set-up.

3.4.2 Energy Requirement

Other than milling, drying poses a chief economic restraint in algae processing, which makes up a predominant share of the total cost (Mohn and Soeder 1978). Drying requires about 3.556 MJ of fuel energy for every kilogram of dry algae (Sander and

Murthy 2010). It was deduced that drying consumed up to 85% of the total energy demand in algae processing (Lardon et al. 2009). Extensive studies have been carried out to explore alternative energy sources for algae drying and milling (Aziz et al. 2013). A comprehensive drying and milling scheme may be improvised for optimum drying speed and disruption efficiency, as well as preservation of algal quality. Besides reducing the energy need, the scheme could also integrate features or devices for heat recycling, and alternative renewable energies such as solar panels or wind turbines to reduce the reliance on fossil fuels and carbon emissions. Industrial drying methods differ in capital expenditure and operational expenditure, particularly because of differing energy demands (Show et al. 2013, 2015). A good way of reducing the energy need and increasing the process efficiency is to incorporate pretreatments or nonmechanical drying methods into the system.

3.4.3 Product Quality

Algae are dried and ground subsequent to processing such as fermentation and transesterification. The processes of drying and milling have several drawbacks. These include high costs of operation and unacceptable product quality. Some of the drying and milling methods are restricted to lipid extraction and not appropriate for recovery of highly vaporized intracellular substances because of the vigorous conditions created during the processing. Elevated pressure, shear stress, or temperature can easily damage such substances (Lee et al. 2017). Prudent selection of drying and milling technology is necessary so as to achieve good quality end products. A work on thermal pretreatment, for instance, concluded that heating at a temperature of 90 °C caused greater damage of cellular walls of *Scenedesmus* sp. (González-Fernández et al. 2012). To sustain functionality of algal products along with high drying rate and disruption yields seems to be a major challenge.

3.4.4 Environmental Impacts

It remains uncertain if the production of biodiesel is environmentally sustainable. It is also unclear which conversion stages need further refinement and optimization. An LCA has been carried out to evaluate the energy balance and possible environmental impacts of the entire process chain (Lardon et al. 2009). Taking a cradle-to-grave approach, the holistic LCA examines the overall process cycle from algae cultivating to biodiesel combustion. The LCA verified the potential of algae as an energy supply and underscored the crucial obligation of reducing the energy and fertilizer requirements.

In another LCA study comparing algal biodiesel production with canola and diesel in terms of costs and emissions, it was deduced that a high rate of production is a crucial factor for viable algal biodiesel (Campbell et al. 2011). Conversely, the potential emissions from the overall algae process chain are expected to be offset by the emission mitigation resulting from enhanced production efficiency and carbon sequestration of algae (Williams and Laurens 2010). An algae scheme producing biodiesel, animal food, and succinic acid was found to be favorable to the environment (Gnansounou and Raman 2016). Thus it was hypothesized that the algae system per se would function as an alternative renewable regime to reduce environmental impacts.

3.4.5 Future Directions

To achieve high production efficiency and lower environmental risk alike, integration of chemical and biological methods could be considered. Microorganisms capable of removing moisture can be cultivated for algal drying purposes (Mazzuca et al. 2015). It has been established that certain extracellular polymeric substances secreted by microorganisms are capable of destabilizing the algae. It follows that a dehydration process with osmotic pressure could be carried out to enhance algae drying (Mazzuca et al. 2015).

3.5 Conclusion

The prospect of algal biomass as feedstock is progressively gaining recognition. Optimizing algae drying and milling would certainly help to lower the cost and render the production viable. At the current rate of development, it is hard to derive a conclusive recommendation for an optimal scheme or ground-breaking technological breakthrough. For realistic applications that are cost-effective and sustainable, the concerns of energy, cost, and environmental impact must be dealt with. As energy-efficient and cost-effective drying and milling are two critical challenges in the processing of algal biofuels, research efforts addressing these challenges have to be strengthened. To leapfrog technological advancement, research collaboration, knowledge sharing, and information dissemination between practitioners, engineers, researchers, and experts in the fields should be intensified.

References

Aarthy, A., Smita, K., Prachi, T., and Sangeetha, S. (2018). An insight on algal cell disruption for biodiesel production. *Asian Journal of Pharmaceutical and Clinical Research* **11** (2): 21–26.

Abomohra, A.E.F., Mostafa, E.S., and Hanelt, D. (2014). Pilot cultivation of the chlorophyte microalga *Scenedesmus obliquus* as a promising feedstock for biofuel. *Biomass and Bioenergy* **64**: 237–244. http://dx.doi.org/10.1016/j.biombioe.2014.03.049.

Adams, J.M.M., Ross, A.B., Anastasakis, K. et al. (2011). Seasonal variation in the chemical composition of the bioenergy feedstock *Laminaria digitata* for thermochemical conversion. *Bioresource Technology* **102** (1): 226–234. http://dx.doi.org/10.1016/j.biortech.2010.06.152.

Agbede, O.O., Babatunde, K.A., Osuolale, F.N., Ogunleye, O.O., Oke, E.O., and Hamed, J.O. (2018). microalgae drying characteristics and energy requirement. Nigerian Society of Chemical Engineers 48th Annual Conference, Abeokuta, Nigeria, November 8–10.

Agerkvist, I. and Enfors, S.O. (1990). Characterization of *E. coli* cell disintegrates from a bead mill and high pressure homogenizers. *Biotechnology and Bioengineering* **36** (11): 1083–1089.

Aghbashlo, M., Kianmehr, M.H., and Samimi-Akhijahani, H. (2008). Influence of drying conditions on the effective moisture diffusivity, energy of activation and energy consumption during the thin-layer drying of berberis fruit (Berberidaceae). *Energy Conversion and Management* **49** (10): 2865–2871.

Al Hattab, M.A. and Ghaly, A.E. (2015). Microalgae oil extraction pre-treatment methods: critical review and comparative analysis. *Journal of Fundamentals of Renewable Energy and Applications* **5** (4): 172. https://doi.org/10.4172/20904541.1000172.

Avinesh, R.B., Adarsha, G., Colin, J.B., and Munish, P. (2015). Comparison of cell disruption methods for improving lipid extraction from Thraustochytrid strains. *Marine Drugs* **13**: 5111–5127. https://doi.org/10.3390/md13085111.

Aziz, M., Takuya, O., and Takao, K. (2013). Enhanced high energy efficient steam drying of Flgae. *Applied Energy* **109**: 163–170. http://dx.doi.org/10.1016/j.apenergy.2013.04.004.

Aziz, M., Takuya, O., Takashi, M. et al. (2015). Enhanced energy utilization system of algae: integrated drying, gasification and combined cycle. *Energy Procedia* **75**: 906–911.

Azizi, K., Moravejia, M.K., and Najafabadi, H.A. (2018). A review on bio-fuel production from microalgal biomass by using pyrolysis method. *Renewable and Sustainable Energy Reviews* **83** (3): 3046–3059.

Balasubramanian, S., Allen, J.D., Kanitkar, A., and Boldor, D. (2011). Oil extraction from *Scenedesmus obliquus* using a continuous microwave system – design, optimization, and quality characterization. *Bioresource Technology* **102** (3): 3396–3403. http://dx.doi.org/10.1016/j.biortech.2010.09.119.

Balasubramanian, R.K., Doan, T.T., and Obbard, J.P. (2013). Factors affecting cellular lipid extraction from marine microalgae. *Chemical Engineering Journal* **215**: 929–936.

Balasundaram, B., Skill, S.C., and Llewellyn, C.A. (2012). A Low energy process for the recovery of bioproducts from cyanobacteria using a ball mill. *Biochemical Engineering Journal* **69**: 48–56.

Baldev, E., Mubarak, A.D., Dhivya, M. et al. (2014). Facile and novel strategy for methods of extraction of biofuel grade lipids from microalgae: an experimental report. *International Journal of Biotechnology for Wellness Industries* **3**: 121–127.

Barros, A.I., Gonçalves, A.L., Simões, M., and Pires, J.C.M. (2015). Harvesting techniques applied to microalgae: a review. *Renewable and Sustainable Energy Reviews* **41**: 1489–1500. http://dx.doi.org/10.1016/j.rser.2014.09.037.

Becker, E.W. and Venkataraman, L.V. (1982). Biotechnology and exploitation of algae – the Indian approach. Eschlorm: Agency for Technical Cooperation.

Bennion, E.P., Daniel, M.G., John, M. et al. (2015). Lifecycle assessment of microalgae to biofuel: comparison of thermochemical processing pathways. *Applied Energy* **154**: 1062–1071. http://dx.doi.org/10.1016/j.apenergy.2014.12.009.

Brink, J. and Marx, S. (2013). Harvesting of Hartbeespoort Dam micro-algal biomass through sand filtration and solar drying. *Fuel* **106**: 67–71. http://dx.doi.org/10.1016/j.fuel.2012.10.034.

Bunge, F., Pietzsch, M., Müller, R., and Syldatk, C. (1992). Mechanical disruption of *Arthrobacter* sp. DSM 3747 in stirred ball mills for the release of hydantoincleaving enzymes. *Chemical Engineering Science* **47**: 225–232.

Campbell, P.K., Beer, T., and Batten, D. (2011). Life cycle assessment of biodiesel production from microalgae in ponds. *Bioresource Technology* **102**: 50–56.

Cao, Y., Liu, W., Xu, X. et al. (2014). Production of free monounsaturated fatty acids by metabolically engineered *Escherichia coli*. *Biotechnology for Biofuels* **7** (1): 48–59. https://doi.org/10.1186/1754-6834-7-59.

Chemat, F., Zill-e-Huma, K., and M. K. (2011). Applications of ultrasound in food technology: processing, preservation and extraction. *Ultrasonics Sonochemistry* **18**: 813–835.

Chen, C.L., Chang, J.S., and Lee, D.J. (2015). Dewatering and drying methods for microalgae. *Drying Technology* **33** (4): 443–454. https://doi.org/10.1080/07373937.2014.997881.

Clark, P.B. and Nujjoo, I. (2000). Ultrasonic sludge pretreatment for enhanced sludge digestion. *Journal of the Chartered Institution of Water and Environment Management* **14** (1): 66–71.

Desmorieux, H. and Decaen, N. (2005). Convective drying of *Spirulina* in thin layer. *Journal of Food Engineering* **66** (4): 497–503. http://dx.doi.org/10.1016/j.jfoodeng.2004.04.021.

Diamante, L.M., Ihns, R., Savage, G.P., and Vanhanen, L. (2010). A new mathematical model for thin layer drying of fruits. *International Journal of Food Science and Technology* **45** (9): 1956–1962.

Dott, R., Genkinger, A., and Afjei, T. (2012). System evaluation of combined solar & heat pump systems. *Energy Procedia* **30**: 562–570. https://doi.org/10.1016/j.egypro.2012.11.066.

Doucha, J. and Livansky, K. (2008). Influence of processing parameters on disintegration of *Chlorella* cells in various types of homogenizers. *Applied Microbiology and Biotechnology* **81**: 431–440.

El Hage, H., Herez, A., Ramadan, M. et al. (2018). An investigation on solar drying: a review with economic and environmental assessment. *Energy* **157**: 815–829. https://doi.org/10.1016/j.energy.2018.05.197.

Eltawil, M.A., Mostafa, M.A., and Abdulrahman, O.A. (2018). Energy analysis of hybrid solar tunnel dryer with PV system and solar collector for drying mint (*Mentha Viridis*). *Journal of Cleaner Production* **181**: 352–364. https://doi.org/10.1016/j.jclepro.2018.01.229.

Fernando, A.H., Maglaya, A.B., and Ubando, A. T. (2016). Optimization of an algae ball mill grinder using artificial neural network. IEEE Region 10 Conference (TENCON), Singapore, November 22–25.

Gnansounou, E. and Raman, J.K. (2016). Life cycle assessment of algae biodiesel and its co-products. *Applied Energy* **161**: 300–308. http://dx.doi.org/10.1016/j.apenergy.2015.10.043.

González-Fernández, C.B., Sialve, N.B., and Steyer, J.P. (2012). Thermal Pretreatment to improve methane production of *Scenedesmus* biomass. *Biomass and Bioenergy* **40**: 105–111. http://dx.doi.org/10.1016/j.biombioe.2012.02.008.

Gouveia, L., Batista, P.A., Nobre, P.B., Marques, A.P., and Moura, P. (2012). Exploring *Scenedesmus obliquus* and *Nannochloropsis* sp. potential as a sustainable raw material for biofuels and high added value compounds. 1-CIAB 1st Congreso Iberoamericano Sobre Biorefinerias, October 24–26.

Greenwell, H.C., Laurens, L.M., Shields, R.J. et al. (2010). Placing microalgae on the biofuels priority list: a review of the technological challenges. *Journal of the Royal Society Interface* **7**: 703–726.

Guine, R.P.F., Francisca, H., and Barroca, M.J. (2012). Mass transfer coefficients for the drying of pumpkin (*Cucurbita moschata*) and dried product quality. *Food and Bioprocess Technology* **5** (1): 176–183.

Guldhe, A., Bhaskar, S., Ismail, R. et al. (2014). Efficacy of drying and cell disruption techniques on lipid recovery from microalgae for biodiesel production. *Fuel* **128**: 46–52. http://dx.doi.org/10.1016/j.fuel.2014.02.059.

Gunerken, E., D'Hondt, E., Eppink, M.H.M. et al. (2015). Cell disruption for microalgae biorefineries. *Biotechnology Advances* **33**: 243–260.

Günerken, E., D'Hondt, E., Eppink, M. et al. (2016). Influence of nitrogen depletion in the growth of *N. oleoabundans* on the release of cellular components after beadmilling. *Bioresource Technology* **214**: 89–95.

Gupta, S., Cox, S., and Abu-Ghannam, N. (2011). Effect of different drying temperatures on the moisture and phytochemical constituents of edible Irish brown seaweed. *LWT – Food Science and Technology* **44** (5): 1266–1272. http://dx.doi.org/10.1016/j.lwt.2010.12.022.

Halim, R., Gladman, B., Danquah, M.K., and Webley, P.A. (2011). Oil extraction from microalgae for biodiesel production. *Bioresource Technology* **102**: 178–185.

Halim, R., Harun, R., Danquah, M.K., and Webley, P.A. (2012). Microalgal cell disruption for biofuel development. *Applied Energy* **91** (1): 116–121.

Halim, R., Rupasinghe, T.W., Tull, D.L., and Webley, P.A. (2013). Mechanical cell disruption for lipid extraction from microalgal biomass. *Bioresource Technology* **140**: 53–63.

Hassebrauck, M. and Ermel, G. (1996). Two examples of thermal drying of sewage sludge. *Water Science and Technology* **33** (12): 235–242. http://dx.doi.org/10.1016/0273-1223(96)00478-7.

Hedenskog, G., Enebo, L., Vendlová, J., and Prokes, B. (1969). Investigation of some methods for increasing the digestibility in vitro of microalgae. *Biotechnology and Bioengineering* **11**: 37–51.

Hognon, C., Delrue, F., and Boissonnet, G. (2015). Energetic and economic evaluation of *Chlamydomonas reinhardtii* hydrothermal liquefaction and pyrolysis through thermochemical models. *Energy* **93** (1): 31–40.

Hopkins, T.R. (1991). Physical and chemical cell disruption for the recovery of intracellular protein. In: *Purification and Analysis of Recombinant Proteins* (eds. R. Seetharam and S. Sharma), 57–84. New York: Marcel Dekker.

Jahanshahi, M., Sun, Y., Santos, E. et al. (2002). Operational intensification by direct product sequestration from cell Disruptates: application of a Pellicular adsorbent in a mechanically integrated disruption-fluidised bed adsorption process. *Biotechnology and Bioengineering* **80**: 201–212.

Kim, J., Yoo, G., Hansol, L. et al. (2013). Methods of downstream processing for the production of biodiesel from microalgae. *Biotechnology Advances* **31**: 862–876.

Kula, M.R. and Schütte, H. (1987). Purification of proteins and the disruption of microbial cells. *Biotechnology Progress* **3**: 31–42.

Kumar, R.R., Rao, P.H., and Arumugam, M. (2015). Lipid extraction methods from microalgae: a comprehensive review. *Frontiers Energy Research* **2**: 1–9.

Kuttruff, H. (1991). *Ultrasonics Fundamentals and Applications*. London: Elsevier Science Publishers Ltd.

Lardon, L., Arnaud, H., Bruno, S. et al. (2009). Life-cycle assessment of biodiesel production from microalgae. *Environmental Science & Technology* **43** (17): 6475–6481. https://doi.org/10.1021/es900705j.

Leach, G., Oliveira, G., and Morais, R. (1998). Spray-drying of *Dunaliella salina* to produce a β-carotene rich powder. *Journal of Industrial Microbiology and Biotechnology* **20** (2): 82–85. http://dx.doi.org/10.1038/sj.jim.2900485.

Lee, A.K., Lewis, D.M., and Ashman, P.J. (2012). Disruption of microalgal cells for the extraction of lipids for biofuels: processes and specific energy requirements. *Biomass and Bioenergy* **46**: 89–101.

Lee, J.Y., Yoo, C., Jun, S.Y. et al. (2010). Comparison of several methods for effective lipid extraction from microalgae. *Bioresource Technology* **101**: S75–S77.

Lee, S.Y., Cho, J.M., Chang, Y.K., and Oh, Y.K. (2017). Cell disruption and lipid extraction for microalgal biorefineries: a review. *Bioresource Technology* **244**: 1317–1328. https://doi.org/10.1016/j.biortech.2017.06.038.

Liapis, A. and Roberto, B. (2014). Freeze drying. In: *Handbook of Industrial Drying*, 4e (ed. A.S. Mujumdar), 259–282. Boca Raton, FL: CRC Press.

Maity, S.K. (2015). Opportunities, recent trends and challenges of integrated biorefinery: part II. *Renewable and Sustainable Energy Reviews* **43**: 1446–1466.

Mata, T.M., Martins, A.A., and Caetano, N.S. (2010). Microalgae for biodiesel production and other applications: a review. *Renewable and Sustainable Energy Reviews* **14**: 217–232.

Mazzuca, S.T., Ibáñez González, M.J., Grima, E.M., and Chisti, Y. (2015). Forward osmosis with waste glycerol for concentrating microalgae slurries. *Algal Research* **8**: 168–173. http://dx.doi.org/10.1016/j.algal.2015.02.008.

Mercer, P. and Armenta, R.E. (2011). Developments in oil extraction from microalgae. *European Journal of Lipid Science and Technology* **113**: 539–547.

Miranda, J.R., Passarinho, P.C., and Gouveia, L. (2012). Bioethanol production from *Scenedesmus obliquus* sugars: the influence of Photobioreactors and culture conditions on biomass production. *Applied Microbiology and Biotechnology* **96**: 555–564.

Mohn, F.H. and Soeder, C.J. (1978). Improved technologies for the harvesting and processing of microalgae and their impact on production costs. *Archiv fur Hydrobiologie, Beihefte Ergebnisse der Limnologie* **1**: 228–253.

Motevali, A., Minaei, S., Khoshtaghaza, M.H., and Amirnejat, H. (2011). Comparison of energy consumption and specific energy requirements of different methods for drying mushroom slices. *Energy* **36** (11): 6433–6441.

Mujumdar, A.S. and Law, C.L. (2010). Drying technology: trends and applications in postharvest processing. *Food and Bioprocess Technology* **3** (6): 843–852.

Mulchandani, K., Kar, J.R., and Singhal, R.S. (2015). Extraction of lipids from *Chlorella saccharophila* using high-pressure homogenization followed by three phase partitioning. *Applied Biochemistry and Biotechnology* **176**: 1613–1626.

Munir, N., Sharif, N., Naz, S. et al. (2013). Harvesting and processing of microalgae biomass fractions for biodiesel production (a review). *Journal of Science, Technology and Development* **23**: 235–243.

Neis, U. (2000). Ultrasound in water, wastewater and sludge treatment. *Sewage Treatment* **21**: 36–39.

Nindo, C.I. and Tang, J. (2007). Refractance window dehydration technology: a novel contact drying method. *Drying Technology* **25** (1): 37–48. http://dx.doi.org/10.1080/07373930601152673.

Northcote, D.H., Goulding, K.J., and Horne, R.W. (1958). The chemical composition and structure of the cell wall of *Chlorella pyrenoidosa*. *The Biochemical Journal* **70**: 391–397.

Olmstead, I.L.D., Kentish, S.E., Scales, P.J., and Martin, G.J.O. (2013a). Low solvent, low temperature method for extracting biodiesel lipids from concentrated microalgal biomass. *Bioresource Technology* **148**: 615–619.

Olmstead, I.L.D., Hill, D.R., Dias, D.A. et al. (2013b). A quantitative analysis of microalgal lipids for optimization of biodiesel and omega-3 production. *Biotechnology and Bioengineering* **110**: 2096–2104.

Ommen, T., Markussen, W.B., and Elmegaard, B. (2014). Heat pumps in combined heat and power systems. *Energy* **76**: 989–1000. https://doi.org/10.1016/j.energy.2014.09.016.

Petrier, C., Jiang, Y., and Lamy, M.F. (1998). Ultrasound and environment: sonochemical destruction of chloroaromatic derivatives. *Environmental Science & Technology* **32**: 1316–1318.

Poblete, R., Cortes, E., Macchiavello, J., and Bakit, J. (2018). Factors influencing solar drying performance of the red algae *Gracilaria chilensis*. *Renewable Energy* **126**: 978–986. https://doi.org/10.1016/j.renene.2018.04.042.

Postma, P.R., Miron, T.L., Olivieri, G. et al. (2015). Mild disintegration of the green microalgae *Chlorella vulgaris* using bead milling. *Bioresource Technology Advances Biofuels Chemical Algae* **184**: 297–304. https://doi.org/10.1016/j.biortech.2014.09.033.

Postma, P.R., Suarez-Garcia, E., Safi, C. et al. (2017). Energy efficient bead milling of microalgae: effect of bead size on disintegration and release of proteins and carbohydrates. *Bioresource Technology* **224**: 670–679.

Pourmortazavi, S.M. and Hajimirsadeghi, S.S. (2007). Supercritical fluid extraction in plant essential and volatile oil analysis. *Journal of Chromatography. A* **1163**: 2–4.

Prabakaran, P. and Ravindran, R.D. (2011). A comparative study on effective cell distruption methods for lipid extraction from microalgae. *Letters in Applied Microbiology* **53**: 150–154.

Prakash, O. and Kumar, A. (2014). Solar greenhouse drying: a review. *Renewable and Sustainable Energy Reviews* **29**: 905–910. https://doi.org/10.1016/j.rser.2013.08.084.

Prakash, P. and Raja, S.N. (2014). Evaluation of protein release rate from mycoprotein – *Fusarium venenatum* by cell disruption method. *International Journal of Pharmacy and Pharmaceutical Sciences* **6**: 491–493.

Raghavi, L.M., Moses, J.A., and Anandharamakrishnan, C. (2018). Refractance window drying of foods: a review. *Journal of Food Engineering* **222**: 267–275.

Ryckebosch, E., Myuylaert, K., and Foubert, I. (2011). Optimization of an analytical procedure for extraction of lipids from microalgae. *Journal of the American Oil Chemists' Society* **89**: 189–198.

Safi, C., Frances, C., Ursu, A.V. et al. (2015). Understanding the effect of cell disruption methods on the diffusion of *Chlorella vulgaris* proteins and pigments in the aqueous phase. *Algal Research* **8**: 61–68.

Sahoo, N.K., Sanjay, K.G., Ismail, R. et al. (2017). Sustainable dewatering and drying of self-flocculating microalgae and study of cake properties. *Journal of Cleaner Production* **159**: 248–256. http://dx.doi.org/10.1016/j.jclepro.2017.05.015.

Sander, K. and Murthy, G.S. (2010). Life cycle analysis of algae biodiesel. *The International Journal of Life Cycle Assessment* **15** (7): 704–714. http://dx.doi.org/10.1007/s11367-010-0194-1.

Scott, S.A., Davey, M.P., Dennis, J.S. et al. (2010). Biodiesel from algae: challenges and prospects. *Current Opinion in Biotechnology* **21**: 277–286.

Shelef, G., Sukenik, A., and Green, M. (1984). Microalgae harvesting and processing: a literature review. Haifa: Technion Research and Development Foundation Ltd.

Shen, Y., Pei, Z., Yuan, W., and Mao, E. (2009). Effect of nitrogen and extraction method on algae lipid yield. *International Journal of Agricultural and Biological Engineering* **2**: 51–57.

Shene, C., Monsalve, M.T., Vergara, D. et al. (2016). High pressure homogenization of *Nannochloropsis oculata* for the extraction of intracellular components: effect of process conditions and culture age. *European Journal of Lipid Science and Technology* **118**: 631–639.

Show, K.Y., Lee, D.J., and Chang, J.S. (2013). Algal biomass dehydration. *Bioresource Technology* **135**: 720–729. http://dx.doi.org/10.1016/j.biortech.2012.08.021.

Show, K.Y., Lee, D.J., Tay, J.H. et al. (2015). Microalgal drying and cell disruption – recent advances. *Bioresource Technology* **184**: 258–266. http://dx.doi.org/10.1016/j.biortech.2014.10.139.

Singh, J. and Gu, S. (2010). Commercialization potential of microalgae for biofuels production. *Renewable and Sustainable Energy Reviews* **14** (9): 2596–2610.

Singh, P., Shrivastava, V., and Kumar, A. (2018). Recent developments in greenhouse solar drying: a review. *Renewable and Sustainable Energy Reviews* **82**: 3250–3262. https://doi.org/10.1016/j.rser.2017.10.020.

Slager, B., Sapounas, A.A., van Henten, E.J., and Hemming, S. (2014). Modelling and evaluation of productivity and economic feasibility of a combined production of tomato and algae in Dutch greenhouses. *Biosystems Engineering* **122**: 149–162. https://doi.org/10.1016/j.biosystemseng.2014.04.008.

Soeder, C.J. (1980). Massive cultivation of microalgae: results and prospects. *Hydrobiology* **72**: 197–209.

Soeder, C.J. and Pabst, W. (1975). Production, properties, preclinical and clinical testing of *Scenedesmus* 276-3a. The PAG Compendium, C-2, 2113. New York: World Mark Press Ltd.

Spiden, E.M., Yap, B.H.J., Hill, D.R.A. et al. (2013). Quantitative evaluation of the ease of rupture of industrially promising microalgae by high pressure homogenization. *Bioresource Technology* **140**: 165–171.

Spiden, E.M., Scales, P.J., Yap, B.H.J. et al. (2015). The effects of acidic and thermal pretreatment on the mechanical rupture of two industrially relevant microalgae: *Chlorella* sp. and *Navicula* sp. *Algal Research* **7**: 5–10.

Syed, I.R., Sukhcharn, S., and Saxena, D.C. (2016). Evaluation of physical and compositional properties of horse-chestnut (*Aesculus indica*) seed. *Journal of Food Processing and Technology* **7** (3): 561.

Taleb, A., Kandilian, R., Touchard, R. et al. (2016). Screening of freshwater and seawater microalgae strains in fully controlled photobioreactors for biodiesel production. *Bioresource Technology* **218**: 480–490.

Tan, J., Low, K.Y., Nik Sulaiman, N.M. et al. (2016). Fuzzy analytical hierarchy process (FAHP) for multi-criteria selection in drying and harvesting process of microalgae system. *Clean Technologies and Environmental Policy* **18**: 2049–2063.

Tunde-Akintunde, T.Y. and Ogunlakin, G.O. (2011). Influence of drying conditions on the effective moisture diffusivity and energy requirements during the drying of pretreated and untreated pumpkin. *Energy Conversion and Management* **52** (2): 1107–1113.

Vassilev, S.V. and Vassileva, C.G. (2016). Composition, properties and challenges of algae biomass for biofuel application: an overview. *Fuel* **181**: 1–33. DOI: http://dx.doi.org/10.1016/j.fuel.2016.04.106.

Villagracia, A.R.C., Andres, P.M., Aristotle, T.U. et al. (2016). Microwave drying characteristics of microalgae (*Chlorella vulgaris*) for biofuel production. *Clean Technologies and Environmental Policy* **18** (8): 2441–2451. https://doi.org/10.1007/s10098-016-1169-0.

Wahlen, B.D., Mohammad, S.R., Kara, G.C. et al. (2017). Managing variability in algal biomass production through drying and stabilization of feedstock blends. *Algal Research* **24**: 9–18. DOI: http://dx.doi.org/10.1016/j.algal.2017.03.005.

Wang, G. and Wang, T. (2012). Characterization of lipid components in two microalgae for biofuel application. *Journal of the American Oil Chemists' Society* **89**: 135–143.

Wang, D.Q., Li, Y.Q., Hu, X.Q. et al. (2015). Combined enzymatic and mechanical cell disruption and lipid extraction of green alga *Neochloris oleoabundans*. *International Journal of Molecular Sciences* **16**: 7707–7722. https://doi.org/10.3390/ijms16047707.

Williams, P.J. and Laurens, L.M. (2010). Microalgae as biodiesel and biomass feedstocks: review and analysis of the biochemistry, energetics and economics. *Energy & Environmental Science* **3**: 554–590.

Xu, L., Derk, W.F., Brilman, J. et al. (2011). Assessment of a dry and a wet route for the production of biofuels from microalgae: energy balance analysis. *Bioresource Technology* **102** (8): 5113–5122. DOI: http://dx.doi.org/10.1016/j.biortech.2011.01.066.

Yap, B.H., Crawford, S.A., Dumsday, G.J. et al. (2014). A mechanistic study of algal cell disruption and its effect on lipid recovery by solvent extraction. *Algal Research* **5**: 112–120.

Zhang, X., Rong, J.F., Chen, H. et al. (2014). Current status and outlook in the application of microalgae in biodiesel production and environmental protection. *Frontiers in Energy Research* **2**: 1–15.

Zheng, H., Yin, J., Gao, Z. et al. (2011a). Disruption of *Chlorella vulgaris* cells for the release of biodiesel-producing lipids: a comparison of grinding, ultrasonication, bead milling, enzymatic Lysis and microwaves. *Applied Biochemistry and Biotechnology* **164**: 1215–1224.

4
Recent Advances in the Use of Greener Extraction Technologies for the Recovery of Valuable Bioactive Compounds from Algae

Marco Garcia-Vaquero[1], Torres Sweeney[2], John O'Doherty[3], and Gaurav Rajauria[3]

[1]*Section of Food and Nutrition, School of Agriculture and Food Science, University College Dublin, Dublin, Ireland*
[2]*School of Veterinary Medicine, Veterinary Sciences Centre, University College Dublin, Dublin, Ireland*
[3]*School of Agriculture and Food Science, University College Dublin, Lyons Research Farm, Celbridge, Ireland*

4.1 Introduction

The main objective of any extraction technique is to maximize the recovery or yield obtained of the target compounds from a sample matrix while preserving the integrity of the molecules of interest and decreasing the extraction of other impurities or undesirable compounds (Tiwari 2015). The development of novel extraction procedures poses a number of challenges as these techniques should be faster and more efficient than conventional techniques, reduce or eliminate the use of organic solvents, and obtain high yields of high-value compounds by selectively extracting these molecules following the principles of green chemistry (Herrero and Ibáñez 2018; Herrero and Ibáñez 2015; Tiwari 2015).

Recent Advances in Micro- and Macroalgal Processing: Food and Health Perspectives, First Edition.
Edited by Gaurav Rajauria and Yvonne V. Yuan.

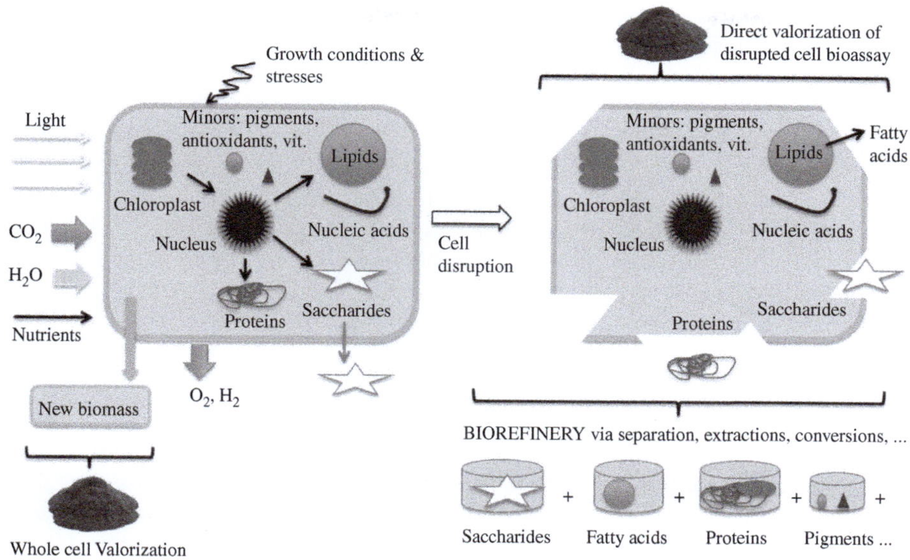

Figure 4.1 Valorization strategies of microalgal biomass, including direct valorization and biorefinery approach. Source: Image reproduced from Hayes et al. (2019) with permission from John Wiley & Sons.

Moreover, resource efficiency is one of the key elements of a sustainable food production and it is in close association with the principles of green chemistry, aiming to reduce the generation of chemical wastes while promoting an efficient use of energy and the biomass (Herrero and Ibáñez 2018). The principles of green chemistry and resource efficiency were applied in the algal industry by the development of the biorefinery approach. The biorefinery concept in the algal industry aims to use processes and technological advances for the conversion of algal biomass into energy and a variety of products, mainly biofuels and added-value co-products such as functional foods and nutraceuticals (Herrero and Ibáñez 2018; Hayes et al. 2019). A schematic representation of a biorefinery approach to recover multiple high-value compounds from algae is presented in Figure 4.1.

Nutraceuticals or functional foods are high-value compounds with additional health benefits beyond basic nutrition (Garcia-Vaquero and Hayes 2016). The market of functional foods and nutraceuticals was estimated to be valued at US$68.60 billion in 2018 and this market is projected to reach a value of US$94.21 billion by 2023 (Markets and Markets 2018). Marine organisms such as algae (seaweed and microalgae) represent a relatively untapped source of nutraceuticals. Algae comprises a diverse group of uni- and multicellular organisms that are able survive in the extreme and variable conditions of the aquatic environments (i.e. changes in salinity, temperature, nutrients, UV irradiation, and CO_2) by producing unique secondary metabolites as reviewed by Garcia-Vaquero et al. (2017b). Compounds synthesized by algae include polysaccharides, proteins-peptides, lipids, polyphenols, and carotenoids (Garcia-Vaquero et al. 2017a). In order to fully utilize algal resources, these molecules should ideally be selectively extracted, minimizing the co-extraction of nondesirable molecules and achieving high yields of compounds by using more environmentally friendly extraction technologies and solvents, aiming to minimize the generation of waste and the use of energy and resources following the principles of green chemistry (Anastas and Warner 2000).

This chapter summarizes the main innovative technologies (pulsed electric fields [PEFs], supercritical fluid extraction (SFE), pressurized liquid extraction (PLE), microwave assisted extraction [MAE], and ultrasound assisted extraction [UAE]) used to generate high-value compounds from algae (macroalgae and microalgae). The concepts of green chemistry applied to these extraction processes are discussed together with the principles, advantages, applications, future trends, and challenges of novel green extraction technologies.

4.2 Green Extraction Technologies and Applications

As previously mentioned, the main objective of any extraction technique is to maximize the yield of the target compounds from a sample matrix while preserving the integrity of the molecules of interest and decreasing the extraction of other undesirable compounds (Tiwari 2015). Conventional protocols commonly involve the extraction of compounds from a solid matrix using solvents, namely solid–liquid extraction techniques such as steam distillation, maceration, and Soxhlet extraction (Tiwari 2015; Wang and Weller 2006). These technologies are time- and solvent-consuming techniques and there is currently an interest to move toward more sustainable practices following the principles of green chemistry.

Chemat et al. (2012) described six principles of green chemistry applied specifically to the generation of natural products: (i) strategic biomass selection (i.e. species, degree of foraging) to ensure the renewal of the natural resources; (ii) use of water or agro-solvents as an alternative to organic solvents; (iii) reduction or recovery of the energy consumed during the process of extraction by implementing innovative technologies; (iv) generation of co-products instead of waste by following the biorefinery concept; (v) application of safe and controlled processes, reducing the unit operations needed during the process of extraction whenever possible; and (vi) generation of intact and biodegradable extracts free of contaminants or solvent residues.

Innovative or emerging technologies including PEFs, SFE, PLE, MAE, and UAE have received great deal of attention in the scientific community in recent years aiming to develop greener extraction protocols.

4.2.1 Pulsed Electric Field (PEF)

PEF is a nonthermal processing technology based on the application of short electric treatments (nano- or milliseconds) to samples placed between two electrodes with variable voltage (100–300 V cm^{-1} or 20–80 kV cm^{-1}) that will determine the intensity of the PEF treatment (Barba et al. 2015; Raso et al. 2016). The application of PEF on biological matrices causes membrane permeabilization or cell electroporation. The increased permeability of the cells after a PEF treatment could be explained due to mechanical, hydrodynamic, osmotic, and viscoelastic instabilities generated on the membranes (Barba et al. 2015; Raso et al. 2016). PEF has also been used as a pretreatment of the matrices to enhance the diffusion and efficiency of later extraction procedures such as pressure extraction (Raso et al. 2016). Moreover, PEF also has gained relevance in other food processing operations to improve food quality, to accelerate heat transfer processes, and to enhance mass transfer efficiency of water from food during the processes of drying, osmotic dehydration, freeze drying, freezing, and thawing processes (Barba et al. 2015; Raso et al. 2016).

4.2.1.1 Advantages and Disadvantages of PEF PEF offers certain advantages for the extraction of bioactive compounds such as an increased mass transfer that allows the recovery of high-value compounds. PEF treatments also help to reduce the energy input and the environmental impacts of the extraction processes compared with other traditional techniques. Moreover, PEF does not require high temperatures and solvents to achieve an efficient extraction, being suitable for the extraction of thermolabile compounds (Barba et al. 2015).

One of the major disadvantages of PEF is the lack of information on the operating protocols and pulses, which is needed to standardize the experimental procedures and increase the reproducibility of the results in order to define the appropriate PEF assisted processing conditions in a commercial set-up (Raso et al. 2016). There have been recent developments aiming to treat large volumes of samples shifting from batch- to flow-processing procedures (Sack et al. 2010; Toepfl 2012) and approx. 30 commercial units are in use worldwide, mainly for the purposes of microbial decontamination of fruit juices and vegetables (Toepfl 2012). Moreover, the variability of the results in the scientific literature can be attributed to differences in equipment and protocols used by the researchers, including pre- and post-treatment conditions, which can considerably influence the mass transfer when extracting compounds using PEF (Raso et al. 2016). For example, Luengo et al. (2014) determined that waiting 1 hour after a PEF treatment was vital to calculate the efficiency of extraction of pigments from microalgae.

4.2.1.2 Applications of PEF Depending on the intensity of the PEF treatment (i.e. intensity of the electric field, single pulse duration, and treatment times) and the biological characteristics of the matrix, the cellular damage could be reversible or irreversible as seen in Figure 4.2.

Reversible electroporation techniques are currently being used as a tool for genetic engineering of microalgae (i.e. to increase oil production) and, in the case of macroalgae for gene transfection and electrofusion, aiming to improve the future use of algal resources (Robin and Golberg 2016). PEF at 4.5 kV cm^{-1} and 5 μs of pulse duration were useful to generate small transient pores (0.8–0.9 nm) in microalgae *Chlamydomonas reinhardtii* (Bodénès et al. 2019). These transition pores allowed the reversible permeabilization of the cell membranes useful for algae milking or extraction of small hydrosoluble molecules while keeping intact the viability of the biomass. Large pores with radius >0.8–0.9 nm were developed by using PEF treatment at 7 kV cm^{-1} and 5 μs of pulse duration. These pores were associated with an irreversible permeabilization of the membrane and cell death, useful for the extraction of larger molecules (Bodénès et al. 2019).

Luengo et al. (2014) obtained high extraction yields of carotenoids and chlorophylls from *Chlorella vulgaris* by inducing an irreversible electroporation of the cells with a PEF treatment (20 kV cm^{-1} for 75 μs). The authors also mentioned that the efficacy of PEF enhancing the extraction of compounds was dependent on the processing parameters and time elapsed between the PEF treatment and the extraction process. The recovery of carotenoids from *C. vulgaris* increased when the compounds were

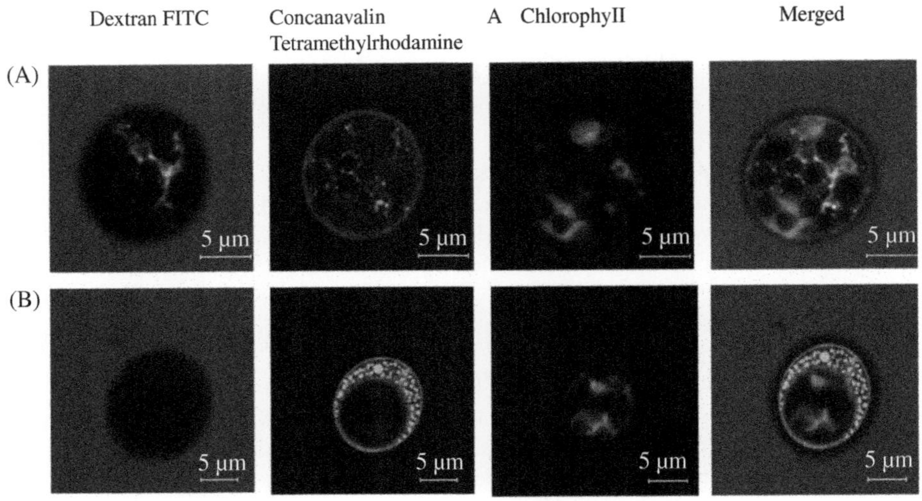

Figure 4.2 Microalgal cells of *Chlamydomonas reinhardtii* visualized using various staining methods (dextran FITC, concanavalin A and chlorophyll) after a pulsed electric fields (PEFs) treatment: (A) irreversible and (B) reversible PEF. Source: Image reproduced from Bodénès et al. (2019) with permission from Elsevier.

extracted 1 hour after the PEF treatment rather than immediately after the treatment. Luengo et al. (2015) reported an increased extraction of lutein from the same microalgae species using PEF (25 kV cm^{-1} and 100 μs) at 25–30 °C compared with the control untreated biomass. Martínez et al. (2017) electroporated *Arthrospira platensis* using PEF (15 kV cm^{-1} for 150 μs) to increase the extraction of c-phycocyanin. An increase in the temperature of extraction from 10 to 40 °C allowed the reduction of the electric strength of the electric field and energy input applied during the process of extraction (Martínez et al. 2017).

There are also a few studies showing the application of PEF combined with other techniques to treat macroalgae. Polikovsky et al. (2016) used PEF at approx. 3 KV cm^{-1} and 0.4 seconds together with hydraulic pressing to increase the selective extraction of proteins from *Ulva* sp. Moreover, the combination of these techniques was also effective to de-ash macroalgal biomass, particularly increasing the extraction of five major elements (K, Mg, Na, P, and S) (Robin et al. 2018).

Despite the promising applications of this technology, some authors suggest that PEF is not competitive or has poor performance in comparison with other techniques for particular applications. Lam et al. (2017) obtained lower release of intracellular proteins (13%) from *C. vulgaris* and *Neochloris oleoabundans* using multiple PEF conditions when compared with the 45–50% of proteins obtained using a bead milling process. A recent study aiming to recover proteins from *Nannochloropsis gaditana* determined that PEF was the least efficient method both in terms of yield recovery and energy cost per unit of released compounds compared with other traditional cell disruption techniques such as high-pressure homogenization and bead milling (Safi et al. 2017). Moreover, PEF processing at 20 kV cm^{-1} and 1–4 ms allowed a selective extraction of water-soluble ionic components and microelements from *Nannochloropsis* sp., but was not effective for the extraction of pigments (Grimi et al. 2014).

Table 4.1 Critical properties of solvents used in supercritical fluid extraction (SFE).

Solvent types	Critical properties			
	Temperature (°C)	Pressure (atm)	Density (g ml^{-1})	Solubility (cal $^{-1/2}$ cm $^{-3/2}$)
Carbon dioxide (CO_2)	31.2	72.9	0.47	7.5
Ethane (C_2H_6)	32.4	48.2	0.2	5.8
Ethene (C_2H_4)	10.1	50.5	0.2	5.8
Methanol (CH_3OH)	−34.4	79.9	0.272	8.9
Nitrous oxide (N_2O)	36.7	71.7	0.46	7.2
n-Butene (C_4H_8)	−139.9	36	0.221	5.2
n-Pentane (C_5H_{12})	−76.5	33.3	0.237	5.1
Sulfur hexafluoride (SF_6)	45.8	37.7	0.73	5.5
Water (H_2O)	101.1	217.6	0.322	13.5

Source: Modified from Herrero et al. (2006) and da Silva et al. (2016).

4.2.2 Supercritical Fluid Extraction (SFE)

The supercritical state of a fluid is achieved when a liquid is forced to pressure and temperature above its critical point and the solvents adopts intermediate properties in between those of a gas and liquid. The critical properties temperature, pressure, density, and solubility of the main solvents are summarized in Table 4.1.

Supercritical fluids have the density of a liquid, viscosity of a gas, and diffusivity between both liquid and gas (Herrero et al. 2006). SFE is an innovative extraction technology that uses supercritical fluids to extract soluble compounds from insoluble matrices (Esquivel-Hernández et al. 2017).

The specificity of SFE relies on the physical properties of the solvent, which can be modulated by increases in temperature and/or pressure depending on the high-value compounds of interest (Esquivel-Hernández et al. 2017). The most commonly used supercritical fluid is carbon dioxide (CO_2), a nontoxic and environmentally friendly liquid that allows the extraction of molecules without exposing them to air, avoiding possible oxidative damages of the extracted compounds (da Silva et al. 2016). Moreover, as seen in Table 4.1, the moderate critical temperature (31.2 °C) and pressure (72.9 atm) of CO_2 makes this solvent gas at room temperature. A substantial elimination of the solvent could be achieved after the process of extraction by returning supercritical CO_2 to its gaseous form at room temperature, obtaining a solvent-free extract. However, supercritical CO_2 has low polarity (solubility parameter, δ of 7.5 cal$^{-1/2}$ cm$^{-3/2}$), and, thus, small amounts of highly polar modifiers or co-solvents (i.e. methanol or ethanol) are needed to increase the yield of extraction of polar molecules (Herrero et al. 2006; Esquivel-Hernández et al. 2017).

During SFE the sample matrix absorbs the supercritical solvent, expanding the cell structures and thus enhancing the mass transfer of the targeted compounds and the flow of solvent through the sample (Esquivel-Hernández et al. 2017). In SFE the molecules are extracted from the sample matrix mainly by convection and diffusion forces or a combination of both depending on the amount of compounds of the sample and the duration of the extraction process (da Silva et al. 2016). A schematic representation of SFE equipment is represented in Figure 4.3.

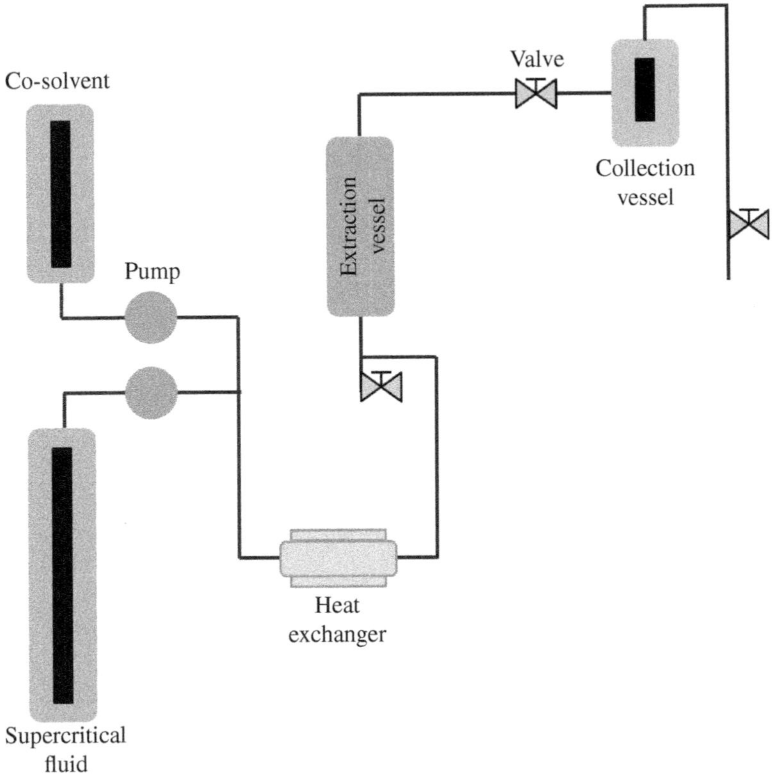

Figure 4.3 Schematic representation of supercritical fluid extraction (SFE) equipment. Source: Image adapted from Esquivel-Hernández et al. (2017).

SFE starts by bringing the fluid to its supercritical state by using pressure and temperature. The solvent is then fed to the extractor and uniformly distributed throughout a fixed bed containing the sample. The solutes are dissolved in the fluid and carried to the separator, experiencing a reduction of pressure and/or an increase of temperature, which transforms the supercritical fluid back into its gaseous state. The solutes are then collected at the bottom of the chamber and the solvent could be recovered (by cooling and/or compressing) or disposed (Esquivel-Hernández et al. 2017).

4.2.2.1 Advantages and Disadvantages of SFE SFE has several advantages over traditional technologies mainly attributed to the physicochemical properties of the supercritical fluids. For instance, the low viscosity and high diffusivity of supercritical fluids enhance the transport of solutes and diffusion of the solvent through the sample, increasing the speed of the extraction process compared with traditional fluids. Moreover, the extraction of several compounds could be improved by adjusting the pressure and/or temperature of the supercritical fluid to modify the density and thus the solubility of the supercritical fluid (da Silva et al. 2016). SFE uses environmentally friendly, low cost, and generally recognized as safe solvents, and it is possible to couple SFE with other analytical tools such as gas or supercritical fluid chromatography (da Silva et al. 2016; Esquivel-Hernández et al. 2017).

However, SFE has some disadvantages such as the high cost of the equipment and the reduced extraction of polar compounds, even with the use of co-solvents. There is also a limited knowledge of the behavior of mixtures containing co-solvents, as these chemicals could change the state of the fluid and be unnoticed during the process of extraction (Esquivel-Hernández et al. 2017; Arsad et al. 2014). Other disadvantages when operating this technology are the need to increase the time of residence of the fluid in contact with the sample to ensure the equilibrium and adequate mass transfer of solutes and other complications when dealing with heavy solutes or high-density supercritical fluids (Arsad et al. 2014).

4.2.2.2 Applications of SFE Supercritical CO_2 is the main SFE technique to extract lipids and pigments from algae, but also other bioactive compounds such as polyphenols. The experimental conditions to target different molecules such as the use of co-solvents and different combinations of temperature, pressure, and time to perform SFE are summarized in Table 4.2.

In general, the extraction of lipids, fatty acids, and various oils is performed without co-solvents and, when needed, the co-solvent of choice used in recent studies is ethanol (see multiple references in Table 4.2). The application of SFE in macroalgae has been mainly explored in the scientific literature to attain high yields of fucoxanthin (Fabrowska et al. 2016; Getachew et al. 2018; Heffernan et al. 2016; Pérez-López et al. 2014; Quitain et al. 2013; Saravana et al. 2017; Sivagnanam et al. 2015). Fucoxanthin is a marine carotenoid present in high concentrations in brown macroalgae, mainly in *Fucus serratus*, with unique chemical features such as the presence of an allenic bond and a 5,6-monoepoxide group in the structure of the molecule (Holdt and Kraan 2011). The unique chemical structure of fucoxanthin together with knowledge on its safety, metabolism, and biological activities (i.e. antiobesity, antidiabetic, antioxidant, anti-inflammatory, and anticancer) have increased the interest of the food industry in this molecule to develop functional foods and nutraceuticals (Gammone and D'Orazio 2015).

Ospina et al. (2017) optimized SFE using CO_2 and ethanol as co-solvent to extract polyphenols and carotenoids from macroalga *Gracilaria mammillaris*. The authors determined that the amount of polyphenols extracted was extremely dependent on the concentration of co-solvent used, while the carotenoid contents were mainly influenced by the pressure applied during SFE. Moreover, fractions obtained at 30 MPa, 60 °C, and 8% of co-solvent had the highest antioxidant activities protecting oil from oxidative damage during accelerated oxidation trials (Ospina et al. 2017). Other authors such as Michalak et al. (2016) also employed SFE to extract multiple compounds from *Polysiphonia nigrescens*, *Ulva clathrata*, and *Cladophora* sp. to obtain metals (macro- and microelements) and other organic compounds such as auxins, cytokinins, and polyphenols, to explore the application of the extracts as plant growth stimulants.

In the case of microalgae, SFE protocols focused mainly on extracting lipids, with important applications for the biofuel industry, and long chain fatty acids with high market and nutritional value such as docosahexaenoic acid (DHA) and eicosapentaenoic acid (EPA). As seen in Table 4.2, SFE has been explored in the recent scientific literature using a huge range of extraction conditions (37–55 °C, 6–75 MPa and 90–240 minutes) aiming to obtain optimum yields of compounds from multiple microalgal species (Feller et al. 2018; Gilbert-López et al. 2017; Kwan et al. 2018; Lorenzen et al. 2017; McKennedy et al. 2016; Nobre et al. 2013; Obeid et al.

Table 4.2 Summary of the extraction conditions used in the recent literature to obtain multiple high-value compounds from algae (macroalgae and microalgae) applying supercritical CO_2.extraction.

	Species	Co-solvent	Temperature (°C)	Pressure (MPa)	Time (minutes)	Targeted compounds	References
Macroalgae	*Saccharina japonica*	–	40	30	180	Oil and fucoxanthin	Getachew et al. (2018)
	Gracilaria mammillaris	Ethanol	40, 50, and 60	10, 20, and 30	240	Polyphenols and carotenoids	Ospina et al. (2017)
	Fucus serratus and*Laminaria digitata*	Ethanol	50	30	105	Fucoxanthin	Heffernan et al. (2016)
	Cladophora glomerata, *Ulva flexuosa*, and *Chara fragilis*	Ethanol	40	30	120	Fucoxanthin, astacene, deinoxanthin, siphonaxanthin, phenols, and carotenoids	Fabrowska et al. (2016)
	Polysiphonia nigrescens, *Ulva clathrata*, and *Cladophora* sp.	–	40	50	300, 360, and 810	Auxins, cytokinins, polyphenols, micro-, and macroelements	Michalak et al. (2016)
	Saccharina japonica and *Sargassum horneri*	Ethanol	45	25	120	Fatty acids, fucoxanthin, and polyphenols	Sivagnanam et al. (2015)
	Sargassum muticum	Ethanol	55	40	120	Fucoxanthin	Pérez-López et al. (2014)
	Undaria pinnatifida	–	25–60	20–40	180	Fucoxanthin	Quitain et al. (2013)

(continued)

Table 4.2 *(continued)*

	Species	Co-solvent	Temperature (°C)	Pressure (MPa)	Time (minutes)	Targeted compounds	References
Microalgae	*Spirulina platensis*	Ethanol and water	50	40	120	Chlorophyll	del Valle et al. (2019)
	Phaeodactylum tricornutum, *Nannochloropsis oculata*, and *Porphyridium cruentum*	–	40	30	120	Lipids and carotenoids	Feller et al. (2018)
	Haematococcus pluvialis	–	45	11.6 and 48.3	240	Astaxanthin and triacylglycerol	Kwan et al. (2018)
	Nannochloropsis oculata and *Chlorella vulgaris*	Ethanol	50	45–75	210	Lipids	Obeid et al. (2018)
	Haematococcus pluvialis	Ethanol	50, 65, and 80	10, 40, and 55	20–80	Asthaxanthin and lutein	Molino et al. (2018)
	Haematococcus pluvialis	–	50 and 65	55	120	Fatty acids, asthaxanthin, and lutein	Sanzo et al. (2018)
	Scenedesmus obliquus	Ethanol and water	50	36	120	Lipids and pigments	Gilbert-López et al. (2017)
	Scenedesmus obliquus and *Scenedesmus obtusiusculus*	–	20	12	540	Lipids	Lorenzen et al. (2017)
	Phaeodactylum tricornutum	–	45	35	25	Lipids	Tommasi et al. (2017)
	Nannochloropsis oculata	Methanol and hexane	37 and 55	5.9 and 7.6	30	Fatty acid methyl esters	McKennedy et al. (2016)
	Scenedesmus obliquus, *Chlorella protothecoides*, and *Nannochloropsis salina*	Ethanol	60	30	90	Oil rich in α-linolenic	Solana et al. (2014)
	Nannochloropsis sp.	Ethanol	40	30	140	Lipids and pigments	Nobre et al. (2013)
	Chlorella vulgaris	–	40	40	45	Lutein	Ruen-ngam et al. (2012)

2018; Sanzo et al. 2018; Solana et al. 2014; Tommasi et al. 2017). Moreover, most of these studies focused on extracting or co-extracting pigments such as chlorophylls (del Valle et al. 2019; Gilbert-López et al. 2017) and high-value carotenoids, i.e. astaxanthin, lutein, and β-carotene (Kwan et al. 2018; Nobre et al. 2013; Ruen-ngam et al. 2012; Sanzo et al. 2018) with important applications as cosmetics and functional foods (Molino et al. 2018). The use of SFE to recover lipids and carotenoids from microalgae have been recently reviewed in detail by Yen et al. (2015) and Gallego et al. (2018).

4.2.3 Pressurized Liquid Extraction (PLE)

PLE is an emerging green technology also known as pressurized solvent extraction or accelerated solvent extraction (Esquivel-Hernández et al. 2017; Gallego et al. 2018). PLE uses the principles of traditional solid–liquid extraction techniques; unlike SFE the solvents are in a liquid state induced by applying temperatures above the boiling point and elevated pressures (3.4–20.4 MPa) (Esquivel-Hernández et al. 2017). Thereby, PLE using water as a solvent (subcritical water extraction, SWE) or subcritical solvent extraction, uses temperatures higher than the boiling point of water (100 °C) and lower than its critical temperature (374 °C), keeping the water in a liquid state during the extraction process by applying high pressures (3.5–20 MPa) (Herrero et al. 2013).

The principle of PLE involves desorption of the compounds of interest from the matrix followed by the diffusion of the molecules through the pores of the sample and collection of the molecules in the solvent (Esquivel-Hernández et al. 2017). A schematic representation of PLE equipment is presented in Figure 4.4.

In a PLE system the sample is placed in an extraction cell containing solvent that is being pushed with a pump. The extraction cell is heated and pressurized before starting the flow of solvent that will be later collected. PLE can operate in a dynamic mode, with a constant flow of solvent through the extraction vessel, or in a static mode by using one or more cycles of extraction. Once the extraction finishes, the extraction cell is purged with nitrogen gas to eliminate the sample residues (Esquivel-Hernández et al. 2017). Pressure and temperature are the main operation parameters that are controlled when performing PLE. The pressure of the fluid has to ensure that the fluid remains in a liquid state, although increments of pressure beyond this objective seem to have little or no effect in the extraction efficiency of the process (Gallego et al. 2018; Herrero et al. 2013). The selection of the appropriate solvent according to the nature of the target compounds is also key to achieve high yields of the target compounds (Gallego et al. 2018).

4.2.3.1 Advantages and Disadvantages of PLE PLE reduces the time of extraction, offers the possibility of automatizing the process, and uses smaller amounts of organic solvents in comparison with traditional technologies (Esquivel-Hernández et al. 2017). These advantages are explained by the increased solubility and decreased viscosity of the fluids under the high temperatures and pressures used in PLE, increasing the mass transfer of solutes and penetration of the solvents in the matrix (Gallego et al. 2018). PLE could also be used with a wide variety of environmentally friendly solvents (i.e. water and ethanol) or mixtures, substituted for organic solvents, to target a wide variety of polar and nonpolar compounds (Esquivel-Hernández et al. 2017). The high

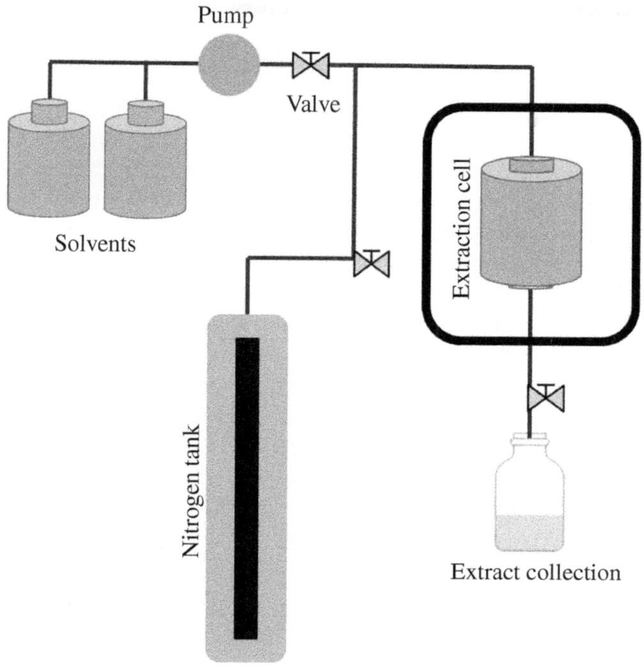

Figure 4.4 Schematic representation of pressurized liquid extraction (PLE) apparatus. Source: Image modified from Sticher (2008).

temperatures applied in PLE weaken the hydrogen bonds of the solvents, reducing the dielectric constant or polarity of the solvent. When using water as a solvent in SWE, the dielectric constant of water changes from being extremely polar (ε of 80) at 25 °C to less polar (ε 25–27) at 250 °C, being similar to that of methanol (ε 33) and ethanol (ε 24) at 25 °C (Herrero et al. 2013; Gallego et al. 2018). Thus, under these conditions water could be used as an alternative solvent to dissolve medium-polar and nonpolar organic compounds in substitution of organic solvents (Herrero et al. 2013).

Despite all these advantages, PLE is an exhaustive and nonselective technique that can obtain both target and nontarget compounds from the sample. This phenomenon can be reduced by the use of adsorbents for the selective retention of residues in the extraction cell. Other disadvantages include the elevated cost of the equipment and the difficulty in maintaining the extraction conditions of the fluids at a large scale, which has hindered the scale-up of this technology at industrial level (Esquivel-Hernández et al. 2017).

4.2.3.2 Applications of PLE PLE has been used to extract multiple compounds from algae in the recent scientific literature. Otero et al. (2019) explored the influence of pure solvents (i.e. hexane, ethyl acetate, and ethanol) and mixtures (ethanol:water) on the recovery of fatty acids and phenolic compounds from the brown alga *Laminaria ochroleuca* using PLE at temperatures ranging from 80 to 160 °C and 10 MPa. Mixtures of ethanol:water showed the highest extraction yields of high-value compounds, while the pure solvents ethyl acetate and ethanol increased the concentration of unsaturated fatty acids, accounting for more than 50% of the lipid fraction of the extract (Otero et al. 2019). PLE was also used in multiple seaweed species (*Ulva intestinalis, Ulva lactuca, Fucus vesiculosus, Dictyota dichotoma, Cystoseira baccata, and Himanthalia elongata*) to produce extracts with strong antioxidant and antibacterial properties (Otero et al. 2018). Plaza et al. (2010) explored the use of PLE to study the antioxidant and antimicrobial activities of extracts from macroalga *H. elongata* and microalga *Synechocystis* sp. The authors identified several fatty acids and volatile compounds including phytol, fucosterol, neophytadiene, or palmitic, palmitoleic, and oleic acids with strong antimicrobial properties. Moreover, the use of PLE with several solvents, combining or not the extraction process with a pretreatment of the biomass, allowed the enrichment and fractionation of neutral lipids such as mono-, di- and triacylglycerols, free fatty acids, and glycolipids from microalga *N. gaditana* (Castejón and Señoráns 2019). Amaro et al. (2018) used PLE at 60 °C and 18 MPa to recover high-value compounds from microalga *Gloeothece* sp. These authors obtained an increase of approximately 3- and 1.5-fold in β-carotene and polyunsaturated fatty acids, respectively, compared with other conventional technologies and UAE. Further detailed extraction protocols and applications of PLE to extract mainly fatty acids and carotenoids from microalgae have been summarized by Esquivel-Hernández et al. (2017).

4.2.4 Microwave Assisted Extraction (MAE)

MAE is a method based on the use of electromagnetic waves with a frequency ranging from 0.1 to 3 GHz. The electromagnetic energy creates ion motion and dipolar rotation of the molecules without affecting their structure. The application of microwaves causes a reorientation of the molecules in the direction of the electric field and, when this field is removed, the thermal agitation turns the molecules to a disordered state, releasing thermal energy (Chemat et al. 2015; Chemat et al. 2017). Thus, microwave heating is generated from the dissipation of electromagnetic waves in an irradiated medium, resulting in faster increases of temperature when compared with conventional heating, in which the energy is transferred between the heating device and the medium (Chemat et al. 2017).

Moisture contents serve as the main target for microwave heating. It evaporates, generating an increased pressure, ruptures of the cell membranes, and leaching of the bioactive compounds (Sosa-Hernández et al. 2018). A scheme of basic MAE equipment is represented in Figure 4.5.

MAE has also experienced recent developments aiming to reduce the time and waste generation during its operation. Recent methods such as solvent-free microwave hydrodistillation (SFME) offer the possibility to reduce or even eliminate the use of solvents; and microwave hydrodiffusion and gravity (MHG) allows the use of microwaves to extract the compounds and atmospheric pressure to collect and later condense the extracted solutes (Chemat et al. 2015; Chemat et al. 2017).

4.2.4.1 Advantages and Disadvantages of MAE MAE achieves several objectives of green chemistry applied to the extraction of bioactive compounds, mainly by increasing the yields of extraction while reducing the use of solvents and time of extraction (Esquivel-Hernández et al. 2017). For example, the aforementioned SFME offers the possibility to perform the extraction without the use of solvents. MAE

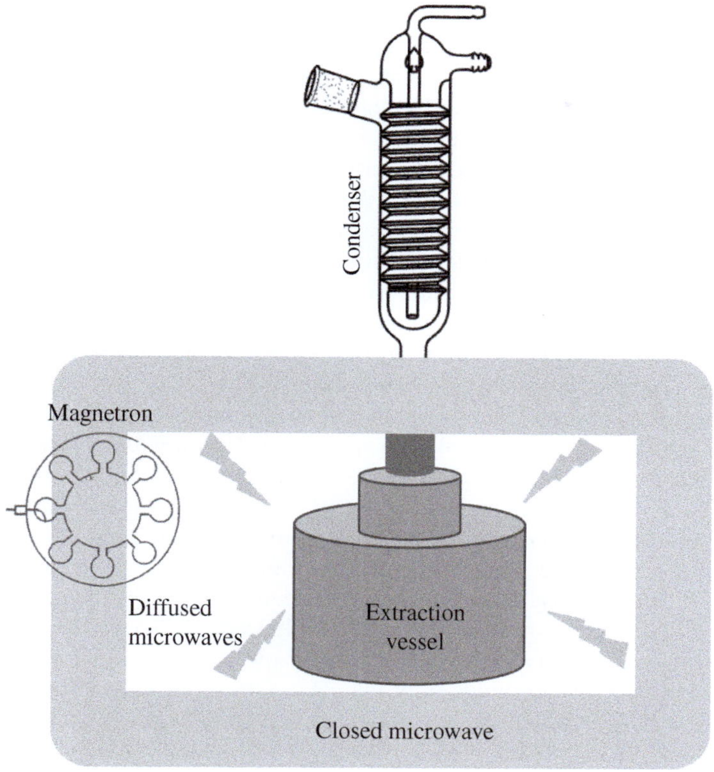

Figure 4.5 Schematic representation of microwave assisted extraction (MAE) equipment. Source: Image adapted from Sticher (2008).

uses a noncontact heat source, increasing the efficiency and selectivity of the heating process while accelerating the mass transfer of solutes and the response to heating control, protecting the products from degradation, and reducing the equipment size and operation units with respect to conventional technologies (Chemat et al. 2015; Esquivel-Hernández et al. 2017). Moreover, MAE offers high reproducibility, the possibility to scale up to industry, and the initial investment in the equipment is lower than in SFE and PLE (Chemat et al. 2015; Esquivel-Hernández et al. 2017).

The main limitations of MAE are the need to separate the solutes extracted from the sample matrix after the process of extraction (i.e. filtration) and the temperature increase of the process means it is not suitable for thermolabile compounds. Also, despite the fact that several units are already being produced at pilot and industrial level, there are several parameters that complicate the scale-up of this technique, such as the difficulty in achieving a uniform heating and dielectric constant, as these parameters will depend on the chemical composition and density of the sample to be treated (Esquivel-Hernández et al. 2017).

4.2.4.2 Applications of MAE MAE is widely used to extract high-value compounds, nutraceuticals, and pharmaceutical-grade constituents from multiple resources including algae. Rodriguez-Jasso et al. (2011) used MAE with pressure

(120 psi) for 1 minute to obtain fucoidan from *F. vesiculosus* and concluded that MAE was an environmentally friendly extraction technique due to the short extraction times, use of noncorrosive solvents, and reduced costs. Yuan et al. (2018a) studied the selective extraction of polysaccharides from the macroalga *Ulva prolifera* using MAE technology. The properties and chemical structure and biological properties of the polysaccharides could be changed during the process of extraction using MAE. Thereby, rhamnose, galacturonic acid, and glucose were the major monosaccharides using MAE at 90 °C and 0.01 M HCl as a solvent, and the glucose and antioxidant activities were higher when the samples were extracted at 150 °C with 0.1 M HCl (Yuan et al. 2018a). Moreover, the use of MAE at 110 °C for 15 minutes resulted in extracts containing higher phenolic contents from *Ascophyllum nodosum*, *Laminaria japonica*, *Lessonia trabeculate*, and *Lessonia nigrecensae* when compared with those obtained using conventional extraction techniques (Yuan et al. 2018b).

In the case of microalgae, multiple parameters have been controlled using MAE to extract oil for biodiesel from several species including *Nannochloropsis* sp. (Bermúdez Menéndez et al. 2014, Xiao et al. 2013), *Scenedesmus* sp. (Balasubramanian et al. 2011; Guldhe et al. 2014; Onumaegbu et al. 2019) and *Dunaliella tertiolecta* (Qv et al. 2014). MAE was used to obtain lipids from *Scenedesmus* sp. at 100 °C, 10 minutes, and 1000 W of microwave power using a solvent mixture of chloroform:ethanol (1:1, v/v) (Guldhe et al. 2014). The authors obtained yields of 28.33% of lipids, higher than the 18.9% obtained when using UAE (Guldhe et al. 2014). The pretreatment of *Scenedesmus quadricauda* with 600 W of microwave power for 8 minutes recovered approximately 49% of lipids from the algal biomass using a solvent mixture of methanol and sulfuric acid (Onumaegbu et al. 2019). MAE at 80 °C, 1 minute, and 300 W with chloroform:methanol (2:1 v/v) was used successfully to recover lipids from *Nannochloropsis oculata*, *Amphora coffeaeformis*, *Chaetoceros gracilis*, and *Isochrysis galbana* (de Moura et al. 2018). When extracting other high-value compounds, Silva et al. (2018) obtained high yields of polysaccharides from *Arthrospira platensis* using a biomass:water ratio of 1:30 w/v, applying MAE treatments of 434 W for 1 minute and waiting for 20 minutes after the application of microwaves to increase the kinetics of extraction. Esquivel-Hernández et al. (2016) operated MAE at 50 °C and 400 W to obtain high yields of tocopherols and carotenoids from *A. platensis*, while the application of higher temperatures (70 °C) at the same microwave power increased the total yield of extract and fatty acids. Oher MAE conditions used to obtain lipids and other high-value compounds from microalgae have been reviewed in detail in the scientific literature (Kapoore et al. 2018).

4.2.5 Ultrasound Assisted Extraction (UAE)

UAE uses sound frequencies above the audible range (>20 kHz) and below microwave frequencies (≤10 MHz) to treat the samples. Ultrasonic treatments can be broadly divided into low-intensity (<1 W cm^{-2}) used as a nondestructive analytical technique for composition, structure, and physical analyses; and high-intensity sonication (10–1000 W cm^{-2}) currently used for the extraction of high-value compounds and other food processing operations (Tiwari 2015; Garcia-Vaquero et al. 2018).

There are several physical and chemical phenomena derived from the application of ultrasounds to the sample such as agitation, vibration, pressure, shock waves, shear forces, microjets, compression-rarefaction, acoustic streaming, cavitation, and radical formation. These effects are mainly associated with the frequency used, being the physical effects more evident at 20–100 kHz, the chemical effects of sonication are mainly the dominant effect when using frequencies between 200 and 500 kHz, whereas acoustic streaming is the main effect at frequencies >1 MHz (Tiwari 2015). In the case of UAE, the main force driving the extraction of bioactive compounds is acoustic cavitation. Ultrasounds propagate through the medium generating compressions and rarefactions of the molecules that induce changes in pressure generating bubbles that grow and collapse in the phenomenon known as acoustic cavitation (Garcia-Vaquero et al. 2018; Tiwari 2015). The temperature and pressure changes associated with cavitation increase the penetration of the solvent and mass transfer of solutes from the cells during the process of extraction due to (i) shear disruption, thinning, and rupture of cell walls, or (ii) pore enlargement that facilitates the hydration and swelling of the matrix. Moreover, the cavitation process also induces microscopic turbulences and agitation of the medium that accelerate the diffusion of high-value compounds from the cells (Tiwari 2015). The ability of ultrasounds to cause cavitation depends on the properties of the ultrasonic waves (i.e. frequency and power used), medium (such as viscosity and surface tension of the solvent), and other extraction conditions (e.g. temperature and pressure) that should be reported and recorded during UAE (Tiwari 2015). The UAE equipment used to date includes the use of ultrasonic baths (see Figure 4.6A) and ultrasonic probes or horns (Figure 4.6B). Recent developments in UAE equipment also include the design of systems that allow a continuous ultrasonic treatment (Tiwari 2015).

UAE baths operating at lower intensities have been widely used to extract high-value compounds for food applications (Garcia-Vaquero et al. 2017aa), but also to increase the dispersion of solutes in the solvent, degas solutions, or cleaning materials (Chemat et al. 2017). High-power ultrasonic probes are gradually displacing ultrasonic baths for the extraction of high-value compounds due to their high efficiency and recovery of molecules, reduced time of extraction, and low energy consumption (Tiwari 2015).

4.2.5.1 Advantages and Disadvantages of UAE UAE is a simple, cost-effective, and efficient alternative to conventional extraction techniques. UAE enhances the

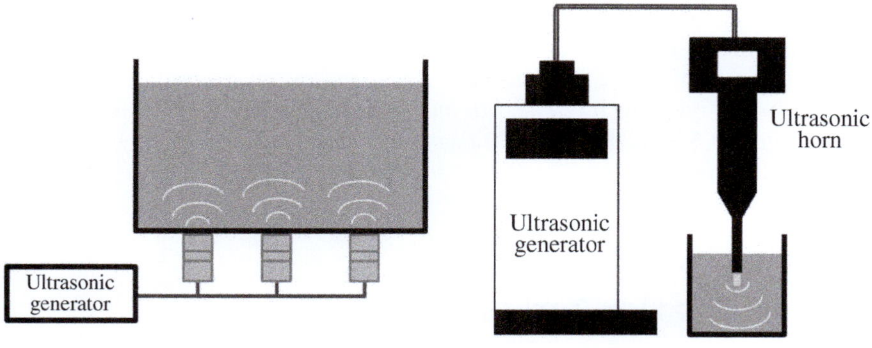

Figure 4.6 Ultrasound assisted extraction (UAE) systems: (A) schematic representation of an ultrasonic bath adapted from Tiwari (2015) and (B) an ultrasonic probe or horn. Source: Adapted from Garcia-Vaquero et al. (2018).

kinetics and mass transfer of solutes in solid–liquid extractions, useful to develop high-yield and low-time extraction protocols (Tiwari 2015). Moreover, the cost of the UAE equipment is lower than other extraction techniques and the operation of UAE allows the use of multiple solvents and mixtures, offering the possibility of a selective extraction of compounds based on the affinity of the molecules for different solvents (Arsad et al. 2014; Tiwari 2015). The shortcomings of this technology include the need for a separation or filtration step to obtain the extract, the attenuation of ultrasonic waves in the dispersed phase, and a gradual decrease of ultrasonic amplitude when increasing the distance from the ultrasonic emitter (Arsad et al. 2014). Furthermore, when using high-intensity ultrasonic probes the temperature of the medium can rise up to 50–85 °C, which could degrade thermolabile compounds (Tiwari 2015).

4.2.5.2 Applications of UAE The application of UAE has been reported to enhance the extraction of multiple algal compounds such as carbohydrates (fucoidan, total glucans, agar, and alginates), carotenoids, proteins, pigments, and phenolic compounds summarized in Table 4.3.

Most of the UAE studies performed in the recent scientific literature have used low-intensity ultrasonic baths (Agregán et al. 2018; Chew et al. 2018; Dang et al. 2017; Eldalatony et al. 2016; Flórez-Fernández et al. 2019; Flórez-Fernández et al. 2017; Garcia-Vaquero et al. 2017a; Gayathri et al. 2018; Hmelkov et al. 2018; Tan et al. 2018). High-power ultrasonic probes are being currently explored in the marine sector to obtain high yields of valuable compounds (Garcia-Vaquero et al. 2018). A recent study optimized UAE to obtain high yields of polysaccharides and antioxidant activities from *Laminaria digitata* (Garcia-Vaquero et al. 2018). A semi-industrial ultra-sonication device (power 500 W and 20 kHz) was used to determine the optimum temperature (°C), time (minutes), and sonication amplitude (%) to achieve high yields of fucoidan (80 °C, 30 minutes, and 40%) and total glucans (52.5 °C, 10 minutes, and 100%) (Garcia-Vaquero et al. 2018). Moreover, the authors emphasized the need to develop protocols to achieve high yields of compounds while preserving intact the biological activities of the compounds that will be later used as nutraceuticals and functional foods (Garcia-Vaquero et al. 2018). An ultrasonic bath was recently used to obtain phenolic compounds and extracts with antioxidant activities from *Hormosira banksia* (Dang et al. 2017). The optimum extraction conditions to achieve high yields of phenolic compounds and antioxidant activities were 30 °C temperature, 60 minutes of extraction, and 60% of ultrasonic power. Using these conditions UAE was found to be more efficient than conventional technologies in terms of time and yields of extraction (Dang et al. 2017). An external clamp-on ultrasonic transducer was used as a pretreatment of microalgal biomass to increase the extraction of lipids for biofuel purposes. The UAE treatment of *C. vulgaris* and cyanobacteria *leptolyngbya* using 750 W of sonication power for 30 minutes doubled the recovery of lipids with respect to non-pretreated biomass (Ellison et al. 2019).

4.3 Combination Techniques

The sequential or simultaneous application of several conventional and/or emerging technologies has been explored recently to increase the efficiency and yields of high-value compounds obtained during the extraction processes. The use of UAE or MAE combined with conventional Soxhlet extraction increased the efficiency of this technology. The application of an ultrasonic probe in a thermostatic bath used to place

Table 4.3 Summary of the extraction conditions used in the recent literature to obtain multiple high-value compounds from algae (macroalgae and microalgae) applying ultrasound assisted extraction (UAE).

Species		UAE conditions	Targeted compounds	References
Macroalgae	*Sargassum muticum*	Ultrasonic bath (1.5 A, 150 W, and 40 Hz) at room temperature (25 °C) for 5–30 minutes	Carbohydrates (alginates)	Flórez-Fernández et al. (2019)
	Ascophyllum nodosum, *Fucus vesiculosus*, and *Bifurcaria bifurcata*	Ultrasonic bath (230–240 W and 40 kHz) at room temperature for 30 minutes	Phenolic compounds	Agregán et al. (2018)
	Gelidium amansii	Ultrasonic bath (30 kHz and 40% amplitude) for 30 minutes	Carbohydrates (agar)	Chew et al. (2018)
	Laminaria digitata, *Laminaria hyperborea*, and *Ascophyllum nodosum*	Ultrasonic horn (500 W and 20 kHz) optimized using 76 °C temperature, 10 minutes, and 100% of ultrasonic amplitude to achieve high yields of polysaccharides and antioxidant activities	Polysaccharides (fucoidan and total glucans)	Garcia-Vaquero et al. (2018)
	Fucus evanescens	Ultrasonic bath (150 W and 35 kHz) at room temperature for 5, 10, 15, 20, and 30 minutes	Total polysaccharides and fucoidan	Hmelkov et al. (2018)
	Hormosira banksii	Ultrasonic bath (250 W and 50 Hz) at 30 °C, 60 minutes, and 60% of power to obtain high yields of phenolic compounds	Phenolic compounds	Dang et al. (2017)
	Sargassum muticum	Ultrasonic bath (150 W and 40 kHz) at room temperature (25 °C) for 5–30 minutes	Polysaccharides (fucoidan)	Flórez-Fernández et al. (2017)
	Himanthalia elongata	Ultrasonic bath (130 W and 40 kHz) for 1 hour. The procedure was repeated twice	Proteins	Garcia-Vaquero et al. (2017ab)
	Chlorella vulgaris and *Leptolyngbya*	External clamp-on ultrasonic transducer (1000 W and 20 kHz) at 750 W of power for 30 minutes obtained high yields of lipids	Lipids	Ellison et al. (2019)

Microalgae	*Chlorella vulgaris* and *Spirulina platensis*	Ultrasonic bath (230–240 W and 40 kHz) at room temperature for 30 minutes	Phenolic compounds	Agregán et al. (2018)
	Chlorella salina	An ultrasonic bath was used to optimize the process of extraction of lutein, with maximum yields obtained at 40 °C, 30 minutes, and 35 kHz of ultrasound frequency	Carotenoids (lutein)	Gayathri et al. (2018)
	Microcystis aeruginosa, *Chlorella pyrenoidosa*, and *Chlamydomonas reinhardtii*	Ultrasonic bath (35 kHz and 0.043 W ml^{-1}) for 18 minutes to induce cell disruption in *Chlamydomonas reinhardtii* and 20 minutes in *Microcystis aeruginosa*. Only 50% of *Chlorella pyrenoidosa* was disrupted after treatments of 360 minutes	Pigments and proteins	Tan et al. (2018)
	Heterochlorella luteoviridis	Ultrasonic horn (50 W cm^{-2} and 20 kHz) at 40–80% of power to increase the extraction of carotenoids. The ultrasonic power did not affect the extraction of lipids	Lipids and carotenoids	Jaeschke et al. (2017)
	Chlamydomonas mexicana	An ultrasonic bath pretreatment at 2.2 kW, 40 KHz, and 50 °C for 15 minutes increased the extraction yields of total reducing sugars	Carbohydrates (reducing sugars)	Eldalatony et al. (2016)

the Soxhlet chamber decreased the number of Soxhlet cycles needed to extract oil compared with to the traditional approaches (Luque de Castro and Priego-Capote 2010). The application of microwave irradiation to the sample compartment of a Soxhlet device increased the yields of extraction of highly retained analytes and enhanced the automatability of the operations with respect to traditional Soxhlet (Luque de Castro and Priego-Capote 2010).

Enzyme assisted extraction (EAE) has been recently used as a pretreatment of the biomass to promote cell wall hydrolysis and increase the accessibility of solvents in the sample when performing the extraction using other techniques such as SFE (da Silva et al. 2016). UAE has also been recently explored combined with SFE to increase the yields and reduce the time and operation costs of extraction (Reátegui et al. 2014). However, the combination of UAE and SFE has certain limitations such as the high acoustic intensity required to induce cavitation when working at high pressure (Reátegui et al. 2014). The simultaneous application of ultrasounds and microwaves resulted in increased extraction yields of oil from multiple vegetable resources (Cravotto et al. 2008). Recently Patel et al. (2019) emphasized the huge improvements in the yield of oils extracted from yeast when using UAE and MAE combined, achieving extracts containing approximately 71% of lipids.

The application of innovative technologies combined with environmentally friendly solvents such as ionic liquids (ILs) is also being explored (da Silva et al. 2016). ILs are anionic and cationic salts with low melting points and liquid state at room temperature. These solvents have low vapor pressure, high thermal stability, and adjustable viscosity and miscibility with water and other organic solvents, allowing their application to extract both polar and nonpolar compounds (da Silva et al. 2016). However, the incomplete physical, chemical, and toxicological data of these solvents is currently the main factor limiting their application (da Silva et al. 2016). The use of IL (1-butyl-3-methylimidazolium tetrafluoroborate) combined with SWE at 175 °C, enhanced the extraction of phenolic compounds (gallic, chlorogenic, gentisic, protocatechuic, caffeic, and syringic acids) and antioxidant activities of the extracts obtained from *Saccharina japonica* compared with the use of SWE alone (Dinh et al. 2018).

4.4 Challenges and Future Perspectives

One of the key elements of a sustainable and green exploitation of natural resources is the reduction of chemical wastes generated while reducing the use of natural resources (Herrero and Ibáñez 2018; Tiwari 2015). Currently most extraction methodologies involve the use of organic or corrosive solvents to obtain high-value compounds. The use of innovative technologies to develop greener extraction protocols is one of the main challenges and key aspects of future development in the field of functional foods and nutraceuticals. The future greener extraction protocols developed should enhance the yields of high-value compounds obtained, reduce the energy input during the extraction process, and reduce or avoid the use of organic solvents (Tiwari 2015). The partial or complete replacement of chemicals during the process of extraction will reduce or eliminate the environmental and health hazards related to the disposal and work with these substances (Herrero and Ibáñez 2018; Tiwari 2015). Within this scenario, the aforementioned pressurized liquids, supercritical fluids, or ILs, together with organic aqueous tunable solvents and deep eutectic solvents, are novel tools that require further study and modeling to create new protocols that enable multiple extraction matrices and access to high-value compounds of a varied chemical nature (Herrero and Ibáñez 2018).

There is also a need to optimize the parameters of extraction when using innovative technologies by targeting increased yields of specific compounds from different matrices (Garcia-Vaquero et al. 2017b). Furthermore, the experimental conditions used during the process of extraction could influence greatly the chemical structure and biological properties of the compounds and, thus, there is a need to monitor the biological activities together with the yields of the compounds of interest to keep intact the biological properties and potential applications of the obtained products (Garcia-Vaquero et al. 2018).

The combination of multiple technologies or the development of multi-unit operation systems will also allow an increase in the yields of extraction and the sequential recovery of multiple high-value compounds from the biomass in agreement with the biorefinery concept (Herrero and Ibáñez 2018; Hayes et al. 2019). Gilbert-López et al. (2017) optimized the conditions for the sequential extraction of high-value compounds from *Scenedesmus obliquus* in three steps: SFE (using CO_2), gas expanded liquids (75% ethanol and 25% supercritical CO_2), and PLE (using water). These authors recovered phenolic compounds, carotenoids, proteins, and sugars with potent antioxidant activities and potential applications in the food industry.

Moreover, the innovative technologies and processes of extraction developed at laboratory scale will need to be scaled up for future industrial applications. These processes require future exploration and optimization, including environmental and economic studies (i.e. life cycle assessment) to offer better, safer, and greener alternatives to the conventional protocols and processes currently used to recover high-value compounds.

Acknowledgments

This work was supported by Science Foundation Ireland (SFI) [grant number: 14/IA/2548].

References

Agregán, R., Munekata, P.E.S., Franco, D. et al. (2018). Antioxidant potential of extracts obtained from macro- (*Ascophyllum nodosum, Fucus vesiculosus* and *Bifurcaria bifurcata*) and micro-algae (*Chlorella vulgaris* and *Spirulina platensis*) assisted by ultrasound. *Medicine* **5** (2): 33.

Amaro, H., Guedes, A., Preto, M. et al. (2018). *Gloeothece* sp. as a nutraceutical source – an improved method of extraction of carotenoids and fatty acids. *Marine Drugs* **16** (9): 327.

Anastas, P.T. and Warner, J.C. (2000). *Green Chemistry: Theory and Practice*, vol. **30**. Oxford: Oxford University Press.

Arsad, A., Danlami, J., Zaini, M.A.A., and Sulaiman, H. (2014). A comparative study of various oil extraction techniques from plants, Reviews in Chemical Engineering. **30** (6): 605–626.

Balasubramanian, S., Allen, J.D., Kanitkar, A., and Boldor, D. (2011). Oil extraction from *Scenedesmus obliquus* using a continuous microwave system – design, optimization, and quality characterization. *Bioresource Technology* **102** (3): 3396–3403.

Barba, F.J., Parniakov, O., Pereira, S.A. et al. (2015). Current applications and new opportunities for the use of pulsed electric fields in food science and industry. *Food Research International* **77**: 773–798. https://doi.org/10.1016/j.foodres.2015.09.015.

Bodénès, P., Bensalem, S., Français, O. et al. (2019). Inducing reversible or irreversible pores in *Chlamydomonas reinhardtii* with electroporation: impact of treatment parameters. *Algal Research* **37**: 124–132. https://doi.org/10.1016/j.algal.2018.11.016.

Castejón, N. and Javier Señoráns, F. (2019). Simultaneous extraction and fractionation of omega-3 acylglycerols and glycolipids from wet microalgal biomass of Nannochloropsis gaditana using pressurized liquids. *Algal Research* **37**: 74–82.

Chemat, F., Vian, M.A., and Cravotto, G. (2012). Green extraction of natural products: concept and principles. *International Journal of Molecular Sciences* **13** (7): 8615–8627.

Chemat, F., Fabiano-Tixier, A.S., Vian, M.A. et al. (2015). Solvent-free extraction of food and natural products. *TrAC Trends in Analytical Chemistry* **71**: 157–168.

Chemat, F., Rombaut, N., Meullemiestre, A. et al. (2017). Review of green food processing techniques. Preservation, transformation, and extraction. *Innovative Food Science & Emerging Technologies* **41**: 357–377.

Chew, K.W., Show, P.L., Yap, Y.J. et al. (2018). Sonication and grinding pre-treatments on Gelidium amansii seaweed for the extraction and characterization of Agarose. *Frontiers of Environmental Science & Engineering* **12** (4): 2. https://doi.org/10.1007/s11783-018-1040-0.

Cravotto, G., Boffa, L., Mantegna, S. et al. (2008). Improved extraction of vegetable oils under high-intensity ultrasound and/or microwaves. *Ultrasonics Sonochemistry* **15** (5): 898–902. https://doi.org/10.1016/j.ultsonch.2007.10.009.

Dang, T.T., Van Vuong, Q., Schreider, M.J. et al. (2017). Optimisation of ultrasound-assisted extraction conditions for phenolic content and antioxidant activities of the alga *Hormosira banksii* using response surface methodology. *Journal of Applied Phycology* **29** (6): 3161–3173.

Dinh, T.V., Saravana, P.S., Woo, H.C., and Chun, B.S. (2018). Ionic liquid-assisted subcritical water enhances the extraction of phenolics from brown seaweed and its antioxidant activity. *Separation and Purification Technology* **196**: 287–299.

Eldalatony, M.M., Kabra, A.N., Hwang, J.-H. et al. (2016). Pretreatment of microalgal biomass for enhanced recovery/extraction of reducing sugars and proteins. *Bioprocess and Biosystems Engineering* **39** (1): 95–103.

Ellison, C.R., Overa, S., and Boldor, D. (2019). Central composite design parameterization of microalgae/cyanobacteria co-culture pretreatment for enhanced lipid extraction using an external clamp-on ultrasonic transducer. *Ultrasonics Sonochemistry* **51**: 496–503.

Esquivel-Hernández, D.A., López, V.H., Rodríguez-Rodríguez, J. et al. (2016). Supercritical carbon dioxide and microwave-assisted extraction of functional lipophilic compounds from *Arthrospira platensis*. *International Journal of Molecular Sciences* **17** (5): 658.

Esquivel-Hernández, D.A., Ibarra-Garza, I.P., Rodríguez-Rodríguez, J. et al. (2017). Green extraction technologies for high-value metabolites from algae: a review. *Biofuels, Bioproducts and Biorefining* **11** (1): 215–231.

Fabrowska, J., Ibañez, E., Łęska, B., and Herrero, M. (2016). Supercritical fluid extraction as a tool to valorize underexploited freshwater green algae. *Algal Research* **19**: 237–245.

Feller, R., Matos, Â.P., Mazzutti, S. et al. (2018). Polyunsaturated ω-3 and ω-6 fatty acids, total carotenoids and antioxidant activity of three marine microalgae extracts obtained by supercritical CO_2 and subcritical n-butane. *The Journal of Supercritical Fluids* **133**: 437–443.

Flórez-Fernández, N., López-García, M., González-Muñoz, M.J. et al. (2017). Ultrasound-assisted extraction of fucoidan from *Sargassum muticum*. *Journal of Applied Phycology* **29** (3): 1553–1561. https://doi.org/10.1007/s10811-016-1043-9.

Flórez-Fernández, N., Domínguez, H., and Torres, M.D. (2019). A green approach for alginate extraction from *Sargassum muticum* brown seaweed using ultrasound-assisted technique. *International Journal of Biological Macromolecules* **124**: 451–459.

Gallego, R., Montero, L., Cifuentes, A. et al. (2018). Green extraction of bioactive compounds from microalgae. *Journal of Analysis and Testing* **2** (2): 109–123. https://doi.org/10.1007/s41664-018-0061-9.

Gammone, M. and D'Orazio, N. (2015). Anti-obesity activity of the marine carotenoid fucoxanthin. *Marine Drugs* **13** (4): 2196–2214.

Garcia-Vaquero, M. and Hayes, M. (2016). Red and green macroalgae for fish and animal feed and human functional food development. *Food Reviews International* **32** (1): 15–45. https://doi.org/10.1080/87559129.2015.1041184.

Garcia-Vaquero, M., Lopez-Alonso, M., and Hayes, M. (2017a). Assessment of the functional properties of protein extracted from the brown seaweed *Himanthalia elongata* (Linnaeus) SF Gray. *Food Research International* **99**: 971–978.

Garcia-Vaquero, M., Gaurav, R., O'Doherty, J.V., and Sweeney, T. (2017b). Polysaccharides from macroalgae: recent advances, innovative technologies and challenges in extraction and purification. *Food Research International* **99**: 1011–1020.

Garcia-Vaquero, M., Rajauria, G., Tiwari, B. et al. (2018). Extraction and yield optimisation of fucose, glucans and associated antioxidant activities from *Laminaria digitata* by applying response surface methodology to high intensity ultrasound-assisted extraction. *Marine Drugs* **16** (8): 257.

Gayathri, S., Rajasree Radhika, S.R., Suman, T.Y., and Aranganathan, L. (2018). Ultrasound-assisted microextraction of β, ε-carotene-3, 3′-diol (lutein) from marine microalgae *Chlorella salina*: effect of different extraction parameters. *Biomass Conversion and Biorefinery* **8** (4): 791–797.

Getachew, A.T., Saravana, P.S., Cho, Y.J. et al. (2018). Concurrent extraction of oil from roasted coffee (*Coffea arabica*) and fucoxanthin from brown seaweed (*Saccharina japonica*) using supercritical carbon dioxide. *Journal of CO_2 Utilization* **25**: 137–146. https://doi.org/10.1016/j.jcou.2018.03.018.

Gilbert-López, B., Mendiola, J.A., van den Broek, L.A.M. et al. (2017). Green compressed fluid technologies for downstream processing of Scenedesmus obliquus in a biorefinery approach. *Algal Research* **24**: 111–121.

Grimi, N., Dubois, A., Marchal, L. et al. (2014). Selective extraction from microalgae Nannochloropsis sp. using different methods of cell disruption. *Bioresource Technology* **153**: 254–259.

Guldhe, A., Singh, B., Rawat, I. et al. (2014). Efficacy of drying and cell disruption techniques on lipid recovery from microalgae for biodiesel production. *Fuel* **128**: 46–52.

Hayes, M., Bastiaens, L., Gouveia, L. et al. (2019). Microalgal bioactive compounds including protein, peptides, and pigments: applications, opportunities, and challenges during biorefinery processes. In: *Novel Proteins for Food, Pharmaceuticals and Agriculture: Sources, Applications and Advances* (ed. M. Hayes), 239–255. Hoboken, NJ: Wiley.

Heffernan, N., Smyth, T.J., FitzGerald, R.J. et al. (2016). Comparison of extraction methods for selected carotenoids from macroalgae and the assessment of their seasonal/spatial variation. *Innovative Food Science & Emerging Technologies* **37**: 221–228.

Herrero, M. and Ibáñez, E. (2015). Green processes and sustainability: an overview on the extraction of high added-value products from seaweeds and microalgae. *The Journal of Supercritical Fluids* **96**: 211–216.

Herrero, M. and Ibáñez, E. (2018). Green extraction processes, biorefineries and sustainability: recovery of high added-value products from natural sources. *The Journal of Supercritical Fluids* **134**: 252–259.

Herrero, M., Cifuentes, A., and Ibáñez, E. (2006). Sub- and supercritical fluid extraction of functional ingredients from different natural sources: plants, food-by-products, algae and microalgae: a review. *Food Chemistry* **98** (1): 136–148. https://doi.org/10.1016/j.foodchem.2005.05.058.

Herrero, M., Castro-Puyana, M., Mendiola, J.A., and Ibáñez, E. (2013). Compressed fluids for the extraction of bioactive compounds. *TrAC Trends in Analytical Chemistry* **43**: 67–83. https://doi.org/10.1016/j.trac.2012.12.008.

Hmelkov, A.B., Zvyagintseva, T.N., Shevchenko, N.M. et al. (2018). Ultrasound-assisted extraction of polysaccharides from brown alga *Fucus evanescens*. Structure and biological activity of the new fucoidan fractions. *Journal of Applied Phycology* **30** (3): 2039–2046. https://doi.org/10.1007/s10811-017-1342-9.

Holdt, S.L. and Kraan, S. (2011). Bioactive compounds in seaweed: functional food applications and legislation. *Journal of Applied Phycology* **23** (3): 543–597. https://doi.org/10.1007/s10811-010-9632-5.

Jaeschke, D.P., Rech, R., Marczak, L.D.F., and Mercali, G.D. (2017). Ultrasound as an alternative technology to extract carotenoids and lipids from *Heterochlorella luteoviridis*. *Bioresource Technology* **224**: 753–757.

Kapoore, R., Butler, T., Pandhal, J., and Vaidyanathan, S. (2018). Microwave-assisted extraction for microalgae: from biofuels to biorefinery. *Biology* **7** (1): 18.

Kwan, T.A., Kwan, S.E., Peccia, J., and Zimmerman, J.B. (2018). Selectively biorefining astaxanthin and triacylglycerol co-products from microalgae with supercritical carbon dioxide extraction. *Bioresource Technology* **269**: 81–88.

Lam, G.P.'t., Postma, P.R., Fernandes, D.A. et al. (2017). Pulsed electric field for protein release of the microalgae *Chlorella vulgaris* and *Neochloris oleoabundans*. *Algal Research* **24**: 181–187. https://doi.org/10.1016/j.algal.2017.03.024.

Lorenzen, J., Igl, N., Tippelt, M. et al. (2017). Extraction of microalgae derived lipids with supercritical carbon dioxide in an industrial relevant pilot plant. *Bioprocess and Biosystems Engineering* **40** (6): 911–918.

Luengo, E., Condón-Abanto, S., Álvarez, I., and Raso, J. (2014). Effect of pulsed electric field treatments on permeabilization and extraction of pigments from *Chlorella vulgaris*. *The Journal of Membrane Biology* **247** (12): 1269–1277. https://doi.org/10.1007/s00232-014-9688-2.

Luengo, E., Martínez, J.M., Bordetas, A. et al. (2015). Influence of the treatment medium temperature on lutein extraction assisted by pulsed electric fields from *Chlorella vulgaris*. *Innovative Food Science & Emerging Technologies* **29**: 15–22. https://doi.org/10.1016/j.ifset.2015.02.012.

Luque de Castro, M.D. and Priego-Capote, F. (2010). Soxhlet extraction: past and present panacea. *Journal of Chromatography A* **1217** (16): 2383–2389. https://doi.org/10.1016/j.chroma.2009.11.027.

Markets and Markets. (2018). Functional food ingredients market by type (probiotics, prebiotics, proteins & amino acids, phytochemical & plant extracts, omega-3 fatty acids, carotenoids, fibers & specialty carbohydrates), application, source, and region – global forecast to 2023. https://www.marketsandmarkets.com/Market-Reports/functional-food-ingredients-market-9242020.html (accessed September 3, 2020).

Martínez, J.M., Luengo, E., Saldaña, G. et al. (2017). C-phycocyanin extraction assisted by pulsed electric field from *Artrosphira platensis*. *Food Research International* **99**: 1042–1047. https://doi.org/10.1016/j.foodres.2016.09.029.

McKennedy, J., Önenç, S., Pala, M., and Maguire, J. (2016). Supercritical carbon dioxide treatment of the microalgae Nannochloropsis oculata for the production of fatty acid methyl esters. *The Journal of Supercritical Fluids* **116**: 264–270.

Menéndez, B., Miguel, J., Arenillas, A. et al. (2014). Optimization of microalgae oil extraction under ultrasound and microwave irradiation. *Journal of Chemical Technology and Biotechnology* **89** (11): 1779–1784. https://doi.org/10.1002/jctb.4272.

Michalak, I., Górka, B., Wieczorek, P.P. et al. (2016). Supercritical fluid extraction of algae enhances levels of biologically active compounds promoting plant growth. *European Journal of Phycology* **51** (3): 243–252.

Molino, A., Mehariya, S., Iovine, A. et al. (2018). Extraction of astaxanthin and lutein from microalga *Haematococcus pluvialis* in the red phase using CO_2 supercritical fluid extraction technology with ethanol as co-solvent. *Marine Drugs* **16** (11): 432.

de Moura, R.R., Etges, B.J., dos Santos, E.O. et al. (2018). Microwave-assisted extraction of lipids from wet microalgae paste: a quick and efficient method. *European Journal of Lipid Science and Technology* **120** (7): 1700419. https://doi.org/10.1002/ejlt.201700419.

Nobre, B.P., Villalobos, F., Barragan, B.E. et al. (2013). A biorefinery from *Nannochloropsis* sp. microalga – extraction of oils and pigments. Production of biohydrogen from the leftover biomass. *Bioresource Technology* **135**: 128–136.

Obeid, S., Beaufils, N., Camy, S. et al. (2018). Supercritical carbon dioxide extraction and fractionation of lipids from freeze-dried microalgae *Nannochloropsis oculata* and *Chlorella vulgaris*. *Algal Research* **34**: 49–56.

Onumaegbu, C., Alaswad, A., Rodriguez, C., and Olabi, A. (2019). Modelling and optimization of wet microalgae *Scenedesmus quadricauda* lipid extraction using microwave pre-treatment method and response surface methodology. *Renewable Energy* **132**: 1323–1331. https://doi.org/10.1016/j.renene.2018.09.008.

Ospina, M., Castro-Vargas, H.I., and Parada-Alfonso, F. (2017). Antioxidant capacity of Colombian seaweeds: 1. Extracts obtained from *Gracilaria mammillaris* by means of supercritical fluid extraction. *The Journal of Supercritical Fluids* **128**: 314–322.

Otero, P., Quintana, S.E., Reglero, G. et al. (2018). Pressurized liquid extraction (PLE) as an innovative green technology for the effective enrichment of Galician algae extracts with high quality fatty acids and antimicrobial and antioxidant properties. *Marine Drugs* **16** (5): 156.

Otero, P., López-Martínez, M.I., and García-Risco, M.R. (2019). Application of pressurized liquid extraction (PLE) to obtain bioactive fatty acids and phenols from *Laminaria ochroleuca* collected in Galicia (NW Spain). *Journal of Pharmaceutical and Biomedical Analysis* **164**: 86–92. https://doi.org/10.1016/j.jpba.2018.09.057.

Patel, A., Arora, N., Pruthi, V., and Pruthi, P.A. (2019). A novel rapid ultrasonication-microwave treatment for total lipid extraction from wet oleaginous yeast biomass for sustainable biodiesel production. *Ultrasonics Sonochemistry* **51**: 504–516.

Pérez-López, P., Balboa, E.M., González-García, S. et al. (2014). Comparative environmental assessment of valorization strategies of the invasive macroalgae *Sargassum muticum*. *Bioresource Technology* **161**: 137–148.

Plaza, M., Santoyo, S., Laura, J. et al. (2010). Screening for bioactive compounds from algae. *Journal of Pharmaceutical and Biomedical Analysis* **51** (2): 450–455.

Polikovsky, M., Fernand, F., Sack, M. et al. (2016). Towards marine biorefineries: selective proteins extractions from marine macroalgae *Ulva* with pulsed electric fields. *Innovative Food Science & Emerging Technologies* **37**: 194–200. https://doi.org/10.1016/j.ifset.2016.03.013.

Quitain, A.T., Kai, T., Sasaki, M., and Goto, M. (2013). Supercritical carbon dioxide extraction of fucoxanthin from *Undaria pinnatifida*. *Journal of Agricultural and Food Chemistry* **61** (24): 5792–5797.

Qv, X.-Y., Zhou, Q.-F., and Jiang, J.-G. (2014). Ultrasound-enhanced and microwave-assisted extraction of lipid from *Dunaliella tertiolecta* and fatty acid profile analysis. *Journal of Separation Science* **37** (20): 2991–2999.

Raso, J., Frey, W., Ferrari, G. et al. (2016). Recommendations guidelines on the key information to be reported in studies of application of PEF technology in food and biotechnological processes. *Innovative Food Science & Emerging Technologies* **37**: 312–321. https://doi.org/10.1016/j.ifset.2016.08.003.

Reátegui, J.L.P., da Fonseca Machado, A.P., Barbero, G.F. et al. (2014). Extraction of antioxidant compounds from blackberry (*Rubus* sp.) bagasse using supercritical CO_2 assisted by ultrasound. *The Journal of Supercritical Fluids* **94**: 223–233.

Robin, A. and Golberg, A. (2016). Pulsed electric fields and electroporation technologies in marine macroalgae biorefineries. In: *Handbook of Electroporation* (ed. D. Miklavčič), 1–16. Cham: Springer.

Robin, A., Sack, M., Israel, A. et al. (2018). Deashing macroalgae biomass by pulsed electric field treatment. *Bioresource Technology* **255**: 131–139. https://doi.org/10.1016/j.biortech.2018.01.089.

Rodriguez-Jasso, R.M., Mussatto, S.I., Pastrana, L. et al. (2011). Microwave-assisted extraction of sulfated polysaccharides (fucoidan) from brown seaweed. *Carbohydrate Polymers* **86** (3): 1137–1144.

Ruen-ngam, D., Shotipruk, A., Pavasant, P. et al. (2012). Selective extraction of lutein from alcohol treated *Chlorella vulgaris* by supercritical CO_2. *Chemical Engineering & Technology* **35** (2): 255–260.

Sack, M., Sigler, J., Frenzel, S. et al. (2010). Research on industrial-scale electroporation devices fostering the extraction of substances from biological tissue. *Food Engineering Reviews* **2** (2): 147–156.

Safi, C., Cabas Rodriguez, L., Mulder, W.J. et al. (2017). Energy consumption and water-soluble protein release by cell wall disruption of *Nannochloropsis gaditana*. *Bioresource Technology* **239**: 204–210. https://doi.org/10.1016/j.biortech.2017.05.012.

Sanzo, G., Mehariya, S., Martino, M. et al. (2018). Supercritical carbon dioxide extraction of astaxanthin, lutein, and fatty acids from *Haematococcus pluvialis* microalgae. *Marine Drugs* **16** (9): 334.

Saravana, P.S., Getachew, A.T., Cho, Y.-J. et al. (2017). Influence of co-solvents on fucoxanthin and phlorotannin recovery from brown seaweed using supercritical CO_2. *The Journal of Supercritical Fluids* **120**: 295–303.

da Silva, R.P.F.F., Rocha-Santos, T.A.P., and Duarte, A.C. (2016). Supercritical fluid extraction of bioactive compounds. *TrAC Trends in Analytical Chemistry* **76**: 40–51. https://doi.org/10.1016/j.trac.2015.11.013.

Silva, A.d.S.e., Teixeira de Magalhães, W., Moreira, L.M. et al. (2018). Microwave-assisted extraction of polysaccharides from *Arthrospira* (*Spirulina*) *platensis* using the concept of green chemistry. *Algal Research* **35**: 178–184. https://doi.org/10.1016/j.algal.2018.08.015.

Sivagnanam, S.P., Yin, S., Choi, J.H. et al. (2015). Biological properties of fucoxanthin in oil recovered from two brown seaweeds using supercritical CO_2 extraction. *Marine Drugs* **13** (6): 3422–3442.

Solana, M., Rizza, C.S., and Bertucco, A. (2014). Exploiting microalgae as a source of essential fatty acids by supercritical fluid extraction of lipids: comparison between *Scenedesmus obliquus*, *Chlorella protothecoides* and *Nannochloropsis salina*. *The Journal of Supercritical Fluids* **92**: 311–318.

Sosa-Hernández, J., Escobedo-Avellaneda, Z., Iqbal, H., and Welti-Chanes, J. (2018). State-of-the-art extraction methodologies for bioactive compounds from algal biome to meet bio-economy challenges and opportunities. *Molecules* **23** (11): 2953.

Sticher, O. (2008). Natural product isolation. *Natural Product Reports* **25** (3): 517–554.

Tan, X., Zhang, D., Parajuli, K. et al. (2018). Comparison of four quantitative techniques for monitoring microalgae disruption by low-frequency ultrasound and acoustic energy efficiency. *Environmental Science & Technology* **52** (5): 3295–3303.

Tiwari, B.K. (2015). Ultrasound: a clean, green extraction technology. *TrAC Trends in Analytical Chemistry* **71**: 100–109.

Toepfl, S. (2012). Pulsed electric field food processing–industrial equipment design and commercial applications. *Stewart Postharvest Review* **8**: 1–7.

Tommasi, E., Cravotto, G., Galletti, P. et al. (2017). Enhanced and selective lipid extraction from the microalga *P. tricornutum* by dimethyl carbonate and supercritical CO_2 using deep eutectic solvents and microwaves as pretreatment. *ACS Sustainable Chemistry & Engineering* **5** (9): 8316–8322.

del Valle, J.M., Martín, Á., Cocero, M.J. et al. (2019). Supercritical CO_2 extraction of solids using aqueous ethanol as static modifier is a two-step mass transfer process. *The Journal of Supercritical Fluids* **143**: 179–190.

Wang, L. and Weller, C.L. (2006). Recent advances in extraction of nutraceuticals from plants. *Trends in Food Science & Technology* **17** (6): 300–312. https://doi.org/10.1016/j.tifs.2005.12.004.

Xiao, X.-H., Yuan, Z.-Q., and Li, G.-K. (2013). Preparation of phytosterols and phytol from edible marine algae by microwave-assisted extraction and high-speed counter-current chromatography. *Separation and Purification Technology* **104**: 284–289. https://doi.org/10.1016/j.seppur.2012.11.032.

Yen, H.-W., Yang, S.-C., Chen, C.-H. et al. (2015). Supercritical fluid extraction of valuable compounds from microalgal biomass. *Bioresource Technology* **184**: 291–296. https://doi.org/10.1016/j.biortech.2014.10.030.

Yuan, Y., Xu, X., Jing, C. et al. (2018a). Microwave assisted hydrothermal extraction of polysaccharides from *Ulva prolifera*: functional properties and bioactivities. *Carbohydrate Polymers* **181**: 902–910. https://doi.org/10.1016/j.carbpol.2017.11.061.

Yuan, Y., Zhang, J., Fan, J. et al. (2018b). Microwave assisted extraction of phenolic compounds from four economic brown macroalgae species and evaluation of their antioxidant activities and inhibitory effects on α-amylase, α-glucosidase, pancreatic lipase and tyrosinase. *Food Research International* **113**: 288–297. https://doi.org/10.1016/j.foodres.2018.07.021.

5 Extraction Technologies for Functional Lipids

Calle Niemi and Francesco G. Gentili
Department of Forest Biomaterials and Technology, Swedish University of Agricultural Sciences, Umeå, Sweden

5.1 Introduction

Lipids are a very diverse group of molecules usually composed of a minor polar hydrophilic part and a nonpolar hydrophobic majority. More than a specific molecular structure, it is hydrophobicity that characterizes the lipids; indeed lipids are soluble in organic solvents but not in water (Mathews et al. 2000; Berlitz et al. 2009). It is worth noting that until the beginning of the twentieth century, lipids or fat were not considered essential dietary components. Only in 1929 did George and Mildred Burr show that fatty acids were essential nutrients after observing that rats fed with a fat-free diet got a deficiency disease (Spector and Kim 2015).

In the past few decades, the function of foods has been shifting from substances consumed mainly to quench hunger, to substances that can potentially promote health and wellness, reducing the risk of diseases; these substances are called functional foods and/or nutraceuticals (Aryee and Boye 2015). The interest in functional foods and/or nutraceuticals is rapidly growing and has a market size that is estimated to reach over US$302 billion by 2022 (Prazad 2016).

Functional lipids can be considered as part of and/or an ingredient of functional foods. Well-known functional lipids are omega-3 polyunsaturated fatty acids (PUFAs) and carotenoids. Even sterols and terpenes can be included as functional lipids. Algae and in particular microalgae are an excellent sources of functional lipids such as PUFAs and carotenoids. Omega-3 PUFAs, especially eicosapentaenoic acid (EPA; 20:5) and docosahexaenoic acid (DHA; 22:6) are found mainly in marine microalgae and in lower amounts in marine macroalgae (Ibanez and Cifuentes 2013; Kadam et al. 2013; Otero et al. 2018). Diatoms (e.g. *Nitzchia* sp. and *Thalassiosira* sp.), haptophytes (e.g. *Pavlova* sp.), and eustigmatophytes (e.g. *Nannochloropsis* sp.) are very good omega-3 PUFA producers (Barba et al. 2015), while some green microalgae (e.g. *Haematococcus pluvialis*, *Chlorella* sp.) are very good carotenoid

Recent Advances in Micro- and Macroalgal Processing: Food and Health Perspectives, First Edition. Edited by Gaurav Rajauria and Yvonne V. Yuan.

producers (Leu and Boussiba 2014). However, to be "harvested" lipids need to be extracted from the algal cells. Indeed several microalgal species have a very thick cell wall made of polysaccharide and cellulose that accounts for about 10% of the algal dry weight (Buono et al. 2014). Often lipid extraction needs more steps represented by cell disruption, which is particularly important for some types of microalgae, and extraction and then fractionation or separation of the functional lipids from the rest of the intracellular compounds. We can divide the lipid extraction methods into two categories: conventional and nonconventional or novel methodologies. A schematic classification of the different extraction methods is summarized in Figure 5.1. The figure indicates the potential steps in the extraction process, going from harvested wet algal biomass to a finalized, functional lipid product. Extraction methods that primarily induce cell disruption are considered a form of pretreatment. An optimal procedure should limit processing steps, to lessen environmental impact and ensure economic viability.

For the purpose of industrial applications for a large-scale functional lipid production, the chapter focuses here on the novel extraction methods that are most promising when it comes to scalability, selectivity, nontoxicity, cost-effectiveness, and environmental sustainability. Minimizing pretreatment in the form of drying and extensive cell disruption procedures should be a goal for the development of industrial processes. Avoiding the need for poorly scalable, overly costly, or toxic fractionation or isolation procedures is also considered a benefit. Reducing environmental impact of the procedure is another focus, with the recent rise in "green" extraction technologies. Figure 5.1 shows a schematic view of the techniques discussed in this section. Extraction techniques that omit as much downstream processing as possible, or at the very least, limit it to scalable and cost-effective forms of processing, are highlighted.

5.2 Conventional Extraction Techniques for Functional Lipids

Conventional extraction techniques are based on the use of organic solvents (Table 5.1) with or without cell disruption as a pretreatment depending on algal cell permeability to the solvent used. The most known and used methods are the method of Folch et al. (1957) and Bligh and Dyer (1959). Both methods use organic solvents – a mixture of chloroform and methanol; however, the method by Folch et al. uses a chloroform:methanol ratio of 2:1 (v/v), while the Bligh and Dyer method uses an increasing stepwise ratio from 1:2 (v/v) to 1:1 (v/v). The choice of solvent system for the extraction of lipids from algae is of pivotal importance because it influences the extraction efficiency, which depends on cell wall permeability and type of organism (Lee et al. 1998). Even though the mixture of chloroform and methanol has generally given the highest extraction yields (Lee et al. 1998; Ryckebosch et al. 2012; Axelsson and Gentili 2014), other solvents and/or mixtures have been tested, especially to replace the chloroform due to its toxicity (The Merck Index 2013). In recent decades, less toxic organic solvents, and/or solvent mixtures such as hexane/isopropanol (3:2, v/v), dichloroethane/methanol (1:1, v/v), dichloroethane/ethanol (1:1, v/v), acetone, diethyl ether, acetone/dichloromethane (1:1, v/v), and methyl-tert-butyl ether/methanol 10:3 (Hara and Radin 1978; Lee et al. 1998; Ryckebosch et al. 2012)

Table 5.1 Comparison of advantages and disadvantages of conventional and novel methods for functional lipid extraction.

Traditional methodologies			Novel methodologies		
	Advantages	**Disadvantages**		**Advantages**	**Disadvantages**
Based on organic solvents	• Inexpensive • Well established • Used at commercial scale	• Toxic • Polluting • Nonselective	Ionic liquid extraction	• Selective • Suitable for functional lipids and foods • Potentially nontoxic	• Costly • Not yet available at large scale
			Supercritical fluid extraction	• Nontoxic • Selective • Suitable for functional lipids and foods • Scalable	• Costly
			Pressurized liquid extraction	• Selective • Less toxic than traditional methodologies	• Costly • Possible thermal degradation of functional lipids and food

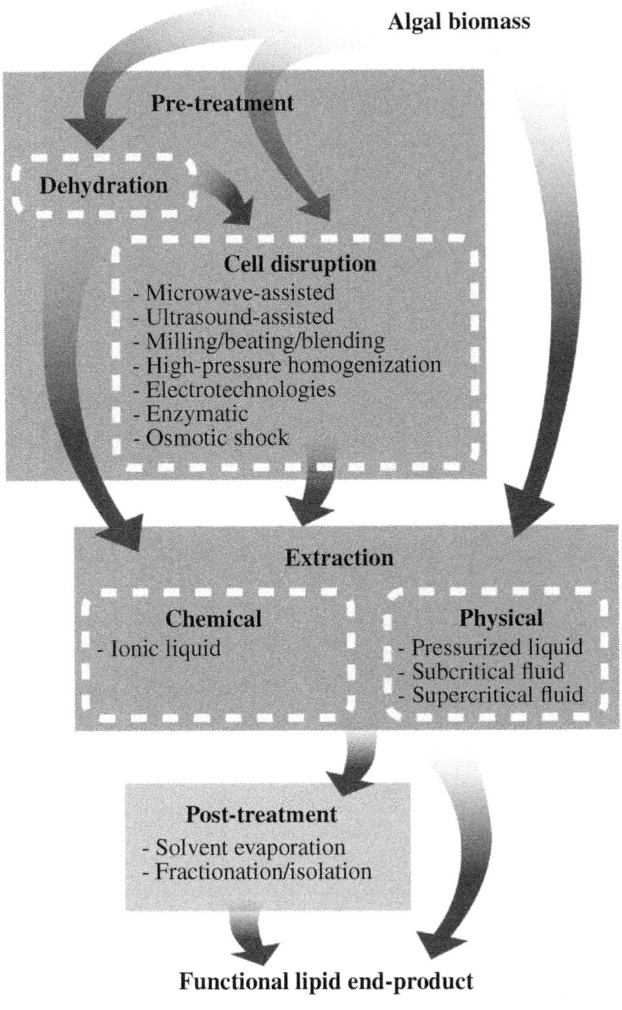

Figure 5.1 Schematic view of novel techniques for the extraction of functional lipids from algae.

have also been tested. The conventional methods can be preceded by a cell disruption step such as French press, bead milling, Potter–Elvehjelm homogenizer, cell homogenizer, autoclave, or microwave (Lee et al. 1998; Axelsson and Gentili 2014; Singh et al. 2019). Often organic solvents are used in a Soxhlet extractor (Ekendahl et al. 2018; Kumar et al. 2018), which is a glass apparatus where the organic solvent is first evaporated then condensed and left to drip over the algal biomass placed in a thimble-holder. The evaporation–condensation cycle of the solvent is repeated several times until the lipids are totally removed from the algal sample.

As described in Figure 5.1 the lipid extraction process can be divided into three steps: pretreatment (dehydration, cell disruption), extraction, and post-treatment (solvent evaporation, fractionation, and purification). Several of the novel methods for algal cell disruption and for extraction have been tested during the past few years/decades. They have been adopted from other research/industrial areas such as microbiological processes of bacteria and yeasts. However, many of these novel methods are in reality a mixture of novel and conventional methods because they still use standard organic solvents to extract the lipids.

5.3 Application of Novel Extraction Technologies for Functional Lipids

There are several novel nonconventional methods that have been developed to extract algal lipids (Table 5.1) and in particular functional algal lipids to maintain their quality and functionality. As shown in Figure 5.1 the novel extraction methods can be divided into three main subgroups: physical, chemical, and enzymatic methods. Several of these methods are an advancement to improve efficiency of lipids yield and work as a pretreatment to extraction systems based on the use of organic solvents.

5.3.1 Algal Cell Disruption Methods

Disruption methods can be seen as extraction pretreatments needed to break down cell walls and cell membranes to release the intracellular compounds. Especially for the extraction of products such as functional lipids, it is very important to choose a disruption method that does not alter the quality of the products. Hence, methods that avoid excess heat, oxidation, and reduce or minimize the use of traditional organic solvents should be the choice for the extraction of functional lipids. Furthermore, a disruption method should improve and facilitate the successive extraction and post-treatment processes.

5.3.1.1 Bead Milling Bead milling is a mechanical cell disruption method where algal cells are broken by direct impact with beads, which can be made of different materials such as glass, zirconia-silica, zirconium oxide, or titanium carbide (Shen et al. 2009; Kumar et al. 2015). Bead milling is a method that can be used for both dry and wet algal biomass. The latter avoids a drying operation, thus reducing the processing costs. During milling the temperature can increase, damaging the quality of functional lipids; to avoid this problem there are bead milling apparatuses with cooling jackets. Bead milling is an energy-intensive method and difficult to scale up (Kumar et al. 2015).

5.3.1.2 Electrotechnologies In the past few years electrotechnologies have been used to extract valuable compounds from algae (Zbinden et al. 2013; Grimi et al. 2014; Goettel et al. 2013; Barba et al. 2015; Geada et al. 2018). Electrotechnology methods include pulsed electric field (PEF), high-voltage electrostatic field (HVEF), and high-voltage electric discharge (HVED). The most used method is the PEF, which is performed by applying multiple short pulses for less than a second (generally in the order of μs to ms) of high-intensity electric fields (20–50 $kV\,cm^{-1}$) between two electrodes. The application of a PEF damages the algal cell membrane producing electropores (holes) in the algae cell membrane so that the cell contents can be efficiently extracted using organic solvents (Zbinden et al. 2013; Goettel et al. 2013;

Parniakov et al. 2015). The energy demand of PEF to obtain a considerable microalgal cell disruption is about 4.8% of the upper heating value of the algae; however, this procedure led to release of the soluble compounds (Goettel et al. 2013). Hence, to extract lipids from microalgae, PEF should be combined with the organic solvents (Zbinden et al. 2013; Parniakov et al. 2015).

Two other electrotechnology methods have been proposed as potentially useful for extraction of functional food additives from microalgae: HVEF and HVED (Barba et al. 2015). HVEF is a nonpulsed electrostatic field treatment while HVED is a pulsed electrical technique where the discharge is produced by two submersed electrodes that release energy directly into the aqueous solution where the cells are present (Grimi et al. 2014; Barba et al. 2015; Delsart et al. 2016). However, in a study on the extraction of pigments (chlorophylls and carotenoids) from *Nannochloropsis* sp., HVED was shown to be rather ineffective (Grimi et al. 2014).

5.3.1.3 Enzymatic Methods Enzyme assisted extraction (EAE) has attracted interest during the past few years (Wang et al. 2015; Zuorro et al. 2016; Kumar et al. 2017; Qiu et al. 2019). EAE has been used alone or in combination with other extraction and/or cell disruption techniques such as high pressure homogenization (HPH) or ultrasound (Liang et al. 2012; Wang et al. 2015). EAE is performed using single enzymes such as, e.g. cellulases or proteinases, or a multi-enzyme mixture, such as cellulase and proteinase, or cellulase and mannanases, or a combination of other hydrolytic enzymes (Huo et al. 2015; Wang et al. 2015; Zuorro et al. 2016; Qiu et al. 2019). On one hand EAE is a rapid, highly specific, and nontoxic method suitable for algal biorefinery; on the other hand, it is a costly technique (Kumar et al. 2017).

5.3.1.4 High Pressure Homogenization (HPH) HPH HPH is a mechanical cell disruption technique that breaks the cell at pressures from 20–275 MPa (Samarasinghe et al. 2012; Grimi et al. 2014; Mulchandani et al. 2015; Wang et al. 2015). HPH has been used together with three-phase partitioning (ammonum sulfate/slurry/t-butanol) for the successful recovery of algal lipids and carotenoids (Mulchandani et al. 2015). When dealing with HPH, the most relevant parameters are the pressure differential across the nozzle and the number of passes through the homogenizer (Samarasinghe et al. 2012). HPH is an efficient method of cell disruption that can be scaled up. However, it has the following drawbacks: high energy consumption, it is nonselective, and it can damage sensitive compounds due to the increase of temperature (Grimi et al. 2014; Barba et al. 2015).

5.3.1.5 Microwaves Microwave assisted extraction (MAE) has been successfully used for the extraction of bioactive molecules from plant materials and macroalgae (Sosa-Hernandez et al. 2018). MAE is a promising method for improving lipid extraction efficiency (Balasubramanian et al. 2011; Kumar et al. 2017; Almeida Nogueira et al. 2018). It has been shown that MAE gave a higher lipid yield at lower temperatures compared with autoclaving and conventional heating (Singh et al. 2019). Compared with conventional methods, MAE is more environmentally friendly, more economical, faster, needs less solvent, and inhibits degradation of thermolabile compounds (Kumar et al. 2017; Sosa-Hernandez et al. 2018). On the other hand, MAE needs filtration or centrifugation to remove the solid residues and efficiency can be very poor for nonpolar compounds (Kumar et al. 2017).

5.3.1.6 Osmotic Shock Osmotic shock is a method of cell disruption that has been successfully tested in different algal strains (Yoo et al. 2012; Byreddy et al. 2015). As pointed out by Naghdi et al. (2016), the main bottleneck of osmotic shock is represented by its dependency on the algal species. In other words, osmotic shock efficiency is species-dependent and it should be tuned for each species. However osmotic shock is a low-cost method using less energy than other methods, but requires longer treatment times (Kumar et al. 2015).

5.3.1.7 Ultrasound Ultrasound is a technique that uses ultrasonic cavitation and acoustic streaming to lyse the algal cells and release the lipids (Byreddy et al. 2015; Kumar et al. 2015; Marrone et al. 2018). Ultrasound has been successfully used to disrupt cells of *Chlorellasp.* and some cyanobacteria species (Prabakaran and Ravindran 2011; Byreddy et al. 2015). Ultrasound is a fast cell disruption method that needs less solvent and better penetrates into the cells; moreover, it is a method suitable for all cell types. However, it has high power consumption, is difficult to scale up, and in the case of a prolonged process, it can damage the chemical structure of the molecules thereby reducing the quality of the products (Byreddy et al. 2015; Kumar et al. 2015, 2017). However, when ultrasound was performed at a low temperature (−4 °C) for 90 minutes it showed very good results in terms of the quality of pigments and fatty acids produced (Wiltshire et al. 2000).

In conclusion, several cell disruption methods are very interesting and promising to help or assist lipid extraction. There are studies using a combination of different cell disruption techniques such as enzymatic hydrolysis and high-pressure homogenization or ultrasound. We should bear in mind that the above-described methods were originally developed to extract lipids and other compounds from plant materials and microorganisms such as bacteria and yeasts and only later have been tested for algae.

Moreover the majority of these methods have been tested at laboratory scale on a few algal strains. Hence future studies should focus on the application of these methods on several different algal strains and then on the upscaling of the most promising and suitable methods.

5.3.2 Novel Extraction Methods

The use of a nontoxic and environmentally friendly solvent plays a pivotal role in the successful development of a novel sustainable functional lipid extraction process. Kumar et al. (2017) describe several different promising solvents that have been recently used or that have potential for the extraction of algal lipids. The described solvents are the following: bio-derived solvents, supercritical CO_2, ionic liquid (IL), switchable solvents, liquid polymers, deep eutectic solvents, natural deep eutectic solvents, fluorous solvents, and supramolecular solvents. Among these solvents IL and supercritical CO_2 are the most studied and have even been used at a larger scale, especially in the case of supercritical $CO_{2.}$

Ideally, the novel extraction method should be selective, scalable, and environmentally friendly avoiding the use of toxic organic solvents as much as possible. In this chapter we have focused on the following novel extraction methods: supercritical fluid extraction (SFE), pressurized liquid extraction (PLE), and ionic liquid extraction (ILE) (Table 5.1).

5.3.2.1 Application of Novel Extraction Technologies for Functional Lipids The current application of more novel extraction techniques is discussed in this section. In contrast to classical lipid extraction techniques, novel methods are often focused on minimizing environmental impact and potential toxicity of the procedure by limiting or eliminating the use of organic solvents. Novel techniques are also generally more selective in nature, and can often be fine-tuned to produce a more specific end-product than can be achieved through traditional means. It should be noted, of course, that an excessive focus on the purity of the end-product is unnecessary, as long as the other components of the product are harmless. As mentioned by King (2014), most functional compounds extracted by SFE that are commercially available contain relatively small quantities of the actual bioactive product, the remaining components being largely inert lipids. An important factor to consider is that bioactive compounds often comprise a very small fraction of the biomass they are derived from, and so it might be unreasonable to expect extremely high purities. However, any method that can produce at least a decent level of selectivity should be considered useful, in order to obtain an enriched bioactive oil extract with functional properties (Satriana et al. 2019). Another factor to consider is that a fractionation process should optimally allow for the separation of the target bioactive compound from the major constituents of the biomass, without compromising either. Some of the more substantial compounds in the biomass can be useful in bulk quantities (largely carbohydrates in plants and algae) but are typically not worth extracting on their own due to high extraction cost and low product value. As such, the combined extraction of bulk products and, for instance, functional lipids is a good strategy for making the process economically viable (Wijngaard et al. 2012).

5.3.2.1.1 Supercritical Fluid Extraction SFE The potential use of supercritical fluids for the purpose of extraction was discovered as early as the 1800s, but the technique started to be investigated in earnest in the mid-1900s (Stahl and Schilz 2004). The principle of SFE is to flush the extraction material with a solvent under a set range of temperatures and pressures, under which the solvent is kept in a supercritical state, meaning that it takes on a set of physical properties that are in-between those of a liquid and a gas (Attard and Hunt 2018; Reverchon and De Marco 2006). The mass transfer properties of the solvent increase under these extreme pressures, rendering the desired compound more soluble in the supercritical fluid solvent than it would normally be. Supercritical CO_2 ($SCCO_2$) is the most common solvent used in SFE, and there are numerous studies on the solubility optima of various substances, including different lipid classes, under different ranges of temperatures and pressures (Bjornsson et al. 2011; Macias-Sanchez et al. 2009; Millao and Uquiche 2016; Pour Hosseini et al. 2017). SFE for the production of microalgal oils has been investigated over the past few decades, albeit with a focus on biodiesel rather than functional lipids (Halim et al. 2012; Mercer and Armenta 2011).

SFE is often used in tandem with column-based fractionation to separate extracted lipids and other substances (Liau et al. 2011; Temelli 2009), but some degree of selectivity can be obtained directly through the use of specific co-solvents (as well as altering co-solvent concentration), temperature, and pressure. For instance, SFE has been shown to be useful in carotenoid and chlorophyll separation, being far more efficient at retrieval of carotenoids than conventional ultrasound assisted extraction (Macias-Sanchez et al. 2009). The authors obtained a carotenoid chlorophyll ratio of 191 with $SCCO_2$ under 300 bar pressure at a temperature of 40 °C, compared with a ratio of 5.65 and 8.93 for the two ultrasound assisted methods tested. Direct fractionation by SFE has the clear benefit of limiting downstream processing of the extract, but it is unlikely that one can obtain a pure extract of a single, specific substance. There are almost always going to be at least trace levels of other compounds present (Reverchon and De Marco 2006), but as mentioned above, the absolute purity of the desired solute is rarely important. The use of a two-step extraction procedure is a strategy that can potentially increase the purity of the extract, by first solubilizing the majority of unwanted compounds at a specific temperature and pressure, before subsequently adjusting the parameters to extract the compound of interest. This method has been demonstrated in extraction of astaxanthin and carotenoids from the red yeast *Phaffia rhodozyma* (Lim et al. 2002). The authors reported an increase in astaxanthin and total carotenoid concentration by 10 and 13 times, respectively, when raising the pressure from 300 to 500 bar at a temperature of 60 °C. Using similar multi-step extraction schemes, some control can be exerted over the purity of the final extract.

The nonpolar nature of CO_2 makes $SCCO_2$ itself a suitable solvent for the semi-selective extraction of triglycerides (Cheng et al. 2011), effectively excluding phospholipids and other more polar lipid classes. This makes $SCCO_2$ a more attractive method for specifically separating triacylglycerols (TGs) from polar lipids than classical solvent methods (Bjornsson et al. 2011). Medium-chain TGs can themselves be considered a functional lipid class, as they have beneficial effects for those who suffer from difficulties in fat metabolism or digestion (Alabdulkarim et al. 2012), and TG extraction from algae with a large concentration of medium-chain TGs can therefore be of value. By using either neat $SCCO_2$, or $SCCO_2$ with a low concentration of ethanol co-solvent, one can first effectively extract TGs, and subsequently extract phospholipids by an increase in ethanol concentration or pressure (Hegel et al. 2011). This is an effective two-step process for separating polar lipids from the residual material after TG extraction (Subra-Paternault et al. 2015). The use of co-solvents does add to the environmental and economic cost of the extraction procedure, however, and would optimally be avoided. As mentioned previously, the pressure under which SFE is carried out affects the solubility of specific lipid subclasses as well. With higher pressures and temperatures, triglycerides with higher degrees of unsaturation are more readily solubilized and therefore more efficiently extracted (Santana et al. 2012). Excessively high temperatures, on the other hand, have been found to reduce the yield of long-chain PUFAs, probably as a result of thermal degradation (Cheung et al. 1998).

A major advantage of extraction using $SCCO_2$ is the lack of a need for solvent evaporation, producing a completely solvent-free end-product provided that no co-solvent is used. CO_2 is also a far less environmentally harmful and toxic solvent than traditional ones, in addition to being readily available and inexpensive. It is even possible to recycle the CO_2, provided the right instrumentation. This makes SFE potentially one of the most environmentally friendly extraction techniques available, although the high pressures under which $SCCO_2$ is formed do add to the energy consumption. Another disadvantage of SFE is the high installation cost, as the machinery required is relatively expensive. There exist pilot-scale facilities for lipid extraction from microalgae (Bjornsson et al. 2011; Lorenzen et al. 2017; Mendiola et al. 2008) already, albeit mostly focused on total oil production rather than any specific functional lipids.

5.3.2.1.2 Pressurized Liquid Extraction PLE PLE relies on the use of elevated temperatures to render the desired substance more soluble, while using high pressure to ensure the solvent remains in liquid form (Kaufmann and Christen 2002). This potentially allows for enhanced extraction speed, when compared with more established methods such as Soxhlet extraction. By using specific solvent mixtures, the selectivity of the PLE procedure can also be fine-tuned (Attard and Hunt 2018). Thus, PLE has been studied for the extraction of bioactive compounds, including various lipid-soluble species. The potential efficiency of using PLE for pigment extraction was demonstrated by Denery et al. (2004), who extracted carotenoids and kavalactones from *H. pluvialis* and *Dunaliella salina*. The authors noted the considerably shorter extraction time (20 minutes, compared with 90 minutes for sonication assisted methods), making the procedure less damaging to thermolabile substances, while simultaneously using lower quantities of solvents.

Heffernan et al. (2014) estimated extraction efficiency and the antioxidant capacity of macroalgal extracts obtained through PLE and a simple maceration extraction procedure using several different solvent systems. The authors found that the total extraction efficiency was lower using PLE, in addition to PLE performing considerably worse when it came to relative antioxidant activity. They suggest the decrease in activity could be due to the elevated temperatures of the PLE (100 °C), causing thermal degradation of antioxidant compounds. The issue of thermal degradation in PLE of antioxidant pigments from microalgae has been further documented by Plaza et al. (2012). They extracted pigments from *Chlorella vulgaris* at four different temperatures from 50 to 200 °C and found a drastic decrease in total pigment levels in the extracts, including chlorophylls *a* and *b* as well as four identified carotenoids, at higher temperatures. Tierney et al. (2013) also concluded that PLE confers little advantage in antioxidant extraction from macroalgae compared with conventional methods, besides shorter extraction times, reduced solvent use, and the fact that the extraction occurs in an oxygen-free environment, preventing oxidation. The authors highlighted the issues of elevated temperatures, as well as the environmental impact of using silicate sand or diatomaceous earth as packing materials to prevent lumping during PLE processes.

In a recent study, Castejón and Señoráns (2019) used a four-step, sequential PLE method to simultaneously extract and fractionate lipids from *Nannochloropsis gaditana*, producing a lipid extract with an enriched EPA fraction of up to 53%. This extract was also derived from wet biomass, thus omitting the need for drying, but the best results required enzymatic pretreatment, leading to potential difficulties in industrial scale-up as well as increased costs. Nonetheless, the study shows the potential of PLE to rapidly produce omega-3 enriched oils, meaning that the procedure could be highly useful for certain classes of functional lipids.

Several groups have pointed out the high capital investment necessary for establishing industrial-scale PLE of algal biomass. Combined with the aforementioned issues with thermal instability of certain functional compounds and the environmental impact of packing materials, it seems that PLE will require further research and some substantial improvement before it becomes a viable avenue for large-scale application.

5.3.2.1.3 Ionic Liquid Extraction ILE ILs have gained a lot of attention, particularly in the past decade, as potential "green" solvents for extraction of functional lipids and other cellular components of value. The use of IL extraction has been studied in microalgae, higher plants, and many other cell and tissue types (Bhan et al. 2017;

Shankar et al. 2017; Zhang et al. 2018). In addition to many ILs being more environmentally friendly and nontoxic than traditional solvents, they can also be used to more selectively isolate specific substances based on the presence of certain functional groups, allowing for specific extraction of – for instance – a desired class of lipids (Clark et al. 2018). Such selectivity cuts down on lengthy and costly separation procedures. ILs containing aromatic rings have been demonstrated by multiple groups to be effective in the isolation of omega-3 PUFAs from fish (Cheong et al. 2011; Li et al. 2009a, 2009b), and could potentially be used for extraction from algal biomass as well, provided there is effective cell disruption. The selectivity of aromatic ILs for omega-3 PUFAs is attributed to π-complexing between the double bonds of the aromatic rings and the double bonds of the PUFAs.

Many ILs can also be used repeatedly without noticeably affecting extraction efficiency, as demonstrated for the 1-ethyl-3-methylimidazolium ethylsulfate [C2mim][EtSO4] and tetrabutylphosphonium propionate [P4444][Prop] ILs (Zhang et al. 2018). The authors saw no discernible loss in efficiency or quality after five re-uses. Another group found that 1-ethyl-3-methylimidazolium dibutylphosphate (EMIM) (DBP) could be reused for astaxanthin extraction a limited number of times, showing some decrease in cell permeabilization efficiency after four re-uses (Desai et al. 2016). Recycling of solvents contributes to the environmental advantages of using ILs over conventional solvents. Further, ILs elicit good extraction efficiency of lipids even in heavily hydrated samples, in contrast to more traditional methods such as Soxhlet extraction (Orr et al. 2015). This circumvents the costly processing step of drying the biomass prior to extraction, and makes them more suitable for extraction from algal biomass, which is by nature very low in dry matter.

The effective cell disruptive capability of many ILs can further reduce the need for processing, as they can outperform costlier and more energy-demanding methods like sonication and MAE (Shankar et al. 2017). Another advantage of IL-mediated extraction techniques is that they generally require relatively low reaction temperatures, sometimes performing well even at room temperature (Chua et al. 2018). Desai et al. (2016) evaluated the extraction of astaxanthin from *H. pluvialis* using a variety of phosphonium and imidazolium-based ILs at different temperatures. They achieved approximately 70% extraction of astaxanthin from *H. pluvialis* cysts at 45 °C, which was lower extraction efficiency than the methanol chloroform control, but requiring considerably lower temperatures.

In cases where the IL solvent itself is not sufficient to cause adequate cell disruption, the use of mechanical disruption methods has been combined with IL extraction to obtain high-efficiency lipid extraction. IL-MAE has been used to extract lipids from microalgae, using the IL butyl-3-methylimidazolium hydrogen sulfate [BMIM][HSO^4], showing a clear improvement over conventional solvent extraction (Pan et al. 2016). Similarly, the diterpenoid andrographolide was extracted from the angiosperm *Andrographis paniculata* using the IL 1-butyl-3-methyl-imidazolium chloride [BMIM][Cl], in conjunction with microwave assisted cell disruption (Bhan et al. 2017). The use of this IL also considerably improved andrographolide-specific extraction as compared with Soxhlet and maceration-based methods. The authors suggest this improved extraction efficiency stems from charge–charge and/or H-bonding interactions between the IL and andrographolide, rendering the terpenoid more soluble in the IL. While not tested on microalgae, this study serves as a good proof-of-concept that it is possible to selectively extract terpenoids using ILE. Several other groups have also indicated that the strong H-bonding of imidazolium-based

IL solvents to cellulose can dissolve intramolecular H-bonds within the cellulose layer of cell walls in different biological materials, thereby weakening the cell wall and enabling cell disruption (Swatloski et al. 2002; Zhang et al. 2014). The amino acid IL cholinium arginate [Ch][Arg] has also been demonstrated to induce cell wall disruption in *Nannochloropsis* sp., the authors again attributing this effect to the strong H-bonding capacity of arginine ions (Chua et al. 2018).

ILs, when chosen carefully, can thus serve the dual function of maximizing extraction yield by disrupting the cells while also conferring selectivity for a desired extraction product. These properties, along with their environmental and economic advantages, make them highly suitable for extraction of relatively low-yield, high-value products such as functional lipids. To the authors' knowledge, there are currently no pilot-scale facilities for ILE from algal biomass, but some do exist for extraction and isolation of bioactive compounds from higher plants (Chen et al. 2017). Industrial application for ILE of algal compounds is yet to be proven, but it seems likely to occur in time, given the many benefits of ILE.

5.4 Future Recommendations

When dealing with the extraction of functional lipids that have both a high metabolic and economic value, the choice of the extraction method should focus on the quality of the final product(s) and on the environmental sustainability of the entire process. Hence, the research should focus on the development of new environmentally friendly solvents, energy efficient processes reducing the pretreatment steps, and finally a selective extraction step to reduce post-treatment processes as much as possible. The majority of the studies found in the literature are performed at laboratory scale and/or at a small scale that produces high-quality data but unfortunately a part of these studies is that they are not relevant at a larger/industrial scale. We are aware that for researchers in academia it is very time- and resource costly to produce data at a larger scale, using pilot facilities that will be more relevant from an application point of view later on at larger/industrial scale. Hence, we believe that close collaborations between academia and industry would generate data of great relevance for the development in the short term of extraction processes for new products based on functional lipids. Of course in the long term, cultivation techniques and molecular tools enabling an increase in the amount of functional lipids will be pivotal to improve algal productivity of functional foods together with easier extraction procedures.

In conclusion, the biorefinery concept should be adapted to the algal sector where the biomass is seen as a whole and not just for a single product. In such a way, it will be possible to use several different fractions generating different products of economic value, such as functional lipids, proteins, and carbohydrates.

Acknowledgments

The authors greatly appreciate the financial support from the EU Interreg Botnia-Atlantica (TransAlgae project).

References

Alabdulkarim, B., Bakeet, Z.A.N., and Arzoo, S. (2012). Role of some functional lipids in preventing diseases and promoting health. *Journal of King Saud University – Science* **24** (4): 319–329. https://doi.org/10.1016/j.jksus.2012.03.001.

Almeida Nogueira, D., da Silveira, J.M., Mendes Vidal, E. et al. (2018). Cell disruption of *Chaetoceros calcitrans* by microwave and ultrasound in lipid extraction. *International Journal of Chemical Engineering* **2018**: 9508723. https://doi.org/10.1155/2018/9508723.

Aryee, A.N.A. and Boye, J.I. (2015). Current and emerging trends in the formulation and manufacture of nutraceuticals and functional food products. In: *Nutraceutical and Functional Food Processing Technology*, 1e (ed. J.I. Boye), 1–63. Hoboken, NJ: Wiley.

Attard, T.M. and Hunt, A.J. (2018). Introduction to high-pressure solvent systems. In: *Supercritical and Other High-Pressure Solvent Systems: For Extraction, Reaction and Material Processing* (eds. T.M. Attard and A.J. Hunt), 1–13. London: The Royal Society of Chemistry.

Axelsson, M. and Gentili, F. (2014). A single-step method for rapid extraction of total lipids from green microalgae. *PLoS One* **9**: e89643.

Balasubramanian, S., Allen, J.D., Kanitkar, A., and Boldor, D. (2011). Oil extraction from *Scenedesmus obliquus* using a continuous microwave system – design, optimization, and quality characterization. *Bioresource Technology* **102**: 3396–3403.

Barba, F.J., Grimi, N., and Vorobiev, E. (2015). New approaches for the use of non-conventional cell disruption technologies to extract potential food additives and nutraceuticals from microalgae. *Food Engineering Reviews* **7**: 45–62.

Berlitz, H.D., Grosch, W., and Schieberle, P. (2009). *Food Chemistry*, 4e, 989. Berlin, Heidelberg: Springer-Verlag.

Bhan, M., Satija, S., Garg, C. et al. (2017). Optimization of ionic liquid-based microwave assisted extraction of a diterpenoid lactone-andrographolide from *Andrographis paniculata* by response surface methodology. *Journal of Molecular Liquids* **229**: 161–166. https://doi.org/10.1016/j.molliq.2016.12.011.

Bjornsson, W.J., MacDougall, K.M., Melanson, J.E. et al. (2011). Pilot-scale supercritical carbon dioxide extractions for the recovery of triacylglycerols from microalgae: a practical tool for algal biofuels research. *Journal of Applied Phycology* **24** (3): 547–555. https://doi.org/10.1007/s10811-011-9756-2.

Bligh, E.G. and Dyer, W.J. (1959). A rapid method of total lipid extraction and purification. *Canadian Journal of Biochemistry and Physiology* **37**: 911–917.

Buono, S., Langellotti, A.L., Martello, A. et al. (2014). Functional ingredients from microalgae. *Food & Function* **5**: 1669–1685.

Byreddy, A.R., Gupta, A., Barrow, C.J., and Puri, M. (2015). Comparison of cell disruption methods for improving lipid extraction from *Thraustochytrid* strains. *Marine Drugs* **13**: 5111–5127.

Castejón, N. and Señoráns, F.J. (2019). Simultaneous extraction and fractionation of omega-3 acylglycerols and glycolipids from wet microalgal biomass of *Nannochloropsis gaditana* using pressurized liquids. *Algal Research* **37**: 74–82. https://doi.org/10.1016/j.algal.2018.11.003.

Chen, F., Zhang, Q., Mo, K. et al. (2017). Optimization of ionic liquid-based homogenate extraction of orientin and vitexin from the flowers of *Trollius chinensis* and its application on a pilot scale. *Separation and Purification Technology* **175**: 147–157. https://doi.org/10.1016/j.seppur.2016.10.062.

Cheng, C.H., Du, T.B., Pi, H.C. et al. (2011). Comparative study of lipid extraction from microalgae by organic solvent and supercritical CO_2. *Bioresource Technology* **102** (21): 10151–10153. https://doi.org/10.1016/j.biortech.2011.08.064.

Cheong, L.Z., Guo, Z., Yang, Z. et al. (2011). Extraction and enrichment of n-3 polyunsaturated fatty acids and ethyl esters through reversible pi-pi complexation with aromatic rings containing ionic liquids. *Journal of Agricultural and Food Chemistry* **59** (16): 8961–8967. https://doi.org/10.1021/jf202043w.

Cheung, P.C.K., Leung, A.Y.H., and Ang, P.O. (1998). Comparison of supercritical carbon dioxide and Soxhlet extraction of lipids from a brown seaweed, *Sargassum hemiphyllum*. *Journal of Agricultural and Food Chemistry* **46** (10): 4228–4232. https://doi.org/10.1021/jf980346h.

Chua, E.T., Brunner, M., Atkin, R. et al. (2018). The ionic liquid cholinium arginate is an efficient solvent for extracting high-value *Nannochloropsis* sp. lipids. *ACS Sustainable Chemistry & Engineering* **7** (2): 2538–2544. https://doi.org/10.1021/acssuschemeng.8b05448.

Clark, K.D., Trujillo-Rodriguez, M.J., and Anderson, J.L. (2018). Advances in the analysis of biological samples using ionic liquids. *Analytical and Bioanalytical Chemistry* **410** (19): 4567–4573. https://doi.org/10.1007/s00216-018-0898-9.

Delsart, C., Grimi, N., Boussetta, N. et al. (2016). Impact of pulsed-electric field and high-voltage electrical discharges on red wine microbial stabilization and quality characteristics. *Journal of Applied Microbiology* **120**: 152–164.

Denery, J.R., Dragull, K., Tang, C.S., and Li, Q.X. (2004). Pressurized fluid extraction of carotenoids from *Haematococcus pluvialis* and *Dunaliella salina* and kavalactones from *Piper methysticum*. *Analytica Chimica Acta* **501** (2): 175–181. https://doi.org/10.1016/j.aca.2003.09.026.

Desai, R.K., Streefland, M., Wijffels, R.H., and Eppink, M.H.M. (2016). Novel astaxanthin extraction from *Haematococcus pluvialis* using cell permeabilising ionic liquids. *Green Chemistry* **18** (5): 1261–1267. https://doi.org/10.1039/c5gc01301a.

Ekendahl, S., Bark, M., Engelbrektsson, J. et al. (2018). Energy-efficient outdoor cultivation of oleaginous microalgae at northern latitudes using waste heat and flue gas from a pulp and paper mill. *Algal Research* **31**: 138–146.

Folch, J., Lees, M., and Stanley, G.H.S. (1957). A simple method for the isolation and purification of total lipides from animal tissues. *The Journal of Biological Chemistry* **226**: 497–509.

Geada, P., Rodrigues, R., Loureiro, L. et al. (2018). Electrotechnologies applied to microalgal biotechnology – applications, techniques and future trends. *Renewable and Sustainable Energy Reviews* **94**: 656–668.

Goettel, M., Eing, C., Gusbeth, C. et al. (2013). Pulsed electric field assisted extraction of intracellular valuables from microalgae. *Algal Research* **2**: 401–408.

Grimi, N., Dubois, A., Marchal, L. et al. (2014). Selective extraction from microalgae *Nannochloropsis* sp. using different methods of cell disruption. *Bioresource Technology* **153**: 254–259.

Halim, R., Danquah, M.K., and Webley, P.A. (2012). Extraction of oil from microalgae for biodiesel production: a review. *Biotechnology Advances* **30** (3): 709–732. https://doi.org/10.1016/j.biotechadv.2012.01.001.

Hara, A. and Radin, N.S. (1978). Lipids extraction of tissues with a low-toxicity solvent. *Analytical Biochemistry* **90**: 420–426.

Heffernan, N., Smyth, T.J., FitzGerald, R.J. et al. (2014). Antioxidant activity and phenolic content of pressurised liquid and solid-liquid extracts from four Irish origin macroalgae. *International Journal of Food Science & Technology* **49** (7): 1765–1772. https://doi.org/10.1111/ijfs.12512.

Hegel, P.E., Camy, S., Destrac, P., and Condoret, J.S. (2011). Influence of pretreatments for extraction of lipids from yeast by using supercritical carbon dioxide and ethanol as cosolvent. *The Journal of Supercritical Fluids* **58** (1): 68–78. https://doi.org/10.1016/j.supflu.2011.04.005.

Huo, S., Wang, Z., Cui, F. et al. (2015). Enzyme-assisted extraction of oil from wet microalgae *Scenedesmus* sp. G4. *Energies* **8**: 8165–8174.

Ibanez, E. and Cifuentes, A. (2013). Benefits of using algae as natural sources of functional ingredients. *Journal of the Science of Food and Agriculture* **93**: 703–709.

Kadam, S.E., Tiwari, B.K., and O'Donnell, C.P. (2013). Application of novel extraction technologies for bioactives from marine algae. *Journal of Agricultural and Food Chemistry* **61**: 4667–4675.

Kaufmann, B. and Christen, P. (2002). Recent extraction techniques for natural products: microwave-assisted extraction and pressurised solvent extraction. *Phytochemical Analysis* **13** (2): 105–113. https://doi.org/10.1002/pca.631.

King, J.W. (2014). Modern supercritical fluid technology for food applications. *Annual Review of Food Science and Technology* **5**: 215–238. https://doi.org/10.1146/annurev-food-030713-092447.

Kumar, R.R., Rao, P.H., and Arumugam, M. (2015). Lipid extraction methods from microalgae: a comprehensive review. *Frontiers in Energy Research* **2**: 61.

Kumar, J.S.P., Kumar Garlapati, V., Dash, A. et al. (2017). A sustainable green solvents and techniques for lipid extraction from microalgae: a review. *Algal Research* **21**: 138–147.

Kumar, V., Nanda, M., Joshi, H.C. et al. (2018). Production of biodiesel and bioethanol using algal biomass harvested from fresh water river. *Renewable Energy* **116**: 606–612.

Lee, S.J., Yoon, B.D., and Oh, H.M. (1998). Rapid method for the determination of lipid from the green alga *Botryococcus braunii*. *Biotechnology Techniques* **12**: 553–556.

Leu, S. and Boussiba, S. (2014). Advances in the production of high-value products by microalgae. *Industrial Biotechnology* **10**: 169–183.

Li, M., Pham, P.J., Pittman, C.U., and Li, T. (2009a). SBA-15-supported ionic liquid compounds containing silver salts: novel mesoporous π-complexing sorbents for separating polyunsaturated fatty acid methyl esters. *Microporous and Mesoporous Materials* **117** (1–2): 436–443. https://doi.org/10.1016/j.micromeso.2008.07.017.

Li, M., Pittman, C.U. Jr., and Li, T. (2009b). Extraction of polyunsaturated fatty acid methyl esters by imidazolium-based ionic liquids containing silver tetrafluoroborate – extraction equilibrium studies. *Talanta* **78** (4–5): 1364–1370. https://doi.org/10.1016/j.talanta.2009.02.011.

Liang, K., Zhang, Q., and Cong, W. (2012). Enzyme-assisted aqueous extraction of lipid from microalgae. *Journal of Agricultural and Food Chemistry* **60**: 11771–11776.

Liau, B.-C., Hong, S.-E., Chang, L.-P. et al. (2011). Separation of sight-protecting zeaxanthin from *Nannochloropsis oculata* by using supercritical fluids extraction coupled with elution chromatography. *Separation and Purification Technology* **78** (1): 1–8. https://doi.org/10.1016/j.seppur.2011.01.008.

Lim, G.B., Lee, S.Y., Lee, E.K. et al. (2002). Separation of astaxanthin from red yeast *Phaffia rhodozyma* by supercritical carbon dioxide extraction. *Biochemical Engineering Journal* **11** (2–3): 181–187. S1369-703x(02)00023-2.

Lorenzen, J., Igl, N., Tippelt, M. et al. (2017). Extraction of microalgae derived lipids with supercritical carbon dioxide in an industrial relevant pilot plant. *Bioprocess and Biosystems Engineering* **40** (6): 911–918. https://doi.org/10.1007/s00449-017-1755-5.

Macias-Sanchez, M.D., Mantell, C., Rodriguez, M. et al. (2009). Comparison of supercritical fluid and ultrasound-assisted extraction of carotenoids and chlorophyll a from *Dunaliella salina*. *Talanta* **77** (3): 948–952. https://doi.org/10.1016/j.talanta.2008.07.032.

Marrone, B.L., Lacey, R.E., Anderson, D.B. et al. (2018). Review of the harvesting and extraction program within the National Alliance for Advanced Biofuels and Bioproducts. *Algal Reseach* **33**: 470–485.

Mathews, C.K., van Holde, K.E., and Ahern, K.G. (2000). *Biochemistry*, 3e. San Francisco, CA: Addison Wesley Longman.

Mendiola, J.A., García-Martínez, D., Rupérez, F.J. et al. (2008). Enrichment of vitamin E from *Spirulina platensis* microalga by SFE. *The Journal of Supercritical Fluids* **43** (3): 484–489. https://doi.org/10.1016/j.supflu.2007.07.021.

Mercer, P. and Armenta, R.E. (2011). Developments in oil extraction from microalgae. *European Journal of Lipid Science and Technology* **113** (5): 539–547. https://doi.org/10.1002/ejlt.201000455.

Millao, S. and Uquiche, E. (2016). Extraction of oil and carotenoids from pelletized microalgae using supercritical carbon dioxide. *The Journal of Supercritical Fluids* **116**: 223–231. https://doi.org/10.1016/j.supflu.2016.05.049.

Mulchandani, K., Kar, J.R., and Singhal, R.S. (2015). Extraction of lipids from using high-pressure homogenization followed by three phase partitioning. *Applied Biochemistry and Biotechnology* **176**: 1613–1626.

Naghdi, F.G., Bai, X., Thomas-Hall, S.R. et al. (2016). Lipid extraction from wet *Chaetoceros muelleri* culture and evaluation of remaining defatted biomass. *Algal Research* **20**: 205–212.

Orr, V.C.A., Plechkova, N.V., Seddon, K.R., and Rehmann, L. (2015). Disruption and wet extraction of the microalgae *Chlorella vulgaris* using room-temperature ionic liquids. *ACS Sustainable Chemistry & Engineering* **4** (2): 591–600. https://doi.org/10.1021/acssuschemeng.5b00967.

Otero, P., Quintana, S.E., Reglero, G. et al. (2018). Pressurized liquid extraction (PLE) as an innovative green technology for the effective enrichment of Galician algae extracts with high quality fatty acids and antimicrobial and antioxidant properties. *Marine Drugs* **16**: 156. https://doi.org/10.3390/md16050156.

Pan, J., Muppaneni, T., Sun, Y. et al. (2016). Microwave-assisted extraction of lipids from microalgae using an ionic liquid solvent [BMIM][HSO4]. *Fuel* **178**: 49–55. https://doi.org/10.1016/j.fuel.2016.03.037.

Parniakov, O., Barba, F.J., Grimi, N. et al. (2015). Pulsed electric field assisted extraction of nutritionally valuable compounds from microalgae *Nannochloropsis* spp. using the binary mixture of organic solvents and water. *Innovative Food Science and Emerging Technologies* **27**: 79–85.

Plaza, M., Santoyo, S., Jaime, L. et al. (2012). Comprehensive characterization of the functional activities of pressurized liquid and ultrasound-assisted extracts from *Chlorella vulgaris*. *LWT - Food Science and Technology* **46** (1): 245–253. https://doi.org/10.1016/j.lwt.2011.09.024.

Pour Hosseini, S.R., Tavakoli, O., and Sarrafzadeh, M.H. (2017). Experimental optimization of SC-CO_2 extraction of carotenoids from *Dunaliella salina*. *The Journal of Supercritical Fluids* **121**: 89–95. https://doi.org/10.1016/j.supflu.2016.11.006.

Prabakaran, P. and Ravindran, A.D. (2011). A comparative study on effective cell disruption methods for lipid extraction from microalgae. *Letters in Applied Microbiology* **53**: 150–154.

Prazad, E. (2016). Nutraceuticals market by type (functional food (probiotics fortified foods, omega fatty acid fortified food, branded ionized salts, branded wheat flour market, and other functional food), functional beverages (fruits and vegetable juices & drinks, dairy & dairy alternative drinks, non-carbonated drinks (bottled water, tea, and coffee, and others (herbal tea, sports drinks, energy drinks), dietary supplements (proteins & peptides, vitamins & minerals, herbals (ayurveda extracts, plant extracts, algal extracts, phytochemicals), and others (fatty acids, fiber) and personal care) – global opportunity analysis and industry forecast, 2014–2022. Allied Market Research Report FO_161815. www.alliedmarketresearch.com (accessed September 3, 2020).

Qiu, C., He, Y., Huang, Z. et al. (2019). Lipid extraction from wet *Nannochloropsis* biomass via enzyme-assisted three phase partitioning. *Bioresource Technology* **284**: 381–390.

Reverchon, E. and De Marco, I. (2006). Supercritical fluid extraction and fractionation of natural matter. *The Journal of Supercritical Fluids* **38** (2): 146–166. https://doi.org/10.1016/j.supflu.2006.03.020.

Ryckebosch, E., Muylaert, K., and Foubert, I. (2012). Optimization of an analytical procedure for extraction of lipids from microalgae. *Journal of the American Oil Chemists' Society* **89**: 189–198.

Samarasinghe, N., Fernando, S., Lacey, R., and Brock Faulkner, W. (2012). Algal cell rupture using high pressure homogenization as a prelude to oil extraction. *Renewable Energy* **48**: 300–308.

Santana, A., Jesus, S., Larrayoz, M.A., and Filho, R.M. (2012). Supercritical carbon dioxide extraction of algal lipids for the biodiesel production. *Procedia Engineering* **42**: 1755–1761. https://doi.org/10.1016/j.proeng.2012.07.569.

Satriana, S., Supardan, M.D., Arpi, N., and Mustapha, W.A.W. (2019). Development of methods used in the extraction of avocado oil. *European Journal of Lipid Science and Technology* **121**: 1800210. https://doi.org/10.1002/ejlt.201800210.

Shankar, M., Chhotaray, P.K., Agrawal, A. et al. (2017). Protic ionic liquid-assisted cell disruption and lipid extraction from fresh water *Chlorella* and *Chlorococcum* microalgae. *Algal Research* **25**: 228–236. https://doi.org/10.1016/j.algal.2017.05.009.

Shen, Y., Pei, Z., Yuan, W., and Mao, E. (2009). Effect of nitrogen and extraction method on algae lipid yield. *International Journal of Agricultural and Biological Engineering* **2**: 51–57.

Singh, R., Kumar, A., and Sharma, Y.C. (2019). Evaluation of various lipid extraction techniques for microalgae and their effect on biochemical components. *Waste and Biomass Valorization* **11**: 2603–2612. https://doi.org/10.1007/s12649-019-00601-4.

Sosa-Hernandez, J.E., Escobedo-Avellaneda, Z., Iqbal, H.M.N., and Welti-Chanes, J. (2018). State of the art extraction methodologies for bioactive compounds from algal biome to meet bio-economy challenges and opportunities. *Molecules* **23**: 2953.

Spector, A.A. and Kim, H.Y. (2015). Discovery of essential fatty acids. *Journal of Lipid Research* **56**: 11–21.

Stahl, E. and Schilz, W. (2004). Extraction with supercritical gases in coupling with thin-layer chromatography. *Fresenius' Zeitschrift für Analytische Chemie* **280** (2): 99–104. https://doi.org/10.1007/bf00592408.

Subra-Paternault, P., ThongDeng, H., Grélard, A., and Cansell, M. (2015). Extraction of phospholipids from scallop by-product using supercritical CO_2/alcohol mixtures. *LWT – Food Science and Technology* **60** (2): 990–998. https://doi.org/10.1016/j.lwt.2014.09.057.

Swatloski, R.P., Spear, S.K., Holbrey, J.D., and Rogers, R.D. (2002). Dissolution of cellose with ionic liquids. *Journal of the American Chemical Society* **124** (18): 4974–4975. https://doi.org/10.1021/ja025790m.

Temelli, F. (2009). Perspectives on supercritical fluid processing of fats and oils. *The Journal of Supercritical Fluids* **47** (3): 583–590. https://doi.org/10.1016/j.supflu.2008.10.014.

The Merck Index (2013). *An Encyclopedia of Chemicals, Drugs, and Biologicals*, 15e (ed. J. O'Neil). Cambridge: The Royal Society of Chemistry.

Tierney, M.S., Smyth, T.J., Hayes, M. et al. (2013). Influence of pressurised liquid extraction and solid-liquid extraction methods on the phenolic content and antioxidant activities of

Irish macroalgae. *International Journal of Food Science & Technology* **48** (4): 860–869. https://doi.org/10.1111/ijfs.12038.

Wang, D., Li, Y., Hu, X. et al. (2015). Combined enzymatic and mechanical cell disruption and lipid extraction of green alga *Neochloris oleoabundans*. *International Journal of Molecular Sciences* **16**: 7707–7722.

Wijngaard, H., Hossain, M.B., Rai, D.K., and Brunton, N. (2012). Techniques to extract bioactive compounds from food by-products of plant origin. *Food Research International* **46** (2): 505–513. https://doi.org/10.1016/j.foodres.2011.09.027.

Wiltshire, K.H., Boersma, M., Möller, A., and Buhtz, H. (2000). Extraction of pigments and fatty acids from the green alga *Scenedesmus obliquus* (Chlorophyceae). *Aquatic Ecology* **34**: 119–126.

Yoo, G., Park, W.K., Kim, C.W. et al. (2012). Direct lipid extraction from wet *Chlamydomonas reinhardtii* biomass using osmotic shock. *Bioresource Technology* **123**: 717–722.

Zbinden, M.D.A., Sturm, B.S.M., Nord, R.D. et al. (2013). Pulsed electric field (PEF) as an intensification pretreatment for greener solvent lipid extraction from microalgae. *Biotechnology and Bioengineering* **110**: 1605–1615.

Zhang, Y., Liu, Z., Li, Y., and Chi, R. (2014). Optimization of ionic liquid-based microwave-assisted extraction of isoflavones from *Radix puerariae* by response surface methodology. *Separation and Purification Technology* **129**: 71–79. https://doi.org/10.1016/j.seppur.2014.03.022.

Zhang, Y., Ward, V., Dennis, D. et al. (2018). Efficient extraction of a eocosahexaenoic acid (DHA) – rich lipid fraction from *Thraustochytrium* sp. using ionic liquid. *Materials (Basel)* **11** (10): 1986. https://doi.org/10.3390/ma11101986.

Zuorro, A., Maffei, G., and Lavecchia, R. (2016). Optimization of enzyme-assisted lipid extraction from *Nannochloropsis* microalgae. *Journal of the Taiwan Institute of Chemical Engineers* **67**: 106–114.

6
Extraction Technologies for Proteins and Peptides

Ariane Tremblay and Lucie Beaulieu
Département des Sciences des aliments, Institut sur la nutrition et les aliments fonctionnels (INAF), Université Laval, Québec, Canada

6.1 Introduction

By 2050, the Food and Agriculture Organization of the United Nations (FAO) expects a world population of 9 billion (Alexandratos and Bruinsma 2012; van der Spiegel et al. 2013). This increasing human population and demand for healthy foods have driven the search for unconventional protein sources to replace animal-derived proteins that contribute as major sources of greenhouse gas emissions (Cole et al. 2015; Marinho et al. 2015; Rioux et al. 2017). Currently considered as underexploited crops, microalgae and macroalgae (seaweed) can be viewed as a sustainable protein source for the future (Bleakley and Hayes 2017). They have been ever more promoted for their protein quality, which is mainly defined by their amino acid composition, digestibility, and health benefit properties (McHugh 2003; Rioux et al. 2017; Wells et al. 2017).

The protein content of algae depends on the species and the season varying according to environmental changes such as salinity, light, temperature, drought, and nutrient supply during the growth phase (Beaulieu et al. 2016; Connan et al. 2007; Fleurence 1999, 2004; Harnedy et al. 2014; Holdt and Kraan 2011; Kim and Wijesekara 2010; Marinho et al. 2015; Martínez and Rico 2002; Tierney et al. 2010). Nonetheless, algae have relatively high levels of proteins. For instance, microalgae produced for human or animal consumption typically are composed of between 60 and 70% proteins (Ritala et al. 2017), while seaweeds have up to 47% protein of dry weight (DW) (Fleurence et al. 1999; Pereira 2011). The protein contents of some species of microalgae and seaweeds are comparable with those found in high-protein vegetables such as soybeans (37% DW protein) and in traditional animal proteins such as meat (43% DW protein), milk (26% DW protein), as well as yeast (39% DW protein) (Bleakley and Hayes 2017; Fleurence et al. 1999; Gouveia et al. 2008; Soto-Sierra et al. 2018; Wells et al. 2017). Microalgae and seaweeds contain all of the essential amino acids at various concentrations (Bleakley and Hayes 2017; Fleurence et al. 2012). For instance, the amino

Recent Advances in Micro- and Macroalgal Processing: Food and Health Perspectives, First Edition.
Edited by Gaurav Rajauria and Yvonne V. Yuan.

acid pattern of microalgae and seaweeds compares favorably with that of other food proteins such as legumes or egg proteins (Becker 2007; Fleurence 2004).

Proteins are present in algae in various cellular compartments as enzymes or as intracellular components or can be bound to pigments and polysaccharides (Stengel et al. 2011). The algal proteins that have been studied the most belong to the class of phycobiliproteins (phycoerythrin, phycocyanins, and allophycocyanins) and lectins, the two main known groups of functionally active proteins (Chojnacka et al. 2012; Fleurence et al. 2018; Pangestuti and Kim 2011, 2015; Stengel et al. 2011). Phycobiliproteins are present in red seaweed and those from microalgae (*Spirulina*) are used as food dyes, cosmetics, and as fluorescent markers in biomedical research (Stengel et al. 2011). The lectins have been isolated from red and green seaweed (Pangestuti and Kim 2015), and, in addition to their affinity for carbohydrates, possess potential antimicrobial, anti-inflammatory, and anticancer activities (Chojnacka et al. 2012). However, algal protein composition, structure, and potential bioactivities remain much less characterized than those of other algal components such as polysaccharides, phenols, and pigments (Harnedy and FitzGerald 2013), even though recent studies have shown that enzymatic hydrolysis of algal extracts generates a new range of peptides with various biological activities (Afify et al. 2018; Beaulieu et al. 2015, 2016; Harnedy and FitzGerald 2011; Samarakoon and Jeon 2012). Algae are a promising food ingredient due to their nutritional composition and richness in bioactive compounds (Batista et al. 2017; Bleakley and Hayes 2017; Henchion et al. 2017; Soto-Sierra et al. 2018; van der Spiegel et al. 2013). Based on their protein content and the degree of purifying, protein products from algae can be classified as whole-cell protein, protein concentrates, isolates, hydrolysates, and bioactive peptides (Soto-Sierra et al. 2018).

The human consumption of seaweed is well established in Asia but still in its infancy in Western countries (Rioux et al. 2017). For the most part, *Porphyra tenera* (nori) is used in the production of sushi (Bleakley and Hayes 2017). Many species of seaweeds have a high aspartic and glutamic acid content, which gives the characteristic umami taste sensation (Mouritsen 2012; Mouritsen et al. 2013). In addition, seaweeds have been successfully incorporated into food products as a functional ingredient. For instance, *Undaria pinnatifida* (wakame) has been incorporated into pasta demonstrating an antioxidant activity at levels up to 10% (Prabhasankar et al. 2009). The presence of 4% *Ascophylum nodosum* in bread has significantly reduced the energy intake of overweight individuals in meals following enriched bread consumption (Hall et al. 2012). The properties of renin-inhibitory peptides from *Palmaria palmata* (dulse) hydrolysates in bread were retained even after the baking process (Fitzgerald et al. 2014b). The integration of *Saccharina longicruris* (sugar kelp) into Camembert-type cheese has displayed a higher angiotensin I-converting enzyme (ACE)-inhibitory activity after 10 days of ripening in comparison with the cheese control (Hell et al. 2017).

Microalgae are consumed as a dietary supplement in the form of powder, capsules, tablets, or liquid, and they have also been incorporated into foods such as pasta, baked goods, snacks, and drinks (Bleakley and Hayes 2017; Liang et al. 2004; Ritala et al. 2017). Another example of an algae-based product launched on the market is a microalgae protein concentrate (PC) from *Chlorella protothecoides* (http://algavia.com/ingredients/proteins/) (Bleakley and Hayes 2017). Indeed, the production of vegan PCs is of growing interest in the food industry (Rioux et al. 2017; Suresh Kumar et al. 2014). However, before considering PCs as ingredients in food formulations,

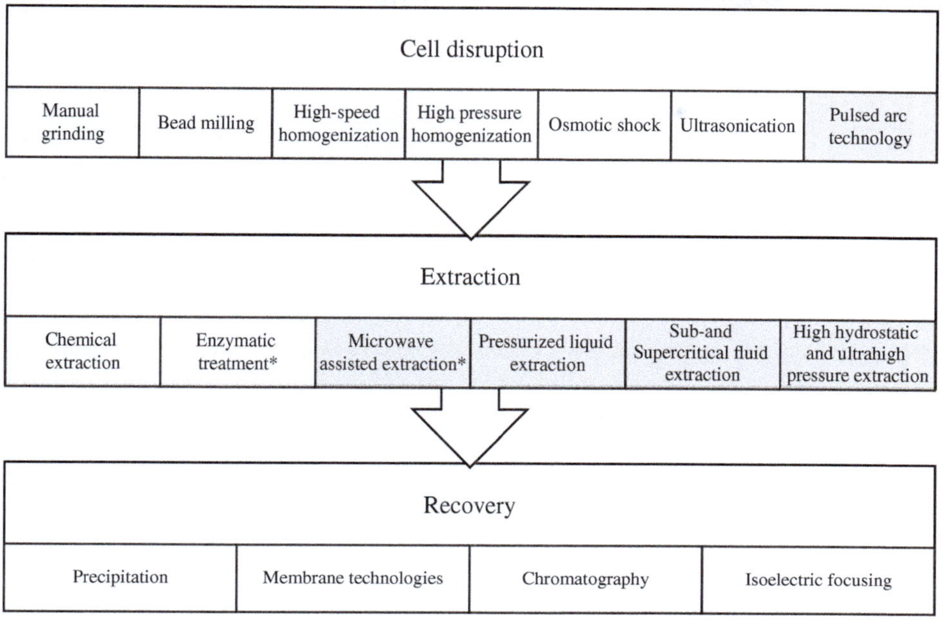

Figure 6.1 Overview of the conventional and emerging methods (highlighted in gray) for protein and peptide extraction from algae. * Both enzymatic treatment and microwave assisted extraction could be considered as cell disruption methods.

food-grade solvents have to be used during the extraction method avoiding chemical residues, which could be toxic (Shannon and Abu-Ghannam 2016). Thus, functionality, bioavailability, bioaccessibility, allergenicity, and toxicity of PCs from algae before and after the incorporation into food matrices are important points, especially taking into account the regulatory issues for functional foods (health claims), which constitute an important challenge for the industry (Barba 2017).

The widespread use of seaweed and microalgae is limited by many environmental factors such as harvesting access, seasonality, and geographical location, but also by the development of scalable production processes of protein isolation (Bleakley and Hayes 2017). Extraction is the most important starting step in isolating these high-value molecules. However, the presence of compounds attached to the cell wall, such as polysaccharides (Fleurence 1999; Joubert and Fleurence 2008; Wijesekara et al. 2017) and polyphenols (Wijesinghe and Jeon 2012) is a limiting factor in protein extraction, as they cannot be easily extracted using typical extraction methods with aqueous solvents (Wijesinghe and Jeon 2012). The protein extraction yield can also be reduced by the rigidity of the cell wall in microalgae (Safi et al. 2014c). Protein digestibility is an important factor to take into consideration in the evaluation of the nutritional value and algal food quality, which can be limited by the presence of compounds such as glycosylated protein, polysaccharides, lectins, and phenolic compounds (Fleurence 1999; Goni et al. 2002; Wong and Cheung 2001). Microalgae and seaweed have poor protein digestibility in their raw form (Bleakley and Hayes 2017). Some studies have suggested that fermenting seaweeds can increase the protein digestibility and the bioavailability of nutrients (Marrion et al. 2003). Hence, there is a need to develop efficient methods to recover proteins and peptides from microalgae and seaweeds. This chapter is an overview of the conventional and emerging extraction techniques for proteins and peptides in microalgae and seaweeds. Figure 6.1 summarizes the methods that are discussed in this chapter.

6.2 Conventional Extraction Techniques for Proteins and Peptides

Algal protein extraction techniques are often preceded by a cell disruption treatment like mechanical grinding, osmotic shock, ultrasonication, or polysaccharidase-aided digestion to improve protein recovery (Harnedy and FitzGerald 2013). Then, proteins are extracted by aqueous, acid and alkaline extraction or enzymatic hydrolysis, followed by centrifugation. A subsequent recovery step is performed using membrane technologies, precipitation, or chromatography (Kadam et al. 2017). It is also possible to generate peptides by enzymatic hydrolysis using proteolytic enzymes following protein extraction (Bondu et al. 2015). Different studies using conventional extraction techniques, presented below, are outlined in Table 6.1.

6.2.1 Cell Disruption Methods

Cell disruption methods involve the destruction of the cell wall in a nonspecific manner to improve the accessibility of the protein molecules. It is a crucial part in the extraction process (Günerken et al. 2015; Harnedy and FitzGerald 2013).

6.2.1.1 Mechanical Grinding Mechanical grinding consists of the application of mechanical forces to break the cell wall (Günerken et al. 2015). To achieve this, diverse techniques are available using simple to sophisticated devices.

6.2.1.1.1 Manual Grinding Manual grinding simply consists of grinding the dry material with a mortar and a pestle. This technique can be performed alone or followed by another cell disruption technique (Barbarino and Lourenço 2005; Fleurence et al. 1995b). A study comparing different cell disruption methods (manual grinding, ultrasonication, alkaline treatment, high-pressure treatment) for five microalgae has reported that this method led to the lowest protein recovery for all species (Safi et al. 2014b).

6.2.1.1.2 Bead Milling Cell disruption is carried out in an apparatus consisting of a shaft equipped with agitators of varied design (disks, rings, or pins) and beads. The agitator shaft and the beads are enclosed in a grinding chamber (Kula and Schutte 1987). Beads entering into collision with one another would cause the disruption of the cells placed between the beads by compaction or shear forces (Melendres et al. 1992). The main operational parameters influencing cell disintegration efficiency are the agitator speed and design, geometry of the grinding chamber, feed rate, bead loading, size and material, time, temperature, and concentration of the suspension (Kula and Schutte 1987). This technique is commonly used for cell disruption of microalgae and seaweeds (Beaulieu et al. 2016; Garcia et al. 2018; Kazir et al. 2019; Postma et al. 2017; Schwenzfeier et al. 2011).

Table 6.1 Conventional methods of algal protein extraction reported in different studies in the literature.

Type of extraction	Algae species	Optimum conditions and reagents	Protein yield	References
Chemical	*Laminaria digitata*	Aqueous polymer two-phase system: PEG 1550 (10% w/v) and K_2CO_3 (15% w/v)	—	Jordan and Vilter (1991)
	Ulva rigida	5% w/v algae in deionized water, then 0.1 M NaOH with 0.5% v/v β-mercaptoethanol	26.80% ± 1.3% of total protein	Fleurence et al. (1995a)
	Ulva rotundata		36.10% ± 1.4% of total protein	
	Ascophyllum nodosum	5% w/v algae in deionized water, then 0.4 M HCl and 0.4 M NaOH	59.76% ± 2.44%	Kadam et al. (2017)
	Ulva sp.	Lysis solution (8 M urea, 2% Tween 20, 1% polyvinyl propelene, 30 mM dithiothreitol)	11.88% ± 0.88% extractable protein (DW)	Wijesekara et al. (2017)
	Ulva sp.	Two cycles of suspension in 10% w/v NaOH and sonication	70 g protein/100 g powder (DW)	Kazir et al. (2019)
	Gracilaria sp.		86 g/100 g powder (DW)	
Enzymatic	*Chondrus crispus*	Carrageenase + cellulase, pH 6.8, 45 °C, 2 hours	—	Fleurence et al. (1995b)
	Gracilaria verrucosa	Agarase + cellulase, pH 6, 55 °C, 2 hours		
	Palmaria palmata	Xylanase, pH 5, 55 °C, 14 hours		
	Palmaria palmata	Celluclast® and Shearzyme®, pH 5, 40 °C, 6 hours	3.3-fold increase compared with control	Joubert and Fleurence (2008)
	Ulva armoricana	Commercial neutral endo-protease, 6% w/dw, 50 °C, 3 hours	1.75-fold increase compared with extraction with water	Hardouin et al. (2016)
	Chlamydomonas reinhardtii	Autolysin, 4 hours, room temperature, then sonication or detergent (LDS buffer)	100% solubilization of extractable protein	Sierra et al. (2017)
	Palmaria palmata	Xylanase (2 mg enzyme/300 g seaweed), 60 °C overnight	—	Bjarnadóttir et al. (2018)

Table 6.1 (*continued*)

Type of extraction	Algae species	Optimum conditions and reagents	Protein yield	References
Miscellaneous	*Palmaria palmata*	Polysaccharidase digestion of milled ovendried seaweed, then sequential aqueous-alkaline extraction: 5% w/v in deionized water and 0.12 mol l^{-1} NaOH with 0.1 g/100 ml N-acetyl-L-cysteine	11.57% ± 0.08% DW (67% yield)	Harnedy and FitzGerald (2013)

6.2.1.1.3 High-Speed Homogenization A high-speed homogenizer is composed of a stator and a rotor, which exist in a wide range of designs. This device allows the stirring at high rpm. Cell disruption mechanisms involved are cavitation (above 8000 rpm) and shear force at the solid–liquid interphase (Günerken et al. 2015; Shirgaonkar et al. 1998).

High-speed homogenization (9000 rpm) has been performed on *Arthrospira platensis* to rupture the cell wall and obtain PCs and isolates for food applications (Pereira et al. 2018). This technique has been also used to disrupt macroalgal cells from *P. palmata* before protein extraction. Two shearing speeds have been tested (15 000 and 24 000 rpm). No significant difference was observed between these two speeds regarding the recovery of water-soluble proteins. However, the total protein recovery was higher with shearing at 24 000 rpm (Harnedy and FitzGerald 2013).

6.2.1.1.4 High-Pressure Homogenization (HPH) HPH is a mechanical process where a liquid dispersion of plant material or cell bio-suspension is forced under pressure (50–300 MPa) to pass through a micrometric disruption chamber (Carullo et al. 2018; Soto-Sierra et al. 2018). As a result, the biological suspension is subjected to the combination of intense shear force, cavitation, and turbulent flow, which induce cell disruption.

Among the cell disruption methods, HPH is one of the most efficient methods for releasing protein from microalgae (Safi et al. 2014b). In comparison with manual grinding, higher levels of protein solubilization have been reported for *Haematococcus pluvialis*, *Nannochloropsis gaditana*, and *Chlorella vulgaris* (Soto-Sierra et al. 2018).

6.2.1.2 Osmotic Shock Osmosis is a physical process where the solvent (water) molecules go through a partially permeable membrane to a region with a higher solute concentration (Safi et al. 2014b). The general procedure for cell disruption by osmotic shock consists of suspending the algal material in deionized water, which allows cell lysis (Fleurence et al. 1995a). The effect of time (3, 7, and 16 hours) and temperature (4 and 22 °C) of this cell disruption method on the protein extraction efficiency from *P. palmata* has been assessed. The highest total protein recoveries were obtained for 7 hours at 4 °C and 16 hours at 22 °C (Harnedy and FitzGerald 2013).

6.2.1.3 Ultrasonication Ultrasound waves are high-frequency sound waves above 20 Hz, which is inaudible for humans. Sound waves must pass through matter, where expansion and compression cycles occur. In a liquid, at sufficient ultrasound frequencies, vapor bubbles are formed during the expansion cycle. The bubbles grow and undergo an implosive collapse, which is known as cavitation. When this phenomenon occurs in a liquid near a solid surface, the cavity collapse generates high-speed streams of liquid, which can damage the solid surfaces and consequently cause cell disruption (Luque-Garcia and de Castro 2003).

The two main devices used for ultrasonication are an ultrasonic bath or ultrasonic probe, the latter being more powerful. The ultrasonic bath involves the immersion of the sample in a water bath. The ultrasonic probe is directly immersed in the fluid and can be used for small samples (Ibañez et al. 2012).

For the seaweeds *Ulva rigida* and *Ulva rotundata*, the use of ultrasound before protein extraction has not significantly increased the protein yield (Fleurence et al. 1995a). However, it was found that an ultrasound treatment using a probe at an amplitude level of 68.4 μm reduced acid and alkali extraction processing times for *A. nodosum*. This pretreatment led to better protein extraction yields versus the acid and alkali treatments alone, with an increment of 540 and 27%, respectively (Kadam et al. 2017). For microalgae, it has been reported that ultrasonication pretreatment gave different results depending on the species. A slight improvement in green microalgae (*H. pluvialis*, *Nannochloropsis oculata*, *C. vulgaris*) protein concentration and a more important increase in *A. platensis* and *Porphyridum cruentum* were noted (Safi et al. 2014b).

6.2.2 Chemical Extraction

Chemical methods include aqueous, acid, and alkaline extractions. Initially this consists of suspending algal powder in deionized water, Tris HCl, or NaOH, stirring the suspension overnight at 4 °C, and centrifuging and collecting the supernatant for measurement of the protein content (Fleurence et al. 1995a). Based on this general procedure, two-phase extraction can be implemented. For example, two-phase acid and alkali treatments have been used to extract proteins from the seaweeds *A. nodosum*, *Ulva* sp., *Laminaria digitata* and from the microalgae *Scenedesmus acutus* (Fleurence et al. 1995a; Jordan and Vilter 1991; Kadam et al. 2017). Adding reducing agents to improve alkaline-soluble protein yields has also been achieved, which reduced disulfide bonds of algal proteins associated with the cell walls (Harnedy and FitzGerald 2013). Thus, to improve the efficiency of algal protein extraction, the addition of selected chemical reagents together with use of cell disruption methods are prerequisite (Bleakley and Hayes 2017). Prior to alkaline-soluble protein extraction, an initial aqueous extraction is usually performed where cells have been disrupted by osmotic shock. As mentioned above, the effect of different cell disruption methods has also been investigated for aqueous extraction proteins from microalgae (Safi et al. 2014b). Indeed, this study has shown that the aqueous media containing the most protein content followed the order: high-pressure cell disruption > chemical treatment > ultrasonication > manual grinding (Safi et al. 2014b).

Conventional methods of algal protein extraction are time-consuming and require large amounts of solvents and are followed by several rounds of centrifugation and recovery using techniques such as ultrafiltration, precipitation, or chromatography (Bleakley and Hayes 2017; Kadam et al. 2017).

6.2.3 Enzymatic Processes

The physical and chemical barriers of the plant material being the key drawbacks of protein extraction, enzymatic processes have received more and more attention as an alternative to chemical and mechanical processes. Indeed, most of the available literature on the application of enzymes for protein extraction suggests that they have improved selectivity, high yields, and enhanced biological properties while using mild reactive conditions with a time saving, and with reduced energy and process costs (Charoensiddhi et al. 2017, 2016; Wijesinghe and Jeon 2012).

The enzymatic treatments depend on the composition of the algae cell walls, which are made up of chemically complex and heterogeneous biomolecules such as sulfated and branched polysaccharides, which are associated with proteins (Kadam et al. 2017; Soto-Sierra et al. 2018). The success of enzyme assisted extraction (EAE) is based on the disruption of algal cell walls by breaking these specific polymers. This requires the use of more than one appropriate enzyme such as carbohydrases and proteases at optimal temperature and pH conditions (Charoensiddhi et al. 2016; Kadam et al. 2017; Soto-Sierra et al. 2018; Wijesinghe and Jeon 2012). An advantage of EAE is that common enzymes that are used in the food industry (neutral and alkaline protease, α-amylase, cellulose, pepsin) can be suitable for the algal cell disruption (Postma et al. 2016).

A review on EAE from seaweed has compared different approaches for recovery of industrially useful bioactive metabolites (Wijesinghe and Jeon 2012). For example, some fractions of red and green seaweeds have demonstrated antiviral and antioxidant activities (Hardouin et al. 2014, 2016). The protein content was increased up to 1.75-fold in *Ulva* sp. extracts produced by EAE compared with an extraction with water (Hardouin et al. 2016). It has also been revealed that extractable protein content and protein profile differ according to the extraction liquid system and the season (Wijesekara et al. 2017). Different enzyme technologies improve the recovery of biological properties with regard to probiotics, antioxidant, ACE inhibitory, anti-inflammatory, and antiviral effects (Charoensiddhi et al. 2017). The development of seaweed-derived bioactive compounds using enzyme technologies presents significant opportunities for novel food applications.

Microalgae cells have been significantly disrupted by the combination of sonication and enzymatic hydrolysis allowing the improvement of the recovery of carbohydrates and proteins (Eldalatony et al. 2016). For instance, this combination of pretreatment enhanced the release of total reducing sugars and dissolved protein fractions up to 53 and 7% compared with sonication alone (14 and 2.3%) in *Chlamydomonas mexicana* microalgae, respectively. In addition, when the total reducing sugar fraction was fermented, the dissolved protein fraction was enriched up to 56% (Eldalatony et al. 2016). Depending on the desired end-product, proteolytic methods could be advantageous or not. To preserve functional properties such as emulsification and/or foaming capacity of extracted protein hydrolysates, protein fragments greater than >10–20 kDa in size should be targeted (Schröder et al. 2017). Otherwise, fractions containing small peptides ranging in size between 2 and 5 kDa can exhibit bioactive properties. In this case, for the production of protein hydrolysates, both the enzymatic hydrolysis and the release of protein fragments can be performed in a single step and bioactive properties can be generated profitably (Kadam et al. 2017; Soto-Sierra et al. 2018). Hence, the enzymatic pretreatment allowed the extraction of proteins from microalgae (*Chlorella* sp., *Scenedesmus* sp.) with antiproliferative effects against several tumor cell lines (Jabeen et al. 2017).

6.2.4 Recovery/Enrichment Techniques

Several downstream processing options are used to extract and purify algal protein products in order to generate high-value ingredients such as PCs, hydrolysates, or bioactive peptides (Soto-Sierra et al. 2018). In general, following cell disintegration (e.g. mechanical grinding and/or enzymatic pretreatment) and extraction steps (aqueous, acid and alkaline or enzymatic hydrolysis), the supernatant enriched in proteins or peptides is collected after centrifugation. The protein and peptides purification are then based on their ionic charges, size, and hydrophobicity (Vijaykrishnaraj and Prabhasankar 2015). Hence, algal protein enrichment methods include precipitation, membrane technologies, chromatographic methods, and dialysis, or combinations of these processes (Bleakley and Hayes 2017; Garcia et al. 2018).

6.2.4.1 Precipitation Selective precipitation of proteins or peptides is based on their solubility and isoelectric point (p*I*). The p*I* refers to a pH-shifting method using a broad range of pH adjustment to allow protein precipitation at their isoelectric point (Safi et al. 2014b; Garcia et al. 2018). Proteins and peptides are less soluble where they have zero net charge, at their p*I*, and can easily approach each other with minimal charge repulsion (Burgess 2009). Precipitation using ammonium sulfate based on the "salting out" involves determining the appropriate ammonium sulfate concentrations experimentally for any proteins or peptides of interest (Burgess 2009).

Supernatants rich in macroalgal proteins and peptides have been brought to 80% ammonium sulfate saturation for protein precipitation (Beaulieu et al. 2015, 2016; Bondu et al. 2015). The average extraction yield varied between 7.89 ± 0.60 and 16.97 ± 0.55 depending on the studied species, with higher yields obtained with red seaweeds (Bondu et al. 2015). Microalgal PCs have been prepared using isoelectric precipitation and ultrafiltration and, when both technologies were compared, lower protein recovery yields were observed using isoelectric precipitation (76 vs. 95%) (Safi et al. 2014b; Soto-Sierra et al. 2018).

6.2.4.2 Membrane Technologies The currently used membrane technologies that could be scaled up to an industrial level are microfiltration, ultrafiltration, nanofiltration, and reverse osmosis (Bleakley and Hayes 2017). Well established in the dairy industry (Kumar et al. 2013), membrane technologies can be promising methods of enriching algal proteins (Bleakley and Hayes 2017). These methods involve continual passing of the algal suspension across a filter on which algal proteins will concentrate until a certain enrichment level is reached (Safi et al. 2014c). The use of selective semi-permeable membranes differing in their polarity and molecular weight allows the separation of a liquid to obtain fractions rich in target molecules (Bleakley and Hayes 2017; Safi et al. 2014b, 2014c, 2017; Garcia et al. 2018).

Different studies have reported that ultrafiltration is a suitable technology for the concentration of proteins extracted from seaweeds allowing the removal of small undesirable compounds such as salts, carbohydrates, and phenols (Bleakley and Hayes 2017; Denis et al. 2009; Kadam et al. 2017). For instance, ultrafiltration was effective for R-phycoerythrin concentration and pre-purification (Denis et al.

2009) as well as for bioactive peptides (Beaulieu et al. 2015, 2016; Bondu et al. 2015). Ultrafiltration has also been performed in order to concentrate proteins from microalgae *C. vulgaris* (Ursu et al. 2014), *H. pluvialis* (Ba et al. 2016), and *Tetraselmis suecica* (Safi et al. 2014a).

6.2.4.3 Chromatographic Techniques In order to increase the protein purity after membrane filtration, chromatography techniques can be used to remove polysaccharides, pigments, and other extract contaminants (Soto-Sierra et al. 2018). Chromatography methods having higher selectivity in comparison with membrane filtration technologies, they are used mainly for the purification of bioactive proteins and peptides based on size exclusion, ion exchange, or affinity principles (Soto-Sierra et al. 2018).

For example, ion exchange chromatography was among the strategies used to isolate and characterize high-value proteins from the green microalga *Tetraselmis* sp. for techno-functional applications in foods (Schwenzfeier et al. 2011). The purification of R-phycoerythrin from the macroalga *Heterosiphonia japonica* has also been successfully achieved using gel filtration combined with ion exchange chromatography by linear ionic strength gradients (Sun et al. 2009). Several bioassay-guided approaches using liquid chromatography techniques combined with mass spectrometry (LC-MS) analysis have allowed identification of bioactive peptide sequences from red macroalgae (Bondu et al. 2015; Fitzgerald et al. 2012, 2014a; Harnedy et al. 2015, 2017).

6.2.4.4 Isoelectric Focusing Proteins and peptides can also be fractionated by liquid-phase isoelectric focusing (IEF) (Beaulieu et al. 2015; Sun et al. 2009). Electrolytes from pH 3 to 10 have been added to macroalgal protein hydrolysate samples in a focusing chamber. Acidic peptides were attracted to the anode (the H_3PO_4 membrane chamber), whereas basic peptides migrated toward the cathode (NaOH) until they reached their zwitterionic state and stabilized at a pH corresponding to their p*I*. In the course of each run, peptide fractions can be collected for further analysis such as LC-MS.

6.2.5 Protein Extraction Methods in Proteomics

Protein dynamics during growth changes can be inferred through proteomic analysis. The first step to any proteomic experiment is the sample preparation and protein extraction, which often fails to extract water-insoluble proteins (Safi et al. 2014b). A study has investigated the use of three protein extraction methods: trichloroacetic acid (TCA)-acetone, phenol, and TRIzol, in the eustigmatophyte alga *Microchloropsis gaditana* CCMP526 for proteomic analysis (Anbarasu et al. 2017). It has been reported that the protein yield was higher using the TCA-acetone and phenol methods in comparison with the TRIzol method in terms of protein abundance. In addition, high-quality protein extracts have been obtained from a reliable phenol extraction protocol using *Scytosiphon gracilis* and *Ectocarpus siliculosus* (Contreras et al. 2008). Proteome imaging and analysis can then be performed by two-dimensional gel electrophoresis and liquid chromatography followed by mass spectrometry (Lopez-Cristoffanini et al. 2015; Tee et al. 2015; Xu et al. 2013; Yotsukura et al. 2009; Zou et al. 2015).

6.3 Emerging Technologies for Proteins and Peptides

Table 6.2 shows all the emerging methods discussed in the present chapter and gives their different advantages and limitations. Another chapter on extraction of biomolecules from seaweeds has compared most of the novel extraction techniques described in the present chapter (Kadam et al. 2015).

6.3.1 Microwave Assisted Extraction (MAE)

MAE has been extensively studied in medicinal plant research because the method allows a shorter time, less solvent, higher extraction rate, moderate capital cost, and can be performed under atmospheric conditions (Kadam et al. 2015; Wijesinghe and Jeon 2012). Microwaves induce the vibration of water molecules within the cell, which causes an increase in the temperature of the intracellular liquids. Then, subsequent evaporation of water applies pressure on the cell walls causing their disruption releasing the intracellular contents into the medium (Michalak and Chojnacka 2014). In MAE, hydrogen bonds are disrupted and dissolved ions can more easily migrate allowing a higher penetration of solvent into the matrix facilitating the extraction of target compounds (Kadam et al. 2015; Michalak and Chojnacka 2014).

Two MAE systems are known, namely closed vessel (multimode) and open vessel (monomode) systems. The former are used for extraction of target compounds at a higher temperature and pressure conditions, while the latter systems are used for extractions carried out at atmospheric pressure conditions (Kaufmann and Christen 2002).

In the literature, the application of MAE for compound extraction from microalgae and seaweeds was mainly used for polysaccharides (fucoidans), pigment (carotenoids), minerals (iodine, bromine), and oil extraction (Ibañez et al. 2012; Kadam et al. 2015; Michalak and Chojnacka 2014).

Due to the high temperature involved in MAE, which would likely make it unsuitable for extraction of proteins in algae (Bleakley and Hayes 2017), some studies have been conducted on this biomass. For instance, a microwave pretreatment has been used on microalgal biomass (*Stigeoclonium* sp. and *Monoraphidium* sp.), which allowed obtaining increased levels of soluble proteins compared with ultrasound treatment (Passos et al. 2015).

6.3.2 Pulsed Arc Technology

Pulsed arc technology includes pulsed electric fields (PEFs) and high-voltage electrical discharges (HVEDs). They are environmentally friendly and energy-efficient disruption techniques (Phong et al. 2018). Most studies on the effectiveness of electrical disruption techniques on algae have been achieved using PEF.

PEF processing uses short (from several nanoseconds to few milliseconds), high-voltage electric pulses (10–50 kV cm^{-1}) and a specific treatment chamber to perforate a cell wall or cell membrane, causing their permeabilization by electroporation (Bleakley and Hayes 2017; Carullo et al. 2018; Kempkes 2016). PEF is a green technology for inactivating microorganisms and extracting of intracellular material of plant cells (Bleakley and Hayes 2017; Kempkes 2016).

Table 6.2 Emerging technologies of algal protein extraction and their different advantages and limitations.

Technique	Mechanism of action	Advantages	Limitations	References
Pulsed electric fields (PEFs)	Permeabilization of cells by electroporation	Environmentally friendly	High maintenance and operating costs	Phong et al. (2018)
		Energy-efficient	Efficiency dependable of the medium composition	Joannes et al. (2015)
		Fast treatment time	Not suitable for scale-up	Günerken et al. (2015)
			Difficulties in operating at large scale	Gonçalves et al. (2013)
Microwave assisted extraction (MAE)	Vibration of water molecules in the cells causing heating then cell disruption	Improved extraction rates and yields	Need of a subsequent separation step to remove the solid residues	Kadam et al. (2015)
		Cost-effective	Not suitable for heat-sensitive compounds	Michalak and Chojnacka (2014)
Supercritical fluid extraction (SFE)	Extraction of compounds in a fluid heated and pressurized above its critical point	Possibility of obtaining solvent-free extracts	Mainly used to extract molecules with low polarity	Ibañez et al. (2012)
			High investment costs	
Pressurized liquid extraction (PLE)	Combination of high pressures and high temperatures to increase the solubility and mass transfer rate of the analytes in the liquid solvent	Environmentally friendly	Less selective than SFE	Ibañez et al. (2012)
		Possibility of automation		
		Short operating time		
Ultrahigh pressure extraction	Use of high pressures to enhance the mass transfer rates of compounds and possibly rupture the algae cell walls	Use of mild processing temperatures	High investment costs	Xi (2017)
		Short extraction time		
		Low solvent consumption		

Applications of PEF to algal processing have emerged in the past two decades in the field of algal cell disintegration to enhance the release of several components. More protein, chlorophyll, and carotenoids have been extracted from *C. vulgaris* with up to 27, 80, and 53%, respectively (Postma et al. 2016). PEF has also been demonstrated to be an effective procedure for extracting proteins from *H. pluvialis* (Coustets et al. 2015), C-phycocyanin from *A. platensis* (Martínez et al. 2017), and proteins from *Nannochloropsis* spp. (Grimi et al. 2014; Parniakov et al. 2015). Recently, PEF has been used for a selective extraction of carbohydrates (36% w/w, of total carbohydrates), whereas the extracted proteins were relatively low and did not exceed 5.2% (w/w) of the total (Carullo et al. 2018).

A selective extraction of proteins from green macroalga *Ulva* by electroporation has been reported with the PEF process (Polikovsky et al. 2016). PEF increased by approx. three times the total protein extraction, increasing the extraction yields of some proteins but damaging others (Polikovsky et al. 2016).

The upscaling of this technology could be limited due to the conductivity and electrode gap, which are two important factors to take into account (Bleakley and Hayes 2017).

6.3.3 Pressurized Liquid Extraction (PLE)

PLE has exhibited great potential for extracting bioactive compounds from plant tissues as well as algal biomass, especially in terms of extraction yield, phenolic content, and antioxidant activity (Boisvert et al. 2015; Ibañez et al. 2012). PLE techniques combine the use of high pressure with high temperatures, which could reach their normal boiling point (Ibañez et al. 2012; Michalak and Chojnacka 2014). PLE techniques may also consist of accelerated solvent extraction (considered as a new version of the Soxhlet apparatus), pressurized hot water extraction, subcritical water extraction (SWE) (see below), near-critical fluid extraction, and enhanced fluidity extraction (Ibañez et al. 2012; Michalak and Chojnacka 2014).

Briefly, the instrumentation includes a solvent reservoir coupled to a high-pressure pump to introduce the solvent into the system, an oven where the extraction takes place through the extraction cell, and a valve to maintain the pressure in the system (Ibañez et al. 2012). Following the preheating step, both the temperature and the pressure are kept constant in the oven. The solvent, filled in the extraction cell, is then collected in a vial and the cell flushed and purged with nitrogen gas (Ibañez et al. 2012).

PLE techniques have been used efficiently in the extraction of algal antioxidants: phenols, carotenoids (fucoxanthin), fatty acids, and fucosterol (Michalak and Chojnacka 2014). The protein content in ethanol extracts obtained by PLE has been evaluated, and was lower than in crude seaweeds (*Ulva lactuca*, *A. nodosum*, and *S. longicruris*) at 4.77, 4.72, and 1.86%, respectively (Boisvert et al. 2015).

The possibility of the automation of PLE-based techniques, along with the reduced extraction time and solvents required, has supported its development (Ibañez et al. 2012).

6.3.4 Sub- and Supercritical Fluid Extraction (SFE)

Nonconventional extraction techniques such as subcritical fluid extraction and SFE are currently being investigated (Kadam et al. 2017). SWE requires using hot water under high pressure to maintain water in the liquid phase while SFE is a method that heats a fluid above its critical point (Barba et al. 2015; Bleakley and Hayes 2017). Under these supercritical conditions, the fluid has similar properties as in its gaseous phase, with the same density as a fluid but with the viscosity of a gas. SFE uses carbon dioxide (CO_2), with low solvent consumption, supporting a green chemistry application (Barba et al. 2015; Bleakley and Hayes 2017).

Nonetheless, high investment costs for equipment are required for SWE and SFE technologies and they have been used in algae so far only for the extraction of nonpolar molecules (Bleakley and Hayes 2017) such as fatty acids, vitamin E, carotenoids, flavonoids, and terpenoids (Ibañez et al. 2012; Kadam et al. 2013, 2015).

6.3.5 High Hydrostatic Pressure (HHP) and Ultra-high Pressure Extraction (UHP)

Nonthermal HHP and ultrahigh pressure in the range of 100–600 MPa have been studied for their impact on proteins and bioactive peptides and vitamin extractability from numerous examples of plant-based biomass (Xi 2017). The high-pressure treatment consists of structural modification (unfolding) of protein to expose the enzyme cleavage sites, which are not accessible to the native proteins. Assistance through HHP during or prior to EAE could be a viable alternative to improve the extraction yield (Bourgougnon 2014). The potential of HHP assisted enzymatic extraction of proteins, polyphenols, and polysaccharides from red seaweeds has been recently demonstrated. The antioxidant activity was highly correlated with polysaccharide (89%) and protein (83%) content for *Solieria chordalis*, and with polyphenol content (65%) for *P. palmata* (Suwal et al. 2019).

6.4 Conclusion and Future Outlook

Algae play an economic role through their use as food, either as basic ingredients or as dietary supplements. They are generally considered nutritive due to their abundance in fibers, minerals, vitamins, polyunsaturated fatty acids (omega-3), and proteins. Modern lifestyle trends, such as the enhanced consumption of vegan, sustainable, and healthy food products, have brought algae to the forefront of protein alternative sources. Algae have also been associated with high-quality proteins in terms of their essential amino acid content and their *in vitro* protein digestibility, which approach those of commonly consumed plants.

There is a broad variety of protein extraction methods and the successful enrichment of algal protein ingredients at a commercial scale depends crucially on efficient cell disruption techniques. Conventional protein extraction methods are often laborious, time-consuming, and may require the use of nonnegligible amounts of solvents. Emerging extraction technologies are thus investigated to overcome the drawbacks of the conventional methods. The most promising methods must be based on important criteria such as being nonthermal and environmentally sustainable (requiring low solvent consumption), and have to be scalable and involve economically viable processes. In addition, based on the extraction of compounds in other food processes, membrane technologies are promising and have to be further investigated as recovery methods in the algae area.

Basic information is thus needed on algal protein extraction methods and this may also support the understanding of the regulation of various proteins in algae by proteomic approaches. All these efforts may lead to new active algae-based food with beneficial health properties which can be seen as functional foods that can reach the growing healthcare and well-being markets.

References

Afify, A.E.-M.M.R., El Baroty, G.S., El Baz, F.K. et al. (2018). *Scenedesmus obliquus*: antioxidant and antiviral activity of proteins hydrolyzed by three enzymes. *Journal of Genetic Engineering and Biotechnology* **16** (2): 399–408. https://doi.org/10.1016/j.jgeb.2018.01.002.

Alexandratos, N. and Bruinsma, J. (2012). World agriculture towards 2030/2050, The 2012 revision. Food. FAO ESA Working Paper No. 12-03. www.fao.org/3/a-ap106e.pdf (accessed Sepember 4, 2020).

Anbarasu, K., Pranali, D., Vineeta, R. et al. (2017). Time for multiple extraction methods in proteomics? A comparison of three protein extraction methods in the eustigmatophyte alga *Microchloropsis gaditana* CCMP526. *OMICS: A Journal of Integrative Biology* **21** (11): 678–683. https://doi.org/10.1089/omi.2017.0128.

Ba, F., Ursu, A.V., Laroche, C., and Djelveh, G. (2016). *Haematococcus pluvialis* soluble proteins: extraction, characterization, concentration/fractionation and emulsifying properties. *Bioresource Technology* **200**: 147–152. https://doi.org/10.1016/j.biortech.2015.10.012.

Barba, F.J. (2017). Microalgae and seaweeds for food applications: challenges and perspectives. *Food Research International* **99**: 969–970. https://doi.org/10.1016/j.foodres.2016.12.022.

Barba, F.J., Grimi, N., and Vorobiev, E. (2015). New approaches for the use of non-conventional cell disruption technologies to extract potential food additives and nutraceuticals from microalgae. *Food Engineering Reviews* **7** (1): 45–62. https://doi.org/10.1007/s12393-014-9095-6.

Barbarino, E. and Lourenço, S.O. (2005). An evaluation of methods for extraction and quantification of protein from marine macro- and microalgae. *Journal of Applied Phycology* **17** (5): 447–460. https://doi.org/10.1007/s10811-005-1641-4.

Batista, A.P., Niccolai, A., Fradinho, P. et al. (2017). Microalgae biomass as an alternative ingredient in cookies: sensory, physical and chemical properties, antioxidant activity and in vitro digestibility. *Algal Research* **26**: 161–171. https://doi.org/10.1016/j.algal.2017.07.017.

Beaulieu, L., Bondu, S., Doiron, K. et al. (2015). Characterization of antibacterial activity from protein hydrolysates of the macroalga *Saccharina longicruris* and identification of peptides implied in bioactivity. *Journal of Functional Foods* **17**: 685–697. https://doi.org/10.1016/j.jff.2015.06.026.

Beaulieu, L., Sirois, M., and Tamigneaux, E. (2016). Evaluation of the *in vitro* biological activity of protein hydrolysates of the edible red alga, *Palmaria palmata* (dulse) harvested from the Gaspe coast and cultivated in tanks. *Journal of Applied Phycology* **28** (5): 3101–3115. https://doi.org/10.1007/s10811-016-0850-3.

Becker, E.W. (2007). Micro-algae as a source of protein. *Biotechnology Advances* **25** (2): 207–210. https://doi.org/10.1016/j.biotechadv.2006.11.002.

Bjarnadóttir, M., Aðalbjörnsson, B.V., Nilsson, A. et al. (2018). *Palmaria palmata* as an alternative protein source: enzymatic protein extraction, amino acid composition, and nitrogen-to-protein conversion factor. *Journal of Applied Phycology* **30** (3): 2061–2070. https://doi.org/10.1007/s10811-017-1351-8.

Bleakley, S. and Hayes, M. (2017). Algal proteins: extraction, application, and challenges concerning production. *Foods* **6** (5): 33. https://doi.org/10.3390/foods6050033.

Boisvert, C., Beaulieu, L., Bonnet, C., and Pelletier, É. (2015). Assessment of the antioxidant and antibacterial activities of three species of edible seaweeds. *Journal of Food Biochemistry* **39** (4): 377–387. https://doi.org/10.1111/jfbc.12146.

Bondu, S., Bonnet, C., Gaubert, J. et al. (2015). Bioassay-guided fractionation approach for determination of protein precursors of proteolytic bioactive metabolites from macroalgae. *Journal of Applied Phycology* **27** (5): 2059–2074. https://doi.org/10.1007/s10811-014-0425-0.

Bourgougnon, N. (2014). *Sea Plants*. San Diego, CA: Elsevier Science.

Burgess, R.R. (2009). Protein precipitation techniques. In: *Methods in Enzymology*, vol. **463** (eds. R.R. Burgess and M.P. Deutscher), 331–342. London: Academic Press https://doi.org/10.1016/S0076-6879(09)63020-2.

Carullo, D., Abera, B.D., Casazza, A.A. et al. (2018). Effect of pulsed electric fields and high pressure homogenization on the aqueous extraction of intracellular compounds from the microalgae *Chlorella vulgaris*. *Algal Research* **31**: 60–69. https://doi.org/10.1016/j.algal.2018.01.017.

Charoensiddhi, S., Lorbeer, A.J., Lahnstein, J. et al. (2016). Enzyme-assisted extraction of carbohydrates from the brown alga *Ecklonia radiata*: effect of enzyme type, pH and buffer on sugar yield and molecular weight profiles. *Process Biochemistry* **51** (10): 1503–1510. https://doi.org/10.1016/j.procbio.2016.07.014.

Charoensiddhi, S., Conlon, M.A., Franco, C.M.M., and Zhang, W. (2017). The development of seaweed-derived bioactive compounds for use as prebiotics and nutraceuticals using enzyme technologies. *Trends in Food Science & Technology* **70**: 20–33. https://doi.org/10.1016/j.tifs.2017.10.002.

Chojnacka, K., Saeid, A., Witkowska, Z., and Tuhy, L. (2012). Biologically active compounds in seaweed extracts – the prospects for the application. *The Open Conference Proceedings Journal* **3**: 20–28.

Cole, A.J., de Nys, R., and Paul, N.A. (2015). Biorecovery of nutrient waste as protein in freshwater macroalgae. *Algal Research* **7**: 58–65. https://doi.org/10.1016/j.algal.2014.12.005.

Connan, S., Deslandes, E., and Gall, E.A. (2007). Influence of day–night and tidal cycles on phenol content and antioxidant capacity in three temperate intertidal brown seaweeds. *Journal of Experimental Marine Biology and Ecology* **349** (2): 359–369. https://doi.org/10.1016/j.jembe.2007.05.028.

Contreras, L., Ritter, A., Dennett, G. et al. (2008). Two-dimensional gel electrophoresis analysis of brown algal protein extracts. *Journal of Phycology* **44** (5): 1315–1321. https://doi.org/10.1111/j.1529-8817.2008.00575.x.

Coustets, M., Joubert-Durigneux, V., Hérault, J. et al. (2015). Optimization of protein electroextraction from microalgae by a flow process. *Bioelectrochemistry* **103**: 74–81. https://doi.org/10.1016/j.bioelechem.2014.08.022.

Denis, C., Massé, A., Fleurence, J., and Jaouen, P. (2009). Concentration and pre-purification with ultrafiltration of a R-phycoerythrin solution extracted from macro-algae *Grateloupia turuturu*: process definition and up-scaling. *Separation and Purification Technology* **69** (1): 37–42. https://doi.org/10.1016/j.seppur.2009.06.017.

Eldalatony, M.M., Kabra, A.N., Hwang, J.-H. et al. (2016). Pretreatment of microalgal biomass for enhanced recovery/extraction of reducing sugars and proteins. *Bioprocess and Biosystems Engineering* **39** (1): 95–103. https://doi.org/10.1007/s00449-015-1493-5.

Fitzgerald, C., Mora-Soler, L., Gallagher, E. et al. (2012). Isolation and characterization of bioactive pro-peptides with in vitro renin inhibitory activities from the macroalga *Palmaria palmata*. *Journal of Agricultural and Food Chemistry* **60** (30): 7421–7427. https://doi.org/10.1021/jf301361c.

Fitzgerald, C., Aluko, R.E., Hossain, M. et al. (2014a). Potential of a renin inhibitory peptide from the red seaweed *Palmaria palmata* as a functional food ingredient following confirmation and characterization of a hypotensive effect in spontaneously hypertensive rats. *Journal of Agricultural and Food Chemistry* **62** (33): 8352–8356. https://doi.org/10.1021/jf500983n.

Fitzgerald, C., Gallagher, E., Doran, L. et al. (2014b). Increasing the health benefits of bread: assessment of the physical and sensory qualities of bread formulated using a renin inhibitory *Palmaria palmata* protein hydrolysate. *LWT – Food Science and Technology* **56** (2): 398–405. https://doi.org/10.1016/j.lwt.2013.11.031.

Fleurence, J. (1999). Seaweed proteins: biochemical, nutritional aspects and potential uses. *Trends in Food Science & Technology* **10** (1): 25–28. https://doi.org/10.1016/S0924-2244(99)00015-1.

Fleurence, J. (2004). *Proteins in Food Processing* (ed. R.Y. Yada). Cambridge: Woodhead Publishing Ltd.

Fleurence, J., Le Coeur, C., Mabeau, S. et al. (1995a). Comparison of different extractive procedures for proteins from the edible seaweeds *Ulva rigida* and *Ulva rotundata*. *Journal of Applied Phycology* **7** (6): 577–582. https://doi.org/10.1007/BF00003945.

Fleurence, J., Massiani, L., Guyader, O., and Mabeau, S. (1995b). Use of enzymatic cell wall degradation for improvement of protein extraction from *Chondrus crispus*, *Gracilaria verrucosa* and *Palmaria palmata*. *Journal of Applied Phycology* **7** (4): 393–397. https://doi.org/10.1007/BF00003796.

Fleurence, J., Chenard, E., and Luçcon, M. (1999). Determination of the nutritional value of proteins obtained from *Ulva armoricana*. *Journal of Applied Phycology* **11** (3): 231–239. https://doi.org/10.1023/A:1008067308100.

Fleurence, J., Morançais, M., Dumay, J. et al. (2012). What are the prospects for using seaweed in human nutrition and for marine animals raised through aquaculture? *Trends in Food Science & Technology* **27** (1): 57–61. https://doi.org/10.1016/j.tifs.2012.03.004.

Fleurence, J., Morançais, M., and Dumay, J. (2018). Seaweed proteins. In: *Proteins in Food Processing*, 2e (ed. R.Y. Yada), 245–262. Cambridge: Woodhead Publishing Ltd.

Garcia, E.S., van Leeuwen, J., Safi, C. et al. (2018). Selective and energy efficient extraction of functional proteins from microalgae for food applications. *Bioresource Technology* **268**: 197–203. https://doi.org/10.1016/j.biortech.2018.07.131.

Gonçalves, A.L., Pires, J.C.M., and Simões, M. (2013). Green fuel production: processes applied to microalgae. *Environmental Chemistry Letters* **11** (4): 315–324. https://doi.org/10.1007/s10311-013-0425-3.

Goni, I., Valdivieso, L., and Gudiel-Urbano, M. (2002). Capacity of edible seaweeds to modify in vitro starch digestibility of wheat bread. *Nahrung/Food* **46** (1): 18. https://doi.org/10.1002/1521-3803(20020101)46:1<18::AID-FOOD18>3.0.CO;2-C.

Gouveia, L., Batista, A.P., Sousa, I. et al. (2008). Microalgae in novel food products. In: *Food Chemistry Research Developments* (eds. N. Konstantinos and P.P. Papadopoulos), 1–37. New York: Nova Science Publishers.

Grimi, N., Dubois, A., Marchal, L. et al. (2014). Selective extraction from microalgae *Nannochloropsis* sp. using different methods of cell disruption. *Bioresource Technology* **153**: 254–259. https://doi.org/10.1016/j.biortech.2013.12.011.

Günerken, E., D'Hondt, E., Eppink, M.H.M. et al. (2015). Cell disruption for microalgae biorefineries. *Biotechnology Advances* **33** (2): 243–260. https://doi.org/10.1016/j

.biotechadv.2015.01.008.

Hall, A.C., Fairclough, A.C., Mahadevan, K., and Paxman, J.R. (2012). *Ascophyllum nodosum* enriched bread reduces subsequent energy intake with no effect on post-prandial glucose and cholesterol in healthy, overweight males. A pilot study. *Appetite* **58** (1): 379–386. https://doi.org/10.1016/j.appet.2011.11.002.

Hardouin, K., Burlot, A.-S., Umami, A. et al. (2014). Biochemical and antiviral activities of enzymatic hydrolysates from different invasive French seaweeds. *Journal of Applied Phycology* **26** (2): 1029–1042. https://doi.org/10.1007/s10811-013-0201-6.

Hardouin, K., Bedoux, G., Burlot, A.-S. et al. (2016). Enzyme-assisted extraction (EAE) for the production of antiviral and antioxidant extracts from the green seaweed *Ulva armoricana* (Ulvales, Ulvophyceae). *Algal Research* **16**: 233–239. https://doi.org/10.1016/j.algal.2016.03.013.

Harnedy, P.A. and FitzGerald, R.J. (2011). Bioactive proteins, peptides, and amino acids from macroalgae. *Journal of Phycology* **47** (2): 218–232. https://doi.org/10.1111/j.1529-8817.2011.00969.x.

Harnedy, P.A. and FitzGerald, R.J. (2013). Extraction of protein from the macroalga *Palmaria palmata*. *LWT – Food Science and Technology* **51** (1): 375–382. https://doi.org/10.1016/j.lwt.2012.09.023.

Harnedy, P.A., Soler-Vila, A., Edwards, M.D., and FitzGerald, R.J. (2014). The effect of time and origin of harvest on the in vitro biological activity of *Palmaria palmata* protein hydrolysates. *Food Research International* **62**: 746–752. https://doi.org/10.1016/j.foodres.2014.04.035.

Harnedy, P.A., O'Keeffe, M.B., and FitzGerald, R.J. (2015). Purification and identification of dipeptidyl peptidase (DPP) IV inhibitory peptides from the macroalga *Palmaria palmata*. *Food Chemistry* **172**: 400–406. https://doi.org/10.1016/j.foodchem.2014.09.083.

Harnedy, P.A., O'Keeffe, M.B., and FitzGerald, R.J. (2017). Fractionation and identification of antioxidant peptides from an enzymatically hydrolysed *Palmaria palmata* protein isolate. *Food Research International* **100**: 416–422. https://doi.org/10.1016/j.foodres.2017.07.037.

Hell, A., Labrie, S., and Beaulieu, L. (2017). Effect of seaweed flakes addition on the development of bioactivities in functional Camembert-type cheese. *International Journal of Food Science and Technology* **53**: 1054–1064. https://doi.org/10.1111/ijfs.13681.

Henchion, M., Hayes, M., Mullen, A. et al. (2017). Future protein supply and demand: strategies and factors influencing a sustainable equilibrium. *Foods* **6** (7): 53. https://doi.org/10.3390/foods6070053.

Holdt, S.L. and Kraan, S. (2011). Bioactive compounds in seaweed: functional food applications and legislation. *Journal of Applied Phycology* **23** (3): 543–597. https://doi.org/10.1007/s10811-010-9632-5.

Ibañez, E., Herrero, M., Mendiola, J.A., and Castro-Puyana, M. (2012). Extraction and characterization of bioactive compounds with health benefits from marine resources: macro and micro algae, cyanobacteria, and invertebrates. In: *Marine Bioactive Compounds: Sources, Characterization and Applications* (ed. M. Hayes), 55–98. Boston, MA: Springer US https://doi.org/10.1007/978-1-4614-1247-2_2.

Jabeen, A., Reeder, B., Hisaindee, S. et al. (2017). Effect of enzymatic pre-treatment of microalgae extracts on their anti-tumor activity. *Biomedical Journal* **40** (6): 339–346. https://doi.org/10.1016/j.bj.2017.10.003.

Joannes, C., Sipaut, C.S., Dayou, J. et al. (2015). The potential of using pulsed electric field (PEF) technology as the cell disruption method to extract lipid from microalgae for biodiesel production. *International Journal of Renewable Energy Research* **5** (2): 598–621.

Jordan, P. and Vilter, H. (1991). Extraction of proteins from material rich in anionic mucilages: partition and fractionation of vanadate-dependent bromoperoxidases from the brown algae *Laminaria digitata* and *L. saccharina* in aqueous polymer two-phase systems. *Biochimica et Biophysica Acta (BBA) – General Subjects* **1073** (1): 98–106. https://doi.org/10.1016/0304-4165(91)90188-M.

Joubert, Y. and Fleurence, J. (2008). Simultaneous extraction of proteins and DNA by an enzymatic treatment of the cell wall of *Palmaria palmata* (Rhodophyta). *Journal of Applied Phycology* **20** (1): 55–61. https://doi.org/10.1007/s10811-007-9180-9.

Kadam, S.U., Tiwari, B.K., and O'Donnell, C.P. (2013). Application of novel extraction technologies for bioactives from marine algae. *Journal of Agricultural and Food Chemistry* **61** (20): 4667–4675. https://doi.org/10.1021/jf400819p.

Kadam, S.U., Álvarez, C., Tiwari, B.K., and O'Donnell, C.P. (2015). Extraction of biomolecules from seaweeds. In: *Seaweed Sustainability* (eds. B.K. Tiwari and D.J. Troy), 243–269. San Diego, CA: Academic Press.

Kadam, S.U., Álvarez, C., Tiwari, B.K., and O'Donnell, C.P. (2017). Extraction and characterization of protein from Irish brown seaweed *Ascophyllum nodosum*. *Food Research International* **99**: 1021–1027. https://doi.org/10.1016/j.foodres.2016.07.018.

Kaufmann, B. and Christen, P. (2002). Recent extraction techniques for natural products: microwave-assisted extraction and pressurised solvent extraction. *Phytochemical Analysis* **13** (2): 105–113. https://doi.org/10.1002/pca.631.

Kazir, M., Abuhassira, Y., Robin, A. et al. (2019). Extraction of proteins from two marine macroalgae, *Ulva* sp. and *Gracilaria* sp., for food application, and evaluating digestibility, amino acid composition and antioxidant properties of the protein concentrates. *Food Hydrocolloids* **87**: 194–203. https://doi.org/10.1016/j.foodhyd.2018.07.047.

Kempkes, M.A. (2016). Pulsed electric fields for algal extraction and predator control. In: *Handbook of Electroporation* (ed. D. Miklavcic), 1–16. Cham: Springer International Publishing.

Kim, S.-K. and Wijesekara, I. (2010). Development and biological activities of marine-derived bioactive peptides: a review. *Journal of Functional Foods* **2** (1): 1–9. https://doi.org/10.1016/j.jff.2010.01.003.

Kula, M.R. and Schutte, H. (1987). Purification of proteins and the disruption of microbial-cells. *Biotechnology Progress* **3** (1): 31–42. https://doi.org/10.1002/btpr.5420030107.

Kumar, P., Sharma, N., Ranjan, R. et al. (2013). Perspective of membrane technology in dairy industry: a review. *Asian-Australasian Journal of Animal Sciences* **26** (9): 1347–1358. https://doi.org/10.5713/ajas.2013.13082.

Liang, S., Liu, X., Chen, F., and Chen, Z. (2004). Current microalgal health food R&D activities in China. In: *Asian Pacific Phycology in the 21st Century: Prospects and Challenges* (ed. P.O. Ang Jr.), 45–48. Dordrecht: Springer.

Lopez-Cristoffanini, C., Zapata, J., Gaillard, F. et al. (2015). Identification of proteins involved in desiccation tolerance in the red seaweed *Pyropia orbicularis* (Rhodophyta, Bangiales). *Proteomics* **15** (23–24): 3954–3968. https://doi.org/10.1002/pmic.201400625.

Luque-Garcia, J.L. and de Castro, L. (2003). Ultrasound: a powerful tool for leaching. *TrAC –Trends in Analytical Chemistry* **22** (1): 41–47. https://doi.org/10.1016/s0165-9936(03)00102-x.

Marinho, G.S., Holdt, S.L., and Angelidaki, I. (2015). Seasonal variations in the amino acid profile and protein nutritional value of *Saccharina latissima* cultivated in a commercial IMTA system. *Journal of Applied Phycology* **27** (5): 1991–2000. https://doi.org/10.1007/s10811-015-0546-0.

Marrion, O., Schwertz, A., Fleurence, J. et al. (2003). Improvement of the digestibility of the proteins of the red alga *Palmaria palmata* by physical processes and fermentation.

Food/Nahrung **47** (5): 339–344. https://doi.org/10.1002/food.200390078.
Martínez, B. and Rico, J.M. (2002). Seasonal variation of p content and major n pools in *Palmaria palmata* (rhodophyta) 1. *Journal of Phycology* **38** (6): 1082–1089. https://doi.org/10.1046/j.1529-8817.2002.01217.x.
Martínez, J.M., Luengo, E., Saldaña, G. et al. (2017). C-phycocyanin extraction assisted by pulsed electric field from *Artrosphira platensis*. *Food Research International* **99**: 1042–1047. https://doi.org/10.1016/j.foodres.2016.09.029.
McHugh, D.J. (2003). A guide to the seaweed industry. FAO Fisheries Technical paper No. 441. www.fao.org/3/a-y4765e.pdf (accessed September 4, 2020).
Melendres, A.V., Unno, H., Shiragami, N., and Honda, H. (1992). A concept of critical velocity for cell disruption by bead mill. *Journal of Chemical Engineering of Japan* **25** (3): 354–356. https://doi.org/10.1252/jcej.25.354.
Michalak, I. and Chojnacka, K. (2014). Algal extracts: technology and advances. *Engineering in Life Sciences* **14** (6): 581–591. https://doi.org/10.1002/elsc.201400139.
Mouritsen, O.G. (2012). The emerging science of gastrophysics and its application to the algal cuisine. *Flavour* **1** (1): 6. https://doi.org/10.1186/2044-7248-1-6.
Mouritsen, O.G., Dawczynski, C., Duelund, L. et al. (2013). On the human consumption of the red seaweed dulse (*Palmaria palmata* (L.) Weber & Mohr). *Journal of Applied Phycology* **25** (6): 1777–1791. https://doi.org/10.1007/s10811-013-0014-7.
Pangestuti, R. and Kim, S.-K. (2011). Biological activities and health benefit effects of natural pigments derived from marine algae. *Journal of Functional Foods* **3** (4): 255–266. https://doi.org/10.1016/j.jff.2011.07.001.
Pangestuti, R. and Kim, S.-K. (2015). Seaweed proteins, peptides, and amino acids. In: *Seaweed Sustainability* (eds. B.K. Tiwari and D.J. Troy), 125–140. San Diego, CA: Academic Press https://doi.org/10.1016/b978-0-12-418697-2.00006-4.
Parniakov, O., Barba, F.J., Grimi, N. et al. (2015). Pulsed electric field and pH assisted selective extraction of intracellular components from microalgae *Nannochloropsis*. *Algal Research* **8**: 128–134. https://doi.org/10.1016/j.algal.2015.01.014.
Passos, F., Carretero, J., and Ferrer, I. (2015). Comparing pretreatment methods for improving microalgae anaerobic digestion: thermal, hydrothermal, microwave and ultrasound. *Chemical Engineering Journal* **279**: 667–672. https://doi.org/10.1016/j.cej.2015.05.065.
Pereira, L. (2011). A review of the nutrient composition of selected edible seaweeds. In: *Seaweed: Ecology, Nutrient Composition and Medicinal Uses* (ed. V.H. Pomin), 15–47. New York: Nova Science Publishers.
Pereira, A.M., Lisboa, C.R., and Costa, J.A.V. (2018). High protein ingredients of microalgal origin: obtainment and functional properties. *Innovative Food Science & Emerging Technologies* **47**: 187–194. https://doi.org/10.1016/j.ifset.2018.02.015.
Phong, W.N., Show, P.L., Ling, T.C. et al. (2018). Mild cell disruption methods for bio-functional proteins recovery from microalgae – recent developments and future perspectives. *Algal Research* **31**: 506–516. https://doi.org/10.1016/j.algal.2017.04.005.
Polikovsky, M., Fernand, F., Sack, M. et al. (2016). Towards marine biorefineries: selective proteins extractions from marine macroalgae *Ulva* with pulsed electric fields. *Innovative Food Science & Emerging Technologies* **37**: 194–200. https://doi.org/10.1016/j.ifset.2016.03.013.
Postma, P.R., 't Lam, G.P., Barbosa, M.J. et al. (2016). Microalgal biorefinery for bulk and high-value products: product extraction within cell disintegration. In: *Handbook of Electroporation* (ed. D. Miklavcic), 1–20. Cham: Springer International Publishing.
Postma, P.R., Suarez-Garcia, E., Safi, C. et al. (2017). Energy efficient bead milling of microalgae: effect of bead size on disintegration and release of proteins and carbohydrates. *Bioresource Technology* **224**: 670–679. https://doi.org/10.1016/j.biortech.2016.11.071.

Prabhasankar, P., Ganesan, P., Bhaskar, N. et al. (2009). Edible Japanese seaweed, wakame (*Undaria pinnatifida*) as an ingredient in pasta: chemical, functional and structural evaluation. *Food Chemistry* **115** (2): 501–508. https://doi.org/10.1016/j.foodchem.2008.12.047.

Rioux, L.-E., Beaulieu, L., and Turgeon, S.L. (2017). Seaweeds: a traditional ingredients for new gastronomic sensation. *Food Hydrocolloids* **68** (Supplement C): 255–265. https://doi.org/10.1016/j.foodhyd.2017.02.005.

Ritala, A., Häkkinen, S.T., Toivari, M., and Wiebe, M.G. (2017). Single cell protein – state-of-the-art, industrial landscape and patents 2001–2016. *Frontiers in Microbiology* **8** (2009) https://www.frontiersin.org/article/10.3389/fmicb.2017.02009.

Safi, C., Liu, D.Z., Yap, B.H.J. et al. (2014a). A two-stage ultrafiltration process for separating multiple components of *Tetraselmis suecica* after cell disruption. *Journal of Applied Phycology* **26** (6): 2379–2387. https://doi.org/10.1007/s10811-014-0271-0.

Safi, C., Ursu, A.V., Laroche, C. et al. (2014b). Aqueous extraction of proteins from microalgae: effect of different cell disruption methods. *Algal Research* **3**: 61–65. https://doi.org/10.1016/j.algal.2013.12.004.

Safi, C., Zebib, B., Merah, O. et al. (2014c). Morphology, composition, production, processing and applications of *Chlorella vulgaris*: a review. *Renewable and Sustainable Energy Reviews* **35**: 265–278. https://doi.org/10.1016/j.rser.2014.04.007.

Safi, C., Olivieri, G., Campos, R.P. et al. (2017). Biorefinery of microalgal soluble proteins by sequential processing and membrane filtration. *Bioresource Technology* **225**: 151–158. https://doi.org/10.1016/j.biortech.2016.11.068.

Samarakoon, K. and Jeon, Y.-J. (2012). Bio-functionalities of proteins derived from marine algae – a review. *Food Research International* **48** (2): 948–960. https://doi.org/10.1016/j.foodres.2012.03.013.

Schröder, A., Berton-Carabin, C., Venema, P., and Cornacchia, L. (2017). Interfacial properties of whey protein and whey protein hydrolysates and their influence on O/W emulsion stability. *Food Hydrocolloids* **73**: 129–140. https://doi.org/10.1016/j.foodhyd.2017.06.001.

Schwenzfeier, A., Wierenga, P.A., and Gruppen, H. (2011). Isolation and characterization of soluble protein from the green microalgae *Tetraselmis* sp. *Bioresource Technology* **102** (19): 9121–9127. https://doi.org/10.1016/j.biortech.2011.07.046.

Shannon, E. and Abu-Ghannam, N. (2016). Antibacterial derivatives of marine algae: an overview of pharmacological mechanisms and applications. *Marine Drugs* **14** (4): 81. http://www.ncbi.nlm.nih.gov/pubmed/27110798.

Shirgaonkar, I.Z., Lothe, R.R., and Pandit, A.B. (1998). Comments on the mechanism of microbial cell disruption in high-pressure and high-speed devices. *Biotechnology Progress* **14** (4): 657–660. https://doi.org/10.1021/bp980052g.

Sierra, L.S., Dixon, C.K., and Wilken, L.R. (2017). Enzymatic cell disruption of the microalgae *Chlamydomonas reinhardtii* for lipid and protein extraction. *Algal Research* **25**: 149–159. https://doi.org/10.1016/j.algal.2017.04.004.

Soto-Sierra, L., Stoykova, P., and Nikolov, Z.L. (2018). Extraction and fractionation of microalgae-based protein products. *Algal Research* **36**: 175–192. https://doi.org/10.1016/j.algal.2018.10.023.

van der Spiegel, M., Noordam, M.Y., and van der Fels-Klerx, H.J. (2013). Safety of novel protein sources (insects, microalgae, seaweed, duckweed, and rapeseed) and legislative aspects for their application in food and feed production. *Comprehensive Reviews in Food Science and Food Safety* **12** (6): 662–678. https://doi.org/10.1111/1541-4337.12032.

Stengel, D.B., Connan, S., and Popper, Z.A. (2011). Algal chemodiversity and bioactivity: sources of natural variability and implications for commercial application. *Biotechnology Advances* **29** (5): 483–501. https://doi.org/10.1016/j.biotechadv.2011.05.016.

Sun, L., Wang, S., Gong, X. et al. (2009). Isolation, purification and characteristics of R-phycoerythrin from a marine macroalga *Heterosiphonia japonica*. *Protein Expression and Purification* **64** (2): 146–154. https://doi.org/10.1016/j.pep.2008.09.013.

Suresh Kumar, K., Ganesan, K., Selvaraj, K., and Subba Rao, P.V. (2014). Studies on the functional properties of protein concentrate of *Kappaphycus alvarezii* (Doty) Doty – an edible seaweed. *Food Chemistry* **153**: 353–360. https://doi.org/10.1016/j.foodchem.2013.12.058.

Suwal, S., Perreault, V., Marciniak, A. et al. (2019). Effect of high hydrostatic pressure and polysaccharidases on the extraction of antioxidant compounds from red macroalgae, *Palmaria palmata* and *Solieria chordalis*. *Journal of Food Engineering* **252**: 53–59. https://doi.org/10.1016/j.jfoodeng.2019.02.014.

Tee, M.Z., Yong, Y.S., Rodrigues, K.F., and Yong, W.T.L. (2015). Growth rate analysis and protein identification of *Kappaphycus alvarezii* (Rhodophyta, Gigartinales) under pH induced stress culture. *Aquaculture Reports* **2**: 112–116. https://doi.org/10.1016/j.aqrep.2015.09.001.

Tierney, M.S., Croft, A.K., and Hayes, M. (2010). A review of antihypertensive and antioxidant activities in macroalgae. *Botanica Marina* **53** (5): 387–408. https://doi.org/10.1515/bot.2010.044.

Ursu, A.-V., Marcati, A., Sayd, T. et al. (2014). Extraction, fractionation and functional properties of proteins from the microalgae *Chlorella vulgaris*. *Bioresource Technology* **157**: 134–139. https://doi.org/10.1016/j.biortech.2014.01.071.

Vijaykrishnaraj, M. and Prabhasankar, P. (2015). Marine protein hydrolysates: their present and future perspectives in food chemistry – a review. *RSC Advances* **5** (44): 34864–34877. https://doi.org/10.1039/C4RA17205A.

Wells, M.L., Potin, P., Craigie, J.S. et al. (2017). Algae as nutritional and functional food sources: revisiting our understanding. *Journal of Applied Phycology* **29** (2): 949–982. https://doi.org/10.1007/s10811-016-0974-5.

Wijesekara, I., Lang, M., Marty, C. et al. (2017). Different extraction procedures and analysis of protein from *Ulva* sp. in Brittany, France. *Journal of Applied Phycology* **29** (5): 2503–2511. https://doi.org/10.1007/s10811-017-1239-7.

Wijesinghe, W.A.J.P. and Jeon, Y.-J. (2012). Enzyme-assistant extraction (EAE) of bioactive components: a useful approach for recovery of industrially important metabolites from seaweeds: a review. *Fitoterapia* **83** (1): 6–12. https://doi.org/10.1016/j.fitote.2011.10.016.

Wong, K. and Cheung, P.C. (2001). Nutritional evaluation of some subtropical red and green seaweeds part II. In vitro protein digestibility and amino acid profiles of protein concentrates. *Food Chemistry* **72** (1): 11–17. https://doi.org/10.1016/S0308-8146(00)00176-X.

Xi, J. (2017). Ultrahigh pressure extraction of bioactive compounds from plants – a review. *Critical Reviews in Food Science and Nutrition* **57** (6): 1097–1106. https://doi.org/10.1080/10408398.2013.874327.

Xu, Y., Chen, C., Ji, D. et al. (2013). Proteomic profile analysis of *Pyropia haitanensis* in response to high-temperature stress. *Journal of Applied Phycology* **26** (1): 607–618. https://doi.org/10.1007/s10811-013-0066-8.

Yotsukura, N., Nagai, K., Kimura, H., and Morimoto, K. (2009). Seasonal changes in proteomic profiles of Japanese kelp: *Saccharina japonica* (Laminariales, Phaeophyceae). *Journal of Applied Phycology* **22** (4): 443–451. https://doi.org/10.1007/s10811-009-9477-y.

Zou, H.X., Pang, Q.Y., Zhang, A.Q. et al. (2015). Excess copper induced proteomic changes in the marine brown algae *Sargassum fusiforme*. *Ecotoxicology and Environmental Safety* **111**: 271–280. https://doi.org/10.1016/j.ecoenv.2014.10.028.

7

Extraction Technologies to Recover Dietary Polyphenols from Macro- and Microalgae

M. Shanmugam[1], Abirami Ramu Ganesan[2], and Gaurav Rajauria[3]

[1]*Research and Development Division (DSIR-Lab), AquAgri Processing Private Limited, Manamadurai, India*

[2]*Department of Food Science and Home Economics, School of Applied Sciences, College of Engineering, Science and Technology, Fiji National University, Nasinu, Fiji Islands*

[3]*School of Agriculture and Food Science, University College Dublin, Lyons Research Farm, Celbridge, Ireland*

7.1 Introduction

A growing interest in a healthier diet and lifestyle has led consumers to increase their intakes of functional food, which has, in turn, promoted the search for new functional ingredients to be added to foods in order to improve nutrition and health (Ajila et al. 2011). Thus, current research is focused on research into natural sources, particularly botanicals, containing nutraceuticals (Sanger et al. 2019). Phytochemicals such as phenols, tannins, alkaloids, saponins, etc. (Li et al. 2011; Ganesan et al. 2019a) have been reported to exert beneficial effects in reducing the risk factors of diet-related chronic diseases including immunomodulatory effects (IgE/antigen), cardiovascular diseases, and osteoporosis, among others (Mokrani and Madani 2016; Barbosa et al. 2018). Phenolic compounds like tannins and alkaloids are one of these phytochemicals able to induce healthy effects (Li et al. 2011). Dietary polyphenols represent a group of secondary metabolites that widely occur in most plants including macro- and microalgae (Singh and Bharate 2006). Among the wide range of polyphenols, the characteristic features of some polyphenols such as phlorotannins, chlorogenic acid, and phloroglucinol are soluble or cell wall-bound complexes; soluble phlorotannins are generally localized in highly refractive and colorless vesicles known as physodes in the Ochraphyta and Phaeophyta (Li et al. 2017). The cell wall-bound phlorotannins

Recent Advances in Micro- and Macroalgal Processing: Food and Health Perspectives, First Edition.
Edited by Gaurav Rajauria and Yvonne V. Yuan.

arise when the physodes fuse with cell walls and the phlorotannins form complexes with the constituent alginic acid.

Generally, Phaeophyta (e.g. *Eisenia bicyclis*) contain more polyphenols than Rhodophyta (e.g. *Hypnea musciformis*) and Chlorophyta (e.g. *Ulva lactuca*, *Ulva fasciata*) varying from 1 to 14% of the dry algal dry mass (Mabeau and Fleurence 1993; Swanson and Druehl 2002). Examples of biological activities of polyphenols have been reported to include antioxidant (Gupta and Abu-Ghannam 2011), antiproliferative (Namvar et al. 2013), antibiotic (Gupta and Abu-Ghannam 2011), antidiabetic (Sanger et al. 2019), anti-HIV (Besednova et al. 2019), antiallergenic (Le et al. 2009), and anti-inflammatory properties (Li et al. 2011). Dietary polyphenols may offer an indirect antioxidant protection *in vivo* by activating endogenous defense systems (e.g. glutathione reductase) and by modulating cellular signaling processes (e.g. signal transduction) as reviewed by Cuong et al. (2019).

Further, the total measurable phenolic content and antioxidant activities of algal extracts are highly dependent upon the method of extraction (Ramluckan et al. 2014). The difference in chemical structures between terrestrial plant tannins and phlorotannins from Phaeophyta is that the molecular skeleton of the latter can consist of eight phenol rings as seen in *Ascophyllum nodosum*, (O'Sullivan et al. 2011), while tannins consist of only three or four rings (Cuong et al. 2019). Phlorotannins consist of phloroglucinol (1,3,5-trihydroxybenzene) monomer units, linked to each other in various ways (Singh and Bharate 2006). Phlorotannins can be classified into fuhalols and phlorethols (ether linkage), fucols (phenyl linkage), fucophloroethols (ether and phenyl linkage), and eckols (dibenzodioxin linkage) (Li et al. 2017). Most polyphenols isolated and identified to date from marine sources are of macroalgal origin (Li et al. 2017).

The significant potential of marine algae as functional foods, sources of nutraceuticals, and ingredients is increasingly being recognized, particularly for the polyphenol fractions (Yuan et al. 2018). To better exploit this potential, there is a need to develop new and enhanced extraction technologies as conventional extraction techniques including solvent extraction are time-consuming and are not eco-friendly owing to the use of organic solvents (Mokrani and Madani 2016). Yields obtained with traditional solvent extraction techniques are also limited compared with the novel extraction technologies described in this review. Therefore, the main objective of this review is to focus on various extraction techniques involved in algal polyphenols and associated factors in the extraction method are discussed in detail.

7.2 Conventional Extraction Techniques for Polyphenols

Extraction with Soxhlet apparatus, solid–liquid extraction (SLE), and liquid–liquid extraction (LLE) are some of the conventional techniques used in extracting polyphenols from macro- and microalgae (Yuan et al. 2018). In classic extraction methods, organic solvents including petroleum ether, hexane, cyclohexane, isooctane, toluene, benzene, diethyl ether, dichloromethane, isopropanol, chloroform, acetone, methanol, ethanol, butanol, etc. have been used to extract and solubilize polyphenols from macroalgae (Godlewska et al. 2017). However, extraction using Soxhlet apparatus is the most frequently practiced owing to its simplicity in operation

(Li et al. 2011). The advantage of this method is safety and the ability to scale up (Ramluckan et al. 2014). According to current trends in nontoxic, safe extraction processes, solvents used for extraction should be inexpensive. The loss of some compounds (e.g. lipids), consumption of large volumes of organic solvents (e.g. more than 50%), high energy and time consumption (e.g. more than 12 hours), and low extraction efficiencies are some of the drawbacks associated with classical methods for polyphenol extraction from macroalgae (Zhang et al. 2019). Thus, emerging technologies have been developed to counteract these issues by using supercritical and subcritical fluid extraction (Herrero et al. 2015), pulsed electric fields (PEFs; Prabhu et al. 2019), high-voltage electrical discharge (Zhang et al. 2019), ultrasound assisted extraction (UAE; Rodsamran and Sothornvit 2019), microwave assisted extraction (MAE; Hannachi et al. 2019), high-pressure processing (HPP and ultra-high-pressure processing (UHPP); Zhang et al. 2019).

7.2.1 Liquid-Liquid Extraction (LLE)

LLE is a commonly used method for the purification of algae-based phenolic compounds (Gall et al. 2015). In this method, the crude seaweed extract was partitioned with different polar solvents followed by filtering to obtain filtrate, which can then be fractionated using solvents of different miscibilities. For example, *Himanthalia elongata* crude liquid methanolic extract was partitioned using ethyl acetate and water in equal proportions, which yielded 310 mg GAE g^{-1} of total phenolic content (TPC) as compared with crude extract of 193 mg GAE g^{-1} (Rajauria et al. 2016). This shows that an extraction mixture consisting of an organic and an aqueous phase shows more compound elution.

7.2.2 Solid-Liquid Extraction (SLE)

Polar solvents such as water, methanol, and ethanol have been broadly utilized for the extraction of polyphenolics from solid algal biomass utilizing conventional SLE (Gümüş Yılmaz et al. 2019). The extraction yield relies upon the solubility of the polyphenols of interest in the chosen solvent or blends of solvents; for example, methanol or ethanol in an aqueous medium to elute phlorotannins (Generalić Mekinić et al. 2019). Furthermore, the chosen solvent(s) greatly affects the availability of phenolic compounds, which are relatively bonded with polysaccharides (Ganesan et al. 2019b), proteins, and peptides (Gümüş Yılmaz et al. 2019). Existing procedures for extraction of phenols from macroalgae incorporate Soxhlet distillation with polar solvents, hydrodistillation using an aqueous medium, and maceration followed by methanol or ethanol (Li et al. 2017; Rajauria et al. 2013). Many Phaeophyceae species showed a better quantity of polyphenol when extracted with 70% of acetone and water, which shows a high degree of polymerization and solubility in this solvent mixture (Generalić Mekinić et al. 2019). Mechanical and chemical procedures including milling, grinding of algal biomass followed by solvent extraction, and distillation are commonly used for phenolic extraction from macroalgae (Yuan and Walsh 2006). The most efficient SLE methodology might be a combination of two solvents, water and highly polar solvents, which is better than a single solvent in the extraction of phenolic compounds. For example, the TPC of *U. fasciata* was

23 mg TAE g^{-1} using methanol as a single solvent (Abirami and Kowsalya 2017) as compared with ethanol and water in a solvent mixture on *Fucus spiralis*, which resulted in 142.81 μg phloroglucinol equivalents (PGE) mg^{-1} (Tierney et al. 2013). This shows that diffusion of solvent and rate of action might influence the extraction quantity of phenolic compounds.. Further, SLE might show different action even with the same species, i.e. *Carpophyllum flexuosum* and *Carpophyllum plumosum* showed 8.6 and 7.5% of TPC, respectively, when extracted sequentially in acidified methanol (50%) with acetone (70%) (Magnusson et al. 2017). These reports showed that ethanol and acetone with water are effective solvents, which gave the maximum phenolic content across all classes. However, these organic solvents are unsafe in terms of environmental issues. For instance, hexane used in the SLE process is categorized by the United States Natural Environmental Protection Agency as a harmful pollutant (US Department of Health and Human Services 1993).

7.3 Innovative Extraction Technologies for Isolation of Polyphenols from Macroalgae

Green technology is the process of utilizing environmentally friendly methods of extraction including high efficiency and time savings (taking less than 15 minutes), low-cost inputs (100 MPa), a high level of recovery (more than 30% of TPC), purity of compounds, and food and environmental safety (Pérez-Larrán et al. 2019) associated with the use of solvents including methanol, petroleum ether, and hexane (Agregan et al. 2019). The use of new extraction techniques such as supercritical fluid extraction (SFE), MAE, UAE, enzyme assisted extraction (EAE), pressurized liquid extraction (PLE) (also known as pressurized fluid extraction (PFE), enhanced solvent extraction (ESE), high-pressure solvent extraction (HPSE), or accelerated solvent extraction (ASE) techniques (O'Sullivan et al. 2013) may provide alternatives to the traditional methods discussed above. These techniques have been successfully used for the extraction of polyphenols applicable in the food and pharmaceutical industries (Kadam et al. 2013) and have been reviewed with a view to their potential adoption in industrial and large-scale operations (Priyadarshini et al. 2019).

7.3.1 Enzyme-Assisted Extraction (EAE)

Macro- and microalgal cell walls are structurally and chemically more complex than cell walls of terrestrial plants and hence bioactive compounds can be extracted through enzyme treatments (Hahn et al. 2012; del Pilar Sánchez-Camargo et al. 2016). Algal cell disruption can be achieved by neutral and alkaline protease, α-amylase, cellulase, and pepsin, and the targeted compounds isolated with optimum conditions (Wijesinghe and Jeon 2012). For instance, the enzyme viscozyme® used in EAE for extraction from tropical seaweeds *Sargassum aquifolium*, *Sargassum ilicifolium*, and *Sargassum polycystum* extracted more phenolic content in *S. aquifolium* and *S. polycystum*, with 7.0 and 8.1% of dry material, respectively. However, the effectiveness of Protamex® was found to be equivalent to methanol 50% (v/v) in extracting the phenolic compound from all three *Sargassum* species (Puspita et al. 2017). Similarly, protease from *Bacillus licheniformis* presented the highest extraction yield of ~7.5 mg GAE g^{-1} total phenol from *Lobophora variegata* at pH 5 and 50 °C compared with Celluclast® 1.5 l with protease ~7 mg GAE g^{-1} (Gümüş Yılmaz et al. 2019). However, higher pH and increase in temperature raise the total yield in the same species, i.e. with pH 8.17 and 60 °C, protease yielded more than 10 mg GAE g^{-1}, and alcalase 2.41 FG ~20 mg GAE g^{-1} in this study. On the other hand, a blend of neutral and alkaline endo-proteases for 3 hours at 50 °C led to 0.4 g DW of TPC in *Ulva armoricana*, with similar values found in control samples without enzyme in the medium yielding 0.3 g DW (Hardouin et al. 2016). Aqueous extract of *Palmaria palmata* showed 0.5 GAE% of TPC but Umamizyme® with protease yielded 1.55 GAE% (Adalbjörnsson and Jónsdóttir 2015). This shows that changing the extraction medium influences the extraction efficiency of the TPC along with the specificity of the enzymes used in EAE (del Pilar Sánchez-Camargo et al. 2016) considered to be essential in polyphenol extraction in algae (Table 7.1; Figure 7.1).

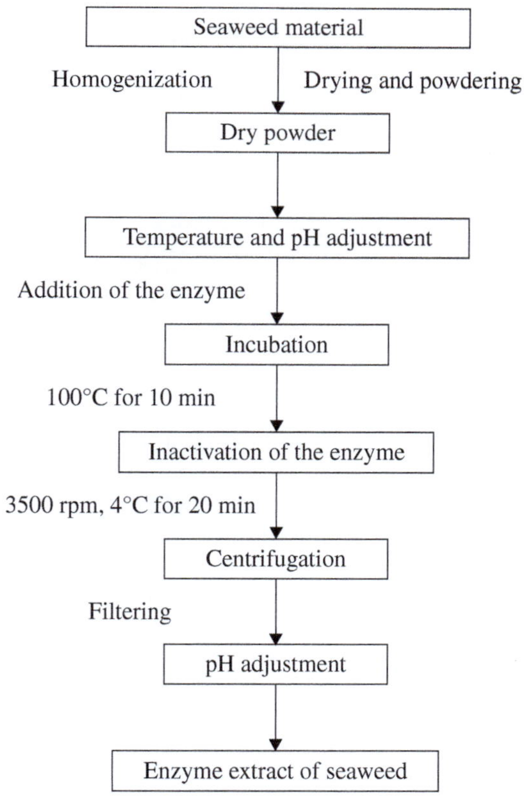

Figure 7.1 Enzyme assisted extraction of polyphenols from seaweeds. Source: Wijesinghe and Jeon (2012).

Table 7.1 Enzyme assisted extraction (EAE) of polyphenols from seaweeds.

Seaweeds	Treated enzyme	Total phenolics	Bioactivity	References
Sargassum horneri	Proteases	199–533	Antioxidant	Heo et al. (2005a)
Sargassum horneri	Carbohydrate hydrolyzes	160–384	Antioxidant	Heo et al. (2005a)
Sargassum fulvellum	Proteases	193–366	Antioxidant	Heo et al. (2005a)
Sargassum fulvellum	Carbohydrate hydrolyses	234–313	Antioxidant	Heo et al. (2005a)
Sargassum coreanum	Proteases	815–996	Antioxidant	Heo et al. (2005a)
Sargassum coreanum	Carbohydrate hydrolyses	746–1123	Antioxidant	Heo et al. (2005a)
Sargassum thunbergii	Proteases	253–416	Antioxidant	Heo et al. (2005a)
Sargassum thunbergii	Carbohydrate hydrolyses	261–386	Antioxidant	Heo et al. (2005a)
Sargassum. thunbergii	Carbohydrases and proteases	—	Antioxidant	Park et al. (2005)
Sargassum horneri	Carbohydrases and proteases	—	Antioxidant	Park et al. (2004)
Sargassum aquifolium	Viscozyme	7.0	Antioxidant	Puspita et al. (2017)
Sargassum aquifolium	Ptotamex	3.5	Antioxidant	Puspita et al. (2017)
Sargassum ilicifolium	Viscozyme	4.0	Antioxidant	Puspita et al. (2017)
Sargassum ilicifolium	Ptotamex	4.2	Antioxidant	Puspita et al. (2017)
Sargassum polycystum	Viscozyme	8.1	Antioxidant	Puspita et al. (2017)
Sargassum polycystum	Ptotamex	5.2	Antioxidant	Puspita et al. (2017)
Ecklonia cava	Proteases	1087–1245	Antioxidant	Heo et al. (2005b)
Ecklonia cava	Carbohydrate hydrolyses	1032–1352	Antioxidant	Heo et al. (2005b)
Ishige okamurae	Proteases	196–420	Antioxidant	Heo et al. (2005b)
Ishige okamurae	Carbohydrate hydrolyses	213–275	Antioxidant	Heo et al. (2005b)
Scytosiphon lomentaria	Proteases	112–207	Antioxidant	Heo et al. (2005b)
Scytosiphon lomentaria	Carbohydrate hydrolyses	114–149	Antioxidant	Heo et al. (2005b)
Ecklonia cava	Carbohydraces		Antioxidant	Heo et al. (2005b)
Hizikia fusiformis	Alcalase and Ultraflo	—	—	Siriwardhana et al. (2008)
Ecklonia cava	Kojizyme	—	Immunomodulation	Ahn et al. (2008)
Palmaria palmate	Protease and carbohydrase	—	Antioxidant	Wang et al. (2010)

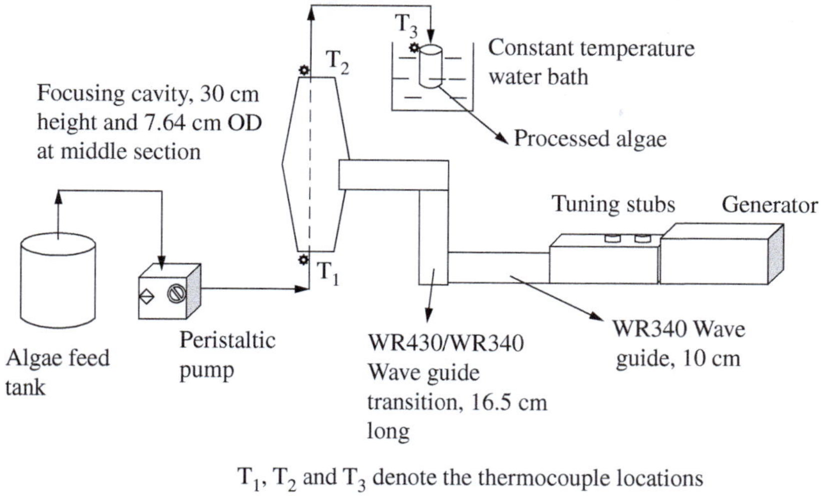

Figure 7.2 Microwave processing system. Source: Balasubramanian et al. (2011).

7.3.2 Microwave Assisted Extraction (MAE)

In this methodology (Figure 7.2), microwaves, the nonionizing electromagnetic or radio wave radiation with frequencies from 300 MHz to 300 GHz with a maximum of 200 W, induce the vibration of water molecules within the cell matrix, thereby increasing the temperature of the intracellular fluids, and intracellular contents are released into the extraction medium as a result of the breakdown of cell walls owing to the pressure exerted on the structures (Hahn et al. 2012). For example, enzyme in combination with microwave showed a better yield of TPC, i.e. MAE with viscozyme used for extraction on *Ecklonia radiata* reported a yield of 4.4 g PGE/100 g DW, which accounts for more than 52% of TPC for 5–30 minutes of time as compared with the conventional method of extraction using acidic medium for 24 hours, which gave 3.4 g PGE/100 g DW (Charoensiddhi et al. 2015). Although temperature and input energy play a role in MAE, solvent used in the system enhances the total quantity of polyphenols. *C. flexuosum* yielded 11.4% PGE/g DW TPC when extracted using water in MAE; the total biomass and the solvent used in this system was 1 : 5 to 1 : 40 with the holding time of 1–20 minutes at a temperature of 135–185 °C. In contrast, ethanol used in a similar MAE system yielded 8.4% PGE/g DW. This study confirms that a higher percentage of solvent in an MAE system gives better results in the ratio of 1 : 30 and 1 : 40 (Magnusson et al. 2017). Similarly, MAE took less time than the traditional method, which takes 4 hours, i.e. *Laminaria japonica* yielded 20.93% TPC with MAE using 70% methanol for 15 minutes at 110 °C, followed by *A. nodosum* (12.46%), *Lessonia nigrescens* (9.28%), and *Lessonia trabeculate* (5.22%) in the same set-up (Yuan et al. 2018). Similarly, varying solvents in the MAE system also led to variation in the final yield of TPC. For example, microwave at 1200 W with a frequency of 2450 MHz in extraction of *S. vestitum* biomass with variation in solvent showed varied results: 70% acetone in MAE had the highest TPC of 74.05 mg GAE·g^{-1}, followed by 30% acetone with 60.73 mg GAE·g^{-1}; further, 70% methanol exhibited 59.13 mg GAE·g^{-1} (Dang et al. 2018). These studies prove that

Table 7.2 Microwave assisted extraction (MAE) of polyphenols from seaweed.

	Microwave operating conditions				
Seaweed species	**Frequency (MHz) and Power (W)**	**Solvent**	**Temp (°C)**	**Time (minutes)**	**References**
Carpophyllum flexuosum	—	Water	160	3	Zhang et al. (2018)
Carpophyllum flexuosum	—	Water	135, 160, and 185	1, 3, 5, 10, 15, 20	Magnusson et al. (2017)
Carpophyllum plumosum	—	Water	160	3	Zhang et al. (2018)
Ecklonia radiata	—	Water	160	3	Zhang et al. (2018)
Enteromorpha prolifera	300–700 —	10–60% EtOH	—	5–40	Ren et al. (2017)
Caulerpa racemosa	100–600 —	20–100 EtOH	20–70	5–60	Li et al. (2012)

MAE (approx. US$5000) is a more economically feasible option compared with SFE (approx. US$26 000), though it does require an additional separation process to remove solid residue from the extraction solvent compared with SFE and it is also not suitable for extracting heat-sensitive compounds such as phloroglucinol (Dinh et al. 2018) Table 7.2.

7.3.3 Pressurized Liquid Extraction (PLE)

The equipment for PLE involves an extraction vessel to which the algal biomass is introduced (Figure 7.3) (Otero et al. 2019). The vessel is then filled with organic solvent (ethanol, methanol, ethyl acetate), and heated using an electric heating jacket. High temperature and pressure are maintained in ranges between 50 and 200 °C and 3.5–20 MPa, respectively, to facilitate rapid extraction (Cikoš et al. 2018). For example, PLE was found to be more efficient if appropriate temperature and solvent were used in the extraction system, i.e. PLE applied on *Sargassum muticum* using ethanol and water in the medium followed by sonication for 10 minutes yielded 29.61 mg GAE g^{-1} at 50 °C as compared with the highest temperature of 125 °C in the PLE system using 100% ethanol, which yielded 93.84 mg GAE g^{-1}, but reducing the ethanol to 50% yielded only 76.62 mg GAE g^{-1} (del Pilar Sánchez-Camargo et al. 2016). This proved that the combined use of high pressures and temperatures in this method provides many advantages over traditional extraction methods such as SLE and LLE, including higher selectivity, shorter extraction time (static extraction 20 minutes), and smaller volumes of organic solvents. Otero et al. (2019) identified that increasing the temperature without changing the pressure yielded more TPC in *Laminaria ochroleuca*, where 10 MPa of pressure given at 80 °C and 160 °C yielded 37.48 and 51.91% of TPC when ethanol and water were used as a solvent in a 1 : 1 ratio; however, ethyl acetate used in this study showed low TPC content (5.25 and 5.29%). These studies show that external pressure causes the solvents (water/ethanol) to rise above their boiling

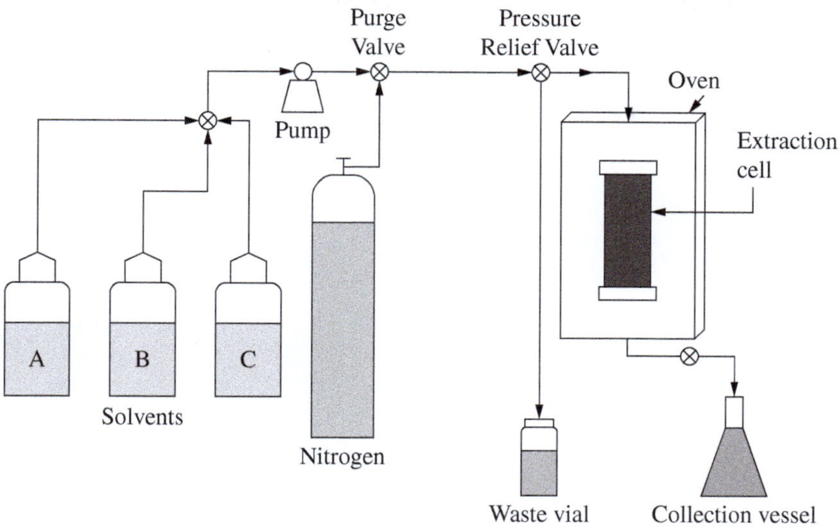

Figure 7.3 Operational schematic principle and mechanism of pressurized liquid extraction (PLE) systems.

points while the increased temperatures reduce the viscosity and surface tension of solvents, helping to distribute the solvent throughout the algal biomass to improve the extraction rate compared with the conventional method of heating in Soxhlet apparatus. However, PLE has not been used on a commercial scale to extract polyphenols from algal biomass owing to its cost. ASE (O'Sullivan et al. 2013), pressurized hot water extraction (PHWE; Saravana et al. 2016), and subcritical water extraction (SWE; Rodríguez-Meizoso et al. 2010) are the variations of PLE and are considered as promising techniques to extract polyphenols from microalgae like *Spirulina platensis* (Herrero et al. 2005). Reported applications of PLE concerning algal biomass are summarized in Table 7.3. Although a wider range of solvents, including ethanol, water, methanol, and ethyl acetate, can be used for PLE extraction, it is not suitable for thermolabile compounds such as phlorotannins, phloroglucinol, etc. (Herrero et al. 2015). According to Plaza et al. (2010a), application of PLE variations PHWE/SWE yielded neo-antioxidants from *Undaria pinnatifida* during the extraction of antioxidants. By using 70% (v/v) ethanol, PLE yielded a greater recovery of total phenolic compounds (10.18% DW) from *S. muticum* with the processing conditions of 6 minutes at 120 °C, static extraction time of 20 minutes and pressure 10.3 MPa (Tanniou et al. 2013) (Table 7.3).

7.3.4 Subcritical Water Extraction (SWE)

This is the most promising technique for the extraction of bioactive compounds including dietary polyphenols. In this method, pressure and temperature are applied to maintain the solvents near their critical region in the liquid state, keeping the solvents below their boiling point (Duarte et al. 2014). SWE operates at high temperatures (50–200 °C) and pressures (0.34–2.06 MPa) for a short period of

Table 7.3 Pressurized liquid extraction (PLE) of polyphenols from micro- and macroalgae.

Seaweed species	Extraction condition	Phenolic compound	Yield (%)	References
Sargassum muticum	Pressure of 10.3 MPa at 120 °C temperature for 6 minutes	Polyphenols	—	Tanniou et al. (2013)
Undaria pinnatifida	Water as solvent	Polyphenol	—	Plaza et al. (2010a)
Himanthalia elongata	Temperatures of 50, 100, 150, and 200 °C for 20 minutes	Bioactive phenols	—	Plaza et al. (2010b)
Dunaliella salina	Temperatures of 40, 100, and 160 °C and times of 5, 17.5, and 30 minutes	Bioactive phenols	—	Herrero et al. (2006)
Asophyllum nodosum	Water as solvent	Phloroglucinol	28.72	Tierney et al. (2013)
Asophyllum nodosum	Ethanol/water as solvent	Phloroglucinol	11.27	Tierney et al. (2013)
Asophyllum nodosum	Acetone/water as solvent	Phloroglucinol	6.83	Tierney et al. (2013)
Pelvetia canaliculata	Water as solvent	Phloroglucinol	28.61	Tierney et al. (2013)
Pelvetia canaliculata	Ethanol/water as solvent	Phloroglucinol	17.33	Tierney et al. (2013)
Pelvetia canaliculata	Acetone/water as solvent	Phloroglucinol	4.32	Tierney et al. (2013)
Fucus spiralis	Water as solvent	Phloroglucinol	27.59	Tierney et al. (2013)
Fucus spiralis	Ethanol/water as solvent	Phloroglucinol	20.48	Tierney et al. (2013)
Fucus spiralis	Acetone/water as solvent	Phloroglucinol	18.99	Tierney et al. (2013)
Ulva intestinalis	Water as solvent	Phloroglucinol	10.88	Tierney et al. (2013)
Ulva intestinalis	Ethanol/water as solvent	Phloroglucinol	4.33	Tierney et al. (2013)
Ulva intestinalis	Acetone/water as solvent	Phloroglucinol	3.95	Tierney et al. (2013)
Fucus serratus	Ethanol/water as solvent	Gallic acid	31.7	Heffernan et al. 2014
Fucus serratus	Methanol/water as solvent	Gallic acid	29.2	Heffernan et al. 2014
Fucus serratus	Hot water extract	Gallic acid	33.4	Heffernan et al. 2014

(continued)

Table 7.3 (*continued*)

Seaweed species	Extraction condition	Phenolic compound	Yield (%)	References
Laminaria digitata	Ethanol/water as solvent	Gallic acid	24.8	Heffernan et al. 2014
Laminaria digitata	Methanol/water as solvent	Gallic acid	28.2	Heffernan et al. 2014
Laminaria digitata	Hot water extract	Gallic acid	29.8	Heffernan et al. 2014
Gracilaria gracilis	Ethanol/water as solvent	Gallic acid	21.8	Heffernan et al. 2014
Gracilaria gracilis	Methanol/water as solvent	Gallic acid	24.5	Heffernan et al. 2014
Gracilaria gracilis	Hot water extract	Gallic acid	36.9	Heffernan et al. 2014
Codium fragile	Ethanol/water as solvent	Gallic acid	26.9	Heffernan et al. 2014
Codium fragile	Methanol/water as solvent	Gallic acid	24.6	Heffernan et al. 2014
Codium fragile	Hot water extract	Gallic acid	30.3	Heffernan et al. 2014

time (5–10 minutes) with a small amount of solvent (Tanniou et al. 2013). Physical and chemical properties of water are changed during the extraction because high temperature and pressure are applied. Consequently, the dielectric constant of water is significantly decreased from 80 (25 °C) to 33 (200 °C), which is close to the dielectric constant of methanol (56; Turner and Ibanez 2011). del Pilar Sanchez Camargo et al. (2017) demonstrated the application of SWE with enzymes as pretreatment for increasing the extraction yield and phlorotannin recovery, but it did not give the best results. Heffernan et al. (2014) reported that among brown, red, and green seaweeds, the brown algae contained the highest amount of polyphenols and, consequently, the highest antioxidant activity. Brown macroalgae generally have a higher content of polyphenols than red and green macroalgae, owing to the presence of phlorotannins, which are not present in the other macroalgae groups (Castro-Puyana et al. 2013). While Tierney et al. (2013) reported that the extracts obtained with conventional methods contained a higher concentration of polyphenols compared with SWE extracts. Dinh et al. (2018) obtained the opposite results. When the dielectric constant decreases with increasing temperature and pressure during SWE, a larger quantity of polyphenols is extracted. Dinh et al. (2018) noticed that phenolic content increased as the temperature rose from 100 °C to 225 °C, but when it reached 250 °C, the phenolic content started to reduce. The same behavior is noticed for the antioxidant activity of the extracts, which showed that phenolic content and antioxidant activity are correlated (Figure 7.4; Table 7.4).

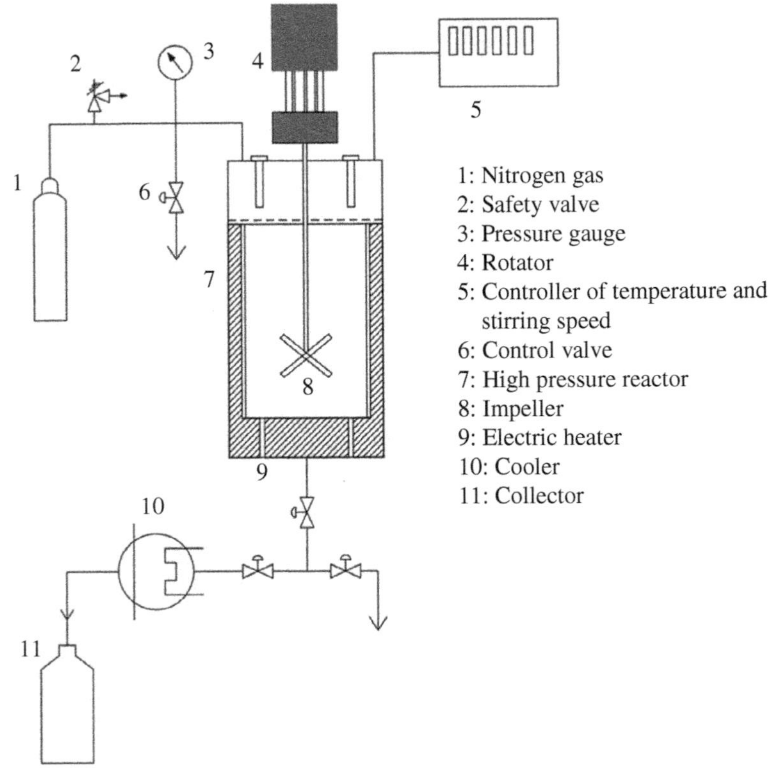

Figure 7.4 Schematic diagram of laboratory-scale subcritical water apparatus. Source: Dinh et al. (2018).

7.3.5 Supercritical Fluid Extraction (SFE)

A typical schematic diagram of an SFE system is presented in Figure 7.5. In SFE, the solvents, most often CO_2, are used at temperatures (30–75 °C) and pressures (8–40 MPa) above their critical points (up to 240 minutes) (Cikoš et al. 2018). In this state, the density of the solvent is similar to that of a liquid (density of SC CO_2 from 290 to 841 kg m^{-3}) (Manna et al. 2015), and the density can be altered by changing the temperature and pressure (327 bar) (Kadam et al. 2013); while changing these factors the TPC yield would change. For instance, the TPC content in *H. musciformis* obtained by SCWE showed a difference as the solid to liquid (S/L) ratio increased along with the temperature. The TPC and total flavonoid content (TFC) of *H. musciformis* content was 39.57 mg GAE g^{-1} and 12.10 mg QE g^{-1}, respectively, with S/L ratio 1 : 50 at 210 °C. However, these results are significant in contrast with conventional extraction of TPC from *H. musciformis*, which yielded 20.19–49.77 mg GAE g^{-1} but TFC was found to be high as 20.65–70.67 mg QE g^{-1} (Pangestuti et al. 2019). The physicochemical properties of water changed during SFE due to the rise in temperature and pressure applied. Subsequently, the dielectric constant of water was found to be diminished from 80 to 33 at 25–200 °C, which is near the dielectric constant of methanol (Cikoš et al. 2018). Further, these changes might

Table 7.4 Subcritical water extraction (SWE) of polyphenols from seaweeds and their bioactivity.

Seaweed species	Ultrasound operating conditions			Bioactivity	References
	Pressure (MPa)	Temp (°C)	Time (minutes)		
Porphyra spp.	10.3	120 and 200	20	Antioxidant	Plaza et al. (2010a)
Gracilaria gracilis	10.3	120	25	Antioxidant	Heffernan et al. (2014)
Sargassum muticum	10.3	50, 125, 200	20	Antioxidant	del Pilar Sanchez Camargo et al. (2017)
Padina pavonica	15	60	10	Antihyaluronidase	Fayad et al. (2017)
Fucus serratus	10.3	120	25	Antioxidant	Heffernan et al. (2014)
Laminaria digitata	10.3	120	25	Antioxidant	Heffernan et al. (2014)
Cystoseira abies-marina	10.3	120 and 200	20	Antioxidant	Plaza et al. (2010a)
Sargassum vulgare	10.3	120 and 200	20	Antioxidant	Plaza et al. (2010a)
Sargassum muticum	10.3	120 and 200	20	Antioxidant	Plaza et al. (2010a)
Undaria pinnatifida	10.3	120 and 200	20	Antioxidant	Plaza et al. (2010a)
Ascophyllum nodosum	10.3	120	—	—	Tierney et al. (2013)
Pelvetia canalicu-lata	10.3	120	5	Antioxidant	Tierney et al. (2013)
Saccharina japonica	5	100–250	5	Antioxidant	Saravana et al. (2016)
Fucus spiralis	10.3	120	—	Antioxidant	Tierney et al. (2013)
Ulva intesti-nalis	10.3	120	—	Antioxidant	Tierney et al. (2013)
Codium fragile	10.3	120	25	Antioxidant	Heffernan et al. (2014)

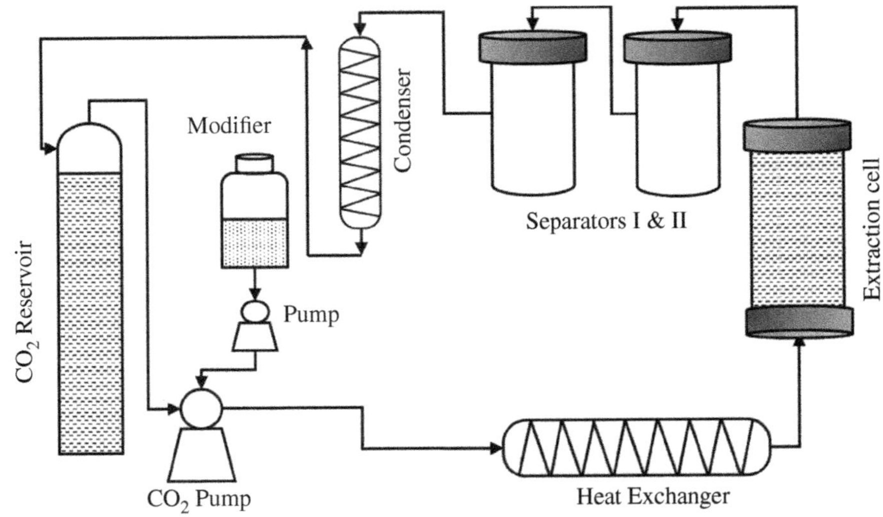

Figure 7.5 Schematic diagram of supercritical fluid extraction (SFE). Source: Kadam et al. (2013).

influence viscosity, and low viscosity and high diffusibility of supercritical fluids result in improved solubilization compared with liquids. The solvent CO_2 in SFE was found to be cost-effective, inert, nonflammable, and demonstrates a great ability to extract volatile compounds as well as polyphenols including carotenoids (Pangestuti et al. 2019). A rapid extraction rate (2–15 minutes), high yield of polyphenols (10–37%) which are not degraded (Dinh et al. 2018), and eco-friendly technology with minimal use of organic solvents are all advantages of SFE; however, the disadvantage with this method is the high costs associated with SFE (Agregan et al. 2019), and that it is not suitable to extract polar substances including many polyphenols such as flavonoids and phloroglucinol. (Table 7.5)

7.3.6 Ultrasound Assisted Extraction (UAE)

With this technique (Figure 7.6), sound waves travel through the solvent to create pressure variations (Han et al. 2011). The acoustic cavitations produced, develop, break down, and change the sound waves into mechanical motion, which causes disruption of cells and the cell wall matrices (Macías-Sánchez et al. 2009). In order to disrupt the algal biomass cell wall matrices UAE must use physical disruption phenomena, which include diffusion of solvent through the cell wall and removal of tissue debris once the wall matrix has been disrupted (Dang et al. 2017). UAE is often used as a pretreatment (ultrasonic shower or ultrasound test instrument) before extraction. UAE is an alternative to the conventional extraction methods discussed above with benefits such as decreased extraction time (less than 30 minutes), energy needs (100–400 W), and improved recovery of solvents due to isothermal condition (Tierney et al. 2013). The improvement in extraction utilizing ultrasound is associated with the impact of acoustic cavitation from the ultrasonic waves (20–1000 kHz) (Parniakov et al. 2015). The ultrasonic waves also exert mechanical impacts in the

Table 7.5 Supercritical CO_2 (SC-CO_2) extraction of polyphenols from seaweeds and their bioactivity.

Seaweed species	Extraction parameters				Bioactivity	References
	Pressure (MPa)	Temperature (°C)	Time (minutes)	Co-solvent (%)		
Gracilaria mammilaris	10, 20, 30	30, 50, 60	240	EtOH (2, 5, 8)	Antioxidant	Ospina et al. (2017)
Undaria pinnatifida	20–40	25–60	180	EtOH (3)	—	Roh et al. (2008)
Undaria pinnatifida	10–40	35–75	10–60	—	—	Klejdus et al. (2010)
Saccharina japonica	20–30	45–55	240	EtOH and water	Antioxidant	Saravana et al. (2017)
Saccharina japonica	25	45	120	EtOH	Antioxidant, antimicrobial, and antihypertensive	Sivagnanam et al. (2015)
Cladophora glomerata	10–30	40–60	120	EtOH (0–15)	Antioxidant	Fabrowska et al. (2016)
Cladophora glomerata	50	40	300, 360, 810	—	Plant growth biostimulant	Michalak et al. (2016)
Ulva flexuosa	10–30	40–60	120	—	Antioxidant	Fabrowska et al. (2016)
Ulva flexuosa ssp. *pilifera*	50	40	300, 360, 810	—	Plant growth biostimulant	Michalak et al. (2016)
Ulva clathrata	50	40	300, 360, 810	—	Plant growth biostimulant	Michalak et al. (2016)
Hypnea spinella	10–40	35–75	10–60	—	—	Klejdus et al. (2010)
Gloiopeltis tenax	30	45	—	—	—	Zheng et al. (2012)

form of cavitation bubbles on the algal biomass and solvent, permitting greater infiltration of solvent into the sample and increased contact surface area (Li et al. 2017). UAE onducted using an ultrasonic bath (220 V, 50 Hz, and 250 W) in ethanol (70%) extract showed a steady increase in TPC noticed in *Hormosira banksia*. When temperature was decreased from 50 to 30 °C and ultrasonic time increased from 20 to 60 minutes, *H. banksia* showed the highest TPC of 22.25 mg g^{-1} at 30 °C for 60 minutes with 80% ultrasound, but increasing the ultrasonication up to 100% decreased the TPC content to 21.85 mg g^{-1} (Dang et al. 2017). Therefore, the extracted compounds of interest rapidly diffuse out from the sample into the solvent. For example, UAE extraction of *Laurencia obtuse* resulted in TPC of 26.23 mg GAE g^{-1} phenolic content

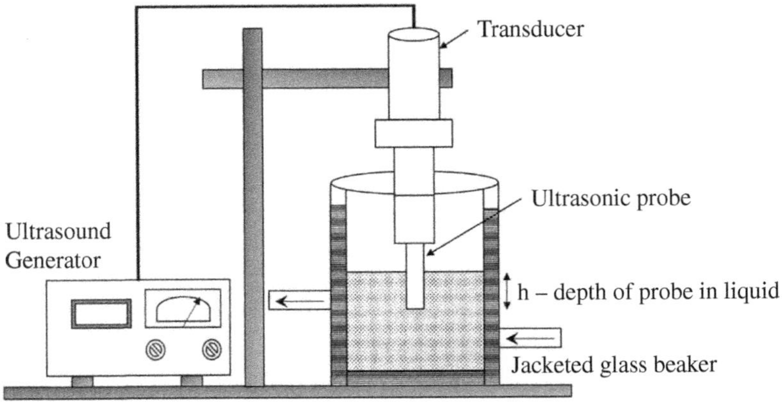

Figure 7.6 Schematic diagram of ultrasound assisted extraction (UAE). Source: Kadam et al. (2013).

when treated under 250 W, 40 kHz frequency ultrasonication with 95% ethanol at 50 °C for 30–60 minutes (Table 7.6); although there was no variation in ultrasonication time the solvent to *L. obtuse* mixture ratio (24.3 : 1) and extraction time (58 minutes) increased the phenolic yield (26.23 mg GAE g^{-1}) and improved the antioxidant activity (120.89 Trolox equivalent antioxidant capacity [TEAC]) (Topuz et al. 2016). However, Dang et al. (2017) reported that ultrasonic power (150–250 W, 50 Hz), time (20–60 minutes), and temperature (30–50 °C) influence the TPC of algae. In this study, increased extraction time (60 minutes) with decreased power of ultrasonication (150 W) and increased power (250 W) had a maximum concentration of TPC at 40 °C with *H. banksii* (23.12 mg GAE g^{-1}) (Dang et al. 2017). But for better total yield of TPC, low power (80% ultrasonication), longer (60 minutes) treatments were found to be effective for polyphenol extraction (22.25 mg g^{-1}) from algal samples including *H. banksii* compared with the conventional method (16.21 mg g^{-1} TPC) (Dang et al. 2017). In some reports, increased temperatures (more than 50 °C) in UAE expanded the solubility, diffusion, and total yield of polyphenols, associated with the ultrasonic waves entering the algal biomass and extracting polyphenols in an assortment of solvents including phlorotannins (Kadam et al. 2013). Specifically, hot water extraction in combination with sonication was reported to be an ideal extraction method for agar-containing Rhodophyta including *Gelidium sesquipedale* to extract polyphenols, reducing the extraction time and increasing the penetration time, while safeguarding the properties of the agar-based concentrate in comparison with hot water treatment (de Oliveira et al., 2019), but the high energy inputs required for UAE (Rodsamran and Sothornvit 2019) appear to be a disadvantage of this method.

7.4 Factors Affecting Extraction

Determination of the optimal pH and solvent mixture is an important factor for the extraction of polyphenols from algal biomass (Barbosa et al. 2017). Water, aqueous methanol, and aqueous mixtures of ethanol, methanol, and acetone are commonly used solvents for the extraction of polyphenols from plant material including algal

Table 7.6 Ultrasound assisted extraction (UAE) of polyphenolic compounds from seaweeds.

Seaweed species	Ultrasonic operating conditions			References
	Ultrasound equipment (Frequency [kHz] and power [W])	Temp (°C)	Time (minutes)	
Laurencia obtuse	Ultrasonic bath (40 and 250)	30–50	30–60	Topuz et al. (2016)
Osmundea pinnatifida	Ultrasonic bath (50/60 and 400)	50	60	Rodrigues et al. (2015)
Hormosira banksii	Ultrasonic bath (50 and 150–250)	10, 40, 50	20, 40, and 60	Dang et al. (2017)
Sargassum muticum	Ultrasonic bath (50/60 and 400)	50	60	Rodrigues et al. (2015)
Ecklonia cava	Ultrasonic bath (40 and 200)	30	360 and 720	Lee et al. (2013)
Ascophyllum nodosum	Ultrasonic probe (20 and 750)	—	15	Kadam et al. (2015a)
Ascophyllum nodosum	Ultrasonic probe (20 and 750)	—	10	Kadam et al. (2015b)
Laminaria hyperborea	Ultrasonic probe (20 and 750)	—	15	Kadam et al. (2015a)
Codium tomentosum	Ultrasonic bath (50/60 and 400)	50	60	Rodrigues et al. (2015)

biomasses (Zenthoefer et al. 2017). During the extraction process, polyphenols often develop complexes and bind with proteins or cell wall carbohydrates (Ganesan et al. 2018) rendering them insoluble in organic solvents. Therefore, this a common problem when trying to develop a general protocol(s) for the extraction of polyphenols from algal biomass (Vázquez-Rodríguez et al. 2020).

7.4.1 pH

The pH is an important factor for the extraction of phenolics due to dissolvability in the solvent mixture (Godlewska et al. 2017). The solvent pH can be determined by the nature of polyphenolic compounds to be extracted and the source of the plant material (López-Pérez et al. 2020). Usually, low pH solvents can prevent the oxidation of phenolics, which is important in the case of extracting polyphenols. For example, at low pH 3 the total phenolic concentration was found to be high (1077 mg l^{-1}), high pH 7 yielded 669 mg l^{-1}, and the least amount was found with pH 10 (616 mg l^{-1} in water extract) (Godlewska et al. 2017). The solvent to be used for the extraction of compounds varies with the source and also the type of phenolic compounds to be extracted

(Rajauria 2018). In fact, an integrated combination of pH and solvent can lead to enhanced extraction of polyphenols as pH determines the solubility of the polyphenols and the solvents address the efficient contact (Ajila et al. 2011). For example, *H. fusiformis* incubated at different pH conditions from pH 2.0 to 12.0 at various times (0–24 hours) showed maximum yield and polyphenols were yielded at pH 12.0 at 34.5 and 7.59 g/100 g DW. At this pH (11 and 12) higher 2,2-diphenyl-1-picrylhydrazyl (DPPH) radical scavenging was recorded in *H. fusiformis* (Siriwardhana et al. 2008).

7.4.2 Solvents

Polyphenolic extracts of algal biomass or terrestrial plants are always a mixture of different classes of phenols, which are selectively soluble in solvents (Dinh et al. 2018). A wide range of solvents including water, acetone, methanol, ethanol, N,N-dimethylformamide, or their mixtures with water have been studied for their extraction efficiency of polyphenols because of their differences in polarities (Hidayati et al. 2020). The use of an alcoholic solution provides satisfactory extraction. For instance, methanol, acetone, and water alone are inefficient solvents for the extraction of total polyphenols from dehydrated algal biomass as the polyphenols are frequently bound to other biomolecules including proteins, cell wall polysaccharides, terpenes, chlorophyll, lipids, and inorganic compounds (Gager et al. 2020). For example, polyphenol fraction of *Cladophora vagabunda* was 212 mg equivalent GAE/100 g in water extract but when using a methanolic extract it was 110 mg/100 g. In the case of *Enteromorpha intestinalis*, the water extract yielded 146 mg/100 g while methanolic extract yielded only 75.5 mg/100 g (Horincar et al. 2011). Advanced extraction techniques including MAE (Dang et al. 2018), PLE (López-Pérez et al. 2020), ultrasonic extraction (Agregan et al. 2019), and SFE (Manna et al. 2015) have aided in overcoming the drawbacks of the traditional methods.

7.5 Challenges and Future Recommendations

Translation of technologies to a commercial scale and the high energy requirement to obtain targeted compounds are the major challenges for modern extraction techniques (Dinh et al. 2018). Other challenges including the high costs of production and lack of specificity of enzymes in EAE, unsuitability of MAE and PLE for handling thermolabile compounds including specific polyphenols (e.g. phloroglucinol and phlorotannins) owing to the high temperatures in use during extractions as discussed above, the high costs associated with SFE, and the high energy inputs of UAE. Future research priorities in these technologies should concentrate on overcoming the challenges of employing these novel technologies on an industrial scale so that the significant benefits to be obtained by improved extraction of polyphenols from algal biomass can be sustainably exploited by industry.

Acknowledgments

The authors are grateful to Mr. Abhiram Seth, Managing Director and Mr. Tanmaye Seth, Director of AquAgri Processing Private Limited for their support and encouragement for the present work.

References

Abirami, R.G. and Kowsalya, S. (2017). Quantification and correlation study on derived phenols and antioxidant activity of seaweeds from gulf of Mannar. *Journal of Herbs, Spices & Medicinal Plants* **23** (1): 9–17.

Adalbjörnsson, B.V. and Jónsdóttir, R. (2015). Enzyme-enhanced extraction of antioxidant ingredients from algae. In: *Natural Products from Marine Algae*, 145–150. New York: Humana Press.

Agregan, R., Munekata, P.E., Franco, D. et al. (2019). Phenolic content and antioxidant activity of extracts from *Bifurcaria bifurcata* alga, obtained by diverse extraction conditions using three different techniques (hydrothermal, ultrasounds and supercritical CO_2). *Environmental Engineering & Management Journal (EEMJ)* **18** (7): 1–9.

Ahn, G., Hwang, I., Park, E. et al. (2008). Immunomodulatory effects of an enzymatic extract from *Ecklonia cava* on murine splenocytes. *Marine Biotechnology* **10** (3): 278–289.

Ajila, C.M., Brar, S.K., Verma, M. et al. (2011). Extraction and analysis of polyphenols: recent trends. *Critical Reviews in Biotechnology* **31** (3): 227–249.

Balasubramanian, S., Allen, J.D., Kanitkar, A., and Boldor, D. (2011). Oil extraction from *Scenedesmus obliquus* using a continuous microwave system–design, optimization, and quality characterization. *Bioresource Technology* **102** (3): 3396–3403.

Barbosa, M., Lopes, G., Ferreres, F. et al. (2017). Phlorotannin extracts from Fucales: marine polyphenols as bioregulators engaged in inflammation-related mediators and enzymes. *Algal Research* **28**: 1–8.

Barbosa, M., Lopes, G., Valentão, P. et al. (2018). Edible seaweeds' phlorotannins in allergy: a natural multi-target approach. *Food Chemistry* **265**: 233–241.

Besednova, N.N., Zvyagintseva, T.N., Kuznetsova, T.A. et al. (2019). Marine algae metabolites as promising therapeutics for the prevention and treatment of HIV/AIDS. *Metabolites* **9** (5): 87.

Castro-Puyana, M., Herrero, M., Mendiola, J.A., and Ibanez, E. (2013). Subcritical water extraction of bioactive components from algae. In: *Functional Ingredients from Algae for Foods and Nutraceuticals* (ed. H. Dominguez), 534–560. Cambridge: Woodhead Publishing.

Charoensiddhi, S., Franco, C., Su, P., and Zhang, W. (2015). Improved antioxidant activities of brown seaweed *Ecklonia radiata* extracts prepared by microwave-assisted enzymatic extraction. *Journal of Applied Phycology* **27** (5): 2049–2058.

Cikoš, A.M., Jokić, S., Šubarić, D., and Jerković, I. (2018). Overview on the application of modern methods for the extraction of bioactive compounds from marine macroalgae. *Marine Drugs* **16** (10): 348.

Cuong, D.X., Hoan, N.X., Dong, D.H. et al. (2019). Tannins: extraction from plants. In: *Tannins-Structural Properties, Biological Properties and Current Knowledge* (ed. A. Aires), 1–20. London: IntechOpen.

Dang, T.T., Van Vuong, Q., Schreider, M.J. et al. (2017). Optimisation of ultrasound-assisted extraction conditions for phenolic content and antioxidant activities of the alga *Hormosira banksii* using response surface methodology. *Journal of Applied Phycology* **29** (6): 3161–3173.

Dang, T.T., Bowyer, M.C., Van Altena, I.A., and Scarlett, C.J. (2018). Optimum conditions of microwave-assisted extraction for phenolic compounds and antioxidant capacity of the brown alga *Sargassum vestitum*. *Separation Science and Technology* **53** (11): 1711–1723.

de Oliveira, J.P., Bruni, G.P., Fabra, M.J. et al. (2019). Development of food packaging bioactive aerogels through the valorization of *Gelidium sesquipedale* seaweed. *Food Hydrocolloids* **89**: 337–350.

Dinh, T.V., Saravana, P.S., Woo, H.C., and Chun, B.S. (2018). Ionic liquid-assisted subcritical water enhances the extraction of phenolics from brown seaweed and its antioxidant activity. *Separation and Purification Technology* **196**: 287–299.

Duarte, K., Justino, C.I.L., Gomes, A.M. et al. (2014). Green analytical methodologies for preparation of extracts and analysis of bioactive compounds. *Comprehensive Analytical Chemistry* **65**: 59–78.

Fabrowska, J., Ibanez, E., Leska, B., and Herrero, M. (2016). Supercritical fluid extraction as a tool to valorize underexploited freshwater green algae. *Algal Research* **19**: 237–245.

Fayad, S., Nehme, R., Tannoury, M. et al. (2017). Macroalga *Padina pavonica* water extracts obtained by pressurized liquid extraction and microwave-assisted extraction inhibit hyaluronidase activity as shown by capillary electophoresis. *Journal of Chromatography. A* **1497**: 19–27.

Gager, L., Connan, S., Molla, M. et al. (2020). Active phlorotannins from seven brown seaweeds commercially harvested in Brittany (France) detected by 1 H NMR and in vitro assays: temporal variation and potential valorization in cosmetic applications. *Journal of Applied Phycology*: 1–12.

Gall, E.A., Lelchat, F., Hupel, M. et al. (2015). Extraction and purification of phlorotannins from brown algae. In: *Natural Products from Marine Algae*, 131–143. New York: Humana Press.

Ganesan, A.R., Shanmugam, M., Palaniappan, S., and Rajauria, G. (2018). Development of edible film from *Acanthophora spicifera*: structural, rheological and functional properties. *Food Bioscience* **23**: 121–128.

Ganesan, A.R., Tiwari, U., and Rajauria, G. (2019a). Seaweed nutraceuticals and their therapeutic role in disease prevention. *Food Science and Human Wellness* **8** (3): 252–263.

Ganesan, A.R., Shanmugam, M., and Bhat, R. (2019b). Quality enhancement of chicken sausage by semi-refined carrageenan. *Journal of Food Processing and Preservation* **43** (7): e13988.

Generalić Mekinić, I., Skroza, D., Šimat, V. et al. (2019). Phenolic content of brown algae (Pheophyceae) species: extraction, identification, and quantification. *Biomolecules* **9** (6): 244.

Godlewska, K., Michalak, I., Tuhy, Ł., and Chojnacka, K. (2017). The influence of pH of extracting water on the composition of seaweed extracts and their beneficial properties on *Lepidium sativum*. *BioMed Research International* **2017**: 1–11.

Gümüş Yılmaz, G., Gómez Pinchetti, J.L., Cifuentes, A. et al. (2019). Comparison of extraction techniques and surfactants for the isolation of Total polyphenols and phlorotannins from the brown algae *Lobophora variegata*. *Analytical Letters*: 1–17.

Gupta, S. and Abu-Ghannam, N. (2011). Recent developments in the application of seaweeds or seaweed extracts as a means for enhancing the safety and quality attributes of foods. *Innovative Food Science & Emerging Technologies* **12** (4): 600–609.

Hahn, T., Lang, S., Ulber, R., and Muffler, K. (2012). Novel procedures for the extraction of fucoidan from brown algae. *Process Biochemistry* **47** (12): 1691–1698.

Han, D., Zhu, T., and Row, K.H. (2011). Ultrasonic extraction of phenolic compounds from *Laminaria japonica aresch* using ionic liquid as extraction solvent. *Bulletin of the Korean Chemical Society* **32** (7): 2212–2216.

Hannachi, H., Benmoussa, H., Saadaoui, E. et al. (2019). Optimization of ultrasound and microwave-assisted extraction of phenolic compounds from olive leaves by response surface methodology. *Research Journal of Biotechnology* **14**: 7.

Hardouin, K., Bedoux, G., Burlot, A.S. et al. (2016). Enzyme-assisted extraction (EAE) for the production of antiviral and antioxidant extracts from the green seaweed *Ulva armoricana* (Ulvales, Ulvophyceae). *Algal Research* **16**: 233–239.

Heffernan, N., Smyth, T.J., FitzGerald, R.J. et al. (2014). Antioxidant activity and phenolic content of pressurized liquid and solid-liquid extracts from four Irish origin macroalgae. *International Journal of Food Science and Technology* **49**: 1765–1772.

Heo, S.J., Cha, S.H., Lee, K.W. et al. (2005a). Antioxidant activities of chlorophyta and phaeophyta from Jeju Island. *Algae* **20** (3): 251–260.

Heo, S.J., Park, P.J., Park, E.J. et al. (2005b). Antioxidant activity of enzymatic extracts from a brown seaweed *Ecklonia cava* by electron spin resonance spectrometry and comet assay. *European Food Research and Technology* **221** (1–2): 41–47.

Herrero, M., Martín-Álvarez, P.J., Señoráns, F.J. et al. (2005). Optimization of accelerated solvent extraction of antioxidants from *Spirulina platensis* microalga. *Food Chemistry* **93** (3): 417–423.

Herrero, M., Jaime, L., Martín-Álvarez, P.J. et al. (2006). Optimization of the extraction of antioxidants from *Dunaliella salina* microalga by pressurized liquids. *Journal of Agricultural and Food Chemistry* **54**: 5597–5603.

Herrero, M., del Pilar Sánchez-Camargo, A., Cifuentes, A., and Ibanez, E. (2015). Plants, seaweeds, microalgae and food by-products as natural sources of functional ingredients obtained using pressurized liquid extraction and supercritical fluid extraction. *TrAC Trends in Analytical Chemistry* **71**: 26–38.

Hidayati, J.R., Yudiati, E., Pringgenies, D. et al. (2020). Comparative study on antioxidant activities, total phenolic compound and pigment contents of tropical *Spirulina platensis, Gracilaria arcuata* and *Ulva lactuca* extracted in different solvents polarity. *E3S Web of Conferences* **147** (3): 03012.

Horincar, V.B., Parfene, G., and Bahrim, G. (2011). Evaluation of bioactive compounds in extracts obtained from three Romanian marine algae species. *Romanian Biotechnological Letters* **16** (6): 71–78.

Kadam, S.U., Tiwari, B.K., and O'Donnell, C.P. (2013). Application of novel extraction technologies for bioactives from marine algae. *Journal of Agricultural and Food Chemistry* **61** (20): 4667–4675.

Kadam, S.U., O'Donnell, C.P., Rai, D.K. et al. (2015a). Laminarin from Irish brown seaweeds *Ascophyllum nodosum* and *Laminaria hyperborea*: ultrasound assisted extraction, characterization and bioactivity. *Marine Drugs* **13**: 4270–4280.

Kadam, S.U., Tiwari, B.K., Smyth, T.J., and O'Donnell, C.P. (2015b). Optimization of ultrasound assisted extraction of bioactive components from brown seaweed *Ascophyllum nodosum* using response surface methodology. *Ultrasonics Sonochemistry* **23**: 308–316.

Klejdus, B., Lojkova, L., Plaza, M. et al. (2010). Hyphenated technique for the extraction and determination of isoflavones in algae: ultrasound-assisted supercritical fluid extraction followed by fast chromatography with tandem mass spectrometry. *Journal of Chromatography. A* **1217**: 7956–7965.

Le, Q.T., Li, Y., Qian, Z.J. et al. (2009). Inhibitory effects of polyphenols isolated from marine alga *Ecklonia cava* on histamine release. *Process Biochemistry* **44** (2): 168–176.

Lee, S.H., Kang, M.C., Moon, S.H. et al. (2013). Potential use of ultrasound in antioxidant extraction from *Ecklonia cava*. *Algae* **28**: 371–378.

Li, Y.X., Wijesekara, I., Li, Y., and Kim, S.K. (2011). Phlorotannins as bioactive agents from brown algae. *Process Biochemistry* **46** (12): 2219–2224.

Li, Z., Wang, B., Zhang, Q. et al. (2012). Preparation and antioxidant property of extract and semipurified fractions of *Caulerpa racemosa*. *Journal of Applied Phycology* **24**: 1527–1536.

Li, Y., Fu, X., Duan, D. et al. (2017). Extraction and identification of phlorotannins from the brown alga, *Sargassum fusiforme* (Harvey) Setchell. *Marine Drugs* **15** (2): 49.

López-Pérez, O., del Olmo, A., Picon, A., and Nuñez, M. (2020). Volatile compounds and odour characteristics during long-term storage of kombu seaweed

(*Laminaria ochroleuca*) preserved by high pressure processing, freezing and salting. *Lebensmittel-Wissenschaft & Technologie* **118**: 108710.

Mabeau, S. and Fleurence, J. (1993). Seaweed in food products: biochemical and nutritional aspects. *Trends in Food Science & Technology* **4** (4): 103–107.

Macías-Sánchez, M.D., Mantell, C., Rodriguez, M.D.L. et al. (2009). Comparison of supercritical fluid and ultrasound-assisted extraction of carotenoids and chlorophyll a from *Dunaliella salina*. *Talanta* **77** (3): 948–952.

Magnusson, M., Yuen, A.K., Zhang, R. et al. (2017). A comparative assessment of microwave assisted (MAE) and conventional solid-liquid (SLE) techniques for the extraction of phloroglucinol from brown seaweed. *Algal Research* **23**: 28–36.

Manna, L., Bugnone, C.A., and Banchero, M. (2015). Valorization of hazelnut, coffee and grape wastes through supercritical fluid extraction of triglycerides and polyphenols. *The Journal of Supercritical Fluids* **104**: 204–211.

Michalak, I., Gorka, B., Wieczorek, P.P. et al. (2016). Supercritical fluid extraction of algae enhances levels of biologically active compounds promoting plant growth. *European Journal of Phycology* **51**: 1–10.

Mokrani, A. and Madani, K. (2016). Effect of solvent, time and temperature on the extraction of phenolic compounds and antioxidant capacity of peach (*Prunus persica* L.) fruit. *Separation and Purification Technology* **162**: 68–76.

Namvar, F., Mohamad, R., Baharara, J. et al. (2013). Antioxidant, antiproliferative, and antiangiogenesis effects of polyphenol-rich seaweed (*Sargassum muticum*). *BioMed Research International* **2013**: 1–9.

Ospina, M., Casto-Vargas, H.I., and Parada-Alfonso, F. (2017). Antioxidant capacity of Colombian seaweeds: 1. Extracts obtained from *Gracilaria mammillaris* by means of supercritical fluid extraction. *Journal of Supercritical Fluids* **128**: 314–322.

O'Sullivan, A.M., O'Callaghan, Y.C., O'grady, M.N. et al. (2011). In vitro and cellular antioxidant activities of seaweed extracts prepared from five brown seaweeds harvested in spring from the west coast of Ireland. *Food Chemistry* **126** (3): 1064–1070.

O'Sullivan, A.M., O'Callaghan, Y.C., O'Grady, M.N. et al. (2013). The effect of solvents on the antioxidant activity in Caco-2 cells of Irish brown seaweed extracts prepared using accelerated solvent extraction (ASE®). *Journal of Functional Foods* **5** (2): 940–948.

Otero, P., López-Martínez, M.I., and García-Risco, M.R. (2019). Application of pressurized liquid extraction (PLE) to obtain bioactive fatty acids and phenols from *Laminaria ochroleuca* collected in Galicia (NW Spain). *Journal of Pharmaceutical and Biomedical Analysis* **164**: 86–92.

Pangestuti, R., Getachew, A.T., Siahaan, E.A., and Chun, B.S. (2019). Characterization of functional materials derived from tropical red seaweed *Hypnea musciformis* produced by subcritical water extraction systems. *Journal of Applied Phycology*: 1–12.

Park, P.J., Shahidi, F., and Jeon, Y.J. (2004). Antioxidant activities of enzymatic extracts from an edible seaweed *Sargassum horneri* using ESR spectrometry. *Journal of Food Lipids* **11**: 15–27.

Park, P. J., Heo, S. J., Park, E. J., Kim, S. K., Byun, H. G., Jeon, B. T., and Jeon, Y. J. (2005). Reactive oxygen scavenging effect of enzymatic extractsfrom Sargassum thunbergii. *Journal of Agricultural and Food Chemistry*, **53** (17), 6666–6672.

Parniakov, O., Apicella, E., Koubaa, M. et al. (2015). Ultrasound-assisted green solvent extraction of high-added value compounds from microalgae Nannochloropsis spp. *Bioresource Technology* **198**: 262–267.

Pérez-Larrán, P., Torres, M.D., Flórez-Fernández, N. et al. (2019). Green technologies for cascade extraction of *Sargassum muticum* bioactives. *Journal of Applied Phycology*: 1–15.

del Pilar Sanchez Camargo, A., Ibanez, E., Cifuentes, A., and Herrero, M. (2017). Bioactives obtained from plants, seaweeds, microalgae and food by-products using pressurized liquid extraction and supercritical fluid extraction. *Comprehensive Analytical Chemistry* **76**: 1–24.

del Pilar Sánchez-Camargo, A., Montero, L., Stiger-Pouvreau, V. et al. (2016). Considerations on the use of enzyme-assisted extraction in combination with pressurized liquids to recover bioactive compounds from algae. *Food Chemistry* **192**: 67–74.

Plaza, M., Amigo-Benavent, M., Del Castillo, M.D. et al. (2010a). Facts about the formation of new antioxidants in natural samples after subcritical water extraction. *Food Research International* **43** (10): 2341–2348.

Plaza, M., Santoyo, S., Jaime, L. et al. (2010b). Screening for bioactive compounds from algae. *Journal of Pharmaceutical and Biomedical Analysis* **2010** (51): 450–455.

Prabhu, M.S., Levkov, K., Livney, Y.D. et al. (2019). High-voltage pulsed electric fields preprocessing enhances extraction of starch, proteins and ash from marine macroalgae *Ulva ohnoi*. *ACS Sustainable Chemistry & Engineering* **7**: 17453–17463.

Priyadarshini, A., Rajauria, G., O'Donnell, C.P., and Tiwari, B.K. (2019). Emerging food processing technologies and factors impacting their industrial adoption. *Critical Reviews in Food Science and Nutrition* **59** (19): 3082–3101.

Puspita, M., Deniel, M., Widowati, I. et al. (2017). Antioxidant and antibacterial activity of solid-liquid and enzyme-assisted extraction of phenolic compound from three species of tropical *Sargassum*. *IOP Conference Series: Earth and Environmental Science* **55** (1): 012057.

Rajauria, G. (2018). Optimization and validation of reverse phase HPLC method for qualitative and quantitative assessment of polyphenols in seaweed. *Journal of Pharmaceutical and Biomedical Analysis* **148**: 230–237.

Rajauria, G., Jaiswal, A.K., Abu-Ghannam, N., and Gupta, S. (2013). Antimicrobial, antioxidant and free radical-scavenging capacity of brown seaweed *Himanthalia elongata* from western coast of Ireland. *Journal of Food Biochemistry* **37** (3): 322–335.

Rajauria, G., Foley, B., and Abu-Ghannam, N. (2016). Identification and characterization of phenolic antioxidant compounds from brown Irish seaweed *Himanthalia elongata* using LC-DAD–ESI-MS/MS. *Innovative Food Science & Emerging Technologies* **37**: 261–268.

Ramluckan, K., Moodley, K.G., and Bux, F. (2014). An evaluation of the efficacy of using selected solvents for the extraction of lipids from algal biomass by the Soxhlet extraction method. *Fuel* **116**: 103–108.

Ren, B., Chen, C., Li, C. et al. (2017). Optimization of microwave-assisted extraction of *Sargassum thunbergii* polysaccharides and its antioxidant and hypoglycemic activities. *Carbohydrate Polymers* **173**: 192–201.

Rodrigues, D., Sousa, S., Silva, A. et al. (2015). Impact of enzyme- and ultrasound-assisted extraction methods on biological properties of red, brown and green seaweeds from the central west coast of Portugal. *Journal of Agricultural and Food Chemistry* **63**: 3177–3188.

Rodríguez-Meizoso, I., Jaime, L., Santoyo, S. et al. (2010). Subcritical water extraction and characterization of bioactive compounds from *Haematococcus pluvialis* microalga. *Journal of Pharmaceutical and Biomedical Analysis* **51** (2): 456–463.

Rodsamran, P. and Sothornvit, R. (2019). Extraction of phenolic compounds from lime peel waste using ultrasonic-assisted and microwave-assisted extractions. *Food Bioscience* **28**: 66–73.

Roh, M.K., Uddin, M.S., and Chun, B.S. (2008). Extraction of fucoxanthin and polyphenol from *Undaria pinnatifida* using supercritical carbon dioxide with co-solvent. *Biotechnology and Bioprocess Engineering* **13**: 724–729.

Sanger, G., Rarung, L.K., Damongilala, L.J. et al. (2019). Phytochemical constituents and antidiabetic activity of edible marine red seaweed (*Halymenia durvilae*). *IOP Conference Series: Earth and Environmental Science* **278** (1): 012069.

Saravana, P.S., Choi, J.H., Park, Y.B. et al. (2016). Evaluation of the chemical composition of brown seaweed (*Saccharina japonica*) hydrolysate by pressurized hot water extraction. *Algal Research* **13**: 246–254.

Saravana, P.S., Tilahun, A., Cho, Y.J. et al. (2017). Influence of co-solvents on fucoxanthin and phlorotannin recovery from brown seaweed using supercritical CO_2. *Journal of Supercritical Fluids* **120**: 295–303.

Singh, I.P. and Bharate, S.B. (2006). Phloroglucinol compounds of natural origin. *Natural Product Reports* **23** (4): 558–591.

Siriwardhana, N., Kim, K.N., Lee, K.W. et al. (2008). Optimisation of hydrophilic antioxidant extraction from *Hizikia fusiformis* by integrating treatments of enzymes, heat and pH control. *International Journal of Food Science & Technology* **43** (4): 587–596.

Sivagnanam, S.P., Yin, S., Choi, J.H. et al. (2015). Biological properties of fucoxanthin in oil recovered from two brown seaweeds using supercritical CO_2 extraction. *Marine Drugs* **13**: 3422–3442.

Swanson, A.K. and Druehl, L.D. (2002). Induction, exudation and the UV protective role of kelp phlorotannins. *Aquatic Botany* **73** (3): 241–253.

Tanniou, A., Esteban Serrano, L., Vandanjon, L. et al. (2013). Green improved processes to extract bioactive phenolic compounds from brown macroalgae using *Sargassum muticum* as model. *Talanta* **104**: 44–52.

Tierney, M.S., Smyth, T.J., Hayes, M. et al. (2013). Influence of pressurised liquid extraction and solid–liquid extraction methods on the phenolic content and antioxidant activities of Irish macroalgae. *International Journal of Food Science & Technology* **48** (4): 860–869.

Topuz, O.K., Gokoglu, N., Yerlikaya, P. et al. (2016). Optimization of antioxidant activity and phenolic compound extraction conditions from red seaweed (*Laurencia obtuse*). *Journal of Aquatic Food Product Technology* **25** (3): 414–422.

Turner, C. and Ibanez, E. (2011). Pressurized hot water extraction and processing. In: *Enhancing Extraction Processes in the Food Industry* (eds. N. Lebovka, E. Vorobiev and F. Chemat), 223–254. Abingdon: Taylor & Francis Group.

US Department of Health and Human Services. (1993). Registry of toxic effects of chemical substances (RTECS, online database). National Toxicology Information Program. Bethesda, MD: National Library of Medicine.

Vázquez-Rodríguez, B., Gutiérrez-Uribe, J.A., Antunes-Ricardo, M. et al. (2020). Ultrasound-assisted extraction of phlorotannins and polysaccharides from *Silvetia compressa* (Phaeophyceae). *Journal of Applied Phycology*: 1–13.

Wang, T., Jónsdóttir, R., Kristinsson, H.G. et al. (2010). Enzyme-enhanced extraction of antioxidant ingredients from red algae *Palmaria palmate*. *LWT – Food Science and Technology* **43**: 1387–1393.

Wijesinghe, W.A.J.P. and Jeon, Y.J. (2012). Enzyme-assistant extraction (EAE) of bioactive components: a useful approach for recovery of industrially important metabolites from seaweeds: a review. *Fitoterapia* **83** (1): 6–12.

Yuan, Y.V. and Walsh, N.A. (2006). Antioxidant and antiproliferative activities of extracts from a variety of edible seaweeds. *Food and Chemical Toxicology* **44** (7): 1144–1150.

Yuan, Y., Zhang, J., Fan, J. et al. (2018). Microwave assisted extraction of phenolic compounds from four economic brown macroalgae species and evaluation of their antioxidant activities and inhibitory effects on α-amylase, α-glucosidase, pancreatic lipase and tyrosinase. *Food Research International* **113**: 288–297.

Zenthoefer, M., Geisen, U., Hofmann-Peiker, K. et al. (2017). Isolation of polyphenols with anticancer activity from the Baltic Sea brown seaweed *Fucus vesiculosus* using bioassay-guided fractionation. *Journal of Applied Phycology* **29** (4): 2021–2037.

Zhang, R., Yuen, A.K.I., Magnusson, M. et al. (2018). A comparative assessment of activity and structure of phlorotannins from the brown seaweed *Carpophyllum flexuosum*. *Algal Research* **29**: 130–141.

Zhang, R., Grimi, N., Marchal, L., and Vorobiev, E. (2019). Application of high-voltage electrical discharges and high-pressure homogenization for recovery of intracellular compounds from microalgae *Parachlorella kessleri*. *Bioprocess and Biosystems Engineering* **42** (1): 29–36.

Zheng, Y., Chen, F., Yao, W.C., and Shi, G. (2012). Chemical composition and antioxidant /antimicrobial activities in supercritical carbon dioxide fluid extract of *Gloiopeltis tenax*. *Marine Drugs* **10** (12): 2634–2647.

8
Extraction Technologies for Bioactive Polysaccharides

Rashida Qari[1] and Rajeev Ravindran[2]
[1]*Department of Maritime Sciences, Bahria University, Karachi, Pakistan*
[2]*School of Agriculture and Food Science, University College Dublin, Dublin, Ireland*

8.1 Introduction

Polysaccharides are high molecular weight substances or polymeric carbohydrate macromolecules composed of many repeated subunits or monosaccharides joined through glycoside bonds or linkages. Polysaccharides are also known as glycans. Polysaccharides have complex structures and perform various functions depending on their structure. If a polysaccharide has the same monosaccharides, it is called a homo-saccharide and if it has different monosaccharides it is called a hetero-saccharide. Based on their function they are divided into two categories. Polysaccharides used for storing energy are called "storage polysaccharides," e.g. starch ($C_6H_{10}O_5$) and glycogen ($C_6H_{10}O_5$)n; and those that send cellular messages and provide support to cells and tissues are called "structural polysaccharides," e.g. cellulose ($C_6H_{10}O_5$)n and chitin ($C_8H_{13}O_5N$)n.

Polysaccharides exist in plants, animals, and microorganisms. Seaweeds or marine algae commonly occurring in the marine environment are the biggest source of natural bioactive polysaccharides (agar, carrageenan, and alginic acid); therefore, a great deal of attention has been directed at isolation and characterization of marine algae polysaccharides owing to their many health benefits (Xu et al. 2017). The present and potential uses of seaweed are as human food, cosmetics, and fertilizers, and for the extraction of industrial gums and chemicals. In Asia seaweeds are used as human food and linked to protection from the major chronic diseases including cardiovascular, cancer, digestive, mental illness, sarcopenia, and some kidney and liver diseases (Fardet and Boirie 2014). All polysaccharides extracted from seaweeds constitute biologically active compounds and have antioxidant, antiallergic, anticoagulant, antiviral, anticancer, anti-inflammatory, and antihyperlipidemic properties.

Recent Advances in Micro- and Macroalgal Processing: Food and Health Perspectives, First Edition.
Edited by Gaurav Rajauria and Yvonne V. Yuan.

Rhodophyta is the division name for red algae. The red color is down to two phycochromoproteids, R-phycoerythrin and R-phycocyanin, which mask the other pigments. The cell wall of red algae contains polygalactose esters and cellulose, sometimes impregnated with calcium carbonate. Most of the world's seaweeds belong to this group. There are over 10 000 species of red algae found worldwide. The main uses of red seaweeds are as food and as sources of two hydrocolloids: agar and carrageenan. There are several red species of seaweeds that are in great demand owing to their products as food items and raw materials, i.e. agar and carrageenan used in the manufacturing of industrial products. In developing countries like India agar is manufactured from *Gelidiella acerosa*, *Gracilaria edulis*, and *Gracilaria crassa* (Kaliaperumal et al. 1992). Approximately 1 million t of seaweeds plants are harvested today for extraction, producing 55 000 t of hydrocolloids, valued at almost US$600 million (McHugh 2003).

Most of the marine multicellular brown algae or Phaeophyceae are a large group of filamentous and macroscopic plants. They have practical applications as a source of structurally and functionally unique polysaccharides, alginic acids, and their salts, i.e. alginates (Shevchenko et al. 2007). There are about 1500–2000 brown seaweed species occurring around the world (FAO 1987). They produce a series of low and high molecular weight carbohydrates and all brown algal cell walls have a fibrillar component formed mainly of cellulose microfibrils that is embedded in an amorphous matrix of acid polysaccharides such as alginic acid linked to each other by proteins (Chandia et al. 2004; Andrade et al. 2003; Kloareg and Quatrano 1988).

8.2 Polysaccharides in Seaweed

Ulvan is a cell wall polysaccharide that is mainly composed of sulfated rhamnose, uronic acids (namely glucuronic acid and iduronic acid) and xylose. The structure of ulvan consists of repeating units of uronic acid linked to a neutral sulfated sugar (Kidgell et al. 2019). This makes ulvan an ideal candidate for the development of new biomaterials for tissue engineering since it has the potential to play modulatory roles in mammalian processes in a similar way to glycosaminoglycans (Dash et al. 2014). Ulvans also find wide applications in the nutraceutical industry as antiviral, antioxidant, anticancer, and immunostimulatory agents (Tanna and Mishra 2019; Thanh et al. 2016). The polysaccharide ulvan is extracted from green seaweeds (Chlorophyta) cell walls (Figure 8.1a). It constitutes 18–29% of the green seaweeds ulva dry weights, used in food, pharma, and cosmetics.

Chemically, agar is a polymer made up of subunits of the sugar galactose and is a component of the cell walls of several species of red seaweeds (Figure 8.1b). Agar is mainly composed of two sugar residues D-galactose (51–53%) and 3,6 anhydrogalactose (46%) with smaller proportions of other monosaccharides and substituent groups (Qari and Siddiqui 1993). Agar is mainly used as a culture medium for various microorganisms, particularly for bacteria; its other less well-known uses include serving as a thickening agent for soups and sauces, in jellies and ice cream, in cosmetics, for clarifying beverages, and for sizing fabrics. Praiboon et al. (2006) reported that agar is known as a water-soluble gel-forming polysaccharide that is extracted from agarophyte members of the Rhodophyta. *Gracilaria* is the third largest genus in the Rhodophyceae, has more than 300 species, and is commercially important in the production of phycocolloid agar (Tseng and Xia 1999; Sahu and Sahoo 2013). The worldwide production of agar was 9600 t valued at US$173 million in 2009, and

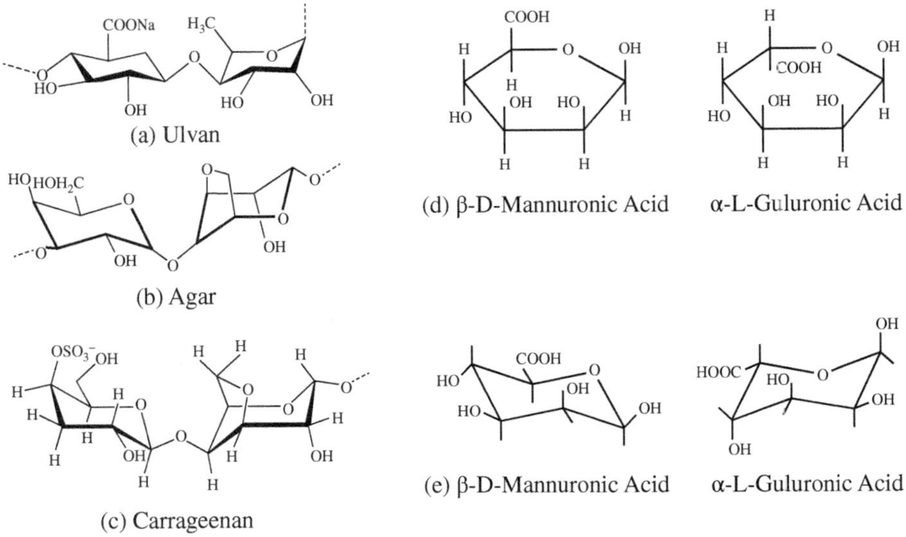

Figure 8.1 Chemical structure of polysaccharides (a) ulvan, (b) agar, (c) carrageenan, (d) monomeric units of alginic acid, and (e) three-dimensional arrangement of the two monomeric units of alginic acid. Sources: Shahidi and Rahman (2018), Sudha et al. (2017), Mampho et al. (2016), FAO (1987).

China, Chile, and Indonesia were the main producers (Bixler and Porse 2010). Species of *Gracilaria* are mainly used for making food-grade agar. Ryther et al. (1975) evaluated numerous species of red seaweeds for their potential growth rates and dry weight yields. They found the genus *Gracilaria* was the most attractive candidate because of its ability to achieve high yields while producing commercially valuable extracts (de Almeida et al. 2011).

Carrageenan is a cell wall polysaccharide complex of D-galactose 3,6-anhydro D-galactose, and monoesterified sulfuric acid obtained from some red seaweeds (Figure 8.1c). It is commonly used as a thickening, suspending, gelling, and stabilizing agent for food products and in other industrial applications as gelatin (Renn 1997). It differs from agar mainly in its higher sulfated fraction and higher ash content (Ramalingam et al. 2003). Carrageenophytes has been commercially grown in the Philippines significantly for the past four decades (Anicia et al. 2013). Pereira et al. (2003) have studied eight species of carrageenophytes collected from the occidental Portuguese coast. Seaweeds are still the leading producer of carrageenan globally (Anicia et al. 2013). Recently Qari et al. (2018) extracted kappa--carrageenan from three species of *Hypnea* (*Hypnea musciformis*, *Hypnea pannosa*, and *Hypnea valentiae*) according to a method adapted from Vandermeulen (1988).

Alginic acid is a major gelling carbohydrate polymer of D-mannuronic acid (M) and L-guluronic acid (G). The classical Haworth formulas for these monomers are shown in Figure 8.1d and Figure 8.1e illustrates a clear picture of the three-dimensional arrangement of the molecules. Alginic acid has considerable technological importance both for its solution properties and as a gelling agent (Tako et al. 2001; Miller 1996). Alginic acid has various chemical and physical properties, and biological activities, therefore it is used for thickening, stabilizing, film-forming, and gel-producing purposes (Arvizu et al. 2007; Khan and Qari 2009, 2012; Khan et al. 2013). Alginic acid has a long history as used in foods and these uses are based mainly on its thickening, gelling, and general colloidal properties. Thickening is useful in sauces, syrups, and toppings for ice cream, etc., pie fillings (it reduces moisture retention by the pastry), cake mixes (it thickens the batter and aids moisture retention), and canned meat and vegetables (it can give either temporary or delayed-action thickening). Its gel formation properties have led to its use in instant milk desserts and jellies, bakery filling cream, fruit pies, animal foods, and reformed fruit. Its general colloidal properties are utilized the addition of sodium alginate to ice cream and water ices, or propylene glycol alginate to stabilize beer foam or the suspended solids in fruit drinks (Sime 1984; King 1983; Littlecott 1982).

The alginate of greatest industrial importance is the sodium salt. Uses are also found for the potassium, ammonium, and calcium salts, as well as alginic acid itself. The only synthetic derivative of alginic acid to find wide use and acceptance as a food additive is propylene glycol alginate. This is formed by reacting propylene oxide with moist alginic acid (FAO 1987). One main use for alginate in the paper industry is surface sizing. It is also used in starch adhesives for making corrugated boards because it stabilizes the viscosity of the adhesive. Alginic acid is insoluble in water but swells when placed in water. This property makes it a useful disintegrating agent in tablets. It is more expensive than the traditional disintegrating agent, starch, but its overall addition to the cost of the tablet is still usually very low. It is a better disintegrating agent than starch so less is required. It can be added during the granulating process, rather than as a powder after granulation, so the processing is easier. The mechanical strength of the final tablet is greater, compared with using starch. Sodium alginate is also used in some liquid medicines to increase viscosity and improve the suspension of solids. Capsules containing sodium alginate and calcium carbonate are used to protect inflamed areas near the entrance to the stomach. Alginic acid extraction described here is based on the method described by Haug (1964) and Whyte (1988).

Laminarin is a polysaccharide widely found in several macroalgal species. Being a storage polysaccharide, laminarin is a homopolymer of glucose bound by (1-3)-β-D-glucopyranose residues with β-(1-6)-intrachain links (Kadam et al. 2015c). Laminarin can be soluble or insoluble in water and other polar solvents; solubility of this polysaccharide is dependent on the level of branching. Seaweed species such as *Laminaria digitata* (kelp), *Laminaria hyperborea*, *Laminaria japonica*, *Saccharina latissima*, and *Fucus vesiculosus* have been reported to contain large quantities of laminarin (Zha et al. 2012). Other species known to have high laminarin content include kelp, which is widely spread in the coastal regions of Ireland, and on the North European and eastern North American coastline. Laminarins have been known to exhibit anticancer activity and are used for the synthesis of hydrogels, which are primarily used to produce artificial tissue (Custódio et al. 2016; Ji and Ji 2014). Meanwhile, fucoidan is a structural polysaccharide found in several species of brown algae. It is a heteropolymer formed by D-uronic acid, D-galactose, D-xylose, and L-fucose sulfate. *Ascophyllum nodosum* is a species of brown algae that has been identified as a rich source of fucoidan. Fucoidan is an important compound in the pharmaceutical industry due to its anti-inflammatory properties (Wang et al. 2008). It has also shown potential as an effective prebiotic agent, which is capable of hosting and aiding the growth of bacteria such as *Lactobacillus* and *Bifidobacterium* in the gut (Shang et al. 2016).

8.3 Conventional Technologies for Polysaccharide Extraction

There are many techniques used for the extraction of polysaccharides, such as the conventional techniques of Soxhlet extraction, maceration, and hydrodistillation. In the Soxhlet technique (Folch et al. 1957) a small amount of dry sample (1 g) is placed in a porous thimble and transferred to an extractor fitted to the Bolt head flask where the solvent passes through. The Bolt head flask contains 100 ml of Folch reagent, a mixture of chloroform and methanol (2:1). The extraction is carried out at 80 °C for 6–8 hours. The process is performed repeatedly until all the quantity of bioactive compound along with the pigment is extracted. The pigments are removed by passing through an activated charcoal column. The solvent is evaporated on a waterbath under a slow stream of inert gas. The residual weight denotes the bioactive compound (lipid) content (Cravotto et al. 2011). In this technique, a long extraction time and large amounts of solvent are needed (Heleno et al. 2016).

The maceration extraction technique is conducted at room temperature. In plants, fresh or dry powder is immersed in a liquid: water, oil, and alcohol for 9–12 hours or overnight, boiled, and then filtered. For lipophilic compounds, oil is used, while water is used to extract hydrophilic compounds. Finally, the macerated mixture is filtered to separate the plant material from the liquid. The residue of the plant is still saturated with solvent, and needs a final press at the end to recover all of the product. The most frequent conventional extraction parameters used for the recovery of brown algae polysaccharides are listed in Table 8.1.

Agar can be extracted using the method described by Whyte et al. (1981). For agar extraction in this study, samples were dried at 70 °C for 24 hours till a constant weight was achieved. The samples were then homogenized with a porcelain pestle and mortar to a powder form, sieved, and stored in a plastic bottle until further analysis. Before the extraction of algae, the dry algal sample was extracted for 60–90 minutes with 400 ml water at 95–100 °C. The resultant mixture was centrifuged at 4000 rpm and the residue was re-extracted with a further 400 ml of water. The combined centrifugates were rotary evaporated to 300 ml, and 1500 ml of ethanol added to precipitate the crude agar. The residue was separated by centrifugation and purified by dissolving the residue in 200 ml water and then the excess ethanol evaporated off by heating on a waterbath. For further purification and strong gelation, the resultant solution was frozen and thawed three times and finally freeze dried.

Agar can also be extracted using the nonalkali method described by Praiboon et al. (2006). In this study the dry algae (30 g) was extracted with 500 ml distilled water at 95–100 °C for 90 minutes. The extracted agar solution was filtered through a muslin cloth. Hot and extracted agar was kept at room temperature until it solidified, then frozen at 20 °C for 48 hours, and thawed in tap water to a hydrogel and then dried. A schematic diagram for the extraction of agar from red seaweeds *Gracilaria* and *Gelidium* is shown in Figure 8.2.

Carrageenan can be extracted using the method outlined by Chapman and Chapman (1980) and Whyte (1988). Here, the sample was cleaned with water and then blot-dried on a paper towel. The first sample was taken in one 1 l dry beaker and treated with 2% NaOH and distilled water. After boiling the slurry for 15 minutes the material was chopped into small pieces by a blender. For filtering the sample four layers of cheesecloth were taped over the mouth of the beaker. The final filtrate extract

Table 8.1 The most frequent conventional extraction parameters used for the recovery of brown algae polysaccharides.

Algae	Polysaccharide	Pretreatment Solvent; time; temperature	Extraction Solvent; time; temperature	Purification	Yield
Sargassum henslowianum	Fucoidan	95% EtOH; 2 × 12 hours	H_2O; 3 × 2 hours; reflux	EtOH Precipitation; dialysis (12 000 Da)	5.1%
Sargassum fusiforme	Fucoidan	95% EtOH; 24 hours; 30 °C	H_2O; 3 hours; 80 °C	EtOH precipitation; dialysis (3,5 kDa)	3.94–11.24%
Ecklonia maximaLaminaria pallidaSplachnidium rugosum	Fucoidan	Ethanol Methanol:chloroform:H_2O (4:2:1); overnight; room temp.	1.0 M HCl; 6 hours; 25 °C 2% $CaCl_2$; 3 hours; 50 °C H_2O; 24 hours; 70 °C 0.15 M HCl; 2 hours; 65 °C 2% $CaCl_2$; 5 hours; 85 °C	EtOH precipitation 10% CTAB	
Cystoseira barbata	Laminarin	Acetone:methanol (7:3); 2 × 24 hours; 30 °C chloroform; 2 × 24 hours; 30 °C	0.1 M HCl; 2 × 2 hours; 60 °C	EtOH precipitation; ultrafiltration (50, 10, and 1 kDa)	7.27%
Cystoseira compressa	Sodium alginate	Acetone; 2 × 24 hours; 25 °C methanol; 2 × 24 hours; 25 °C	0.1 M HCl; 2 hours; 60 °C 3% Na_2CO_3; 2 hours; 60 °C	EtOH precipitation; dialysis (3.5 kDa)	Fucoidan – 5.2%
Dictyopteris divaricata	Polysaccharides	/	H_2O; 5–7 hours; 80–100 °C; water to solid ratio 90–110 ml g^{-1}	EtOH precipitation	3.05%
Sargassum latifolium	Sodium alginate	/	2% citric acid; 2 hours; room temperature 3% Na_2CO_3; 1–3 hours; 25–45 °C	EtOH precipitation	18.89–40.43%

Fucus serratusFucus vesiculosusAscophyllum nodosum	Fucoidan	85% EtOH; overnight; room temp.	0.1 M HCl; 4 hours; 80 °C 1% $CaCl_2$; overnight; 4 °C	EtOH precipitation	*F. serratus* – 4.2–7.5%*F. vesiculo-sus* – 8.1–12.2%*A. nodosum* – 6.5–8.9%
Dictyopteris membranaceaPadina pavonica	Sodium alginate	Methanol-dichloromethane (1:1); 3 × 48 hours; room temp. petroleum ether; Soxhlet acetone; Soxhlet	2% $CaCl_2$; 3 × 3 hours 1 M Na_2CO_3; 2 hours	EtOH precipitation	*D. mem-branaceae* – 18.93%*P. pavonica* – 66.72%
Cystoseira sedoides	Fucoidan sodium alginate	Acetone; 24 hours; 25 °C 80% EtOH; 24 hours; 25 °C 80% EtOH; 24 hours; 78 °C	2% $CaCl_2$; 7 hours; 70 °C 2% Na_2CO_3; 70 °C	Dialysis (7 kDa)	Fucoidan – 4.2% alginate – 11%
Cystoseira myrica	Polysaccharides	Petroleum ether acetone	H_2O; 8 hours; 80 °C	EtOH precipitation; 10% CTAB; dialysis	5.3%
Cystoseira criniteCystoseira compressaCystoseira sedoides	Fucoidan	Methanol-dichloromethane (1:1); 3 × 48 hours; room temp.	2% $CaCl_2$; 3 × 3 hours	Dialysis (30 kDa)	2.8–3.7%

Source: Dobrinčić et al. (2020).

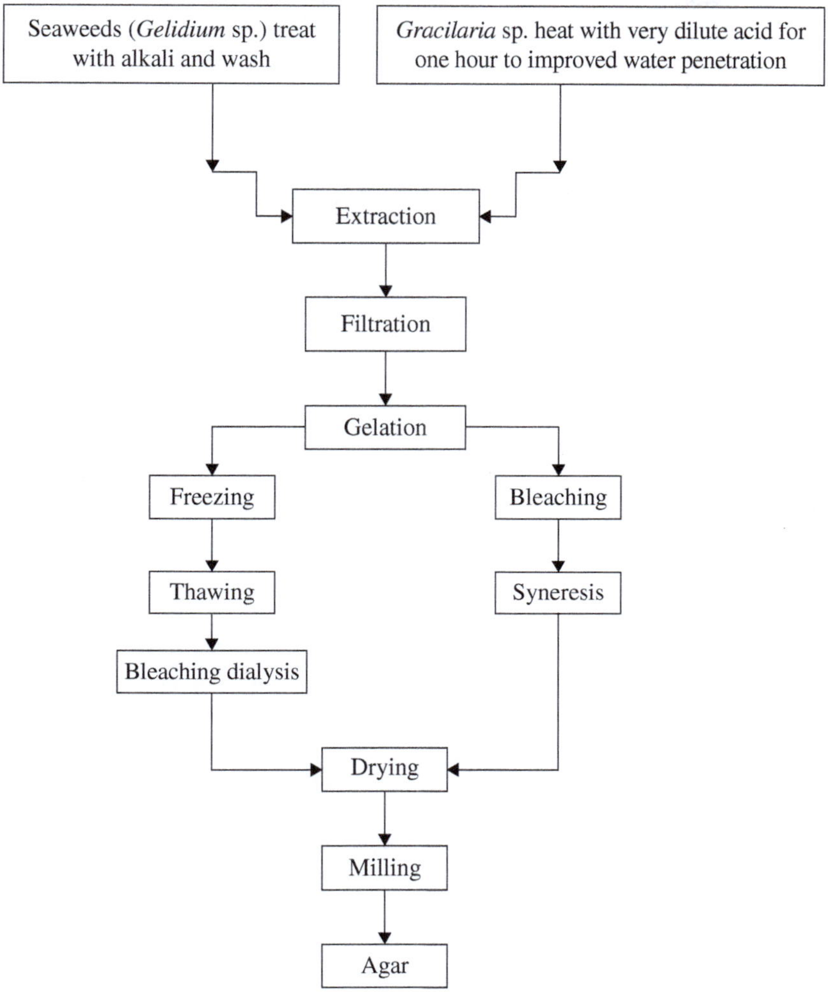

Figure 8.2 The schematic diagram for the extraction of agar. Source: Armisen and Galatas (1987).

was placed in dialysis tubing and then cooled on ice. The schematic diagram for the extraction of carrageenan is shown in Figure 8.3.

Another carrageenan extraction method is outlined in Vandermeulen (1988). A small handful of frozen seaweed was taken and placed into a 1-l clean beaker of water. The plants were cleaned off with the water then blot-dried on a paper towel. For extraction 10 g of the clean seaweeds were weighed out and 7 ml of 2% NaOH/KOH and 343 ml distilled water added. The beaker was placed onto a hot plate and the slurry boiled for 15 minutes. A large watch glass was placed on top to prevent water loss and then the mixture was stirred with a glass rod to stop the extract from foaming out of the beaker. After 15 minutes the contents of the beaker were poured into a blender. A short burst of power was applied to chop the material into small pieces (about 4 mm diameter). The blender was washed with 150 ml of very hot distilled water and this

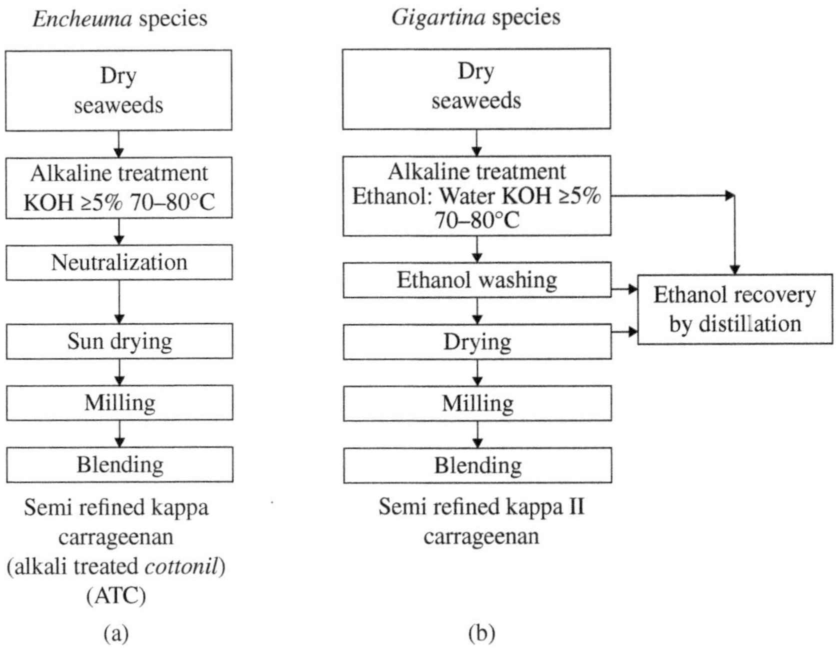

Figure 8.3 Schematic diagram for the extraction of carrageenan. Source: Hernández-Carmona et al. (2013)

was added to the beaker. The mixture was simmered for another 15 minutes, stirring to keep the froth down. For filtering the sample four layers of cheesecloth were taped over the mouth of the beaker. Before the filtrate cooled approx. 100 ml was poured into a large fluted filter paper in a glass funnel. The final filtrate was clear and the beakers were cooled on ice to about room temperature if the final filtrate was still warm. Next 100 ml of ice-cold isopropyl alcohol was added while stirring with a glass rod. The carrageenan precipitate was stuck to the glass rod.

Hydrodistillation is performed with distilled water and is used to extract the volatile fraction in food. This method usually takes 6–8 hours and organic solvents are not involved. In this technique, three main physicochemical processes are involved (i) hydrodiffusion, (ii) hydrolysis, and (iii) decomposition by heat. High temperature can degrade the compounds. The volatile and nonvolatile organic compounds can be extracted and physically separated in one step.

The Haug (1964) and Whyte (1988) methods are used most commonly for alginic acid extraction. A schematic of the process of alginic acid extraction in brown seaweed is presented in Figure 8.4. The sample of seaweed (10 g) and 1% aqueous calcium chloride (300 ml) were taken in a 1 l beaker and kept on a hot plate while stirring the contents continuously with a high torque electric stirrer at 60 °C for 15 minutes. The mixture was then centrifuged at 2000 rpm for 5 minutes. The supernatant was discarded and the seaweed residue returned to the 1 l beaker for re-extraction with a further portion of hot aqueous calcium chloride. The residues were combined and washed with water and diluted acid HCl (0.05 M). The centrifuge bottles were filled with distilled water up to the ¾ point and then mixed thoroughly before centrifugation for 5 minutes. The supernatant was discarded and the bottles filled with HCl

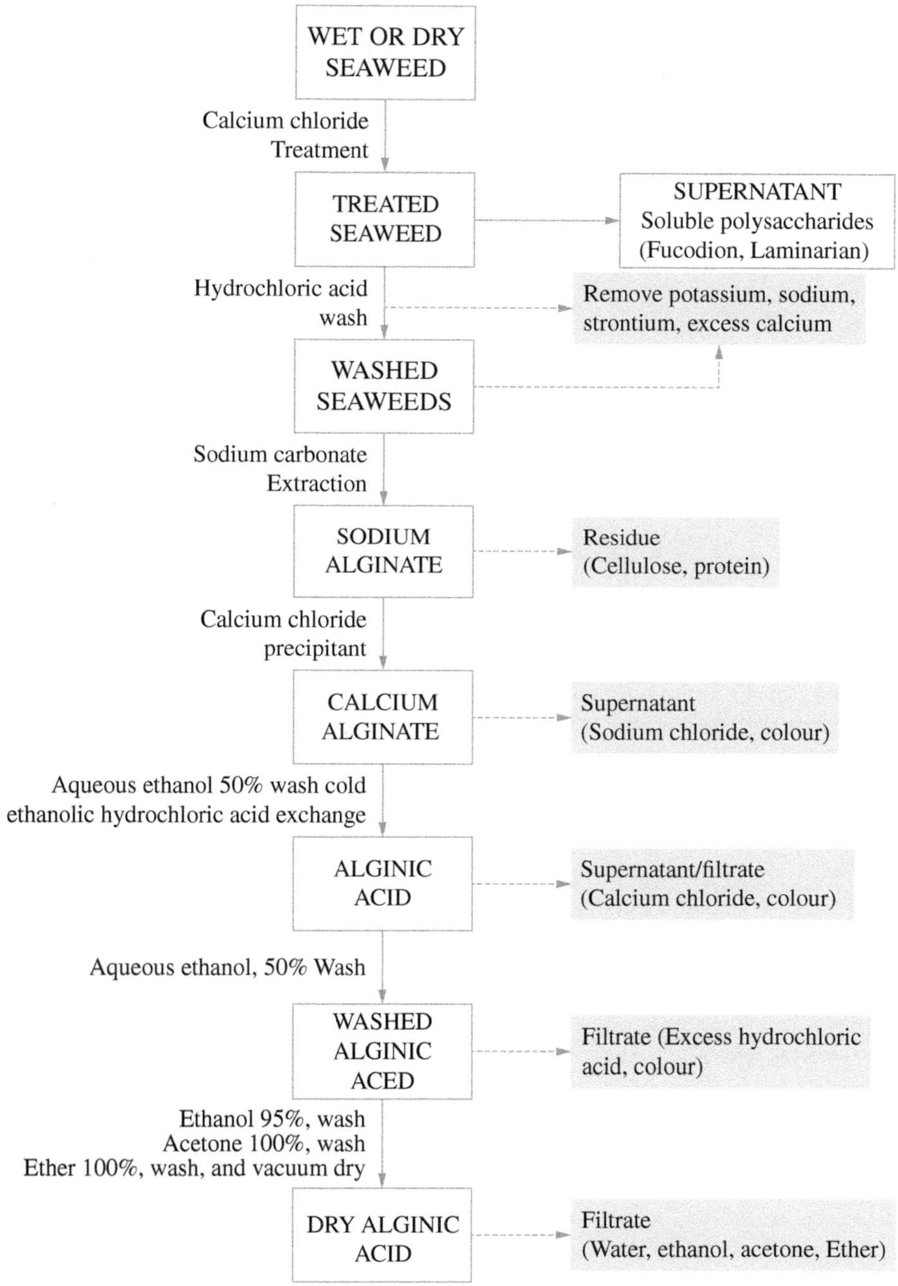

Figure 8.4 Schematic diagram for the extraction of alginic acid in brown seaweed.

(0.05 M) up to the ¾ point. Again the contents were mixed and centrifuged. The residual seaweed was twice more with HCl and the supernatant discarded each time.

The residue of the above sample was returned to a 1 l beaker and treated with 300 ml aqueous sodium carbonate (0.5%). The contents were stirred continuously and heated at 45 °C for 30 minutes. The mixture was centrifuged twice and the supernatant saved. The alginate solution was poured slowly with stirring by glass rod into the 100 ml aqueous calcium chloride (25%) in a 2 l beaker and stirring continued for an additional 10 minutes. The precipitated calcium alginate was centrifuged and the supernatants discarded.

The calcium alginate was transferred for filtration to pre-weighed filter paper under vacuum. The calcium alginate was washed first with 50% 200 ml ethanol and then 300 ml cold HCl (1 M). The product alginic acid that was still on the filter paper was washed with (50%) aqueous ethanol until free from chloride. The filtrate was tested with one drop of silver nitrate solution until no formation of chloride precipitate was evident. It was washed with 95% 200 ml ethanol, acetone, and 100 ml diethyl ether for solvent exchange, and dried under vacuum in a desiccator for 15 minutes. Finally, the product was weighed and the percentage yield of partially purified alginic acid was calculated. The alginic acid yield (in weight percentage) is defined as:

$$\text{Yield (\%)} = \left(\frac{\textit{Dried mass of extracted final alginic acid product}}{\textit{Dried algal mass before acid extraction}} \right) \times 100$$

For the assessment of purity 25 ml standardized aqueous sodium hydroxide (0.1 M) was added to 200 mg dry alginic acid powder in a 100 ml beaker and stirred on a hotplate at 30 °C until the total dissolution of acid. The excess alkali was back-titrated with standardized HCl (0.1 M) and phenolphthalein used as an indicator (red to colorless). Finally, the alginic acid purity was calculated and 1 ml sodium hydroxide was equivalent to 0.0194 g alginic acid in the hydrated form.

Fucoidan or fucans are a group of polysaccharides found in the cell wall of brown algae composed of sulfate L-fucose with less than 10% of other monosaccharides. These polysaccharides are extracted using hot water or an acid solution. Fucoidan is produced as a complex heterogeneous polysaccharide. A schematic diagram of polysaccharide laminarin and fucoidan extraction and purification from macroalgal biomass is depicted in Figure 8.5. Fucoidan is a complex sulfated polysaccharide found in abundance in brown macroalgae. It mainly comprises repeating units of sulfated fucose with additional sugars in lesser quantities such as xylose, galactose, and uronic acids. Depending on the species fucoidans may have straight chains, branched structures, or both. The molecular weight of this compound varies from species to species and has been reported over a wide range typically from 20–200 kDa. Low molecular weight fucoidans may be categorized as those with a molecular weight that falls within the range of 400–5000 Da (Tsai et al. 2017). Fucoidan was originally discovered in 1913 by Kylin, who termed it "fucoidin" and reported it to be a polymer of fucose (Kylin 1913). Researchers have shown great interest in the structural, biological, and other potential properties of fucoidan since then. Several extraction methods for fucoidan from various species have been devised over the years. The major sources of fucoidan for extraction include brown macroalgal species, namely, mozuku, kombu, limu moui, bladderwrack, wakame, and hijiki (Senthilkumar et al. 2013).

Ulvan is one of the main sulfated polysaccharides extracted from the cell wall of green seaweeds belonging to the members of the Ulvales, mainly *Ulva* sp. Ulvan may

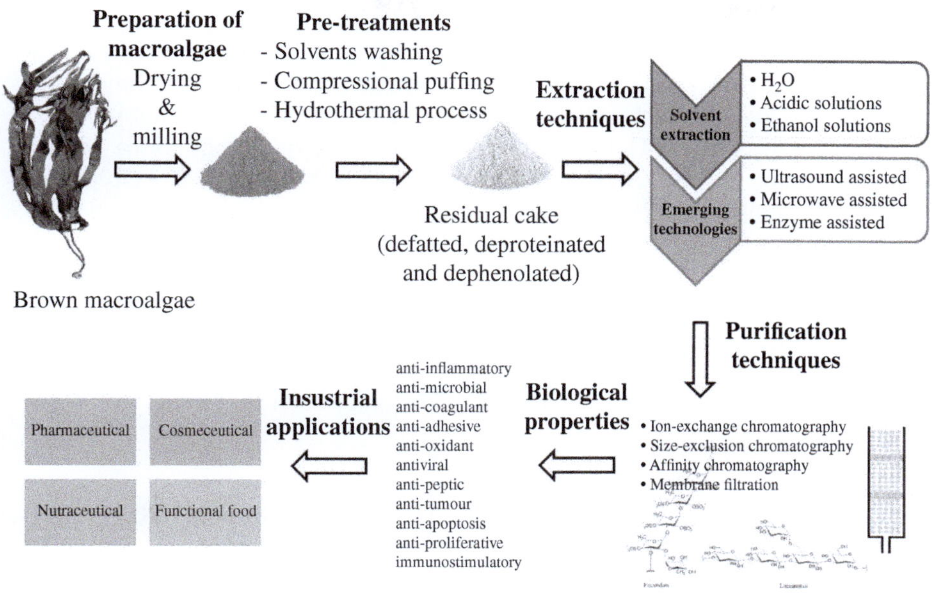

Figure 8.5 Schematic diagram of polysaccharide extraction and purification from macroalgal biomass. Source: Garcia-Vaquero et al. (2017).

constitute 18–29% of green seaweed dry weight, depending on the seaweed species, taxonomic origins, season, growth conditions, postharvest stabilization treatment, and extraction procedures. Recent findings demonstrated that ulvan is an attractive polysaccharide with different biological and medicinal properties; hence, it is suitable for a wide range of applications including food, pharmacy, and cosmetics. Among the biological activities, its anticancer, antioxidant, antihyperlipidemic, and anticoagulant properties are the most widely studied areas. In this contribution, we have presented a general view of the occurrence of ulvan and its major biological activities. For the determination of viscosity of alginic acid the method of Whyte et al. (1981) was followed. The viscosity of 1% solution was determined at 20 °C by using an Ubbelohde type viscometer.

The gelation temperature (Whyte and Englar 1979) was determined by using a hot 1% aqueous solution of carrageenan (10 ml) poured into a test tube. The tube was then clamped in a 1 l beaker containing 900 ml of boiling water, which was stirred constantly by a bar magnet. A precision thermometer (0.1 °C divisions) was positioned off in the center of a test tube and the cooling rate regulated to approximately 0.25 °C per minute. After the 50 °C temperature was attained glass beads (diameter: 3 mm) were introduced periodically at the surface of the solution and the gel temperature recorded when the bead just failed to sink. The method proved to be reproducible to +0.1 °C.

For the determination of gel melting point (Whyte and Englar 1979) a hot 1% aqueous solution of carrageenan (10 ml) was poured into a test tube and a glass rod of the same diameter as the thermometer was then immersed into the solution in an off-center location and the gel was allowed to set overnight at room temperature. The rod was then carefully replaced by the precision thermometer and the test tube was clamped in a waterbath heated at 1 °C per minute. The melting point was recorded when a 3-mm diameter color glass bead, placed just below the surface of the gel, sank.

The relative density and viscosity of gel (carrageenan) were determined by the method of Whyte and Englar (1979). The relative density of 1% solution was determined simply by using R.D. bottles of 25 ml. The viscosity, in centipoises, of a 1% aqueous solution of carrageenan was measured at 65 °C by using an Ubbelohde type viscometer manufactured by Techino Nominal. To determine the gel strength or texture it is necessary to know the maximum load required to rupture the gel matrix in the immediate vicinity of the applied load g cm^{-2}. Nowadays Fourier-transform infrared spectroscopy (FTIR) is used to obtain an infrared spectrum of absorption or emission for any polysaccharide. It is concluded that the extraction technologies for bioactive polysaccharides involve various methods and techniques. To improve these techniques monitoring of times and toxicity is necessary for good results.

8.4 Advanced Technologies for Polysaccharide Extraction

8.4.1 Microwave Assisted Extraction (MAE)

In the MAE technique, nonionizing radiation that falls within the frequency range of 300 MHz and 300 GHz is employed to derive polysaccharides from macroalgae (Jammet et al. 1988). Exposing seaweed to microwave generates heat from within due to dipole rotation or conduction of ions present. Hence, MAE of polysaccharides from seaweed is usually conducted in the presence of a polar solvent such as water or dilute acid (Dobrinčić et al. 2020). The cell wall is broken down by rapid internal heating leading to the release of intracellular components. Microwave extraction measures to derive algal polysaccharides are generally employed in conjunction with other factors such as pressure, time, solid to liquid ratio, etc. (Rodriguez-Jasso et al. 2011). These parameters can be optimized to derive the desired yield and/or product quality.

While several researchers have employed microwaves to extract various compounds from terrestrial and marine plants alike, a majority of studies have been focused on deriving fucoidan from macroalgal species. Yuan and Macquarrie (2015) performed an interesting study to determine the effect of extraction time and temperature on the composition and sulfate content in fucoidan derived from *A. nodosum*. Accordingly, higher temperatures (150 °C) resulted in fucoidan that was rich in glucuronic acid, while lower temperatures (90 °C) yielded the same polysaccharide but with higher fucose content. This extraction procedure required short time frames and relatively low volumes of solvent. Furthermore, the temperature has a detrimental effect on the molecular weight of the fucoidan extracted. This decreases the yield obtained after the extraction process (Kadam et al. 2015a). Another bottleneck of using a microwave as an extraction measure is the variability in temperature measurements due to the presence of high-intensity electromagnetic fields (Rodriguez-Jasso et al. 2011). As well as fucoidan, carrageenan and alginate have also been extracted efficiently employing microwaves in aqueous organic solvents in less time compared with conventional extraction methods (Youssouf et al. 2017).

8.4.2 Ultrasound Assisted Extraction (UAE)

In this type of extraction technique, the biomass is exposed to ultrasound frequency (>20 KHz) in an aqueous environment. This results in cavitation where bubbles form, and expand and contract with the propagation of ultrasound waves until they collapse generating enormous amounts of heat and pressure (up to 5000 K and 1000 atm) in a localized area. The implosion of the bubbles in proximity to cell walls leads to their disruption and release of intracellular contents into the solvent (Ravindran et al. 2017). UAE can be performed at low temperatures and can be ideal for temperature-sensitive components that need to be extracted. Reduced operating time, low solvent consumption, high yields, and low energy requirements are some of the promising features of UAE. Factors that influence UAE include extraction time, solvents to solid ratio, ultrasound power, and nature of the compound to be extracted (Alboofetileh et al. 2019).

Several researchers have investigated the application of ultrasound extraction as a feasible technique to obtain polysaccharides from seaweed (Garcia-Vaquero et al. 2017, 2018, 2020). A typical UAE of polysaccharide and further purification has been represented in Figure 8.6. Li et al. (2013) successfully optimized conditions to extract polysaccharides from *Sargassum fusiforme* and reported a higher antioxidant activity for the extracts in comparison with conventional extraction. Meanwhile, Youssouf et al. (2017) conducted a study employing UAE for the extraction of alginates and carrageenan from *Kappaphycus alvarezii* and *Euchema denticulatum* taking into

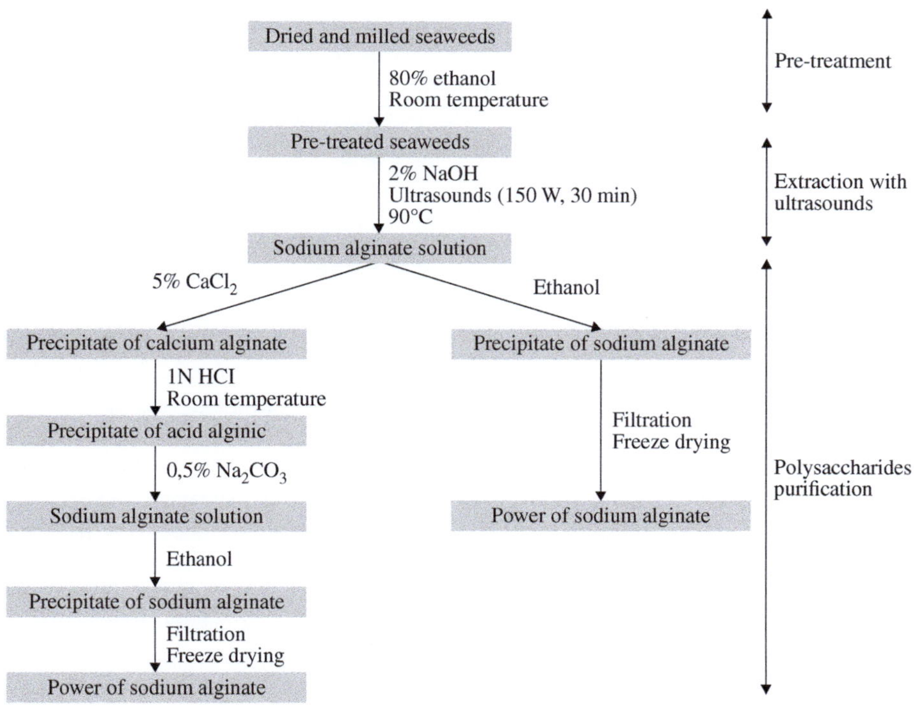

Figure 8.6 Essential steps involved in the ultrasound-assisted extraction and purification of alginates from seaweed. Source: Youssouf et al. (2017).

consideration external factors such as pH, temperature, time, solid to solvent ratio, and ultrasound power. pH was found to be an important factor in the extraction of polysaccharides from seaweed biomass indicating alkaline conditions better suited UAE of polysaccharides. This was particularly relevant in the case of alginates where the polysaccharide was converted into sodium alginate in the presence of alkali. They were able to reduce the extraction time to 30 minutes when compared with conventional measures with higher yields. Furthermore, the chemical structure and molecular mass distribution were unaffected by the UAE. Interestingly, Kadam et al. (2015b) devised an efficient method employing ultrasonication to extract laminarin from *A. nodosum* and *L. hyperborea*. Water and dilute HCl were employed as the extraction solvents in this study. Subsequently, UAE assisted by an acidic environment resulted in higher laminarin yields from both macroalgal species as compared with using water for extraction.

8.4.3 Pressurized Liquid Extraction (PLE)

PLE is a novel technique that utilizes a combination of high temperature and pressure to derive component biomolecules from biomass. Extraction is performed in the absence of oxygen and light and requires low volumes of solvent. Elevated temperatures result in higher solubility of the substrate as well as increased diffusion into the solvent while higher pressure maintains the solvent at boiling point (Saravana et al. 2016). Some of the most common examples of PLE include subcritical water extraction (SWE), hot water extraction, accelerated solvent extraction, etc. (Dobrinčić et al. 2020). Meanwhile, the compressional–puffing–hydrothermal extraction process is also a novel technique that employs heat and pressure to modify the physicochemical nature of biomass. The puffing process is achieved by rapidly increasing the atmospheric temperature while coupling it with the reduction of pressure in a vessel that contains superheated water. This results in the expansion of gas within the seaweed matrix resulting in disruption of internal structures and release of contents. This extraction technique was successfully tested by Huang et al. (2016) for the procurement of fucoidan from *Sargassum glaucescens*.

As mentioned earlier, SWE is a form of PLE that has been reported to efficiently extract polysaccharides from macroalgae. Saravana et al. (2018) successfully optimized SWE for the extraction of crude fucoidan from *Saccharina japonica*. In this study, five parameters, namely temperature, pressure, solid to liquid ratio, agitation speed, and reaction time, were optimized to obtained maximized yields from fucoidan. While a higher yield for fucoidan was observed when implementing SWE, the final product obtained also contained a higher amount of impurities as compared with conventional extraction methods. Hot buffer extraction is a modification of PLE where, as the name suggests, a hot buffer is used to obtain polysaccharides from the macroalgal matrix. This method is a simple and straightforward technique where temperature, pH, and solid to liquid ratio are altered to maximize polysaccharide yield (Hifney et al. 2016). Meanwhile, hydrothermal extraction was extensively researched by Garcia-Vaquero et al. (2019) to determine the best conditions for maximizing polysaccharide yield among other products. Accordingly, they reported that mild temperature conditions ranging from 85–100 °C were suited for the extraction of glucans (laminarins) from macroalgal species such as *A. nodosum* and *L. hyperborea*.

8.4.4 Enzyme Assisted Extraction (EAE)

EAE, as the name suggests, involves enzymes that degrade the cell walls of macroalgae to release the internal components. This technology can improve extraction efficiency concerning cost, yield, time, environmental impact, and safety for food applications (Garcia-Vaquero et al. 2017). Polysaccharides such as fucoidan are tightly bound with structural carbohydrates such as cellulose and proteins. Application of carbohydrate-digesting enzymes and proteases digests the cellulose–protein networks, which weakens the cell wall leading to the release of polysaccharides such as fucoidan and alginate without degradation (Charoensiddhi et al. 2016). In EAE, factors that influence the yield and quality of the polysaccharide obtained include controllable parameters such as pH, temperature, agitation, solid to liquid ratio, and enzyme loading (Lakmal et al. 2015). Advantages of this extraction technique include a low solvent requirement, low cost of operation, higher yield of the target compound, environment friendly, etc. Meanwhile, enzymes are very sensitive to the conditions in the reaction environment, meaning that this method requires stringent process control measures. Furthermore, the target compounds are at risk of being digested by the enzymes used in the process considering that they have the potential to degrade polysaccharides (Habeebullah et al. 2020). Some of the important commercial enzymes used for the extraction of bioactive polysaccharides from seaweed matrices include viscozyme, celluclast, termamyl, ultraflo, etc. (Dobrinčić et al. 2020). EAE does affect the molecular weight of the polysaccharides extracted from macroalgae. Accordingly, Charoensiddhi et al. (2016) observed that maintaining the pH of the extraction process at 4.5 yielded low molecular weight components.

8.5 Conclusion

There is a high demand for potential ingredients that can be used for the preparation of functional foods. Algal polysaccharides have garnered considerable attention due to their wide spectra of biological activities. These polysaccharides are finding wide applications in several industrial processes pertaining to food, pharmaceuticals, cosmetics, etc. This calls for efficient extraction processes to derive these compounds from seaweed matrices without disrupting their bioactive properties. While conventional extraction methods use polar and nonpolar solvents, acids and alkali, etc., novel measures have emerged that involve the application of state-of-the-art technology such as ultrasound, microwaves, pressurized liquids, and enzyme assisted measures. The application of novel technologies has proven to reduce costs while increasing yields and ease of the overall process. However, the practical usage of such technologies has remained in the confines of the laboratory and is yet to be explored on a larger scale.

References

Alboofetileh, M., Rezaei, M., Tabarsa, M., and You, S. (2019). Ultrasound-assisted extraction of sulfated polysaccharide from *Nizamuddinia zanardinii*: process optimization, structural characterization, and biological properties. *Journal of Food Process Engineering* **42** (2): e12979. https://doi.org/10.1111/jfpe.12979.

de Almeida, C.L.F., Falcão, H.d.S., Lima, G.R.d.M. et al. (2011). Bioactivities from marine algae of the genus *Gracilaria. International Journal of Molecular Sciences* **12** (7): 4550–4573.

Andrade, L.R., Salgado, L.T., Farina, M., and AmadoFilho, G.M. (2003). Sem of soluble polysaccharides extracted from the cell walls of the marine brown algae *Padina gymnospora. Microscopy and Microanalysis* **9** (2): 246.

Anicia, Q.H., Marco Nemesio, E.M., and Milagrosa, R.M. (2013). Commercial production of carrageenophytes in the Philippines: ensuring long term sustainability for the industry. *Journal of Applied Phycology* **25** (3): 733–742.

Armisen, R. and Galatas, F. (1987). Production, properties and uses of agar. In: *Production and Utilization of Products from Commercial Seaweeds* (ed. D.J. McHugh), 1–57. Rome: FAO.

Arvizu, D.L., Rodriguez, Y.E., Hernandez, G., and Murillo, J.I. (2007). Chemical constituents of *Eisenia arborea* Areschoug from Baja California Sur, Mexico. *Investigaciones Marinas* **35** (2): 63–69.

Bixler, H.J. and Porse, H. (2010). A decade of change in the seaweed hydrocolloids industry. *Journal of Applied Phycology* **23**: 321–335.

Chandia, N.P., Matsuhiro, B., Mejias, E., and Moenne, A. (2004). Alginic acid in *lessonia vadosa*: partial hydrolysis and elicitor properties of the polymannuronic acid fraction. *Journal of Applied Phycology* **16**: 127–133.

Chapman, V.J. and Chapman, D.J. (1980). *Seaweed and their Uses*. London/New York: Chapman and Hall.

Charoensiddhi, S., Lorbeer, A.J., Lahnstein, J. et al. (2016). Enzyme-assisted extraction of carbohydrates from the brown alga *Ecklonia radiata*: effect of enzyme type, pH and buffer on sugar yield and molecular weight profiles. *Process Biochemistry* **51** (10): 1503–1510.

Cravotto, G., Stefano Mantegna, S., and Mantegna, S. (2011). Extraction of kiwi seed oil: Soxhlet versus four different non-conventional technique. *Natural Product Research* **25** (10): 974–981.

Custódio, C.A., Reis, R.L., and Mano, J.o.F. (2016). Photo-cross-linked laminarin-based hydrogels for biomedical applications. *Biomacromolecules* **17** (5): 1602–1609.

Dash, M., Samal, S., Bartoli, C. et al. (2014). Biofunctionalization of Ulvan scaffolds for bone tissue engineering. *ACS Applied Materials & Interfaces* **6** https://doi.org/10.1021/am404912c.

Dobrinčić, A., Balbino, S., Zorić, Z. et al. (2020). Advanced technologies for the extraction of marine brown algal polysaccharides. *Marine Drugs* **18** (3): 168.

FAO (1987). Production and utilization of products from commercial seaweeds. In: *Production, Properties and Uses of Alginates*. FAO Fisheries technical paper No. 288 (ed. D.J. McHugh). Rome: FAO.

Fardet, A. and Boirie, A. (2014). Associations between food and beverage groups and major diet-related chronic diseases: an exhaustive review of pooled/meta-analyses and systematic reviews. *Nutrition Reviews* **72** (12): 741–762.

Folch, J., Lees, M., and Sloane-Slanely, G.H. (1957). A simple method for the isolation and purification of total lipids from animal tissues. *The Journal of Biological Chemistry* **226**: 497–509.

Garcia-Vaquero, M., Rajauria, G., O'Doherty, J.V., and Sweeney, T. (2017). Polysaccharides from macroalgae: recent advances, innovative technologies and challenges in extraction and purification. *Food Research International* **99**: 1011–1020.

Garcia-Vaquero, M., Rajauria, G., Tiwari, B. et al. (2018). Extraction and yield optimisation of fucose, glucans and associated antioxidant activities from *Laminaria digitata* by applying response surface methodology to high intensity ultrasound-assisted extraction. *Marine Drugs* **16**: 257.

Garcia-Vaquero, M., O'Doherty, J.V., Tiwari, B.K. et al. (2019). Enhancing the extraction of polysaccharides and antioxidants from macroalgae using sequential hydrothermal-assisted extraction followed by ultrasound and thermal technologies. *Marine Drugs* **17** (8): 457.

Garcia-Vaquero, M., Ummat, V., Tiwari, B., and Rajauria, G. (2020). Exploring ultrasound, microwave and ultrasound–microwave assisted extraction technologies to increase the extraction of bioactive compounds and antioxidants from brown macroalgae. *Marine Drugs* **18** (3): 172.

Habeebullah, S.F.K., Alagarsamy, S., Sattari, Z. et al. (2020). Enzyme-assisted extraction of bioactive compounds from brown seaweeds and characterization. *Journal of Applied Phycology* **32**: 115.

Haug, A. (1964). Composition and properties of alginates. Report of the Norwegian Institute of Seaweed Research, No.30. Oslo: Norwegian Institute of Seaweed Research.

Heleno, S.A., Lage, M.A.P., Barros, L. et al. (2016). Optimization of microwave-assisted extraction of ergosterol from *Agaricus bisporus* L. by-products using response surface methodology. *Food and Bioproducts Processing* **100**: 25–35.

Hernández-Carmona, G., Freile-Pelegrín, Y., and Hernández-Garibay, E. (2013). Conventional and alternative technologies for theextraction of algal polysaccharides. In: *FunctionalIngredients from Algae for Foods and Nutraceuticals* (ed. Dominguez, H.), 475–516. Cambridge, UK, Woodhead Publishing.

Hifney, A.F., Fawzy, M.A., Abdel-Gawad, K.M., and Gomaa, M. (2016). Industrial optimization of fucoidan extraction from *Sargassum* sp. and its potential antioxidant and emulsifying activities. *Food Hydrocolloids* **54**: 77–88.

Huang, C.-Y., Wu, S.-J., Yang, W.-N. et al. (2016). Antioxidant activities of crude extracts of fucoidan extracted from *Sargassum glaucescens* by a compressional-puffing-hydrothermal extraction process. *Food Chemistry* **197**: 1121–1129.

Jammet, H., Bernhardt, J., Bosnjakovic, B.F. et al. (1988). Guidelines on limits of exposure to radiofrequency electromagnetic fields in the frequency range from 100 kHz to 300 GHz. *Health Physics* **54** (1): 115–123.

Ji, C.F. and Ji, Y.B. (2014). Laminarin-induced apoptosis in human colon cancer LoVo cells. *Oncology Letters* **7** (5): 1728–1732.

Kadam, S.U., Álvarez, C., Tiwari, B.K., and O'Donnell, C.P. (2015a). Chapter 9). Extraction of biomolecules from seaweeds. In: *Seaweed Sustainability* (eds. B.K. Tiwari and D.J. Troy), 243–269. San Diego, CA: Academic Press.

Kadam, S.U., O'Donnell, C.P., Rai, D.K. et al. (2015b). Laminarin from Irish brown seaweeds *Ascophyllum nodosum* and *Laminaria hyperborea*: ultrasound assisted extraction, characterization and bioactivity. *Marine Drugs* **13** (7): 4270–4280.

Kadam, S.U., Tiwari, B.K., and O'Donnell, C.P. (2015c). Extraction, structure and biofunctional activities of laminarin from brown algae. *International Journal of Food Science & Technology* **50** (1): 24–31.

Kaliaperumal, N., Kalimuthu, S., and Ramalingam, J.R. (1992). Studies on the agar content in *Gracilaria arcuata* var. *arcuata* and *G. corticata* var. *cylindrical. Seaweed Research and Utilisation* **15** (1 & 2): 191–195.

Khan, F. and Qari, R. (2009). Seasonal; variation in water soluble polysaccharides alginic acid extracted from *Sargassum boveanum* J. Agardh (Phaeophyta, Sargassaceae) along the different shore of Karachi coast, Pakistan. *International Journal of Biology and Biotechnology* **6** (4): 277–281.

Khan, F. and Qari, R. (2012). Variation in biomass, biochemical composition and alginic acid content in two brown seaweeds *Spatoglossum variable* Kutz and *Stoechospermum marginatum* Agardh. *International Journal of Phycology and Phycochemistry* **8** (1): 59–68.

Khan, F., Abbas, Q., and Qari, R. (2013). Alginic acid yield, biochemical composition and biomass in brown seaweed species of cape Monze shore, Karachi. In: *Climate Change Impact on Ecosystem* (eds. J. Sundaresan, S. Sreekesh, A. Ramanathan, et al.), 220. India: Scientific Publisher.

Kidgell, J.T., Magnusson, M., de Nys, R., and Glasson, C.R.K. (2019). Ulvan: a systematic review of extraction, composition and function. *Algal Research* **39**: 101422.

King, A.H. (1983). Brown seaweed extracts (alginates). In: *Food Hydrocollids* (ed. M. Glicksman), 115–188. Boca Raton, FL: CRC Press.

Kloareg, B. and Quatrano, R.S. (1988). Structure of the cell walls of marine algae and ecophysiological functions of the matrix polysaccharides. *Oceanography and Marine Biology: An Annual Review* **26**: 259–315.

Kylin, H. (1913). Biochemistry of sea algae. *Hoppe-Seyler's Zeitschrift fur Physiologische Chemiei* **83** (171197): 3.

Lakmal, H., Lee, J., and Jeon, Y. (2015). Enzyme-assisted extraction of a marine algal polysaccharide, fucoidan and bioactivities. In: *Polysaccharides: Bioactivity and Biotechnology* (eds. K.G. Ramawat and J.M. Mérillon), 1065–1077. Cham: Springer International Publishing.

Li, C., Wang, C., Wang, S. et al. (2013). Optimization of ultrasonic-assisted extraction technology of *Sargassum fusiforme* polysaccharides and evaluation of their antioxidant activity. *Food Science and Technology Research* **19** (2): 157–162.

Littlecott, G.W. (1982). Food gels – the role of alginates. *Food Technology in Australia* **34**: 412–418.

Mampho, C., Pandey, P., Ramontja, J., Fosso-Kankeu, E., and Waanders, F. (2016). Synthesis and characterization of superabsorbent hydrogels based on natural polymers: kappa carrageenan. Proceedings of the International Conference on Advances in Science, Engineering, Technology and Natural Resources (ICASETNR), Parys, South Africa

McHugh, D.J. (2003). A guide to the seaweed industry. FAO Fisheries Technical Paper, No. 441. Rome: FAO.

Miller, I.J. (1996). Alginate composition of some New Zealand brown seaweeds. *Phytochemistry* **41**: 1315–1317.

Pereira, L., Sousa, A., Coelho, H. et al. (2003). Use of FTIR, FT-Raman and 13C-NMR spectroscopy for identification of some seaweed phycocolloids. *Biomolecular Engineering* **20**: 223–228.

Praiboon, J., Chirapart, A., akakabe, Y. et al. (2006). Physical and chemical characterization of agar polysaccharides extracted from the Thai and Japanese species of *Gracilaria. Science Asia* **1**: 11–17.

Qari, R. and Siddiqui, S.A. (1993). Biochemical composition and yield of agar from the *Gracilaria corticata* of Karachi, Pakistan. *Journal of Marine Biology* **2**: 77–81.

Qari, R., Abbas, O., and Khan, A.R. (2018). Carrageenan content in three species of *Hypnea* (*H. musciformis* Wulfen J. V. Lamouroux, *H. pannosa* J. Agardh and *H. valentiae* Turner Montagne) of Karachi coast. *International Journal of Marine Science* **8** (11): 89–100.

Ramalingam, J.R., Kaliaperumal, N., and Kalimuthu, S. (2003). Commercial scale production of carrageenan from red algae. *Seaweed Research and Utilisation* **25** (1 and 2): 37–46.

Ravindran, R., Jaiswal, S., Abu-Ghannam, N., and Jaiswal, A.K. (2017). Evaluation of ultrasound assisted potassium permanganate pre-treatment of spent coffee waste. *Bioresource Technology* **224**: 680–687.

Renn, D. (1997). Biotechnology and the red seaweed polysaccharide industry: status, needs and prospects. *Trends in Biotechnology* **15** (1): 9–14.

Rodriguez-Jasso, R.M., Mussatto, S.I., Pastrana, L. et al. (2011). Microwave-assisted extraction of sulfated polysaccharides (fucoidan) from brown seaweed. *Carbohydrate Polymers* **86** (3): 1137–1144.

Ryther, J.C., Goldman, C.E., Gifford, C.E., and Huguenin, J.E. (1975). Physical models of integrated waste recycling marine polyculture systems. *Aquaculture* **5**: 163–177.

Sahu, N. and Sahoo, D. (2013). Study of morphology and agar contents in some important *Gracilaria* species of Indian coasts. *AJPS* **4**: 52–59.

Saravana, P.S., Cho, Y.-J., Park, Y.-B. et al. (2016). Structural, antioxidant, and emulsifying activities of fucoidan from *Saccharina japonica* using pressurized liquid extraction. *Carbohydrate Polymers* **153**: 518–525.

Saravana, P.S., Tilahun, A., Gerenew, C. et al. (2018). Subcritical water extraction of fucoidan from *Saccharina japonica*: optimization, characterization and biological studies. *Journal of Applied Phycology* **30** (1): 579–590.

Senthilkumar, K., Manivasagan, P., Venkatesan, J., and Kim, S.-K. (2013). Brown seaweed fucoidan: biological activity and apoptosis, growth signaling mechanism in cancer. *International Journal of Biological Macromolecules* **60**: 366–374.

Shahidi, F. and Rahman, M.J. (2018). Bioactives in seaweeds, algae, and fungi and their role in health promotion. *Journal of Food Bioactives* **2**: 58–81.

Shang, Q., Shan, X., Cai, C. et al. (2016). Dietary fucoidan modulates the gut microbiota in mice by increasing the abundance of Lactobacillus and Ruminococcaceae. *Food & Function* **7** (7): 3224–3232.

Shevchenko, N.M., Anastyuk, S.D., Gerasimenko, N.I. et al. (2007). Polyssacharides and lipid composition of the brown seaweed *Laminaria gurjanovea*. *Russian Journal of Bioorganic Chemistry* **33** (1): 88–98.

Sime, W.J. (1984). The practical utilization of alginates in food gelling system. In: *Gums and Stabilizers for the Food Industry*, vol. **2** (eds. G.O. Phillips, P.J. Wedlock and P.A. Williams), 177–188. Oxford: Permegon.

Sudha, P.N., Sangeetha, K., and Gomathi, T. (2017). Introduction to marine biopolymers. In: *Industrial Applications of Marine Biopolymers* (ed. P.N. Sudha), 608. Boca Raton, FL: CRC Press.

Tako, M., Kiyuna, S., Uechi, S., and Hongo, F. (2001). Isolation and characterization of alginic acid from commercially cultured *Nemacystus decipiens* (Itomozuku). *Bioscience, Biotechnology, and Biochemistry* **65** (3): 654–657.

Tanna, B. and Mishra, A. (2019). Nutraceutical potential of seaweed polysaccharides: structure, bioactivity, safety, and toxicity. *Comprehensive Reviews in Food Science and Food Safety* **18** (3): 817–831.

Thanh, T.T., Quach, T.M., Nguyen, T.N. et al. (2016). Structure and cytotoxic activity of ulvan extracted from green seaweed *Ulva lactuca*. *International Journal of Biological Macromolecules* **93** (Pt A): 695–702.

Tsai, H.-L., Tai, C.-J., Huang, C.-W. et al. (2017). Efficacy of low-molecular-weight fucoidan as a supplemental therapy in metastatic colorectal cancer patients: a double-blind randomized controlled trial. *Marine Drugs* **15** (4): 122. https://doi.org/10.3390/md15040122.

Tseng, C.K. and Xia, B.M. (1999). On the *Gracilaria* in the western Pacific and the south eastern Asia region. *Botanica Marina* **42**: 209–217.

Vandermeulen, H. (1988). Crude extraction and testing of carrageenan. In: *Experimental Phycology – a Laboratory Manual* (eds. C.S. Lobban, D.J. Chapman and B.P. Kremer), 164–167. Cambridge: Cambridge University Press.

Wang, Y., Xu, Z., Bach, S.J., and McAllister, T.A. (2008). Effects of phlorotannins from *Ascophyllum nodosum* (brown seaweed) on in vitro ruminal digestion of mixed forage or barley grain. *Animal Feed Science and Technology* **145** (1): 375–395.

Whyte, J.N. (1988). Extraction of alginic acid from brown seaweed. In: *Experimental Phycology – a Laboratory Mannual* (eds. C.S. Lobban, D.J. Chapman and B.P. Kremer), 168–183. Cambridge: Cambridge University Press.

Whyte, J.N.C. and Englar, J.R. (1979). Agar elaborated by *Gracilaria* sp. from the coast of British Columbia. Part 1. Properties of agar isolated from algae collected at Bamfield Inlet, Wiseman's Bay and Nuttan Bay. Fisheries and Marine Service Technical Report, No. 860, Vancouver, BC.

Whyte, J.N.C., Englar, J.R., Saunders, R.G., and Landsay, J.C. (1981). Seasonal variation in the biomass, quantity & quality of agar from the reproductive and vegetative stages of *Gracilaria* (Verrucosa type). *Botanica Marina* **24**: 493–501.

Xu, S.-Y., Huang, X., and Cheong, K.-L. (2017). Recent advances in marine algae polysaccharides: isolation, structure, and activities. *Marine Drugs* **15** (12): 388. https://doi.org/10.3390/md 15120388.

Youssouf, L., Lallemand, L., Giraud, P. et al. (2017). Ultrasound-assisted extraction and structural characterization by NMR of alginates and carrageenans from seaweeds. *Carbohydrate Polymers* **166**: 55–63.

Yuan, Y. and Macquarrie, D. (2015). Microwave assisted extraction of sulfated polysaccharides (fucoidan) from *Ascophyllum nodosum* and its antioxidant activity. *Carbohydrate Polymers* **129**: 101–107.

Zha, X.-Q., Xiao, J.-J., Zhang, H.-N. et al. (2012). Polysaccharides in *Laminaria japonica* (LP): extraction, physicochemical properties and their hypolipidemic activities in diet-induced mouse model of atherosclerosis. *Food Chemistry* **134** (1): 244–252.

Section II

Biological Properties of Algal Derived Compounds

9
Potential Biological Activities Associated with Algal Derived Compounds

Yvonne V. Yuan
School of Nutrition, Ryerson University,, Toronto, Ontario, Canada

9.1 Introduction

Edible marine macroalgae include Ochrophyta (comprising those of the Phaeophyceae class [brown (B)]), Chlorophyta (the Chlorophyceae class [green (G)]), and Rhodophyta (the Rhodophyceae class [red (R)]) phyla or divisions, with species valorized and therefore, wild-harvested or cultivated, as sources of hydrocolloids (e.g. agar-agar, alginates, carrageenans), other soluble (e.g. Floridean starch, fucoidans) and insoluble dietary fibers (e.g. cellulose, mannans, xylans), proteins, minerals, vitamins, long-chain n-3 polyunsaturated fatty acids (PUFAs) as well as a variety of potentially biologically active, and thereby, nutraceutical, cosmeceutical, or pharmacognosic compounds such as the mycosporine-like amino acids (MAAs), fucoidans, carotenes and xanthophylls, tocols, polyphenols, phenolic acids, phlorotannins, and lignans (Tou et al. 2019; Athukorala et al. 2016; Athukorala and Yuan 2013; Plaza et al. 2008; Yuan 2007, 2008). The diversity of unicellular edible microalgae is reflected in the Dinoflagellata (marine and freshwater dinoflagellates or plankton), Cryptophyta (freshwater microalgae, but also in marine and brackish waters), Raphidophyta (marine and freshwater microalgae), and Cyanophyta (blue-green algae, e.g. Cyanophyceae) phyla or divisions (Tou et al. 2019; Garcia et al. 2017).

Marine macroalgae (i.e. seaweeds or sea vegetables) as well as marine, freshwater, and brackish microalgae have a long and ancient history in the diets of coastal peoples and their cultures and are growing in importance for health-seeking and environmentally sustainable cuisines for today's consumers. The primacy of edible seaweeds such as the kelps "arame" (*Eisenia bicyclis*), "hijiki" (*Hizikia fusiformis*), "kombu" (*Laminaria digitata*), "wakame" in Japanese, or "sea mustard" (*Undaria pinnatifida*) in Korean cuisines; "sea tangle" or "hai dai" (*Laminaria japonica*) in Korean or Chinese cuisines; red seaweeds such as "nori" or "kim/gim" (*Pyropia tenera* or *Pyropia*

Recent Advances in Micro- and Macroalgal Processing: Food and Health Perspectives, First Edition.
Edited by Gaurav Rajauria and Yvonne V. Yuan.

yezoensis) in Japanese or Korean cuisines; "Ceylon moss" (*Gracilaria edulis*) in Southwest and -east Asian cuisines; "sol" or "dulse/dillisk/dilleasc/creathnach" (*Palmaria palmata*) in Icelandic, Scottish, Irish, Norwegian, Atlantic Canadian, or American cuisines; "maërl" or "margo" (*Lithothamnion coralliodides* and *Phymatolithon calcareum*) as fertilizer in France or the UK; and green seaweeds including "limu pālahalaha" (*Ulva fasciata*) in Hawaiian cuisine is well recognized (Tou et al. 2019; Mac Monagail et al. 2017; Yuan 2007, 2008). Moreover, seaweeds are also known to play a role in the cuisines of numerous East and Southeast Asian (e.g. Vietnam, Indonesia, Philippines) cultures, as well as in Pacific (e.g. New Zealand Maori), Caribbean (e.g. Jamaica, Saint Lucia, Grenadines), Central (e.g. Belize, Honduras, Panama) and South American cultures (e.g. Chile, Argentina, Brazil, Peru, Venezuela). On the other hand, seaweeds are not as commonplace in North American or European cultures, with some notable exceptions as above, as well as Mexico, Norway, Wales, and more recently France. These coastal cultures have incorporated macro- and microalgae as well as seaweed extracts, primarily as hydrocolloids, throughout the diet in salads, soups, stews, sushi wraps, condiments, gelled desserts (i.e. seaweed pie on Prince Edward Island, Canada; agar-agar almond jello in China), and beverages (i.e. Irish moss drink in the Caribbean) (Tou et al. 2019; Yuan 2007, 2008; Robledo and Freile Pelegrín 1997).

Microalgae, whether wild-harvested or cultivated, have been incorporated into macrobiotic diets and used as dietary supplements for nutritional (i.e. protein, long-chain n-3 PUFAs, carotenes, and xanthophylls, carbohydrates) or functional food and nutraceutical benefits in modern times (Tou et al. 2019; Khan et al. 2018; Garcia et al. 2017; Lordan et al. 2011). On the other hand, various microalgae also have an ancient history of use: Aztecs harvested *Spirulina platensis* (or *Arthrospira platensis* (Cyanophyceae)) from Lake Texcoco as "tecuitlatl" to consume with corn or tortillas; consumption of *S. platensis* harvested from Lake Kossorom, Chad known as "dihé"; consumption of *Nostoc commune* (Cyanophyceae) in China known as "fah-tsai" or "facai"; or consumption of *Spirogyra varians* (Charophyta Division, Zygnematophyceae Class) in Thailand known as "tao" or "water silk," "pond silk," or "mermaid's tree" (Tou et al. 2019; Garcia et al. 2017).

Over the past two decades in particular, there has been a steadily growing body of knowledge in the scientific literature and patent applications focused on not only the potential nutritional, bioactive, and thereby, functional food and nutraceutical, cosmeceutical, and pharmacognosic benefits of macro- and microalgae, but also the potential bioactivities of macro- and microalgal tissue extracts and extractable constituents *in vitro* (i.e. bench-top chemistry, cell culture),and *in vivo* from animal model studies, case control, and epidemiological studies in reducing chronic disease risk factors (Yoshinaga et al. 2018; Nishihira et al. 2017; Hitoe and Shimoda 2017; Yang et al. 2010; Ceccoli et al. 2008; Kim et al. 2008; de la Coba et al. 2006). Key areas of investigation continue to be chemical characterization of unique micro- and macroalgal specimens collected and isolated from terrestrial as well as freshwater, brackish, and marine environments due to the influence of oxidative stress on these algae from exposure to varying nutrient levels, temperatures, tides, and/or desiccation and UV irradiation. Oxidative stress experienced by these photosynthetic organisms can ultimately influence growth rates, metabolism, and synthesis of secondary metabolites, with many of the latter compounds of interest as potential nutraceuticals, cosmeceuticals, or pharmacognosics. While bench-top and *in vitro* cell culture studies are key to understanding the mechanisms of action of extracts and/or their constituent purified compounds, the *in vivo* bioaccessibility and ultimately bioavailability and metabolism of these molecules is key to determining their potential to influence and protect human health. A particularly intriguing avenue of investigation is evaluating the efficacy of UV-absorbing compounds from micro- and macroalgae as potential nutraceuticals, antioxidants, and sunscreen molecules in cosmeceuticals (Ceccoli et al. 2008; de la Coba et al. 2006; Schmid et al. 2006). In-depth reviews of not only the chemistry, isolation, and potential bioactivities of kelp fucoidans of industrial importance (Athukorala and Yuan 2013), but also red macroalgal MAAs as potential cosmeceuticals (Yuan and Athukorala 2012) have been published in recent years. The reader is also encouraged to refer to the in-depth discussions focused on, not only the bioactivities of macro- and microalgal carotenes and xanthophylls in Chapter 12, but also the advancements in macro- and microalgal constituents including sulfated polysaccharides and chlorophylls, etc. as functional foods and nutraceuticals in Chapter 18, as well as pharmaceuticals and cosmetics in Chapter 19. Thus, this chapter reviews the evidence underlying the biological activities of selected macro- and microalgal constituents and the proposed mechanisms of action in reducing diet-related chronic disease risk factors.

9.2 Antioxidant and Anticarcinogenic Activities of Macro- and Microalgal Constituents

Humans are constantly exposed to free radical species, whether through endogenous oxidative metabolic pathways or exogenous oxidative stressors such as infection, radiation, exposure to xenobiotics as well as diet-related chronic disease risk factors such as inflammation, obesity, types I and II diabetes mellitus, carcinogenesis, and cardiovascular diseases. Thus, similar to the endogenous antioxidant systems needed to combat oxidative stress experienced by macro- and microalgae, it is vital that humans maintain their antioxidant protection mechanisms whether antioxidant enzyme systems (e.g. glutathione [GSH] peroxidase, GSH reductase, catalase (CAT), superoxide dismutase (SOD), etc.), or biologically active antioxidant molecules (Yuan 2007). The basis of antioxidant activity is any molecule that can delay the onset (i.e. initiation) or interrupt the progression (i.e. propagation) of an oxidizable substrate (e.g. proteins, lipids, nucleic acids, etc.). Thus, antioxidant activity may involve hydrogen atom transfer (HAT) or single electron transfer (SET); these two mechanisms generally occur simultaneously and can be influenced by the structure and chemistry of the antioxidant molecule in question, as well as the polarity and pH of the assay system being studied.

As photosynthetic organisms subject to oxidative stress including desiccation and UV irradiation, macro- and microalgae require an extensive endogenous antioxidant capacity. Many of these antioxidant molecules are intracellular in nature (e.g. L-ascorbic acid, GSH, carotenes, xanthophylls, phenolic acids, MAAs, etc.), but can also be found in extracellular compartments such as the phlorotannins excreted by kelps into surrounding seawater, or the UV-absorbing pigments knowns as scytonemins present in the extracellular polysaccharide sheath (EPS) of certain Cyanobacteria (Pathak et al. 2019a,b; Athukorala et al. 2016; Rastogi et al. 2013; Yuan 2007). Antioxidative and UV-protective functions of micro- and macroalgal constituents and secondary metabolites can be inferred from studies with algae exposed to varying levels of photosynthetically active radiation (PAR, 400–700 nm), UVA (400–320 nm) and UVB (320–280 nm), wherein tissue levels of ascorbate, carotenoids, sytonemins, and MAAs were increased in algae exposed to greater UV radiation compared with specimens in the shade, or harvested from greater depths (Athukorala et al. 2016; Rastogi et al. 2013; Yuan et al. 2009; Sinha et al. 2007).

9.2.1 Mycosporine-like Amino Acids (MAAs)

MAAs are characterized by an aminocyclo-hexenone or -hexenimine core conjugated with the nitrogen moiety of an amino acid or alcohol (Sinha et al. 2007; Figure 9.1). These colorless, water-soluble, secondary metabolites are typically <400 Da in size, although glycosylated derivatives have been isolated with molecular masses of 508 and 612 Da (Nazifi et al. 2013). The conjugated double-bond structure within MAAs allows these molecules to exhibit absorption maxima from 310 to 362 nm. MAAs have been found to be most abundant in Rhodophyta species (e.g. *P. palmata*, *Chondrus crispus*, *Mastocarpus stellatus*, *Gracilaria* sp., *Gelidium* sp.), compared with Chlorophyta (e.g. *Caulerpa* sp., *Prasiola* sp., *Codium* sp.) and Pheophyta (e.g. *Desmarestia* sp., *Halopteris scoparia*, *Padina crassa*) macroalgal species (Athukorala et al. 2016; Sinha et al. 2007), and are also reported in numerous microalgal Cyanobacteria species (e.g. *Euhalothece* sp., *Microcoleus chthonoplastes*, *N. commune*, *Gloeocapsa* sp., *Scytonema* sp.; Nazifi et al. 2013; Sinha et al. 2007; Kedar et al. 2002; Karsten 2002). The most prevalent MAAs, namely mycosporine-glycine, asterina-330, shinorine, palythinol, porphyra-334, palythene, palythine, and usujirene, are depicted in Figure 9.1, in addition to two glycosylated derivatives. When the MAA profiles of two specimens of *P. palmata*, wild-harvested from locations varying in UV exposure (west vs. east coasts of Grand Manan Island, New Brunswick, Canada), were determined by liquid chromatography/mass spectrometry (LC/MS), both the low-UV and high-UV exposed samples contained palythine, shinorine, asterina-330, palythinol, and porphyra-334; however, usujirene was present only in the high-UV exposed specimen (Yuan et al. 2009). Interestingly, the antioxidant activity of aqueous methanolic extracts of the low-UV and high-UV *P. palmata*, as oxygen radical absorbance capacity (ORAC) assayed using the stable free radical 2,20-azo-bis(2-amidinopropane)dihydrochloride (AAPH) were 36.42 and 38.78 μmol Trolox (6-hydroxy 2,5,7,8-tetramethylchroman-2-carboxylic acid) g^{-1} extract, respectively; whereas the potential anticarcinogenic bioactivities of these extracts against B16-F1 murine skin melanoma cells were manifested by 68.5 and 91.9% inhibition of cell proliferation, respectively, at concentrations of 0.375–6.0 mg extract ml^{-1} culture medium. The greater antiproliferative activity of the high-UV *P. palmata* extract was ascribed to the presence of the least polar MAA, usujirene, which may have been passively absorbed through the murine skin melanoma cell membranes enhancing the antiproliferative effects of this extract (Yuan et al. 2009). The MAA profiles of low-UV and high-UV exposed wild-harvested and cultivated specimens of the carrageenophyte *C. crispus* (Irish moss) were confirmed by LC/MS/MS to comprise palythine, asterina-330, shinorine, palythinol, and porphyra-334 (Athukorala et al. 2016). Palythine, asterina-330, palythinol, and porphyra-334 were present in greater amounts in the aqueous methanolic extracts from high-UV exposed *C. crispus* versus the low-UV specimen. It was noteworthy that while the MAA profile of the cultivated *C. crispus* was similar to that of the wild-harvested specimens, the amounts

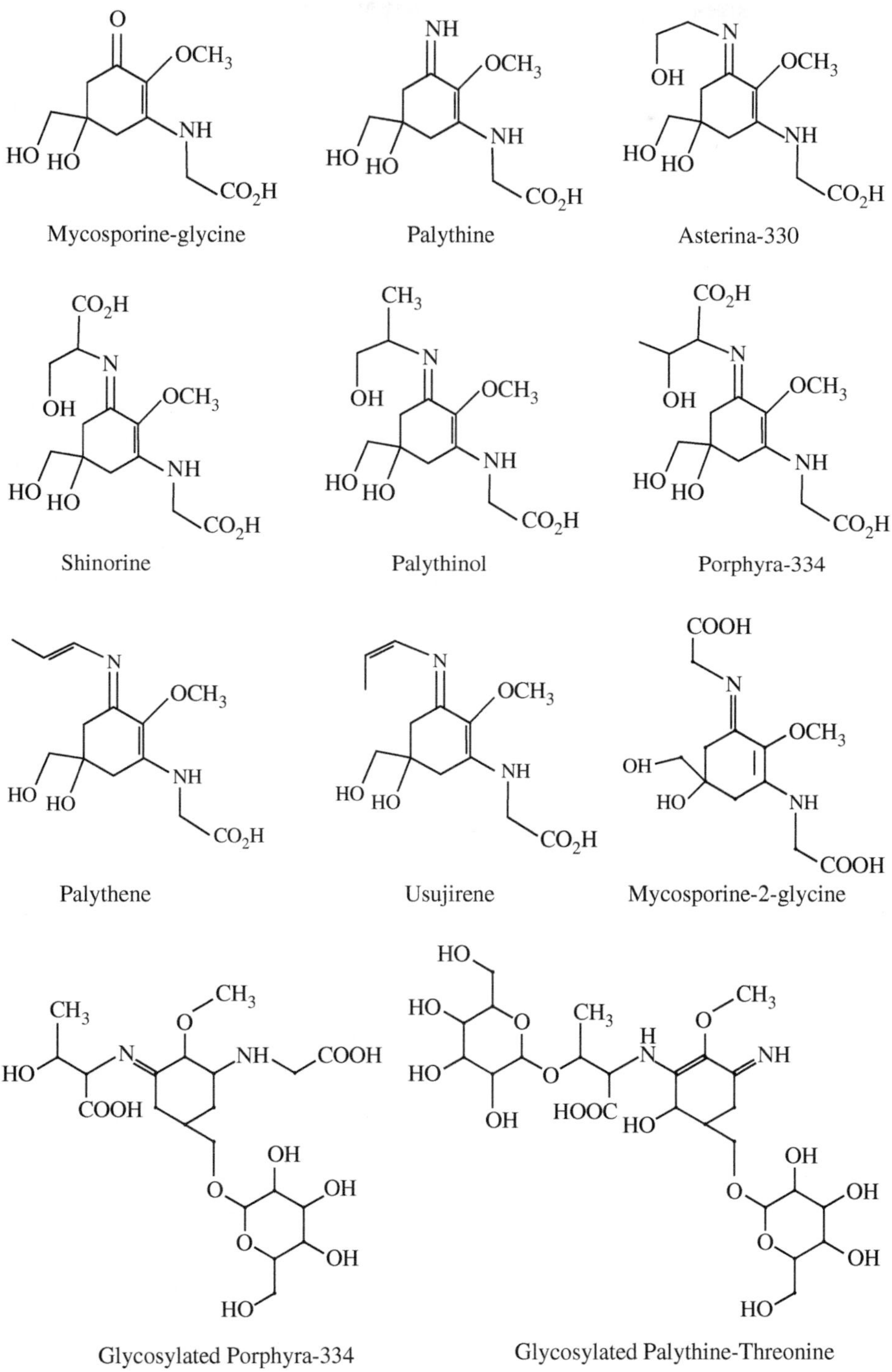

Figure 9.1 Mycosporine-like amino acids (MAAs) identified in macroalgal Rhodophyta and microalgal Cyanobacteria. Source: Athukorala et al. (2016); Nazifi et al. (2013); Yuan et al. (2009); Sinha et al. (2007); Kedar et al. (2002)

(as peak area counts) of specific MAAs were greatly enhanced: palythine ×3.2-fold, asterina-330 ×1.8-fold, and shinorine ×9.7-fold (Athukorala et al. 2016). When the antioxidant activities of these same extracts were evaluated using two different assays: reducing activity as a measure of SET and ORAC as a measure of HAT, the reducing activities for the low-UV, high-UV, and cultivated *C. crispus* extracts were 1.02, 0.79, and 2.06 mg ascorbic acid equivalents g^{-1} extract, respectively, whereas the ORAC activities were 21.6, 14.2, and 33.0 μmol Trolox equivalents g^{-1} extract, respectively. The relatively weak reducing activities of extracts from sundried, stored, and lyophilized macroalgae such as these was not surprising given that sundrying has been reported to markedly reduce labile antioxidant molecules including L-ascorbate. On the other hand, the enhanced HAT capacity of the cultivated *C. crispus* extract compared with the wild-harvested specimens may be associated with hydrogen ion abstraction from the cycloheximine ring of shinorine at C-4, C-6, or the methylene group at C-9 of the glycine residue with resonance stabilization from the carbon ring double-bond structure (Figure 9.1). It is also possible that palythine and asterina could exhibit HAT efficacy as has been reported for other extracts containing MAA mixtures (Athukorala et al. 2016). The potential anticarcinogenic bioactivities of the *C. crispus* extracts exhibited dose-dependent inhibition of cell proliferation between 0.125 and 4 mg ml^{-1} extract for both HeLa (adherent, cervical adenocarcinoma) and U-937 (suspended, histiocytic lymphoma) cell lines. The EC_{50} efficacies of the extracts were: low-UV = 0.457, high-UV = 1.06, and for cultivated *C. crispus* = 1.73 mg ml^{-1} for HeLa cells and high-UV = 0.772, low-UV = 0.344, and for cultivated *C. crispus* = 1.99 mg ml^{-1} for U-937 cells. HeLa cells incubated with the cultivated *C. crispus* extract exhibited morphological changes consistent with apoptosis (i.e. shrinkage and rounding) as well as increased caspase-3/7 activities and a greater proportion of cells in sub G_1 arrest (Athukorala et al. 2016). Caspase-3/7 activation is known to be responsible for cleavage of cell cycle regulators, which can induce cell cycle arrest, ultimately resulting in induction of apoptosis (i.e. programmed type I cell death).

The anticarcinogenic biological activities of MAAs have been associated with cell membrane permeation by low-polarity or lipophilic constituents as above, or with *Gracilaria cervicornis* extracts against HeLa cells with an EC_{50} of 0.075 mg ml^{-1} (Moo-puc et al. 2009). Other researchers have reported a dose-dependent, saturable, active transport of shinorine across human skin carcinoma A341 cell membranes leading to antiproliferative effects (Mason et al. 1998). It is noteworthy however, that the EC_{50} values outlined above represent low antiproliferative efficacies compared with the US National Cancer Institute standard of $EC_{50} \leq 30$ μg ml^{-1} extract for cancer cells; this is perhaps not unexpected given the variety of potential MAAs and other extracted constituents in the algal extracts studied (Athukorala et al. 2016; Moo-puc et al. 2009).

Taken together, the *in vitro* and cell cycle studies discussed above may provide insight into the results of a case control study with pre- and post-menopausal women in Korea, which revealed that average intake and frequency of Gim (*Porphyra* sp. [R]) consumption was inversely associated with breast cancer risk (Yang et al. 2010). Notably, this study found no such associations with Miyeok (*U. pinnatifida* [B]) consumption and breast cancer disease risk. Indeed, one of the first functional food applications for edible macroalgae dates back to the Ebers papyrus of approx. 1534 BCE Egypt, for use in the treatment or prevention of breast cancer. Moreover, epidemiological data support hypotheses of reduced diet-related chronic disease risks including breast cancer and colorectal risk in East and Southeast Asian populations known to consume macroalgae regularly in the diet compared with North American and Western European cultures (Athukorala et al. 2016).

The UV-protective function of macro- and microalgal MAAs is clear from their absorption maxima from 310 to 362 nm, which overlaps with UVB irradiation. It is noteworthy that a cyanobacterial ancestor or a cyanobacterium is regarded as the source of the enzymes needed to synthesize MAAs via the Shikimic acid pathway (Pathak et al. 2019a). MAAs are biosynthesized via 3-dehydroquinic acid and 4-deoxygadusol (4-DG). 4-DG occurs as resonance tautomers in equilibrium, followed by conjugation with an amino acid such as glycine to form the oxocarbonyl MAA mycosporine-glycine (Figure 9.1). Mycosporine-glycine can then be converted to an imino-MAA such as shinorine or porphyra-334 (Yuan 2007). Interestingly, tyrosine, which is a feedback inhibitor of the Shikimic acid pathway, could inhibit MAA biosynthesis in *Chlorogloeopsis* sp. (Pathak et al. 2019a). The antioxidant capacity of MAAs can be inferred from the strong antioxidant activity of 4-DG. When UVB-resistant Chlorophyta *Enallax coelastroides*, *Scenedesmus* sp., and *Scotiella chlorelloidea*, and UVB-sensitive Chlorophyta *Ankistrodesmus spiralis*, *Chlorella minutissima*, *Chlorella sorokiniana*, and *Pseudococcomyxa* sp. cultures were exposed to PAR and UVB irradiation for 90 minutes, asterina-330, shinorine, palythine, porphyra-334, and mycosporine-glycine were isolated and identified in a species-dependent manner (Xiong et al. 1999). These authors also identified two novel unidentified compounds, one with an absorbance maxima of 302 nm (in *C. sorokiniana* and *Scenedesmus* sp.) and the other at 292 nm (in *Scenedesmus* sp.). MAA accumulation was induced by both artificial and solar UVB irradiation in both the UVB-resistant and -sensitive species (Xiong et al. 1999). Mycosporine-2-glycine (Figure 9.1) was isolated and identified for the first time in a cyanobacterium *Euhalothece* sp. specimen harvested from a gypsum crust in a hypersaline saltern pond in Eilat, Israel (Kedar et al. 2002). While mycosporine-2-glycine was the major MAA, another with an absorbance maxima at 362 nm and mass of 330 Da was also reported. This cyanobacterium is noted for inhabiting the upper layer of a gypsum crust on the bottom of a hypersaline saltern pond under high light intensities of full daylight (Kedar et al. 2002).

Nazifi et al. (2013) identified two unique glycosylated MAAs from the terrestrial cyanobacterium *N. commune*. This cyanobacterium is noted to occur as colonies that experience not only frequent anhydrobiosis, i.e. cycles of desiccation and wetting from rain, but also direct solar/UV radiation; thus, this species has adapted several adaptation strategies against these environmental and oxidative stressors, including EPS and UV-absorbing molecules. In wild-harvested *N. commune* colonies from Ishikawa, Japan, aqueous extracts were reported to contain three novel MAAs: a glycosylated porphyra-334 with a hexose moiety (λ_{max} 334 nm, 508 Da), a glycosylated palythine-threonine with two hexose moieties (λ_{max} 322 nm, 612 Da; Figure 9.1), and another glycosylated palythine-threonine with a single hexose moiety (λ_{max} 322 nm, 450 Da). The 612-Da MAA accounted for approx. 60% of MAAs (Nazifi et al. 2013). The HAT antioxidant activities of the purified MAAs from 2,2′-azino-bis(3-ethyl-benzthiazoline-6-sulfonic acid) cation free radical ($ABTS^+$) studies revealed IC_{50} values of 58 mM for 508-Da MAA and 16 mM for the 612-Da MAA, compared with IC_{50} values of 0.28 and 0.25 mM for ascorbic acid and Trolox, respectively. From time course evaluations from 10 minutes to 2 hours, these MAAs were identified as slow-acting free radical quenchers compared with the fast-acting control antioxidants (Nazifi et al. 2013). Interestingly, when chromatography of the *N.*

commune water extracts was performed, MAA fractions accounted for only 45% of total antioxidant activity (including 20% attributed to the 612-Da MAA), which is not surprising given the potential presence of other aqueous small molecule antioxidants such as ascorbic acid, GSH, etc. These authors hypothesized the glycosylation of porphyra-334 and palythine-threonine MAAs to be a unique adaptation of this terrestrial cyanobacterium subjected to frequent anhydrobiosis.

Karsten (2002) reported the MAA profiles of benthic, filamentous cyanobacterium *M. chthonoplastes* specimens collected from intertidal marine sediment of the Ebre Delta, the Mediterranean Sea, Spain (EBD); an intertidal marine, mangrove flat at Towra Point in Sydney, Australia (TOW) and brackish sediment from Poel Island, Baltic Sea, Germany (WIS). All specimens contained shinorine at 4.88, 0.69, and 1.84 mg g^{-1} fresh weight, respectively; the latter specimen was the only one to contain an unknown MAA with λ_{max} 346 nm at 0.68 mg g^{-1} fresh weight; the former two specimens contained another unknown MAA with λ_{max} 332 nm at 3.31 and 8.66 mg g^{-1} fresh weight, respectively. MAA biosynthesis by *M. chthonoplastes* was influenced by increased salinity from 5 to 60 PSU (practical salinity units) in that EBD exhibited unchanged MAA-332, but decreased shinorine; TOW exhibited increased total MAAs due to increased MAA-332 by 3× with constant small amounts of shinorine; and WIS exhibited increased total MAAs comprising increased shinorine by 34× and MAA-346 by 4×. MAA biosynthesis by *M. chthonoplastes* was also influenced by UVB irradiation (280–320 nm with a 18:6 light:dark ratio) in that EBD exhibited an approx. 3× increase in shinorine and MAA-332 at 32 PSU; TOW exhibited a 14× increase in shinorine and 3× increase in MAA-332 at 32 PSU; whereas WIS did not survive the UVB irradiation treatments (Karsten 2002). Thus, taken together, these lines of evidence, as discussed above, indicate that MAAs function as UV protectants as well as osmolytes.

Further industrial exploitation of the antioxidant activities and UV protection by MAAs in sunscreens is evidenced by the issuance of multiple patents as early as 1987, "Sunscreen compositions and compounds for use therein" by Bird et al. (1987), and more recently focusing on individual MAAs, namely shinorine (de la Coba et al. 2006) and porphyra-334 (Aguilera et al. 2006) as antioxidants. Extracts from red macroalgae such as *C. crispus* were part of the formulation contained in an international patent application for anti-aging skin cream use (Ceccoli et al. 2008).

9.2.2 Scytonemins

Cyanobacteria are known to synthesize other UV-absorbing molecules in addition to MAAs, namely scytonemins and pterins (Pathak et al. 2019a,b; Hanaya and Yamamoto 2013; Rastogi et al. 2013; Bultel-Poncé et al. 2004; Karsten 2002; Matsunaga et al. 1993). Scytonemin is characterized as a dimer of indolic and phenolic subunits linked through an olefinic carbon atom (Figure 9.2), and is a highly stable, yellow-brown, lipid-soluble pigment located in the EPS of several cyanobacterial species, including *Rivularia* sp. (Rastogi et al. 2013), *Scytonema* sp. (Bultel-Poncé et al. 2004), *N. commune*, *Nostoc punctiforme*, *Anabaena* sp., *Lyngbya* sp., *Chlorogleopsis* sp., and *Nodularia* sp. (Pathak et al. 2019a). *In vivo* scytonemin has been reported to have a λ_{max} of 370 nm, and when purified, a λ_{max} of 386 nm, with absorbances recorded at 252, 278, and 300 nm, which suggests photoprotection against both UVA and UVB wavelengths (Pathak et al. 2019b). Moreover, scytonemin exists in both reduced and

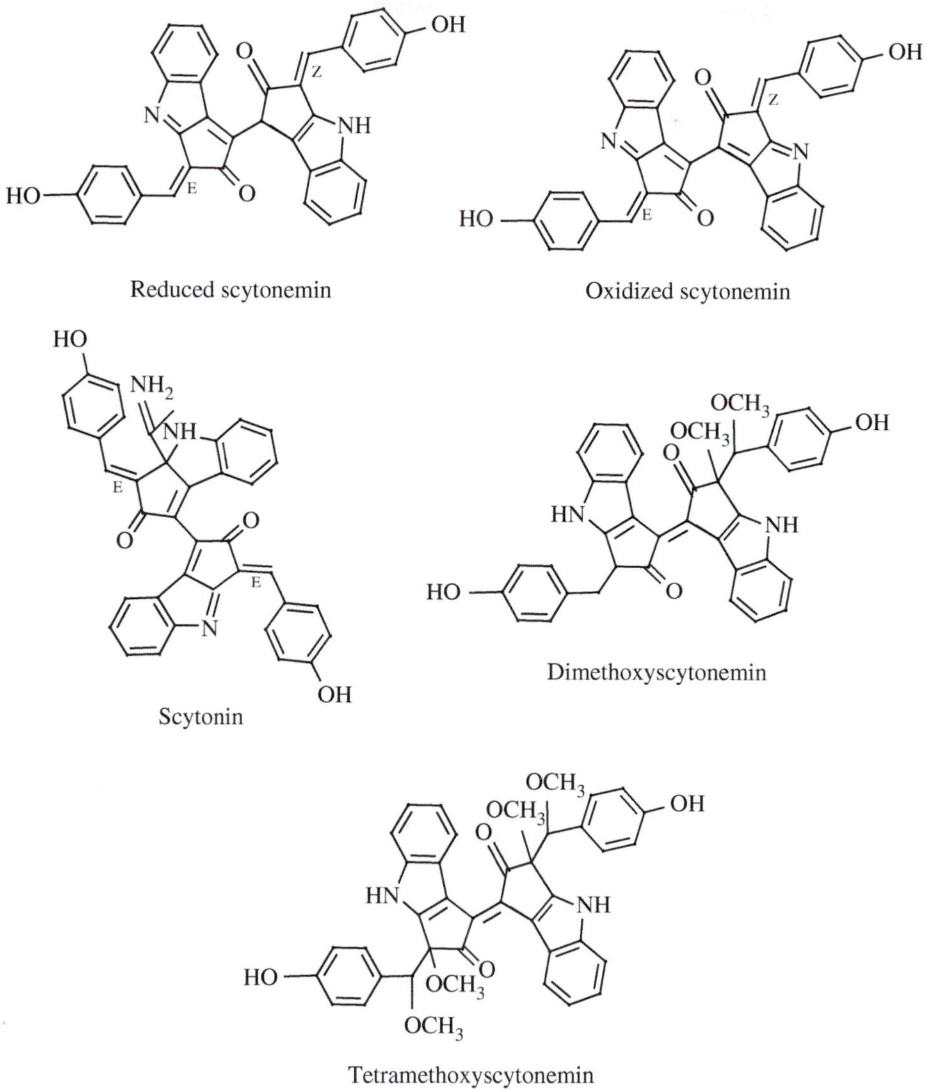

Figure 9.2 Scytonemins identified in microalgal Cyanobacteria. Source: Pathak et al. (2019a,b); Rastogi et al. (2013); Bultel-Poncé et al. (2004).

oxidized states with molecular masses of 546 and 544 Da, respectively (Figure 9.2). Tyrosine and tryptophan derivatives were identified as precursors in scytonemin biosynthesis, potentially involving the acyloin reaction as a key step (Pathak et al. 2019b).

When the cyanobacterium *Scytonema* sp. (a terrestrial, filamentous, sheathed species), isolated from a fresh water pond in Anand, Gujarat, India, was exposed to PAR, PAR + UVA and PAR + UVA + UVB irradiation, synthesis of both forms of scytonemin was upregulated in cultures, particularly when PAR was combined with UVA and the combination of UVA + UVB (Rastogi et al. 2014). Interestingly, heat stress on cultures exposed to PAR + UVA + UVB irradiation revealed increased total scytonemin biosynthesis at 35 °C. A protective effect of scytonemin against UV irradiation induced oxidative stress and reactive oxygen species (ROS) induced thymine-dimer (cyclobutane pyrimidine dimer, CPD) formation was observed as significant decreases in both intracellular ROS and CPD in *Scytonema* sp. cells. Thus, scytonemin was reported to exhibit an antioxidant capacity of 20.8%, compared with ascorbic acid alone at 45.8%, and a combination of scytonemin + ascorbic acid at 58.7% (Rastogi et al. 2014). When Bultel-Poncé et al. (2004) analyzed the scytonemin profile of *Scytonema* sp. isolated in the dry state from the Mitaraka Inselberg (isolated hills arising from surrounding plains), French Guyana, characterized by exposed granite under intense solar radiation, they reported three unique pigments: tetramethoxyscytonemin ($C_{40}H_{34}N_2O_8$; 671.24 Da), which was purple; dimethoxyscytonemin ($C_{38}H_{28}N_2O_6$; 609.20 Da), which was dark red in color; and scytonin ($C_{31}H_{22}N_2O_6$; 519.16 Da), which was brown in color (Figure 9.2). These scytonemin derivatives arise from the condensation of tryptophanyl- and tyrosinyl-subunits with a unique linkage between subunits (Bultel-Poncé et al. 2004). These three scytonemin derivatives were determined to be non-cytotoxic against KB cells at concentrations up to 0.01 mM. Matsui et al. (2012) isolated scytonemin from the terrestrial cyanobacterium *N. commune* wild-harvested from a field on the Kakuma campus of Kanazawa University, Japan, and reported that the EPS sheath pigment represented approx. 0.04% of the dry weight of *N. commune* colonies. Purified scytonemin exhibited HAT antioxidant radical scavenging activity against $ABTS^+$ with an IC_{50} of 567 μM compared with an IC_{50} of 300 μM for the control Trolox; scytonemin was determined to be a slow-acting radical scavenger acting over a 2-hour incubation period (Matsui et al. 2012). When an ethanol extract of the *N. commune* colonies was chromatographed, the scytonemin fraction accounted for 10% of $ABTS^+$ radical quenching, with the remaining antioxidant activity attributed to chlorophyll and carotenoids. Thus, the scytonemin pigment functions both as a UV radiation protectant and antioxidant molecule in this cyanobacterium, which is subject to anhydrobiosis in its natural habitat. The UV protection and antioxidant activities of these unique molecules is supported by the extensive conjugated double-bond structures of scytonemin and its derivatives as illustrated in Figure 9.2. Moreover, scytonemin has been reported to exhibit efficacy in inhibiting cell cycle kinases, namely a serine/threonine kinase, which has a role in the regulation of the G2/M transition in the cell cycle (Stevenson et al. 2002). Scytonemin inhibited growth-factor-induced cell proliferation of rheumatoid synovial fibroblasts, endothelial cell growth factor-induced human umbilical vein endothelial cells, and fetal bovine serum-stimulated normal human lung fibroblasts over a dose range of 100 nM to 30 μM. Moreover, scytonemin was efficacious in inducing apoptosis in Jurkat T cells (a T cell lymphoma cell line) between 1 and 30 μM (Stevenson et al. 2002).

9.2.3 Pterins

Pterins (2-aminopteridin-4(3*H*)-one) derivatives are synthesized from guanosine triphosphate (Hanaya and Yamamoto 2013). Biopterin (Figure 9.3, where R = H) and its glycosides have been isolated from various Cyanobacteria including biopterin, where R = α-D-glucopyranosyl was identified in *Anacystis nidulans*, *Oscillatoria* sp., *S. platensis* (*A. platensis*), *Synechococcus* sp.; or where R = β-D-ribofuranosyl

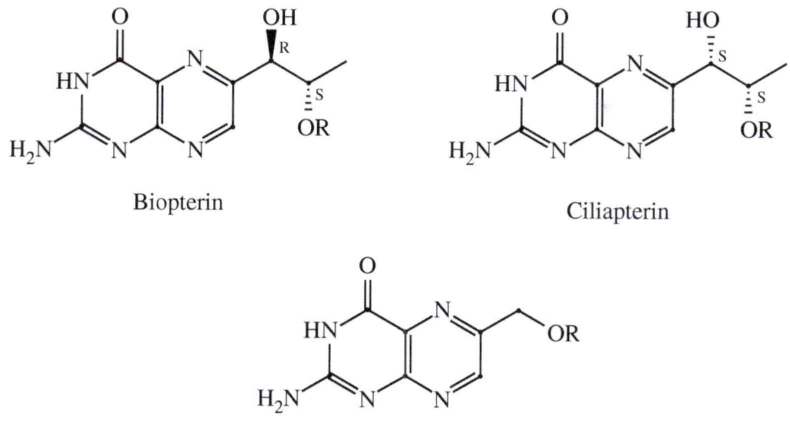

Figure 9.3 Biopterin and related pterin glycosides identified in microalgal Cyanobacteria. Source: Hanaya and Yamamoto (2013); Matsunaga et al. (1993).

was identified in *S. platensis* (*A. platensis*; Matsunaga et al. 1993; Hanaya and Yamamoto 2013). Ciliapterin (Figure 9.3, where R = H) and its glycosides (where R = D-glucopyranosyl, or D-mannopyranosyl, or D-xylopyranosyl) were identified in the cyanobacterium *Alphanizomenon flos-aquae*. 6-Hydroxymethylpterin glycosides (Figure 9.3, where R = D-glucopyranosyl, or 4-O-methyl-α-D-glucopyranosyl-uronic acid-(1→6)-β-D-galactopyranosyl) were identified in the cyanobacterium *Synechocysts* sp. (Hanaya and Yamamoto, 2013). It is noteworthy that biopterin has been identified in human urine as well as Cyanobacteria. While pterin glycosides have been reported to help photostabilize phycocyanin, their physiological function has not been clarified (Hanaya and Yamamoto 2013). On the other hand, Matsunaga et al. (1993) reported increased intracellular biopterin glycoside levels in the planktonic cyanobacterium *Oscillatoria* sp. exposed to UVA irradiation (320–390 nm). A UV-protective role and thereby antioxidant capacity for biopterins can be inferred from the conjugated double-bond structure of these unique biomolecules, as well as the biopterin glucoside λ_{max} of 362 nm (Figure 9.3; Pathak et al. 2019b).

9.2.4 Carotenes and Xanthophylls

While chlorophylls are the major photosynthetic pigments in macro- and microalgae, carotenoids (i.e. carotenes and xanthophylls) are also considered to be secondary photosynthetic pigments. Carotenes (e.g. α- and β-carotene) and their oxygenated derivatives, xanthophylls (e.g. astaxanthin, fucoxanthin, siphonaxanthin, siphonein; Figure 9.4) are key players in the photosynthetic apparatus and contribute to not only light-harvesting, but also the photoprotective and antioxidant capacity of algae. When Ranga Rao et al. (2015) determined the ketocarotenoid astaxanthin (3,3′-dihydroxy-β,β’- carotene-4,4′-dione; ASX, Figure 9.4) and astaxanthin ester (ASXE) content of the freshwater, eukaryotic microalga *Haematococcus pluvialis*

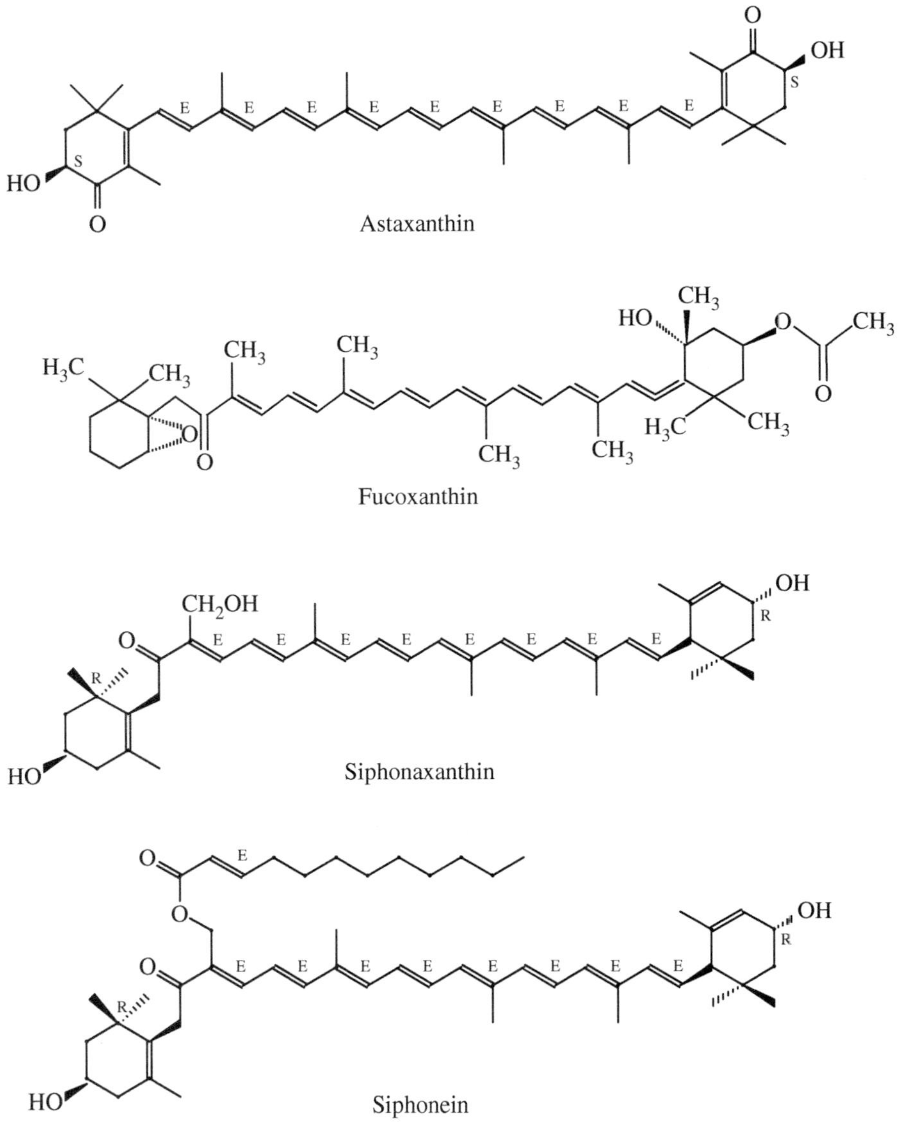

Figure 9.4 Xanthophylls identified in macro- and microalgae. Source: Ranga Rao et al. (2015, 2010); Goiris et al. (2012); Ganesan et al. (2011).

(Chlorophyta division, Chlorophyceae class), the biomass contained approx. 2.35% total carotenoids, comprising 2% free ASX and 78% ASXE of total carotenoids on a dry weight basis. The ASXE composition of *H. pluvialis* is typically composed of 70% mono- and 15–20% di-esters of fatty acids including C16:0, C17 and its −1, −2 unsaturated counterparts, and C18 and its −1, −2, −3, −4 unsaturated counterparts (Ranga Rao et al. 2015). When Wistar rats (200–220 g body wt.) were treated with the liver carcinogen carbon tetrachloride ($2\,g\,kg^{-1}$ body wt.) and fed ASX and ASXEs at 100 and $250\,\mu g\,kg^{-1}$ body wt. for 2 weeks, ASX and ASXE treatment prevented increased serum levels of serum glutamate pyruvate transaminase, serum glutamate oxaloacetate transaminase, and alkaline phosphatases as biomarkers of CCl_4-induced liver damage. Liver antioxidant enzymes (i.e. catalase, GSH peroxidase, SOD) and GSH, which were decreased by 30–50% in CCl_4-treated controls, were restored by ASX or even elevated by ASXE treatments. Thus, ASX and ASXE were hepatoprotective and exerted antioxidant protection against a known liver carcinogen (Ranga Rao et al. 2015).

When Goiris et al. (2012) evaluated the carotenoid contents and antioxidant activities of 32 commercially sourced microalgae, carotenoid contents of aqueous ethanol extracts varied considerably even within the same species: *Chaetoceros calcitrans* = 2.33; *Chlorella vulgaris* = 0.25–3.04; *Isochrysis* sp. = 3.08–7.75; *Nannochloropsis* sp. = 1.65–2.17; *Phaeodactylum tricornutum* = 2.26–6.14; *Tetraselmis* sp. = 2.88–4.27 mg g^{-1} dry weight. The antioxidant activities as HAT ($ABTS^+$ radical quenching) and SET (ferric reducing potential) capacities were similarly variable: *C. calcitrans* = 24.2 μmol Trolox equivalents g^{-1} dry weight versus 4.7 μmol Trolox equivalents g^{-1} dry weight; *C. vulgaris* = 5.4–59.6 μmol Trolox equivalents g^{-1} dry weight versus 30.6–6.4 μmol Trolox equivalents g^{-1} dry weight; *Isochrysis* sp. = 34.9–22.5 μmol Trolox equivalents g^{-1} dry weight versus 46.7–53.7 μmol Trolox equivalents g^{-1} dry weight; *Nannochloropsis* sp. = 20.2–25.8 μmol Trolox equivalents g^{-1} dry weight versus 40.7–40.8 μmol Trolox equivalents g^{-1} dry weight; *P. tricornutum* = 4.6–48.9 μmol Trolox equivalents g^{-1} dry weight versus 34.9–89.7 μmol Trolox equivalents g^{-1} dry weight; *Tetraselmis* sp. = 69.4–56.5 μmol Trolox equivalents g^{-1} dry weight versus 46.6–11.4 μmol Trolox equivalents g^{-1} dry weight, respectively (Goiris et al. 2012). The variability in the HAT versus SET antioxidant activities of the microalgal aqueous ethanolic extracts could be attributed to the mixture of extracted compounds comprising the hydrophobic carotenes and xanthophylls as well as phenolics. Taken together, *Tetraselmis suecica*, *Nannochloropsis oleoabundans*, *Isochrysis* sp., *C. vulgaris*, and *P. tricornutum* exhibited the greatest antioxidant activities as sources of natural antioxidants of interest to the food and nutraceutical industries. It is noteworthy that an ethanol extract of *C. calcitrans*, which is native to Malaysia, was efficacious in inhibiting the proliferation of two human breast cancer cell lines, the IC_{50} of the extract was 3.0 and 12.0 μg ml^{-1} for MCF-7 and MCF-10A cells after 24 hours and 2.7 and 3.3 μg ml^{-1}, respectively, after 72 hours (Ebrahimi Nigjeh et al. 2013). Moreover, the *C. calcitrans* extract was reported to induce apoptosis in MCF-7 cells as evidenced by rounding and shrunken cells detached from a monolayer, with membrane blebbing and formation of apoptotic bodies. Cell cycle analyses revealed that the $subG_1$ population of MCF-7 cells increased from 0.4% in untreated control cells to 2.3% after incubation with 3 μg ml^{-1} *C. calcitrans* extract for 24 hours, increasing to 55.8 and 72.8% at 48 and 72 hours, respectively. It is noteworthy that the *C. calcitrans* extract induced apoptosis through activation of caspase-7 (Ebrahimi Nigjeh et al. 2013).

Apoptosis of human leukemia HL-60 cells was also induced when cells were incubated with purified xanthophylls including ASX and fucoxanthin ($C_{42}H_{58}O_6$, λ_{max} = 447 nm, 658.91 Da) extracted from a macroalgal kelp *U. pinnatifida*, and siphonaxanthin ($C_{40}H_{56}O_4$, λ_{max} = 449 nm, 600.9 Da) and siphonein extracted from the Chlorophyta *Codium fragile* (Figure 9.4; Ganesan et al. 2011). Xanthophylls reduced HL-60 cell viability in a dose-dependent manner at 5, 10, and 20 μM: siphonaxanthin was the most inhibitory, followed by fucoxanthin < ASX < siphonein, which is the esterified form of siphonaxanthin (Figure 9.4). Siphonaxanthin was inhibitory to HL-60 cells as early as 6 hours at 20 μM, reaching 95% inhibition at 24 hours; whereas fucoxanthin was not inhibitory until 12 hours at 10 and 20 μM, reaching 60.5% inhibition at 24 hours with 20 μM. Siphonaxanthin and fucoxanthin were observed to induce apoptosis via activation of caspase-3 in HL-60 cells. Thus, these xanthophylls could potentially have applications as nutraceuticals, or as chemopreventative and/or chemotherapeutic agents.

9.3 Antiobesogenic Biological Activities of Macroalgal Constituents

The potential efficacy and utility of xanthophylls in chronic disease risk factor reduction is strengthened by evidence of cellular uptake of siphonaxanthin and fucoxanthin by HL-60 cells incubated with 10 μM xanthophylls for 2 and 6 hours (Ganesan et al. 2011). In a double-blind placebo-controlled clinical trial with mildly obese male and female Japanese subjects (defined as a BMI > 25, but <30 kg m^{-2}; abdominal circumference of at least 85 cm for males and 90 cm for females) aged 20– 59 years of age, fucoxanthin treatment resulted in decreased relative body weight and BMI as well as decreased relative visceral fat area with 3 mg day^{-1} fucoxanthin, although body fat ratio, fat mass, lean mass, muscle mass, and basal metabolic rate were not changed (Hitoe and Shimoda 2017). On the other hand, treatment with 1 mg day^{-1} fucoxanthin did result in decreased absolute and relative total fat areas and relative subcutaneous fat area compared with before treatment. Interestingly, the 3 mg day^{-1} fucoxanthin treatment resulted in significantly reduced diastolic (114 versus 127 mmHg) and systolic blood pressures (66 versus 80 mmHg) compared with the placebo, respectively, albeit both values remained within the normal range. The 3 mg day^{-1} fucoxanthin treatment significantly reduced low-density lipoprotein (LDL)-cholesterol levels compared with the untreated placebo group (Hitoe and Shimoda 2017). Fucoxanthin has been previously reported to reduce lipid accumulation in obese KKAy mice fed on 0.4% fucoxanthin diets. This xanthophyll has been reported to exert antiobesogenic effects through suppression of lipid absorption, increased β-oxidation and increased expression of lipid-metabolizing enzymes (Hitoe and Shimoda 2017).

All-*trans*-fucoxanthin, an orange-colored carotenoid, has been reported to be a major xanthophyll carotenoid in *H. fusiformis* (B) along with two *cis*-isomers (Yan et al. 1999). The structure of fucoxanthin differs from other carotenoids in that there is a double allenic carbon at C-7′ near one of the two hydroxyl groups in its structure, which may confer additional stability and resonance stabilization within the conjugated double-bond structure of this molecule (Figure 9.4). Thus, it is noteworthy that fucoxanthin exhibited strong HAT antioxidant activity against the 1,1-diphenyl-2-picrylhydrazyl (DPPH•) stable free radical as a free radical scavenger *in vitro* (Yan et al. 1999).

9.4 Antidiabetic Biological Activities of Macroalgal Constituents

The polysaccharide fractions of macroalgae include the laminarins, alginates, and fucans of the Phaeophyceae as well as agaran, agaropectin, κ-, λ-, and ι-carrageenans from the Rhodophyceae. The laminarins represent low molecular

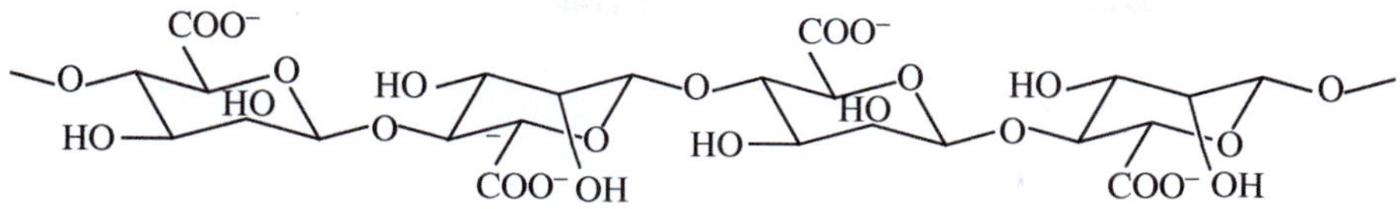

poly (D-mannuronic acid) segment of alginate

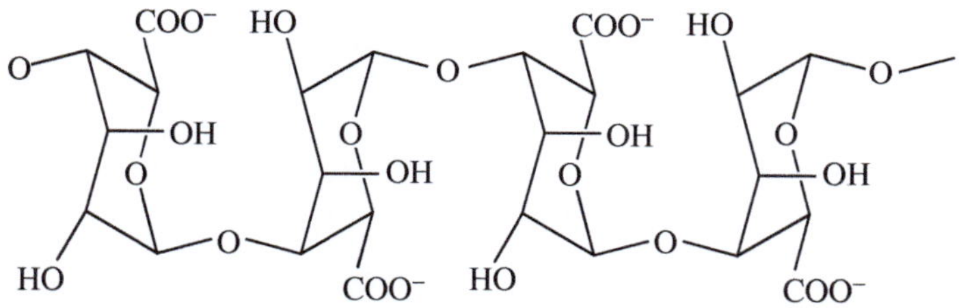

poly (L-guluronic acid) segment of alginate

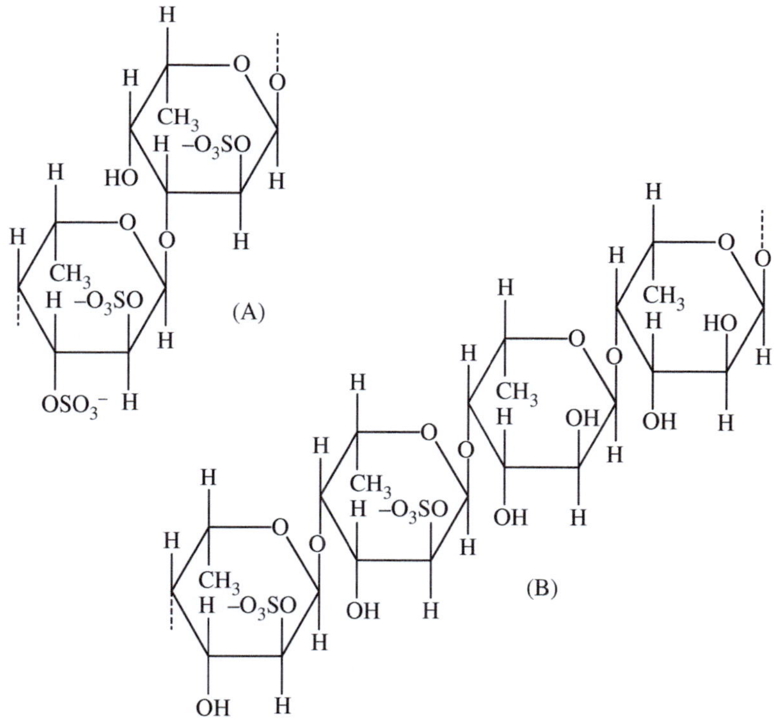

Fucoidan and sulphated fucan

Figure 9.5 Alginates, fucoidans, and sulfated fucans from Phaeophyceae macroalgae. Source: Athukorala and Yuan (2013); Yuan et al. (2009).

weight storage β-glucans as a polysaccharide store, i.e. (1,3)-β-D-glucans comprising (1,3)-β-D-glucopyranosyl residues with C6-O-branching in the main chain and some β-(1,6)-intrachain links of Phaeophyceae. Alginates, which comprise the major polyuronide matrix component of *Phaeophyceae* sp., consist of alternating sequences of β-(1,4)-D-mannuronic acid and α-(1,4)-L-guluronic acid with 20–30 uronic acid residues (Figure 9.5; Athukorala and Yuan 2013). Fucans comprise the fucoidans, xylofucoglycouronans, and glycouronogalactofucans. Fucoidans contain (1,2)-α-L-fucose-4-sulfate with branching or sulfate esters on C3 with small amounts of D-xylose, galactose, mannose, and uronic acids (Figure 9.5); xylofucoglycouronans (also referred to as Ascophyllans) contain a backbone of poly-β-(1,4)-D-mannuronic acid with branches of 3-O-D-xylosyl-L-fucose-4-sulfate or uronic acid; whereas glycouronogalactofucans comprise linear chains of (1,4)-D-galactose with branching at C5 with L-fucosyl-3-sulfate or uronic acid (Yuan 2008). Fucoidans are bound to alginates and are therefore a cheap by-product from alginate isolation as a potential functional food and nutraceutical ingredient.

In a randomized, placebo-controlled clinical trial with type II diabetes mellitus patients (9 males, 11 females; 40–70 years of age; BMI < 35 $kg\,m^{-2}$; fasting glucose >150 $mg\,dl^{-1}$ [150–300 $mg\,dl^{-1}$]), treatment with 48 $g\,d^{-1}$ equal parts of *L. japonica* (sea tangle) and *U. pinnatifida* (sea mustard) kelps for 4 weeks resulted in significantly reduced fasting blood glucose (152 $mg\,dl^{-1}$), as well postprandial blood glucose (203 $mg\,dl^{-1}$) levels (Kim et al. 2008). Although there was no change in plasma total cholesterol, levels of triacylglycerols and LDL-cholesterol were decreased by kelp treatment, while high-density lipoprotein (HDL)-cholesterol levels were increased. Kelp treatment of patients also decreased red blood cell lipid peroxidation products as thiobarbituric acid reactive substances, while red blood cell CAT and GSH peroxidase antioxidant enzyme activities were greatly increased, albeit SOD activity was not different (Kim et al. 2008). Thus, kelp derived polysaccharides were observed to increase the dietary fiber intake of the treatment group by 2.5× compared with the placebo group. Moreover, kelp supplementation of the diet had a positive effect on glycemic control in type II diabetes mellitus patients and was also efficacious in decreasing plasma lipids and incidents of oxidative stress, and thereby, may decrease diet-related chronic disease risk of cardiovascular disease.

9.5 Prebiotic Biological Activities of Macroalgal Constituents

Further evidence of biological activities of kelp constituents as functional foods was demonstrated when Yoshinaga et al. (2018) reported the intestinal effects of a 2-week dietary supplementation with 4 g *U. pinnatifida* in 22 healthy Japanese females aged 20–49 years. Kelp supplementation increased total dietary fiber as expected; also increased were intestinal indices including defecation frequency from 4.6 to 5.6 times $week^{-1}$, defecation days from 4 to 5 d/$week^{-1}$; as well as stool volume from 9 to 13 pieces $week^{-1}$. Moreover, terminal restriction fragment length polymorphism analyses revealed that the fraction of bifidobacteria (i.e. *Bifidobacterium longum*) in fecal bacteria increased with kelp intake; in addition, the relative abundance of Actinobacteria was increased, while that of Bacteroides was decreased in feces (Yoshinaga et al. 2018). Thus, dietary kelp supplementation exhibited efficacy as a source of prebiotics, given that fucoidans can interact with the gut microbiome.

9.6 Immune System Biological Activities of Macroalgal Constituents

In a double-blind, placebo-controlled clinical trial with healthy Japanese men and women (10 males, 48 females) aged 35–65 years, BMI approx. 20 kg m^{-2} for both sexes, dietary supplementation with 0.8 g kelp day^{-1} *Kjellmaniella crassifolia* (Gagome) powder containing 200 mg dietary fiber, composed of 80 mg fucoidan, for 2 months, increased natural killer (NK) cell activities slightly from 18.8% in the placebo group to 19.4% with kelp supplementation (Nishihira et al. 2017). While serum IgM concentrations were not affected by kelp supplementation, IgA concentrations were increased at 8 weeks' treatment. As well, when evaluating Th-1-type cytokine levels, while interleukin (IL)-12 was not different, there was a slight increase in interferon (IFN)-γ that did not reach significance at 4 weeks' treatment. Serum IgM levels have been noted as a biomarker of early-phase immunoglobulin profiles, whereas IgA levels have been regarded as biomarkers of gut immunity (Nishihira et al. 2017). Compared with Yoshinaga et al. (2018) above, who used 4 g *U. pinnatifida* supplementation, these subjects given a lower dose of kelp did not exhibit any changes to serum total cholesterol, LDL- or HDL-cholesterol, triacylglycerols, glucose levels, or defecation frequency and volumes, which is not unexpected. This lower dosage of *K. crassifolia* was also chosen to minimize any potential iodine toxicity (Nishihira et al. 2017). Thus, a relatively modest diet supplementation with *K. crassifolia* was efficacious in enhancing/activating the immune system via effects on NK cell activities, and IgA and IFN-γ enhancement. Moreover, taken together, the kelp supplementation studies discussed above provide evidence to support the historic traditional consumption of *K. crassifolia* harvested in Northern Japan.

9.7 Conclusion and Future Work

It is clear that edible Rhodophyceae, Chlorophyceae, and Phaeophyceae species of macroalgae and Cyanobacteria of microalgae may exert a variety of biological activities to reduce the risk of diet-related chronic diseases including cancers, cardiovascular diseases, diabetes mellitus, and activate the immune system. Thus, macro- and microalgae and their constituents can a play a role as functional foods and nutraceuticals, or even cosmeceuticals and pharmacognosics. While there is a need for further *in vitro* and mechanistic studies, particularly with purified compounds, the efficacy of macro- and microalgal biological activities needs to be substantiated with *in vivo* studies and ultimately with clinical trials to elucidate the mechanisms of observed beneficial effects. Moreover, because micro- and macroalgae are photosynthetically active organisms and algal composition is known to vary seasonally and with harvest location, this information needs to be recorded and reported in the literature for wild-harvested specimens, or the relevant culture conditions defined for cultivated specimens to allow for easier comparison between studies.

Acknowledgments

The work of the author was supported by funding from the Faculty of Community Services of Ryerson University.

References

Aguilera, J., de la Coba, F., and López Figueroa, F. (2006). Use of micosporine type amino acid (porphyra-334) as an antioxidant. Spanish Patent No. ES2301293B1.

Athukorala, Y. and Yuan, Y.V. (2013). Fucoidans from marine brown macroalgae: isolation, identification and potential biological activities. Chapter 24. In: *Marine Nutraceuticals: Prospects and Perspectives* (ed. S.-K. Kim), 393–435. Boca Raton, FL: CRC Taylor & Francis Press Inc.

Athukorala, Y., Trang, S., Kwok, C., and Yuan, Y.V. (2016). Antiproliferative and antioxidant activities and mycosporine-like amino acid profiles of wild-harvested and cultivated edible Canadian marine red macroalgae. *Molecules* **21** (1): 119. https://doi.org/10.3390/molecules21010119.

Bird, G., Fitzmaurice, N., Dunlap, W.C. et al. (1987). Sunscreen compositions and compounds for use therein. U.S. Patent No. 5000946A.

Bultel-Poncé, V., Felix-Theodose, F., Sarthou, C. et al. (2004). New pigments from the terrestrial cyanobacterium *Scytonema* sp. collected on the Mitaraka Inselberg, French Guyana. *Journal of Natural Products* **67**: 678–681.

Ceccoli, J., Costello, B., and Pillai, S. (2008). Marine extracts and biofermentations for use in cosmetics. US Patent No. 8,202,519 B2.

de la Coba, F., Aguilera, J., and López Figueroa, F. (2006). Use of a mycosporin-type amino acid (shinorine) as an antioxidant. International Patent No. 2007/026038 A3.

Ebrahimi Nigjeh, S., Yusoff, F.M., Mohamed Alitheen, N.B. et al. (2013). Cytotoxic effect of ethanol extract of microalga, *Chaetoceros calcitrans*, and its mechanisms in inducing apoptosis in human breast cancer cell line. *BioMed Research International*. https://doi.org/10.1155/2016/8693826.

Ganesan, P., Noda, K., Manabe, Y. et al. (2011). Siphonaxanthin, a marine carotenoid from green algae, effectively induces apoptosis in human leukemia (HL-60) cells. *Biochemica et Biophysica Acta* **1810**: 497–503.

Garcia, J.L., de Vicente, M., and Galán, B. (2017). Microalgae, old sustainable food and fashion nutraceuticals. *Microbial Biotechnology* **10** (5): 1017–1024.

Goiris, K., Muylaert, K., Fraeye, I. et al. (2012). Antioxidant potential of microalgae in relation to their phenolic and carotenoid content. *Journal of Applied Phycology*. https://doi.org/doi:101007/s1081-012-9804-6.

Hanaya, T. and Yamamoto, H. (2013). Synthesis of biopterin and related pterin glycosides. *International Union of Biochemistry and Molecular Biology* **65** (4): 300–309.

Hitoe, S. and Shimoda, H. (2017). Seaweed fucoxanthin supplementation improves obesity parameters in mildly obese Japanese subjects. *Functional Foods in Health and Disease* **7** (4): 246–262.

Karsten, U. (2002). Effects of salinity and ultraviolet radiation on the concentration of mycosporine-like amino acids in various isolates of the benthic cyanobacterium *Microcoleus chthonoplastes*. *Phycological Research* **50**: 129–134.

Kedar, L., Kashman, Y., and Oren, A. (2002). Mycosporine-2-glycine is the major mycosporine-like amino acid in a unicellular cyanobacterium (*Euhalothece* sp.) isolated from a gypsum crust in a hypersaline saltern pond. *FEMS Microbiology Letters* **208**: 233–237.

Khan, M.I., Shin, J.H., and Kim, J.D. (2018). The promising future of microalgae: current status, challenges, and optimization of a sustainable and renewable industry for biofuels, feed, and other products. *Microbial Cell Factories* **17** (1): 36. https://doi.org/10.1186/s12934-018-0879-x.

Kim, M.S., Kim, J.Y., Choi, W.H., and Lee, S.S. (2008). Effects of seaweed supplementation on blood glucose concentration, lipid profile, and antioxidant enzyme activities in patients with type 2 diabetes mellitus. *Nutrition Research and Practice* **2** (2): 62–67.

Lordan, S., Ross, R.P., and Stanton, C. (2011). Marine bioactives as functional food ingredients: potential to reduce the incidence of chronic diseases. *Marine Drugs* **9**: 1056–1100.

Mac Monagail, M., Cornish, L., Morrison, L. et al. (2017). Sustainable harvesting of wild seaweed resources. *European Journal of Phycology* **52** (4): 371–390. https://doi.org/10.1080/09670262.2017.1365273.

Mason, D.S., Schafer, F., Shick, J.M., and Dunlap, W.C. (1998). Ultraviolet radiation-absorbing mycosporine-like amino acids (MAAs) are acquired from their diet by medaka fish (*Oryzias latipes*) but not by SKH-1 hairless mice. *Comparative Biochemistry and Physiology Pt. A* **120**: 587–598.

Matsui, K., Nazifi, E., Hirai, Y. et al. (2012). The cyanobacterial UV-absorbing pigment scytonemin displays radical-scavenging activity. *The Journal of General and Applied Microbiology* **58**: 137–144. https://doi.org/10.2323/jgam.58.137.

Matsunaga, T., Burgess, J.G., Yamada, N. et al. (1993). An ultraviolet (UV-A) absorbing biopterin glucoside from the marine planktonic cyanobacterium *Oscillatoria* sp. *Applied Microbial and Cell Physiology* **39**: 250–253.

Moo-Puc, R., Robledo, D., and Freile-Pelegrín, Y. (2009). In vitro cytotoxic and antiproliferative activities of marine macroalgae from Yucatán, Mexico. *Ciencias Marinas* **35**: 345–358.

Nazifi, E., Wada, N., Yamaba, M. et al. (2013). Glycosylated porphyra-334 and palythine-threonine from the terrestrial cyanobacterium *Nostoc commune*. *Marine Drugs* **11** (9): 3124–3154. https://doi.org/10.3390/md11093124.

Nishihira, J., Nishimura, M., Sugawara, M., and Kudo, M. (2017). Double-blind, parallel group, placebo-controlled study of *Kjellmaniella crassifolia* Miyabe (Gagome) in human: the potential of Gagome to activate the immune system. *Functional Foods in Health and Disease* **7** (10): 758–772.

Pathak, J., Ahmed, H., Rajneesh et al. (2019a). Genetic regulation of scytonemin and mycosporine-like amino acids (MAAs) biosynthesis in cyanobacteria. *Plant Gene* **17**: 100172.

Pathak, J., Ahmed, H., Rajneesh et al. (2019b). Mechanisms of photoprotection in cyanobacteria. In: *Cyanobacteria from Basic Science to Applications* (eds. A.K. Mishra, D.N. Tiwari and A.N. Rai), 145–171. London: Academic Press.

Plaza, M., Cifuentes, A., and Ibáñez, E. (2008). In the search of new functional food ingredients from algae. *Trends in Food Science and Technology* **19**: 31–39.

Ranga Rao, A., Raghunath Reddy, R.L., Baskaran, V. et al. (2010). Characterization of microalgal carotenoids by mass spectrometry and their bioavailability and antioxidant properties elucidated in rat model. *Journal of Agricultural and Food Chemistry* **58**: 8553–8559.

Ranga Rao, A., Sarada, R., Shylaja, M.D., and Ravishankar, G.A. (2015). Evaluation of hepatoprotective and antioxidant activity of astaxanthin and astaxanthin esters from microalga – *Haematococcus pluvialis*. *Journal of Food Science Technology* **52** (10): 6703–6710.

Rastogi, R.P., Sinha, R.P., and Incharoensakdi, A. (2013). Partial characterization, UV-induction and photoprotective function of sunscreen pigment, scytonemin from *Rivularia* sp. HKAR-4. *Chemosphere* **93**: 1874–1878.

Rastogi, R.P., Sonani, R.R., and Madamwar, D. (2014). The high-energy radiation protectant extracellular sheath pigment scytonemin and its reduced counterpart in the cyanobacterium *Scytonema* sp. R77DM. *Bioresource Technology* **171**: 396–400.

Robledo, D. and Freile Pelegrín, Y. (1997). Chemical and mineral composition of six potentially edible seaweed species of Yucatán. *Botanica Marina* **40**: 301–306.

Schmid, D., Schürch, C., and Zülli, F. (2006). Mycosporine-like amino acids from red algae protect against premature skin-aging. *European Cosmetics* **9**: 1–4.

Sinha, R.P., Singh, S.P., and Häder, D.P. (2007). Database on mycosporines and mycosporine-like amino acids (MAAs) in fungi, cyanobacteria, macroalgae, phytoplankton and animals. *Journal of Photochemistry and Photobiology B* **89** (1): 29–35.

Stevenson, C.S., Capper, E.A., Roshak, A.K. et al. (2002). The identification and characterization of the marine natural product scytonemin as a novel antiproliferative pharmacocore. *The Journal of Pharmacology and Experimental Therapeutics* **303** (2): 858–866.

Tou, J., Oldaker, C., and Yuan, Y.V. (2019). Novel marine sources of nutraceuticals and functional foods: the marine crustacean Krill, macro- and microalgae. Chapter 119. In: *Encyclopedia of Marine Biotechnology* (ed. S.-K. Kim). Chichester: Wiley.

Xiong, F., Kopecky, J., and Nedbal, L. (1999). The occurrence of UV-B absorbing mycosporine-like amino acids in freshwater and terrestrial microalgae (Chlorophyta). *Aquatic Botany* **63**: 37–49.

Yan, X., Chuda, Y., Suzuki, M., and Nagata, T. (1999). Fucoxanthin as the major antioxidant in *Hijikia fusiformis*, a common edible seaweed. *Bioscience, Biotechnology, and Biochemistry* **63**: 605–607.

Yang, Y.J., Nam, S.-J., Kong, G., and Kim, M.K. (2010). A case-control study on seaweed consumption and the risk of breast cancer. *British Journal of Nutrition* **103**: 1345–1353.

Yoshinaga, K., Maruya, R., Koikeda, T., and Nakano, T. (2018). Effects of *Undaria pinnatifida* (wakame) on the human intestinal environment. *Functional Foods in Health and Disease* **8** (10): 477–493.

Yuan, Y.V. (2007). Antioxidants from edible seaweeds. Chapter 19. In: *Antioxidant Measurement and Applications* (eds. F. Shahidi and C.-T. Ho), 268–301. Washington, DC: ACS, Oxford University Press.

Yuan, Y.V. (2008). Marine algal constituents. Chapter 11. In: *Marine Nutraceuticals and Functional Foods* (eds. C. Barrow and F. Shahidi), 259–296. Boca Raton, FL: CRC Taylor & Francis Press Inc.

Yuan, Y.V. and Athukorala, Y. (2012). Red algal mycosporine-like amino acids (MAAs) as potential cosmeceuticals. Chapter 12. In: *Marine Cosmeceuticals: Trends and Prospects* (ed. S.-K. Kim), 143–167. Boca Raton, FL: CRC Taylor & Francis Press Inc.

Yuan, Y.V., Westcott, N.D., Hu, C., and Kitts, D.D. (2009). Mycosporine-like amino acid composition of the edible red alga, *Palmaria palmata* (dulse) harvested from the west and east coasts of Grand Manan Island, New Brunswick. *Food Chemistry* **112**: 321–328.

10
Algal Polysaccharides and Their Biological Properties

Kit-Leong Cheong, Valentina Jesumani, Bilal Muhammad Khan, Yang Liu, and Hong Du

Guangdong Provincial Key Laboratory of Marine Biotechnology, STU-UNIVPM Joint Algal Research Center, Department of Biology, College of Science, Shantou University, Shantou, China

10.1 Introduction

The biodiversity in oceans, which cover a large area (70%) of our planet, is reported to be higher than that represented by tropical rainforests (Ebada et al. 2008). Marine organisms are a major source of food and are gaining a lot of interest from the scientific community for their potential role in the health and pharmaceutical industries. Algae, or seaweeds, represent one of the most abundant groups of marine organisms. They are rich in functional metabolites including peptides, proteins, amino acids, lipids, vitamins, mineral salts, polyphenols, and polysaccharides (Brown et al. 2014). Seaweeds are an integral component of numerous dishes in Asia (Rioux et al. 2017), and their consumption is routinely associated with reduced frequency of diet-related chronic diseases including cancer, and cardiovascular and heart diseases (Brown et al. 2014; Mohamed et al. 2012).

In fact, collection and/or cultivation of seaweed is common in many parts of the world with the final goal of polysaccharide extraction (Stiger-Pouvreau et al. 2016). With 27% of worldwide annual wild seaweed harvesting and 72% of the global annual harvest from cultivated seaweed, China stands as the global leader in seaweed production (Duarte et al. 2017; Wei et al. 2013). Other countries on the list of top 10 global annual wild seaweed harvesters in descending order of productivity are Chile, Norway, Japan, Russia, Ireland, Mexico, Iceland, and France, though Asia leads the rest of the world in terms of seaweed cultivation (Stiger-Pouvreau et al. 2016). Furthermore, the genera *Porphyra* (Rhodophyta), *Eucheuma* (Rhodophyta), *Gracilaria* (Rhodophyta), *Laminaria* (Phaeophyta), and *Undaria* (Phaeophyta) account for 76% of the total seaweed aquaculture production (Milledge and Harvey 2016).

Recent Advances in Micro- and Macroalgal Processing: Food and Health Perspectives, First Edition.
Edited by Gaurav Rajauria and Yvonne V. Yuan.

Polysaccharides, as long-chain polymers of monosaccharide units linked via glycosidic bonds, are essentially polymeric carbohydrates. They can be linear or highly branched, and yield their constituent monosaccharide or oligosaccharide subunits upon hydrolysis. Polysaccharides have found utility in a number of industrial applications for the production of emulsifiers, stabilizers, thickeners in beverages, processed foods, and animal feeds (Kraan 2012). Seaweeds are a rich source of polysaccharides in the form of muco-, storage-, and cell wall (structural)-polysaccharides (Chandini et al. 2008). The most widely extracted algal polysaccharides are structural in nature having numerous functional characteristics (Usov and Zelinsky 2013).

Marine algal polysaccharides (MAP) differ from their terrestrial counterparts in that they are all essentially sulfated (Aquino et al. 2011). Phycocolloids, algal polysaccharides with gelling ability, including agar, carrageenan, and alginates, frequently undergo large-scale production (Bixler and Porse 2011). Such polysaccharides find utility in the manufacturing sector for the production of pharmaceuticals, cosmetics, and food, and the bioactivities of numerous related nongelling polysaccharides are under investigation (Rinaudo 2007).

A number of potential biological activities including anticancer, antioxidant, antiviral, and anticoagulant potency have been attributed to MAP (De Jesus Raposo et al. 2015). The chemical characteristics of polysaccharides including molecular size, type, constituent monosaccharide subunits, and glycosidic bonds have been found to influence their biological activities (Ahmadi et al. 2015; De Jesus Raposo et al. 2015; Deniaud-Bouët et al. 2017; Hamed et al. 2015). The chemical structure of an individual polysaccharide may differ according to algal species, life cycle stage, nutrient availability, harvesting season, habitat, as well as extraction protocols (Pomin 2011; Synytsya et al. 2015). Knowledge of their physical and chemical properties is essential for their effective use in functional food and related industries (Xu et al. 2017) as well as to enable chemical modifications that would improve their bioactivities (Usov and Zelinsky 2013). In addition, the choice of extraction solvents used and the extraction procedure employed may also impact the final bioactivities of the polysaccharide. The regulatory approval of polysaccharides and fractions thereof for use in pharmaceuticals, dermatological preparations, nutraceuticals, and similar marketable applications is, hitherto, hindered by an absence of standardized extraction procedures (Ale and Meyer 2013).

This chapter deals with chemical and structural characteristics of algal polysaccharides along with the extraction and purification regimes in vogue for the same. Moreover, the biological activities and industrial applications of these polysaccharides will also be discussed (see Figure 10.1). Without any doubt, seaweed polysaccharides are highly potent with respect to numerous industrial and commercial undertakings. But an understanding of their physical and chemical nature and an appropriate choice of extraction and purification procedure are of utmost importance for the final product to produce the desired effects.

10.2 Structure of Marine Algae Polysaccharides

The chemical constituents of marine algae vary with the taxonomy of the algae. Polysaccharides are one of the main components of marine algae, and the biological activities of MAP may be linked with particular structural features. Therefore,

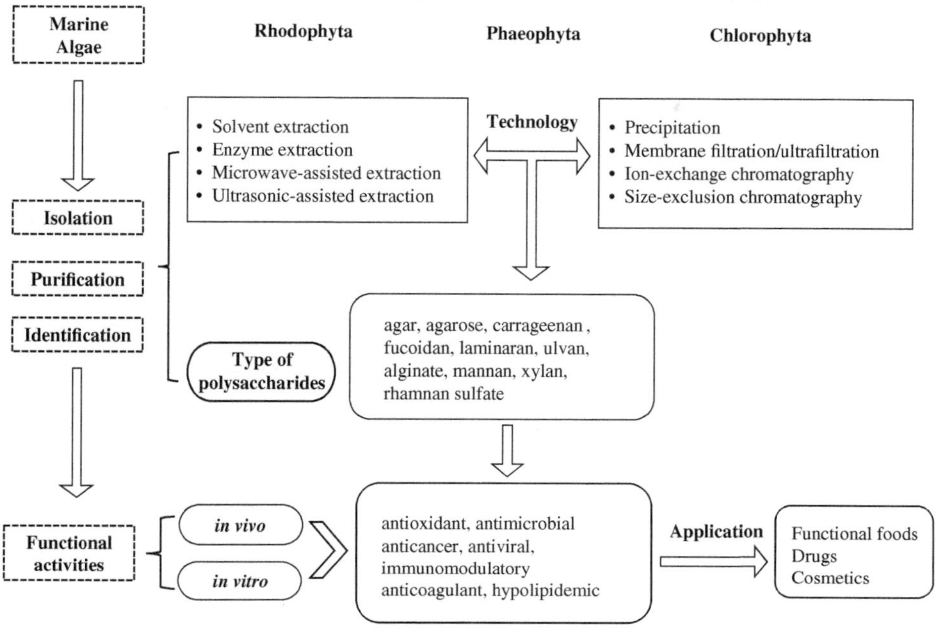

Figure 10.1 Schematic diagram of isolation, purification, potential functional activities, and applications of marine algal polysaccharides

elucidation of the chemical structure of MAP is mandatory and could improve elucidation of the beneficial properties and chemical modifications.

The most common polysaccharides of Phaeophyta include alginates, fucoidans, and laminarans, while Rhodophyta contain agars, carrageenans, and xylans, and Chlorophyta contain ulvan and sulfated rhamnan (Table 10.1).

Table 10.1 Polysaccharides reported in Phaeophyta, Rhodophyta, and Chlorophyta.

Type of polysaccharide	Phaeophyta	Rhodophyta	Chlorophyta
Agars	—[a]	√[b]	—
Alginates	√	—	—
Carrageenans	—	√	—
Cellulose	√	√	√
Fucoidans	√	—	—
Laminarans	√	—	—
Mannans	—	√	√
Sulfated galactans	—	√	√
Sulfated rhamnans	—	—	√
Ulvans	—	—	√
Xylans	—	√	—

[a] Undetected.
[b] Detected.

10.2.1 Agar

Agar is found in red algae and is the collective term used to describe a mixture of gelling polysaccharides. The naming of agar is arbitrary, with agarans, agarose, agaroids, agaropectin, or porphyran being used to describe different agar components with different purities, conformations, and side chain substitutions (such as methoxyl group, sulfate ester group, and pyruvic acid acetal group) (Lee et al. 2017).

Agaropectin shows complex patterns of substitution such as sulfate and/or methyl groups at different positions, and/or pyruvic acid acetals at O-4,6 of the β-D-galactopyranose residues (Duarte et al. 2004; Pérez Recalde et al. 2016). Whereas agarose has a linear backbone with repeating sugar units of 3-linked β-D-galactopyranose and 4-linked α-3,6-anhydro-L-galactose (Figure 10.2) and is purified from agar as a result of the removal of agarapectin, porphyran (a highly substituted form of agarose) is mainly obtained from *Porphyra* spp. such as *Porphyra haitanensis*, *Porphyra suborbiculata*, *Porphyra tenera*, and *Porphyra yezoensis* (Bhatia et al. 2013). Porphyran is structurally related to agarose, with the repetition moieties of 4-linked α-L-galactopyranose-6-sulfate and 3-linked β-D-galactopyranose residues (Correc et al. 2011).

10.2.2 Alginates

Alginates or alginic acid polymers occur as a cellular wall matrix in brown algae. Alginates constitute a family of linear polysaccharides, consisting of (1→4) linked β-D-mannuronic acid (M) and α-L-guluronic acid (G) residues. Alginates were determined to be a true block copolymer arranged in a nonregular repeating unit (Draget and Taylor 2011). The residues typically occurred as poly M-blocks, poly G-blocks, and MG-blocks (stretches of blocks of predominantly alternating monomers) (Figure 10.3) (Stokke et al. 1991). It has been shown that the physical properties such as gel strength and solubility of alginates depend on the relative proportions of these three types of blocks (Draget and Taylor 2011). The alginate yield of extracted *Sargassum fluitans* was found to be 45% of the dry weight of the biomass (Davis et al. 2003). A previous report showed that alginates extracted from *Laminaria digitata*, *Laminaria hyperborea*, *Saccharina latissimi*, and *Alaria esculenta* accounted for 34.6, 33.2, 28.5, and 37.4% of the dry weight of biomass, respectively (Schiener et al. 2015).

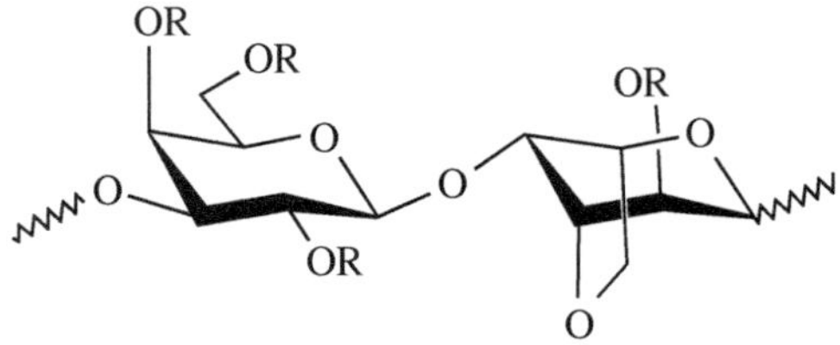

Figure 10.2 Chemical structures of agar repeating units of 3-linked β-D-galactopyranose and 4-linked α-3,6-anhydro-L-galactose. R can be H or side chain substituents such as methoxyl group, sulfate ester group, and pyruvic acid acetal group. Source: from Lee et al. (2017).

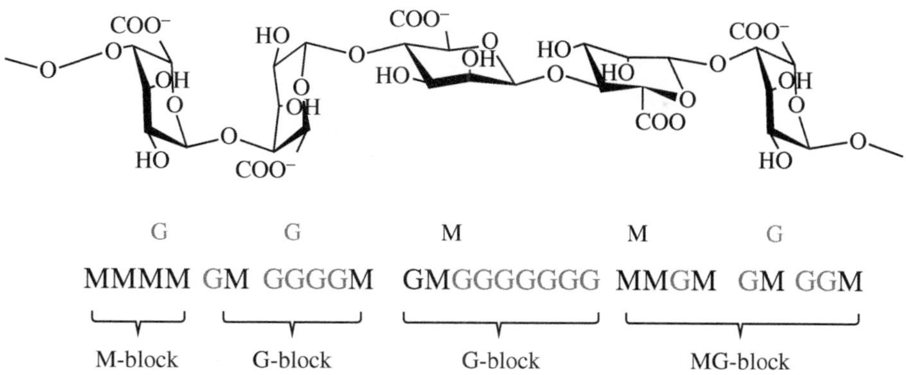

Figure 10.3 Structural characteristics of alginates and block distribution. M: β-D-mannuronic acid residue; G: α-L-guluronic acid residue. Source: from Draget and Taylor (2011).

10.2.3 Carrageenan

Carrageenans are derived from certain species of red seaweeds of the class Rhodophyceae including *Chondrus crispus*, *Kappaphycus alvarezii*, *Euchema cottonii*, *Hypnea musciformis*, etc. Carrageenans are mixtures of sulfated galactans with 15–40% of ester-sulfate content and a relatively high molecular weight above 100 kDa (Viebke et al. 1995). The structure of carrageenans is formed by alternate units of D-galactose and 3,6-anhydro-galactose with sulfate ester moieties, which are linked by α-1,3-glucosidic and β-1,4-glycosidic linkages (Campo et al. 2009). In general, carrageenans are classified into three common forms, designated as kappa-, iota-, and lambda-carrageenan. Structures of these carrageenans are shown in Figure 10.4. The differences among them are in the position and number of sulfate groups on the galactose unit. Kappa-carrageenan is composed of alternate units of 3-linked 4-sulfate-β-D-galactopyranose and 4-linked anhydro-galactose. Iota-carrageenan and lambda-carrageenan have a similar structure to κ-carrageenan but with two and three sulfate groups, respectively (De Ruiter and Rudolph 1997).

10.2.4 Cellulose

Cellulose is present in the primary cell wall of marine algae. The structure of cellulose is a linear (1→4)-linked β-D-glucan and it consists of more than 10 000 β-1,4-linked D-glucose units (Figure 10.5). It exists as a mixture of two crystalline forms, one is α-cellulose, with a one-chain triclinic structure; the other is β-cellulose, with a two-chain monoclinic structure (Sugiyama et al. 2008). Cellulose obtained from algae showed a porous web-like or sponge-like structure and had a high level of crystallinity that is considerably different from terrestrial plant cellulose (Strømme et al. 2002). There was little variation in the yields of cellulose from brown algae (9–10%, such as *Dictyota dichotoma* and *Sargassum tenerrimum*), while green algae (1.5–11%, *Codium dwarkense* and *Caulerpa taxifolia*) and red algae (1.2–13.5%, *Gracilaria dura* and *Gelidiella acerosa*) were more variable (Siddhanta et al. 2011).

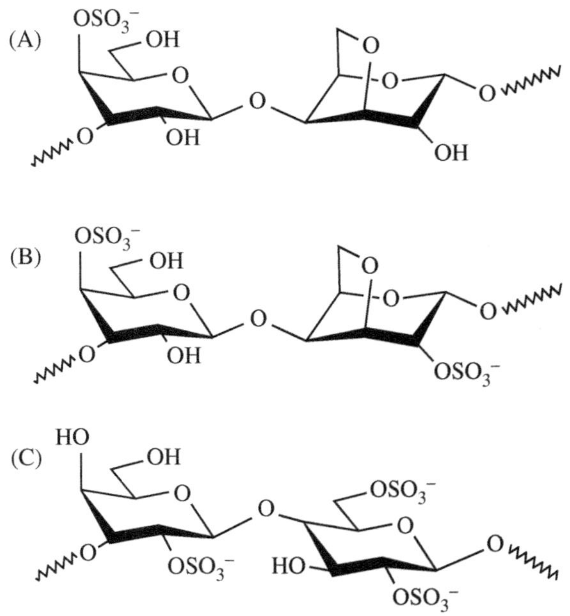

Figure 10.4 Major repeating disaccharides of (A) kappa-carrageenan, (B) iota-carrageenan, and (C) lambda-carrageenan. Source: from De Ruiter and Rudolph (1997).

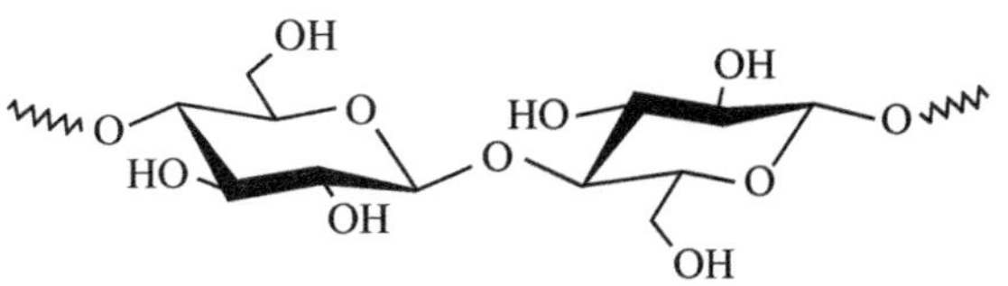

Figure 10.5 Chemical structure of cellulose derived from marine algae. Source: from Sanandiya (2009).

10.2.5 Fucoidans

Fucoidans are fucose-enriched and sulfated polysaccharides, and mainly found in brown algae. The structure of fucoidans generally consist of a backbone of α-(1→3)-L-fucopyranose (6-deoxy-L-galactose) residues or of alternating α-(1→3) and α-(1→4)-linked L-fucopyranose, with various substitutions such as sulfate, acetate, uronic acid groups (Figure 10.6) (Ale and Meyer 2013). Fucoidans often contain minor amounts of xylose, glucose, galactose, and rhamnose as well as glucuronic acid, phenolic compounds, phosphorus, and minerals (Ale and Meyer 2013). It is noteworthy that fucoidans are commonly bound to alginates and are thus an inexpensive by-product of alginate isolation.

Fucoidans isolated from different algal species may differ considerably in their chemical structure, monosaccharide composition, and substitution groups. The fucoidans from *Laminaria saccharina*, *Cladosiphon okamuranus*, and *Lessonia vadosa*

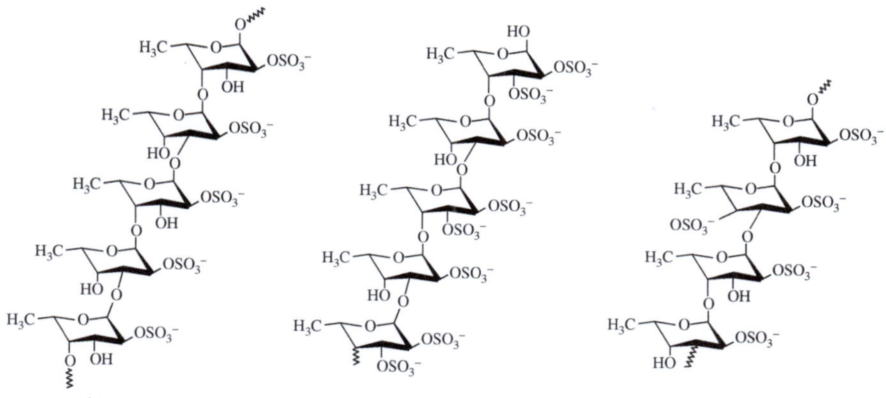

Figure 10.6 Typical structure of fucoidan obtained from some brown seaweed species in the order of Fucales. The L-fucopyranose backbone of the fucoidan extracted from *Fucus serratus* (A), *Ascophyllum nodosum* (B), and *Fucus vesiculosus* (C), respectively. Source: from Ale et al. (2011).

contain linear α-(1→3)-L-fucopyranose residues, with some containing 2-sulfate substituents (Chandía and Matsuhiro 2008; Nagaoka et al. 1999), whereas fucoidans isolated from *Sargassum horneri*, *Fucus evanescens*, and *Fucus serratus* contain alternating (1→3)- and (1→4)-linked α-L-fucopyranose, which may be substituted with sulfate groups on C-2 and C-4 positions (Bilan et al. 2004; Ermakova et al. 2011).

Fucoidans rich in galactose and fucose can be obtained from *Laminaria japonica* (Chen et al. 2017a), *Adenocystis utricularis* (Trinchero et al. 2009), and *Padina australis* (Yuguchi et al. 2016). Fucoidans from *Sargassum* species and *Fucus vesiculosus* contained varying amounts of fucose, galactose, xylose, and glucuronic acid (Ale et al. 2011a).

10.2.6 Laminarans

Laminarans (or laminarins) were first discovered in *Laminaria* species and appear to be the reserve or storage polysaccharides of brown algae. Laminaran is a β-glucan that consists of a backbone of β-1,3-linked-glucose residues with branching β-1,6-glucose residues; the proportion of β-1,6 to β-1,3 appears to be roughly 1:3 (Maeda and Nisizawa 1968). There are two types of laminaran chains (mannitol chain and glucose chain), which differ in their reducing ends: the mannitol chains end with a mannitol residue, whereas glucose chains end with a glucose residue (Figure 10.7). Laminaran is a low molecular weight polysaccharide, approximately 4–10 kDa and has an average polymerization degree of 25 glucose units (Kadam et al. 2015b). For example, the laminaran isolated from brown algae *L. hyperborea* had a molecular weight ranging from 3042 to 5052 Da, corresponding to a degree of polymerization (DP) of 20–31 (Rioux et al. 2010). Laminarans from *Eisenia bicyclis* with a ratio of 1.3:1.6 bonds of 1.5:1, had molecular weights of 5 kDa (Ermakova et al. 2013).

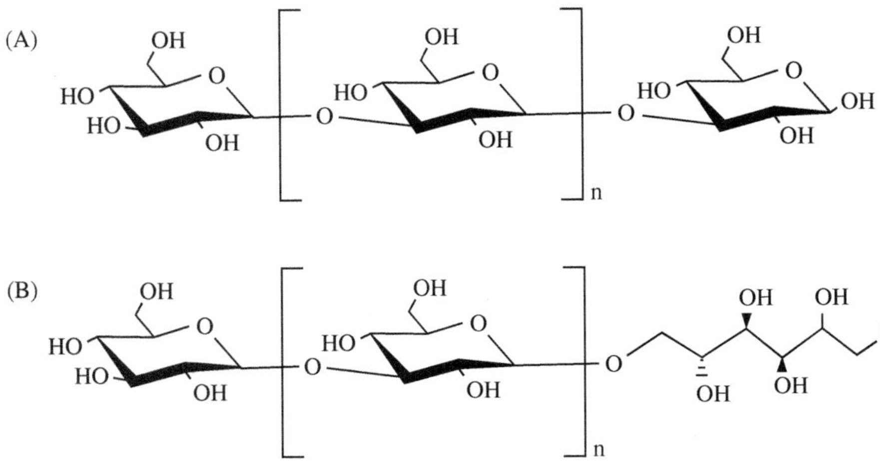

Figure 10.7 Chemical structures of glucose (A) and mannitol chains (B) of laminaran. Source: from Kadam et al. (2015).

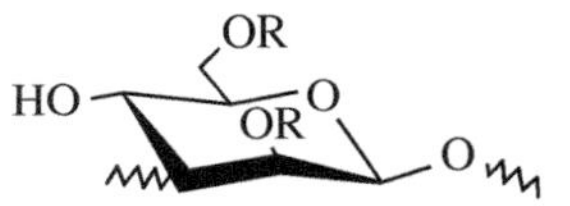

Figure 10.8 The structure of mannan derived from red seaweed *Nothogenia fastigiata* and carrying sulfate groups. Similar substitution pattern to that of green seaweed *Codium vermilara*. R can be H or side chain substituents sulfate group. Source: from Erra-Balsells et al. (2000).

10.2.7 Mannans

Mannans are similar to cellulose and are located in the primary cell walls of marine algae. The linear type of α-1,3-linked-mannan is mainly found in Rhodophyceae (Figure 10.8). For example, α-mannan has been isolated from red algae such as *Nothogenia fastigiata*, *Liagora valida*, and *Nemalion helminthoides* (Kolender et al. 1997; Pérez Recalde et al. 2009). This linear mannan was partially sulfated on C-2 of the mannose units and also substituted on C-6 with single residues of β-xylose (Pérez Recalde et al. 2009), and found in red algae *Chondrophycus papillosus* and *Chondrophycus flagelliferus*. Likewise, mixed-linkage mannans (including α-1,3-linked and β-1,4-linked-mannan) were found in the Chlorophyceae *Codium vermilara*, *Codium fragile*, and *Acetabularia acetabulum* (Dunn et al. 2007; Estevez et al. 2009; Fernández et al. 2012). If only a small extent of β-1,4-linked-mannan were substituted, then these side chains would hinder their ability to form high tensile strength microfibrils, but might enhance their ability to form a flexible network (Dunn et al. 2007). Different relative amounts of mannan are found in the algae; that is, 4% (w/w) seaweed dry weight in *C. vermilara* and 31% (w/w) in *C. fragile* (Estevez et al. 2009; Fernández et al. 2012).

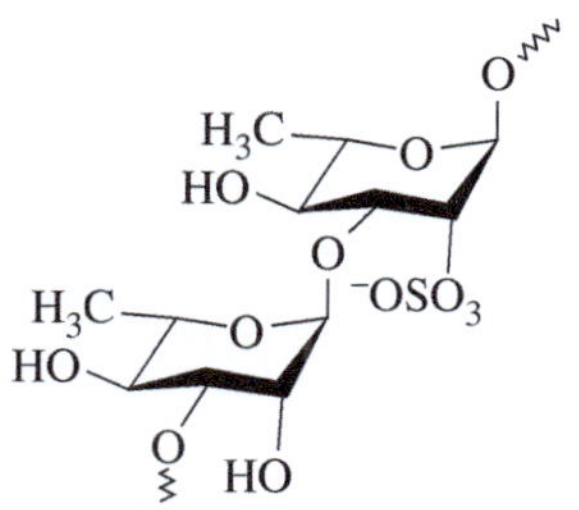

Figure 10.9 Typical chemical structure of rhamnan sulfate isolated from *Monostroma* species. Source: from Li et al. (2011).

10.2.8 Sulfated Rhamnans

Chemical structures of sulfated rhamnans from *Monostroma nitidum* consisted of α-(1→3)-linked rhamnose residues with a sulfate group substituted at C-2 (Figure 10.9) (Harada and Maeda 1998). Another sulfated rhamnan isolated from *M. nitidum* consisted of α-(1→3)- and α-(1→2)-linked rhamnose residues in a molar ratio of 2:1; sulfation was mainly substituted at C-3 or C-4 in the α-(1→3)- and α-(1→2)-linked rhamnose residues (Lee et al. 2010). A similar branched and sulfated hetero-rhamnan with molecular weight of 513 kDa is a major polysaccharide found in *Monostroma latissimum* (Li et al. 2011).

10.2.9 Ulvans

Ulvans are a complex sulfated polysaccharide found in the Chlorophyceae genera *Ulva* and *Enteromorpha* (Lahaye and Robic 2007). The ulvan content in the algae may be as high as approx. 30% of algal biomass (Costa et al. 2012). The main monosaccharide subunits in ulvan are glucose, glucuronic acid, rhamnose, xylose, iduronic acid, and sulfate in different proportions. The two major structures of ulvans correspond to the disaccharide repeating units, one is composed of O-3-sulfate rhamnose and glucuronic acid, designated as β-D-GlcA-(1→4)-L-Rha3S; and in the other, iduronic acid replaces glucuronic acid, designated as α-L-IdoA-(1→4)-L-Rha3S (Figure 10.10) (Lahaye et al. 1997, 1998). The sulfate groups in ulvan structures are mainly located at C-2 and C-3 of 3- and 2-linked rhamnose residues, respectively. Similar structures of branched and sulfated heterorhamnans were isolated from *Gayralia oxysperma* (Cassolato et al. 2008). The variation in monosaccharide composition may in fact reflect different origins, the different locations, or seasons when green algae were harvested. The ulvan isolated from *Ulva lactuca* collected in Tunisia contained xylose (Yaich et al. 2013), while *U. lactuca* collected in the South China Sea contained xylose and glucose (Tian et al. 2015).

10.2.10 Xylans

Xylans are hemicelluloses mainly found in Rhodophyceae of the orders *Nemaliales* and *Palmariales* (Pérez Recalde et al. 2009). The chemical structures of water-soluble

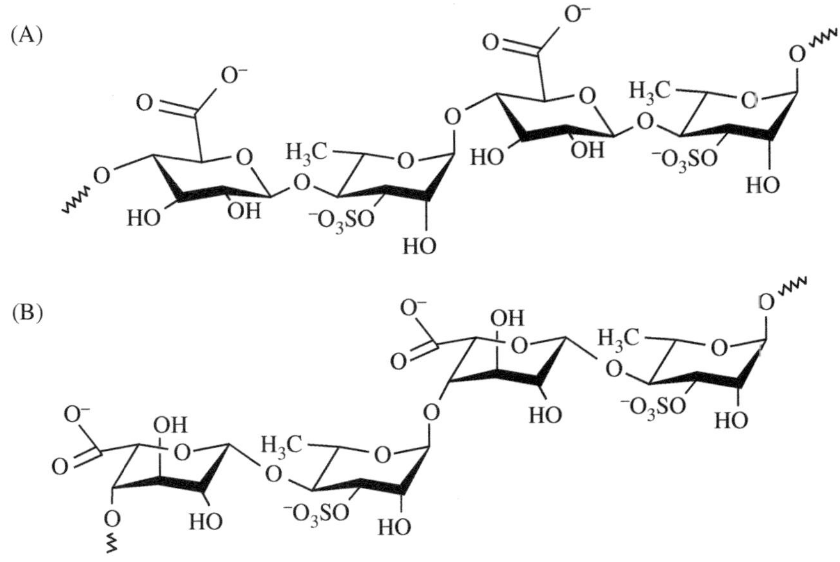

Figure 10.10 Structure of the main repeating disaccharide units in ulvans. (A) Glucuronic acid and O-3-sulfate rhamnose; and (B) iduronic acid and O-3-sulfate rhamnose. Source: from Jiao et al. (2011).

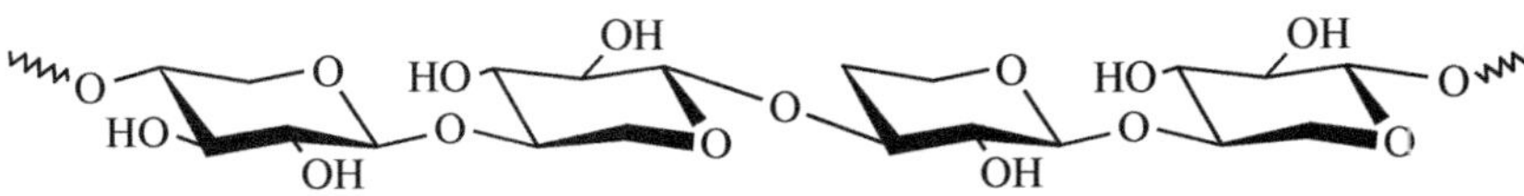

Figure 10.11 Linear β-(1→3), β-(1→4)-linked mixed polymer of xylan. Source: from Viana et al. (2011).

xylans are neutral linear β-(1→3), β-(1→4)-linked xylose residues with substitutions including α-arabinofuranose and α-glucuronic acids (Figure 10.11) (Viana et al. 2011). Some water-insoluble xylans of the same type remain in the cell wall and are only extracted by alkaline solvents (Deniaud et al. 2003). A linear β-(1→4)-linked xylan was obtained from red algae *Scinaia hatei* (from the order *Nemaliales*) by alkali extraction (Mandal et al. 2010). In addition, β-(1→3)-xylans are part of the fibrillar components of the cell walls of some green algae, such as *Bryopsidales* (Ciancia et al. 2012).

10.3 Isolation and Purification of Polysaccharides from Algae

Polysaccharides from marine algae can be isolated and purified using different techniques, each with its own pros and cons. The ultimate selection of an appropriate extraction as well as purification method depends upon the solubility characteristics, scale of production, and final use of the isolated polysaccharide. The extraction of polysaccharides is commonly preceded by a number of pretreatments so that the polysaccharides are obtained in their pure form.

The first step involves cleaning of the algal biomass in sea- or distilled water for the removal of epiphytes and sand particles. The cleaned biomass is then dried in an oven (40–60 °C) or freeze dryer prior to grinding. Algal biomass needs to be powdered in order to attain the maximum possible surface to volume ratio in the course of extraction (Hahn et al. 2012; Imbs et al. 2016).

As a common pretreatment measure, the dried biomass is washed in acetone (Dore et al. 2013) or in a concoction of methanol, chloroform, and water mixed in a volumetric ratio of 4:2:1 (Ale et al. 2011b; Lim et al. 2014). Likewise, acetone mixed with ethanol (Shan et al. 2016) or a number of treatments with ethanol at varying temperatures (Imbs et al. 2016; Yuan and Macquarrie 2015) can also be used for algal biomass pretreatment. The strongly bound intracellular constituents including phenols, chlorophyll, proteins, mannitol, and lipids are removed from polysaccharides as a result of these alcoholic pretreatments (Hahn et al. 2012). Another recently described pretreatment, a compressional–puffing–hydrothermal procedure, involves a temperature treatment at 140, 180, and 220 °C under atmospheric pressure, and afterwards rapidly reducing pressure in the ultra-heated water-holding container, thereby allowing cellular structure break down preceding extraction (Huang et al. 2016).

10.3.1 Isolation

The aforementioned preparation and pretreatments aid in optimum polysaccharide extraction from the algal biomass. A number of procedures are reported in the literature for this purpose including solvent extraction, microwave assisted and ultrasonic assisted extraction, and enzymatic extraction (Table 10.2). This section details the procedure and effectiveness of these extraction processes in relation to polysaccharide isolation from pretreated algal biomass.

10.3.1.1 Extraction with Solvents Solvent extraction is the most widely used method for polysaccharide extraction from algae. Polysaccharide extraction from dried, pretreated algal biomass is usually carried out with various solvents, for many hours, at temperatures ranging from ambient to 120 °C (Garcia-Vaquero et al. 2017). Aqueous extraction (Shan et al. 2016; Vijayabaskar et al. 2012; Wang et al. 2012b) and extraction with ethyl alcohol (Foley et al. 2011) are the most commonly employed extraction techniques in this regard, while extraction with marginally acidic solutions (low-molarity HCl solutions) has also been reported (Dinesh et al. 2016; Imbs et al. 2016; Lorbeer et al. 2015; Menshova et al. 2015). For example, the brown algae *Alaria angusta* (20 g) was extracted twice with 0.1 mol l^{-1} HCl for 2 hoursat 60 °C, and lyophilized to yield a crude polysaccharide (1.03 g) (Menshova et al. 2015).

Specific treatments ensue after the preliminary extraction in order to obtain the desired compounds from the polysaccharide mix. For precipitation of polysaccharides from this mixture, treatments with organic solvents (ethyl alcohol) or surfactants (cetyltrimethylammonium bromide) are commonly employed (Hahn et al. 2012; Kadam et al. 2015b). After precipitation, a single- or multi-step ethanolic precipitation can be employed for further precipitation or dialysis of the polysaccharides to ensure removal of salts and other impurities (Garcia-Vaquero et al. 2017).

Table 10.2 Algal polysaccharides isolated using different extraction procedures.

Algae	Polysaccharide	Extraction media and protocol	Reference
Silvetia babingtonii, *Fucus evanescens*, and *Coccophora langsdorfii* (Fucales)	Fucoidan	HCl (1 mol l^{-1}, 60 °C, pH 2–3, 3 hours, twice) followed by concentration, dialysis, and freeze drying	Anastyuk et al. (2012b) and Imbs et al. (2016)
Laminaria cichorioides and *Costaria costata* (Laminariales)			Anastyuk et al. (2010, 2012a)
Sargassum henslowian, *Fucus vesiculosus*	Fucoidan	HCl (0.03 mol l^{-1}, 90 °C, 4 hours) followed by filtration and ethanol (60%) precipitation. The final pellet was freeze dried	Ale et al. (2012)
Ascophyllum nodosum	Fucoidan	Ethanol (80%, 20 °C, 12 hours) followed by the same treatment at 70 °C. The pellet was treated twice at 20 and 70 °C with H_2O (7 hours). The pooled supernatants were treated with $CaCl_2$ (2 mol l^{-1}, 5 hours), centrifuged and the pellet dialyzed (1 kDa) and freeze dried	Foley et al. (2011)
Ascophyllum nodosum, *Fucus vesiculous*	Laminarin, galactofucans	$CaCl_2$ (1%, 85 °C, 4 hours) followed by centrifugation (16 887× *g*, 20 minutes). The supernatant was precipitated with ethanol (1 hours) and reprecipitated with ethanol (−20 °C, 48 hours). The pellets were dialyzed (15 kDa) and freeze dried	Kim (2012)
Sargassum swartzii	Sulfated polysaccharides	H_2O (90–95 °C, 16 hours) followed by filtration and concentration. The extract was precipitated with ethanol, centrifuged, and the pellet dehydrated with CH_3OCH_3	Vijayabaskar et al. (2012)
Laminaria japonica	Fucoidan	H_2O (120 °C, 3 hours) followed by filtration and addition of $MgCl_2$ and ethanol (85%) and filtered again. The new filtrate was dialyzed (3.6 kDa, 24 hours), precipitated with ethanol (95%, 3×). The pellet was dried (80 °C)	Wang et al. (2012a)

Table 10.2 *(continued)*

Algae	Polysaccharide	Extraction media and protocol	Reference
Sargassum vulgare	Fucoidan	Protease in NaCl (0.25 mol l^{-1}, pH 8, 60 °C, 24 hours) followed by filtration, precipitation with acetone (0.3, 0.5, 1, and 1.5 volumes) and collection of precipitates generated by the different volumes for freeze drying	Dore et al. (2013)
Sargassum binderi	Fucoidan	$CaCl_2$ (2%, 85 °C, 24 hours, 6×). The combined supernatants were treated with 10% $CH_3(CH_2)15N(Br)(CH_3)_3$, followed by centrifugation (3000 × *g*, 10 minutes) and the pellet washed several times with H_2O and ethanol (20%) and dialyzed (2 kDa)	Lim et al. (2014)
Laminaria hyperborea, Ascophyllum nodosum	Laminarin	Sonication 15 minutes at 20 °C with HCl (0.1 mol l^{-1}) and water, followed by centrifugation and precipitation of the supernatant with ethanol (4 °C, overnight). The mixture was centrifuged and the pellet freeze dried	Kadam et al. (2015b)
Alaria angusta	Galactofucan	HCl (0.1 mol l^{-1}, 60 °C, 2 hours, 2×) followed by centrifugation, dialysis of supernatant, and freeze drying	Menshova et al. (2015)
Ascophyllum nodosum	Fucoidan	Microwave treatment (120 °C, 15 minutes) with biomass in HCl (0.1 mol l^{-1}). The mixture was dried (80 °C), redissolved in $CaCl_2$ (2%, 4 °C, overnight) followed by centrifugation and ethanol precipitation of the supernatant	Yuan and Macquarrie (2015)
Sargassum fusiforme	Fucoidan	H_2O (100 °C) followed by concentration and centrifugation. The supernatant was precipitated with ethanol (95%) and the pellet treated with $CaCl_2$ (2%) and freeze dried	Cong et al. (2016)

Table 10.2 (*continued*)

Algae	Polysaccharide	Extraction media and protocol	Reference
Sargassum swartzii	Fucoidan	HCl (0.05 mol l^{-1}, 20 °C, 24 hours, 2×). Supernatants mixed with $CaCl_2$ (4%, 4 °C, overnight) followed by centrifugation and ethanol precipitation of supernatant and dialysis of the pellet	Dinesh et al. (2016)
Sargassum galaucescens	Fucoidan	H_2O (85 °C, 1 hours) followed by centrifugation (3870 × *g*, 10 minutes). The supernatant was precipitated with ethanol (20% to precipitate alginic acid) and then 50% followed by centrifugation and drying (40 °C)	Huang et al. (2016)
Coccophora langsdorfii	Laminarin, fucoidan, and alginates	HCl (0.1 mol l^{-1}, 20 °C, 2×) and the supernatant neutralized with $NaHCO_3$ (3%) to pH 5.7–6.1, followed by concentration, dialysis, and freeze drying	Imbs et al. (2016)
Sargassum sp., *Fucus vesiculosus*, *Ascophyllum nodosum*, *Lessonia nigrescence*, *Kjellmaniella crassifolia*, *Costaria costata*	Fucoidan	H_2O (80 °C, 3 hours, 3×), followed by centrifugation (5000 rpm, 10 minutes). Supernatants were precipitated with ethanol (80%) and the pellet washed in several steps with ethanol-acetone and centrifuged each time until final dialysis and freeze drying	Shan et al. (2016)

Table is adapted with permission from Garcia-Vaquero et al. (2017).

Hot water extraction is the most commonly used technique for algal polysaccharide isolation (Zhang et al. 2010), and is regarded as a widely held and expedient procedure in this regard (Savage 2012). This procedure, however, has certain shortcomings as it requires operation at extreme temperatures, is extremely time-consuming, and above all, its extraction efficiency is quite low (Xu et al. 2017). For example, *P. haitanensis* was extracted by hot water at 90 °C for 2 hours, and the yield of polysaccharide was 4.1% (Xu et al. 2019). It is for this reason that new extraction methodologies have been developed in order to achieve greater efficiency in relation to yield, extraction time, and working budget, and to lower the environmental hazards associated with such extraction by reducing the energy requirements of the whole operation (Barba et al. 2015; Kadam et al. 2013).

10.3.1.2 Microwave Assisted Extraction A number of desired compounds have been isolated from plants (Vinatoru et al. 2017) as well as algae (Gilbert-López et al. 2016) using microwave assisted extraction including polysaccharides, flavonoids, terpenoids, alkaloids, and tannins. This technique has also been successfully employed for polysaccharide extraction from algal biomass; for example, fucoidan has been isolated from *F. vesiculosus* (Rodriguez-Jasso et al. 2011), *Undaria pinnatifida* (Quitain et al. 2013), and *Ascophyllum nodosum* (Yuan and Macquarrie 2015) using this technique. The spectral frequency of microwaves is 300–300 000 MHz representing electromagnetic energy created by the coupling of electrical and magnetic fields. Response surface methodology has been used to optimize the parameters (irradiation time, microwave power, temperature, and solid : liquid ratio) of microwave assisted extraction (Sousa et al. 2010).

This method is clearly advantageous over conventional methods of organic solvent extraction because it lowers the energy requirement, cost, and extraction time, and at the same time increases the efficiency of extraction (Hahn et al. 2012). For example, in contrast to a lengthier extraction time of 3 hours required for conventional extraction protocols, a much shorter duration of 15 minutes has been reported for extraction of fucoidan using microwave assisted extraction (Yuan and Macquarrie 2015). Moreover, valued lower molecular weight (5–30 kDa) products have been reportedly produced from previously isolated fucoidans using this technique (You et al. 2010). Microwave assisted extraction, however, can affect the quality of the extracted polysaccharide as a result of degradation due to high temperatures. Heat-sensitivity of certain compounds might accrue damage because this technique generates heat in the course of extraction (Michalak and Chojnacka 2014). A variation in the viscosity and molecular weights of polysaccharides extracted using this method, for example, could be observed depending on the temperatures maintained during the process (Tsubaki et al. 2016). Hence, a consideration of microwave parameters in relation to their effects on polysaccharide degradation, sulfate content, molecular weights, monosaccharide composition, and viscosity is warranted beforehand (Rodriguez-Jasso et al. 2011).

10.3.1.3 Ultrasonic Assisted Extraction Unlike microwave assisted extraction, ultrasonic assisted extraction does not rely on heat generation for the extraction of polysaccharides. In ultrasonic assisted extraction, disruption of cell walls and reduction in particle size to facilitate solvent–compound interactions is achieved by transformation of soundwaves into mechanical energy brought about by induction of pressure variations generating growing and collapsing cavitation as soundwaves migrate through the medium (Michalak and Chojnacka 2014; Ying et al. 2011). This technique is growing in popularity and is used extensively for polysaccharide extraction from dried algal biomass (Kadam et al. 2013, 2015b; Wijesekara et al. 2011). Previously isolated polysaccharides from *Porphyridium cruentum* have also been subjected to this treatment resulting in the production of lower molecular weight compounds with improved physicochemical and biological characteristics (Sun et al. 2012).

In comparison with traditional solvent extraction techniques, ultrasonic assisted extraction has obvious advantages including higher yield and reduced extraction time (Kadam et al. 2015a). For example, the ultrasound assisted extraction of brown algae, *F. evanescens* was carried at room temperature for 15 minutes while hot water extraction use extraction at 60 °C for 6 hours (Hmelkov et al. 2018).

Moreover, this technique can easily be scaled up for industrial application and its operating cost is much lower than the other modern isolation procedures

(Garcia-Vaquero et al. 2017). Similarly, it offers lower solvent consumption, higher automation level, and can be combined with other techniques like superfluid assisted extraction and microwave assisted extraction (Ibañez et al. 2012).

10.3.1.4 Enzymatic Extraction The growing popularity of enzymatic extraction is due to the ability of enzymes used in the process to hydrolyze algal cell walls and to disrupt intricate internal storage compounds thereby releasing intracellular polysaccharides (Rodrigues et al. 2015; Wijesinghe and Jeon 2012a). With regard to chemical and structural characteristics, algal cells are far more complex than land plants (Garcia-Vaquero et al. 2017). An appropriate enzyme mixture as well as optimum activity conditions, particularly temperature and pH, are the prerequisites for suitable product recovery (Jeon et al. 2011). Agarase (EC 3.2.1.81), amyloglucosidase (EC 3.2.1.3), alcalase™, protamex™, carrageenanase (EC 3.2.1.83), kojizyme™, cellucast™, neutrase™, viscozyme™, termamyl™, umamizyme™, flavourzyme™, ultraflo-Max™, and xylanase (EC 3.2.1.8) are the main commercially available enzymes currently being widely used in enzymatic extraction (Heo et al. 2005; Jeon et al. 2011; Kang et al. 2011). These enzymes have been reported to show optimum catalytic activity at pH 3.8–8.0 and a temperature of 40–60 °C (Jeon et al. 2011).

Enzymatic extraction is superior to conventional solvent mediated extractions because of its high specificity and catalytic efficiency, and mild reaction conditions (Kulshreshtha et al. 2015). This technique has also been reported to increase polysaccharide yield from algal biomass (Hardouin et al. 2016). For example, Hardouin et al. (2014) have compared the use of carbohydrases (cellulase, xylanase, β-glucanase, and arabinase), and traditional water extraction of *Ulva* sp. They got higher dry matter yields (51%) when using the carbohydrases compared with water extraction (28.8%) (Hardouin et al. 2014). Moreover, due to their environmentally friendly nature and nontoxicity, and since the enzymes used are essentially food-grade and the process can easily be scaled up (Michalak and Chojnacka 2014), this technique offers an advantageous alternative for polysaccharide extraction for food uses. The high cost of the enzymes used, nonetheless, limits use in industrial operations (Hahn et al. 2012; Michalak and Chojnacka 2014).

10.3.2 Purification

The polysaccharides after being extracted are essentially a mixture with variable monosaccharide composition and sulfate content in addition to small quantities of proteins and phenolics, which might possess their own bioactivities (Ale et al. 2011). Hence, purification of the extracted polysaccharides is necessary in order to ascertain their biological importance and/or to produce the product in its pure form. Prior to ascertaining their biological activities, the extracted polysaccharides are frequently subjected to one or more purifications in order to obtain extracts abundantly enriched with desired polysaccharides (Jin et al. 2013; Wang et al. 2012b).

10.3.2.1 Membrane Filtration Membrane filtration is employed in order to fractionate polysaccharides on the basis of their molecular weights. A number of "molecular weight cut-off" membranes are commercially available (Xie et al. 2014), with the potential to be used for algal polysaccharide separation. In fact, various types of membrane filtrations such as reverse osmosis, nanofiltration, and ultrafiltration are the focus of consideration as potential industrial separation techniques for MAP (Patel et al. 2013). Current literature describes the main utility of this technique as a means for salt removal from the extracted polysaccharides in one or more filtration steps (Anastyuk et al. 2010). Membrane filtration has been successfully used for the separation of laminarin from fucoidan, and for fractionation of other polysaccharides from algae (Hjelland et al. 2012).

Since large volumes can be separated using filtration processes and such processes can easily be automated, they work well in relation to preliminary industrial-scale extractions and purifications (Patel et al. 2013). However, reduction in performance due to excessive membrane-fouling, requirements for elevated energy inputs, and a recurrent need to clean or replace the membrane thwart their wide use (Marcati et al. 2014). It is pertinent to mention that diafiltration (Patel et al. 2013) or successive ultrafiltration in combination with diafiltration using membranes with declining molecular weight cut-off (Marcati et al. 2014), nonetheless, have been recommended for countering fouling and improving membrane-efficiency.

10.3.2.2 Ion-Exchange Chromatography Ion-exchange chromatography separates molecules on the basis of their respective charges. It is a commonly used technique in a wide range of laboratory and industrial applications. An alteration in the concentration and/or pH of the elution buffer elutes molecules of charged solute adsorbed on an immobilized resin comprising oppositely charged ion-exchange groups (Rieman and Walton 2013). The reasons for the widespread applicability of this technique include elevated performance, enhanced resolution, lower running cost, huge sample-handling capability, and automation.

This type of chromatographic separation is particularly suited to experiments wherein neutral or acidic polysaccharides are to be separated from negatively charged polysaccharides through gradient salt elution or alterations in pH (Anastyuka et al. 2017; Shi et al. 2018; Usoltseva et al. 2016). A diethylaminoethyl-A25 anion-exchange column has been successfully employed for the fractionation of *L. japonica* water-extracted samples where gradient elution was performed with 0.7–0.8 $mol\,l^{-1}$ NaCl yielding fucoidan (Peng et al. 2012).

Likewise, sulfated polysaccharides, with net-negative charge, can be purified using the anion-exchange chromatographic technique wherein immobilized positively charged resins are used for the adsorption of solute molecules (Garcia-Vaquero et al. 2017). For instance, the linkages of sulfate ester groups to the carbohydrate backbone in fucoidans confer a strong anionic charge to them, which is stable even at lower pH values. Anion-exchange chromatography, hence, can be employed for the purification of fucoidans and other negatively charged polysaccharides. In fact, fucoidan has been purified using this technique using a linear salt (NaCl) gradient (Dinesh et al. 2016; Imbs et al. 2016; Menshova et al. 2015; Wang et al. 2012a) as well as stepwise NaCl gradient (Anastyuk et al. 2012b; Cong et al. 2016). The degree of sulfation of various fucoidan fractions can be utilized for their further separation through anion-exchange chromatography. With stronger interactions with the immobilized resin, highly sulfated fucoidan fractions generally necessitate elevated salt concentrations for their elution (Garcia-Vaquero et al. 2017). Fucoidan fractions exhibiting diverse physicochemical characteristics can, therefore, be conveniently purified using anion-exchange chromatography (Hahn et al. 2012).

10.3.2.3 Size-Exclusion Chromatography A porous matrix composed of physically and chemically stable inert constituents is utilized for the separation of analytes on the basis of size differences, as they pass through it, in a chromatographic technique known as size-exclusion chromatography. This technique has been extensively employed for the separation and purification of polysaccharides from a wide range of algal species (Arman and Qader 2012; Tong et al. 2017) including *Saccharina japonica*, *L. saccharina*, *M. nitidum*, and *Gracilariopsis lemaneiformis*. In contrast to ion-exchange chromatography, separation in size-exclusion chromatography is not directly affected by composition of the elution buffer as this technique does not rely upon a binding between analytes and the separation matrix (Garcia-Vaquero et al. 2017). A noteworthy advantage of this chromatographic technique, therefore, lies in its flexibility in the use of elution buffer best suited for the preservation or additional decontamination of the analyte after it has been separated by ion-exchange chromatography or another process (Mori and Barth 2013).

Size-exclusion chromatography also offers an extended diversity in the choice of column being used. Similarly, the columns can either be used individually (one column at a time) such as PL-Aquagel-OH™, Sepharose™ CL-6B, Superdex™ 200, or Sephacryl™ S-300 (Cong et al. 2016; Wang et al. 2012b), or in combination such as TSK-gel™ G4000 SW-XL, and TSK-gel G3000 SW-XL (Foley et al. 2011). This technique can be utilized for molecular weight-dependent fractionation of fucoidans and laminarins (Garcia-Vaquero et al. 2017) as well as for desalination of analytes purified via highly saline buffers during anion-exchange chromatography (Hahn et al. 2012).

10.3.2.4 Affinity Chromatography Reversible interactions between analytes and a particular immobilized ligand form the basis for affinity chromatographic separation wherein a diverse range of compounds are purified based on their bio-functionality or distinct chemical structure (Dunlap 2013). In contrast to nonspecific ionic interactions in ion-exchange chromatography, separation in affinity chromatography is based on highly specific interactions between biomolecules. Some illustrations of affinity chromatographic separation comprise specific interactions between antibody–antigen, enzyme–substrate, and enzyme–inhibitor.

This technique has been successfully utilized for the separation and purification of various algal polysaccharides. For instance, immobilized cationic dyes, toluidine and methylene blue (Hahn et al. 2016), and toluidine blue and thionine acetate (Zayed et al. 2016), have been effectively used for specific purification of anionic sulfated polysaccharides including fucoidan, carrageenan, and, sulfated rhamnan. In addition, fucoidan has been purified from brown algae with purity levels surpassing that of the commercial fucoidan from Sigma-Aldrich (95%) using a combination of toluidine blue and altered amino-derivatized sepabeads (Hahn et al. 2016).

10.4 Health-Promoting Activities of MAP

MAP have various applications and humans have used macroalgae for millennia due to their macro- and micronutrients. With advances in research, the polysaccharides derived from marine algae are distinctive from the polysaccharides found in terrestrial plants. The bioactivities of polysaccharides are potentially related to their chemical and physical structures (Cheong et al. 2015). Indeed, the unique polysaccharides obtained from macroalgae such as agars, alginates, carrageenans, fucoidans, ulvans, and laminarans, have been reported to exhibit unique and effective bioactivities associated with their distinctive structural features (Table 10.3). These understandings help the researchers to study the application of seaweeds in various fields.

Several preclinical studies have reported that MAP possess a range of biological activities such as antioxidant, anticoagulant, anticancer, antiviral, antiallergenic, antiadhesive, antiangiogenic, and anti-inflammatory activities (Cardoso et al. 2016; Kadam et al. 2015b; Posocco et al. 2015; Ruocco et al. 2016; Wang et al. 2014). The potent activities of seaweed polysaccharides could play an important role in formulating products in the nutraceutical, pharmaceutical, and cosmeceutical industries. For example, carrageenan and porphyran are important ingredients in some cosmeceutical products as thickening agents due to their gelling properties, while their chemical structure is related to antioxidant and antiwrinkle properties (Cheong et al. 2018). Meanwhile, fucoidan shows promising features as a marine drug in reducing the risk of several cancers including lung, breast, and colon cancers (Atashrazm et al. 2015). Food products, nutraceutical products, or food supplements containing MAP are useful for health promotion and disease risk reduction.

In recent years, there has been growing interest in the application of MAP in health-related fields. In this part, we focus on the ongoing review on MAP and their biological activities including antitumor, antioxidant, immunemodulatory, antihypolipidemic, anticoagulant, anti-infection, and antiproliferative effects.

10.4.1 Antioxidant Activity

The metabolism of oxygen produces reactive oxygen species (ROS) including hydrogen peroxide, superoxide anion, and hydroxyl radicals, which may contribute to various oxidative stress-induced diseases such as cancer, diabetes, cardiovascular, and neuro-degenerative diseases (Xu et al. 2017). Further, several studies have reported that oxidative stress is responsible for causing various types of tumor (Benz and Yau 2008; Valko et al. 2006). Oxidative stress can trigger carcinogenesis by mutating nuclear or mitochondrial DNA, or by damaging the structures of intracellular lipids and proteins. A growing tumor mass may exaggerate intracellular and extracellular oxidative stress, which can transiently or permanently modify its malignant features (Benz and Yau 2008).

The detrimental effects of ROS responsible for inducing diseases and signaling transductions of oxidative stress that lead to damage of the connective tissues are shown in Figure 10.12 (Priyan Shanura Fernando et al. 2019). Enzymes such as superoxide dismutase (SOD) and catalase (CAT) help in scavenging ROS in cells. The Forkhead homebox type-O (FoxO) is one of the key transcription factors that regulate the antioxidant defense in response to oxidative stress (Daitoku et al. 2011). Sirtuin 1 mediates the FoxO deacetylation and its activation is vital (Daitoku et al. 2011). However, phosphorylation by protein kinase B (AKT) could inactivate FoxO transcription factors, which in turn affect SOD and CAT production (Yiu et al. 2010). Thus, antioxidants play an important role in resistance to oxidative stress and the damage induced by external and internal factors including pathogens, pollutants, peroxide, and hydroxyl radicals generated during normal cellular metabolism (Priyan Shanura Fernando et al. 2019).

Table 10.3 List of some bioactive algal polysaccharides with health-promoting activities.

Bioactivity	Polysaccharides	Sources	Reference
Antitumor	Fucoidan, laminaran, carrageenan, mannan	Brown seaweeds (*Saccharina japonica, Alaria angusta, Undaria pinnatifida, Dictyopteris delicatula, Dictyota menstrualis, Laminaria saccharina, Ecklonia cava, Ascophyllum nodosum, Sargassum* spp.), green seaweeds (*Caulerpa prolifera, Monostroma nitidum*), red seaweeds (*Gracilariopsis lemaneiformis*)	Palanisamy et al. (2017b), Ermakova et al. (2011, 2013), Marudhupandi et al. (2015), and Vishchuk et al. (2013)
Immunomodulatory	Fucoidan, carrageenan	Brown seaweeds (*Cladosiphon okamuranus, Hizikia fusiforme, Fucus vesiculosus, Laminaria japonica, Fucus evanescens, Macrocystis pyrifera, Undaria pinnatifida, Ascophyllum nodosum*), red seaweeds (*Kappaphycus striatus, Porphyra haitanensis*)	Fang et al. (2015), Jeong et al. (2015), Khil'chenko et al. (2011), and Zhang et al. (2015)
Anticoagulant	Carrageenan, sulfated rhamnan, fucoidan	Brown seaweeds (*Dictyota cervicornis, Ecklonia cava, Dictyota menstrualis, Laminaria saccharina, Monostroma latissimum*), green seaweeds (*Caulerpa cupressoides, Codium fragile, Codium vermilara, Monostroma latissimum, Ulva fasciata*), red seaweeds (*Agardhiella subulata*)	Athukorala et al. (2006, 2007), Li et al. (2011), and Zoysa et al. (2008)
Antihypolipedemic	Fucoidan, ulvan	Brown seaweeds (*Sargassum polycystum, Sargassum wightii, Laminaria japonica, Fucus vesiculosus, Apostichopus japonicus, Monostroma nitidum, Cystoseira crinite*), green seaweeds (*Ulva lactuca, Ulva pertusa, Enteromorpha prolifera*), red seaweeds (*Gyrodinium impudium*)	Ben Gara et al. (2017), Minh Hien et al. (2015), and Teng et al. (2013)

Table 10.3 (*continued*)

Bioactivity	Polysaccharides	Sources	Reference
Antioxidant	Fucoidan, agar, carrageenan, sulfated rhamnan	Brown seaweeds (*Fucus vesiculosus, Dictyopteris delicatula, Dictyota cervicornis, Laminaria japonica, Sargassum* spp., *Undaria pinnitafida, Turbinaria conoides, Saccharina latissimi*), red seaweeds (*Gracilaria birdiae, Gracilaria chouae, Corallina officinalis, Solieria filiformis*), green seaweeds (*Ulva* spp.)	Huang et al. (2016), Khan et al. (2019), Li et al. (2018), Qi and Sun (2015), and Suresh et al. (2013)
Antiviral	Mannans, sulfated rhamnan, xylan, carrageenan	Brown seaweeds (*Laminaria angustata, Sphacelaria indica, Cystoseira indica*), red seaweeds (*Grateloupia indica, Sebdenia polydactyla, Grateloupia filicinia*), green seaweeds (*Ulva lactuca*)	Elizondo-Gonzalez et al. (2012), Lopes et al. (2017), Pujol et al. (2012), Thuy et al. (2015), Wang et al. (2017a), and Yue et al. (2017)
Antimicrobial	Fucoidan, laminaran	Brown seaweeds (*Laminaria japonica, Spatoglossum asperum Sargassum spp*), red Seaweeds (*Gracilaria corticata, Porphyridium cruentum, Gracilaria ornate*)	Kadam et al. (2015a), Liu et al. (2017a), Marudhupandi and Kumar (2013), and Palanisamy et al. (2017a)

ROS can regulate nuclear factor kappa-B (NF-κB) activation through activating and inactivating the IκB kinases (IKK) complex leading to an effect on the downstream targets via oxidation and phosphorylation. After the dimer is released from IκB to the nucleus, related transcriptional factors are regulated by ROS through the NF-κB signaling pathway (Geoffrey et al. 2006). Meanwhile, ROS accumulation is implicated in activating signal transduction pathways and has been shown to phosphorylate cell surface receptors, which in turn activate the mitogen-activated protein kinase (MAPK) signaling pathway, leading to sustained activation of the Jun N-terminal kinase (JNK) and p38 pathways (Visalini and Piva 2010).

In vitro experiments of antioxidant activities are generally determined by 2,2-diphenyl-1-picrylhydrazyl (DPPH) radical scavenging, lipid peroxide inhibition, ferric reducing antioxidant power, nitric oxide (NO) scavenging, 2,2-azino-bis(3-ethylbenzothiazoline sulfonic acid) (ABTS) radical scavenging (Huang et al. 2016), superoxide radical and hydroxyl radical scavenging assays (Karadag et al. 2009).

The antioxidant mechanism of sulfated polysaccharides is to form stable macromolecular radicals through the sulfate groups owing to electron delocalization on the molecule structure (Chen et al. 2009). This may be attributed to the free radical accepting an electron from the lone-pair electron of sulfate groups to form a stable free radical ion, e.g. the electron transfer from the sulfate group of sulfated polysaccharide to the free radical to form a stable free radical ion (Chen et al. 2009).

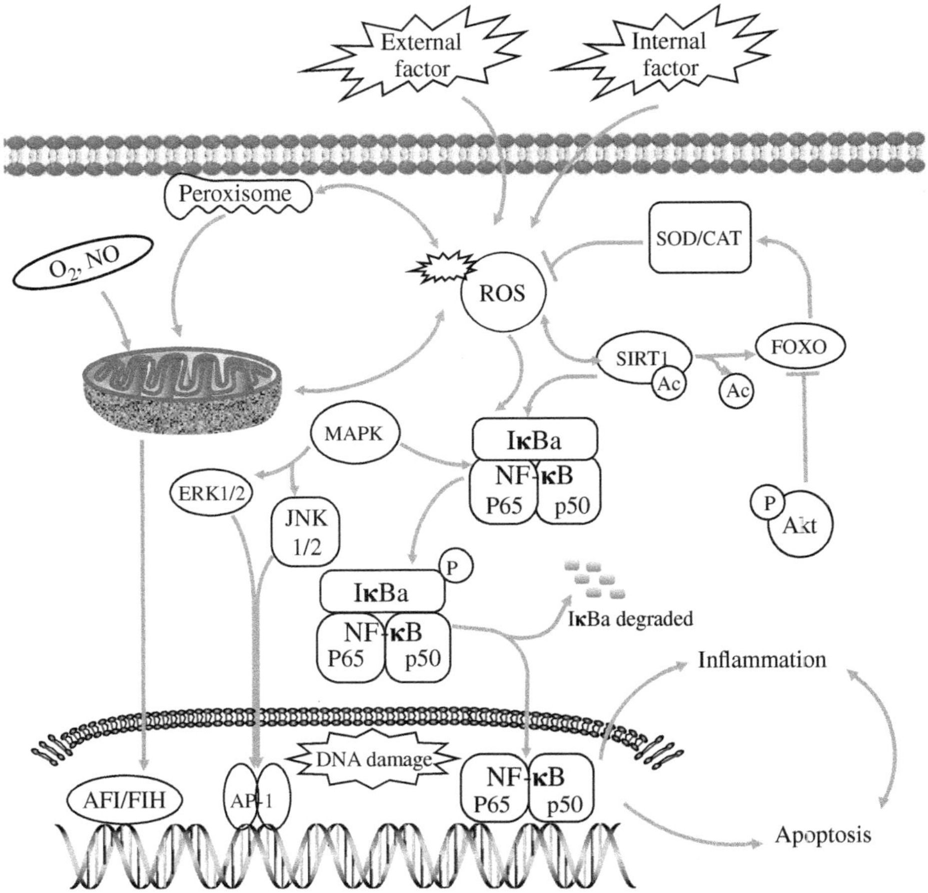

Figure 10.12 Reactive oxygen species-induced tissue damage. Summarized signaling pathways involved in oxidative stress-induced pathologic events diseases including neurodegeneration, cancer, kidney disease, cardiovascular diseases, and diabetes. Source: from Ray et al. (2015).

In the view of Kim et al. (2007) the fucoidan from *Sargassum fulvellum* showed stronger scavenging activity of NO than butylated hydroxyanisole (Kim et al. 2007). Crude fucoidan extracted from *Sargassum glaucescens* showed antioxidant activity with concentration dependence (Huang et al. 2016). The half maximal inhibitory concentration (IC_{50}) value on DPPH radical scavenging activity and ferrous ion chelating effect were 4.30 and 0.65 mg ml^{-1}, respectively. It also exhibited reducing power in a dose-dependent manner (Huang et al. 2016). Fucoidan from *Sargassum plagiophyllum* showed the maximum inhibition of 36.60, 42.12, and 32.12% on DPPH scavenging, hydroxyl, and superoxide radical scavenging activity, respectively, at the concentration of 5 mg ml^{-1} (Suresh et al. 2013). Sulfated polysaccharides from *Solieria filiformis* also possess DPPH radical scavenging ability and molybdate ion reducing ability with an IC_{50} value of 1.77 and 2.01 mg ml^{-1}, respectively, while chelating ferrous ability with maximum activity of 38.98% chelation at 4 mg ml^{-1}. All these antioxidant activities are exhibited in a dose-dependent manner (Sousa et al. 2016).

Antioxidant properties of polysaccharides such as carrageenans and ulvans also depend on their sulfate content (Ngo and Kim 2013). Jimenez-Escrig et al. (2015) studied the antioxidant activity of polysaccharide extracted from *S. latissima*. This study suggested that polysaccharide showed ABTS radical scavenging ability and the acid-soluble fractions that contain fucans exhibited greater antioxidant activity than alginate and laminaran extracted from *Turbinaria conoides* seaweed (Jimenez-Escrig et al. 2015). The fucoidan extracted from *Sargassum polycystum* exhibited potent antioxidant activities in a concentration-dependent manner (Palanisamy et al. 2017a).

In our previous study, the antioxidant activity of *Gelidium amansii* polysaccharides can be enhanced after digestion by agarase (Xu et al. 2018). These findings were similar to the report of Kang et al. (2014), who explained that Celluclast-degraded agaro-oligosaccharides exhibited ABTS and DPPH radical scavenging, which was possibly dependent on the degree of the hydrolysis (Kang et al. 2014). In general, the antioxidant activity of the marine algae discussed above showed maximum activity with degraded polysaccharide of low molecular weight, which suggests that the antioxidant activity is highly related to molecular weight.

A *Sargassum fusiforme* polysaccharide displayed protective properties on cyclophosphamide-induced immune suppressed mice (Wang et al. 2013). The hepatic SOD and glutathione levels of the cyclophosphamide-induced immune suppressed mice were significantly decreased, while administration of *S. fusiforme* polysaccharide (200 mg kg^{-1} body weight) significantly increased the SOD and glutathione (GSH) activities. Zhang et al. (2003) reported that a *P. haitanensis* porphyran could increase total antioxidant capacity and the activity of SOD and glutathione peroxidase in aging mice tested in all the organs (Zhang et al. 2003). The levels of serum SOD and glutathione peroxidase in a MAP-treated group (250 mg kg^{-1} body weight) increased considerably by 51.2 and 99.6% compared with the control group (Wang et al. 2017b). Similar results were also reported with ulvan, which significantly decreased malondialdehyde, and increased CAT and SOD compared with the hyperlipidemic group. These results suggested that ulvan can decrease the effect of oxidative stress via regulating antioxidant enzymes and lipid metabolism (Li et al. 2018).

Qi et al. (2005) compared the *in vitro* antioxidant activity of natural ulvan and chemically modfied ulvan, i.e. high sulfate content derivatives of ulvan prepared with sulfur trioxide/N,N-dimethylformamide in formamide. The molecules of these derivatives with –OH groups substituted by $-OSO_3H$ groups exhibited stronger antioxidant activity. Results showed that at the concentration of 23 μg ml^{-1}, natural ulvan showed a 75.1% scavenging effect of superoxide radical, whereas high sulfate content ulvan showed 94.3% at the same concentration. The high sulfate ulvan showed a stronger scavenging effect on hydroxyl radical with the EC_{50} of 0.46 mg ml^{-1} than natural ulvan. But the influence of sulfate content on reducing power was not significant (Qi et al. 2005). Similarly, *in vivo* antioxidant activity also confirmed that high sulfate content ulvan demonstrated stronger antioxidant activity *in vivo* than ulvan, and especially increased the levels of SOD and GSH-Px in the liver at the dose of 250 and 125 mg kg^{-1}, respectively (Qi and Sun 2015).

10.4.2 Immunomodulatory Activity

Polysaccharides can activate the immune system by interacting with and triggering several signal pathways (Xu et al. 2017). The most important cells of the innate immune system are the macrophages. The macrophages play a significant role in modulating the adaptive immune response. which includes phagocytosis, functioning of antigen-presenting cells, and activation of T lymphocytes (Iwasaki and Medzhitov 2010). A schematic presentation of the cellular and molecular events of the immune system activated by MAP is shown in Figure 10.13.

A polysaccharide extracted from *P. haitanensis*, a red algae, can increase the phagocytic cell action in RAW264.7 macrophages (Liu et al. 2017b). This polysaccharide increased NO production by inducing the signaling pathways such as Janus kinase and the JNK in RAW264.7 macrophages. Results showed that sulfated polysaccharide from *P. haitanensis* plays key roles in immune-regulation and increases the levels of serum cytokines (interleukins [ILs]-10 and tumor necrosis factor [TNF]-α) (Liu et al. 2017b).

A fucoidan extracted from a brown alga, *Hizikia fusiforme*, increases the production of NO and induces the expression of nitric oxide synthase in RAW264.7 macrophages (Jeong et al. 2015). The *in vitro* immune-modulating activity of polysaccharide extracted from *H. fusiforme* showed a potential stimulating effect on murine macrophage and splenocytes (Jeong et al. 2015). It also induced the production of NO and proinflammatory cytokines in RAW 264.7 cells and splenocytes (Jeong et al. 2015).

Significant stimulation of macrophages was displayed by the polysaccharide isolated from *L. japonica*, a brown alga (Fang et al. 2015). It also enhanced cytokine production, including TNF-α, IL-1β, IL-6, and -10. This polysaccharide showed promising effects on the phosphorylation of extracellular signal regulated kinase (ERK1/2), JNK1/2, and P38 (Fang et al. 2015). A unique water-soluble homogeneous polysaccharide from *L. japonica* exhibited potential in immunostimulation through the activation of toll-like receptor 4 of MAPK and NF-κB signaling pathways (Fang et al. 2015).

Fucoidan extracted from *F. evanescens*, a brown alga, increased the stimulation and maturation of dendritic cells, which is significant in the function of immune systems (Khil'chenko et al. 2011). This study proposed that fucoidan induced the maturation of dendritic cells facilitated by the production of TNF-α and activated the MAPK p38, phosphoinositide-3 kinase, and glycogen synthase kinase 3 signaling pathways.

Zhang et al. (2015) described the activation of mouse NK cells stimulated by fucoidans obtained from *A. nodosum*, *Macrocystis pyrifera*, *U. pinnatifida*, and *Fucus vesuculosus*. The fucoidan extracted from *U. pinnatifida* exhibited its potential effects as a result of increased NK cells (Zhang et al. 2015). Jeong et al. (2012) reported that fucoidan showed cytoprotective ability on dendritic cells against 5-fluorouracil in cell viability and size. The 5-fluorouracil is as an anticancer drug used in the treatment of several types of cancer but it has the side effect of damaging immune cells and, thus, results in decreased immune function in 5-fluorouracil-treated patients. However, results indicated that fucoidan might have the ability to retain the immunity of cancer patients (Jeong et al. 2012).

Sulfated polysaccharides extracted from marine macroalgae may be able to inhibit the adhesion of *Helicobacter pylori* and also the reduction of biofilm formation (Besednova et al. 2015). The effect of MAP on infection produced by *H. pylori* was correlated to their activities on cells of innate and adaptive immunity. MAP could

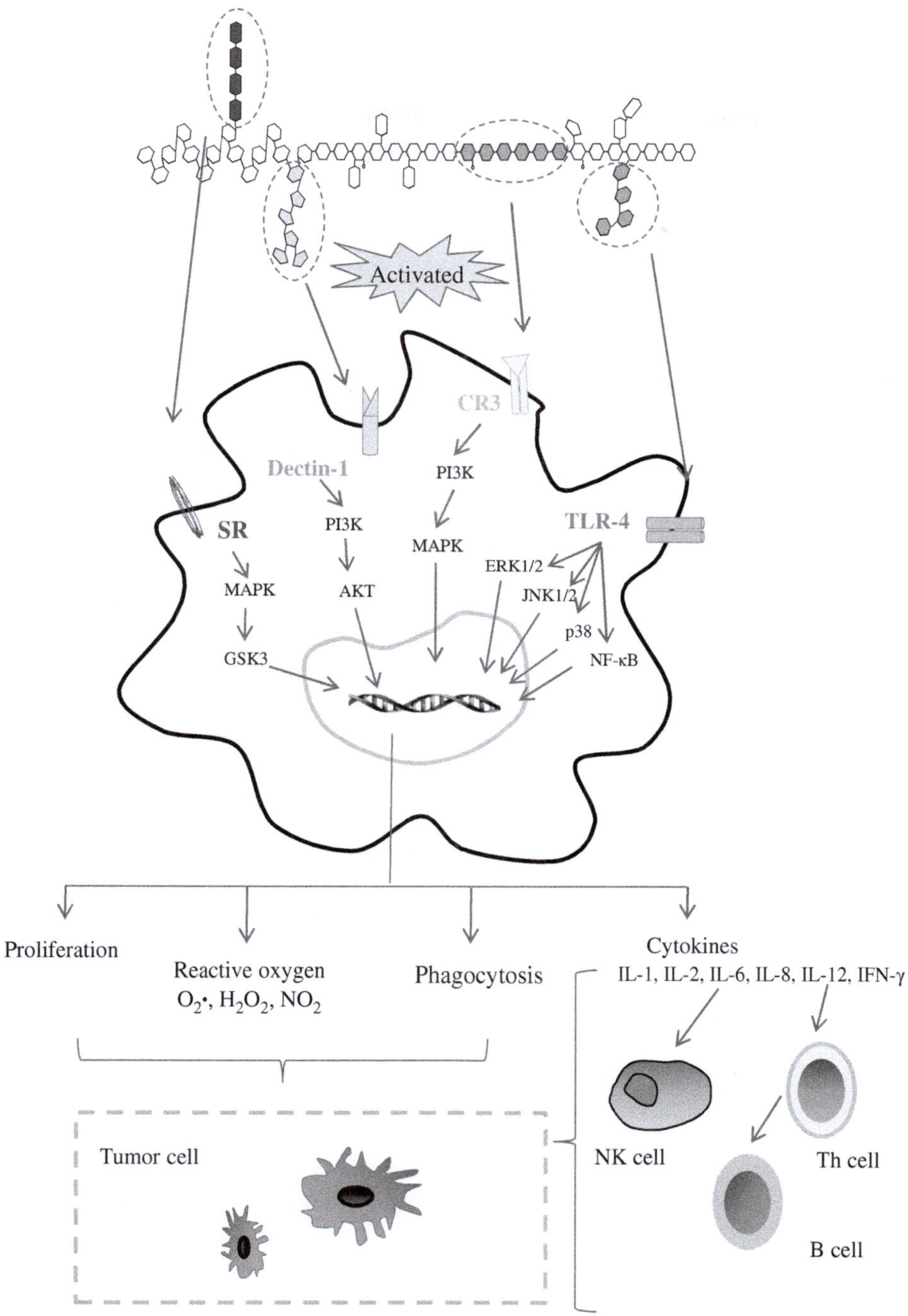

Figure 10.13 Schematic presentation of the immune system activated by marine algae polysaccharides after interaction of several molecular events. Akt: protein kinase B; CR3: complement receptor 3; ERK1/2: extracellular signal regulated kinase 1/2; GSK3: glycogen synthase kinase 3-β; IFN: interferon; IL: interleukin; JNK1/2: c-Jun N-terminal kinase 1/2; MAPK: mitogen-activated protein kinase; PAK: p21-activated kinase; PI3K: phosphatidylinositol-3 kinase; SR: scavenger receptor; TLR-4: toll-like receptor 4; and TNF-α: tumor necrosis factor-α. Source: Reproduced with permission from Xu et al. (2017), published by Marine Drugs.

act at the membrane level by modulating the activity of key signal transduction and also could alter the early phases of activation of immune-competent cells (Besednova et al. 2015).

Since there is no evidence regardig the sensitivity, toxicity, and concentration effect of polysaccharides, it is important to study the toxicological and potential harmful effects of polysaccharide on human cells and *in vivo*.

10.4.3 Anticancer Activity

Cancer is a disease where the cells divide rapidly, spread into neighboring tissues, and form tumors. Cancer is one of the main causes of death worldwide, so there is a need to find potential anticancer drugs, which remains an ultimate challenge. The aim of the treatment is to kill the cancer-causing cells without damaging the normal cells. Therefore, there is a need to find compounds with antitumor properties that can act on specific cell with less adverse effects. Algal polysaccharides have been broadly considered as anticancer agents (Andrade et al. 2018). In order to review the data available in the references, selected MAP with good *in vitro* anticancer activities are shown in Table 10.4.

Treatment with sulfated polysaccharides from *Sargassum vulgare* inhibited the proliferation of HeLa and B16 cells, without damaging the endothelial cells (Guerra Dore et al. 2013). Extracted carrageenan oligosaccharides from the red alga *Kappaphycus striatus* inhibited transplantable sarcoma cell growth, induced phagocytic cell action, improved the production of antibodies and proliferation of lymphocytes, and also enhanced the activity of NK cells and cytokine levels such as IL-2 and TNF-α (Hu et al. 2006). These results suggested that the examined oligosaccharides exhibited antitumor property by stimulating the immune system (Hu et al. 2006).

An important approach in the progress of anticancer drug development is arresting the cell cycle. Sulfated polysaccharides from *G. oxysperma* exhibited antitumor activity by arresting the cell cycle, through the p53/p21 pathway (Ropellato et al. 2015). Fucoidan extracted from *F. vesiculosus* also arrested the cell cycle in G1 phase and also reduced the HCT116 human colorectal carcinoma cell viability by 60% in a dose-dependent manner (Park et al. 2017). Another important strategy in cancer therapy is the activation of apoptosis. Palanisamy et al. (2017b) studied the effect of fucoidan on an MCF-7 human breast cancer cell line and the results showed that fucoidan extracted from *S. polycystum* exhibited strong anticancer activity. Antiproliferative ability of fucoidan was revealed at 50 μg ml^{-1} in human breast cancer cells and it also induced apoptosis-mediated cell death in cancer cells (Palanisamy et al. 2017b). Glycoprotein isolated from *L. japonica* exhibited anticancer activity against HT-29 cells by stimulation of apoptosis and degradation of DNA through caspase-3, poly(adenosine diphosphate-ribose) polymerase (Go et al. 2010).

Kang et al. (2016) demonstrated that the *G. lemaneiformis* carrageenan exhibited antitumor ability and was thereby demonstrated to be an active antitumor candidate (Kang et al. 2016). Usoltseva et al. (2016) reported that the laminaran and the fucoidan extracted from the brown alga *A. angusta* did not show any significant cytotoxicity on HT-29, T-47D, and SK-MEL-28 cell lines *in vitro*. The fucoidan fraction inhibited the proliferation of HT-29 and T-47D cancer cells, while laminaran inhibited the proliferation of HT-29 cancer cells (Usoltseva et al. 2016).

Table 10.4 *In vitro* anticancer activity of fucoidans.

Sources	Type of cancer	Cell line	Inhibition %	Reference
Sargassum polycystum	Breast	MCF-7	90% at 150 μg ml^{-1}	Palanisamy et al. (2017b)
Turbinaria conoides	Lung	A549	73% at 500 μg ml^{-1}	Marudhupandi et al. (2015)
Fucus evanescens	Melanoma	RPMI-7951	55% at 200 μg ml^{-1}	Vishchuk et al. (2013)
	Breast	T-47D	25% at 200 μg ml^{-1}	Vishchuk et al. (2013)
Costaria costata	Colon	DLD-1	55% at 100 μg ml^{-1}	Ermakova et al. (2011)
	Melanoma	SK-MEL-28	20% at 100 μg ml^{-1}	Ermakova et al. (2011)
Undaria pinnatifida	Breast	T-47D	46% at 200 μg ml^{-1}	Vishchuk et al. (2011)
	Melanoma	SK-MEL-28	34% at 200 μg ml^{-1}	Vishchuk et al. (2011)
	Melanoma	RPMI-7951	40% at 200 μg ml^{-1}	Vishchuk et al. (2013)
	Breast	T-47D	60% at 200 μg ml^{-1}	Vishchuk et al. (2013)
	Alveolar	A549	40% at 800 μg ml^{-1}	Synytsya et al. (2010)
	Cervical	HeLa	70% at 800 μg ml^{-1}	Synytsya et al. (2010)
	Hepatocellular	HepG2	30% at 800 μg ml^{-1}	Synytsya et al. (2010)
	Prostate	PC-3	30% at 800 μg ml^{-1}	Synytsya et al. (2010)
Sargassum sp.	Melanoma	B16	56% at 100 μg ml^{-1}	Ale et al. 2011a
	Lung	Lewis	40% at 1 mg ml^{-1}	Ale et al. 2011a
Fucus vesiculosus	Melanoma	B16	50% at 500 μg ml^{-1}	Wang et al. (2018)
	Prostate	DU-145	90% at 1 mg ml^{-1}	Rui et al. (2017)
	Colon	HCT-116	50% at 150 μg ml^{-1}	Chen et al. (2017b) and Park et al. (2017)
	Colon	HCT-15	62% at 100 μg ml^{-1}	Hyun et al. (2009)
	Colon	HCT-116	36% at 20 μg ml^{-1}	Kim et al. (2010)
	Colon	HT-29	65% at 20 μg ml^{-1}	Kim et al. (2010)
Saccharina japonica	Breast	T-47D	46% at 200 μg ml^{-1}	Vishchuk et al. (2011)
	Melanoma	SK-MEL-28	34% at 200 μg ml^{-1}	Ermakova et al. (2011)
Ecklonia cava	Colon	DLD-1	50% at 100 μg ml^{-1}	Ermakova et al. (2011)
	Melanoma	SK-MEL-28	30% at 100 μg ml^{-1}	Ermakova et al. (2011)
Eisenia bicyclis	Colon	DLD-1	49% at 100 μg ml^{-1}	Ermakova et al. (2013)
	Melanoma	SK-MEL-28	12% at 100 μg ml^{-1}	Ermakova et al. (2013)
Sargassum horneri	Colon	DLD-1	44% at 100 μg ml^{-1}	Ermakova et al. (2011)
	Melanoma	SK-MEL-28	15% at 100 μg ml^{-1}	Ermakova et al. (2011)

10.4.4 Antiviral Activity

The unique structure and complex life cycle of viruses have made the demand for the discovery of antiviral drugs important. Different viruses including human immunodeficiency virus type 1 (HIV-1) developing resistance to available antiviral agents has become a considering obstacle to treating these viral infections (De Clercq 2002). The use of algae derived polysaccharides as a source of antiviral agents was introduced by Gerber and colleagues in 1958 when they revealed the inhibition of mumps and influenza B virus by MAP (Gerber et al. 1958). Numerous studies have reported the

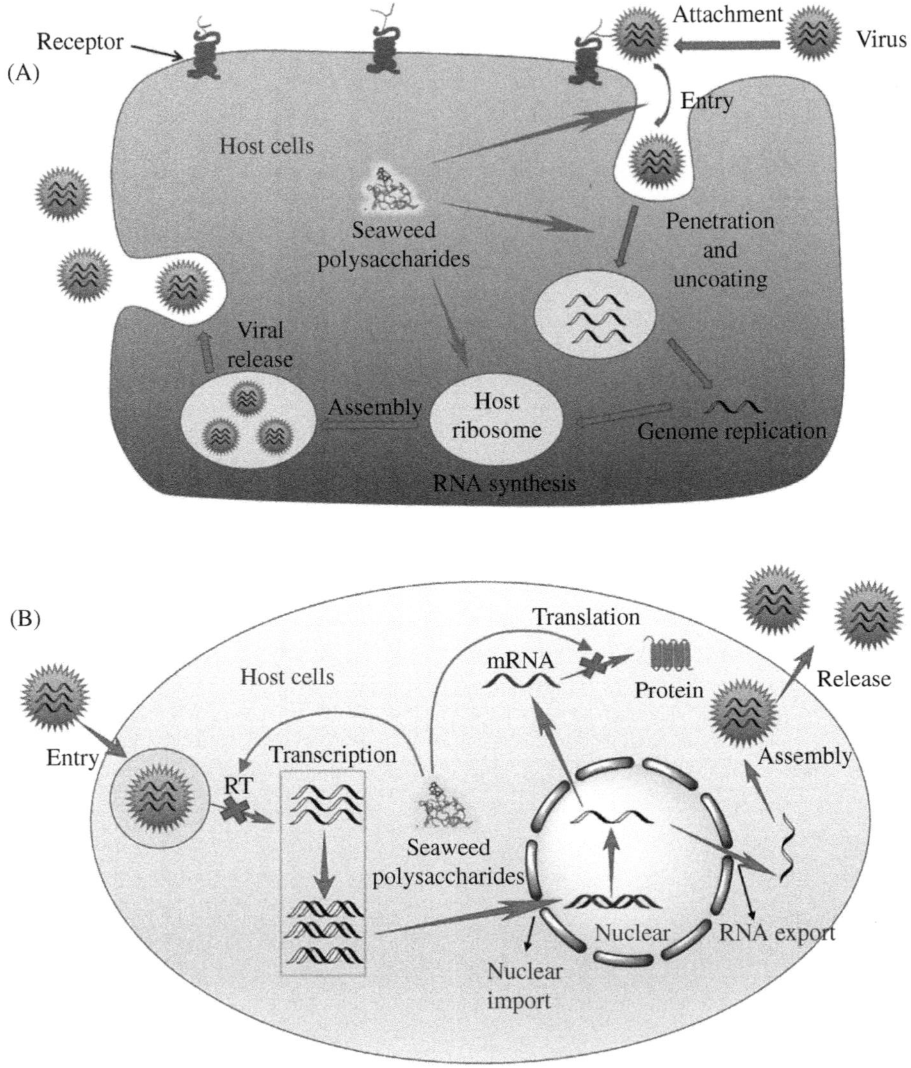

Figure 10.14 Marine algae polysaccharides exert antiviral activities by interfering at different stages of the viral infection process (a) and the mechanism of inhibition of virus replication and transcription (b). Source: figure is adapted with permission from Shi et al. (2017).

potential of polysaccharide fractions extracted from marine algae for their antiviral properties against herpes simplex virus (HSV) and other viruses (Ahmadi et al. 2015; Lopes et al. 2017; Ray et al. 2015). MAP possess unique structures and exert antiviral effects by interfering with different stages of the viral infection process (Bouhlal et al. 2011) (Figure 10.14). MAP also have been found to prevent the viral replication and transcription processes after infection of a host cell; the possible mechanisms are inhibition of intracellular molecules and direct inhibition of viral replication enzymes (Aguilar-Briseño et al. 2015; Fabregas et al. 1999) (Figure 10.14). The advantages of using the MAP are based on their high bioavailability, their low cost, and low initiation

Table 10.5 List of some polysaccharides derived from marine algae with antiviral activity.

Sources	Polysaccharides	Virus	Results (IC_{50})	Reference
Sargassum mcclurei	Fucoidan	HIV[a]	0.96 μg ml^{-1}	Thuy et al. (2015)
Sargassum polycystum	Fucoidan	HIV	0.34 μg ml^{-1}	Thuy et al. (2015)
Turbinara ornata	Fucoidan	HIV	0.39 μg ml^{-1}	Thuy et al. (2015)
Enteromorpha compressa	Ulvan	HSV-1[b]	153 μg ml^{-1}	Lopes et al. (2017)
Grateloupia indica	Sulfated galactans	Dengue virus	0.18 μg ml^{-1}	Pujol et al. (2012)
Scinaia hatei	Xylomannans	Dengue virus	1.1 μg ml^{-1}	Pujol et al. (2012)
Stoechospermum marginatum	Fucans	Dengue virus	6.3 μg ml^{-1}	Pujol et al. (2012)
Sphacelaria indica	Xylogalactofucan	HSV-1	1.3 μg ml^{-1}	Bandyopadhyay et al. (2011)
Scinaia hatei	Sulfated xylomannan	HSV-1 HSV-2	0.6–1.53 μg ml^{-1} 2–1.2 μg ml^{-1}	Ray et al. (2015)
Sargassum swartzii	Fucoidan	HIV-1	1.56 μg ml^{-1}	Dinesh et al. (2016)
Cladosiphon okamuranus	Fucoidan	Newcastle disease virus	0.75 μg ml^{-1}	Elizondo-Gonzalez et al. (2012)
Kjellmaniella crassifolia	Fucoidan	H1N1	34.4 μg ml^{-1}	Wang et al. (2017a)
Gigartina skottsbergii	Carrageenan	BoHV-1[c] SuHV-1[d]	0.52 μg ml^{-1} 10.42 μg ml^{-1}	Diogo et al. (2015)
Laminaria japonica	Acidic polysaccharide	Enterovirus 71	32.6 μg ml^{-1}	Yue et al. (2017)

[a] HIV: human immunodeficiency virus.
[b] HSV: herpes simplex virus.
[c] BoHV: bovine herpesvirus.
[d] SuHV: suid herpesvirus.

of resistance (Wang et al. 2012c). Therefore, MAP are of interest for drugs in general and pharmaceutical discovery of antiviral drugs. In order to review the data available in the references, selected MAP with good antiviral activities are shown in Table 10.5.

Antiviral activities of carrageenans are associated with their molecular weights and the existence of sulfation groups (Wang et al. 2012c). Sun et al. (2017) have conducted experiments on several low molecular weight polysaccharides extracted from *Grateloupia filicinia* and studied their antiviral activity against Avian Leucosis Virus Subgroup J *in vitro* ([ALV-J]; (Sun et al. 2017)). Results showed that lower molecular weight polysaccharides from *G. filicinia* proved to be a strong inhibitor of ALV-J, especially the polysaccharide with molecular weight 8.7 kDa at 200 μg ml^{-1}, which possesses a stronger inhibition. Therefore, lower molecular weight polysaccharides from *G. filicina* might be a worthy choice for ALV-J prevention and treatment (Sun et al. 2017). Moreover, antiviral activity is highly influenced by the sulfate content. The activity was suppressed and enhanced by desulfation and oversulfation of xylomannan in studying the propagation of HSV-1 in Vero cells (Vavilala and D'Souza 2015). Bandyopadhyay et al. (2011) extracted the xylogalactofucan and sulfated polysaccharides from *Sphacelaria indica* and revealed the high anti-HSV *in vitro*. The IC_{50} values of these polysaccharides against HSV were in the range of 0.6–10 μg ml^{-1}. The study proposed that antiviral activity was reliant on the polysaccharide sulfate content (Bandyopadhyay et al. 2011). The *in vivo* antiviral activity of modified carrageenans such as low molecular weight carrageenans (3, 5, and 10 kDa) along with acetylated and sulfated derivatives in mice was examined and revealed that all the carrageenans showed potent inhibition of influenza virus (Tang et al. 2014) at the dose of 30 mg kg^{-1}. In addition, the low molecular weight κ-carrageenan with a sulfation degree of 2.4 and an acetylation degree of 1.0 showed significant antiviral activity (Tang et al. 2014).

Fucoidans extracted from *Sargassum mcclurei*, *S. polycystum*, and *Turbinara ornata* showed potential antiviral effects on HIV at doses of 0.34–0.39 μg ml^{-1} with no cytotoxicity for Vero cell cultures (Thuy et al. 2015). Notably, fucoidan and sulfated fucans showed extremely effective antiviral activities against infections of HSV, H1N1, dengue virus, and Newcastle disease virus at the related doses as summarized in Table 10.5.

Carrageenans are selective inhibitors of HSV and act mainly by suppressing the attachment or introduction of virus into the host cells (Cosenza et al. 2015). Diogo et al. (2015) evaluated the effect of two viral pathogens of veterinary concern along with lambda-carrageenan. The lambda-carrageenan showed effective antiviral ability toward animal viruses that belongs to the Alphaherpesvirinae subfamily, bovine herpesvirus type 1 (BoHV-1) strain Cooper, and suid herpesvirus type 1 (SuHV-1) strain Bartha. For BoHV-1, the IC_{50} was 0.52 μg ml^{-1}, while for SuHV-1 it was 10.42 μg ml^{-1}. Moreover, no cytotoxic effect was observed even when the concentration was increased to 1000 μg ml^{-1} in soluble form. These results demonstrated that lambda-carrageenan might be used as prospective antiviral agents in the veterinary field (Diogo et al. 2015).

Alginate is extracted from brown seaweeds such as *Fucus spiralis*, *F. serratus*, *Bifurcaria bifurcata*, and *L. digitata* has been extensively used as a thickener and gelling agent in the food, cosmetic, and pharmaceutical industries (Wang et al. 2012c). Bandyopadhyay et al. (2011) reported that an alginate from *S. indica* expresses a strong antiviral effect toward HSV with an IC_{50} in the range of 0.6 μg ml^{-1} (Bandyopadhyay et al. 2011).

Chiu et al. (2012) confirmed the antiviral activity of sulfated polysaccharides from *U. lactuca* against Japanese encephalitis virus in Vero cells. The entry of virus into the cells could be hindered by blocking the Japanese encephalitis virus adsorption by sulfated polysaccharide at the concentration of 3 μg ml^{-1} (Chiu et al. 2012). Matsuhiro et al. (2005) revealed the antiviral ability of a sulfated galactan extracted from the red seaweed *Schizymenia binderi* and showed a specific antiviral effect toward HSV types 1 and 2 with less cytotoxicity (Vero cells at a concentration up to 1000 μg ml^{-1}) (Matsuhiro et al. 2005).

10.4.5 Antihyperlipidemic Activity

Hyperlipidemia is a lifestyle disorder that affects human health and may lead to various cardiovascular disorders (Hall et al. 2002). The diagnosis of hyperlipidemia is dependent on an abnormal rise in serum lipid that includes a rise in total triglyceride (TG), total cholesterol (TC), and low-density lipoprotein cholesterol (LDL-C), and the lowering of high-density lipoprotein cholesterol (HDL-C; Boullart et al. 2012). Antihyperlipidemic drugs, such as statins and fibrates, used to adjust the dysfunction of the lipid metabolism may have adverse effects such as asymptomatic elevations in serum creatine kinase levels and severity of muscle injury (myalgia, myositis, and rhabdomyolysis) or have contraindications to statin therapy, including lactation, pregnancy, and active liver disease (Pedro-Botet et al. 2016). Therefore, the interest in dietary fiber or polysaccharides especially derived from marine algae that can have an equivalent lipid-lowering effect without any side effects has increased in recent years.

Supplementation of ulvan extracted from *Ulva pertusa* 250 mg kg^{-1} body weight to Kunming mice, male/female, weighing from 18 to 22 g, fed with a high cholesterol diet for 21 days showed reduction in TC and LDL-C in serum but insignificant effects on serum TG (Qi et al. 2012).

Sulfated polysaccharides extracted from *Enteromorpha prolifera* exhibit lipid-lowering properties in hyperlipidemic animal models (Teng et al. 2013). The hypolipidemic activity of crude sulfated polysaccharides was analyzed in Sprague–Dawley rats fed with a high-fat diet containing 10% (w/w) lard, 15% (w/w) egg yolk powder, 1% (w/w) cholesterol, and commercial diet to 100% (w/w). The hypolipidemic activity included reduction of body weight, TC, TG, LDL, and also decreased liver weights, increased fecal fat, and plasma HDL-C within 6 weeks of the feeding test (Teng et al. 2013). Thus, *E. prolifera* polysaccharide might be a suitable substitute for hypolipidemic sources in humans due to its antihypolipidemic properties (Teng et al. 2013).

Sulfated polysaccharides from *M. nitidum* were purified and studied for bioactivity *in vitro* (Minh Hien et al. 2015). These sulfated polysaccharides stimulated the lipid-loaded hepatocytes and lowered the cellular lipid concentrations more than the controls. Reduction in cellular lipid concentrations was also revealed by quantitative polymerase chain reaction analysis indicating reduced cholesterol synthesis gene expression (such as CYP7A1, LDL-R, and HMG-CoA) and increased expression of the gene responsible for degradation of cholesterol, uptake of LDL, and peroxisomal β-oxidation (Minh Hien et al. 2015). These sulfated polysaccharides also suppressed the expression of genes related to NO synthase, TNF-α, IL-6, IL-8, and visfatin in lipid-loaded hepatocytes (Minh Hien et al. 2015).

Ben Gara et al. (2017) have investigated the potential of sulfated polysaccharide extracted from the Phaeophyta *Cystoseira crinita* to act as a potential hyperlipidemic agent in rats fed with a high-fat diet (Ben Gara et al. 2017). The lipase activity was measured using the amount of 4-methylumbelliferone released by lipase and showed the inhibitory activity of the polysaccharides (100 μg ml^{-1}) on pancreatic lipase. The *in vivo* studies explained the lipase activity of the polysaccharides administered in high-fat diet rats. It inhibited the enzymes (lipase) responsible for lipid metabolism in plasma and small intestine and also considerably reduced the LDL-C and TG levels and increased the HDL-C in blood and subsequently reduced the bodyweight (Ben Gara et al. 2017).

10.4.6 Anticoagulant Activity

Disorders in blood clotting could lead to a greater risk of hemorrhage (bleeding) or thrombosis (clotting). The cardiovascular diseases such as heart diseases and stroke that are associated with clotting are the leading cause of death (Shobharani et al. 2014). Anticoagulants are the substances used to stop blood from coagulating. Heparin is a sulfated polysaccharide present in mammalian tissues and has been used as an anticoagulant for many years (Lindahl 2000). However, heparin has many disadvantages such as difficulties in production, chemical dissimilarities, unpredictable physiological activities, and thrombocytopenia, hemorrhage, as well as serious contraindications (Shobharani et al. 2014). Hence it is necessary to find an alternative to heparin. Sulfated polysaccharides from marine seaweeds that have a similar structure to heparin have also shown anticoagulant activity (Shobharani et al. 2014). Anticoagulant activity was tested by common coagulation examinations such as activated partial thromboplastin time (APTT), thrombin time, and prothrombin time (Wijesinghe and Jeon 2012b).

Athukorala et al. (2006) purified the fucose-containing sulfated polysaccharide from *Ecklonia cava* and evaluated it for its anticoagulant activity including APTT, thrombin time, and prothrombin time. The APTT assay revealed that the purified fucose-containing sulfated polysaccharide showed similar activity at 0.7 $\mu g\,ml^{-1}$ when compared with heparin at the same concentration. Activated coagulation factor assay results demonstrated the inhibition of serine proteases II, X, and VII of the coagulation cascade (Athukorala et al. 2006). Further, Athukorala et al. (2007) evaluated the anticoagulant activity of 22 different algal species and significant anticoagulant activity with high APTT was observed in the fucoidan (molecular weight larger than 30 kDa) extracted from the brown seaweed, *Sargassum horneri* (Athukorala et al. 2007).

Faggio et al. (2016) have assessed the prospective use of sulfated polysaccharides extracted from *Ulva fasciata* and *Agardhiella subulata* as anticoagulant drugs and in which the activity was measured by APTT and prothrombin time tests. Sulfated polysaccharides at 10 $mg\,ml^{-1}$ affected the coagulation cascade by extending the prothrombin time and APTT, and without any cytotoxicity on human red blood cells (Faggio et al. 2016). Li et al. (2011) evaluated the sulfated rhamnan (with a molecular weight of 513 kDa) from *M. latissimum* and found that it demonstrated high anticoagulant activity as estimated by APTT and thrombin time at the concentration of 2–8 $\mu g\,ml^{-1}$ (Li et al. 2011). Further Li et al. (2012) prepared low molecular weight polysaccharide rhamnan by mild acid hydrolysis, named it LMWP, and purified the polysaccharide with a molecular weight of about 33.6 kDa. LMWP at the concentration of 50 $\mu g\,ml^{-1}$ successfully extended the clotting time and also acted as a potential inhibitor of thrombin, which is mediated by heparin cofactor II. The investigation confirmed that LMWP is a sulfated polysaccharide with a unique anticoagulant activity (Li et al. 2012).

Zoysa et al. (2008) isolated the fucose-containing sulfated polysaccharide from *S. fulvellum* using diethylaminoethyl (DEAE) cellulose anion-exchange followed by Sepharose® 4B chromatography. These workers also reported that the sulfated polysaccharide showed a relative clotting factor of 27.47 at concentrations of 180 $\mu g\,ml^{-1}$ (Zoysa et al. 2008).

10.4.7 Antimicrobial Activity

MAP such as alginates, fucoidans, and laminarins have demonstrated good antibacterial activities against bacteria (Vavilala and D'Souza 2015). For example, laminarin-rich extracts prepared using ultrasound and acid solvents had minimum inhibitory concentrations of 13.1 mg ml^{-1} for *Escherichia coli* and *Salmonella typhimurium* and 6.6 and 3.3 mg ml^{-1} for *Staphylococcus aureus* and *Listeria monocytogenes* (Kadam et al. 2015a). The polysaccharides kill the bacteria by damaging the cell membrane (Pérez et al. 2016). This is proposed to be due to the polysaccharides attaching themselves to glycoprotein receptors present on the bacteria cell wall, and thereby causing increased penetrability of cytoplasmic membrane and protein leakage (Pérez et al. 2016). Cytoplasmic membrane permeability was usually determined by the method of Hancock with the membrane-potential-sensitive cyanine dye diSC35, while the protein leakage was determined according to Bradford's method (Feng et al. 2010).

The antibacterial activity also depends on the molecular weight, monosaccharide composition, linkage type, and sulfation pattern of the MAP (Pérez et al. 2016). The antibacterial activity of fucoidans from *L. japonica* was determined using both the liquid turbidity method and plate smearing method (Liu et al. 2017a). The native fucoidans did not show any antibacterial activity against *E. coli* and *S. aureus*. In contrast, the depolymerized fucoidans at the concentration of 5 mg ml^{-1} showed excellent antibacterial activity against *E. coli* and *S. aureus* by destroying membrane integrity. Recently the antibacterial activity of fucoidan extracted from *Spatoglossum asperum* against *Aeromonos hydrophila* was also studied by agar bioassay and agar well diffusion assay (Palanisamy et al. 2017a). The maximum zone of inhibition was 33 mm at 150 μg ml^{-1} of fucoidan concentration in agar bioassay and agar well diffusion assay, and the minimum inhibitory concentration was found to be 100 μg ml^{-1} fucoidan concentration (Palanisamy et al. 2017a). Similarly, fucoidan extracted from *S. polycystum* between the concentrations of 31.25 and 250 μg ml^{-1} inhibited the replication of *Vibrio harveyi*, *S. aureus*, *E. coli*, *Pseudomonas aeruginosa*, and *Salmonella typhi* (Marudhupandi and Kumar 2013).

10.5 Conclusion and Future Trends

Marine algae are one of the major producers of biomass in the oceans and represent a potential source of unique bioactive compounds, especially polysaccharides. Today, marine algae resources have the potential of yielding natural bioproducts with unique carbon skeletons and unique biological properties. In many locations, cultivation methods are being extensively studied, such as unique seaweeds from different areas to evaluate the potential biological activities related to health and chronic disease risk reduction.

The various applications of MAP pave the way in developing potential therapeutic areas including antiviral, antimicrobial, anticoagulant, anticarcinogenic, antihypolipidemic, anticoagulant, and antimicrobial. Several studies have proved that potential bioactivities and favorable effects of MAP show their potential usage in a broad spectrum of applications in foods, pharmaceutical, cosmeceutical, and nutraceutical industries; however, there are still studies needed, in particular, to determine the bioavailability or bioaccessibility of these polysaccharides. More investigations for enhancing the yield and lowering the extraction costs, standardization of analytical methods used for quality control, detailed chemical-physical characterization, determination of the structural and bioactivity relationship as well as safety evaluation are needed.

References

Aguilar-Briseño, J., Cruz-Suarez, L., Sassi, J.-F. et al. (2015). Sulphated polysaccharides from *Ulva clathrata* and *Cladosiphon okamuranus* seaweeds both inhibit viral attachment/entry and cell-cell fusion, in NDV infection. *Marine Drugs* **13** (2): 697–712.

Ahmadi, A., Zorofchian, M.S., Abubakar, S., and Zandi, K. (2015). Antiviral potential of algae polysaccharides isolated from marine sources: a review. *BioMed Research International* **2015** (4): 825203.

Ale, M.T. and Meyer, A.S. (2013). Fucoidans from brown seaweeds: an update on structures, extraction techniques and use of enzymes as tools for structural elucidation. *RSC Advances* **3** (22): 8131–8141.

Ale, M.T., Mikkelsen, J.D., and Meyer, A.S. (2011). Important determinants for fucoidan bioactivity: a critical review of structure-function relations and extraction methods for fucose-containing sulfated polysaccharides from brown seaweeds. *Marine Drugs* **9** (10): 2106–2130.

Ale, M.T., Maruyama, H., Tamauchi, H. et al. (2011a). Fucoidan from *Sargassum* sp. and *Fucus vesiculosus* reduces cell viability of lung carcinoma and melanoma cells *in vitro* and activates natural killer cells in mice *in vivo*. *International Journal of Biological Macromolecules* **49** (3): 331–336.

Ale, M.T., Maruyama, H., Tamauchi, H. et al. (2011b). Fucose-containing sulfated polysaccharides from brown seaweeds inhibit proliferation of melanoma cells and induce apoptosis by activation of caspase-3 in vitro. *Marine Drugs* **9** (12): 2605–2621.

Ale, M.T., Mikkelsen, J.D., and Meyer, A.S. (2012). Designed optimization of a single-step extraction of fucose-containing sulfated polysaccharides from *Sargassum* sp. *Journal of Applied Phycology* **24** (4): 715–723.

Anastyuk, S.D., Shevchenko, N.M., Nazarenko, E.L. et al. (2010). Structural analysis of a highly sulfated fucan from the brown alga *Laminaria cichorioides* by tandem MALDI and ESI mass spectrometry. *Carbohydrate Research* **345** (15): 2206–2212.

Anastyuk, S.D., Imbs, T.I., Shevchenko, N.M. et al. (2012a). ESIMS analysis of fucoidan preparations from *Costaria costata*, extracted from alga at different life-stages. *Carbohydrate Polymers* **90** (2): 993–1002.

Anastyuk, S.D., Shevchenko, N.M., Dmitrenok, P.S., and Zvyagintseva, T.N. (2012b). Structural similarities of fucoidans from brown algae *Silvetia babingtonii* and *Fucus evanescens*, determined by tandem MALDI-TOF mass spectrometry. *Carbohydrate Research* **358** (9): 78–81.

Anastyuka, S.D., Shevchenko, N.M., Usoltseva, R.V. et al. (2017). Structural features and anticancer activity *in vitro* of fucoidan derivatives from brown alga *Saccharina cichorioides*. *Carbohydrate Polymers* **157**: 1503–1510.

Andrade, K.A.M., Lauritano, C., Romano, G., and Ianora, A. (2018). Marine microalgae with anti-cancer properties. *Marine Drugs* **16** (5): 165.

Aquino, R.S., Grativol, C., and Mourão, P.A. (2011). Rising from the sea: correlations between sulfated polysaccharides and salinity in plants. *PLoS One* **6** (4): e18862.

Arman, M. and Qader, S.A.U. (2012). Structural analysis of kappa-carrageenan isolated from *Hypnea musciformis* (red algae) and evaluation as an elicitor of plant defense mechanism. *Carbohydrate Polymers* **88** (4): 1264–1271.

Atashrazm, F., Lowenthal, R., Woods, G. et al. (2015). Fucoidan and cancer: a multifunctional molecule with anti-tumor potential. *Marine Drugs* **13** (4): 2327–2346.

Athukorala, Y., Jung, W.-K., Vasanthan, T., and Jeon, Y.-J. (2006). An anticoagulative polysaccharide from an enzymatic hydrolysate of *Ecklonia cava*. *Carbohydrate Polymers* **66** (2): 184–191.

Athukorala, Y., Lee, K.W., Kim, S.K., and Jeon, Y.J. (2007). Anticoagulant activity of marine green and brown algae collected from Jeju Island in Korea. *Bioresource Technology* **98** (9): 1711–1716.

Bandyopadhyay, S.S., Navid, M.H., Ghosh, T. et al. (2011). Structural features and in vitro antiviral activities of sulfated polysaccharides from *Sphacelaria indica*. *Phytochemistry* **72** (2–3): 276–283.

Barba, F.J., Grimi, N., and Vorobiev, E. (2015). New approaches for the use of non-conventional cell disruption technologies to extract potential food additives and nutraceuticals from microalgae. *Food Engineering Reviews* **7** (1): 45–62.

Ben Gara, A., Kolsi, R.B., Chaaben, R. et al. (2017). Inhibition of key digestive enzymes related to hyperlipidemia and protection of liver-kidney functions by *Cystoseira crinita* sulphated polysaccharide in high-fat diet-fed rats. *Biomedicine & Pharmacotherapy* **85**: 517–526.

Benz, C.C. and Yau, C. (2008). Ageing, oxidative stress and cancer: paradigms in parallax. *Nature Reviews Cancer* **8**: 875–879.

Besednova, N.N., Zaporozhets, T.S., Somova, L.M., and Kuznetsova, T.A. (2015). Review: prospects for the use of extracts and polysaccharides from marine algae to prevent and treat the diseases caused by *Helicobacter pylori*. *Helicobacter* **20** (2): 89–97.

Bhatia, S., Rathee, P., Sharma, K. et al. (2013). Immuno-modulation effect of sulphated polysaccharide (porphyran) from *Porphyra vietnamensis*. *International Journal of Biological Macromolecules* **57**: 50–56.

Bilan, M.I., Grachev, A.A., Ustuzhanina, N.E. et al. (2004). A highly regular fraction of a fucoidan from the brown seaweed *Fucus distichus* L. *Carbohydrate Research* **339** (3): 511–517.

Bixler, H.J. and Porse, H. (2011). A decade of change in the seaweed hydrocolloids industry. *Journal of Applied Phycology* **23** (3): 321–335.

Bouhlal, R., Haslin, C., Chermann, J.C. et al. (2011). Antiviral activities of sulfated polysaccharides isolated from *Sphaerococcus coronopifolius* (Rhodophytha, Gigartinales) and *Boergeseniella thuyoides* (Rhodophyta, Ceramiales). *Marine Drugs* **9** (7): 1187–1209.

Boullart, A.C.I., Graaf, J.D., and Stalenhoef, A.F. (2012). Serum triglycerides and risk of cardiovascular disease. *Biochimica et Biophysica Acta (BBA) – Molecular and Cell Biology of Lipids* **1821** (5): 867–875.

Brown, E.M., Allsopp, P.J., Magee, P.J. et al. (2014). Seaweed and human health. *Nutrition Reviews* **72** (3): 205–216.

Campo, V.L., Kawano, D.F., Silva, D.B.d., and Carvalho, I. (2009). Carrageenans: biological properties, chemical modifications and structural analysis – a review. *Carbohydrate Polymers* **77** (2): 167–180.

Cardoso, M.J., Costa, R.R., and Mano, J.F. (2016). Marine origin polysaccharides in drug delivery systems. *Marine Drugs* **14** (2): 34.

Cassolato, J.E.F., Noseda, M.D., Pujol, C.A. et al. (2008). Chemical structure and antiviral activity of the sulfated heterorhamnan isolated from the green seaweed *Gayralia oxysperma*. *Carbohydrate Research* **343** (18): 3085–3095.

Chandía, N.P. and Matsuhiro, B. (2008). Characterization of a fucoidan from *Lessonia vadosa* (Phaeophyta) and its anticoagulant and elicitor properties. *International Journal of Biological Macromolecules* **42** (3): 235–240.

Chandini, S.K., Ganesan, P., and Bhaskar, N. (2008). In vitro antioxidant activities of three selected brown seaweeds of India. *Food Chemistry* **107** (2): 707–713.

Chen, S.K., Tsai, M.L., Huang, J.R., and Chen, R.H. (2009). *In vitro* antioxidant activities of low-molecular-weight polysaccharides with various functional groups. *Journal of Agricultural and Food Chemistry* **57** (7): 2699–2704.

Chen, A., Lan, Y., Liu, J. et al. (2017a). The structure property and endothelial protective activity of fucoidan from *Laminaria japonica*. *International Journal of Biological Macromolecules* **105**: 1421–1429.

Chen, L.-M., Liu, P.-Y., Chen, Y.-A. et al. (2017b). Oligo-fucoidan prevents IL-6 and CCL2 production and cooperates with p53 to suppress ATM signaling and tumor progression. *Scientific Reports* **7** (1): 11864.

Cheong, K.L., Wu, D.T., Zhao, J., and Li, S.P. (2015). A rapid and accurate method for the quantitative estimation of natural polysaccharides and their fractions using high performance size exclusion chromatography coupled with multi-angle laser light scattering and refractive index detector. *Journal of Chromatography A* **1400**: 98–106.

Cheong, K.-L., Qiu, H.-M., Du, H. et al. (2018). Oligosaccharides derived from red seaweed: production, properties, and potential health and cosmetic applications. *Molecules* **23** (10): 2451.

Chiu, Y.-H., Chan, Y.-L., Li, T.-L., and Wu, C.-J. (2012). Inhibition of Japanese encephalitis virus infection by the sulfated polysaccharide extracts from *Ulva lactuca*. *Marine Biotechnology* **14** (4): 468–478.

Ciancia, M., Alberghina, J., Arata, P.X. et al. (2012). Characterization of cell wall polysaccharides of the coencocytic green seaweed *Bryopsis plumosa* (Bryopsidaceae, Chlorophyta) from the Argentine coast. *Journal of Phycology* **48** (2): 326–335.

Cong, Q., Chen, H., Liao, W. et al. (2016). Structural characterization and effect on anti-angiogenic activity of a fucoidan from *Sargassum fusiforme*. *Carbohydrate Polymers* **136**: 899–907.

Correc, G., Hehemann, J.-H., Czjzek, M., and Helbert, W. (2011). Structural analysis of the degradation products of porphyran digested by *Zobellia galactanivorans* β-porphyranase A. *Carbohydrate Polymers* **83** (1): 277–283.

Cosenza, V.A., Navarro, D.A., Pujol, C.A. et al. (2015). Partial and total C-6 oxidation of gelling carrageenans. Modulation of the antiviral activity with the anionic character. *Carbohydrate Polymers* **128**: 199–206.

Costa, C., Alves, A., Pinto, P.R. et al. (2012). Characterization of ulvan extracts to assess the effect of different steps in the extraction procedure. *Carbohydrate Polymers* **88** (2): 537–546.

Daitoku, H., Sakamaki, J.I., and Fukamizu, A. (2011). Regulation of FoxO transcription factors by acetylation and protein–protein interactions. *Biochimica et Biophysica Acta –Molecular Cell Research* **1813** (11): 1954–1960.

Davis, T.A., Llanes, F., Volesky, B., and Mucci, A. (2003). Metal selectivity of *Sargassum* spp. and their alginates in relation to their α-L-guluronic acid content and conformation. *Environmental Science & Technology* **37** (2): 261–267.

De Clercq, E. (2002). Strategies in the design of antiviral drugs. *Nature Reviews Drug Discovery* **1** (1): 13–25.

De Jesus Raposo, M.F., De Morais, A.M.B., and De Morais, R.M.S.C. (2015). Marine polysaccharides from algae with potential biomedical applications. *Marine Drugs* **13** (5): 2967–3028.

De Ruiter, G.A. and Rudolph, B. (1997). Carrageenan biotechnology. *Trends in Food Science & Technology* **8** (12): 389–395.

Deniaud, E., Fleurence, J., and Lahaye, M. (2003). Interactions of the mix-linked β-(1,3)/β-(1,4)-D-xylans in the cell walls of *Palmaria palmata* (Rhodophyta). *Journal of Phycology* **39** (1): 74–82.

Deniaud-Bouët, E., Hardouin, K., Potin, P. et al. (2017). A review about brown algal cell walls and fucose-containing sulfated polysaccharides: cell wall context, biomedical properties and key research challenges. *Carbohydrate Polymers* **175**: 395–408.

Dinesh, S., Menon, T., Hanna, L.E. et al. (2016). In vitro anti-HIV-1 activity of fucoidan from *Sargassum swartzii*. *International Journal of Biological Macromolecules* **82**: 83–88.

Diogo, J.V., Galdo Novo, S., Gonzalez, M.J. et al. (2015). Antiviral activity of lambda-carrageenan prepared from red seaweed (*Gigartina skottsbergii*) against BoHV-1 and SuHV-1. *Research in Veterinary Science* **98**: 142–144.

Dore, C.M.P.G., Alves, M.G.d.C.F., Will, L.S.E.P. et al. (2013). A sulfated polysaccharide, fucans, isolated from brown algae *Sargassum vulgare* with anticoagulant, antithrombotic, antioxidant and anti-inflammatory effects. *Carbohydrate Polymers* **91** (1): 467–475.

Draget, K.I. and Taylor, C. (2011). Chemical, physical and biological properties of alginates and their biomedical implications. *Food Hydrocolloids* **25** (2): 251–256.

Duarte, C.M., Wu, J., Xiao, X. et al. (2017). Can seaweed farming play a role in climate change mitigation and adaptation? *Frontiers in Marine Science* **April**: 100.

Duarte, M.E.R., Cauduro, J.P., Noseda, D.G. et al. (2004). The structure of the agaran sulfate from *Acanthophora spicifera* (Rhodomelaceae, Ceramiales) and its antiviral activity. Relation between structure and antiviral activity in agarans. *Carbohydrate Research* **339** (2): 335–347.

Dunlap, R. (2013). *Immobilized Biochemicals and Affinity Chromatography*, vol. **42**. Cham: Springer Science & Business Media.

Dunn, E.K., Shoue, D.A., Huang, X. et al. (2007). Spectroscopic and biochemical analysis of regions of the cell wall of the unicellular 'mannan weed', *Acetabularia acetabulum*. *Plant and Cell Physiology* **48** (1): 122–133.

Ebada, S.S., Edrada, R.A., Lin, W., and Proksch, P. (2008). Methods for isolation, purification and structural elucidation of bioactive secondary metabolites from marine invertebrates. *Nature Protocols* **3**: 1820–1831.

Elizondo-Gonzalez, R., Cruz-Suarez, L.E., Ricque-Marie, D. et al. (2012). *In vitro* characterization of the antiviral activity of fucoidan from *Cladosiphon okamuranus* against Newcastle disease virus. *Virology Journal* **9** (1): 307.

Ermakova, S., Sokolova, R., Kim, S.M. et al. (2011). Fucoidans from brown seaweeds *Sargassum hornery*, *Eclonia cava*, *Costaria costata*: structural characteristics and anticancer activity. *Applied Biochemistry and Biotechnology* **164** (6): 841–850.

Ermakova, S., Men'Shova, R., Vishchuk, O. et al. (2013). Water-soluble polysaccharides from the brown alga *Eisenia bicyclis*: structural characteristics and antitumor activity. *Algal Research* **2** (1): 51–58.

Erra-Balsells, R., Kolender, A.A., Matulewicz, M.a.C. et al. (2000). Matrix-assisted ultraviolet laser-desorption ionization time-of-flight mass spectrometry of sulfated mannans from the red seaweed *Nothogenia fastigiata*. *Carbohydrate Research* **329** (1): 157–167.

Estevez, J.M., Fernández, P.V., Kasulin, L. et al. (2009). Chemical and in situ characterization of macromolecular components of the cell walls from the green seaweed *Codium fragile*. *Glycobiology* **19** (3): 212–228.

Fabregas, J., Garcı´ a, D., Fernandez-Alonso, M. et al. (1999). *In vitro* inhibition of the replication of haemorrhagic septicaemia virus (VHSV) and African swine fever virus (ASFV) by extracts from marine microalgae. *Antiviral Research* **44** (1): 67–73.

Faggio, C., Pagano, M., Dottore, A. et al. (2016). Evaluation of anticoagulant activity of two algal polysaccharides. *Natural Product Research* **30** (17): 1934–1937.

Fang, Q., Wang, J.-F., Zha, X.-Q. et al. (2015). Immunomodulatory activity on macrophage of a purified polysaccharide extracted from *Laminaria japonica*. *Carbohydrate Polymers* **134**: 66–73.

Feng, H., Ying, Y., Yang, G., and Yu, L. (2010). Studies on antibacterial activity and antibacterial mechanism of a novel polysaccharide from *Streptomyces virginia* H03. *Food Control* **21** (9): 1257–1262.

Fernández, P.V., Estevez, J.M., Cerezo, A.S., and Ciancia, M. (2012). Sulfated β-D-mannan from green seaweed *Codium vermilara. Carbohydrate Polymers* **87** (1): 916–919.

Foley, S.A., Eva, S., Barbara, M. et al. (2011). An unfractionated fucoidan from *Ascophyllum nodosum*: extraction, characterization, and apoptotic effects *in vitro. Journal of Natural Products* **74** (9): 1851–1861.

Garcia-Vaquero, M., Rajauria, G., O'Doherty, J., and Sweeney, T. (2017). Polysaccharides from macroalgae: recent advances, innovative technologies and challenges in extraction and purification. *Food Research International* **99**: 1011–1020.

Geoffrey, G., Sylvie, L.P., and Jacques, P. (2006). NF-κB activation by reactive oxygen species: fifteen years later. *Biochemical Pharmacology* **72** (11): 1493–1505.

Gerber, P., Dutcher, J.D., Adams, E.V., and Sherman, J.H. (1958). Protective effect of seaweed extracts for chicken embryos infected with influenza B or mumps virus. *Proceedings of the Society for Experimental Biology and Medicine* **99** (3): 590–593.

Gilbert-López, B., Barranco, A., Herrero, M. et al. (2016). Development of new green processes for the recovery of bioactives from *Phaeodactylum tricornutum. Food Research International*: 1056–1065.

Go, H., Hye-Jung, H., and Nam, T.-J. (2010). A glycoprotein from *Laminaria japonica* induces apoptosis in HT-29 colon cancer cells. *Toxicology in Vitro* **24** (6): 1546–1553.

Guerra Dore, C.M.P., Faustino Alves, M.G.C., Santos, N.D. et al. (2013). Antiangiogenic activity and direct antitumor effect from a sulfated polysaccharide isolated from seaweed. *Microvascular Research* **88**: 12–18.

Hahn, T., Lang, S., Ulber, R., and Muffler, K. (2012). Novel procedures for the extraction of fucoidan from brown algae. *Process Biochemistry* **47** (12): 1691–1698.

Hahn, T., Zayed, A., Kovacheva, M. et al. (2016). Dye affinity chromatography for fast and simple purification of fucoidan from marine brown algae. *Engineering in Life Sciences* **16** (1): 78–87.

Hall, J.E., Crook, E.D., Jones, D.W. et al. (2002). Mechanisms of obesity-associated cardiovascular and renal disease. *American Journal of the Medical Sciences* **324** (3): 127–137.

Hamed, I., Özogul, F., Özogul, Y., and Regenstein, J.M. (2015). Marine bioactive compounds and their health benefits: a review. *Comprehensive Reviews in Food Science and Food Safety* **14** (4): 446–465.

Harada, N. and Maeda, M. (1998). Chemical structure of antithrombin-active rhamnan sulfate from *Monostrom nitidum. Bioscience, Biotechnology, and Biochemistry* **62** (9): 1647–1652.

Hardouin, K., Burlot, A.-S., Umami, A. et al. (2014). Biochemical and antiviral activities of enzymatic hydrolysates from different invasive French seaweeds. *Journal of Applied Phycology* **26** (2): 1029–1042.

Hardouin, K., Bedoux, G., Burlot, A.S. et al. (2016). Enzyme-assisted extraction (EAE) for the production of antiviral and antioxidant extracts from the green seaweed *Ulva armoricana* (Ulvales, Ulvophyceae). *Algal Research* **16**: 233–239.

Heo, S.-J., Park, E.-J., Lee, K.-W., and Jeon, Y.-J. (2005). Antioxidant activities of enzymatic extracts from brown seaweeds. *Bioresource Technology* **96** (14): 1613–1623.

Hjelland, F., Andersen, A.H., and Yang, H.S. (2012). Process for isolating fucoidan and laminarin from live, harvested seaweed. Google Patents.

Hmelkov, A.B., Zvyagintseva, T.N., Shevchenko, N.M. et al. (2018). Ultrasound-assisted extraction of polysaccharides from brown alga *Fucus evanescens.* Structure and biological activity of the new fucoidan fractions. *Journal of Applied Phycology* **30** (3): 2039–2046.

Hu, X., Jiang, X., Aubree, E. et al. (2006). Preparation and *in vivo* antitumor activity of *ι*-carrageenan oligosaccharides. *Pharmaceutical Biology* **44** (9): 646–650.

Huang, C.Y., Wu, S.J., Yang, W.N. et al. (2016). Antioxidant activities of crude extracts of fucoidan extracted from *Sargassum glaucescens* by a compressional-puffing-hydrothermal extraction process. *Food Chemistry* **197** (Pt B): 1121–1129.

Hyun, J.-H., Kim, S.-C., Kang, J.-I. et al. (2009). Apoptosis inducing activity of fucoidan in HCT-15 colon carcinoma cells. *Biological and Pharmaceutical Bulletin* **32** (10): 1760–1764.

Ibáñez, E., Herrero, M., Mendiola, J.A., and Castro-Puyana, M. (2012). Extraction and characterization of bioactive compounds with health benefits from marine resources: macro and micro algae, cyanobacteria, and invertebrates. In: *Marine Bioactive Compounds: Sources, Characterization and Applications* (ed. M. Hayes), 55–98. Boston, MA: Springer US.

Imbs, T.I., Ermakova, S.P., Malyarenko, O.S. et al. (2016). Structural elucidation of polysaccharide fractions from the brown alga *Coccophora langsdorfii* and in vitro investigation of their anticancer activity. *Carbohydrate Polymers* **135**: 162–168.

Iwasaki, A. and Medzhitov, R. (2010). Regulation of adaptive immunity by the innate immune system. *Science* **327** (5963): 291.

Jeon, Y.J., Wijesinghe, W.P., and Kim, S.K. (2011). Enzyme-assisted extraction and recovery of bioactive components from seaweeds. In: *Handbook of Marine Macroalgae: Biotechnology and Applied Phycology* (ed. S. Kim), 221–228. Hoboken, NJ: Wiley.

Jeong, B.-E., Ko, E.-J., and Joo, H.-G. (2012). Cytoprotective effects of fucoidan, an algae-derived polysaccharide on 5-fluorouracil-treated dendritic cells. *Food and Chemical Toxicology* **50** (5): 1480–1484.

Jeong, S.C., Jeong, Y.T., Lee, S.M., and Kim, J.H. (2015). Immune-modulating activities of polysaccharides extracted from brown algae *Hizikia fusiforme*. *Bioscience, Biotechnology, and Biochemistry* **79** (8): 1362–1365.

Jiao, G., Yu, G., Zhang, J., and Ewart, H.S. (2011). Chemical structures and bioactivities of sulfated polysaccharides from marine algae. *Marine Drugs* **9** (2): 196–223.

Jimenez-Escrig, A., Gomez-Ordonez, E., and Ruperez, P. (2015). Infrared characterisation, monosaccharide profile and antioxidant activity of chemical fractionated polysaccharides from the edible seaweed sugar kombu (*Saccharina latissima*). *International Journal of Food Science and Technology* **50** (2): 340–346.

Jin, W., Zhang, Q., Wang, J., and Zhang, W. (2013). A comparative study of the anticoagulant activities of eleven fucoidans. *Carbohydrate Polymers* **91** (1): 1–6.

Kadam, S.U., Tiwari, B.K., and O'Donnell, C.P. (2013). Application of novel extraction technologies for bioactives from marine algae. *Journal of Agricultural and Food Chemistry* **61** (20): 4667–4675.

Kadam, S.U., O'Donnell, C.P., Rai, D.K. et al. (2015a). Laminarin from Irish brown seaweeds *Ascophyllum nodosum* and *Laminaria hyperborea*: ultrasound assisted extraction, characterization and bioactivity. *Marine Drugs* **13** (7): 4270–4280.

Kadam, S.U., Tiwari, B.K., and O'Donnell, C.P. (2015b). Extraction, structure and biofunctional activities of laminarin from brown algae. *International Journal of Food Science & Technology* **50** (1): 24–31.

Kang, O.L., Ghani, M., Hassan, O. et al. (2014). Novel agaro-oligosaccharide production through enzymatic hydrolysis: physicochemical properties and antioxidant activities. *Food Hydrocolloids* **42**: 304–308.

Kang, S.M., Kim, K.N., Lee, S.H. et al. (2011). Anti-inflammatory activity of polysaccharide purified from AMG-assistant extract of *Ecklonia cava* in LPS-stimulated RAW 264.7 macrophages. *Carbohydrate Polymers* **85** (1): 80–85.

Kang, Y., Li, H., Wu, J. et al. (2016). Transcriptome profiling reveals the antitumor mechanism of polysaccharide from marine algae *Gracilariopsis lemaneiformis*. *PLoS One* **11** (6): e0158279.

Karadag, A., Ozcelik, B., and Saner, S. (2009). Review of methods to determine antioxidant capacities. *Food Analytical Methods* **2** (1): 41–60.

Khan, B.M., Qiu, H.M., Wang, X.F. et al. (2019). Physicochemical characterization of *Gracilaria chouae* sulfated polysaccharides and their antioxidant potential. *International Journal of Biological Macromolecules* **134**: 255–261.

Khil'chenko, S.R., Zaporozhets, T.S., Shevchenko, N.M. et al. (2011). Immunostimulatory activity of fucoidan from the brown alga *Fucus evanescens*: role of sulfates and acetates. *Journal of Carbohydrate Chemistry* **30** (4–6): 291–305.

Kim, K. (2012). Seasonal variation of seaweed components and novel biological function of fucoidan extracted from brown algae in Quebec (Doctoral dissertation, Université Laval). Kinetin on potato yields. *Journal of the Science of Food and Agriculture* **28**: 121–125.

Kim, S.-H., Choi, D.-S., Athukorala, Y. et al. (2007). Antioxidant activity of sulfated polysaccharides isolated from *Sargassum fulvellum*. *Preventive Nutrition and Food Science* **12** (2): 65–73.

Kim, E.J., Park, S.Y., Lee, J.-Y., and Park, J.H.Y. (2010). Fucoidan present in brown algae induces apoptosis of human colon cancer cells. *BMC Gastroenterology* **10** (1): 96.

Kolender, A.A., Pujol, C.A., Damonte, E.B. et al. (1997). The system of sulfated α-(1 → 3)-linked d-mannans from the red seaweed *Nothogenia fastigiata*: structures, antiherpetic and anticoagulant properties. *Carbohydrate Research* **304** (1): 53–60.

Kraan, S. (2012). Algal polysaccharides, novel applications and outlook. In: *Carbohydrates – Comprehensive Studies on Glycobiology and Glycotechnology* (ed. C.-F. Chang), 489–532. London: IntechOpen Limited.

Kulshreshtha, G., Burlot, A.-S., Marty, C. et al. (2015). Enzyme-assisted extraction of bioactive material from *Chondrus crispus* and *Codium fragile* and its effect on herpes simplex virus (HSV-1). *Marine Drugs* **13** (1): 558–580.

Lahaye, M. and Robic, A. (2007). Structure and functional properties of ulvan, a polysaccharide from green seaweeds. *Biomacromolecules* **8** (6): 1765–1774.

Lahaye, M., Brunel, M., and Bonnin, E. (1997). Fine chemical structure analysis of oligosaccharides produced by an ulvan-lyase degradation of the water-soluble cell-wall polysaccharides from *Ulva* sp. (Ulvales, Chlorophyta). *Carbohydrate Research* **304** (3–4): 325–333.

Lahaye, M., Inizan, F., and Vigouroux, J. (1998). NMR analysis of the chemical structure of ulvan and of ulvan-boron complex formation. *Carbohydrate Polymers* **36** (2–3): 239–249.

Lee, J.-B., Koizumi, S., Hayashi, K., and Hayashi, T. (2010). Structure of rhamnan sulfate from the green alga *Monostroma nitidum* and its anti-herpetic effect. *Carbohydrate Polymers* **81** (3): 572–577.

Lee, W.-K., Lim, Y.-Y., Leow, A.T.-C. et al. (2017). Biosynthesis of agar in red seaweeds: a review. *Carbohydrate Polymers* **164**: 23–30.

Li, H., Mao, W., Zhang, X. et al. (2011). Structural characterization of an anticoagulant-active sulfated polysaccharide isolated from green alga *Monostroma latissimum*. *Carbohydrate Polymers* **85** (2): 394–400.

Li, H., Mao, W., Hou, Y. et al. (2012). Preparation, structure and anticoagulant activity of a low molecular weight fraction produced by mild acid hydrolysis of sulfated rhamnan from *Monostroma latissimum*. *Bioresource Technology* **114**: 414–418.

Li, W., Jiang, N., Li, B. et al. (2018). Antioxidant activity of purified ulvan in hyperlipidemic mice. *International Journal of Biological Macromolecules* **113**: 971–975.

Lim, S.J., Aida, W.M.W., Maskat, M.Y. et al. (2014). Isolation and antioxidant capacity of fucoidan from selected Malaysian seaweeds. *Food Hydrocolloids* **42**: 280–288.

Lindahl, U. (2000). 'Heparin' – from anticoagulant drug into the new biology. *Glycoconjugate Journal* **17** (7): 597–605.

Liu, M., Liu, Y., Cao, M.-J. et al. (2017a). Antibacterial activity and mechanisms of depolymerized fucoidans isolated from *Laminaria japonica*. *Carbohydrate Polymers* **172**: 294–305.

Liu, Q.-M., Xu, S.-S., Li, L. et al. (2017b). In vitro and in vivo immunomodulatory activity of sulfated polysaccharide from *Porphyra haitanensis*. *Carbohydrate Polymers* **165**: 189–196.

Lopes, N., Ray, S., Espada, S.F. et al. (2017). Green seaweed *Enteromorpha compressa* (Chlorophyta, Ulvaceae) derived sulphated polysaccharides inhibit herpes simplex virus. *International Journal of Biological Macromolecules* **102**: 605–612.

Lorbeer, A.J., Lahnstein, J., Bulone, V. et al. (2015). Multiple-response optimization of the acidic treatment of the brown alga *Ecklonia radiata* for the sequential extraction of fucoidan and alginate. *Bioresource Technology* **197**: 302–309.

Maeda, M. and Nisizawa, K. (1968). Fine structure of laminaran of *Eisenia bicyclis*. *The Journal of Biochemistry* **63** (2): 199–206.

Mandal, P., Pujol, C.A., Damonte, E.B. et al. (2010). Xylans from *Scinaia hatei*: structural features, sulfation and anti-HSV activity. *International Journal of Biological Macromolecules* **46** (2): 173–178.

Marcati, A., Ursu, A.V., Laroche, C. et al. (2014). Extraction and fractionation of polysaccharides and B-phycoerythrin from the microalga *Porphyridium cruentum* by membrane technology. *Algal Research* **5**: 258–263.

Marudhupandi, T. and Kumar, T.T.A. (2013). Antibacterial effect of fucoidan from *Sargassum wightii* against the chosen human bacterial pathogens. *International Current Pharmaceutical Journal* **2** (10): 156–158.

Marudhupandi, T., Ajith Kumar, T.T., Lakshmanasenthil, S. et al. (2015). *In vitro* anticancer activity of fucoidan from *Turbinaria conoides* against A549 cell lines. *International Journal of Biological Macromolecules* **72** (72): 919–923.

Matsuhiro, B., Conte, A.F., Damonte, E.B. et al. (2005). Structural analysis and antiviral activity of a sulfated galactan from the red seaweed *Schizymenia binderi* (Gigartinales, Rhodophyta). *Carbohydrate Research* **340** (15): 2392–2402.

Menshova, R.V., Anastyuk, S.D., Ermakova, S.P. et al. (2015). Structure and anticancer activity in vitro of sulfated galactofucan from brown alga *Alaria angusta*. *Carbohydrate Polymers* **132**: 118–125.

Michalak, I. and Chojnacka, K. (2014). Algal extracts: technology and advances. *Engineering in Life Sciences* **14** (6): 581–591.

Milledge, J.J. and Harvey, P.J. (2016). Potential process 'hurdles' in the use of macroalgae as feedstock for biofuel production in the British Isles. *Journal of Chemical Technology and Biotechnology* **91** (8): 2221–2234.

Minh Hien, H., Kim, J.-Y., Lee, J.H. et al. (2015). Antioxidative, hypolipidemic, and anti-inflammatory activities of sulfated polysaccharides from *Monostroma nitidum*. *Food Science and Biotechnology* **24** (1): 199–205.

Mohamed, S., Hashim, S.N., and Rahman, H.A. (2012). Seaweeds: a sustainable functional food for complementary and alternative therapy. *Trends in Food Science & Technology* **23** (2): 83–96.

Mori, S. and Barth, H.G. (2013). *Size Exclusion Chromatography*. Cham: Springer Science & Business Media.

Nagaoka, M., Shibata, H., Kimura-Takagi, I. et al. (1999). Structural study of fucoidan from *Cladosiphon okamuranus* tokida. *Glycoconjugate Journal* **16** (1): 19–26.

Ngo, D.H. and Kim, S.K. (2013). Sulfated polysaccharides as bioactive agents from marine algae. *International Journal of Biological Macromolecules* **62**: 70–75.

Palanisamy, S., Vinosha, M., Marudhupandi, T. et al. (2017a). *In vitro* antioxidant and antibacterial activity of sulfated polysaccharides isolated from *Spatoglossum asperum*. *Carbohydrate Polymers* **170**: 296–304.

Palanisamy, S., Vinosha, M., Marudhupandi, T. et al. (2017b). Isolation of fucoidan from *Sargassum polycystum* brown algae: structural characterization, in vitro antioxidant and anticancer activity. *International Journal of Biological Macromolecules* **102**: 405–412.

Park, H.Y., Park, S.-H., Jeong, J.-W. et al. (2017). Induction of p53-independent apoptosis and G1 cell cycle arrest by fucoidan in HCT116 human colorectal carcinoma cells. *Marine Drugs* **15** (6).

Patel, A.K., Laroche, C., Marcati, A. et al. (2013). Separation and fractionation of exopolysaccharides from *Porphyridium cruentum*. *Bioresource Technology* **145**: 345–350.

Pedro-Botet, J., Millán Núñez-Cortés, J., Chillarón, J.J. et al. (2016). Severity of statin-induced adverse effects on muscle and associated conditions: data from the DAMA study. *Expert Opinion on Drug Safety* **15** (12): 1583–1587.

Peng, Z., Liu, M., Fang, Z. et al. (2012). Composition and cytotoxicity of a novel polysaccharide from brown alga (*Laminaria japonica*). *Carbohydrate Polymers* **89** (4): 1022–1026.

Pérez, M., Falqué, E., and Domínguez, H. (2016). Antimicrobial action of compounds from marine seaweed. *Marine Drugs* **14** (3): 52.

Pérez Recalde, M., Noseda, M.D., Pujol, C.A. et al. (2009). Sulfated mannans from the red seaweed *Nemalion helminthoides* of the South Atlantic. *Phytochemistry* **70** (8): 1062–1068.

Pérez Recalde, M., Canelón, D.J., Compagnone, R.S. et al. (2016). Carrageenan and agaran structures from the red seaweed *Gymnogongrus tenuis*. *Carbohydrate Polymers* **136**: 1370–1378.

Pomin, V.H. (2011). Structure and use of algal sulfated fucans and galactans. In: *Handbook of Marine Macroalgae: Biotechnology and Applied Phycology* (ed. S.-K. Kim), 229–261. Hoboken, NJ: Wiley Blackwell.

Posocco, B., Dreussi, E., Santa, J.D. et al. (2015). Polysaccharides for the delivery of antitumor drugs. *Materials* **8** (5): 2569–2615.

Priyan Shanura Fernando, I., Kim, K.-N., Kim, D., and Jeon, Y.-J. (2019). Algal polysaccharides: potential bioactive substances for cosmeceutical applications. *Critical Reviews in Biotechnology* **39** (1): 99–113.

Pujol, C.A., Ray, S., Ray, B., and Damonte, E.B. (2012). Antiviral activity against dengue virus of diverse classes of algal sulfated polysaccharides. *International Journal of Biological Macromolecules* **51** (4): 412–416.

Qi, H. and Sun, Y. (2015). Antioxidant activity of high sulfate content derivative of ulvan in hyperlipidemic rats. *International Journal of Biological Macromolecules* **76**: 326–329.

Qi, H., Zhang, Q., Zhao, T. et al. (2005). Antioxidant activity of different sulfate content derivatives of polysaccharide extracted from *Ulva pertusa* (Chlorophyta) *in vitro*. *International Journal of Biological Macromolecules* **37** (4): 195–199.

Qi, H., Liu, X., Zhang, J. et al. (2012). Synthesis and antihyperlipidemic activity of acetylated derivative of ulvan from *Ulva pertusa*. *International Journal of Biological Macromolecules* **50** (1): 270–272.

Quitain, A.T., Kai, T., Sasaki, M., and Goto, M. (2013). Microwave-hydrothermal extraction and degradation of fucoidan from supercritical carbon dioxide deoiled *Undaria pinnatifida*. *Industrial & Engineering Chemistry Research* **52** (23): 7940–7946.

Ray, S., Pujol, C.A., Damonte, E.B., and Ray, B. (2015). Additionally sulfated xylomannan sulfates from *Scinaia hatei* and their antiviral activities. *Carbohydrate Polymers* **131**: 315–321.

Rieman, W. and Walton, H.F. (2013). *Ion Exchange in Analytical Chemistry: International Series of Monographs in Analytical Chemistry*. London: Elsevier.

Rinaudo, M. (2007). Seaweed polysaccharides. In: *Comprehensive Glycoscience – From Chemistry to Systems Biology*, vol. **2** (ed. J.P. Kamerling), 691–735. London: Elsevier.

Rioux, L.E., Turgeon, S.L., and Beaulieu, M. (2010). Structural characterization of laminaran and galactofucan extracted from the brown seaweed *Saccharina longicruris*. *Phytochemistry* **71** (13): 1586–1595.

Rioux, L.-E., Beaulieu, L., and Turgeon, S.L. (2017). Seaweeds: a traditional ingredients for new gastronomic sensation. *Food Hydrocolloids* **68**: 255–265.

Rodrigues, D., Sousa, S.R., Silva, A. et al. (2015). Impact of enzyme-and ultrasound-assisted extraction methods on biological properties of red, brown, and green seaweeds from the central west coast of Portugal. *Journal of Agricultural and Food Chemistry* **63** (12): 3177–3188.

Rodriguez-Jasso, R.M., Mussatto, S.I., Pastrana, L. et al. (2011). Microwave-assisted extraction of sulfated polysaccharides (fucoidan) from brown seaweed. *Carbohydrate Polymers* **86** (3): 1137–1144.

Ropellato, J., Carvalho, M.M., Ferreira, L.G. et al. (2015). Sulfated heterorhamnans from the green seaweed *Gayralia oxysperma*: partial depolymerization, chemical structure and antitumor activity. *Carbohydrate Polymers* **117**: 476–485.

Rui, X., Pan, H.-F., Shao, S.-L., and Xu, X.-M. (2017). Anti-tumor and anti-angiogenic effects of fucoidan on prostate cancer: possible JAK-STAT3 pathway. *BMC Complementary and Alternative Medicine* **17** (1): 378.

Ruocco, N., Costantini, S., Guariniello, S., and Costantini, M. (2016). Polysaccharides from the marine environment with pharmacological, cosmeceutical and nutraceutical potential. *Molecules* **21** (5): 551.

Sanandiya, N.D. (2009). Profiling of cellulose content in Indian seaweed species. *Bioresource Technology* **100** (24): 6669–6673.

Savage, P.E. (2012). Algae under pressure and in hot water. *Science* **338** (6110): 1039–1040.

Schiener, P., Black, K.D., Stanley, M.S., and Green, D.H. (2015). The seasonal variation in the chemical composition of the kelp species *Laminaria digitata*, *Laminaria hyperborea*, *Saccharina latissima*, and *Alaria esculenta*. *Journal of Applied Phycology* **27** (1): 363–373.

Shan, X., Liu, X., Hao, J. et al. (2016). In vitro and in vivo hypoglycemic effects of brown algal fucoidans. *International Journal of Biological Macromolecules* **82**: 249–255.

Shi, F., Yan, X., Cheong, K.L., and Liu, Y. (2018). Extraction, purification, and characterization of polysaccharides from marine algae *Gracilaria lemaneiformis* with anti-tumor activity. *Process Biochemistry* **73**: 197–203.

Shi, Q., Wang, A., Lu, Z. et al. (2017). Overview on the antiviral activities and mechanisms of marine polysaccharides from seaweeds. *Carbohydrate Research* **453–454**: 1–9.

Shobharani, P., Nanishankar, V.H., Halami, P.M., and Sachindra, N.M. (2014). Antioxidant and anticoagulant activity of polyphenol and polysaccharides from fermented *Sargassum* sp. *International Journal of Biological Macromolecules* **65** (5): 542–548.

Siddhanta, A.K., Chhatbar, M.U., Mehta, G.K. et al. (2011). The cellulose contents of Indian seaweeds. *Journal of Applied Phycology* **23** (5): 919–923.

Sousa, A.M.M., Alves, V.D., Morais, S. et al. (2010). Agar extraction from integrated multitrophic aquacultured *Gracilaria vermiculophylla*: evaluation of a microwave-assisted process using response surface methodology. *Bioresource Technology* **101** (9): 3258–3267.

Sousa, W.M., Silva, R.O., Bezerra, F.F. et al. (2016). Sulfated polysaccharide fraction from marine algae *Solieria filiformis*: structural characterization, gastroprotective and antioxidant effects. *Carbohydrate Polymers* **152**: 140–148.

Stiger-Pouvreau, V., Bourgougnon, N., and Deslandes, E. (2016). Carbohydrates from seaweeds. In: *Seaweed in Health and Disease Prevention* (eds. J. Fleurence and I. Levine), 223–274. Boston, MA: Academic Press.

Stokke, B.T., Smidsroed, O., Bruheim, P., and Skjaak-Braek, G. (1991). Distribution of uronate residues in alginate chains in relation to alginate gelling properties. *Macromolecules* **24** (16): 4637–4645.

Strømme, M., Mihranyan, A., and Ek, R. (2002). What to do with all these algae? *Materials Letters* **57** (3): 569–572.

Sugiyama, J., Persson, J., and Chanzy, H. (2008). Combined infrared and electron diffraction study of the polymorphism of native celluloses. *Macromolecules* **24** (4): 2461–2466.

Sun, L., Ling, W., and Yan, Z. (2012). Immunomodulation and antitumor activities of different-molecular-weight polysaccharides from *Porphyridium cruentum*. *Carbohydrate Polymers* **87** (2): 1206–1210.

Sun, Y., Chen, X., Cheng, Z. et al. (2017). Degradation of polysaccharides from *Grateloupia filicina* and their antiviral activity to avian leucosis virus subgroup. *Journal of Marine Drugs* **15** (11): 345.

Suresh, V., Senthilkumar, N., Thangam, R. et al. (2013). Separation, purification and preliminary characterization of sulfated polysaccharides from *Sargassum plagiophyllum* and its *in vitro* anticancer and antioxidant activity. *Process Biochemistry* **48** (2): 364–373.

Synytsya, A., Woojung, K., Sungmin, K. et al. (2010). Structure and antitumour activity of fucoidan isolated from sporophyll of Korean brown seaweed *Undaria pinnatifida*. *Carbohydrate Polymers* **81** (1): 41–48.

Synytsya, A., Čopíková, J., Kim, W.J., and Park, Y.I. (2015). Cell wall polysaccharides of marine algae. In: *Springer Handbook of Marine Biotechnology* (ed. S.-K. Kim), 543–590. New York: Springer.

Tang, F., Chen, F., and Li, F. (2014). Preparation and potential *in vivo* anti-influenza virus activity of low molecular-weight κ-carrageenans and their derivatives. *Journal of Applied Polymer Science* **127** (3): 2110–2115.

Teng, Z.L., Qian, L., and Zhou, Y. (2013). Hypolipidemic activity of the polysaccharides from *Enteromorpha prolifera*. *International Journal of Biological Macromolecules* **62**: 254–256.

Thuy, T.T.T., Ly, B.M., Van, T.T.T. et al. (2015). Anti-HIV activity of fucoidans from three brown seaweed species. *Carbohydrate Polymers* **115**: 122–128.

Tian, H., Yin, X., Zeng, Q. et al. (2015). Isolation, structure, and surfactant properties of polysaccharides from *Ulva lactuca* L. from South China Sea. *International Journal of Biological Macromolecules* **79**: 577–582.

Tong, D., Chen, G., Yi, S. et al. (2017). Antioxidant and immunostimulating activities in vitro of sulfated polysaccharides isolated from *Gracilaria rubra*. *Journal of Functional Foods* **28**: 64–75.

Trinchero, J., Ponce, N.M.A., Córdoba, O.L. et al. (2009). Antiretroviral activity of fucoidans extracted from the brown seaweed *Adenocystis utricularis*. *Phytotherapy Research* **23** (5): 707–712.

Tsubaki, S., Oono, K., Hiraoka, M. et al. (2016). Microwave-assisted hydrothermal extraction of sulfated polysaccharides from *Ulva* spp. and *Monostroma latissimum*. *Food Chemistry* **210**: 311–316.

Usoltseva, R.V., Anastyuk, S.D., Shevchenko, N.M. et al. (2016). The comparison of structure and anticancer activity *in vitro* of polysaccharides from brown algae *Alaria marginata* and *A. angusta*. *Carbohydrate Polymers* **153**: 258–265.

Usov, A. and Zelinsky, N. (2013). Chemical structures of algal polysaccharides. In: *Functional Ingredients from Algae for Foods and Nutraceuticals* (ed. H. Domínguez), 23–86. Cambridge: Woodhead Publishing.

Valko, M., Rhodes, C.J., Moncol, J. et al. (2006). Free radicals, metals and antioxidants in oxidative stress-induced cancer. *Chemico-Biological Interactions* **160** (1): 1–40.

Vavilala, S.L. and D'Souza, J.S. (2015). *Algal Polysaccharides and their Biological Applications*. Weinheim: Wiley-VCH Verlag GmbH & Co. KGaA.

Viana, A.G., Noseda, M.D., Gonçalves, A.G. et al. (2011). β-D-(1→4), β-D-(1→3) 'mixed linkage' xylans from red seaweeds of the order Nemaliales and Palmariales. *Carbohydrate Research* **346** (8): 1023–1028.

Viebke, C., Borgström, J., and Piculell, L. (1995). Characterisation of kappa- and iota-carrageenan coils and helices by MALLS/GPC. *Carbohydrate Polymers* **27** (2): 145–154.

Vijayabaskar, P., Vaseela, N., and Thirumaran, G. (2012). Potential antibacterial and antioxidant properties of a sulfated polysaccharide from the brown marine algae *Sargassum swartzii*. *Chinese Journal of Natural Medicines* **10** (6): 421–428.

Vinatoru, M., Mason, T.J., and Calinescu, I. (2017). Ultrasonically assisted extraction (UAE) and microwave assisted extraction (MAE) of functional compounds from plant materials. *TrAC Trends in Analytical Chemistry* **97**: 159–178.

Visalini, M. and Piva, T.J. (2010). The UV response of the skin: a review of the MAPK, NF-κB and TNF-α signal transduction pathways. *Archives of Dermatological Research* **302** (1): 5–17.

Vishchuk, O.S., Ermakova, S.P., and Zvyagintseva, T.N. (2011). Sulfated polysaccharides from brown seaweeds *Saccharina japonica* and *Undaria pinnatifida*: isolation, structural characteristics, and antitumor activity. *Carbohydrate Research* **346** (17): 2769–2776.

Vishchuk, O.S., Ermakova, S.P., and Zvyagintseva, T.N. (2013). The fucoidans from brown algae of Far-Eastern seas: anti-tumor activity and structure–function relationship. *Food Chemistry* **141** (2): 1211–1217.

Wang, J., Wang, F., Yun, H. et al. (2012a). Effect and mechanism of fucoidan derivatives from *Laminaria japonica* in experimental adenine-induced chronic kidney disease. *Journal of Ethnopharmacology* **139** (3): 807–813.

Wang, L., Wang, X., Wu, H., and Liu, R. (2014). Overview on biological activities and molecular characteristics of sulfated polysaccharides from marine green algae in recent years. *Marine Drugs* **12** (9): 4984–5020.

Wang, P., Zhao, X., Lv, Y. et al. (2012b). Analysis of structural heterogeneity of fucoidan from *Hizikia fusiforme* by ES-CID-MS/MS. *Carbohydrate Polymers* **90** (1): 602–607.

Wang, W., Wang, S.X., and Guan, H.S. (2012c). The antiviral activities and mechanisms of marine polysaccharides: an overview. *Marine Drugs* **10** (12): 2795–2816.

Wang, W., Lu, J.-B., Wang, C. et al. (2013). Effects of *Sargassum fusiforme* polysaccharides on antioxidant activities and intestinal functions in mice. *International Journal of Biological Macromolecules* **58**: 127–132.

Wang, W., Wu, J., Zhang, X. et al. (2017a). Inhibition of influenza A virus infection by fucoidan targeting viral neuraminidase and cellular EGFR pathway. *Scientific Reports* **7**: 40760.

Wang, X., Li, W., Xiao, L. et al. (2017b). *In vivo* antihyperlipidemic and antioxidant activity of porphyran in hyperlipidemic mice. *Carbohydrate Polymers* **174**: 417–420.

Wang, Z.J., Zheng, L., Yang, J.M. et al. (2018). Proteomic analyses for profiling regulated proteins/enzymes by *Fucus vesiculosus* fucoidan in B16 melanoma cells: a combination of enzyme kinetics functional study. *International Journal of Biological Macromolecules* **112**: 667–674.

Wei, N., Quarterman, J., and Jin, Y.-S. (2013). Marine macroalgae: an untapped resource for producing fuels and chemicals. *Trends in Biotechnology* **31** (2): 70–77.

Wijesekara, I., Pangestuti, R., and Kim, S.-K. (2011). Biological activities and potential health benefits of sulfated polysaccharides derived from marine algae. *Carbohydrate Polymers* **84** (1): 14–21.

Wijesinghe, W. and Jeon, Y.-J. (2012a). Enzyme-assistant extraction (EAE) of bioactive components: a useful approach for recovery of industrially important metabolites from seaweeds: a review. *Fitoterapia* **83** (1): 6–12.

Wijesinghe, W.A.J.P. and Jeon, Y.J. (2012b). Biological activities and potential industrial applications of fucose rich sulfated polysaccharides and fucoidans isolated from brown seaweeds: a review. *Carbohydrate Polymers* **88** (1): 13–20.

Xie, J.H., Shen, M.Y., Nie, S.P. et al. (2014). Separation of water-soluble polysaccharides from *Cyclocarya paliurus* by ultrafiltration process. *Carbohydrate Polymers* **101** (1): 479–483.

Xu, S.Y., Huang, X.S., and Cheong, K.L. (2017). Recent advances in marine algae polysaccharides: isolation, structure, and activities. *Marine Drugs* **15** (12): 16.

Xu, S.-Y., Kan, J., Hu, Z. et al. (2018). Quantification of neoagaro-oligosaccharide production through enzymatic hydrolysis and its anti-oxidant activities. *Molecules* **23** (6): 1354.

Xu, S.-Y., Aweya, J.J., Li, N. et al. (2019). Microbial catabolism of *Porphyra haitanensis* polysaccharides by human gut microbiota. *Food Chemistry* **289**: 177–186.

Yaich, H., Garna, H., Besbes, S. et al. (2013). Effect of extraction conditions on the yield and purity of ulvan extracted from *Ulva lactuca*. *Food Hydrocolloids* **31** (2): 375–382.

Ying, Z., Han, X., and Li, J. (2011). Ultrasound-assisted extraction of polysaccharides from mulberry leaves. *Food Chemistry* **127** (3): 1273–1279.

Yiu, W.H., Mead, P.A., Jun, H.S. et al. (2010). Oxidative stress mediates nephropathy in type Ia glycogen storage disease. *Laboratory Investigation* **90**: 620.

You, S., Yang, C., Lee, H., and Lee, B. (2010). Molecular characteristics of partially hydrolyzed fucoidans from sporophyll of *Undaria Pinnatifida* and their *in vitro* anticancer activity. *Food Chemistry* **119** (2): 554–559.

Yuan, Y. and Macquarrie, D. (2015). Microwave assisted extraction of sulfated polysaccharides (fucoidan) from *Ascophyllum nodosum* and its antioxidant activity. *Carbohydrate Polymers* **129**: 101–107.

Yue, Y., Li, Z., Li, P. et al. (2017). Antiviral activity of a polysaccharide from *Laminaria japonica* against enterovirus 71. *Biomedicine & Pharmacotherapy* **96**: 256–262.

Yuguchi, Y., Tran, V.T.T., Bui, L.M. et al. (2016). Primary structure, conformation in aqueous solution, and intestinal immunomodulating activity of fucoidan from two brown seaweed species *Sargassum crassifolium* and *Padina australis*. *Carbohydrate Polymers* **147**: 69–78.

Zayed, A., Muffler, K., Hahn, T. et al. (2016). Physicochemical and biological characterization of fucoidan from *Fucus vesiculosus* purified by dye affinity chromatography. *Marine Drugs* **14** (4): 79.

Zhang, Q., Li, N., Zhou, G. et al. (2003). *In vivo* antioxidant activity of polysaccharide fraction from *Porphyra haitanesis* (Rhodephyta) in aging mice. *Pharmacological Research* **48** (2): 151–155.

Zhang, Z., Wang, F., Wang, X. et al. (2010). Extraction of the polysaccharides from five algae and their potential antioxidant activity in vitro. *Carbohydrate Polymers* **82** (1): 118–121.

Zhang, W., Oda, T., Yu, Q., and Jin, J.-O. (2015). Fucoidan from *Macrocystis pyrifera* has powerful immune-modulatory effects compared to three other fucoidans. *Marine Drugs* **13** (3): 1084–1104.

Zoysa, M.D., Nikapitiya, C., Jeon, Y.J. et al. (2008). Anticoagulant activity of sulfated polysaccharide isolated from fermented brown seaweed *Sargassum fulvellum*. *Journal of Applied Phycology* **20** (1): 67–74.

11 Marine Algal Derived Phenolic Compounds and their Biological Activities for Medicinal and Cosmetic Applications

Leslie Gager, Fanny Lalegerie, Solène Connan, and Valérie Stiger-Pouvreau
Univ Brest, CNRS, IRD, Ifremer, LEMAR, Plouzane, France

11.1 Introduction

The search for natural food ingredients to replace synthetic and controversial molecules, such as the synthetic antioxidants and colorants which could be toxic for the environment and human health, is growing (Carocho et al. 2014). Terrestrial resources are widely explored but marine resources, such as algae, are not yet fully valorized. Algae are photosynthetic organisms belonging to a polyphyletic group including microscopic and large algae, i.e. microalgae and seaweeds, respectively. Moreover, the term "algae" refers to organisms that perform photosynthesis through the chlorophyll *a* pigment, have a simple vegetative form called a thallus, and need water for their life cycle to be complete (Lee 1999). In this way, algae involve a majority of eukaryotic but also prokaryotic organisms. Macroalgae can be classified into three different groups: brown algae (Ochrophyta, which include the Phaeophyceae class), red algae (Rhodophyta) and green algae (Chlorophyta). Cyanobacteria are also referred to as algae; it is the only prokaryotic group, at the base of the living organisms, and Cyanobacteria are known as blue-green algae (Figure 11.1; Stengel et al. 2011). Microalgae, or phytoplankton, are photosynthetic, single-celled organisms or a colony <0.2 mm long, living either floating in the ocean or attached

*Leslie Gager and Fanny Lalegerie contributed equally to this work.

Recent Advances in Micro- and Macroalgal Processing: Food and Health Perspectives, First Edition.
Edited by Gaurav Rajauria and Yvonne V. Yuan.

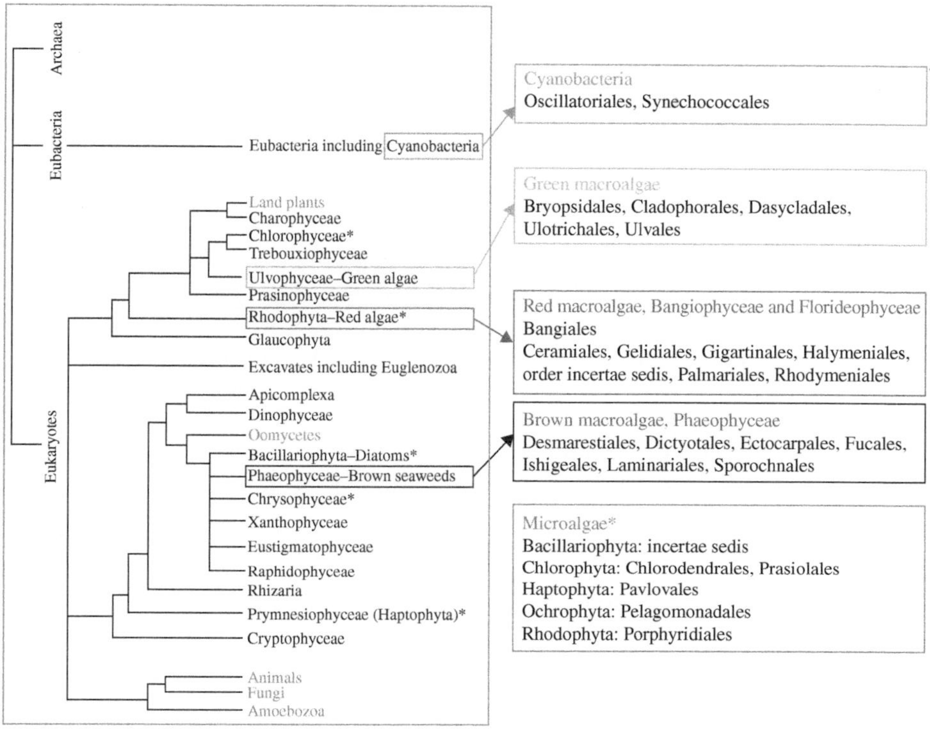

Figure 11.1 Phylogenetic tree showing the taxonomical position of each algal group cited in this chapter together with their taxonomical orders. * near microalgae refers to * near classes of microalgae on the phylogenetic tree. Source: Adapted from Stengel et al. 2011.

to a substrate (Lee 1999). Among the microalgae are found different groups such as the Chlorophyta; the Rhodophyta; the Haptophyta, with a flagellum, sometimes a haptonema, and organic scales; the silicoflagellates, with a siliceous endoskeleton; the diatoms (Bacillariophyta), characterized by a silica cover called a "frustule"; and the dinoflagellates, with or without an outer cellulosic cover (theca) (Lee 1999).

The distinctions between the taxonomic algal groups involve differences over and above size or pigmentation: algae differ considerably at the structural and biochemical levels (Lee 1999). Adaptive diversification of algae for more than 2.45 billion years to optimize their competitive survival in a variety of ecological niches has led to a co-evolution of a range of different biochemical compounds including secondary metabolites (Baurain et al. 2010; Stengel et al. 2011). Indeed, algae contain a panel of bioactive compounds showing valorization potential in various industries, such as the food (i.e. functional foods and nutraceuticals), agriculture, pharmaceutic or cosmetic sectors (Sanjeewa et al. 2016; Wijesinghe and Jeon 2011). Among those algal molecules, phenolic compounds are present in all algal groups. Some phenolics found in terrestrial plants are also found in algae, including caffeic acid and catechin (Onofrejová et al. 2010; Rodríguez-Bernaldo de Quirós et al. 2010; Farvin and Jacobsen 2013), or isoforms of tocopherol, commonly referred to as vitamin E (Farvin and Jacobsen 2013). However, the presence of flavonoids such as anthocyanins in algae is still not conclusive (Stengel et al. 2011). Phenolic compounds can be primary metabolites essential for the survival or structural integrity of algae, as for example, phlorotannins found in brown seaweeds, which are an integral part of the cell wall composition (Deniaud-Bouët et al. 2017). These phlorotannins are also secondary metabolites playing a defensive role against environmental stresses such as herbivorous grazing (Geiselman and McConnell 1981), epiphyte settlement (Jennings and Steinberg 1997), or UV radiation (Swanson and Druehl 2002). Because of the rich and varied compositions of algae (Bourgougnon and Stiger-Pouvreau 2011; Ibañez et al. 2012; Abirami et al. 2018), there is a growing interest in algal research as they may have positive effects on human health (Shalaby 2011). For example, the search is increasing for natural molecules to replace synthetic and controversial preservatives (Gupta and Abu-Ghannam 2011b; Chakraborty et al. 2015) or synthetic antioxidants (Chen et al. 1992). In this sense, algae are excellent candidates to be considered as a functional foods (Rodríguez-Bernaldo de Quirós et al. 2010).

This chapter presents the chemical structures of phenolic compounds that are produced by marine Cyanobacteria, micro- and macroalgae, as well as their isolation methods and biological activities with a focus on the dietary, medical, well-being, and cosmetic sectors. As brown seaweeds are the most studied marine algae, perhaps because they contain high levels of phenolic compounds, we focus mainly on these organisms in this chapter, although other algal groups are also discussed. Finally, we discuss the potential commercial applications to health and dietary sectors of these extraordinary diverse marine compounds.

11.2 Types and Structures of Phenolic Compounds from Algae

Phenolic compounds comprise one or more hydroxyl groups (–OH) directly bonded to an aromatic hydrocarbon group (Waterman and Mole 1994), and include a wide range of compounds, from simple molecules such as phenolic acids to more complex polyphenols such as the phlorotannins encountered in brown seaweeds (Buikema et al. 1979; Ragan and Glombitza 1986; Machu et al. 2015; Gómez-Guzmán et al. 2018). Phenolic compounds tend to be alcohol- or water-soluble, since they frequently occur as glycosides, and are located in vacuoles. As all phenolic compounds contain at least one aromatic ring, they all show intense absorption in the UV region of the spectrum (Harborne 1984).

Although phenolics are present in all algal groups, the most widely studied phenolic compounds in marine algae are the phlorotannins isolated from the marine brown algae class Phaeophyceae (Arnold and Targett 2002), which can accumulate high levels of phenolic compounds up to nearly 30% of their dry weight (DW) (Ragan and Glombitza 1986; Murray et al. 2018a). Some phenolic compounds may be halogenated, nitrogenous, or sulfated (La Barre et al. 2010), conferring different biological activities (Cabrita et al. 2010; La Barre et al. 2010). For example, bromophenols, halogenated monomeric phenolics, are common to all algal groups. Interestingly, they have also been detected in many kinds of seafood (e.g. prawns, crustaceans, mollusks; reviewed in Whitfield et al. 1999) or polychaetes and may contribute to the flavor of marine fish (Whitfield et al. 1999). In this review, we describe phenolic compounds that are produced by each taxonomical group of marine algae. Figure 11.2 illustrates examples

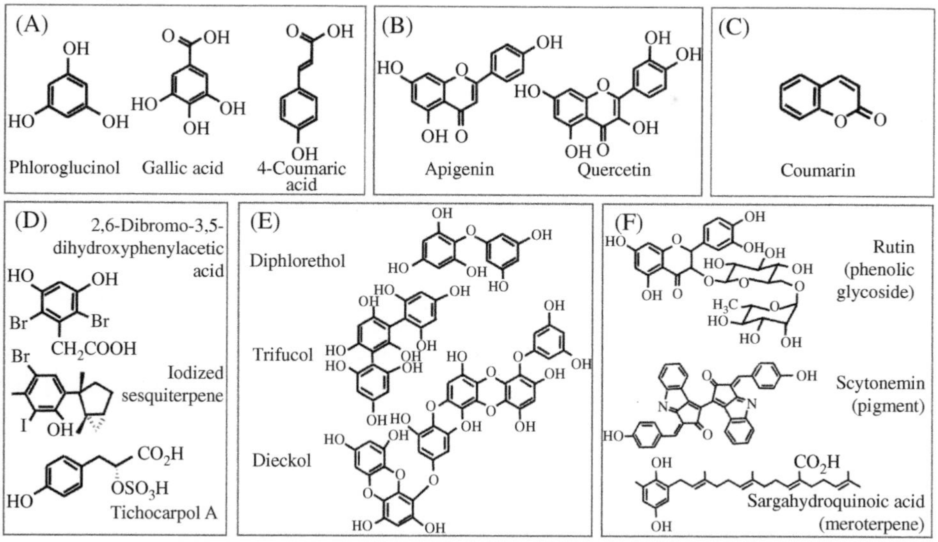

Figure 11.2 Examples of chemical structures of the different types of phenolic compounds produced by marine algae. (A) Phloroglucinol and phenolic acids, (B) flavonoids (flavone and flavonol), (C) coumarin, (D) halogenated and sulfated compounds, (E) phlorotannins (phlorethol, trifucol, eckol), (F) complex molecules (phenolic glycoside, pigment, meroterpene). Sources: De Nanteuil and Mastagli 1981; Whitfield et al. 1999; Yoshie-Stark et al. 2003; Goiris et al. 2014; Kornprobst 2014; Kirke et al. 2017.

of these compounds that have been isolated from the different algal groups including green, red, and brown macroalgae, Cyanobacteria, and microalgae (De Nanteuil and Mastagli 1981; Whitfield et al. 1999; Yoshie-Stark et al. 2003; Goiris et al. 2014; Kornprobst 2014; Kirke et al. 2017).

11.2.1 Phenolic Compounds from Marine Cyanobacteria and Microalgae

As the phenolic content is very low in microalgae and Cyanobacteria compared with macroalgae (<5 mg gallic acid equivalents [GAE] g^{-1} DW in microalgae; Ahmed et al. 2014), these compounds have not been well studied. Many research papers have just reported the phenolic content of algal extracts, with only a few devoted to their structural elucidation. Moreover, while a few research papers are focused on marine microalgae and Cyanobacteria (e.g. Goiris et al. 2014; Chlipala et al. 2010; Choi et al. 2010), the majority are dedicated to freshwater species including *Spongiochloris spongiosa*, *Arthrospira platensis*, *Anabaena doliolum*, *Nostoc* sp., *Cylindrospermum* sp., *Botryococcus braunii* (e.g. Klejdus et al. 2009; Tibbetts et al. 2015). Goiris et al. (2014) identified phloroglucinol, phenolic acids (mainly p-coumaric and ferulic acids), and flavone (apigenin) in the cyanobacterium *A. platensis*, and, together with these compounds, isoflavones (daidzein, genistein) and a flavonol (quercetin) in four marine phytoplankton species of different lineages (*Diacronema lutheri* –

Haptophyta, *Phaeodactylum tricornutum* – Bacillariophyta, *Tetraselmis suecica* – Chlorophyta, and *Porphyridium purpureum* – Rhodophyta), with *D. lutheri* being the most diverse in terms of phenolic composition. Many bromophenols have been also identified in marine Cyanobacteria, such as *Lyngbya majuscula*, *Phormidium nigroviride*, and *Schizothrix calcicola*, which contained bromophenol substituted with a macrodilactone, namely aplysiatoxins and derivatives (reviewed by Kornprobst 2014). Cyanobacterial cytotoxins exhibited in part a phenolic structure such as nhatrangins isolated from *Leptolyngbya majuscula* (Chlipala et al. 2010). Some bromophenols could also be sulfated, such as in *L. crossbyana*, which contains brominated and sulfated polyphenyl ethers, named crossbyanols A–D (Choi et al. 2010). Microalgal phenolic compounds with more complex structures are the chrysophaentin group (chrysophaentins A–H), which comprise linear and cyclic polyhalogenated bisdiarylbutenes isolated from the Chrysophyta *Chrysophaeum taylori* (Plaza et al. 2010a). Finally, a well-known phenolic compound specific to Cyanobacteria is scytonemin, which is a photoprotective pigment (García-Pichel and Castenholz 1991; Proteau et al. 1993).

11.2.2 Phenolic Compounds from Green and Red Macroalgae

Green and red seaweeds contain phenolic compounds, but generally in low concentrations compared with brown seaweeds (Mabeau and Fleurence 1993; Hardouin et al. 2014). First, red seaweeds contain bromoditerpenes (Briand et al. 1997; Ciavatta et al. 2001; Etahiri et al. 2001; Awad 2004) and meroditerpenes, particularly in *Callophycus serratus* (Lane et al. 2009; Paige-Stout et al. 2010; Woolner et al. 2018). The genus *Laurencia* (divided now into *Laurencia* and *Osmundea*), belonging to the Rhodomelaceae, is known for its richness in sesquiterpene derivatives (among papers, see Davyt et al. 2001; Masuda et al. 2002; Kladi et al. 2007; Cassano et al. 2008; Soares 2015). Many bromophenols have also been identified in other Rhodomelaceae genera including *Osmundaria*, *Polysiphonia*, *Rhodomela*, and *Symphyocladia* (Zhao et al. 2004; Wang et al. 2005; De Carvalho et al. 2006; Li et al. 2008a; Liu et al. 2011). More recently, new bromophenols derived from catechol have been isolated from *Symphyocladia latiuscula* (Xu et al. 2019). Specific phenolic compounds can also be found, such as tichocarpol in *Tichocarpus crinitus* (Ishii et al. 2004), halogenated phloroglucinol in *Rhabdonia verticillata* (Blackman and Matthews 1982), alkaloids with a phenol, such as hordenine in *Mastocarpus stellatus* or *Phyllophora crispa* (Güven et al. 1970; Barwell et al. 1989), or bromophycolides in *C. serratus* (Kubanek et al. 2006; Lane et al. 2009). Some authors also classify mycosporine-like amino acids (MAAs) as phenolic compounds (Stengel et al. 2011; Freile-Pelegrin and Robledo 2014). Mainly identified in red algae or Cyanobacteria (but also in lower levels in green algae), MAAs are formed by an aminocyclohexenimine or aminocyclohexenone ring to which are added different groups (Sinha et al. 2007). Nevertheless, we did not take into consideration MAAs as phenolic compounds as they do not possess an aromatic cycle.

In green seaweeds from the class Ulvophyceae, including the three genera *Caulerpa*, *Dasycladus*, and *Halimeda*, some bromophenols such as dibromophenols or simple bromated compounds have been detected (Whitfield et al. 1999). Other nontypical phenolic compounds have also been characterized, such as coumarins and trihydroxycoumarin, in green seaweeds such as *Caulerpa* spp. or *Dasycladus vermicularis* (Pérez-Rodríguez et al. 2001, 2003). In this latter species, Kurth et al. (2015)

also described a sulfated, hydroxylated coumarin derivative as a storage metabolite in its activated defense against fouling organisms. Examples of phenolic compounds found in green seaweeds include avrainvilleol and different bromophenols (2- or 4-), dibromophenols (2,4- and 2,6-), and 2,4,6-tribromophenol (Whitfield et al. 1999). Salicylic acid, also known as 2-hydroxybenzoic acid, was isolated from the green and calcareous *Halimeda incrassata* (Novoa et al. 2011). In this last species, ferulic acid could also be detected, albeit in a minor quantity of 8 $ng\,g^{-1}$ fresh weight (FW) (Novoa et al. 2011). Simple bromated polyphenolic compounds, together with flavonoids and catechins, were isolated from *Halimeda opuntia* and *Halimeda macroloba* (Yoshie et al. 2002). More precisely, epigallocatechin was identified in *H. macroloba*. In another work, *Halimeda monile* was reported to be a source of natural antioxidants including cinnamic, gallic, and caffeic acids (Mancini-Filho et al. 2009). Moreover, some vanillic acid derivatives with sulfate groups were described in another green macroalga, *Cladophora socialis* (Feng et al. 2007).

11.2.3 Phenolic Compounds from Brown Macroalgae

In brown seaweeds, the main phenolic compounds are the phlorotannins. These molecules are produced via the polymerization of the phloroglucinol monomer (1,3,5-trihydroxybenzene). Phlorotannins are synthesized through the acetate–malonate pathway (Targett and Arnold 1998; Shibata et al. 2004), with a molecular size ranging from 126 Da to 650 kDa (Ragan and Glombitza 1986; Ahn et al. 2007). It seems that PKS1, a type III polyketide synthase, is responsible for the synthesis of phlorotannins (Meslet-Cladiere et al. 2013). Phlorotannins constitute a heterogeneous group of molecules characterized by linkages between phloroglucinol units and the number of hydroxyl groups present on the molecule. Thus, they can be classified into four classes depending on the chemical bonds between monomers: fuhalols and phlorethols with ether linkages (Aryl-O-Aryl), fucols with phenyl linkages (Aryl-Aryl), fucophlorethols with ether and phenyl linkages, and finally eckols and carmalols with dibenzodioxin linkages (Singh and Bharate 2006; La Barre et al. 2010; Stiger-Pouvreau et al. 2014; Ar Gall et al. 2015; Lemesheva and Tarakhovskaya 2018). Creis et al. (2018) classified phlorotannins into six groups with the addition of isofuhalols with para- and meta-oriented ether bonds, added to the previous list.

Generally, phlorotannins are considered to be the main phenolic compounds of brown seaweeds. Nevertheless, other aromatic derivatives have also been identified, such as colpol isolated from *Colpomenia sinuosa* or phloroglucinol coupled with fatty acids including palmitic or stearic acid observed in *Zonaria farlowii* (Kornprobst 2014). Halogenated and sulfated compounds are also produced by brown seaweeds. Shibata et al. (2006) reported that the molecules excreted from *Eisenia bicyclis* and *Ecklonia kurome* mainly consisted of three bromophenols (2,4-dibromophenol, 2,4,6-tribromophenol, and dibromo-iodophenol), but not phloroglucinol or phlorotannins.

Some terpenes combined with aromatic derivatives have been reported in brown algae, similar to red and green algae (Kornprobst 2014). Algal species from the genera *Dictyopteris*, *Cystoseira*, *Sargassum*, or *Halidrys* exhibited some meroterpenes, i.e. a coupling of hydroquinone and linear terpenic chains (Kornprobst 2014). For example, a meromonoterpene was described in *Sporochnus bolleanus*; and merosesquiterpenes such as zonarol and isozonarol were found in *Dictyopteris* spp. Finally, meroditerpenes were detected in *Taonia* and *Stypopodium* (Gil et al. 1995), *Cystoseira* (Jégou et al. 2012), *Halidrys* (Culioli et al. 2008), *Bifurcaria*, and *Sargassum* species (Kornprobst 2014).

11.2.4 Variability of Phenolic Content in Space and Time

The phenolic content of algae is not linear all through the year and all around the world. Many parameters, i.e. abiotic and biotic, influence the production of phenolic compounds. Figure 11.3 summarizes all the abiotic and biotic factors that can influence the production of phenolic compounds in all taxonomical groups presented in this review, together with the different sectors of applications of those compounds, with references for each algal class of concern.

In the Phaeophyceae, phlorotannin levels vary from 5–300 mg phloroglucinol equivalents g^{-1} DW (Murray et al. 2018a), depending on the species (Stiger-Pouvreau et al. 2014), grazing (Pavia and Brock 2000; Svensson et al. 2007), epiphytism (Jennings and Steinberg 1997), ontogenic stages (Stiger et al. 2004; Plouguerné et al. 2006), latitude (Targett et al. 1992; Tanniou et al. 2014), depth and nutrients (Le Lann et al. 2012), seasons (Connan et al. 2004; Kamiya et al. 2010), or other environmental parameters

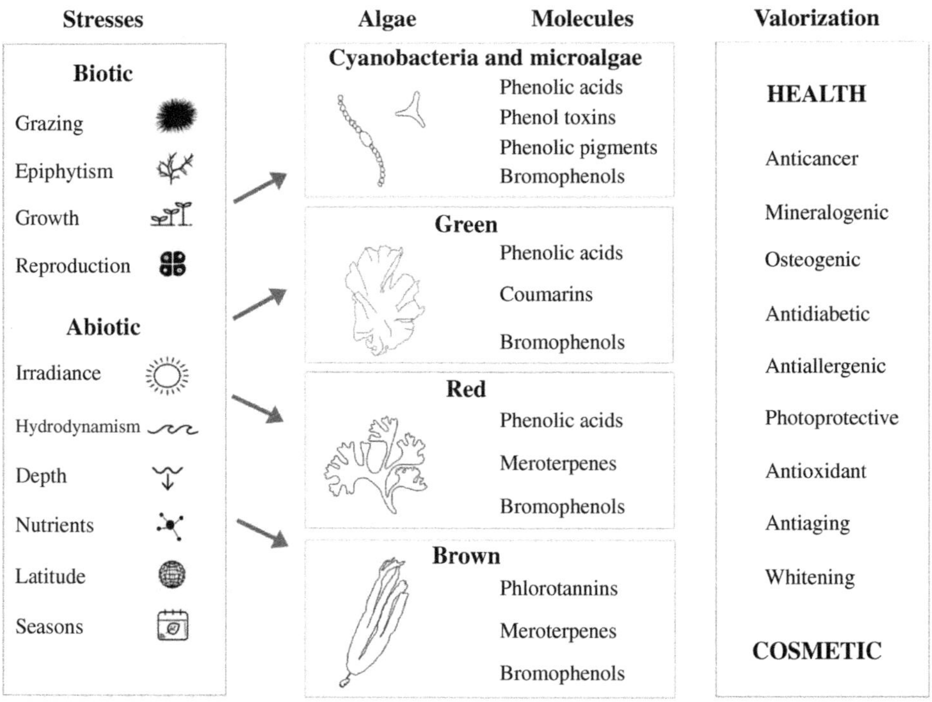

Figure 11.3 Conceptual model showing the impacts of several environmental parameters that influence the production and content of phenolic compounds in all algal groups presented in this review, along with potential bioactive properties of interest for the health and well-being sectors.

such as irradiance and UV radiation (Pavia and Brock 2000; Swanson and Druehl 2002), or hydrodynamism (Plouguerné et al. 2006; Le Lann et al. 2012).

In the same way, phenolic content in microalgae and green lineages varies from ng g^{-1} DW to <5 mg GAE g^{-1} DW for Cyanobacteria and microalgae depending on algal species and culture conditions (Klejdus et al. 2010; Ahmed et al. 2014; Goiris et al. 2014) and 4–60 mg GAE g^{-1} DW for green and red species (Cox et al. 2010; Machu et al. 2015).

11.3 Isolation and Purification of Phenolic Compounds from Algae

11.3.1 Importance of the Pretreatment of the Biomass

To maximize the phenolic extraction yield, microalgal and cyanobacterial biomasses are pretreated, which consists mainly of cell disruption (Parniakov et al. 2015). Different disruption mechanisms have been developed with their use depending on the microalgal group due to their differences in cell wall composition. These mechanisms have mainly been implemented during the extraction of valuable compounds of microalgae such as lipids as opposed to phenolic compounds (Prabakaran and Ravindran 2011). Two main mechanisms are employed: either physical or chemical (reviewed notably in Günerken et al. 2015 and D'Hondt et al. 2017). The physical methods consist of thermal (high, mild, or freezing temperatures, sometimes through a thermal cycle) treatment and/or mechanical disruption. Cryogrinding is an example of thermal treatment with liquid nitrogen (−196 °C) used for microalgae (Serive et al. 2012) but also macroalgae (Vandanjon et al. 2016). Mechanical pretreatment disrupts the cells using bead milling or high pressure (such as the French press; D'Hondt et al. 2017). The use of microwaves is also increasing and its utility has been demonstrated for pigment extraction from diatoms especially chlorophyll *a*, β,β-carotene, and fucoxanthin (Pasquet et al. 2011). The most extensively used disruption method used for phenolic studies is actually ultrasonication (Kepekçi and Saygideger 2012; Goiris et al. 2014; Parniakov et al. 2015). Chemical cell disruption has been widely studied as it can be more selective than physical methods; however, this pretreatment is included with the extraction itself and is thus discussed under extraction procedures below.

Extraction of phenolics from macroalgae can be directly performed on fresh algae, but often extraction cannot be immediately carried out; for example, after seaweed sampling in isolated areas. To prevent the degradation of the compounds, different storage conditions and treatments are available including freezing, freeze drying, sun-, or oven drying. Le Lann et al. (2008) studied several storage condition treatments on two brown Fucales. They reported that oven- and greenhouse drying reduced by around 50% the phenolic contents, respectively, for *Sargassum muticum* and *Bifurcaria bifurcata*, to the high temperatures. Freeze drying and freezing at −20 °C appeared to be good alternatives to conserve extracts mostly for thermosensitive compounds such as phenolic compounds. Indeed, Chan et al. (1997) reported that contact with air and high temperatures during sun- and oven drying impacted the nutritional composition of *Sargassum hemiphyllum*. *Ecklonia cava* extracts exhibited a higher yield of phlorotannins after freeze drying than sun drying (Chowdhury et al. 2011).

11.3.2 Extraction Procedures

Prior to the extraction of active compounds, another important step may include the grinding of seaweed: by reducing the particle size, the surface area in contact with the solvent is increased and thus the extraction rate (Abu-Ghannam and Rajauria 2013). Seaweeds are often ground or crushed using mechanical force such as a blender when mixed with solvent, manually or using a hammer-mill or Wylie Mill using a mesh screen of known size (Michalak and Chojnacka 2014).

Protocols for the extraction of phenolic compounds are widely variable. Historically, and still today, maceration or grinding were used with various solvent mixtures to obtain extracts enriched in phenolics from all algal groups (Stiger-Pouvreau et al. 2014). Thus, the amount of phenolic compounds obtained by solid/liquid extraction depended on the solvent used (often methanol diluted with water) but also on the temperature, extraction time, or pH (Koivikko et al. 2005; Leyton et al. 2016; Creis et al. 2018). Creis et al. (2018) reviewed solid/liquid extraction of phlorotannins with different parameters including type of solvent, temperature, or time. Similarly, when Stiger-Pouvreau et al. (2014), Ar Gall et al. (2015), and Le Lann et al. (2016) reviewed protocols for extraction of brown seaweeds, and Surget et al. (2016, 2017) for green seaweeds, these authors presented solid/liquid extraction protocols followed by a liquid/liquid purification procedure, which resulted in concentrated and very active phenolic fractions. However, these classical extraction protocols are time- and energy-consuming (Ibañez et al. 2012). Thus, in recent years, new extraction techniques have been developed, with an increased interest in green and thereby food-safe extractions, in particular for the valorization of polyphenols as bioactive compounds for dietary or human health (Wijesinghe and Jeon 2012a).

According to Chemat et al. (2012), "green extractions are based on the discovery and design of extraction processes which will reduce energy consumption, allow use of alternative solvents and renewable natural products, and ensure a safe and high quality product." First, the solvents can be changed to less hazardous choices such as water or ethanol or a mix of both solvents as demonstrated by Prat et al. (2016), or the use of deep eutectic solvents (DESs; that is, eutectic mixtures of Lewis or Brønsted acids and bases, which can contain a variety of anionic and/or cationic species) can also be an alternative to organic solvents and have the potential to extract phenolic compounds (Ruesgas-Ramón et al. 2017). The most common DESs are formed by combining choline chloride with most often urea, ethylene glycol, or glycerol (Ruesgas-Ramón et al. 2017). Table 11.1 outlines different green extractions for obtaining brown seaweed extracts rich in phlorotannins. Reviews from Esquivel-Hernández et al. (2017), Cikoš et al. (2018), and Gallego et al. (2018) highlighted the main green extraction technologies for algae, which included supercritical fluid extraction (SFE), microwave assisted extraction (MAE), pressurized liquid extraction (PLE), and ultrasound assisted extraction (UAE). All of these methods have many advantages, such as shorter times, less solvent required, and higher extraction rates. Enzyme assisted extraction (EAE) (Wijesinghe and Jeon 2012b; Kadam et al. 2015b), centrifugal partition chromatography (CPC) (Tanniou et al. 2013), liquid biphasic systems (LBSs; Chia et al. 2018), or ionic liquids (IL; Vo Dinh et al. 2018) were also investigated as green extraction protocols to extract phlorotannins.

The use of EAE for marine algae has rarely been reported. Wang et al. (2010) reported a positive effect of proteases, e.g. Protamex® and Flavourzyme®

Table 11.1 Examples of green extractions to obtain extracts enriched in phlorotannins from brown seaweeds

Green extraction	Species	References
PLE	*Alaria esculenta, Asperococcus bullosus, Bifurcaria bifurcata, Cystoseira tamariscifolia, Desmarestia ligulata, Dictyota dichotoma, Fucus ceranoides, Halidrys siliquosa, Saccorhiza polyschides*	Zubia et al. (2009)
	Ascophyllum nodosum	O'Sullivan et al. (2013), Tierney et al. (2013b)
	Fucus spiralis	Tierney et al. (2013a), Tierney et al. (2013b)
	Fucus serratus	Zubia et al. (2009), O'Sullivan et al. (2013), Heffernan et al. (2014)
	Himanthalia elongata	Plaza et al. (2010a, b)
	Laminaria digitata	Heffernan et al. (2014)
	Padina pavonica	Fayad et al. (2017)
	Pelvetia canaliculata	Tierney et al. (2013b)
	Saccharina japonica	Vo Dinh et al. (2018)
	Sargassum muticum	Tanniou et al. (2013), Pilar Sánchez-Camargo et al. (2016)
	Undaria pinnatifida	Onofrejová et al. (2010)
MAE	*Ascophyllum nodosum, Saccharina japonica, Lessonia trabeculata, Lessonia nigrescens*	Yuan et al. (2018)
	Carpophyllum flexuosum, Carpophyllum plumosum	Magnusson et al. (2017), Zhang et al. (2018)
	Ecklonia radiata	Charoensiddhi et al. (2015), Magnusson et al. (2017), Zhang et al. (2018)
	Padina pavonica	Fayad et al. (2017)
	Saccharina japonica	He et al. (2013)
	Sargassum vestitum	Dang et al. (2018)
EAE	*Ecklonia radiata*	Charoensiddhi et al. (2015)
	Sargassum aquifolium, Sargassum ilicifolium S. polycystum	Puspita et al. (2017)
	Sargassum muticum	Rodrigues et al. (2015), Vandanjon et al. (2016), Pilar Sánchez-Camargo et al. (2016)

Table 11.1 (*continued*)

Green extraction	Species	References
UAE	*Ascophyllum nodosum*	Kadam et al. (2015b), Moreira et al. (2017), Agregán et al. (2017a)
	Ecklonia cava	Lee et al. (2013)
	Fucus vesiculosus, *Bifurcaria bifurcata*	Agregán et al. (2017a)
	Sargassum muticum	Rodrigues et al. (2015)
SFE	*Saccharina japonica*	Saravana et al. (2017)
	Sargassum muticum	Tanniou et al. (2013), Conde et al. (2015)
CPC	*Ecklonia cava*	Lee et al. (2014, 2015)
	Ishige okamurae	Kim et al. (2016)
	Sargassum muticum	Tanniou et al. (2013)
LBS	*Padina australis*, *Sargassum binderi*	Chia et al. (2018)
IL	*Saccharina japonica*	Vo Dinh et al. (2018)

PLE = pressurized liquid extraction, MAE = microwave assisted extraction, EAE = enzyme assisted extraction, UAE = ultrasound assisted extraction, SFE = supercritical fluid extraction, CPC = centrifugal partition chromatography, LBS = liquid biphasic system, IL = ionic liquid.

(Novozymes; www.novozymes.com), on the extraction of polyphenols from the red macroalga *Palmaria palmata*. On the other hand, Hardouin et al. (2014), working with three abundant macroalgal species in Brittany, *S. muticum*, *Solieria chordalis*, and *Ulva* sp., reported that enzymatic hydrolysis was not efficient for the extraction of phenolic compounds compared with the extraction without enzymatic hydrolysis, but it did improve the isolation of proteins and polysaccharides. In addition to conventional chemical methods (the use of acids, alkali, or different solvents) new extraction protocols have been developed for use with macro-, microalgae, and Cyanobacteria, including the use of supercritical fluids such as CO_2 tested to extract benzoic acid derivatives, hydroxybenzaldehydes, and cinnamic acid derivatives from *S. spongiosa*, *Arthrospira* (*Spirulina*) *platensis*, *Trichormus* (*Anabaena*) *doliolum*, *Nostoc* sp., and *Cylindrospermum* sp. (Klejdus et al. 2009); the use of supercritical CO_2 was sometimes coupled with ultrasonication tested to extract isoflavones on *S. muticum*, *Sargassum vulgare*, *Hypnea spinella*, *Porphyra* sp., *Undaria pinnatifida*, *Chondrus crispus*, *Halopythis incurva*, *S. spongiosa*, *Scenedesmus* sp., and *Nostoc* sp. (Klejdus et al. 2010). On the other hand, IL such as the co-solvent 1-ethyl-3-methyl imidazolium methyl sulfate and methanol have not yet been applied to extraction of phenolic compounds but they seem promising and are already used for lipids (Young et al. 2010).

When using SFE protocols, the main drawback with CO_2 has been its low polarity, which is not conducive to phlorotannin extraction (Kadam et al. 2015a). Nevertheless, to increase SFE solvation power, polar modifiers (e.g. methanol or ethanol) have been used to increase the polarity of the supercritical fluid to extract these phenolic compounds (Ibañez et al. 2012; Tanniou et al. 2013). Some work has nevertheless been done to extract phenolic compounds from algae; for example, Tanniou et al.

(2013), Conde et al. (2015), and Saravana et al. (2017) focused on phenolic compounds from *S. muticum* and *Saccharina japonica*. While PLE (e.g. high temperature combined with high pressure) can extract a wide spectrum of compounds such as phenols, this technique is less selective and requires more purification steps (Ibañez et al. 2012; Kadam et al. 2015a). For example, to extract phenolics from *A. platensis*, Esquivel-Hernández et al. (2017) advised the use of MAE or PLE followed by SFE. Further advantages and disadvantages of these different extraction techniques have been reviewed by Kadam et al. (2015a). Da Silva et al. (2017) compared different extraction methodologies for phenolic and flavonoid yields from the Cyanobacteria *A. platensis*: HPTE, i.e. high pressure and high temperature, which is equivalent to PLE, compared with UAE and MAE. They concluded that PLE using ethanol at 90 °C and 2.5 bar in a stirred reactor was the most efficient method to extract a higher polyphenol yield (~3.5 mg of GAE g^{-1} DW), whereas flavonoids were better extracted using MAE with ethanol at 60 W for 60 minutes (~2.8 mg of catechin equivalent g^{-1} DW). LBS is also another alternative extraction compared with conventional extraction. There are several types of LBS, such as a mix of polymer/salt, alcohol/salt, or polymer/polymer (Chia et al. 2018). In Chia et al. (2018), they focused on the extraction of phlorotannins with an alcohol/salt LBS method on *Padina australis* and *Sargassum aquifolium* (*S. binderi*) and found the best combination of alcohol/salt to be 2-propanol and ammonium sulfate for the phlorotannin extraction. CPC or centrifugal partition extraction (CPE) can be also used to extract phenolic compounds from seaweeds (Tanniou et al. 2013; Lee et al. 2014, 2015; Kim et al. 2016). According to Tanniou et al. (2013), CPC used with the solvent mix of ethyl acetate and water (50 : 50) obtained the best yield in phenolic compounds compared with SFE and PLE (22.90, 3.45, and approx. 10% DW, respectively). The best stable free radical scavenging activities were also highlighted with CPC (IC_{50} of 0.52 mg ml^{-1} for CPC, 28.31 mg ml^{-1} for SFE, and 0.80 mg ml^{-1} for PLE with the 2,2-diphenyl-1-picrylhydrazyl (DPPH) assay). Lee et al. (2014, 2015) have succeeded in extracting phlorotannins from the brown alga *E. cava* (dieckol, phlorofucofuroeckol-A, 2,7-phloroglucinol-6,6-bioeckol, and pyrogallol-phloroglucinol-6,6-bioeckol) with the CPC method with a two-phase solvent system comprising n-hexane:ethyl acetate:methanol:water (2:7:3:7, v/v). Another study extracted phlorotannins from *Ishige okamurae* with the CPC using the same solvent system as Lee et al. (2014, 2015) but with a different ratio 0.5:10:4:6 (v/v) (Kim et al. 2016).

11.3.3 Quantification and Analyses of Phenolic Compounds

The quantification and analyses of algal polyphenols are further complicated by the difficulty of separating and isolating them from other compounds naturally occurring *in vivo* (Freile-Pelegrin and Robledo 2014). Polyphenols are generally quantified using different spectrophotometric methods based on reaction of a colored reagent with the phenolic functional group(s). Those methods are summarized, especially for phlorotannins, in the recent review of Ford et al. (2019). The most common assay is the Folin–Ciocalteu method (Waterman and Mole 1994), based on phosphotungstic-phosphomolybdic compounds as the color reagents and phloroglucinol (for brown seaweeds) or gallic acid (for green and red seaweeds) as the reference standards for calibration. However, colorimetric assays are nonspecific and thus detect all phenolic hydroxyl groups in the extract, desired or otherwise

(Stiger-Pouvreau et al. 2014; Kirke et al. 2017). Another colorimetric method using aluminum chloride has been used for flavonoid quantification (Safafar et al. 2015; Da Silva et al. 2017). These colorimetric methods provide little information about the chemical composition of the phenolic content. In this sense, purification steps are needed to obtain more concentrated extracts and information on the chemical composition of phlorotannins, and/or to characterize their chemical structures. Different methods exist to separate/purify phenolics, such as liquid/liquid extraction, solid phase extraction (SPE), ultrafiltration, dialysis, thin layer chromatography (TLC), and high pressure liquid chromatography (HPLC) (Le Lann et al. 2012; Stiger-Pouvreau et al. 2014; Creis et al. 2018). These methods separate molecules according to their polarity or size, in order to enrich fractions or to isolate individual compounds (Vandanjon et al. 2017). Following separation, phenolic compounds can be identified or characterized by Fourier transform infrared spectroscopy (FT-IR), nuclear magnetic resonance (NMR), and/or mass spectrometry (MS). Combined with HPLC, these detection methods offer a rapid way to identify and quantify these molecules (Ferreres et al. 2012; Steevensz et al. 2012; Goiris et al. 2014; Karthik et al. 2016; Le Lann et al. 2016; Rajauria et al. 2016; Agregán et al. 2017b; Rajauria 2018; Gonçalves-Fernández et al. 2019). However, for phlorotannins, their structural characterization and identification is difficult due to their complexity, polymeric nature, instability, rapid oxidation, and their ability to complex with other molecules (Stiger-Pouvreau et al. 2014).

11.4 Biological Properties of Phenolic Compounds in Health, Well-Being, and Cosmetics

Due to their great diversity, phenolics have demonstrated many different bioactivities *in vitro* and *in vivo* (Cornish and Garbary 2010; Thomas and Kim 2011; Wijesinghe and Jeon 2011, 2012a; Catarino et al. 2018). For microalgae and Cyanobacteria, where phenolics are minor constituents (<0.1 mg g^{-1} DW; Goiris et al. 2014), biological activities have often been demonstrated with crude or purified extracts but only a few examples have been published on biological activities of purified and structurally identified phenolic compounds, such as benzoic and cinnamic acid derivatives (Stevenson et al. 2002; Choi et al. 2010; Plaza et al. 2010a; Davison and Bewley 2019). Phlorotannins are among the most studied phenolic compounds, with many reports focused on their biological properties as opposed to other algal phenolic compounds (Gupta and Abu-Ghannam 2011a; Li et al. 2011; Thomas and Kim 2011; Wijesinghe and Jeon 2011; Imbs and Zvyagintseva 2018).

11.4.1 Antioxidant Properties

In normal conditions, organisms are able to regulate their metabolism to maintain very low levels of reactive oxygen species (ROS) or more common free radicals that possess a single electron, i.e. unpaired, which are involved in many cellular functions including respiration (Apak et al. 2016). Thus, production of ROS and their elimination are well balanced via endogenous antioxidant enzyme systems and molecules. However, in some circumstances, including in response to environmental pressures or oxidative stress, this balance may be disrupted, and consequently, these unstable molecules are produced in excess (Wijesinghe and Jeon 2012a; Lushchak 2014). In particular, oxidative stress plays a critical role in the pathogenesis of various chronic diseases including cancers, atherosclerosis, ischemic injury, inflammation, and neurodegenerative disorders (Kang et al. 2005; Reuter et al. 2010). Therefore, the body requires antioxidants, i.e. molecules whose role is to scavenge or quench free radicals, inhibit initiation of peroxidation, and prevent or reduce cell damage from ROS and other reactive species (Surh 2005). Dietary sources of antioxidants may be natural or artificial, although in recent years, the importance of replacing artificial antioxidants with natural ingredients has increased considerably, for increased safety and improved human health (Gupta and Abu-Ghannam 2011b; Farvin and Jacobsen 2013; Chakraborty et al. 2015). Synthetic antioxidants such as BHA (butylated hydroxyanisole) or BHT (butylated hydroxytoluene) are widely used in the food industry (Gupta and Abu-Ghannam 2011b), but they have been reported to be cytotoxic and to exert a carcinogenic effect (Chen et al. 1992). In this sense, natural phenolics from seaweeds have been reported to act as antioxidants and they seem to be a good alternative to synthetics (Agregán et al. 2018). It has been widely demonstrated that phenolic or phlorotannin levels of seaweed extracts are correlated with antioxidant activity (Jiménez-Escrig et al. 2001; Connan et al. 2004; Duan et al. 2006; Matanjun et al. 2008) and that this activity depended on their structure, and, especially for phlorotannins, on the degree of polymerization of phloroglucinol (Nakamura et al. 1996; Kirke et al. 2017).

Studies evaluating antioxidant activity can be divided into two major groups: those using methods based on single electron transfer (SET) and those based on hydrogen atom transfer (HAT) (Huang and Prior 2005; Apak et al. 2016). Oxygen radical absorbance capacity (ORAC), inhibition of lipoperoxidation, or β-carotene assays are examples of HAT assays, while ferric reducing antioxidant power (FRAP), 2,2-diphenyl-1-picrylhydrazyl ($DPPH^{\bullet}$), Trolox equivalent antioxidant capacity (TEAC), or 2,2′-azino-bis(3-ethylbenzothiazoline-6-sulfonic acid) ($ABTS^{+}$) assays are SET methods (Sun et al. 2018). Brown seaweed phlorotannins such as dieckol or fucophlorethol have been reported to possess high antioxidant activity, often with a higher activity than other polyphenols such as flavonoids derived from terrestrial plants (e.g. Agregán et al. 2017a). Phlorotannins were also reported to have higher antioxidant activities than other phenolics such as phenolic acids from red or green algae; although other studies have reported high phenolic contents and antioxidant activities in some red species, including *Chondria baileyana* (Zubia et al. 2007), *Polysiphonia stricta* (Duan et al. 2006), *S. latiuscula* (Zhang et al. 2007), or *Mastocarpus stellatus* (Farvin and Jacobsen 2013) for red algae, and *Avrainvillea longicaulis* (Zubia et al. 2007), *H. incrassata* (Fallarero et al. 2003), *Ulva prolifera* (Cho et al. 2011), *Ulva compressa* (Cho et al. 2010; Paiva et al. 2016), *Capsosiphon fulvescens* (Cho et al. 2010), *Ulva rigida* (Paiva et al. 2016), and *Caulerpa* spp. (Santoso et al. 2004; Cavas and Yurdakoc 2005; Matanjun et al. 2008) for green species.

There have been several reviews of papers demonstrating antioxidant activities of brown seaweed extracts (Wijesinghe and Jeon 2011; Balboa et al. 2013; Murray et al. 2018a; Qin 2018) and also isolated phlorotannins (Nakamura et al. 1996) using *in vitro* assays. As results can be variable, it is important to perform different assays (SET and HAT) to validate the potential antioxidant activity as the observed differences may be down to the reaction conditions and duration (Audibert et al. 2010). The antioxidant activities of individual phlorotannins have rarely been explored except for some isolated from *E. cava* and *E. bicyclis* (Murray et al. 2018b). Recently, Hermund et al. (2018) analyzed the antioxidant capacity of enriched fractions of *Fucus vesiculosus* using chromatography with an electrochemical detector followed by MS. They measured the ability of individual fractions to donate an electron and provided information on their antioxidant capacity using an online cyclic voltammetry approach. They showed that low molecular weight phlorotannins such as an isomer of fucophlorethol with three phloroglucinol units exhibited higher antioxidant capacities, but a decreasing capacity when phlorotannins were polymerized such as fucophlorethol with six or seven phloroglucinol units (Murray et al. 2018b). Although those phlorotannins have exhibited a strong *in vitro* efficacy, their activity is unclear in humans, although some studies have been performed on cell lines (Kang et al. 2005, 2012b; Heo and Jeon 2009; Pinteus et al. 2017). For example, Pinteus et al. (2017) reported that *Fucus spiralis* fractions, obtained with methanol or dichloromethane, decreased H_2O_2 levels (responsible for antioxidant stress) in human cells (MCF-7) by 50.64 and 46.71%, respectively. Similar results were found for other cell lines including murine hippocampus cell line (HT22), Chinese hamster lung fibroblast line (V79-4), cells of a monkey kidney fibroblast line (Vero) by Kang et al. (2005, 2012a) and Heo and Jeon (2009), respectively, and with other brown seaweeds *E. cava* and *I. okamurae*. In brown algae, including *Carpodesmia crinita*, meroterpenes (i.e. a coupling of hydroquinone and linear terpenic chains) such as tetraprenyltoluquinone derivatives, tetra- or triprenyltoluquinol derivatives also demonstrated antioxidant activities with *in vitro* assays (Fisch et al. 2003).

Even if the direct consumption of algae for their natural antioxidants is recommended (Cornish and Garbary 2010), the literature on the direct beneficial human health effects of marine algal polyphenols is sparse as showed previously with many *in vitro* assays, and a few experiments have been conducted using *in vitro* assays simulating the human digestion system (reviewed in Murray et al. 2018b and Qin 2018). Indeed, while the antioxidant benefits associated with the consumption of various terrestrial plants from epidemiological studies have long been accepted, there are relatively few studies on the potential impact of consumption of algae on human health (e.g. Scalbert et al. 2005).

With regard to the potential application of algal polyphenols in the cosmetics or cosmeceuticals sectors, antioxidant activities have also been evaluated studying creams and oils (Balboa et al. 2014; Poyato et al. 2016). Balboa et al. (2014) evaluated the antioxidant activity of *S. muticum* and *Ulva lactuca* extracts in model emulsions and oils after 35 days storage at 50 °C. They measured the peroxide value (PV), which quantified hydroperoxides (primary oxidation) and the p-anisidine values (PA), which measured the production of aldehydes (secondary oxidation) during oxidation of fats or oils from the extract/emulsion. The total oxidation value (TOTOX), which is calculated as 2PV + PA (Wan et al. 2009), was used to estimate the oxidative deterioration of lipids, as well as the primary and secondary oxidation products. After 34 days of storage, the seaweed extract, i.e. from the brown seaweed *S. muticum* and the green seaweed *U. lactuca*, inhibited lipid oxidation evaluated by the PV and the amount of volatile compounds (their presence reflects a degradation of lipids) more effectively in avocado cream (93.96%), than in shower oil (58.58%) and in massage oil (13.90%). Another study evaluated the oxidative stability of a skin care emulsion with a *F. vesiculosus* extract (Poyato et al. 2016): when the extract was included in the emulsion, the color changed more extensively when the cream was exposed under high temperature than the unheated control. Similar to Balboa et al. (2014), water and acetone extracts of *F. vesiculosus* showed protective effects against oxidation, more precisely thermooxidation, i.e. oxidation induced by temperature, but only the water extract showed protection against photoxidation, i.e. oxidation induced by light (Poyato et al. 2016). Taken together, the literature indicates that algal polyphenols and, in particular, the phlorotannins, exhibit strong SET and HAT antioxidant activities *in vitro*. The next steps should endeavor to demonstrate this activity *in vivo*.

11.4.2 Antiallergenic and Anti-inflammatory Properties

Allergic and hypersensitivity reactions represent significant health challenges worldwide and the complexity, frequency, and severity of reactions continue to be concerns due to a variety of factors (environment, genetics, hygiene, diet, etc.) known to have an impact on their development (Singh et al. 2011; Pawankar 2014). They constitute systemic immune responses to various allergens, which encompass skin, food, and respiratory allergies and hypersensitivities. The molecular and cellular mechanisms responsible for these allergies are complex, and patients with asthma and allergies frequently experience a reduced quality of life due to co-existing disorders, including diabetes, obesity, and cardiovascular disease (Pawankar 2014). In particular, asthma is a complex inflammatory disease of the airways that affects approximately 300 million people worldwide (Lambrecht and Hammad 2015).

In response to an allergen, allergic individuals synthesize large amounts of antigen-specific immunoglobulin E (IgE) antibodies (Bousquet et al. 2008). The IgE binds to granulocytes (eosinophils and basophils) or mast cells (also known as mastocytes), which then degranulate and cause the release of mediators such as histamines, β-hexosaminidase, and eicosanoids, which are responsible for allergic reactions (anaphylactic shock) or inflammatory responses (Larsen et al. 2016). Allergic symptoms can be difficult to control in all patients with pharmacotherapies such as norepinephrine alone (Larsen et al. 2016). Allergy desensitization (immunotherapy) is another way to fight against this chronic health condition by attempting to change or lessen the response to allergen exposure and, thereby, building immunological tolerance (Larsen et al. 2016). The search for molecules with antiallergenic and anti-inflammatory potential constitutes a major opportunity. Currently, few algal polyphenols are used for their antiallergenic activities, the majority being polyphenols, such as epigallocatechin derivatives from terrestrial plants including Japanese or Taiwanese tea (*Camellia sinensis*) (Maeda-Yamamoto and Tachibana 2012). The proposed mechanisms of action of these terrestrial polyphenols are notably the suppression of tyrosine phosphorylation of cellular protein kinase, and the suppression of myosin light chain phosphorylation (Maeda-Yamamoto and Tachibana 2012). Recently, an ethanol extract of the brown macroalga *Scytosiphon* sp. showed great antiallergenic activity ($IC_{50} = 0.67\,mg\,ml^{-1}$) similar to the positive control epigallocatechin gallate (EGCG) ($IC_{50} = 0.56\,mg\,ml^{-1}$) using an enzyme assay (Chen et al. 2015).

In order to test the antiallergenicity of a compound, experiments are generally performed on rodent (RBL-2H3, murine model) or human (KU812) mast cells (Girish and Kemparaju 2007; Shim et al. 2009; Ahn et al. 2015; Chen et al. 2015). Degranulation studies, measurement of the level of histamine, β-hexosaminidase or eicosanoids, and investigation of the activity of enzymes involved in the allergic reaction (such as hyaluronidase [HA], phospholipase A2 [PLA2], cyclooxygenases

[COX-1 and COX-2], and lipooxygenase [LOX]) are different methodologies to test the antiallergenic or anti-inflammatory efficacy of a seaweed extract (Girish and Kemparaju 2007; Chen et al. 2015). The regulation of IgE receptors on rodent or human mast cells is another methodology that permits the elucidation of the mechanism of the antiallergenic molecules (Shim et al. 2009; Ahn et al. 2015). Several studies, mainly on brown seaweeds, have reported an antiallergenic effect of phlorotannins in crude or purified extracts, or isolates that seem to be promising molecules against allergies and inflammation (Sugiura et al. 2006b; Samee et al. 2009; Shim et al. 2009; Sugiura et al. 2009; Sugiura et al. 2012). First, crude methanolic extracts of *E. cava*, *Eisenia arborea*, *Sargassum ringgoldianum*, *Ishige foliacea*, *I. okamurae*, *Sargassum thunbergii*, and *Sargassum micracanthum* exhibited antiallergenic activities by inhibiting the degranulation of mast cells (decreasing histamine release; Sugiura et al. 2006b). The antiallergenic activities of *E. cava* extracts were confirmed by Shim et al. (2009) in a study of the regulation of IgE receptors. Moreover, Sugiura et al. (2009) demonstrated that a methanol chloroform extract of *E. arborea* decreased the quantity of eicosanoids, leukotrienes, and prostaglandins (produced by stimulating the cells using antigen–antibody reaction on RBL-2H3 cells) responsible for inflammation. These authors also reported that an extract from *Ecklonia stolonifera* inhibited β-hexosaminidase release and enzymes involved in the inflammatory response (HA, COX-2, LOX, PLA2) in mast cells, linked to the extract phlorotannin content (Sugiura et al. 2012). Samee et al. (2009) reported that an ethanol extract from *Sargassum tenerrimum* exhibited antihyaluronidase activities performed with a colorimetric assay. The results obtained by Chen et al. (2015) also indicated that a *Scytosiphon* sp. hydroethanolic extract enriched in phlorotannins had a higher antihyaluronidase activity than the typical antiallergic drug disodium cromoglycate (DSCG).

Several ethanolic extracts containing phenolics derived from red algae also presented antiallergenic activities. For example, Chen et al. (2015) screened the antiallergenic activity of five algal species including the red macroalga *Porphyra* sp., and reported an antiallergenic activity from its ethanolic extract but 10× lower than the positive control (IC_{50} = 6.86 and 0.56 mg ml^{-1}, respectively). Moreover, an *in vivo* study in female C57BL/6 mice sensitized and stimulated by ovalbumin, an egg white allergen, reported for the first time that the red macroalga *Chondrophycus undulatus* exhibited therapeutic potential for fighting bronchial asthma notably because of its inhibitory activities on all aspects of the asthmatic inflammation process (Jung et al. 2009). Methanolic extracts from the green macroalga *Codium fragile* exhibited anti-inflammatory effects on lipopolysaccharide-stimulated murine macrophage RAW 264.7 cells, in attenuating edema and erythema values in cell incubation tests with a *C. fragile* methanol extract (Kang et al. 2012b). In another study, Khan et al. (2008) demonstrated that mouse ear edema and erythema (induced by phorbol myristate acetate) were both suppressed by a topical application to the inner side of the mouse ear of methanolic extracts from the brown seaweed *U. pinnatifida* and the green macroalga *Ulva linza*.

Similar to the above discussion on algal crude extracts of phenolic compounds, purified fractions with a high phenolic content were promising for antiallergenic properties; for example, Barbosa et al. (2018) reported that *Fucus serratus* and *Fucus guiryi* fractions inhibited β-hexosaminidase and histamine release from RBL-2H3 cells. The effects of these extracts were partly explained by their phlorotannin contents. In another study from the same laboratory, fractions from *F. guiryi*, *F. serratus*,

F. spiralis, and *F. vesiculosus* also inhibited LOX in a cell-free system (Barbosa et al. 2017). A purified diethyl ether fraction from *Sargassum fusiforme* exhibited antiallergenic activities on *in vitro* and *in vivo* models (Sugiura et al. 2016): the mouse ear swelling induced by three different sensitizers reduced from 47 to 61% at a dose of 0.1 mg per mouse upon oral administration of seaweed fractions enriched in phlorotannins. Moreover, this extract also exhibited an inhibitory effect on PLA2, COX-2, and LOX activities with enzyme assays and the strongest inhibition of HA activity.

Isolated phlorotannins have also been reported to exhibit antiallergenic activities: Sugiura et al. (2006a) reported that phlorotannins (i.e. 6-6′-bioeckol, 6,8′-bioeckol and 8,8′-bioeckol, and phlorofucofuroeckol-A and -B) isolated from *E. arborea* had antiallergenic effects determined by inhibition of histamine release from RBL cells stimulated by the antigen–antibody reaction. Phlorofucofuroeckol-B (PFF-B) had the strongest activity: 2.8-fold greater than other inhibitors such as epigallocatechin gallate (EGCG) (Sugiura et al. 2006a, 2007). These authors reported that the antiallergenic activities of the phlorotannins was positively associated with molecular weight and the number of hydroxyl groups as demonstrated with PFF-B. Phlorotannins (i.e. eckol, PFF-A, dieckol and 8,8′-bioeckol) from *E. bicyclis* exhibited similar activities with an inhibition of eicosanoids such as PLA_2, LOX and COX determined with an *in vitro* assay (Shibata et al. 2003). Li et al. (2008b) isolated three phlorotannins from *E. cava* with antiallergenic activities: eckol showed the strongest activity followed by PFF-A and fucodiphlorethol G (FG) assessed using histamine and β-hexosaminidase release from mast cells. Other phlorotannins with antiallergenic activities were isolated from *E. cava*, ranked in increasing order of activity: 6,6′-bioeckol (6B); dieckol; 1-(3′,5′-dihydroxyphenoxy)-7-′(2″,4″,6-trihydroxyphenoxy)-2,4,9-trihydroxydibenzo-1,4-dioxin (DTTD); and phloroglucinol. They showed inhibition of histamine and β-hexosaminidase release by RBL-2H3 and KU812 cells (Le et al. 2009). Ahn et al. (2015) also reported that dieckol from *E. cava* exhibited antiallergenic activities with *in vitro* and *in vivo* assays. Finally, fucophlorethol C, isolated from *Dactylosiphon bullosus*, exhibited inhibition of LOX with an *in vitro* assay (Kurihara et al. 2015); the authors concluded that free phenolic hydroxyl groups were important for the anti allergenic activity associated with blocking the activity of the LOX. A meroditerpene extracted from *Stypopodium flabelliforme*, epitaondiol, exhibited anti-inflammatory activities via decreased eicosanoids release and PLA2 activity in human neutrophils (Gil et al. 1995).

Red seaweeds are also rich in anti-inflammatory compounds, such as the bromophenol metabolites vidalol A and B in *Vidalia obtusaloba*, which showed significant reduction in edema (58–82%) when applied topically to phorbol ester-induced swelling of mouse ears and significant inhibition of the PLA2 in an enzyme assay (Wiemer et al. 1991), or catechol from *Porphyra dentata*, which inhibited the production of nitric oxide (NO), a signaling molecule that plays a key role in the pathogenesis of inflammation (Kazlowska et al. 2010). The inhibitory capacity of phenolic compounds against bee venom derived PLA2 activity in enzyme tests was also highlighted in green algae; for example, Mayer et al. (1993) isolated two sesquiterpenes: bromohydroquinone cymopol from *Caulerpa prolifera* and cyclocymopol from *Cymopolia barbata*, which exhibited inhibition of PLA2 in enzyme tests. Interestingly, Silva et al. (2017) reviewed all the PLA2 inhibitors from marine organisms and discussed that algae represent a good potential source of these inhibitors.

11.4.3 Antidiabetic, Antiobesity Properties and Cardiovascular Protection

Worldwide, obesity and diabetes are considered two of the most prevalent metabolic diseases (Wild et al. 2004; James et al. 2012). According to the World Health Organization (WHO), worldwide obesity has nearly tripled since 1975 and the number of people with diabetes has risen from 108 million in 1980 to 422 million in 2014. Diabetes or diabetes mellitus comprises three major diagnoses, the most common of which is type II diabetes, then type I diabetes, and, finally, gestational diabetes, which is temporary occurring during pregnancy (American Diabetes Association 2010). Type I diabetes is characterized as an autoimmune disease marked by insulin hyposecretion, thus causing an increase in blood glucose content, resulting in metabolic damage. On the other hand, patients with type II diabetes are unable to produce enough insulin or are not able to use their endogenous insulin effectively (American Diabetes Association 2010). The severity of diabetes is linked to the development of chronic complications, which may affect many organs including the kidneys, the cardiovascular system, vision, and neuropathies of the extremities (Forbes and Cooper 2013). Diabetes can induce hyperglycemia and dyslipidemia and, thus, contributes to cardiovascular diseases and thereby high rates of mortality and morbidity (Thomas and Foody 2007). Current treatments for type II diabetes comprise long-term drug intake which can be accompanied by unpleasant side effects such as nausea and vomiting (Meier 2012). There are different treatments for type I diabetes (Atkinson and Eisenbarth 2001) and type II diabetes (Olokoba et al. 2012; Kahn et al. 2014). The most common treatment is the injection/inhalation of insulin, which inhibits glucose production through gluconeogenesis and stimulates glucose uptake and lipid synthesis (Sonksen and Sonksen 2000; Edgerton et al. 2017). Another treatment is the use of α-glucosidase and α-amylase inhibitors to delay digestion of carbohydrates and thereby the release of glucose into the circulation (Lee et al. 2010; Hwang et al. 2015). Inhibiting the activity of these two enzymes can control postprandial hyperglycemia, and reduce the risk of diabetic complications (Abirami et al. 2018). The third treatment method comprises aldose reductase inhibitors, which have a considerable therapeutic potential since they prevent the transformation of glucose into sorbitol (as part of the polyol pathway of glucose metabolism), which is responsible for diabetic complications (eye and nerve damage) (Wang et al. 2005). Additionally, the improvement of dyslipidemia is one of the key protective activities of treatments to reduce cardiovascular disease risk as a co-morbidity of diabetes (Thompson 2004; Hunter and Hegele 2017).

Gupta and Abu-Ghannam (2011a) and Murray et al. (2018b, c) reviewed studies evaluating phenolic extracts from *Alaria esculenta*, *E. cava*, *E. stolonifera*, *I. okamurae*, *F. vesiculosus*, and *Ascophyllum nodosum*, which showed antihyperglycemic effects. Yuan et al. (2018) validated this activity with extracts from *A. nodosum*, *Saccharina japonica*, *Lessonia trabeculata*, and *L. nigrescens* showing inhibition of enzymes involved in diabetes, i.e. α-amylase, α-glucosidase, and pancreatic lipase. Phlorotannins isolated from *I. okamurae* (diphlorethohydroxycarmalol), *E. bicyclis* (phlorofucofuroeckol-A, dieckol, 8,8′-bieckol), and *E. cava* (dieckol) showed the same enzymatic inhibitory activities (Murray et al. 2018b, c). Antihyperlipidemic effects have also been reported for phlorotannins isolated from *E. cava* (dieckol) and *E. stolonifera* (phloroglucinol, eckol, dieckol, dioxinodehydroeckol, phlorofucofuroeckol-A) (Murray et al. 2018c). Phlorotannins are therefore potential antihyperlipidemic agents in humans, but differences have been observed between humans and animal models associated with bioavailability and dosing of these potential bioactive agents (Murray et al. 2018b).

Bromophenols from red algae also have strong potential in the treatment of diabetes; for example, five bromophenols (2,2′,3,6,6′-pentabromo-3′,4,4′,5-tetrahydroxydibenzyl ether, bis(2,3,6-tribromo-4,5-dihydroxyphenyl)methane, 2,2′,3,5′,6-pentabromo-3′,4,4′,5-tetrahydroxydiphenyl-methane, 2,3,6-tribromo-4,5-dihydroxymethylbenzene, and 2,3,6-tribromo-4,5-dihydroxybenzaldehyde) from *S. latiuscula* exhibited significant aldose reductase inhibitory activities (Wang et al. 2005); one bromophenol (bis(2,3-dibromo-4,5-dihydroxybenzyl) ether) purified and identified from *Polyopes lancifolius* was an α-glucosidase inhibitor (Kim et al. 2010); and four bromophenol derivatives (2,2′,3,3′-tetrabromo-4,4′,5,5′-tetrahydroxydiphenylmethane, 3-bromo-4,5-bis(2,3-dibromo-4,5-dihydroxybenzyl) pyrocatechol, bis(2,3-dibromo-4,5-dihydroxybenzyl) ether, and 2,2′,3-tribromo-3′,4,4′,5-tetrahydroxy-6′-ethyloxymethyldiphenylmethane) from *Rhodomela confervoides* (Shi et al. 2008) exhibited significant inhibitory activities against protein tyrosine phosphatase 1B (PTP1B), a protein that regulates the insulin signaling pathway. A crude ethanol extract from the green macroalga *U. rigida* also reduced plasma glucose levels in rats (Celikler et al. 2009). In their review of the antiobesity potential of marine organisms, Lauritano and Ianora (2016) discussed that marine algae are potential therapeutical agents for the treatment of type I and type II diabetes. Microalgae and Cyanobacteria have been identified as promising candidates to potentially reduce the risk of diabetes and cardiovascular diseases (De Jesus Raposo and De Morais 2015; Lauritano and Ianora 2016) with their phenolic compounds thought to play a role in these effects (Aboulthana et al. 2018). On the other hand, Sun et al. (2010) identified algal carotenoids and unsaturated fatty acids as the main contributors to their strong antiglycative capacities that inhibit the formation of advanced glycation end-products (AGEs) such as methylglyoxal and similar aldehydes, but not phenolics.

Hypertension is one of the most important independent risk factors for cardiovascular diseases (World Health Organization and International Society of Hypertension Writing Group 2003). One way to treat hypertension is the use of an angiotensin I-converting enzyme (ACE) inhibitor (Ondetti and Cushman 1982). Indeed, ACE is a proteinase that catalyzes the conversion of angiotensin I to angiotensin II, the latter being a potent vasoconstrictor involved in the pathogenesis of hypertension (Ondetti and Cushman 1982). Thus, limiting its action reduces the risk of hypertension (Ondetti and Cushman 1982). The ability to exert antioxidant activities can also suggest antihypertensive activity due to the fact that great concentrations of oxidant molecules such as ROS causes cell damage and induces the progression of atherosclerosis (Gómez-Guzmán et al. 2018). Some ethanol extracts from *F. spiralis*, or phlorotannins such as phlorofucofuroeckol-A, dieckol, and eckol from *E. cava* and *E. stolonifera* showed great inhibitory activities against ACE (Jung et al. 2006; Gómez-Guzmán et al. 2018). Nevertheless, only limited *in vivo* experiments have confirmed these activities (reviewed in Gómez-Guzmán et al. 2018). Some red algae have also been reported to exhibit a strong ACE inhibitory activity, such as phenolic-rich ethanolic extracts of *Gelidium amansii*, which exhibited 50% ACE inhibition (Jung et al. 2006), *Fushitsunagia catenata*, or *Ahnfeltiopsis flabelliformis* with an ACE inhibition greater than 90% (Cha et al. 2006). For green seaweeds, Taboada et al. (2010) reported that *Ulva* species are better suited for diets directed to reduce the low-density lipoprotein (LDL)-cholesterol in plasma, and that their consumption decreased the risk of cardiovascular diseases in rodents.

11.4.4 Antiproliferative and Anticancer Properties

The challenges in curing many chronic diseases, such as the many forms of cancer, as well as the cytotoxicity and unpleasant side effects of many chemotherapeutic drugs have stimulated research into the development of new drugs from natural sources (Rocha et al. 2018). A large variety of seaweed extracts, particularly those enriched in phenolic compounds and also some isolated phlorotannins, have been reported to exhibit cytotoxic activities against a variety of tumoral cells *in vitro* (Rocha et al. 2018). Phenolic compounds have been reported as being potentially promising in the treatment of lymphoma and leukemia; for example, Zubia et al. (2009) demonstrated cytotoxic activities of crude extracts from *B. bifurcata*, *Carpodesmia tamariscifolia*, *Desmarestia ligulata*, *Dictyota dichotoma*, and *Halidrys siliquosa* against the Daudi cell line (Burkitt's lymphoma), as well as against Jurkat and K562 cells (human leukemia). An ethyl acetate extract of *S. fusiforme* induced apoptosis in human leukemia U937 cells and an extract enriched in phlorotannins from *S. japonica* exhibited antiproliferative activity in a murine leukemic cell line (P388) (in Zubia et al. 2009). Moreover, a merosesquiterpene isolated from *Dictyopteris* sp., chromazonarol, exhibited antiproliferative activities against P388 leukemia cells (Barrero et al. 1999). For green algae, Harada and Kamei (1998) reported that low molecular weight polar compounds extracted from *Cladophoropsis vaucheriaeformis* exhibited antiproliferative activities against murine leukemia L1210 cells.

Many studies have also demonstrated that phenolic compounds could be antiproliferative against colorectal cancer; for example, chloroform, ethyl acetate, and methanol fractions of *Cystoseira compressa* exhibited antiproliferative activities against the colon carcinoma cell line HCT15 (Mhadhebi et al. 2012); a phenolic-rich extract from the red macroalga *P. palmata* inhibited the proliferation of Caco-2 human colon cancer cells (Nwosu et al. 2011); and an enzymatic extract from *E. cava* obtained with an exo, 4-alpha-D-glucosidase, enriched in phlorotannins, inhibited cell proliferation of a murine colon cancer cell line (CT-26) (Athukorala et al. 2006). An ethanolic extract from *S. fusiforme* induced apoptosis in cancer cells via upregulating tumor necrosis factor-α (TNF-α) expression and also reduced pre-neoplastic lesions in the colon, which progress into colorectal cancers in F344 male rats (Son et al. 2018). Ryu et al. (2013) also demonstrated the cytotoxic effects of a hydroethanolic extract from the green alga *Ulva fasciata* on HCT 116 colon cancer cells, by activating apoptotic enzymes such as the caspase family. An isolated dibrominated phenolic compound from the red alga *Polysiphonia lanosa* exhibited high cytotoxic activity against human colon adeno-carcinoma DLD-1 cells (Shoeib et al. 2004), and chromazonarol, a merosesquiterpene from *Dictyopteris* sp., exhibited antiproliferative activities against HT-29 colon cancer cells (Barrero et al. 1999).

From a general point of view, phloroglucinol-based polyphenols isolated from brown marine seaweeds, with a focus on *E. cava*, have exhibited antioxidant activities acting as chemopreventive agents against breast cancer cells and are reviewed by Pádua et al. (2015). According to Imbs and Zvyagintseva (2018), phloroglucinol suppressed the metastasic ability of breast cancer cells. A methanol ethyl acetate extract of *Sargassum angustifolium* (Vaseghi et al. 2018), and chloroform, ethyl acetate, or methanol fractions of *C. compressa* enriched in phenolic compounds (Mhadhebi et al. 2012) exhibited antiproliferative activities against MCF7 breast cancer cells. The phlorotannins (dioxinodehydroeckol and 1-(3′,5′-dihydroxyphenoxy)-7-(2″,4″,6-trihydroxyphenoxy)-2,4,9-trihydroxydibenzo-

1,4-dioxin) from *E. cava* also exhibited an antiproliferative effect on MCF-7 cells (Kong et al. 2009; Thomas and Kim 2011).

A phenolic-rich aqueous-methanol soluble extract from *P. palmata* at concentrations between 0.5 and 5.0 mg ml^{-1} in culture (Yuan et al. 2005) and fractions from *S. angustifolium* (Vaseghi et al. 2018) inhibited the proliferation of HeLa cervical cancer cells. A bromophenol isolated from *Rhodomela confervoides* (3-bromo-4,5-dihydroxy benzoic acid methyl ester) exhibited antiproliferative activities against three tumor cell lines with the highest activity against human epithelial tumor cell KB, a subline of the HeLa cell line (Lijun et al. 2005). Furthermore, phlorotannins from *S. japonica* exhibited antiproliferative activities against BEL-7402 human hepatocellular carcinoma cells (cited in Zubia et al. 2009). Mancini-Filho et al. (2009) demonstrated that free phenolic acids (FPAs), i.e. salicylic, cinnamic, gallic, and caffeic acids, extracted from *Halimeda monile* could modulate the antioxidant enzymes and decreased oxidative status in the liver of rats, treated daily for 20 days with FPA (at different concentrations) incorporated within the food of animals. With their *in vivo* experiment with rats with induced hepatic injury, authors showed thereby that FPA protected the expression of superoxide dismutase (SOD) and catalase (CAT), essential hepatic enzymes, in rats under experimental CCl4-induced cirrhosis injury (Mancini-Filho et al. 2009).

A phlorotannin-rich extract of *C. compressa* exhibited antiproliferative activities against the A549 pulmonary adenocarcinoma cell line (Mhadhebi et al. 2012) and purified fractions of *Sargassum oligocystum* exhibited antiproliferative activities against the GLC4-Adr human lung carcinoma cell line resistant to adriamycin, a powerful anticancer drug (Praiboon et al. 2018). Chromazonarol, a merosesquiterpene isolated from *Dictyopteris* sp., exhibited antiproliferative activities against P549 lung cancer cells (Barrero et al. 1999). Finally, Pereira et al. (2011) tested the antiproliferative activity of six meroditerpenoids, tested at different concentrations, from 6.25 to 25 μM or 12.5–50 μM depending on the isolated compound, from *S. flabelliforme* against different cell lines: human (Caco-2 and SH-SY5Y) and nonhuman cancer lines (RBL-2H3 and RAW.267), together with noncancer cells (V79). The authors demonstrated that three meroditerpenoids, i.e. epitaondiol, epitaondiol monoacetate, and stypotriol triacetate, were efficient against the human neuroblastoma (SH-SY5Y; nearly 100% of inhibition of cell proliferation); this cell line representing the most susceptible cell line.

11.4.5 Antimicrobial and Antiparasite Properties

Increasing resistance of clinically important bacteria to current antibiotics is a major problem worldwide (Neu 1992). For example, *Staphylococcus aureus*, a pathogen responsible for life-threatening infections including bacteremia, endocarditis, osteomyelitis, and pneumonia, is resistant to methicillin and is thus often referred to as methicillin-resistant *Staphylococcus aureus* (MRSA) or other current beta-lactam antibiotics from the penicillin family (Neu 1992). Thus, there is a great interest in identifying novel natural antibiotics. In this sense, macroalgal polyphenols may be promising molecules with antimicrobial properties (Bennamara et al. 1999; Sandsdalen et al. 2003; Choi et al. 2010; Pereira et al. 2011; Eom et al. 2012; Eom et al. 2013; Kim et al. 2018), from untapped sources, compared with terrestrial plants (Ríos and Recio 2005 as a review). Several methods are used to assess the antimicrobial activities of algal extracts including *in vitro* assays such as diffusion agar tests, growth inhibition assays, minimum inhibitory concentration determination, or *in vivo* assays such as tests on shrimp or fish feed, which were less numerous (reviewed by Pérez et al. 2016), with methanol identified as the best extractive solvent for active constituents (Cox et al. 2010; Jaswir et al. 2014; Moubayed et al. 2017).

Eight phlorotannins (i.e. phloroglucinol, eckol, fucofuroeckol-A, phlorofucofuroeckol-A or PFF, dioxinodehyroeckol, 8,8′-bioeckol, 7-phloroeckol, and dieckol) isolated from *E. bicyclis*, *Ecklonia cava*, *E. kurome*, and *E. stolonifera* exhibited antimicrobial activities against food-borne pathogenic bacteria (*Campylobacter jejuni*, *Escherichia coli*, *Salmonella enteritidis*, *Salmonella typhimurium*, *Vibrio parahaemolyticus*), antibiotic-resistant bacteria (MRSA), and foot fungus (*Tinera pedis*) (reviewed by Eom et al. 2012). Eom et al. (2013) confirmed the antibacterial activities against MRSA of six phlorotannins isolated from *E. bicyclis* (eckol, fucofuroeckol-A, 7-phloroeckol, dioxinodehydroeckol, PFF, and dieckol). According to Kim et al. (2018), three phlorotannins (fucofuroeckol-A, PFF, and dioxinodehydroeckol) exhibited strong inhibition of *Listeria monocytogenes*, the food-borne pathogen responsible for listeriosis. Fucophlorethol from *F. vesiculosus* also exhibited antibacterial effects against *Proteus mirabilis*, *Pseudomonas aeruginosa*, *Staphylcoccus epidermidis*, *S. aureus*, and *E. coli* (Sandsdalen et al. 2003). A merodíterpenoid from the brown alga *Cystoseira tamariscifolia*, methoxybifurcarenone, exhibited antibacterial activities against *E. coli* and *Agrobacterium tumefaciens* (Bennamara et al. 1999). Pereira et al. (2011) reported that meroditerpenoids from *S. flabelliforme*, i.e. epitaondiol monoacetate, stypotriol triacetate, and stypodiol, exhibited antibacterial activities against *S. aureus*, *Micrococcus luteus*, *Enterococcus faecalis*, *Bacillus cereus*, *P. mirabilis*, and *S. typhimurium*. The Cyanobacteria *Leptolyngbya crossbyana* was reported to contain crossbyanols, which are brominated and sulfated polyphenyl ethers, which exhibited antibacterial activity especially against MRSA (Choi et al. 2010).

In the skincare or dermatology sector, acne or acne vulgaris is a common skin disease or condition affecting adolescents and adults, which is a complex and multifactorial skin pathogenesis (Tan et al. 2001). *Staphylococcus epidermidis*, *S. aureus*, and *P. aeruginosa* are often responsible for acne conditions (Wang et al. 2017). These authors reported that an ethyl acetate fraction from *Fucus evanescens* exhibited strong antibacterial activity against *Propionibacterium acnes*, often present in acne vulgaris, and also against MRSA. Lee et al. (2014) also reported that fucofuroeckol-A inhibited acne-related bacteria (*P. acnes*). Kok et al. (2016) studied a methanol fraction of *Sargassum polycystum* and reported an *in vitro* inhibitory activity against *P. acnes*.

Interest in antifungal activities of phenolic compounds has also been demonstrated; for example, extracts from brown macroalgae *Cystoseira sedoides*, *C. crinita*, and *Dictyopteris membranacea* exhibited antifungal activities against yeast *Candida albicans*, *Candida glabrata*, *Candida krusei*, *Candida dubliniensis*, and *Candida kefyr* (Mhadhebi et al. 2012). Purified phlorotannins from *Cystoseira nodicaulis*, *Cystoseira usneoides*, and *F. spiralis* exhibited fungistatic and fungicidal activities against *C. albicans* and dermatophytes, i.e. *Epidermophyton floccosum* and *Trichophyton rubrum* (Lopes et al. 2013). Kim et al. (2018) reported antifungal activity against *C. albicans* due to fucofuroeckol-A isolated from *E. bicyclis*. A meroditerpenoid from *C. tamariscifolia*, methoxybifurcarenone, also exhibited antifungal activities but against different species, which included tomato pathogenic fungi, *Botrytis cinerea*, *Fusarium oxysporum* f.sp. *lycopersici*, and *Verticillium alboatrum* (Bennamara et al. 1999).

Bromophenols from red algae have also been reported to exhibit antimicrobial and antifungal activities; for example, Barreto and Meyer (2006) reported that lanosol derivatives, a bromophenol common in the Rhodomelaceae, have antimicrobial activity against various terrestrial and marine bacteria together with fungi. The bromophenol 3-bromo-4,5-dihydroxy-benzaldehyde isolated from *R. confervoides* demonstrated antibacterial activities against *S. aureus* and *P. aeruginosa* (Lijun et al. 2005). Some bromophenols, 2,5-dibromo-3,4-dihydroxy-6-(2,3,6-tribromo-4,5-dihydroxybenzyl) benzyl methyl ether and 2,2′,3,3′-tetrabromo-4,4′,5,5′-tetrahydroxydiphenylmethane, isolated from, respectively, *S. latiuscula* (Xu et al. 2014) and *Odonthalia corymbifera* (Oh et al. 2008) were reported to exhibit antifungal activities against the pathogenic yeast *C. albicans*. Some bromophycolides isolated from *C. serratus* (Lane et al. 2009; Paige-Stout et al. 2010) have been reported to exhibit antimalaria properties due to their macrolide structure.

11.4.6 Antiviral Activities

Viral diseases are caused by infectious agents that enter the cells of organisms to reproduce (Koonin and Starokadomskyy 2016). They may then go on to cause illnesses or diseases, which can be more or less severe, ranging from a common cold due to rhinovirus, to the human immunodeficiency virus (HIV) giving rise to acquired immunodeficiency syndrome (AIDS) (Moir et al. 2011). Viral diseases may be transmitted from one individual to another through aerosol droplets or saliva (influenza virus), unprotected sexual intercourse (herpes simplex virus [HSV], and human papillomavirus [HPV]), or vectors such as mosquitoes and animals (dengue, chikungunya, ebola, or rabies viruses) (Koonin and Starokadomskyy 2016). In some cases, viral diseases can be highly contagious leading to outbreaks, epidemics, or even pandemics.

HIV, which is responsible for AIDS, is one of the most studied viruses to date (Moir et al. 2011). The exploration for potential drug treatments has increased the development of new generation anti-HIV therapeutics (Flexner 2007). Thus, phlorotannins 6,6′-bioeckol, 8,8′-bieckol, and 8,4″-dieckol from *E. cava* may be potential inhibitory substances for HIV type 1 (HIV-1) infections (Thomas and Kim 2011). Karadeniz et al. (2014a) validated 8-4″-dieckol as a potential candidate for inhibition of HIV-1 with especially an inhibition of the HIV-1 reverse transcriptase. A review by Karadeniz et al. (2015a) discussed the inhibitory activities of a phlorotannin, diphlorethohydroxycarmalol, isolated from *I. okamurae* against HIV-1. This Phaeophyta species is also a potential source of antivirals against influenza A virus, due to the production of phlorofucofuroeckol (Ryu et al. 2011). Soares et al. (2007) reported that while three meroditerpenoids from *Stypopodium zonale* did not inhibit the transcriptase reverse enzyme of HIV-1, they may act on other phases of the virus replication cycle.

Genital HPV infection is the most common sexually transmitted infection and may lead to cervical cancer (Muñoz et al. 2006). Eckol, dieckol, 8-8′-bieckol, 6-6′bioeckol, and phlorofucofuroeckol-A (PFF-A), isolated from *E. bicyclis*, exhibited reductions of HPV strains HPV16PV and HPV18PV *in vitro* (Kim and Kwak 2015). Dieckol and PFF-A also exhibited antiviral activities against murine norovirus, which was responsible for epidemics with symptoms including vomiting, diarrhea, mild fever, abdominal cramping, and nausea (Eom et al. 2015).

Human metapneumovirus (HMPV) is an important agent of severe upper respiratory infections (Mazzoncini et al. 2010). Mendes et al. (2011) reported that the meroditerpenoids epitaondiol and atomaric acid isolated from *Stypopodium zonale* inhibited more than 90% of *in vitro* HMPV replication. These two meroditerpenoids and peroxylactone of 5′a-desmethyl-5′-acetylatomaric acid extracted from this same species inhibited HSV type 1 (HSV-1) replication (Soares et al. 2007).

11.4.7 Mineralogenic and Osteogenic Activities

The formation and remodeling of bone tissue is regulated by the osteoblast cells that form bone tissue and the osteoclasts which resorb it (Raisz 2001). In some individuals, male or female, aging and numerous pathological processes induce a decrease in the bone formation and an increase in bone resorption leading to osteoporosis, which is characterized by a decrease in bone mass (Riggs et al. 1998; Habauzit and Horcajada 2007; Yamaguchi 2013). Osteoporosis is widely recognized as a major public health concern worldwide particularly, as populations advance in age (Johnell and Kanis 2006; Hernlund et al. 2013; Yamaguchi 2013). In osteoporosis, it has been shown that oxidative stress plays an important role (Wauquier et al. 2009); for example, Arai et al. (2007) reported that ROS may be responsible for the development of bone loss and that the activity of antioxidant enzymes, such as SOD, is a marker of oxidative stress in menopausal women. Several studies have demonstrated that natural compounds with antioxidant activity, including green tea, vitamins, quinones, and polyphenols may influence bone mineralization/remodeling (Karadeniz et al. 2015b; Córdoba et al. 2014; Córdoba et al. 2015; Watson and Schönlau 2015). In particular, polyphenols could be effective candidates for the prevention of osteoporosis by preventing bone loss through the inhibition of oxidative stress; more precisely, these compounds activated the proliferation and differentiation of osteoblasts in culture (Habauzit and Horcajada 2007; Woo et al. 2010; Karadeniz et al. 2014b; Karadeniz et al. 2015b).

Surget et al. (2016) demonstrated the efficacy of phenolic compounds including phenolic acids from two green seaweeds, *C. fragile* and *Cladophora rupestris*, for *in vitro* pro-mineralogenic and *in vivo* pro-osteogenic properties. In their work, bone derived teleost VSa13 cells exposed to purified phenolic fractions exhibited an increase in extracellular matrix (ECM) mineralization, potentially by promoting cell differentiation. This *in vitro* work was accompanied by an *in vivo* assay with developing zebrafish larvae (Laizé et al. 2014). The mineralized area of the operculum, a dermal bone derived from neural crest cells, was increased in fish exposed to the purified phenolic fractions, at similar levels promoted by the positive control. Similar pro-mineralogenic effects were observed when human fetal lung fibroblast MRC-5 cells (Ryu et al. 2009) and human osteosarcoma MG-63 cells were treated with phlorotannins from the brown seaweed *E. cava* (Ryu et al. 2009; Yeo et al. 2012). Ryu et al. (2009) identified two phlorotannins responsible for the pro-mineralogenic activity *in vitro*: dieckol and 1-(3,5-dihydroxyphenoxy)-7-(2,4,6-trihydroxyphenoxy)-2,4,9-trihydroxydibenzo-1,4-dioxin.

With respect to bone building and tissue regeneration, studies have shown that phlorotannins could stimulate the differentiation of osteoblasts by enhanced alkaline phosphatase (ALP) activity, collagen, and mineralization in the noncytotoxic concentration range, which makes them interesting for applications related to bone regeneration (Córdoba et al. 2014, 2015; Watson and Schönlau 2015). In particular, phlorotannins from *E. cava* increased ALP activity, mineralization, total protein, and collagen synthesis in human osteosarcoma cells (MG-63 cells) (Ryu et al. 2009; Ali and Hasan 2012; Yeo et al. 2012; Karadeniz et al. 2015b), suggesting that they may act as regulators of osteoblast differentiation and bone formation. Additionally, Yoon et al. (2013) demonstrated that the meroditerpene sargachromanol D, isolated from the brown macroalga *Sargassum siliquastrum*, inhibited production of inflammatory cytokines, which play a major role in osteoclastogenesis, leading to the bone resorption frequently associated with osteoporosis. Sargachromanol D acted as an inhibitor of osteoclast formation and could be an alternative nutraceutical or treatment in the prevention of or to reduce osteolysis or osteoporosis (Yoon et al. 2013). Other biological activities, i.e. anti-inflammatory, and anticarcinogenic activities were observed for this meroditerpene extracted from Sargassaceae species (Birringer et al. 2018). Nevertheless, the noncytotoxicity of these compounds to tissues/cells/organisms is vital for the recommended use of such compounds in humans.

11.4.8 Photoprotective Properties

Exposure to ultraviolet (UV) radiation from sunlight, in particular the UVB (280-320 nm) and UVA (320-400 nm) wavelengths, can be damaging to the skin causing sunburn, photoaging, or even skin cancer due to skin cell DNA damage (Parrish et al. 1982; Brash et al. 1991). To reduce exposure to and penetration of UV radiation, sunscreens or sunblocking agents are recommended to be applied on the skin (Singh and Kumar 2018). While synthetic photoprotective molecules such as para-aminobenzoic acid (PABA) can be found on the current market, the discovery and development of products containing natural sunscreen molecules is growing due to concerns about the harmful potential of the synthetics such as an increase of phototoxic/photoirritation or photoallergic responses and, longer-term, an increased risk of skin cancers or photoageing (Nash and Tanner 2014).

The most important consideration in the development of a new photoprotective product is safety. Brunt and Burgess (2017) and Pangestuti et al. (2018) reviewed publications which showed that phlorotannins may be good candidates as photoprotective molecules. Indeed, the ethyl acetate fraction enriched in phlorotannins of *H. siliquosa* appeared to be a broad-spectrum UV absorber (absorbing both UVB and UVA wavelengths) in *in vitro* assays with calculation of a sun protection factor (Le Lann et al. 2016). In other work, protection against photo-oxidative stress induced by UVB radiation was evaluated using assays including inhibition of tyrosinase and melanin synthesis, radical scavenging properties in cell cultures, cell viability, DNA damage, and *in vitro* microscopic analyses for dead cells (Heo et al. 2009). Phlorotannins isolated from *E. cava*, particularly dieckol, inhibited melanogenesis and reduced UVB radiation-induced cell damage. *In vivo* studies were also conducted with zebrafish embryos treated with phlorotannins isolated from *E. cava*, which showed a reduction in UVB damage (Ko et al. 2011; Cha et al. 2012).

On the other hand, as photosynthetic organisms subjected to UV radiation and thereby damage themselves, accumulation of UV-absorbing compounds such as bromophenols or coumarins was reported in green algae, including *U. lactuca* (Flodin et al. 1999), *U. pertusa* (Han and Han 2005), *Dasycladus vermicularis* (Pérez-Rodríguez et al. 2003), and *Prasiola stipitata* (Gröniger and Häder 2002). Moreover, scytonemin, a polyphenolic pigment, protects Cyanobacteria against UV radiation (García-Pichel and Castenholz 1991; Proteau et al. 1993). Thus, algal polyphenols may be useful as chemopreventive agents to reduce the risk of UVB induced skin carcinogenesis (Hwang et al. 2006). Although only a few *in vivo* tests have yet been conducted (Ko et al. 2011; Cha et al. 2012), cosmetic products have already been developed from these molecules to protect the skin.

11.4.9 Biological Properties Specific to Cosmetics or Cosmeceuticals

11.4.9.1 Anti-aging Properties Anti-aging skin care is a large and growing segment of the cosmetic and cosmeceutical markets, with an annual growth rate close to 10%, when the global skin care sector growth rate is less than 8% (Brandt et al. 2011). Aging is a complex phenomenon involving intrinsic (genetic) and extrinsic causes, including exposure to sun or smoking (Ramos-e-Silva et al. 2013). One visible effect of aging is the appearance of wrinkles due to changes in skin thickness and elasticity of fibers (Sanjeewa et al. 2016). According to Couteau and Coiffard (2016), there are three types of wrinkles: crinkles, nonpermanent wrinkles linked to the degradation of the elastic fibers of the dermis; glyphic wrinkles, which are permanent and accentuate the cutaneous micro-relief; and facial linear wrinkles, which are permanent wrinkles corresponding to expression lines. Different mechanisms can be used to fight wrinkles: stimulating collagen and hyaluronic acid synthesis, or inhibition of matrix metalloproteinase (MMP) (collagenase), elastase, or hyaluronidase (Ramos-e-Silva et al. 2013). Thus, extracts from macroalgae could be tested to determine their efficacy in inhibition of enzymes implicated in the aging process.

MMPs are endopeptidases able to degrade extracellular matrix (ECM) proteins, which form the skin matrix and are responsible for the firmness, strength, and elasticity of the skin (Ramos-e-Silva et al. 2013); with aging, MMP levels are reported to decrease. Isolated phlorotannins (eckol, dieckol) from *E. bicyclis* and *E. kurome*, *E. stolonifera*, and *E. cava* exhibited MMP-1 (collagenase), MMP-2 (gelatinase), or MMP-9 (gelatinase) inhibition in cell models (Joe et al. 2006; Kim et al. 2006). Riani et al. (2018) demonstrated an anticollagenase activity of a *Sargassum plagiophyllum* extract *in vitro*.

Hyaluronidase is an enzyme responsible for the depolymerization of hyaluronic acid, an important polysaccharide present in the ECM of the skin and responsible for water retention and tissue regeneration (Meyer 1947). This enzyme is also involved in allergenic effects (see the paragraph on antiallergy properties above). In the review of Sanjeewa et al. (2016), hyaluronidase inhibition was observed with phlorotannins isolated from *F. spiralis*, *C. nodicaulis*, *C. usneoides*, and *C. tamariscifolia* (Ferreres et al. 2012) and also from *Eisenia kurome* and *E. bicyclis* (Shibata et al. 2002). Shibata et al. (2002) hypothesized that the structure of the phlorotannins has an important role because acetylation of the phenolic hydroxyl group reduced the inhibitory effect. Fayad et al. (2017) reported similar antihyaluronidase activities in an *Eisenia bicylis* phlorotannin fraction and an extract from *Padina pavonica* using capillary electrophoresis-based enzymatic assays.

Elastase is a proteinase capable of degrading elastin, which is an important ECM protein providing elasticity of the skin (Tsuji et al. 2001). According to Puspita et al. (2017), an enriched phenolic compound fraction of *S. muticum*, extracted using different commercial enzymes, exhibited elastase inhibition activities in an *in vitro* assay. Tyrosinase is a metalloenzyme oxidase which catalyzes melanin synthesis (Solano et al. 2006). Molecules that inhibit this enzyme are potential candidates for antiwrinkle applications but also for whitening skin (Lin et al. 2008; Sanjeewa et al. 2016) (see below).

11.4.9.2 Whitening Properties With aging and chronic UV exposure, hyperpigmentation is unavoidable, with the emergence of brown melanin pigmentation patches or spots on the skin (Gilchrest et al. 1979). Depigmenting or whitening/lightening molecules such as arbutin (hydroquinone-O-beta-D-glucopyranoside) and derivatives, kojic acid and derivatives, and flavonoids have been investigated to remove those localized brown patches as skin whitening/lightening is a common practice, particularly in Asia (Lin et al. 2008; Sanjeewa et al. 2016). Tyrosinase has a key role in pigmentation as this enzyme catalyzes melanin synthesis in melanocytes with conversion of L-tyrosine to dihydroxyphenylalanine (L-DOPA), followed by the oxidation of L-DOPA to dopaquinone with polymerization to finally yield melanin (Slominski et al. 2004; Lin et al. 2008). Consequently, tyrosinase inhibitors have been explored for their antipigmentation properties and as potential agents to reduce brown patches (Solano et al. 2006; Lin et al. 2008).

The most common method to evaluate tyrosinase inhibition is spectrophotometrically using mushroom tyrosinase (see references in Sanjeewa et al. 2016). Several studies using crude extracts of brown seaweeds containing phlorotannins have shown tyrosinase inhibition *in vitro* using the mushroom enzyme test: an acetone extract of *A. nodosum* (Jiménez et al. 2010), a methanolic extract of *E. stolonifera* (Kang et al. 2004), ethanolic extracts of *E. cava*, and *S. siliquastrum* (Yoon et al. 2009). However, opposite outcomes have also been reported, as with an ethanolic extract of *Sargassum polycystum*, which did not inhibit tyrosinase activity in the mushroom enzyme assay (Chan et al. 2011). In the crude extracts above, the inhibitory activities were linked to phenolic compounds, but other molecules likely existed in the crude extracts as well. An ethyl acetate fraction from *E. cava*, rich in phenolics, exhibited close to 80% tyrosinase inhibition at 50 $\mu g \cdot ml^{-1}$ (Yoon et al. 2009).

Isolated phlorotannins have also been reported to inhibit tyrosinase activity when using the *in vitro* mushroom enzyme-based assay; for example, Heo et al. (2009) reported tyrosinase inhibition by phlorotannins isolated from *E. cava*, with dieckol having the greatest effect on tyrosinase, compared with the positive control kojic acid, phloroglucinol, and eckol. Dioxinodehydroeckol and 7-phloroeckol purified from the same algal species have also been reported to inhibit tyrosinase (Yoon et al. 2009). Moreover, phloroglucinol and 7-phloroeckol were identified as noncompetitive tyrosinase inhibitors (Yoon et al. 2009). Similarly, Kang et al. (2004) reported the tyrosinase inhibitory activity of isolated phlorotannins from *E. stolonifera* with the greatest efficacies for dieckol followed by eckol, phloroglucinol, eckstolonol, and phlorofucofureckol A. These authors also demonstrated that eckol, phlorofucofuroeckol-A, and dieckol were noncompetitive inhibitors for the oxidation of the substrate catalyzed by tyrosinase, while phloroglucinol and eckstolonol were competitive inhibitors.

11.4.9.3 Hair Growth Properties A review paper by Sanjeewa et al. (2016) discussed how dieckol and 7-phloroeckol from *E. cava* induced hair growth with a proliferation of dermal papilla cells (which play a critical role in regulating hair follicle development and regeneration) and an inhibition of 5α-reductase enzyme activity (a marker for hair loss prevention). Shin et al. (2016) reported similar effects in *ex vivo* human hair follicle cultures treated with enriched phenolic compound fractions or purified phenolic compounds isolated from *E. cava* (dieckol, phlorofurofucoeckol A), but found no activity with the purified compounds. These authors discussed that the effects of phenolic compounds varied depending on cell type and test conditions such as *in vitro*, *in vivo*, or *ex vivo* as expected (Shin et al. 2016). Moreover, a combination of several phlorotannins might be more effective than a single molecule.

11.5 Potential Commercial Applications

Due to their large range of biological activities as discussed above, algal phenolic compounds are potential candidates for many industrial applications such as functional foods and nutraceuticals, pharmaceuticals, and functional cosmetic or cosmeceuticals (Plaza et al. 2008).

11.5.1 Interest in Health and Nutraceutical Ingredients

Although the commercial use of seaweeds for their antioxidant properties remains in its infancy (Cornish and Garbary 2010), epidemiological data as well as accumulating evidence suggest that algal phenolic compounds may influence several health parameters or risk factors of diet-related chronic diseases: glycemic control, lipid or inflammation levels, antimicrobial inhibition, cardiovascular disorders, and proliferation of cancer as discussed above.

Some products are already on the market for different aspects of health. For example, Seanol® (Botamedi Inc., Korea) is a phlorotannin extract from *E. cava*, which is included in the composition of supplements to provide antioxidant protection. It is also available as a hydrogel application to enhance mineralization and regeneration of bone and antibacterial agents to reduce the risk of infection (Douglas et al. 2016). HealSea™ (Diana Naturals, France), is an extract from *F. vesiculosus* sold for cardiovascular health purposes (cited in Stiger-Pouvreau and Guérard 2018).

Several patents exist demonstrating different potential applications of phlorotannins in health; for example, antibiotic preparations included phlorotannins derived from *E. bicyclis* (Kim et al. 2012) or *Ecklonia* species (Ginnaga et al. 2002). Phlorotannins from *E. cava* have also been used in a preparation to prevent influenza (Cho 2016). Phlorotannins from both *E. stolonifera* and *E. cava* were included in a preparation for hepatoprotection related to alcoholic hepatic damage (Kim 2011). The antidiabetic activity of a commercial extract of *F. vesiculosus* and *A. nodosum* (InSea^{2}™, INNOVACTIV, Canada; innovactiv.com) has been reported in a human trial. More precisely, after the ingestion of 250 mg of InSea^{2}, 30 minutes before a consumption of 50 g of carbohydrates, the authors demonstrated a reduction of 12% in the insulin content and InSea^{2} was also responsible of an increase in almost 8% of the insulin sensitivity of patients (Catarino et al. 2018).

Several studies have highlighted the potential therapeutic use of algal antioxidants, as dietary supplements for bone diseases such as osteoporosis or as nanocoatings to functionalize biomaterials, i.e. make a biomaterial functional, and improve current bone implants (Córdoba et al. 2014, 2015; Karadeniz et al. 2015b; Watson and Schönlau 2015). Rao and Rao (2015) discussed a commercially available nutritional supplement, Greens+™, which contains polyphenols as a mixture of flavonoids from terrestrial plants in this work, but which are also found in some algae, combined with minerals and vitamins, which act to increase the antioxidant capacity of the preparation, and thereby potentially reduce oxidative stress associated with bone loss. These authors suggested that such a preparation could be a viable and efficient option to assist with bone formation.

Studies have reported the supplementation of bioceramic-based medical scaffolds with phenolic compounds such as phlorotannins from the brown alga *E. cava* with an aim to increase bone tissue regeneration or increase bone density (Yeo et al. 2012; Córdoba et al. 2014, 2015; Watson and Schönlau 2015). Purified polyphenolic extracts that exhibit multiple biological activities without cytotoxicity could play a role in reducing cellular oxidative stress and thereby potentially promote bone mineralization (Yeo et al. 2012; Córdoba et al. 2015; Surget et al. 2017). These natural compounds have potential applications in nutraceuticals or functional foods in the prevention of bone loss but also in medicine, to complement existing treatments of osteoporosis (Wauquier et al. 2009; Rao and Rao 2015). Senthilkumar et al. (2014) discussed examples of marine derived osteogenic compounds/molecules including algal phenolic compounds such as including symbioimine from the marine dinoflagellate *Symbiodinium* sp. that showed excellent clinical potential as discussed above.

11.5.2 Interest in Cosmetics and Cosmeceutical Ingredients

Innovative bioactive molecules are constantly being researched and developed in the cosmetics sector. To date, terrestrial organisms such as *Aloe vera* have been intensely valorized, but the demand for marine sources is increasing (Eshun and He 2004). Seaweeds are already widely valorized by the cosmetic industry with their applications widespread (reviewed in Couteau and Coiffard 2016; Stiger-Pouvreau and Guérard 2018); marine phenolic compounds are currently used in the cosmetics industry in moisturizers, sunscreens, antiwrinkle preparations, whitening agents, or to replace synthetic preservatives with antimicrobial properties (see examples below).

Antioxidant ingredients would potentially provide protection against pro-oxidative reactions in or on human skin but could also stabilize a cosmetic cream; for example, Balboa et al. (2014) reported that phenolic-enriched extracts from *S. muticum* incorporated into a skin cream inhibited lipid oxidation in the cream during 34 days of storage. Another extract from the same seaweed was included in a sunscreen and protected against lipid oxidation with no variation in the cream color (Balboa et al. 2017). Liu et al. (2018) described a facial cleansing formula containing an *S. muticum* extract and reported that glycerol and 1,2-propanediol extracts improved the stability of the emulsion and demonstrated a role for algal compounds in cosmetics. The inclusion of a methanol extract of *E. cava* in a Supersill® emulsion (a mix of cyclopentasiloxane, dimethicone, and PEG-10 dimethicone crosspolymer; CNTEC Inc.) resulted in a stable emulsion with no change in appearance, color, or odor over 4 weeks (Choi et al. 2013). Currently, on the market, extracts of brown seaweed enriched in phlorotannins can already be found; for example, PHYACTYL® (Gelyma, France; www.gelyma.com), is an *S. muticum* water extract that is purported to protect against free radicals, UV radiation, and provides skin detoxification (Pellegrini et al. 2003a). Another active algal extract from Gelyma (SEA HEATHER®) combines water extracts from *Cystoseira amentacea*, *Cladocora caespitosa*, and *Corymbia brachycarpa* and is identified as protecting against oxidation, inflammation, and DNA damage (Pellegrini et al. 2003b).

Celtalga Extract (Spain; www.celtalga.com/es/algas-industria-cosmetica) produces *A. nodosum*, *B. bifurcata*, and *S. muticum* ethanol extracts available for use by cosmetic companies; they advertise that these extracts exhibit antioxidant properties (Sineiro Torres et al. 2013).

Several skin-lightening cosmetic ingredients rich in phlorotannins can already be found on the market, such as LIGHTOCEANE® (Gelyma, France; www.gelyma.com), which is a skin lightener containing an extract from *Halidrys siliquosa*, which decreased tyrosinase activity and melanin synthesis in water (Pellegrini and Pellegrini 2003). A patent describing the methodology to obtain an extract from *Agarum cribrosum* active against skin pigmentation has been filed in France and the patent has been expanded to the world (Paufique 2003). On the other hand, instead of whitening or lightening properties, BRONZ'ALG® (Gelyma, France; www.gelyma.com) was formulated to help maintain an even suntan; the product combines a *Bifurcaria bifurcata* aqueous extract with acetyl-tyrosine to upregulate the major genes of the melanogenesis pathways as well as protect against free radicals and UV radiation (Pellegrini et al. 2016).

Anti-aging characteristics are among the most active research areas in the cosmetics industry, and extracts enriched in phlorotannins are currently found on the market for this purpose. One example is FIRM'ACT® (Gelyma, France; www.gelyma.com), which combines *Himanthalia elongata* and *F. vesiculosus* extracts with a *Saccharomyces cerevisiae* extract to fight against genetic and environmental skin aging risk factors. To protect against skin irritation and to moisturize the skin, EFFICIENSA® and SEAVIE® (Gelyma, France; www.gelyma.com) are products containing *Pelvetia canaliculata* and *F. serratus* extracts, respectively (Pellegrini et al. 2003c). Another French company (SEPPIC, France; www.seppic.com) produces lipidic and water extracts enriched in phenolic compounds from the marine brown seaweed *F. vesiculosus* (OLEAPHYCOL FV and SUPERPHYCOL-D™ BG PF, respectively).

Phenolic compounds from green algae are also used as ingredients in some cosmetic skincare products such as CODIAVELANE® BG PF (SEPPIC, France; www.seppic.com), which contains an active ingredient extracted from *Codium tomentosum* to be used for its long-lasting hydration. As this green macroalga is rich in polyphenolic antioxidants, the Italian company EME Estetica produces an extract from the same algal species (PRO AGE SERUM; www.eme-estetica.com), that is used by the LOWE company within its Kiemè cosmetic line (http://lo-we.it/en/product-category/kieme) for its purported skin nourishing and moisturizing properties, and also to stimulate circulation, oxygenate the skin, and counteract aging. An extract from another *Codium* species (*C. fragile*) is also used as a moisturizer and cell protector ingredient in MIRUAL® (Gelyma, France; www.gelyma.com). The Spanish company Lipotec S.A.U. uses *U. lactuca* aqueous extracts (ACTIPHYTE™ sea lettuce; www.lipotec.com) for their radical scavenging and anti-inflammatory activities in cosmetic products.

11.6 Conclusions and Future Trends

Phenolics from marine algae form a class of diverse compounds, ranging from simple compounds such as phloroglucinol and coumaric acid, to more complex polyphenols such as phlorotannins, phenolic glycosides, or meroterpenes as described above and illustrated in Figure 11.2. As a consequence of this wide variety of structures, phenolic compounds have numerous biological activities suggesting future prospects in the functional food and nutraceutical sectors to support health and well-being, as well as the cosmetic and cosmeceutical sectors. Among other biological activities, phenolic compounds have been reported to act as antioxidant, anti-inflammatory, antidiabetic, and antimicrobial agents, or in risk factor reduction for diet-related chronic diseases such as the development of some cancers. Algal polyphenols are currently underexploited compared with those from terrestrial plants, and thereby represent a promising resource because of the increased interest of industries in the use of natural ingredients to replace synthetic and controversial molecules. To date, much of the literature has been focused on brown algal phlorotannins, which have the highest levels of phenolic compounds. However, studying all algal phyla could lead to the discovery of more bioactive phenolic compounds. Indeed, although microalgae, and red or green macroalgae generally have lower levels of phenolic compounds, some can be very active even at small concentrations and could offer novel opportunities for industry. The occurrence of phenolic compounds in algae is extremely variable due to variations in a number of biotic (e.g. grazing or pathogen infestation) and abiotic extrinsic factors (e.g. temperature, light, nutrients). To valorize them at an industrial scale, it is therefore important to understand that environmental conditions can influence the production of phenolic compounds.

Furthermore, phenolic compounds are difficult to isolate due to their ability to complex with others molecules. Until now, the majority of studies have focused on the activities of crude extracts and more rarely on purified compounds. In recent years, new extraction techniques were thus developed to obtain active phenolic compounds, with an increased trend for green extractions that could help to enhance the value of polyphenols as bioactive compounds for dietary or human health. Phenolic compounds are often quantified by conventional colorimetric methods, taking into account all compounds with phenolic hydroxyl groups as a whole due to the difficulty of separating and isolating phenolics from other compounds. Consequently, the content of phenolic compounds is generally overestimated, as shown by Jégou et al. (2015), who used qNMR to better quantify phenolic content in *C. tamariscifolia*, a phloroglucinol-producing species. The development of new methods to quickly identify and quantify specific compound or some class of phenolic compounds in particular, is then necessary. In this sense, HPLC seems to be a good method, but it is not yet well developed due to the instability of phenolics and their ability to bond with others molecules (Stiger-Pouvreau et al. 2014), together with the lack of standards of different polymerization degrees.

Finally, even if some studies suggest that algae could be eaten for their antioxidant capacities, more research is needed to evaluate the impact of an algal overconsumption (with the problem of iodine, for example, for the consumption of species that contain a large quantity of it) or the effect of isolated phenolic compounds after ingesting algae. Indeed, a synergy between phenolic compounds and other molecules present in algae may be observed, synergy that may be responsible for some activities measured *in vitro* on crude extracts but not found in isolated compounds. Conversely, an isolated phenolic compound with interesting activity may be, once ingested into the organism, no longer active or exhibit other unexpected undesirable activities. In this sense, most of the reported activities have been measured through *in vitro* tests, but *in vivo* approaches are needed to validate the potential of algal phenolic compounds for human health. However, it is recognized that algal derived phenolic compounds play a major role as active ingredient for health and food products.

Acknowledgments

This review is part of the PhD thesis work carried out by the two first authors, LG and FL, within the Laboratory of Marine Environmental Science (LEMAR UMR 6539) set at the IUEM (UBO). They were supported by a grant from UBO and a research project RIV-AGE2.0 (financed by the Brittany region, the Finistère Department, and Brest metropole) for LG, and from UBO and the Brittany Region for FL. Both PhD students contributed equally to this review, similar to their co-supervisors SC and VSP.

References

Abirami, A., Uthra, S., and Arumugam, M. (2018). Nutritional value of seaweeds and their potential pharmacological role of polyphenolics substances: a review. *Journal of Emerging Technologies and Innovative Research* **5**: 930–939.

Aboulthana, W.M., El-Feky, A.M., Ibrahim, N.E.S. et al. (2018). Evaluation of the pancreatoprotective effect of *Nannochloropsis oculata* extract against Streptozotocin-induced diabetes in rats. *Journal of Applied Pharmaceutical Science* **8**: 046–058. https://doi.org/10.7324/JAPS.2018.8607.

Abu-Ghannam, N. and Rajauria, G. (2013). Antimicrobial activity of compounds isolated from algae. In: *Functional Ingredients from Algae for Foods and Nutraceuticals* (ed. H. Dominguez), 287–306. Cambridge: Woodhead Publishing https://doi.org/10.1533/9780857098689.2.287.

Agregán, R., Munekata, P.E., Domínguez, R. et al. (2017a). Proximate composition, phenolic content and *in vitro* antioxidant activity of aqueous extracts of the seaweeds *Ascophyllum nodosum*, *Bifurcaria bifurcata* and *Fucus vesiculosus*. Effect of addition of the extracts on the oxidative stability of canola oil under accelerated storage conditions. *Food Research International* **99**: 986–994. https://doi.org/10.1016/j.foodres.2016.11.009.

Agregán, R., Munekata, P.E.S., Franco, D. et al. (2017b). Phenolic compounds from three brown seaweed species using LC-DAD–ESI-MS/MS. *Food Research International* **99**: 979–985. https://doi.org/10.1016/j.foodres.2017.03.043.

Agregán, R., Munekata, P.E.S., Franco, D. et al. (2018). Antioxidant potential of extracts obtained from macro- (*Ascophyllum nodosum, Fucus vesiculosus* and *Bifurcaria bifurcata*) and micro-algae (*Chlorella vulgaris* and *Spirulina plantensis*) assisted by ultrasound. *Medicine* **5**: 1–9. https://doi.org/10.3390/medicines5020033.

Ahmed, F., Fanning, K., Netzel, M. et al. (2014). Profiling of carotenoids and antioxidant capacity of microalgae from subtropical coastal and brackish waters. *Food Chemistry* **165**: 300–306. https://doi.org/10.1016/j.foodchem.2014.05.107.

Ahn, G.N., Kim, K.N., Cha, S.H. et al. (2007). Antioxidant activities of phlorotannins purified from *Ecklonia cava* on free radical scavenging using ESR and H_2O_2-mediated DNA damage. *European Food Research and Technology* **226**: 71–79. https://doi.org/10.1007/s00217-006-0510-y.

Ahn, G., Amagai, Y., Matsuda, A. et al. (2015). Dieckol, a phlorotannin of *Ecklonia cava*, suppresses IgE-mediated mast cell activation and passive cutaneous anaphylactic reaction. *Experimental Dermatology* **24**: 968–970. https://doi.org/10.1111/exd.12814.

Ali, T.F. and Hasan, T. (2012). Phlorotannin-incorporated mesenchymal stem cells and their promising role in osteogenesis imperfecta. *Journal of Medical Hypotheses and Ideas* **6**: 85–89. https://doi.org/10.1016/j.jmhi.2012.09.002.

American Diabetes Association (2010). Diagnosis and classification of diabetes mellitus. *Diabetes Care* **33**: S62–S69. https://doi.org/10.2337/dc10-S062.

Apak, R., Özyürek, M., Güçlü, K., and Çapanoğlu, E. (2016). Antioxidant activity/capacity measurement. 1. Classification, physiochemical principles, mechanisms and electron transfer (ET)-based assays. *Journal of Agricultural and Food Chemistry* **64**: 997–1027. https://doi.org/10.1021/acs.jafc.5b04739.

Ar Gall, E., Lelchat, F., Hupel, M. et al. (2015). Extraction and purification of phlorotannins from brown algae. In: *Natural Products from Marine Algae* (eds. D.B. Stengel and S. Connan), 131–143. New York: Humana Press https://doi.org/10.1007/978-1-4939-2684-8_7.

Arai, M., Shibata, Y., Pugdee, K. et al. (2007). Effects of reactive oxygen species (ROS) on antioxidant system and osteoblastic differentiation in MC3T3-E1 cells. *IUBMB Life* **59**: 27–33. https://doi.org/10.1080/15216540601156188.

Arnold, T.M. and Targett, N.M. (2002). Marine tannins: the importance of a mechanistic framework for predicting ecological roles. *Journal of Chemical Ecology* **28**: 1919–1934. https://doi.org/10.1023/A:1020737609151.

Athukorala, Y., Kim, K.-N., and Jeon, Y.-J. (2006). Antiproliferative and antioxidant properties of an enzymatic hydrolysate from brown alga, *Ecklonia cava*. *Food and Chemical Toxicology* **44**: 1065–1074. https://doi.org/10.1016/j.fct.2006.01.011.

Atkinson, M.A. and Eisenbarth, G.S. (2001). Type 1 diabetes: new perspectives on disease pathogenesis and treatment. *The Lancet* **358**: 221–229.

Audibert, L., Fauchon, M., Blanc, N. et al. (2010). Phenolic compounds in the brown seaweed *Ascophyllum nodosum*: distribution and radical-scavenging activities. *Phytochemical Analysis* **21**: 399–405. https://doi.org/10.1002/pca.1210.

Awad, N.E. (2004). Bioactive brominated diterpenes from the marine red alga *Jania rubens* (L.) Lamx. *Phytotherapy Research: An International Journal Devoted to Pharmacological and Toxicological Evaluation of Natural Product Derivatives* **18**: 275–279. https://doi.org/10.1002/ptr.1273.

Balboa, E.M., Conde, E., Moure, A. et al. (2013). *In vitro* antioxidant properties of crude extracts and compounds from brown algae. *Food Chemistry* **138**: 1764–1785. https://doi.org/10.1016/j.foodchem.2012.11.026.

Balboa, E.M., Soto, M.L., Nogueira, D.R. et al. (2014). Potential of antioxidant extracts produced by aqueous processing of renewable resources for the formulation of cosmetics. *Industrial Crops and Products* **58**: 104–110. https://doi.org/10.1016/j.indcrop.2014.03.041.

Balboa, E., Conde, E., Constenla, A. et al. (2017). Sensory evaluation and oxidative stability of a Suncream formulated with thermal spring waters from Ourense (NW Spain) and *Sargassum muticum* extracts. *Cosmetics* **4**: 19. https://doi.org/10.3390/cosmetics4020019.

Barbosa, M., Lopes, G., Ferreres, F. et al. (2017). Phlorotannin extracts from Fucales: marine polyphenols as bioregulators engaged in inflammation-related mediators and enzymes. *Algal Research* **28**: 1–8. https://doi.org/10.1016/j.algal.2017.09.009.

Barbosa, M., Lopes, G., Valentão, P. et al. (2018). Edible seaweeds' phlorotannins in allergy: a natural multi-target approach. *Food Chemistry* **265**: 233–241. https://doi.org/10.1016/j.foodchem.2018.05.074.

Barrero, A.F., Alvarez-Manzaneda, E.J., Herrador, M.M. et al. (1999). Synthesis and antitumoral activities of marine ent-chromazonarol and related compounds. *Bioorganic and Medicinal Chemistry Letters* **9**: 2325–2328. https://doi.org/10.1016/S0960-894X(99)00382-0.

Barreto, M. and Meyer, J.J.M. (2006). Isolation and antimicrobial activity of a lanosol derivative from *Osmundaria serrata* (Rhodophyta) and a visual exploration of its biofilm covering. *South African Journal of Botany* **72**: 521–528. https://doi.org/10.1016/j.sajb.2006.01.006.

Barwell, C.J., Canham, C.A., and Guiry, M.D. (1989). Hordenine content of the marine alga *Mastocarpus stellatus* and the algal food product carrageen. *Phytotherapy Research* **3**: 67–69. https://doi.org/10.1002/ptr.2650030207.

Baurain, D., Brinkmann, H., Petersen, J. et al. (2010). Phylogenomic evidence for separate acquisition of plastids in Cryptophytes, Haptophytes, and Stramenopiles. *Molecular Biology and Evolution* **27**: 1698–1709. https://doi.org/10.1093/molbev/msq059.

Bennamara, A., Abourriche, A., Berrada, M. et al. (1999). Methoxybifurcarenone: an antifungal and antibacterial meroditerpenoid from the brown alga *Cystoseira tamariscifolia*. *Phytochemistry* **52**: 37–40. https://doi.org/10.1016/S0031-9422(99)00040-0.

Birringer, M., Siems, K., Maxones, A. et al. (2018). Natural 6-hydroxy-chromanols and -chromenols: structural diversity, biosynthetic pathways and health implications. *RSC Advances* **8**: 4803–4841. https://doi.org/10.1039/c7ra11819h.

Blackman, A.J. and Matthews, D.J. (1982). Halogenated phloroglucinols from *Rhabdonia verticillata*. *Phytochemistry* **21**: 2141–2142. https://doi.org/10.1016/0031-9422(82)83072-0.

Bourgougnon, N. and Stiger-Pouvreau, V. (2011). Chemodiversity and bioactivity within red and Brown macroalgae along the French coasts, Metropole and overseas Departments and territories. In: *Handbook of Marine Macroalgae: Biotechnology and Applied Phycology* (ed. S.-K. Kim), 58–105. Chichester: Wiley https://doi.org/10.1002/9781119977087.ch4.

Bousquet, J., Khaltaev, N., Cruz, A.A. et al. (2008). Allergic rhinitis and its impact on asthma (ARIA) 2008. *Allergy* **63**: 8–160.

Brandt, F.S., Cazzaniga, A., and Hann, M. (2011). Cosmeceuticals: current trends and market analysis. *Seminars in Cutaneous Medicine and Surgery* **30**: 141–143.

Brash, D.E., Rudolph, J.A., Simon, J.A. et al. (1991). A role for sunlight in skin cancer: UV-induced p53 mutations in squamous cell carcinoma. *Proceedings of the National Academy of Sciences* **88**: 10124–10128. https://doi.org/10.1073/pnas.88.22.10124.

Briand, A., Kornprobst, J.M., Al-Easa, H.S. et al. (1997). (−)-Paniculatol, a new ent-labdane bromoditerpene from *Laurencia paniculata*. *Tetrahedron Letters* **38**: 3399–3400. https://doi.org/10.1016/S0040-4039(97)00629-1.

Brunt, E.G. and Burgess, J.G. (2017). The promise of marine molecules as cosmetic active ingredients. *International Journal of Cosmetic Science* **40**: 1–15. https://doi.org/10.1111/ics.12435.

Buikema, A.L., McGinniss, M.J., and Cairns, J. (1979). Phenolics in aquatic ecosystems: a selected review of recent literature. *Marine Environmental Research* **2**: 87–181. https://doi.org/10.1016/0141-1136(79)90006-0.

Cabrita, M.T., Vale, C., and Rauter, A.P. (2010). Halogenated compounds from marine algae. *Marine Drugs* **8**: 2301–2307. https://doi.org/10.3390/md8082301.

Carocho, M., Barreiro, M.F., Morales, P., and Ferreira, I.C. (2014). Adding molecules to food, pros and cons: a review on synthetic and natural food additives. *Comprehensive Reviews in Food Science and Food Safety* **13** (4): 377–399.

Cassano, V., De-Paula, J.C., Fujii, M.T. et al. (2008). Sesquiterpenes from the introduced red seaweed *Laurencia caduciramulosa* (Rhodomelaceae, Ceramiales). *Biochemical Systematics and Ecology* **36**: 223–226. https://doi.org/10.1016/j.bse.2007.07.005.

Catarino, M.D., Silva, A.M.S., and Cardoso, S.M. (2018). Phycochemical constituents and biological activities of *Fucus* spp. *Marine Drugs* **16**: 249. https://doi.org/10.3390/md16080249.

Cavas, L. and Yurdakoc, K. (2005). A comparative study: assessment of the antioxidant system in the invasive green alga *Caulerpa racemosa* and some macrophytes from the Mediterranean. *Journal of Experimental Marine Biology and Ecology* **321**: 35–41. https://doi.org/10.1016/j.jembe.2004.12.035.

Celikler, S., Tas, S., Vatan, O. et al. (2009). Anti-hyperglycemic and antigenotoxic potential of *Ulva rigida* ethanolic extract in the experimental diabetes mellitus. *Food and Chemical Toxicology* **47**: 1837–1840.

Cha, S.H., Lee, K.W., and Jeon, Y.J. (2006). Screening of extracts from red algae in Jeju for potentials marine angiotensin-I converting enzyme (ACE) inhibitory activity. *Algae* **21**: 343–348. https://doi.org/10.4490/ALGAE.2006.21.3.343.

Cha, S.H., Ko, C.I., Kim, D., and Jeon, Y.J. (2012). Protective effects of phlorotannins against ultraviolet B radiation in zebrafish (*Danio rerio*). *Veterinary Dermatology* **23**: 51–e12. https://doi.org/10.1111/j.1365-3164.2011.01009.x.

Chakraborty, K., Joseph, D., and Praveen, N.K. (2015). Antioxidant activities and phenolic contents of three red seaweeds (division: Rhodophyta) harvested from the Gulf of Mannar of Peninsular India. *Journal of Food Science and Technology* **52**: 1924–1935. https://doi.org/10.1007/s13197-013-1189-2.

Chan, J.C.-C., Cheung, P.C.-K., and Ang, P.O. (1997). Comparative studies on the effect of three drying methods on the nutritional composition of seaweed *Sargassum hemiphyllum* (turn.). *Journal of Agricultural and Food Chemistry* **45**: 3056–3059. https://doi.org/10.1021/jf9701749.

Chan, Y.Y., Kim, K.H., and Cheah, S.H. (2011). Inhibitory effects of *Sargassum polycystum* on tyrosinase activity and melanin formation in B16F10 murine melanoma cells. *Journal of Ethnopharmacology* **137**: 1183–1188. https://doi.org/10.1016/j.jep.2011.07.050.

Charoensiddhi, S., Franco, C., Su, P., and Zhang, W. (2015). Improved antioxidant activities of brown seaweed *Ecklonia radiata* extracts prepared by microwave-assisted enzymatic extraction. *Journal of Applied Phycology* **27**: 2049–2058. https://doi.org/10.1007/s10811-014-0476-2.

Chemat, F., Vian, M.A., and Cravotto, G. (2012). Green extraction of natural products: concept and principles. *International Journal of Molecular Sciences* **13**: 8615–8627. https://doi.org/10.3390/ijms13078615.

Chen, C.H., Pearson, A.M., and Gray, J.I. (1992). Effects of synthetic antioxidants (BHA, BHT and PG) on the mutagenicity of IQ-like compounds. *Food Chemistry* **43**: 177–183. https://doi.org/10.1016/0308-8146(92)90170-7.

Chen, Y., Lin, H., Li, Z., and Mou, Q. (2015). The anti-allergic activity of polyphenol extracted from five marine algae. *Journal of Ocean University of China* **14**: 681–684. https://doi.org/10.1007/s11802-015-2601-5.

Chia, S.R., Show, P.L., Phang, S.M. et al. (2018). Sustainable approach in phlorotannin recovery from macroalgae. *Journal of Bioscience and Bioengineering* **126**: 220–225. https://doi.org/10.1016/j.jbiosc.2018.02.015.

Chlipala, G.E., Tri, P.H., Hung, N.V. et al. (2010). Nhatrangins A and B, aplysiatoxin-related metabolites from the marine cyanobacterium *Lyngbya majuscula* from Vietnam. *Journal of Natural Products* **73**: 784–787. https://doi.org/10.1021/np100002q.

Cho, T.O. (2016). Composition comprising extract of *Ecklonia cava* or phlorotannin compounds isolated from thereof for preventing or treating influenza. Patent KR20180052258A.

Cho, M.L., Kang, I.J., Won, M.H. et al. (2010). The antioxidant properties of ethanol extracts and their solvent-partitioned fractions from various green seaweeds. *Journal of Medicinal Food* **13**: 1232–1239. https://doi.org/10.1089/jmf.2010.1124.

Cho, M.L., Lee, H.-S., Kang, I.J. et al. (2011). Antioxidant properties of extract and fractions from *Enteromorpha prolifera*, a type of green seaweed. *Food Chemistry* **127**: 999–1006. https://doi.org/10.1016/j.foodchem.2011.01.072.

Choi, H., Engene, N., Smith, J.E. et al. (2010). Crossbyanols A–D, toxic brominated polyphenyl ethers from the Hawai'ian bloom-forming cyanobacterium *Leptolyngbya crossbyana*. *Journal of Natural Products* **73**: 517–522. https://doi.org/10.1021/np900661g.

Choi, J., Lee, K., Lee, B. et al. (2013). Safety, functionality and stability tests of *Ecklonia cava* extract for dermal application. *Toxicology and Environmental Health Sciences* **6**: 1–6. https://doi.org/10.1007/s13530-014-0189-6.

Chowdhury, M.T.H., Bangoura, I., Kang, J.Y. et al. (2011). Distribution of phlorotannins in the brown alga *Ecklonia cava* and comparison of pretreatments for extraction. *Fisheries and Aquatic Sciences* **14**: 198–204. https://doi.org/10.5657/FAS.2011.0198.

Ciavatta, M.L., Wahidulla, S., D'Souza, L. et al. (2001). New bromotriterpene polyethers from the Indian alga *Chondria armata*. *Tetrahedron* **57**: 617–623. https://doi.org/10.1016/S0040-4020(00)01031-0.

Cikoš, A.M., Jokić, S., Šubarić, D., and Jerković, I. (2018). Overview on the application of modern methods for the extraction of bioactive compounds from marine macroalgae. *Marine Drugs* **16**: 348. https://doi.org/10.3390/md16100348.

Conde, E., Moure, A., and Domínguez, H. (2015). Supercritical CO_2 extraction of fatty acids, phenolics and fucoxanthin from freeze-dried *Sargassum muticum*. *Journal of Applied Phycology* **27**: 957–964. https://doi.org/10.1007/s10811-014-0389-0.

Connan, S., Goulard, F., Stiger, V. et al. (2004). Interspecific and temporal variation in phlorotannin levels in an assemblage of brown algae. *Botanica Marina* **47**: 410–416. https://doi.org/10.1515/BOT.2004.057.

Córdoba, A., Satué, M., Gómez-Florit, M. et al. (2014). Flavonoid-modified surfaces: multifunctional bioactive biomaterials with Osteopromotive, anti-inflammatory, and anti-fibrotic potential. *Advanced Healthcare Materials* **4**: 540–549. https://doi.org/10.1002/adhm.201400587.

Córdoba, A., Monjo, M., Hierro-Oliva, M. et al. (2015). Bioinspired quercitrin nanocoatings: a fluorescence-based method for their surface quantification, and their effect on stem cell adhesion and differentiation to the osteoblastic lineage. *ACS Applied Materials and Interfaces* **7**: 16857–16864. https://doi.org/10.1021/acsami.5b05044.

Cornish, M.L. and Garbary, D.J. (2010). Antioxidants from macroalgae: potential applications in human health and nutrition. *Algae* **25**: 155–171. https://doi.org/10.4490/algae.2010.25.4.155.

Couteau, C. and Coiffard, L. (2016). Seaweed application in cosmetics. In: *Seaweed in Health and Disease Prevention* (eds. J. Fleurence and I. Levine), 423–441. London: Academic Press https://doi.org/10.1016/B978-0-12-802772-1.00014-2.

Cox, S., Abu-Ghannam, N., and Gupta, S. (2010). An assessment of the antioxidant and antimicrobial activity of six species of edible Irish seaweeds. *International Food Research Journal* **17**: 205–220. https://doi.org/10.21427/D7HC92.

Creis, E., Ar Gall, E., and Potin, P. (2018). Ubiquitous phlorotannins prospects and perspectives. In: *Blue Biotechnology: Production and Use of Marine Molecules* (eds. S. La Barre and S. Bates), 67–117. Weinheim: Wiley-VCH Verlag GmbH & Co https://doi.org/10.1002/9783527801718.ch3.

Culioli, G., Ortalo-Magné, A., Valls, R. et al. (2008). Antifouling activity of meroditerpenoids from the marine brown alga *Halidrys siliquosa*. *Journal of Natural Products* **71**: 1121–1126. https://doi.org/10.1021/np070110k.

Da Silva, M.F., Casazza, A.A., Ferrari, P.F. et al. (2017). Recovery of phenolic compounds of food concern from *Arthrospira platensis* by green extraction techniques. *Algal Research* **25**: 391–401.

Dang, T.T., Bowyer, M.C., Van Altena, I.A., and Scarlett, C.J. (2018). Optimum conditions of microwave-assisted extraction for phenolic compounds and antioxidant capacity of the brown alga *Sargassum vestitum*. *Separation Science and Technology* **53**: 1711–1723. https://doi.org/10.1080/01496395.2017.1414845.

Davison, J.R. and Bewley, C.A. (2019). Antimicrobial chrysophaentin analogs identified from laboratory cultures of the marine microalga *Chrysophaeum taylorii*. *Journal of Natural Products* **82**: 148–153. https://doi.org/10.1021/acs.jnatprod.8b00858.

Davyt, D., Fernandez, R., Suescun, L. et al. (2001). New sesquiterpene derivatives from the red alga *Laurencia scoparia*. Isolation, structure determination, and anthelmintic activity. *Journal of Natural Products* **64**: 1552–1555. https://doi.org/10.1021/np0102307.

De Carvalho, L.R., Guimarães, S.M., and Roque, N.F. (2006). Sulfated bromophenols from *Osmundaria obtusiloba* (C. Agardh) R.E. Norris (Rhodophyta, Ceramiales). *Brazilian Journal of Botany* **29**: 453–459. https://doi.org/10.1590/S0100-84042006000300012.

De Jesus Raposo, M.F. and De Morais, A.M.M.B. (2015). Microalgae for the prevention of cardiovascular disease and stroke. *Life Sciences* **125**: 32–41. https://doi.org/10.1016/j.lfs.2014.09.018.

De Nanteuil, G. and Mastagli, P. (1981). A bromophenol in the red alga *Halopitys incurvus*. *Phytochemistry* **20**: 1750–1751.

Deniaud-Bouët, E., Hardouin, K., Potin, P. et al. (2017). A review about brown algal cell walls and fucose-containing sulfated polysaccharides: cell wall context, biomedical properties and key research challenges. *Carbohydrate Polymers* **175**: 395–408. https://doi.org/10.1016/j.carbpol.2017.07.082.

D'Hondt, E., Martin-Juarez, J., Bolado, S. et al. (2017). Cell disruption technologies. In: *Microalgae-Based Biofuels and Bioproducts* (eds. C. Gonzalez-Fernandez and R. Muñoz), 133–154. Cambridge: Woodhead Publishing.

Douglas, T.E.L., Dokupil, A., Reczyńska, K. et al. (2016). Enrichment of enzymatically mineralized gellan gum hydrogels with phlorotannin-rich *Ecklonia cava* extract Seanol® to endow antibacterial properties and promote mineralization. *Biomedical Materials* **11**: 045015. https://doi.org/10.1088/1748-6041/11/4/04501.

Duan, X.J., Zhang, W.W., Li, X.M., and Wang, B.G. (2006). Evaluation of antioxidant property of extract and fractions obtained from a red alga, *Polysiphonia urceolata*. *Food Chemistry* **95**: 37–43. https://doi.org/10.1016/j.foodchem.2004.12.015.

Edgerton, D.S., Kraft, G., Smith, M. et al. (2017). Insulin's direct hepatic effect explains the inhibition of glucose production caused by insulin secretion. *JCI Insight* **2**: e91863. https://doi.org/10.1172/jci.insight.91863.

Eom, S.H., Kim, Y.M., and Kim, S.K. (2012). Antimicrobial effect of phlorotannins from marine brown algae. *Food and Chemical Toxicology* **50**: 3251–3255. https://doi.org/10.1016/j.fct.2012.06.028.

Eom, S.H., Kim, D.H., Lee, S.H. et al. (2013). *In vitro* antibacterial activity and synergistic antibiotic effects of phlorotannins isolated from *Eisenia bicyclis* against methicillin-resistant *Saureus*. *Phytotherapy Research* **27**: 1260–1264. https://doi.org/10.1002/ptr.4851.

Eom, S.H., Moon, S.Y., Lee, D.S. et al. (2015). *In vitro* antiviral activity of dieckol and phlorofucofuroeckol-A isolated from edible brown alga *Eisenia bicyclis* against murine norovirus. *Algae* **30**: 241–246. https://doi.org/10.4490/algae.2015.30.3.241.

Eshun, K. and He, Q. (2004). *Aloe vera*: a valuable ingredient for the food, pharmaceutical and cosmetic industries – a review. *Critical Reviews in Food Science and Nutrition* **44**: 91–96.

Esquivel-Hernández, D.A., Ibarra-Garza, I.P., Rodríguez-Rodríguez, J. et al. (2017). Green extraction technologies for high-value metabolites from algae: a review. *Biofuels, Bioproducts and Biorefining* **11**: 215–231. https://doi.org/10.1002/bbb.1735.

Etahiri, S., Bultel-Poncé, V., Caux, C., and Guyot, M. (2001). New bromoditerpenes from the red alga *Sphaerococcus coronopifolius*. *Journal of Natural Products* **64**: 1024–1027. https://doi.org/10.1021/np0002684.

Fallarero, A., Loikkanen, J.J., Mansito, P.T. et al. (2003). Effects of aqueous extracts of *Halimeda incrassata* (Ellis) Lamouroux and *Bryothamnion triquetrum* (S.G. Gmelin) Howe on hydrogen peroxide and methyl mercury-induced oxidative stress in GT1-7 mouse hypothalamic immortalized cells. *Phytomedicine* **10**: 39–47.

Farvin, S.K.H. and Jacobsen, C. (2013). Phenolic compounds and antioxidant activities of selected species of seaweeds from Danish coast. *Food Chemistry* **138**: 1670–1681. https://doi.org/10.1016/j.foodchem.2012.10.078.

Fayad, S., Nehmé, R., Tannoury, M. et al. (2017). Macroalga *Padina pavonica* water extracts obtained by pressurized liquid extraction and microwave-assisted extraction inhibit hyaluronidase activity as shown by capillary electrophoresis. *Journal of Chromatography A* **1497**: 19–27. https://doi.org/10.1016/j.chroma.2017.03.033.

Feng, Y., Carroll, A.R., Addepalli, R. et al. (2007). Vanillic acid derivatives from the green algae *Cladophora socialis* as potent protein tyrosine phosphatase 1B inhibitors. *Journal of Natural Products* **70**: 1790–1792. https://doi.org/10.1021/np070225o.

Ferreres, F., Lopes, G., Gil-Izquierdo, A. et al. (2012). Phlorotannin extracts from Fucales characterized by HPLC-DAD-ESI-MS^n: approaches to hyaluronidase inhibitory capacity and antioxidant properties. *Marine Drugs* **10**: 2766–2781. https://doi.org/10.3390/md10122766.

Fisch, K.M., Böhm, V., Wright, A.D., and König, G.M. (2003). Antioxidative meroterpenoids from the brown alga *Cystoseira crinita*. *Journal of Natural Products* **66**: 968–975. https://doi.org/10.1021/np030082f.

Flexner, C. (2007). HIV drug development: the next 25 years. *Nature Reviews Drug Discovery* **6**: 959–966. https://doi.org/10.1038/nrd2336.

Flodin, C., Helidoniotis, F., and Whitfield, F.B. (1999). Seasonal variation in bromophenol content and bromoperoxidase activity in *Ulva lactuca*. *Phytochemistry* **51**: 135–138. https://doi.org/10.1016/S0031-9422(98)00668-2.

Forbes, J.M. and Cooper, M.E. (2013). Mechanisms of diabetic complications. *Physiological Reviews* **93**: 137–188. https://doi.org/10.1152/physrev.00045.2011.

Ford, L., Theodoridou, K., Sheldrake, G.N., and Walsh, P.J. (2019). A critical review of analytical methods used for the chemical characterisation and quantification of phlorotannin compounds in brown seaweeds. *Phytochemical Analysis*: 1–13. https://doi.org/10.1002/pca.2851.

Freile-Pelegrin, Y. and Robledo, D. (2014). Bioactive phenolic compounds from algae. In: *Bioactive Compounds from Marine Foods: Plant and Animal Sources* (eds. B. Herandez-Ledesma and M. Herrero), 113–129. Chichester: Wiley https://doi.org/10.1002/9781118412893/ch6.

Gallego, R., Montero, L., Cifuentes, A. et al. (2018). Green extraction of bioactive compounds from microalgae. *Journal of Analysis and Testing* **2**: 1–15. https://doi.org/10.1007/s41664-018-0061-9.

Garcia-Pichel, F. and Castenholz, R.W. (1991). Characterization and biological implications of scytonemin, a cyanobacterial sheath pigment. *Journal of Phycology* **27**: 395–409. https://doi.org/10.1111/j.0022-3646.1991.00395.x.

Geiselman, J.A. and McConnell, O.J. (1981). Polyphenols in brown algae *Fucus vesiculosus* and *Ascophyllum nodosum*: chemical defenses against the marine herbivorous snail, *Littorina littorea*. *Journal of Chemical Ecology* **7**: 1115–1133. https://doi.org/10.1007/BF00987632.

Gil, B., Ferrándiz, M.L., Sanz, M.J. et al. (1995). Inhibition of inflammatory responses by epitaondiol and other marine natural products. *Life Sciences* **57**: 1–6. https://doi.org/10.1016/0024-3205(95)00260-D.

Gilchrest, B.A., Blog, F.B., and Szabo, G. (1979). Effects of aging and chronic sun exposure on melanocytes in human skin. *Journal of Investigative Dermatology* **73**: 141–143. https://doi.org/10.1111/1523-1747.ep12581580.

Ginnaga. A., Hirayama, I., Iwamura, Y., Nagayama, K., Nakamura, T., and Kiminori, N. (2002). Antibacterial agent based on phlorotannins. Patent JP2003277203.

Girish, K.S. and Kemparaju, K. (2007). The magic glue hyaluronan and its eraser hyaluronidase: a biological overview. *Life Sciences* **80**: 1921–1943. https://doi.org/10.1016/j.lfs.2007.02.037.

Goiris, K., Muylaert, K., Voorspoels, S. et al. (2014). Detection of flavonoids in microalgae from different evolutionary lineages. *Journal of Phycology* **50**: 483–492. https://doi.org/10.1111/jpy.12180.

Gómez-Guzmán, M., Rodríguez-Nogales, A., Algieri, F., and Gálvez, J. (2018). Potential role of seaweed polyphenols in cardiovascular-associated disorders. *Marine Drugs* **16**: 1–21. https://doi.org/10.3390/md16080250.

Gonçalves-Fernández, C., Sineiro, J., Moreira, R., and Gualillo, O. (2019). Extraction and characterization of phlorotannin-enriched fractions from the Atlantic seaweed *Bifurcaria bifurcata* and evaluation of their cytotoxic activity in murine cell line. *Journal of Applied Phycology* **31**: 2573–2583. https://doi.org/10.1007/s10811-018-1729-2.

Gröniger, A. and Häder, D.P. (2002). Induction of the synthesis of an UV-absorbing substance in the green alga *Prasiola stipitata*. *Journal of Photochemistry and Photobiology B: Biology* **66**: 54–59. https://doi.org/10.1016/S1011-1344(01)00275-5.

Günerken, E., D'Hondt, E., Eppink, M.H.M. et al. (2015). Cell disruption for microalgae biorefineries. *Biotechnology Advances* **33**: 243–260. https://doi.org/10.1016/j.biotechadv.2015.01.008.

Gupta, S. and Abu-Ghannam, N. (2011a). Bioactive potential and possible health effects of edible brown seaweeds. *Trends in Food Science and Technology* **22**: 315–326. https://doi.org/10.1016/j.tifs.2011.03.011.

Gupta, S. and Abu-Ghannam, N. (2011b). Recent developments in the application of seaweeds or seaweed extracts as a means for enhancing the safety and quality attributes of foods. *Innovative Food Science and Emerging Technologies* **12**: 600–609. https://doi.org/10.1016/j.ifset.2011.07.004.

Güven, K.C., Bora, A., and Sunam, G. (1970). Hordenine from the algae *Phyllophora nervosa*. *Phytochemistry* **9**: 1893. https://doi.org/10.1016/S0031-9422(00)85613-7.

Habauzit, V. and Horcajada, M.-N. (2007). Phenolic phytochemicals and bone. *Phytochemistry Reviews* **7**: 313–344. https://doi.org/10.1007/s11101-007-9078-9.

Han, Y.-S. and Han, T. (2005). UV-B induction of UV-B protection in *Ulva pertusa* (Chlorophyta). *Journal of Phycology* **41**: 523–530. https://doi.org/10.1111/j.1529-8817.2005.00072.x.

Harada, H. and Kamei, Y. (1998). Dose-dependent selective cytotoxicity of extracts from marine green alga, *Cladophoropsis vaucheriaeformis*, against mouse leukemia L1201 cells. *Biological and Pharmaceutical Bulletin* **21**: 386–389.

Harborne, J.B. (1984). Phenolic compounds. In: *Phytochemical Methods: A Guide to Modern Techniques of Plant Analysis* (ed. J.B. Harborne), 37–99. Heidelberg: Springer https://doi.org/10.1007/978-94-009-5570-7_2.

Hardouin, K., Burlot, A.S., Umami, A. et al. (2014). Biochemical and antiviral activities of enzymatic hydrolysates from different invasive French seaweeds. *Journal of Applied Phycology* **26**: 1029–1042. https://doi.org/10.1007/s10811-013-0201-6.

He, Z., Chen, Y., Chen, Y. et al. (2013). Optimization of the microwave-assisted extraction of phlorotannins from *Saccharina japonica* Aresh and evaluation of the inhibitory effects of phlorotannin-containing extracts on HepG2 cancer cells. *Chinese Journal of Oceanology and Limnology* **31**: 1045–1054. https://doi.org/10.1007/s00343-013-2321-x.

Heffernan, N., Smyth, T.J., Fitzgerald, R.J. et al. (2014). Antioxidant activity and phenolic content of pressurised liquid and solid-liquid extracts from four Irish origin macroalgae. *International Journal of Food Science and Technology* **49**: 1765–1772. https://doi.org/10.1111/ijfs.12512.

Heo, S.J. and Jeon, Y.J. (2009). Evaluation of diphlorethohydroxycarmalol isolated from *Ishige okamurae* for radical scavenging activity and its protective effect against H_2O_2-induced cell damage. *Process Biochemistry* **44**: 412–418. https://doi.org/10.1016/j.procbio.2008.12.005.

Heo, S.J., Ko, S.C., Cha, S.H. et al. (2009). Effect of phlorotannins isolated from *Ecklonia cava* on melanogenesis and their protective effect against photo-oxidative stress induced by UV-B radiation. *Toxicology in Vitro* **23**: 1123–1130. https://doi.org/10.1016/j.tiv.2009.05.013.

Hermund, D.B., Plaza, M., Turner, C. et al. (2018). Structure dependent antioxidant capacity of phlorotannins from Icelandic *Fucus vesiculosus* by UHPLC-DAD-ECD-QTOFMS. *Food Chemistry* **240**: 904–909. https://doi.org/10.1016/j.foodchem.2017.08.032.

Hernlund, E., Svedbom, A., Ivergård, M. et al. (2013). Osteoporosis in the European Union: medical management, epidemiology and economic burden. *Archives of Osteoporosis* **8**: 1–2. https://doi.org/10.1007/s11657-013-0136-1.

Huang, D. and Prior, R.L. (2005). The chemistry behind antioxidant capacity assays. *Journal of Agricultural and Food Chemistry* **53**: 1841–1856. https://doi.org/10.1021/jf030723c.

Hunter, P.M. and Hegele, R.A. (2017). Functional foods and dietary supplements for the management of dyslipidaemia. *Nature Reviews Endocrinology* **13**: 278.

Hwang, H., Chen, T., Nines, R.G. et al. (2006). Photochemoprevention of UVB-induced skin carcinogenesis in SKH-1 mice by brown algae polyphenols. *International Journal of Cancer* **119**: 2742–2749. https://doi.org/10.1002/ijc.22147.

Hwang, P.-A., Hung, Y.-L., Tsai, Y.-K. et al. (2015). The brown seaweed *Sargassum hemiphyllum* exhibits α-amylase and α-glucosidase inhibitory activity and enhances insulin release *in vitro*. *Cytotechnology* **67**: 653–660. https://doi.org/10.1007/s10616-014-9745-9.

Ibañez, E., Herrero, M., Mendiola, J., and Castro-Puyana, M. (2012). Extraction and characterization of bioactive compounds with health benefits from marine resources: macro and micro algae, cyanobacteria, and invertebrates. In: *Marine Bioactive Compounds: Sources, Characterization and Applications* (ed. M. Hayes), 55–98. Springer US Science and Business Media https://doi.org/10.1007/978-1-4614-1247-2.

Imbs, T.I. and Zvyagintseva, T.N. (2018). Phlorotannins are Polyphenolic metabolites of Brown algae. *Russian Journal of Marine Biology* **44**: 263–273. https://doi.org/10.1134/S106307401804003X.

Ishii, T., Okino, T., Suzuki, M., and Machiguchi, Y. (2004). Tichocarpols a and B, two novel phenylpropanoids with feeding-deterrent activity from the red alga *Tichocarpus crinitus*. *Journal of Natural Products* **67**: 1764–1766. https://doi.org/10.1021/np0498509.

James, P.T., Leach, R., Kalamara, E., and Shayeghi, M. (2012). The worldwide obesity epidemic. *Obesity Research* **9**: 228S–233S. https://doi.org/10.1038/oby.2001.123.

Jaswir, I., Tope, T., Raus, R. et al. (2014). Study on anti-bacterial potentials of some Malaysian brown seaweeds. *Food Hydrocolloids* **42**: 275–279. https://doi.org/10.1016/j.foodhyd.2014.03.008.

Jégou, C., Culioli, G., and Stiger-Pouvreau, V. (2012). Meroditerpene from *Cystoseira nodicaulis* and its taxonomic significance. *Biochemical Systematics and Ecology* **44**: 202–204. https://doi.org/10.1016/j.bse.2012.05.003.

Jégou, C., Kervarec, N., Cérantola, S. et al. (2015). NMR use to quantify phlorotannins. The case of *Cystoseira tamariscifolia*, a phloroglucinol-producing brown macroalga in Brittany (France). *Talanta* **135**: 1–6. https://doi.org/10.1016/j.talanta.2014.11.059.

Jennings, J.G. and Steinberg, P.D. (1997). Phlorotannins versus other factors affecting epiphyte abundance on the kelp *Ecklonia radiata*. *Oecologia* **109**: 461–473. https://doi.org/10.1007/s004420050106.

Jiménez, J.T., O'Connell, S., Lyons, H. et al. (2010). Antioxidant, antimicrobial, and tyrosinase inhibition activities of acetone extract of *Ascophyllum nodosum*. *Chemical Papers* **64**: 434–442. https://doi.org/10.2478/s11696-010-0024-8.

Jiménez-Escrig, A., Jiménez-Jiménez, I., Pulido, R., and Saura-Calixto, F. (2001). Antioxidant activity of fresh and processed edible seaweeds. *Journal of the Science of Food and Agriculture* **81**: 530–534. https://doi.org/10.1002/jsfa.842.

Joe, M.J., Kim, S.N., Choi, H.Y. et al. (2006). The inhibitory effects of eckol and dieckol from *Ecklonia stolonifera* on the expression of matrix metalloproteinase-1 in human dermal fibroblasts. *Biological and Pharmaceutical Bulletin* **29**: 1735–1739. https://doi.org/10.1248/bpb.29.1735.

Johnell, O. and Kanis, J.A. (2006). An estimate of the worldwide prevalence and disability associated with osteoporotic fractures. *Osteoporosis International* **17**: 1726–1733. https://doi.org/10.1007/s00198-006-0172-4.

Jung, H.A., Hyun, S.K., Kim, H.R., and Choi, J.S. (2006). Angiotensin-converting enzyme I inhibitory activity of phlorotannins from *Ecklonia stolonifera*. *Fisheries Science* **72**: 1292–1299. https://doi.org/10.1111/j.1444-2906.2006.01288.x.

Jung, W.K., Choi, I., Oh, S. et al. (2009). Anti-asthmatic effect of marine red alga (*Laurencia undulata*) polyphenolic extracts in a murine model of asthma. *Food and Chemical Toxicology* **47**: 293–297. https://doi.org/10.1016/j.fct.2008.11.012.

Kadam, S.U., Álvarez, C., Tiwari, B.K., and O'Donnell, C.P. (2015a). Extraction of biomolecules from seaweeds. In: *Seaweed Sustainability* (eds. B.K. Tiwari and D.J. Troy), 243–269. London: Academic Press.

Kadam, S.U., Tiwari, B.K., Smyth, T.J., and O'Donnell, C.P. (2015b). Optimization of ultrasound assisted extraction of bioactive components from brown seaweed *Ascophyllum nodosum* using response surface methodology. *Ultrasonics Sonochemistry* **23**: 308–316. https://doi.org/10.1016/J.ULTSONCH.2014.10.007.

Kahn, S.E., Cooper, M.E., and Del Prato, S. (2014). Pathophysiology and treatment of type 2 diabetes: perspectives on the past, present, and future. *The Lancet* **383**: 1068–1083.

Kamiya, M., Nishio, T., Yokoyama, A. et al. (2010). Seasonal variation of phlorotannin in Sargassacean species from the coast of the sea of Japan. *Phycological Research* **58**: 53–61. https://doi.org/10.1111/j.1440-1835.2009.00558.x.

Kang, H.S., Kim, H.R., Byun, D. et al. (2004). Tyrosinase inhibitors isolated from the edible brown alga *Ecklonia stolonifera*. *Marine Science and Technology Bulletin* **14**: 49–56. https://doi.org/10.1007/BF02975886.

Kang, K.A., Lee, K.H., Chae, S. et al. (2005). Eckol isolated from *Ecklonia cava* attenuates oxidative stress induced cell damage in lung fibroblast cells. *FEBS Letters* **579**: 6295–6304. https://doi.org/10.1016/j.febslet.2005.10.008.

Kang, S.M., Cha, S.H., Ko, J.Y. et al. (2012a). Neuroprotective effects of phlorotannins isolated from a brown alga, *Ecklonia cava*, against H_2O_2-induced oxidative stress in murine hippocampal HT22 cells. *Environmental Toxicology and Pharmacology* **34**: 96–105. https://doi.org/10.1016/j.etap.2012.03.006.

Kang, C.H., Choi, Y.H., Park, S.Y., and Kim, G.Y. (2012b). Anti-inflammatory effects of methanol extract of *Codium fragile* in lipopolysaccharide-stimulated RAW 264.7 cells. *Journal of Medicinal Food* **15**: 44–50. https://doi.org/10.1089/jmf.2010.1540.

Karadeniz, F., Kang, K.H., Park, J.W. et al. (2014a). Anti-HIV-1 activity of phlorotannin derivative 8,4‴-dieckol from Korean brown alga *Ecklonia cava*. *Bioscience, Biotechnology, and Biochemistry* **78**: 1151–1158. https://doi.org/10.1080/09168451.2014.923282.

Karadeniz, F., Kim, J.-A., Ahn, B.-N. et al. (2014b). Effect of *Salicornia herbacea* on osteoblastogenesis and adipogenesis *in Vitro*. *Marine Drugs* **12**: 5132–5147. https://doi.org/10.3390/md12105132.

Karadeniz, F., Karagozlu, M.Z., and Kim, S.K. (2015a). Antiviral activities of marine algal extracts. In: *Marine Algae Extracts: Processes, Products, and Applications* (eds. S.-K. Kim and K. Chojnacka), 371–380. Weinheim: Wiley-VCH Verlag GmbH & Co https://doi.org/10.1002/9783527679577.ch23.

Karadeniz, F., Ahn, B.-N., Kim, J.-A. et al. (2015b). Phlorotannins suppress adipogenesis in pre-adipocytes while enhancing osteoblastogenesis in pre-osteoblasts. *Archives of Pharmacal Research* **38**: 2172–2182. https://doi.org/10.1007/s12272-015-0637-0.

Karthik, R., Manigandan, V., Sheeba, R. et al. (2016). Structural characterization and comparative biomedical properties of phloroglucinol from Indian brown seaweeds. *Journal of Applied Phycology* **28**: 3561–3573. https://doi.org/10.1007/s10811-016-0851-2.

Kazlowska, K., Hsu, T., Hou, C.C. et al. (2010). Anti-inflammatory properties of phenolic compounds and crude extract from *Porphyra dentata*. *Journal of Ethnopharmacology* **128**: 123–130. https://doi.org/10.1016/j.jep.2009.12.037.

Kepekçi, R.A. and Saygideger, S.D. (2012). Enhancement of phenolic compound production in *Spirulina platensis* by two-step batch mode cultivation. *Journal of Applied Phycology* **24**: 897–905. https://doi.org/10.1007/s10811-011-9710-3.

Khan, M.N.A., Choi, J.S., Lee, M.C. et al. (2008). Anti-inflammatory activities of methanol extracts from various seaweed species. *Journal of Environmental Biology* **29**: 465–469.

Kim, E.B. and Kwak, J.H. (2015). Antiviral phlorotannin from *Eisenia bicyclis* against human papilloma virus *in vitro*. *Planta Medica* **81**: PW_22. https://doi.org/10.1055/s-0035-1565646.

Kim, H.J., Dasagrandhi, C., Kim, S.H. et al. (2018). *In Vitro* antibacterial activity of phlorotannins from edible brown algae, *Eisenia bicyclis* against streptomycin-resistant *Listeria monocytogenes*. *Indian Journal of Microbiology* **58**: 105–108. https://doi.org/10.1007/s12088-017-0693-x.

Kim, H.-H., Kim, H.-S., Ko, J.-Y. et al. (2016). A single-step isolation of useful antioxidant compounds from *Ishige okamurae* by using centrifugal partition chromatography. *Fisheries and Aquatic Sciences* **19**: 1–7. https://doi.org/10.1186/S41240-016-0023-Y.

Kim, H.R. (2011). Ethanol fraction, ethyl acetate fraction, and phlorotannins separated from *Ecklonia stolonifera* or *E. cava* for the hepatoprotection on alcoholic hepatic damage and use thereof as hepatoprotection? Patent KR101301190B1.

Kim, K.Y., Nguyen, T.H., Kurihara, H., and Kim, S.M. (2010). α-Glucosidase inhibitory activity of bromophenol purified from the red alga *Polyopes lancifolia*. *Journal of Food Science* **75**: H145–H150. https://doi.org/10.1111/j.1750-3841.2010.01629.x.

Kim, M.M., Van Ta, Q., Mendis, E. et al. (2006). Phlorotannins in *Ecklonia cava* extract inhibit matrix metalloproteinase activity. *Life Sciences* **79**: 1436–1443. https://doi.org/10.1016/j.lfs.2006.04.022.

Kim S.K., Kim, Y.M., Lee M.S., and Eom, S.H. (2012). Antiobiotic composition including phlorotannin compound derived from *Eisenia bicyclis* as effective component. Patent US20130338217A1.

Kirke, D.A., Smyth, T.J., Rai, D.K. et al. (2017). The chemical and antioxidant stability of isolated low molecular weight phlorotannins. *Food Chemistry* **221**: 1104–1112. https://doi.org/10.1016/j.foodchem.2016.11.050.

Kladi, M., Vagias, C., Papazafiri, P. et al. (2007). New sesquiterpenes from the red alga *Laurencia microcladia*. *Tetrahedron* **63**: 7606–7611. https://doi.org/10.1016/j.tet.2007.05.051.

Klejdus, B., Kopecký, J., Benešová, L., and Vacek, J. (2009). Solid-phase/supercritical-fluid extraction for liquid chromatography of phenolic compounds in freshwater microalgae and selected cyanobacterial species. *Journal of Chromatography A* **1216**: 763–771. https://doi.org/10.1016/j.chroma.2008.11.096.

Klejdus, B., Lojková, L., Plaza, M. et al. (2010). Hyphenated technique for the extraction and determination of isoflavones in algae: ultrasound-assisted supercritical fluid extraction followed by fast chromatography with tandem mass spectrometry. *Journal of Chromatography A* **1217**: 7956–7965. https://doi.org/10.1016/j.chroma.2010.07.020.

Ko, S.C., Cha, S.H., Heo, S.J. et al. (2011). Protective effect of *Ecklonia cava* on UVB-induced oxidative stress: in vitro and in vivo zebrafish model. *Journal of Applied Phycology* **23**: 697–708. https://doi.org/10.1007/s10811-010-9565-z.

Koivikko, R., Loponen, J., Honkanen, T., and Jormalainen, V. (2005). Contents of soluble, cell-wall-bound and exuded phlorotannins in the brown alga *Fucus vesiculosus*, with implications on their ecological functions. *Journal of Chemical Ecology* **31**: 195–212.

Kok, J.M.L., Jee, J.M., Chew, L.Y., and Wong, C.L. (2016). The potential of the brown seaweed *Sargassum polycystum* against acne vulgaris. *Journal of Applied Phycology* **28**: 3127–3133. https://doi.org/10.1007/s10811-016-0825-4.

Kong, C.-S., Kim, J.-A., Yoon, N.-Y., and Kim, S.-K. (2009). Induction of apoptosis by phloroglucinol derivative from *Ecklonia cava* in MCF-7 human breast cancer cells. *Food and Chemical Toxicology* **47**: 1653–1658. https://doi.org/10.1016/j.fct.2009.04.013.

Koonin, E.V. and Starokadomskyy, P. (2016). Are viruses alive? The replicator paradigm sheds decisive light on an old but misguided question. *Studies in history and philosophy of science part C: Studies in history and philosophy of biological and biomedical sciences* **59**: 125–134.

Kornprobst, J.M. (2014). *Encyclopedia of Marine Natural Products*, 2e. Weinheim: Wiley-VCH Verlag GmbH & Co.

Kubanek, J., Prusak, A.C., Snell, T.W. et al. (2006). Bromophycolides C–I from the Fijian red alga *Callophycus serratus*. *Journal of Natural Products* **69**: 731–735. https://doi.org/10.1021/np050463o.

Kurihara, H., Konno, R., and Takahashi, K. (2015). Fucophlorethol C, a phlorotannin as a lipoxygenase inhibitor. *Bioscience, Biotechnology, and Biochemistry* **79**: 1954–1956. https://doi.org/10.1080/09168451.2015.1062716.

Kurth, C., Welling, M., and Pohnert, G. (2015). Sulfated phenolic acids from Dasycladales siphonous green algae. *Phytochemistry* **117**: 417–423. https://doi.org/10.1016/j.phytochem.2015.07.010.

La Barre, S., Potin, P., Leblanc, C., and Delage, L. (2010). The halogenated metabolism of brown algae (Phaeophyta), its biological importance and its environmental significance. *Marine Drugs* **8**: 988–1010. https://doi.org/10.3390/md8040988.

Laizé, V., Gavaia, P.J., and Cancela, M.L. (2014). Fish: a suitable system to model human bone disorders and discover drugs with osteogenic or osteotoxic activities. *Drug Discovery Today* **13**: 29–37. https://doi.org/10.1016/j.ddmod.2014.08.001.

Lambrecht, B.N. and Hammad, H. (2015). The immunology of asthma. *Nature Immunology* **16**: 45–56. https://doi.org/10.1038/ni.3049.

Lane, A.L., Stout, E.P., Lin, A.S. et al. (2009). Antimalarial bromophycolides J–Q from the Fijian red alga *Callophycus serratus*. *The Journal of Organic Chemistry* **74**: 2736–2742. https://doi.org/10.1021/jo900008w.

Larsen, J.N., Broge, L., and Jacobi, H. (2016). Allergy immunotherapy: the future of allergy treatment. *Drug Discovery Today* **21**: 26–37. https://doi.org/10.1016/j.drudis.2015.07.010.

Lauritano, C. and Ianora, A. (2016). Marine organisms with anti-diabetes properties. *Marine Drugs* **14**: 220–234. https://doi.org/10.3390/md14120220.

Le Lann, K., Jégou, C., and Stiger-Pouvreau, V. (2008). Effect of different conditioning treatments on total phenolic content and antioxidant activities in two Sargassacean species: comparison of the frondose *Sargassum muticum* (Yendo) Fensholt and the cylindrical *Bifurcaria bifurcata* R. Ross. *Phycological Research* **56**: 238–245. https://doi.org/10.1111/j.1440-1835.2008.00505.x.

Le Lann, K., Ferret, C., Vanmee, E. et al. (2012). Total phenolic, size-fractionated phenolics and fucoxanthin content of tropical Sargassaceae (Fucales, Phaeophyceae) from the South Pacific Ocean: spatial and specific variability. *Phycological Research* **60**: 37–50. https://doi.org/10.1111/j.1440-1835.2011.00634.x.

Le Lann, K., Surget, G., Couteau, C. et al. (2016). Sunscreen, antioxidant, and bactericide capacities of phlorotannins from the brown macroalga *Halidrys siliquosa*. *Journal of Applied Phycology* **28**: 3547–3559. https://doi.org/10.1007/s10811-016-0853-0.

Le, Q.T., Li, Y., Qian, Z.J. et al. (2009). Inhibitory effects of polyphenols isolated from marine alga *Ecklonia cava* on histamine release. *Process Biochemistry* **44**: 168–176. https://doi.org/10.1016/j.procbio.2008.10.002.

Lee, J.H., Eom, S.H., Lee, E.H. et al. (2014). *In vitro* antibacterial and synergistic effect of phlorotannins isolated from edible brown seaweed *Eisenia bicyclis* against acne-related bacteria. *Algae* **29**: 47–55. https://doi.org/10.4490/algae.2014.29.1.047.

Lee, J.-H., Ko, J.-Y., Oh, J.-Y. et al. (2015). Evaluation of phlorofucofuroeckol-A isolated from *Ecklonia cava* (Phaeophyta) on anti-lipid peroxidation *in vitro* and *in vivo*. *Algae* **30**: 313–323. https://doi.org/10.4490/algae.2015.30.4.313.

Lee, R.E. (1999). *Phycology*, 3e. Cambridge: Cambridge University Press.

Lee, S.-H., Park, M.-H., Heo, S.-J. et al. (2010). Dieckol isolated from *Ecklonia cava* inhibits α-glucosidase and α-amylase *in vitro* and alleviates postprandial hyperglycemia in streptozotocin-induced diabetic mice. *Food and Chemical Toxicology* **48**: 2633–2637. https://doi.org/10.1016/j.fct.2010.06.032.

Lee, S.-H., Kang, M.-C., Moon, S.-H. et al. (2013). Potential use of ultrasound in antioxidant extraction from *Ecklonia cava*. *Algae* **28**: 371–378. https://doi.org/10.4490/algae.2013.28.4.371.

Lemesheva, V. and Tarakhovskaya, E. (2018). Physiological functions of phlorotannins. *Biological Communications* **63**: 70–76. https://doi.org/10.21638/spbu03.2018.108.

Leyton, A., Pezoa-Conte, R., Barriga, A. et al. (2016). Identification and efficient extraction method of phlorotannins from the brown seaweed *Macrocystis pyrifera* using an orthogonal experimental design. *Algal Research* **16**: 201–208. https://doi.org/10.1016/j.algal.2016.03.019.

Li, K., Li, X.M., Ji, N.Y., and Wang, B.G. (2008a). Bromophenols from the marine red alga *Polysiphonia urceolata* with DPPH radical scavenging activity. *Journal of Natural Products* **71**: 28–30. https://doi.org/10.1021/np070281p.

Li, Y., Lee, S.H., Le, Q.T. et al. (2008b). Anti-allergic effects of phlorotannins on histamine release via binding inhibition between IgE and Fc epsilonRI. *Journal of Agricultural and Food Chemistry* **56**: 12073–12080.

Li, Y.X., Wijesekara, I., Li, Y., and Kim, S.K. (2011). Phlorotannins as bioactive agents from brown algae. *Process Biochemistry* **46**: 2219–2224.

Lijun, H., Nianjun, X., Jiangong, S. et al. (2005). Isolation and pharmacological activities of bromophenols from *Rhodomela confervoides*. *Chinese Journal of Oceanology and Limnology* **23**: 226–229. https://doi.org/10.1007/BF02894243.

Lin, J.W., Chiang, H.M., Lin, Y.C., and Wen, K.C. (2008). Natural products with skin-whitening effects. *Journal of Food and Drug Analysis* **16**: 1–10.

Liu, M., Hansen, P.E., and Lin, X. (2011). Bromophenols in marine algae and their bioactivities. *Marine Drugs* **9**: 1273–1292. https://doi.org/10.3390/md9071273.

Liu, N., Fu, X., Duan, D. et al. (2018). Evaluation of bioactivity of phenolic compounds from the brown seaweed of *Sargassum fusiforme* and development of their stable emulsion. *Journal of Applied Phycology* **30**: 1955–1970. https://doi.org/10.1007/s10811-017-1383-0.

Lopes, G., Pinto, E., Andrade, P.B., and Valentão, P. (2013). Antifungal activity of phlorotannins against dermatophytes and yeasts: approaches to the mechanism of action and influence on *Candida albicans* virulence factor. *PLoS One* **8**: e72203. https://doi.org/10.1371/journal.pone.0072203.

Lushchak, V.I. (2014). Free radicals, reactive oxygen species, oxidative stress and its classification. *Chemico-Biological Interactions* **224**: 164–175. https://doi.org/10.1016/j.cbi.2014.10.016.

Mabeau, S. and Fleurence, J. (1993). Seaweed in food products: biochemical and nutritional aspects. *Trends in Food Science and Technology* **4**: 103–107. https://doi.org/10.1016/0924-2244(93)90091-N.

Machu, L., Misurcova, L., Vavra Ambrozova, J. et al. (2015). Phenolic content and antioxidant capacity in algal food products. *Molecules* **20**: 1118–1133. https://doi.org/10.3390/molecules20011118.

Maeda-Yamamoto, M. and Tachibana, H. (2012). Anti-allergic action of *O*-methylated EGCG in green tea cultivar benifuuki. *Journal of Food and Drug Analysis* **20**: 313–317.

Magnusson, M., Yuen, A.K.L., Zhang, R. et al. (2017). A comparative assessment of microwave assisted (MAE) and conventional solid-liquid (SLE) techniques for the extraction of phloroglucinol from brown seaweed. *Algal Research* **23**: 28–36. https://doi.org/10.1016/j.algal.2017.01.002.

Mancini-Filho, J., Novoa, A.V., González, A.E.B. et al. (2009). Free phenolic acids from the seaweed *Halimeda monile* with antioxidant effect protecting against liver injury. *Zeitschrift für Naturforschung. Section C* **64**: 657–663. https://doi.org/10.1515/znc-2009-9-1009.

Masuda, M., Kawaguchi, S., Abe, T. et al. (2002). Additional analysis of chemical diversity of the red algal genus *Laurencia* (Rhodomelaceae) from Japan. *Phycological Research* **50**: 135–144. https://doi.org/10.1046/j.1440-1835.2002.00267.x.

Matanjun, P., Mohamed, S., Mustapha, N.M. et al. (2008). Antioxidant activities and phenolics content of eight species of seaweeds from North Borneo. *Journal of Applied Phycology* **20**: 367–373. https://doi.org/10.1007/s10811-007-9264-6.

Mayer, A.M.S., Paul, V.J., Fenical, W. et al. (1993). Phospolipase A2 inhibitors from marine algae. In: *Fourteenth International Seaweed Symposium* (eds. A.R.O. Chapman, M.T. Brown and M. Lahaye), 521–529. Dordrecht: Springer.

Mazzoncini, J.P. Jr., Crowell, C.B., and Kang, C.S. (2010). Human Metapneumovirus: an emerging respiratory pathogen. *The Journal of Emergency Medicine* **38**: 456–459.

Meier, J.J. (2012). GLP-1 receptor agonists for individualized treatment of type 2 diabetes mellitus. *Nature Reviews Endocrinology* **8**: 728–742. https://doi.org/10.1038/nrendo.2012.140.

Mendes, G., Soares, A.R., Sigiliano, L. et al. (2011). *In vitro* anti-HMPV activity of meroditerpenoids from marine alga *Stypopodium zonale* (Dictyotales). *Molecules* **16**: 8437–8450. https://doi.org/10.3390/molecules16108437.

Meslet-Cladiere, L., Delage, L., Leroux, C.J.-J. et al. (2013). Structure/function analysis of a type III polyketide synthase in the brown alga *Ectocarpus siliculosus* reveals a biochemical pathway in phlorotannin monomer biosynthesis. *The Plant Cell* **25**: 3089–3103. https://doi.org/10.1105/tpc.113.111336.

Meyer, K. (1947). The biological significance of hyaluronic acid and hyaluronidase. *Physiological Reviews* **27**: 335–359.

Mhadhebi, L., Dellai, A., Clary-Laroche, A. et al. (2012). Anti-inflammatory and antiproliferative activities of *Cystoseira compressa. Drug Development Research* **73**: 82–89. https://doi.org/10.1002/ddr.20491.

Michalak, I. and Chojnacka, K. (2014). Review, algal extracts: technology and advances. *Engineering in Life Science* **14**: 581–591. https://doi.org/10.1002/elsc.201400139.

Moir, S., Chun, T.W., and Fauci, A.S. (2011). Pathogenic mechanisms of HIV disease. *Annual Review of Pathology: Mechanisms of Disease* **6**: 223–248.

Moreira, R., Sineiro, J., Chenlo, F. et al. (2017). Aqueous extracts of *Ascophyllum nodosum* obtained by ultrasound-assisted extraction: effects of drying temperature of seaweed on the properties of extracts. *Journal of Applied Phycology* **29**: 3191–3200. https://doi.org/10.1007/s10811-017-1159-6.

Moubayed, N.M.S., Al Houri, J.H., Al Khulaifi, M.M., and Al Farraj, D.A. (2017). Antimicrobial, antioxidant properties and chemical composition of seaweeds collected from Saudi Arabia (Red Sea and Arabian Gulf). *Saudi Journal of Biological Science* **24**: 162–169. https://doi.org/10.1016/j.sjbs.2016.05.018.

Muñoz, N., Castellsagué, X., de González, A.B., and Gissmann, L. (2006). HPV in the etiology of human cancer. *Vaccine* **24**: S1–S10.

Murray, M., Dordevic, A.L., Ryan, L., and Bonham, M.P. (2018a). Phlorotannins and macroalgal polyphenols: potential as functional food ingredients and role in health promotion. In: *Functional Food and Human Health* (eds. V. Rani and U. Yadav), 27–58. Singapore: Springer https://doi.org/10.1007/978-981-13-1123-9.

Murray, M., Dordevic, A., Ryan, L., and Bonham, M. (2018b). An emerging trend in functional foods for the prevention of cardiovascular disease and diabetes: marine algal polyphenols. *Critical Reviews in Food Science and Nutrition* **58**: 1342–1358. https://doi.org/10.1016/j.jsames.2009.03.003.

Murray, M., Dordevic, A.L., Bonham, M.P., and Ryan, L. (2018c). Do marine algal polyphenols have antidiabetic, antihyperlipidemic or anti-inflammatory effects in humans? A systematic review. *Critical Reviews in Food Science and Nutrition* **58**: 2039–2054. https://doi.org/10.1080/10408398.2017.1301876.

Nakamura, T., Nagayama, K., Uchida, K., and Tanaka, R. (1996). Antioxidant activity of phlorotannins isolated from the brown alga *Eisenia bicyclis. Fisheries Science* **62**: 923–926. https://doi.org/10.2331/fishsci.62.923.

Nash, J.F. and Tanner, P.R. (2014). Relevance of UV filter/sunscreen product photostability to human safety. *Photodermatology, Photoimmunology & Photomedicine* **30**: 88–95.

Neu, H.C. (1992). The crisis in antibiotic resistance. *Science* **257**: 1064–1073. https://doi.org/10.1126/science.257.5073.1064.

Novoa, A.V., Andrade-Wartha, E.R.S., Fallarero Linares, A. et al. (2011). Antioxidant activity and possible bioactive components in hydrophilic and lipophilic fractions from the seaweed *Halimeda incrassata. Brazilian Journal of Pharmacognozy* **21**: 53–57. https://doi.org/10.1590/S0102-695X2011005000010.

Nwosu, F., Morris, J., Lund, V.A. et al. (2011). Anti-proliferative and potential anti-diabetic effects of phenolic-rich extracts from edible marine algae. *Food Chemistry* **126**: 1006–1012. https://doi.org/10.1016/j.foodchem.2010.11.111.

Oh, K.B., Lee, J.H., Chung, S.C. et al. (2008). Antimicrobial activities of the bromophenols from the red alga *Odonthalia corymbifera* and some synthetic derivatives. *Bioorganic and Medicinal Chemistry Letters* **18**: 104–108. https://doi.org/10.1016/j.bmcl.2007.11.003.

Olokoba, A.B., Obateru, O.A., and Olokoba, L.B. (2012). Type 2 diabetes mellitus: a review of current trends. *Oman Medical Journal* **27**: 269–273. https://doi.org/10.5001/omj.2012.68.

Ondetti, M.A. and Cushman, D.W. (1982). Enzymes of the renin-angiotensin system and their inhibitors. *Annual Review of Biochemistry* **51**: 283–308.

Onofrejová, L., Vašíčková, J., Klejdus, B. et al. (2010). Bioactive phenols in algae: the application of pressurized-liquid and solid-phase extraction techniques. *Journal of Pharmaceutical and Biomedical Analysis* **51**: 464–470. https://doi.org/10.1016/j.jpba.2009.03.027.

O'Sullivan, A.M., O'Callaghan, Y.C., O'Grady, M.N. et al. (2013). The effect of solvents on the antioxidant activity in Caco-2 cells of Irish brown seaweed extracts prepared using accelerated solvent extraction (ASE®). *Journal of Functional Foods* **5**: 940–948. https://doi.org/10.1016/j.jff.2013.02.007.

Pádua, D., Rocha, E., Gargiulo, D., and Ramos, A.A. (2015). Bioactive compounds from brown seaweeds: Phloroglucinol, fucoxanthin and fucoidan as promising therapeutic agents against breast cancer. *Phytochemistry Letters* **14**: 91–98. https://doi.org/10.1016/j.phytol.2015.09.007.

Paige-Stout, E., Prudhomme, J., Roch, K.L. et al. (2010). Unusual antimalarial meroditerpenes from tropical red macroalgae. *Bioorganic and Medicinal Chemistry Letters* **20**: 5662–5665. https://doi.org/10.1016/j.bmcl.2010.08.031.

Paiva, L., Lima, E., Neto, A.I. et al. (2016). Health-promoting ingredients from four selected Azorean macroalgae. *Food Research International* **89**: 432–438. https://doi.org/10.1016/j.foodres.2016.08.007.

Pangestuti, R., Siahaan, E., and Kim, S.K. (2018). Photoprotective substances derived from marine algae. *Marine Drugs* **16**: 399. https://doi.org/10.3390/md16110399.

Parniakov, O., Apicella, E., Koubaa, M. et al. (2015). Ultrasound-assisted green solvent extraction of high-added value compounds from microalgae *Nannochloropsis* spp. *Bioresource Technology* **198**: 262–267. https://doi.org/10.1016/j.biortech.2015.09.020.

Parrish, J.A., Jaenicke, K.F., and Anderson, R.R. (1982). Erythema and melanogenesis action spectra of normal human skin. *Photochemistry and Photobiology* **36**: 187–191. https://doi.org/10.1111/j.1751-1097.1982.tb04362.x.

Pasquet, V., Chérouvrier, J.R., Farhat, F. et al. (2011). Study on the microalgal pigments extraction process: performance of microwave assisted extraction. *Process Biochemistry* **46**: 59–67. https://doi.org/10.1016/j.procbio.2010.07.009.

Paufique, J. (2003). Method for obtaining an active principle from *Agarum cribosum*, particularly for prevention of pigmentation. Patent WO2003061618 A1.

Pavia, H. and Brock, E. (2000). Extrinsic factors influencing phlorotannin production in the brown alga *Ascophyllum nodosum*. *Marine Ecology Progress Series* **193**: 285–294. https://doi.org/10.3354/meps193285.

Pawankar, R. (2014). Allergic diseases and asthma: a global public health concern and a call to action. *World Allergy Organization Journal* **7**: 12. https://doi.org/10.1186/1939-4551-7-12.

Pellegrini, L., Pellegrini, M., and André, G. (2003b). Extrait d'algue marine du genre *Cystoseira* et utilisation dans les produits de soins. Patent FR2838341 A1.

Pellegrini, L., Pellegrini, M., and Villar, C. (2016). Utilisation d'au moins un extrait de macroalgue pour augmenter la synthèse de melanine dans les melanocytes. Patent FR3032351 A1.

Pellegrini, M. and Pellegrini, L. (2003). Utilisation d'un extrait d'une algue brune du genre *Halidrys* dans les domaines cosmétiques et/ou dermatologiques. Patent FR2942136 A1.

Pellegrini, M., André, G., and Pellegrini, L. (2003a). Compositions cosmetiques ou dermopharmaceutiques renfermant un extrait de macroalgue marine comme principe actif anti-oxydant et/ou anti-pollution. Patent FR2838342 A1.

Pellegrini, M., Pellegrini, L., and André, G. (2003c). Utilisation d'un extrait d'algue brune dans les domaines cosmétique et dermatologique. Patent FR2838340 A1.

Pereira, D.M., Cheel, J., Areche, C. et al. (2011). Anti-proliferative activity of meroditerpenoids isolated from the brown alga *Stypopodium flabelliforme* against several cancer cell lines. *Marine Drugs* **9**: 852–862. https://doi.org/10.3390/md9050852.

Pérez, J., Falqué, E., and Domínguez, H. (2016). Antimicrobial action of compounds from marine seaweed. *Marine Drugs* **14**: 52. https://doi.org/10.3390/md14030052.

Pérez-Rodríguez, E., Aguilera, J., Gomez, I., and Figueroa, F.L. (2001). Excretion of coumarins by the Mediterranean green alga *Dasycladus vermicularis* in response to environmental stress. *Marine Biology* **139**: 633–639. https://doi.org/10.1007/s002270100588.

Pérez-Rodríguez, E., Aguilera, J., and Figueroa, F.L. (2003). Tissular localization of coumarins in the green alga *Dasycladus vermicularis* (Scopoli) Krasser: a photoprotective role? *Journal of Experimental Botany* **54**: 1093–1100. https://doi.org/10.1093/jxb/erg111.

Pilar Sánchez-Camargo, A., Montero, L., Stiger-Pouvreau, V. et al. (2016). Considerations on the use of enzyme-assisted extraction in combination with pressurized liquids to recover bioactive compounds from algae. *Food Chemistry* **192**: 67–74. https://doi.org/10.1016/j.foodchem.2015.06.098.

Pinteus, S., Silva, J., Alves, C. et al. (2017). Antioxidant and cytoprotective activities of *Fucus spiralis* seaweed on a human cell *in vitro* model. *International Journal of Molecular Sciences* **18**: 1–14. https://doi.org/10.3390/ijms18020292.

Plaza, M., Cifuentes, A., and Ibañez, E. (2008). In the search of new functional food ingredients from algae. *Trends in Food Science and Technology* **19**: 31–39. https://doi.org/10.1016/j.tifs.2007.07.012.

Plaza, A., Keffer, J.L., Bifulco, G. et al. (2010a). Chrysophaentins A–H, antibacterial bisdiarylbutene macrocycles that inhibit the bacterial cell division protein FtsZ. *Journal of the American Chemical Society* **132**: 9069–9077. https://doi.org/10.1021/ja102100h.

Plaza, M., Santoyo, S., Jaime, L. et al. (2010b). Screening for bioactive compounds from algae. *Journal of Pharmaceutical and Biomedical Analysis* **51**: 450–455. https://doi.org/10.1016/j.jpba.2009.03.016.

Plouguerné, E., Le Lann, K., Connan, S. et al. (2006). Spatial and seasonal variation in density, reproductive status, length and phenolic content of the invasive brown macroalga *Sargassum muticum* (Yendo) Fensholt along the coast of Western Brittany (France). *Aquatic Botany* **85**: 337–344. https://doi.org/10.1016/j.aquabot.2006.06.011.

Poyato, C., Thomsen, B.R., Hermund, D.B. et al. (2016). Antioxidant effect of water and acetone extracts of *Fucus vesiculosus* on oxidative stability of skin care emulsions. *European Journal of Lipid Science and Technology* **118**: 1–11. https://doi.org/10.1002/ejlt.201600072.

Prabakaran, P. and Ravindran, A.D. (2011). A comparative study on effective cell disruption methods for lipid extraction from microalgae. *Letters in Applied Microbiology* **53**: 150–154. https://doi.org/10.1111/j.1472-765X.2011.03082.x.

Praiboon, J., Palakas, S., Noiraksa, T., and Miyashita, K. (2018). Seasonal variation in nutritional composition and anti-proliferative activity of brown seaweed, *Sargassum oligocystum*. *Journal of Applied Phycology* **30**: 101–111. https://doi.org/10.1007/s10811-017-1248-6.

Prat, D., Wells, A., Hayler, J. et al. (2016). CHEM21 selection guide of classical- and less classical-solvents. *Green Chemistry* **18**: 288–296. https://doi.org/10.1039/C5GC01008J.

Proteau, P.J., Gerwick, W.H., Garcia-Pichel, F., and Castenholz, R. (1993). The structure of scytonemin, an ultraviolet sunscreen pigment from the shealths of cyanobacteria. *Experientia* **49**: 825–829. https://doi.org/10.1007/BF01923559.

Puspita, M., Déniel, M., Widowati, I. et al. (2017). Total phenolic content and biological activities of enzymatic extracts from *Sargassum muticum* (Yendo) Fensholt. *Journal of Applied Phycology* **29**: 2521–2537. https://doi.org/10.1007/s10811-017-1086-6.

Qin, Y. (2018). *Bioactive Seaweeds for Food Applications: Natural Ingredients for Healthy Diets*, 1e. Jiaxing: Elsevier.

Ragan, M.A. and Glombitza, K.W. (1986). Phlorotannins, brown algal polyphenols. In: *Progress in Phycological Research* (eds. F.E. Round and D.J. Chapman), 129–241. Biopress Ltd: Bristol.

Raisz, L.G. (2001). Pathogenesis of postmenopausal osteoporosis. *Reviews in Endocrine & Metabolic Disorders* **2**: 5–12.

Rajauria, G. (2018). Optimization and validation of reverse phase HPLC method for qualitative and quantitative assessment of polyphenols in seaweed. *Journal of Pharmaceutical and Biomedical Analysis* **148**: 230–237. https://doi.org/10.1016/j.jpba.2017.10.002.

Rajauria, G., Foley, B., and Abu-Ghannam, N. (2016). Identification and characterization of phenolic antioxidant compounds from brown Irish seaweed *Himanthalia elongata* using LC-DAD–ESI-MS/MS. *Innovative Food Science and Emerging Technologies* **37**: 261–268. https://doi.org/10.1016/j.ifset.2016.02.005.

Ramos-e-Silva, M., Celem, L.R., Ramos-e-Silva, S., and Fucci-da-Costa, A.P. (2013). Anti-aging cosmetics: facts and controversies. *Clinics in Dermatology* **31**: 750–758.

Rao, L.G. and Rao, A.V. (2015). Oxidative stress and antioxidants in the risk of osteoporosis—role of phytochemical antioxidants lycopene and polyphenol-containing nutritional supplements. In: *Phytochemicals, Isolation, Characterisation and Role in Human Health* (eds. A.V. Rao and L.G. Rao), 247–260. Rijeka: InTech https://doi.org/10.1080/19390210802414295.

Reuter, S., Gupta, S.C., Chaturvedi, M.M., and Aggarwal, B.B. (2010). Oxidative stress, inflammation, and cancer: how are they linked? *Free Radical Biology and Medicine* **49**: 1603–1616. https://doi.org/10.1016/j.freeradbiomed.2010.09.006.

Riani, M.K.L., Anwar, E., and Nurhayati, T. (2018). Antioxidant and anti-collagenase activity of *Sargassum plagyophyllum* extract as an anti-wrinkle cosmetic ingredient. *Pharmacognosy* **10**: 932–936. https://doi.org/10.5530/pj.2018.5.157.

Riggs, B.L., Khosla, S., and Melton, L.J. (1998). A unitary model for involutional osteoporosis: Estrogen deficiency causes both type I and type II osteoporosis in postmenopausal women and contributes to bone loss in aging men. *Journal of Bone and Mineral Research* **13**: 763–773. https://doi.org/10.1359/jbmr.1998.13.5.763.

Ríos, J.L. and Recio, M.C. (2005). Medicinal plants and antimicrobial activity. *Journal of Ethnopharmacology* **100**: 80–84. https://doi.org/10.1016/j.jep.2005.04.025.

Rocha, D., Seca, A., and Pinto, D. (2018). Seaweed secondary metabolites *in vitro* and *in vivo* anticancer activity. *Marine Drugs* **16**: 410. https://doi.org/10.3390/md16110410.

Rodrigues, D., Sousa, S., Silva, A. et al. (2015). Impact of enzyme- and ultrasound-assisted extraction methods on biological properties of red, brown, and green seaweeds from the central west coast of Portugal. *Journal of Agricultural and Food Chemistry* **63**: 3177–3188. https://doi.org/10.1021/jf504220e.

Rodríguez-Bernaldo de Quirós, A., Lage-Yusty, M.A., and López-Hernández, J. (2010). Determination of phenolic compounds in macroalgae for human consumption. *Food Chemistry* **121**: 634–638. https://doi.org/10.1016/j.foodchem.2009.12.078.

Ruesgas-Ramón, M., Figueroa-Espinoza, M.C., and Durand, E. (2017). Application of deep eutectic solvents (DES) for phenolic compounds extraction: overview, challenges, and opportunities. *Journal of Agricultural and Food Chemistry* **65**: 3591–3601. https://doi.org/10.1021/acs.jafc.7b01054.

Ryu, B., Li, Y., Qian, Z.-J. et al. (2009). Differentiation of human osteosarcoma cells by isolated phlorotannins is subtly linked to COX-2, iNOS, MMPs, and MAPK signaling: implication for chronic articular disease. *Chemico-Biological Interactions* **179**: 192–201. https://doi.org/10.1016/j.cbi.2009.01.006.

Ryu, Y.B., Jeong, H.J., Yoon, S.Y. et al. (2011). Influenza virus neuraminidase inhibitory activity of phlorotannins from the edible brown alga *Ecklonia cava*. *Journal of Agricultural and Food Chemistry* **59**: 6467–6473. https://doi.org/10.1021/jf2007248.

Ryu, M.J., Kim, A.D., Kang, K.A. et al. (2013). The green algae *Ulva fasciata* Delile extract induces apoptotic cell death in human colon cancer cells. *In Vitro Cellular and Developmental Biology – Animal* **49**: 74–81. https://doi.org/10.1007/s11626-012-9547-3.

Safafar, H., Van Wagenen, J., Møller, P., and Jacobsen, C. (2015). Carotenoids, phenolic compounds and tocopherols contribute to the antioxidative properties of some microalgae species grown on industrial wastewater. *Marine Drugs* **13**: 7339–7356. https://doi.org/10.3390/md13127069.

Samee, H., Li, Z., Lin, H. et al. (2009). Anti-allergic effects of ethanol extracts from brown seaweeds. *Journal of Zhejiang University Science B* **10**: 147–153. https://doi.org/10.1016/j.cpc.2016.07.012.

Sandsdalen, E., Haug, T., Stenvag, K., and Styrvold, O. (2003). The antibacterial effect of a polyhydroxylated fucophlorethol from the marine brown alga, *Fucus vesiculosus*. *World Journal of Microbiology and Biotechnology* **19**: 777–782. https://doi.org/10.1023/A.

Sanjeewa, K.K.A., Kim, E.A., Son, K.T., and Jeon, Y.J. (2016). Bioactive properties and potentials cosmeceutical applications of phlorotannins isolated from brown seaweeds: a review. *Journal of Photochemistry and Photobiology B: Biology* **162**: 100–105. https://doi.org/10.1016/j.jphotobiol.2016.06.027.

Santoso, J., Yoshie-Stark, Y., and Suzuki, T. (2004). Anti-oxidant activity of methanol extracts from Indonesian seaweeds in an oil emulsion model. *Fisheries Science* **70**: 183–188. https://doi.org/10.1111/j.1444-2906.2003.00787.x.

Saravana, P.S., Tilahun, A., Cho, Y.-J. et al. (2017). Influence of co-solvents on fucoxanthin and phlorotannin recovery from brown seaweed using supercritical CO_2. *Journal of Supercritical Fluids* **120**: 295–303. https://doi.org/10.1016/j.supflu.2016.05.037.

Scalbert, A., Manach, C., Morand, C. et al. (2005). Dietary polyphenols and the prevention of diseases. *Critical Reviews in Food Science and Nutrition* **45**: 287–306. https://doi.org/10.1080/1040869059096.

Senthilkumar, K., Venkatesan, J., and Kim, S.-K. (2014). Marine derived natural products for osteoporosis. *Biomedicine & Preventive Nutrition* **4**: 1–7. https://doi.org/10.1016/j.bionut.2013.12.005.

Serive, B., Kaas, R., Bérard, J.-B. et al. (2012). Selection and optimization of a method for efficient metabolites extraction from microalgae. *Bioresource Technology* **124**: 311–320. https://doi.org/10.1016/j.biortech.2012.07.105.

Shalaby, E. (2011). Algae as promising organisms for environment and health. *Plant Signaling & Behavior* **6**: 1338–1350. https://doi.org/10.4161/psb.6.9.16779.

Shi, D., Xu, F., He, J. et al. (2008). Inhibition of bromophenols against PTP1B and anti-hyperglycemic effect of *Rhodomela confervoides* extract in diabetic rats. *Science Bulletin* **53**: 2476–2479. https://doi.org/10.1007/s11434-008-0353-y.

Shibata, T., Fujimoto, K., Nagayama, K. et al. (2002). Inhibitory activity of brown algal phlorotannins against hyaluronidase. *International Journal of Food Science and Technology* **37**: 703–709. https://doi.org/10.1046/j.1365-2621.2002.00603.x.

Shibata, T., Nagayama, K., Tanaka, R. et al. (2003). Inhibitory effects of brown algal phlorotannins on secretory phospholipase A2s, lipoxygenases and cyclooxygenases. *Journal of Applied Phycology* **15**: 61–66. https://doi.org/10.1023/A:1022972221002.

Shibata, T., Kawaguchi, S., Hama, Y. et al. (2004). Local and chemical distribution of phlorotannins in brown algae. *Journal of Applied Phycology* **16**: 291–296.

Shibata, T., Hama, Y., Miyasaki, T. et al. (2006). Extracellular secretion of phenolic substances from living brown algae. *Journal of Applied Phycology* **18**: 787–794. https://doi.org/10.1007/s10811-006-9094-y.

Shim, S.Y., Quang-To, L., Lee, S.H., and Kim, S.K. (2009). *Ecklonia cava* extract suppresses the high-affinity IgE receptor, F epsilonRI expression. *Food and Chemical Toxicology* **47**: 555–560. https://doi.org/10.1016/j.fct.2008.12.012.

Shin, H., Cho, A.R., Kim, D.Y. et al. (2016). Enhancement of human hair growth using *Ecklonia cava* polyphenols. *Annals of Dermatology* **28**: 15–21. https://doi.org/10.5021/ad.2016.28.1.15.

Shoeib, N.A., Bibby, M.C., Blunden, G. et al. (2004). *In vitro* cytotoxic activities of the major bromophenols of the red alga *Polysiphonia lanosa* and some novel synthetic isomers. *Journal of Natural Products* **67**: 1445–1449. https://doi.org/10.1021/np0305268.

Silva, T.C., Pereira, D.M., Valentão, P., and Andrade, P.B. (2017). Phospholipase A2 inhibitors of marine origin. In: *Natural Products Targeting Clinically Relevant Enzymes* (eds. P.B. Andrade, P. Valentão and D.M. Pereira), 69–92. Weinheim: Wiley-VCH Verlag GmbH & Co.

Sineiro Torres, J., Sánchez Guerrero, M., and Nüñez García, M. J. (2013). Antioxidant extract from brown macroalgae and preparation process. Patent ES2441469B2.

Singh, I.P. and Bharate, S.B. (2006). Phloroglucinol compounds of natural origin. *Natural Product Reports* **23**: 558–591. https://doi.org/10.1039/b600518g.

Singh, G. and Kumar, J. (2018). Artificial and natural photoprotective compounds. In: *Sunscreens: Source, Formulations, Efficacy and Recommendations* (ed. R.P. Rastogi), 153–199. Hauppauge, NY: Nova Science Pub Inc.

Singh, A., Holvoet, S., and Mercenier, A. (2011). Dietary polyphenols in the prevention and treatment of allergic diseases: polyphenols alleviate allergic inflammation. *Clinical and Experimental Allergy* **41**: 1346–1359. https://doi.org/10.1111/j.1365-2222.2011.03773.x.

Sinha, R.P., Singh, S.P., and Häder, D.-P. (2007). Database on mycosporines and mycosporine-like amino acids (MAAs) in fungi, cyanobacteria, macroalgae, phytoplankton and animals. *Journal of Photochemistry and Photobiology B: Biology* **89**: 29–35. https://doi.org/10.1016/j.jphotobiol.2007.07.006.

Slominski, A., Tobin, D.J., Shibahara, S., and Wortsman, J. (2004). Melanin pigmentation in mammalian skin and its hormonal regulation. *Physiological Reviews* **84**: 1155–1228.

Soares, A.R. (2015). Extraction, isolation, and identification of sesquiterpenes from *Laurencia* species. In: *Natural Products from Marine Algae: Methods and Protocols* (eds. D.B. Stengel and S. Connan), 225–252. New York: Springer https://doi.org/10.1007/978-1-4939-2684-8_14.

Soares, A.R., Abrantes, J.L., Souza, T.M.L. et al. (2007). *In vitro* antiviral effect of meroditerpenes isolated from the Brazilian seaweed *Stypopodium zonale* (Dictyotales). *Planta Medica* **73**: 1221–1224. https://doi.org/10.1055/s-2007-981589.

Solano, F., Briganti, S., Picardo, M., and Ghanem, G. (2006). Hypopigmenting agents: an updated review on biological, chemical and clinical aspects. *Pigment Cell Research* **19**: 550–571.

Son, Y.S., Ullah, H.M.A., Elfadl, A.K. et al. (2018). Inhibition of formation of azoxymethane-induced colonic aberrant crypt foci in rats by edible green algae *Capsosiphon fulvescens* and brown algae *Hizikia fusiforme*. *In Vivo* **32**: 101–108. https://doi.org/10.21873/invivo.11210.

Sonksen, P. and Sonksen, J. (2000). Insulin: understanding its action in health and disease. *British Journal of Anaesthesia* **85**: 69–79.

Steevensz, A.J., MacKinnon, S.L., Hankinson, R. et al. (2012). Profiling phlorotannins in brown macroalgae by liquid chromatography-high resolution mass spectrometry: phlorotannins in seaweed by LC-HRMS. *Phytochemical Analysis* **23**: 547–553. https://doi.org/10.1002/pca.2354.

Stengel, D.B., Connan, S., and Popper, Z.A. (2011). Algal chemodiversity and bioactivity: sources of natural variability and implications for commercial application. *Biotechnology Advances* **29**: 483–501. https://doi.org/10.1016/j.biotechadv.2011.05.016.

Stevenson, C.S., Capper, E.A., Roshak, A.K. et al. (2002). The identification and characterization of the marine natural product scytonemin as a novel antiproliferative pharmacophore. *Journal of Pharmacology and Experimental Therapeutics* **303**: 858–866. https://doi.org/10.1124/jpet.102.036350.

Stiger, V., Deslandes, E., and Payri, C.E. (2004). Phenolic contents of two brown algae, *Turbinaria ornata* and *Sargassum mangarevense* on Tahiti (French Polynesia): interspecific, ontogenic and spatio-temporal variations. *Botanica Marina* **47**: 402–409. https://doi.org/10.1515/BOT.2004.058.

Stiger-Pouvreau, V. and Guérard, F. (2018). Bio-inspired molecules extracted from marine macroalgae: a new generation of active ingredients for cosmetics and human health. In: *Blue Biotechnology: Production and Use of Marine Molecules* (eds. S. La Barre and S. Bates), 709–746. Weinheim: Wiley-VCH Verlag GmbH & Co.

Stiger-Pouvreau, V., Jégou, C., Cérantola, S. et al. (2014). Phlorotannins in Sargassaceae species from Brittany (France). *Advances in Botanical Research* **71**: 379–411. https://doi.org/10.1016/B978-0-12-408062-1.00013-5.

Sugiura, Y., Matsuda, K., Yamada, Y. et al. (2006a). Isolation of a new anti-allergic phlorotannin, phlorofucofuroeckol-B, from an edible brown alga, *Eisenia arborea*. *Bioscience, Biotechnology, and Biochemistry* **70**: 2807–2811. https://doi.org/10.1271/bbb.60417.

Sugiura, Y., Takeuchi, Y., Kakinuma, M., and Amano, H. (2006b). Inhibitory effects of seaweeds on histamine release from rat basophile leukemia cells (RBL-2H3). *Fisheries Science* **72**: 1286–1291. https://doi.org/10.1111/j.1444-2906.2006.01287.x.

Sugiura, Y., Matsuda, K., Yamada, Y. et al. (2007). Anti-allergic phlorotannins from the edible brown alga, *Eisenia arborea*. *Food Science and Technology Research* **13**: 54–60. https://doi.org/10.3136/fstr.13.54.

Sugiura, Y., Matsuda, K., Okamoto, T. et al. (2009). The inhibitory effects of components from a brown alga, *Eisenia arborea*, on degranulation of mast cells and eicosanoid synthesis. *Journal of Functional Foods* **1**: 387–393. https://doi.org/10.1016/j.jff.2009.08.002.

Sugiura, Y., Torii, T., Tanaka, R., and Matsushita, T. (2012). Inhibitory effect of extracts from the brown alga, *Ecklonia stolonifera*, on enzymes responsible for allergic reactions and degranulation in RBL-2H3 cells. *Food Science and Technology Research* **18**: 467–471. https://doi.org/10.3136/fstr.18.467.

Sugiura, Y., Kinoshita, Y., Abe, M. et al. (2016). Suppressive effects of the diethyl ether fraction from a brown alga *Sargassum fusiforme* on allergic and inflammatory reactions. *Fisheries Science* **82**: 369–377. https://doi.org/10.1007/s12562-016-0969-9.

Sun, Y., Yang, C., and Tsao, R. (2018). Nomenclature and general classification of antioxidant activity/capacity assays. In: *Measurement of Antioxidant Activity & Capacity:*

Recent Trends and Applications (eds. R. Apak, E. Capanoglu and F. Shahidi), 1–19. Chichester: Wiley.

Sun, Z., Peng, X., Liu, J. et al. (2010). Inhibitory effects of microalgal extracts on the formation of advanced glycation endproducts (AGEs). *Food Chemistry* **120**: 261–267. https://doi.org/10.1016/j.foodchem.2009.10.018.

Surget, G., Roberto, V.P., Le Lann, K. et al. (2016). Marine green macroalgae: a source of natural compounds with mineralogenic and antioxidant activities. *Journal of Applied Phycology* **29**: 575–584. https://doi.org/10.1007/s10811-016-0968-3.

Surget, G., Le Lann, K., Delebecq, G. et al. (2017). Seasonal phenology and metabolomics of the introduced red macroalga *Gracilaria vermiculophylla*, monitored in the bay of Brest (France). *Journal of Applied Phycology* **29**: 2651–2666. https://doi.org/10.1007/s10811-017-1060-3.

Surh, Y.J. (2005). Transcriptional regulation of cellular antioxidant defense mechanisms. In: *Oxidative Stress, Inflammation, and Health* (eds. Y.J. Surh and L. Packer), 21–40. Boca Raton, FL: CRC Press.

Svensson, C.J., Pavia, H., and Toth, G.B. (2007). Do plant density, nutrient availability, and herbivore grazing interact to affect phlorotannin plasticity in the brown seaweed *Ascophyllum nodosum*? *Marine Biology* **151**: 2177–2181. https://doi.org/10.1007/s00227-007-0649-5.

Swanson, A.K. and Druehl, L.D. (2002). Induction, exudation and the UV protective role of kelp phlorotannins. *Aquatic Botany* **73**: 241–253. https://doi.org/10.1016/S0304-3770(02)00035-9.

Taboada, C., Millán, R., and Míguez, I. (2010). Composition, nutritional aspects and effect on serum parameters of marine algae *Ulva rigida*. *Science of Food and Agriculture* **90**: 445–449. https://doi.org/10.1002/jsfa.3836.

Tan, J.K.L., Vasey, K., and Fung, K.Y. (2001). Beliefs and perceptions of patients with acne. *Journal of the American Academy of Dermatology* **44**: 439–444.

Tanniou, A., Serrano Leon, E., Vandanjon, L. et al. (2013). Green improved processes to extract bioactive phenolic compounds from brown macroalgae using *Sargassum muticum* as model. *Talanta* **104**: 44–52. https://doi.org/10.1016/j.talanta.2012.10.088.

Tanniou, A., Vandanjon, L., Incera, M. et al. (2014). Assessment of the spatial variability of phenolic contents and associated bioactivities in the invasive alga *Sargassum muticum* sampled along its European range from Norway to Portugal. *Journal of Applied Phycology* **26**: 1215–1230. https://doi.org/10.1007/s10811-013-0198-x.

Targett, N.M. and Arnold, T.M. (1998). Minireview – predicting the effects of brown algal phlorotannins on marine herbivores in tropical and temperate oceans. *Journal of Phycology* **34**: 195–205. https://doi.org/10.1046/j.1529-8817.1998.340195.x.

Targett, N.M., Coen, L.D., Boettcher, A.A., and Tanner, C.E. (1992). Biogeographic comparisons of marine algal polyphenolics: evidence against a latitudinal trend. *Oecologia* **89**: 464–470. https://doi.org/10.1007/BF00317150.

Thomas, J.E. and Foody, J.M. (2007). The pathophysiology of cardiovascular disease in diabetes mellitus and the future of therapy. *Journal of the Cardiometabolic Syndrome* **2**: 108–113.

Thomas, N.V. and Kim, S.K. (2011). Potential pharmacological applications of polyphenolic derivatives from marine brown algae. *Environmental Toxicology and Pharmacology* **32**: 325–335. https://doi.org/10.1016/j.etap.2011.09.004.

Thompson, G.R. (2004). Management of dyslipidaemia. *Heart* **90**: 949–955.

Tibbetts, S.M., Milley, J.E., and Lall, S.P. (2015). Chemical composition and nutritional properties of freshwater and marine microalgal biomass cultured in photobioreactors. *Journal of Applied Phycology* **27**: 1109–1119.

Tierney, M.S., Soler-Vila, A., Croft, A.K., and Hayes, M. (2013a). Antioxidant activity of the brown macroalgae *Fucus spiralis* Linnaeus harvested from the west coast of Ireland. *Current Research Journal of Biological Sciences* **5**: 81–90.

Tierney, M.S., Smyth, T.J., Hayes, M. et al. (2013b). Influence of pressurised liquid extraction and solid-liquid extraction methods on the phenolic content and antioxidant activities of Irish macroalgae. *International Journal of Food Science and Technology* **48**: 860–869. https://doi.org/10.1111/ijfs.12038.

Tsuji, N., Moriwaki, S., Suzuki, Y. et al. (2001). The role of elastases secreted by fibroblasts in wrinkle formation: implication through selective inhibition of elastase activity. *Photochemistry and Photobiology* **74**: 283–290. https://doi.org/10.1562/0031-8655(2001)0740283TROESB2.0.CO2.

Vandanjon, L., Vallet, L., Le Glatin, T. et al. (2016). Valorization of the macroalgae *Sargassum muticum* by enzymatic hydrolysis, interest of surfactants to improve the extraction of phlorotannins and polysaccharides. *Journal of Marine Biology and Aquaculture* **2**: 1–7. https://doi.org/10.15436/2381-0750.16.014.

Vandanjon, L., Hersant, C., Tanniou, A. et al. (2017). Comparison of different membrane filtration systems for recovering active phenolic compounds from the European spread macroalga *Sargassum muticum*. *Journal of Marine Biology and Aquaculture* **3**: 1–7. https://doi.org/10.15436/2381-0750.17.1224.

Vaseghi, G., Sharifi, M., Dana, N. et al. (2018). Cytotoxicity of *Sargassum angustifolium* partitions against breast and cervical cancer cell lines. *Advanced Biomedical Research* **7**: 1–6. https://doi.org/10.4103/abr.abr.

Vo Dinh, T., Saravana, P.S., Woo, H.C., and Chun, B.S. (2018). Ionic liquid-assisted subcritical water enhances the extraction of phenolics from brown seaweed and its antioxidant activity. *Separation and Purification Technology* **196**: 287–299. https://doi.org/10.1016/j.seppur.2017.06.009.

Wan, T.W., Bahruddin, S., and Boey, P.L. (2009). Determination of TOTOX value in palm oleins using a FI-potentiometric analyzer. *Food Chemistry* **113**: 285–290. https://doi.org/10.1016/j.foodchem.2008.06.082.

Wang, W., Okada, Y., Shi, H. et al. (2005). Structures and aldose reductase inhibitory effects of bromophenols from the red alga *Symphyocladia latiuscula*. *Journal of Natural Products* **68**: 620–622. https://doi.org/10.1021/np040199j.

Wang, T., Jónsdóttir, R., Kristinsson, H.G. et al. (2010). Enzyme-enhanced extraction of antioxidant ingredients from red algae *Palmaria palmata*. *LWT - Food Science and Technology* **43**: 1387–1393. https://doi.org/10.1016/j.lwt.2010.05.010.

Wang, H.M.D., Li, X.C., Lee, D.J., and Chang, J.S. (2017). Potential biomedical applications of marine algae. *Bioresource Technology* **244**: 1407–1415. https://doi.org/10.1016/j.biortech.2017.05.198.

Waterman, P.G. and Mole, S. (1994). *Methods in Ecology: Analysis of Phenolic Plant Metabolites*. Oxford: Blackwell Scientific Publications.

Watson, R.R. and Schönlau, F. (2015). Nutraceutical and antioxidant effects of a delphinidin-rich maqui berry extract Delphinol®: a review. *Minerva Cardioangiologica* **63**: 1–12.

Wauquier, F., Leotoing, L., Coxam, V. et al. (2009). Oxidative stress in bone remodelling and disease. *Trends in Molecular Medicine* **15**: 468–477. https://doi.org/10.1016/j.molmed.2009.08.004.

Whitfield, F.B., Helidoniotis, F., Shaw, K.J., and Svoronos, D. (1999). Distribution of bromophenols in species of marine algae from eastern Australia. *Journal of Agricultural and Food Chemistry* **47**: 2367–2373. https://doi.org/10.1021/jf981080h.

Wiemer, D.F., Idler, D.D., and Fenical, W. (1991). Vidalols A and B, new anti-inflammatory bromophenols from the Caribbean marine red alga *Vidalia obtusaloba*. *Experientia* **47**: 851–853. https://doi.org/10.1007/BF01922471.

Wijesinghe, W.A.J.P. and Jeon, Y.J. (2011). Biological activities and potential cosmeceutical applications of bioactive components from brown seaweeds: a review. *Phytochemistry Reviews* **10**: 431–443. https://doi.org/10.1007/s11101-011-9214-4.

Wijesinghe, W.A.J.P. and Jeon, Y.J. (2012a). Exploiting biological activities of brown seaweed *Ecklonia cava* for potential industrial applications: a review. *International Journal of Food Sciences and Nutrition* **63**: 225–235. https://doi.org/10.3109/09637486.2011.619965.

Wijesinghe, W.A.J.P. and Jeon, Y.J. (2012b). Enzyme-assistant extraction (EAE) of bioactive components: a useful approach for recovery of industrially important metabolites from seaweeds: a review. *Fitoterapia* **83**: 6–12. https://doi.org/10.1016/j.fitote.2011.10.016.

Wild, S., Roglic, G., Green, A. et al. (2004). Global prevalence of diabetes. *Diabetes Care* **27**: 1047–1053. https://doi.org/10.2337/diacare.27.5.1047.

Woo, J.-T., Yonezawa, T., and Nagai, K. (2010). Phytochemicals that stimulate osteoblastic differentiation and bone formation. *Journal of Oral Biosciences* **52**: 15–21. https://doi.org/10.2330/joralbiosci.52.15.

Woolner, V.H., Gordon, R.M.A., Miller, J.H. et al. (2018). Halogenated meroditerpenoids from a south pacific collection of the red alga *Callophycus serratus*. *Journal of Natural Products* **81**: 2446–2454. https://doi.org/10.1021/acs.jnatprod.8b00487.

World Health Organization and International Society of Hypertension Writing Group (2003). 2003 World Health Organization (WHO)/International Society of Hypertension (ISH) statement on management of hypertension. *Journal of Hypertension* **21**: 1983–1992.

Xu, X., Yin, L., Gao, J. et al. (2014). Antifungal bromophenols from marine red algae *Symphyocladia latiuscula*. *Chemistry and Biodiversity* **11**: 807–811. https://doi.org/10.1002/cbdv.201300239.

Xu, X., Yang, H., Khalil, Z.G. et al. (2019). Bromocatechol conjugates from a Chinese marine red alga, *Symphyocladia latiuscula*. *Phytochemistry* **158**: 20–25. https://doi.org/10.1016/j.phytochem.2018.10.026.

Yamaguchi, M. (2013). Marine alga *Sargassum horneri* component and bone homeostasis: role in osteoporosis prevention. *International Journal of Food Science, Nutrition and Dietetics* **2**: 9–14.

Yeo, M., Jung, W.-K., and Kim, G. (2012). Fabrication, characterisation and biological activity of phlorotannin-conjugated PCL/β-TCP composite scaffolds for bone tissue regeneration. *Journal of Materials Chemistry* **22**: 3568. https://doi.org/10.1039/c2jm14725d.

Yoon, N.Y., Eom, T.K., Kim, M.M., and Kim, S.K. (2009). Inhibitory effect of phlorotannins isolated from *Ecklonia cava* on mushroom tyrosinase activity and melanin formation in mouse B16F10 melanoma cells. *Journal of Agricultural and Food Chemistry* **57**: 4124–4129. https://doi.org/10.1021/jf900006f.

Yoon, W.-J., Kim, K.-N., Heo, S.-J. et al. (2013). Sargachromanol G inhibits osteoclastogenesis by suppressing the activation NF-κB and MAPKs in RANKL-induced RAW 264.7 cells. *Biochemical and Biophysical Research Communications* **434**: 892–897. https://doi.org/10.1016/j.bbrc.2013.04.046.

Yoshie, Y., Wang, W., Hsieh, Y.P., and Suzuki, T. (2002). Compositional difference of phenolic compounds between two seaweeds, *Halimeda* spp. *Journal of Tokyo University of Fisheries* **88**: 21–24.

Yoshie-Stark, Y., Hsieh, Y.-P., and Suzuki, T. (2003). Distribution of flavonoids and related compounds from seaweeds in Japan. *Journal of Tokyo University of Fisheries* **89**: 1–6.

Young, G., Nippgen, F., Titterbrandt, S., and Cooney, M.J. (2010). Lipid extraction from biomass using co-solvent mixtures of ionic liquids and polar covalent molecules. *Separation and Purification Technology* **72**: 118–121. https://doi.org/10.1016/j.seppur.2010.01.009.

Yuan, Y.V., Carrington, M.F., and Walsh, N.A. (2005). Extracts from dulse (*Palmaria palmata*) are effective antioxidants and inhibitors of cell proliferation in vitro. *Food and Chemical Toxicology* **43**: 1073–1081. https://doi.org/10.1016/j.fct.2005.02.012.

Yuan, Y., Zhang, J., Fan, J. et al. (2018). Microwave assisted extraction of phenolic compounds from four economic brown macroalgae species and evaluation of their antioxidant activities and inhibitory effects on α-amylase, α-glucosidase, pancreatic lipase and tyrosinase. *Food Research International* **113**: 288–297. https://doi.org/10.1016/j.foodres.2018.07.021.

Zhang, R., Yuen, A.K.L., Magnusson, M. et al. (2018). A comparative assessment of the activity and structure of phlorotannins from the brown seaweed *Carpophyllum flexuosum*. *Algal Research* **29**: 130–141. https://doi.org/10.1016/j.algal.2017.11.027.

Zhang, W.W., Duan, X.J., Huang, H.L. et al. (2007). Evaluation of 28 marine algae from the Qingdao coast for antioxidative capacity and determination of antioxidant efficiency and total phenolic content of fractions and subfractions derived from *Symphyocladia latiuscula* (Rhodomelaceae). *Journal of Applied Phycology* **19**: 97–108. https://doi.org/10.1007/s10811-006-9115-x.

Zhao, J., Fan, X., Wang, S. et al. (2004). Bromophenol derivatives from the red alga *Rhodomela confervoides*. *Journal of Natural Products* **67**: 1032–1035. https://doi.org/10.1021/np030546+.

Zubia, M., Robledo, D., and Freile-Pelegrin, Y. (2007). Antioxidant activities in tropical marine macroalgae from the Yucatan Peninsula, Mexico. *Journal of Applied Phycology* **19**: 449–458. https://doi.org/10.1007/s10811-006-9152-5.

Zubia, M., Fabre, M.S., Kerjean, V. et al. (2009). Antioxidant and antitumoural activities of some Phaeophyta from Brittany coasts. *Food Chemistry* **116**: 693–701. https://doi.org/10.1016/j.foodchem.2009.03.025.

12
Algal Carotenoids: Recovery and their Potential in Disease Prevention

V. Sivamurugan[1], D. Radhika[2], Abirami Ramu Ganesan[3], and S. Murugesan[†4]

[1]*Postgraduate and Research Department of Chemistry, Pachaiyappa's College, Chennai, India*
[2]*Postgraduate and Research Department of Zoology, V.O. Chidambaram College, Tuticorin, India*
[3]*Department of Food Science and Home Economics, School of Applied Sciences, College of Engineering, Science and Technology, Fiji National University, Samabula, Fiji Islands*
[4]*Unit of Algal Biotechnology & Bio-nanotechnology, Postgraduate and Research Department of Botany, Pachaiyappa's College, Chennai, India* [†]*Corresponding author E mail: smurugesan5@gmail.com*

12.1 Introduction

Carotenoids, one of the major classes of isoprenoid or tetraterpenoid plant pigments derived from microalgae, have application as ingredients in functional foods, nutraceuticals, or, potentially, pharmaceutical products that may reduce the risk of various diet-related chronic diseases, including neurodegenerative diseases (Meléndez-Martínez 2019). Although humans are unable to synthesize carotenoids, a carotenoid-rich diet may contribute to improved health by decreasing the occurrence of diet-related chronic diseases like vitamin A deficiency, and decrease morbidity and mortality rates (Meléndez-Martínez 2019). Currently, there is increased interest among consumers in functional foods or nutraceuticals containing natural-sourced bioactive compounds. Products obtained from marine algae have found application in nutrition, animal feed, fertilizer, as well as pharmaceuticals (Kadam and Prabhasankar 2010).

Among the known 600 carotenoids, fewer than 10% are precursors of vitamin A (Corol et al. 2002). However, three macular carotenoids are available through dietary carotenoids for the human circulation system, i.e. lutein, zeaxanthin, and meso-zeaxanthin, which are also found in the macula of the human eye (Abdel-Aal

Recent Advances in Micro- and Macroalgal Processing: Food and Health Perspectives, First Edition. Edited by Gaurav Rajauria and Yvonne V. Yuan.

et al. 2013). Deposition of carotenoids in the human eye macula is essential to protect the retina and epithelium from harmful damage caused by UV irradiation (Abdel-Aal et al. 2013). Other carotenoids like lutein play a major role in constructing structural components. The carotenoid pigments contain nearly 700 distinctive structures and biological activities (Stafsnes et al. 2010). Carotenoid compounds contain a range of yellow, orange, or red pigments present in chloroplasts of terrestrial plants and marine organisms (Henríquez et al. 2016).

There are three main classes of photosynthetic pigments within algae: chlorophylls, carotenoids, and phycobilins. Algae have been found to be plentiful sources of carotenoids including carotene (Jaswir et al. 2011), which contains a conjugated double-bond structure in the hydrocarbon backbone (containing alternate double and single bonds in the structure). Among the group of carotenoids, carotenes have a carbon and hydrogen backbone in their structure, and xanthophylls consist of oxygenated derivatives with hydroxyl, ketone, and aldehydic functional groups. Therefore, carotenes and xanthophylls are collectively known as the carotenoid family.

Carotenoids have a unique chemical structure that allows them to have two key roles in land plants and algae (Goodwin and Britton 1988). Most carotenoids absorb UV light (200–800 nm), which allows the absorption of light energy for photosynthesis and the protection of chlorophyll from photo damage (Koka and Song 1978). The carotenoid profile provides important information about the photo acclimation and photo protection responses to light stress (Koka and Song 1978). Among the pigments such as chlorophylls, anthocyanins, and porphyrins present in algae, carotenoids have an essential role in protecting cells against photosensitized oxidation (Palozza and Krinsky 1992).

Changes in lifestyle, consumption patterns, and nutrition affect the global population worldwide. Undesirable pollution levels, and frequent contact with xenobiotics and radiation, have become immense hazards to human life, and these are the leading causes of several metabolic diseases (Uchiyama and Okada 2008). During metabolism, free radicals and reactive oxygen species (ROS) and/or reactive nitrogen species (RNS) may be produced by normal respiration and metabolism processes including peroxidation, which may cause DNA damage (Zhang et al. 2014; Griendling et al. 2016; Long et al. 2017). DNA damage may be associated with mutations leading to genome instability and thereby carcinogenesis (Raposo et al. 2015).

Many scientific reports have reported beneficial effects of carotenoids on human health in numerous ways, including antioxidant (Xia et al. 2013), antimicrobial (Pushpa and Purushothama 2010), anti-inflammatory (Soontornchaiboon et al., 2012), and anticancer activities (Zhang et al. 2014). For example, β-carotene could be a main dietary supplement of vitamin A, which improves the antioxidant activity in the body, and supplementation with β-carotene has demonstrated suppressive effects on carcinogenesis (Meléndez-Martínez 2019). In addition, another commercially important carotenoid derivative is astaxanthin, a ketocarotenoid belonging to the xanthophyll group that can be exploited as a powerful antioxidant, with anti-inflammatory and anticancer activity. Another carotenoid pigment, fucoxanthin, is an important member of the xanthophyll family, and is a predominant carotenoid found in brown algae known for anticancer, antidiabetic, antioxidant, anti-inflammatory, and antiangiogenic activities (Koyande et al. 2019). These seaweed carotenoids are identified as critical pharmaceutical compounds, which demonstrate promising impact against cell proliferation (Sathasivam and Ki 2018). Chemoprevention is the most fundamental treatment for controlling cancer development; on the other hand, molecular study has showed that using carotenoids is a striking approach to cancer prevention (Wang et al. 2019).

Therefore, this chapter deals with the chemistry of algal carotenoids and their elucidation through different methods and techniques with special emphasis on their applications for metabolic disorders; for example, in prevention of oxidation of human cells and cancer cells, their protective role in the human macula and pancreas, and their bactericidal and wound healing effects. As the demand for natural carotenoids is increasing globally, the commercial market value of various algal carotenoids is also discussed in this chapter.

12.2 Types and Structure of Carotenoids in Microalgae

12.2.1 General Occurrence

The carotenoids are classified according to their chemical structure. Some carotenes contain only carbon and hydrogen, for instance, α-carotene, β-carotene, and lycopene; and some contain oxygen-based functional groups such as alcohol, ketone, and aldehyde moieties, for example, lutein and zeaxanthin (Qian et al. 2012). The scaffold of carotenoids is made of four isoprene units linked to form a conjugated polyene backbone and they are frequently referred to as tetraterpenes, a subclass of terpenes (Shinichi 2011). Xanthophylls are an oxygenated form of carotenes; the majority of the xanthophylls contain carbonyl and hydroxyl groups and a few xanthophylls containing an epoxide ring have also been reported (Shinichi 2011).

The derivatives of carotenoids, e.g. lutein, are known as lipochromes or chromolipids because they exist in plants as a mixture with chlorophylls to form fat-soluble pigments within the thylakoids of the plastids, i.e. chloroplasts and chromoplasts (D'Alessandro and Filho 2016). These derivatives act as photosensitizers that assist with photosynthesis. Xanthophylls are found in chloroplasts of brown algae, which give them a brown or green color. The color of carotenoids ranges from yellow to red depending on the extent of the polyene conjugation. According to X-ray crystallographic analyses, the double bonds in the polyenes are in an all-trans configuration ("E" isomer) and carotenoids represent cis-configuration ("Z" isomers).

12.2.2 Carotenoids Isolated from Seaweeds

The carotenoids isolated from marine algal sources and their biological activities have been summarized in Table 12.1, and the chemical structures of carotenoids and xanthophylls are given Figures 12.1 and 12.2, respectively. Astaxanthin, β-carotene, lutein, canthaxanthin, lycopene, fucoxanthin and zeaxanthin are commercially available carotenoids around the world (Spolaore et al. 2006; Kim et al. 2012; Borowitzka 2013; Mahfuzur et al. 2016). Among these, β-carotene imparts a red, yellow, or orange color to plants, algae, and animals (Becker 2004; Sathasivam et al. 2018). For this reason, the large-scale isolation and extraction of carotenoids is a major business prospect for the healthcare and cosmetic industries (Milledge 2012). As a result,

Table 12.1 Biological functions, common algal sources, health benefits, and applications of chief carotenoids

Carotenoid	Common algal sources	Functions, health benefits, and applications	References
Lycopene	*Chlorella marina* (Renju et al. 2014)	In prostatic hyperplasia and prostate cancer Autophagy	Graydon et al. (2007), Schwarz et al. (2008), Chen et al. (2016), and Zhang et al. (2014) Buyuklu et al. (2014)
β-Carotene	*Synechococcus* sp., *Dunaliella salina*, *Chlorella vulgaris*, *Botryococcus braunii*, *Synechocystis* sp., *Phormidium* sp. *HE10JO*, *Arthrospira maxima*, *Dunaliella* sp., *Chlorella fusca*, *Selenastrum capricornutum*, *Pandorina morum*, *Botryococcus sudeticus* and *Chlorococcum* sp. (Othman et al. 2017)	Pro-vitamin A function In colorectal cancer Prevention of acute and chronic coronary syndromes Prevent night blindness Antioxidant property and prevents liver fibrosis	Sathasivam and Junta Wong (2013), Sathasivam et al. (2014, 2018), and Aust et al. (2005)
Astaxanthin	*Haematococcus pluvialis*, *Chlorella zofingiensis*, *Neochloris oleoabundans* (Reyes et al. 2016)	In benign prostatic hyperplasia and prostate and liver tumors Anti-inflammatory properties Active against liver neoplasma Strong antioxidant property Cardiovascular health Decrease glucose tolerance Enhance serum insulin levels and autophagy	Raposo et al. (2015), Cerón et al. (2007), Lemoine and Sehoefs (2010), Guerin et al. (2003), Uchiyama et al. (2002), Uchiyama and Okada, (2008), and Shen and Mizushima (2014)
Zeaxanthin	*Synechococcus* sp., *Nannochloropsis oculata*, *Chlorella ellipsoidea*, *Dunaliella salina*, *Synechocystis* sp. *Mougeotia* sp.	In the prevention of acute and chronic coronary syndromes Helps to maintain a normal visual function, in the prevention of cataracts To prevent macular degeneration associated with age and active against liver neoplasma	Raposo et al. (2015), Lidebjer et al. (2007), Le and Xiao-Ming (2010), and Olmedilla et al. (2001)

Lutein	*Scenedesmus almeriensis*, *Chlorella vulgaris*, *Scenedesmus obliquus*, *Dunaliella salina*, *Mougeotia* sp., *Chlorella protothecoides*, *Scenedesmus almeriensis* and *Galdieria sulphuraria*, *Neochloris oleoabundans* (Reyes et al. 2016; Othman et al. 2017)	In the prevention of acute, chronic coronary syndromes and stroke Helps to maintain a normal visual function In the prevention of cataracts To prevent macular degeneration associated with age In the prevention of retinitis To avoid gastric infection by *Helicobacter pylori* Antioxidant property and anticancer activity	Minhas et al. (2016), Graziani et al. (2013), and Sanchez et al. (2008)
Violaxanthin	*Mantoniella squamata* (Goss 2003)	Anti-inflammatory activity	Cha et al. (2008) and Soontornchaiboon et al. (2012)
Fucoxanthin	*Odontella aurita* (Xia et al. 2013), *Isochrysis* sp. (Crupi et al. 2013), *Phaeodactylum tricornutum* (Kim et al. 2012), *Dunaliella tertiolecta* (Xu et al. 2016), *Himanthalia elongata* (Rajauria and Abu-Ghannam 2013), *Eisenia bicyclis* (Kim et al. 2011), *Cylindrotheca closterium* (Erdogan et al. 2016), *Undaria pinnatifida* (Grasa-Lopez et al. 2016), *Laminaria japonica* (Wang et al. 2005)	Antiobesity Antioxidant property Antidiabetic Antineuroinflammation and autophagy	Kim et al. (2012), Xia et al. (2013), Dambek et al. (2012), and Zhao et al. (2017)
Canthaxanthin	*Neochloris oleoabundans* (Reyes et al. 2016)	Create a tan color Antioxidant property In the prevention of acute and chronic coronary syndromes and stroke In the prevention of cataracts To prevent macular degeneration associated with age In the prevention of retinitis and to avoid gastric infection by *H. pylori*	Abe et al. (2007) and Cha et al. (2008)

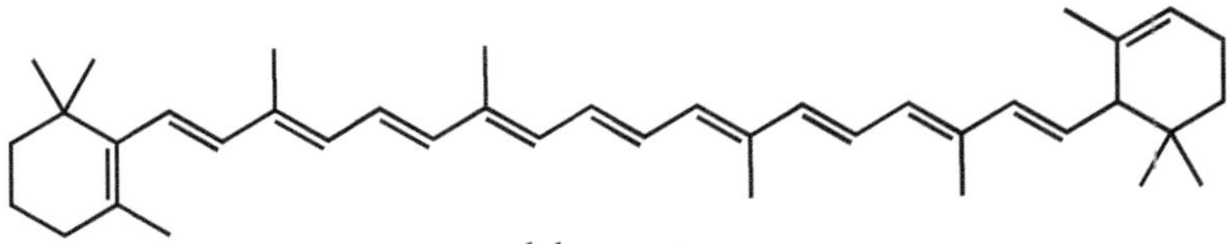

alpha–carotene

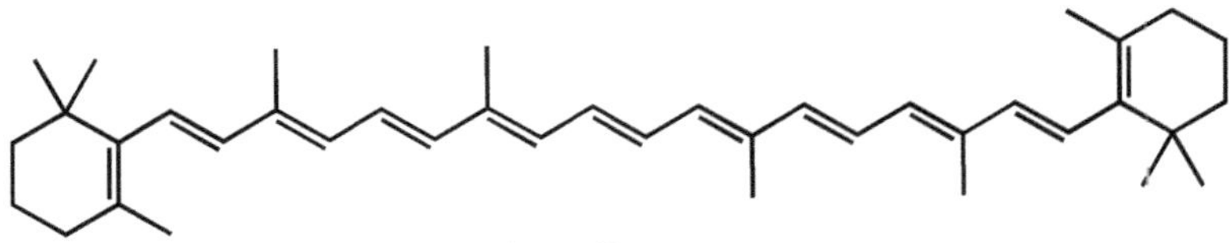

beta–Carotene

Figure 12.1 Structure of carotenes isolated from seaweeds

many international organizations have started identifyng diverse types of carotenoids for innumerable applications.

Seaweeds, especially microalgae contain a wide range of carotenoids, with the most prominent being astaxanthin, β-carotene and fucoxanthin. Seaweeds may be a potential novel source of carotenoids, which have a number of potent biological activities (Abe et al. 2007; Cerón et al. 2007; Shinichi 2011; Chan et al. 2013; Asker and Awad 2019). The Rhodophyta (red algae) contain α- and β-carotene as well as oxygenated derivatives. The chief pigments, such as peridinin, dinoxanthin and fucoxanthin are found in the Pyrrophyta. The Chrysophyta contain epoxy, allenic and acetylenic-carotenoids. Eutreptielanone is identified from the Euglenophyta. The major carotenoids found in the Chloromonadophyta are diadinoxanthin, heteroxanthin, and vaucheriaxanthin (Goodwin and Britton 1988; Goodwin 1992). Microalgae are established to be the best source of light-harvesting pigments. In order to meet the commercial demand for carotenoids, the cultivation of microalgae can be undertaken as an objective for mass cultivation (Becker 2004; Cysewski and Lorenz 2004; Cerón et al. 2007).

Microalgae are sources of carotenoids, predominantly strains of the Chlorophyta such as *Dunaliella salina*, *Haematococcus pluvialis*, and diverse species of *Chlorella* (Zhang et al. 2014). There is a developing interest in natural substitutes for chemical ingredients in the cosmetics business and therefore the widespread analysis of various microalgae strains could lead to wonderful resource materials (Gateau et al. 2016). The composition and production efficiency of carotenoids in algae are noticeably influenced by environmental conditions (D'Alessandro and Filho 2016) such as salinity and nutrients available within the culture medium (Bocanegra et al. 2004; Fazeli et al. 2006; Abe et al. 2007).

The green microalgae are sources of xanthophylls such as xanthin, violaxanthin, and lutein, and carotenes such as α-carotene, β-carotene, and others (Soontornchaiboon et al. 2012; Hillol et al. 2012; Chan et al. 2013). For example, *Chlorella* sp. contain lutein (93%), α-carotene (2.6%) and β-carotene (1.3%), zeaxanthin (1.3%), xanthophylls (0.2%), and β-cryptoxanthin (0.2%) (Inbaraj et al. 2006). One of the methods for *Spirulina* production utilizes heterotrophic fermentation reactors containing sugars without light (Lu et al. 2011); whereas a mixture of sodium bicarbonate and air to provide CO_2 is used to culture *Chlorella vulgaris* and *Spirulina* in autotrophic

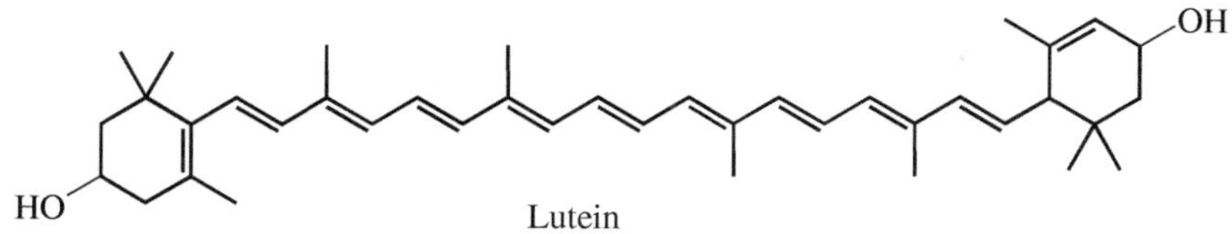

Lutein

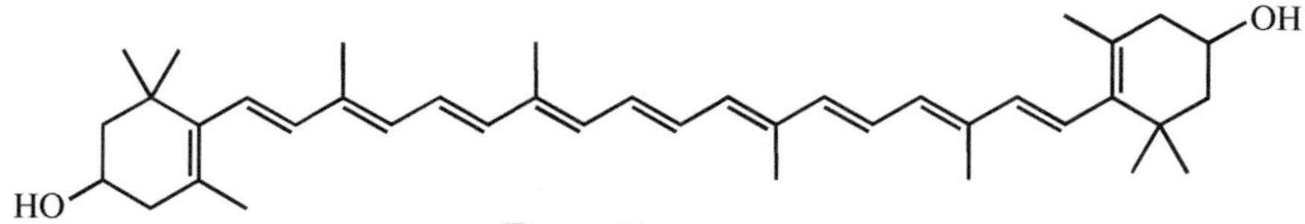

Zeaxanthin

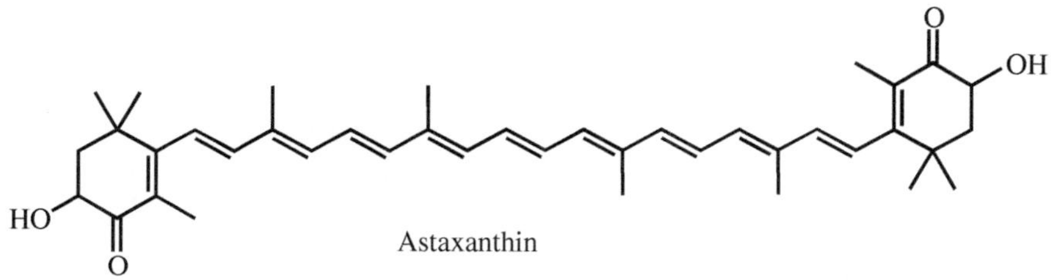

Astaxanthin

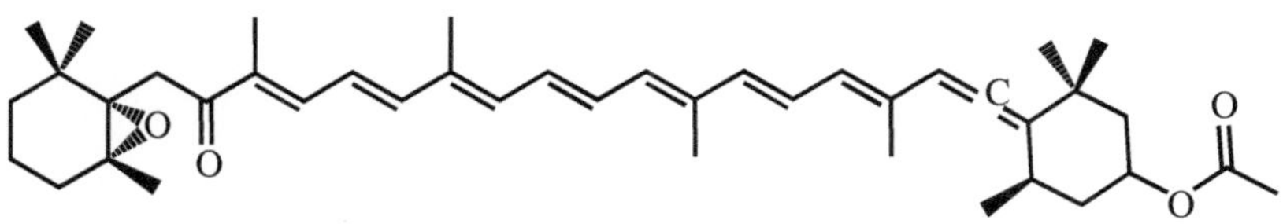

Fucoxanthin

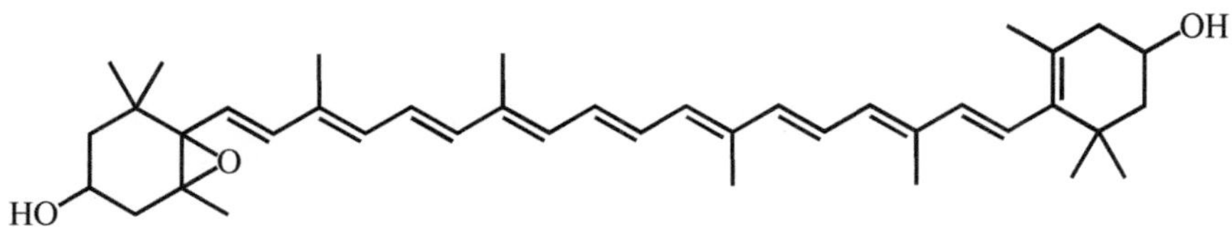

Antheraxanthin

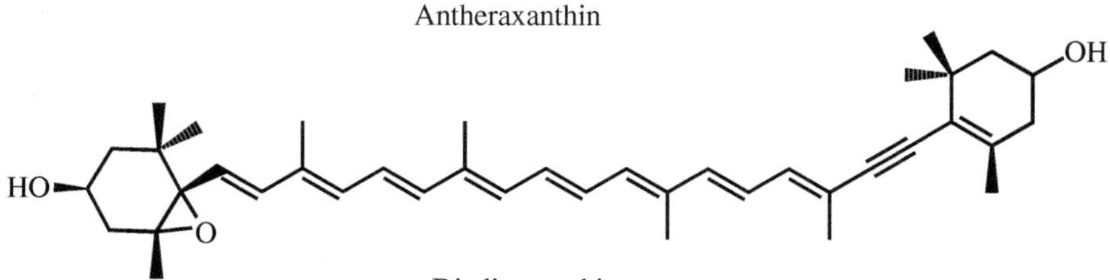

Diadinoxanthin

Figure 12.2 Structures of xanthophylls isolated from seaweeds

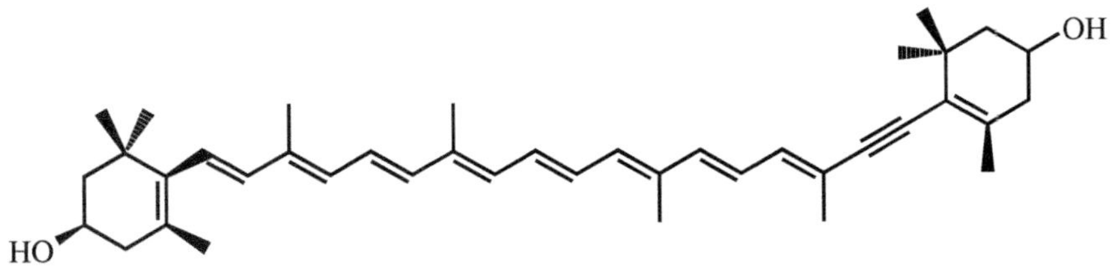

Diatoxanthin

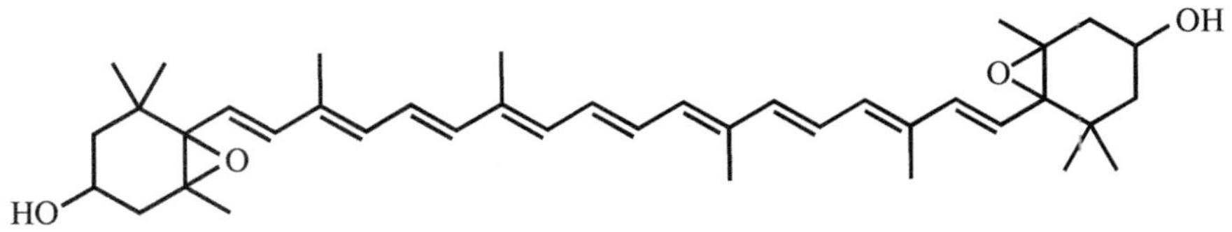

Violaxanthin

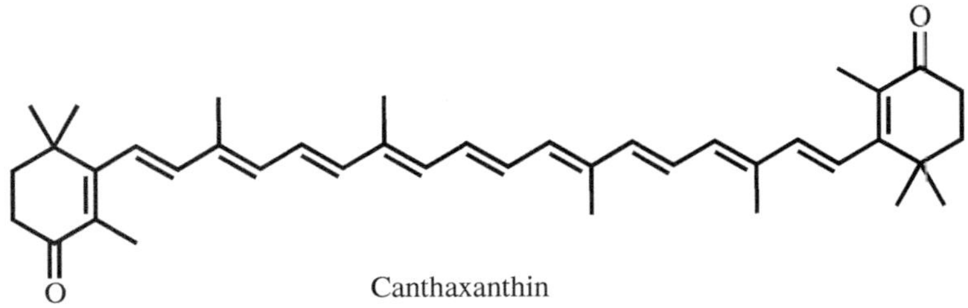

Canthaxanthin

Figure 12.2 (*Continued*)

processes (Chen et al. 2016). While, historically these algae were harvested in Japan, more recently *Chlorella* has gained commercial importance in China as well. Industrially, it presents higher yields of carotenoids than *Spirulina*. On the other hand, the production method must be cautiously restricted to prevent contamination from other carotenoids (Chen et al. 2016).

The commercial production of β-carotene is mostly contributed by the microalga *D. salina*. When contrasted with terrestrial plants, the microalgae are able to deliver more than 3 mg g^{-1} of lutein (Sathasivam et al. 2014). Carotenoids such as canthaxanthin, astaxanthin, and β-carotene have been found in *Botryococcus braunii*. The pigment profile of *Botryococcus* sp. showed lutein (41.57%) and β-carotene (37.96%) as the major carotenoids (Dayananda et al. 2010).

Astaxanthin is another commercially important carotenoid that can be mostly produced by *Haematococcus*. Fucoxanthin is mainly isolated from *Fucus sp.*, *Dictyota sp.*, and *Laminaria sp.* (Peng et al. 2011). The kingdom of microalgae is a plentiful source of a broad range of natural products with various applications in the food, pharmaceutical, and cosmetic industries (Dufossé et al. 2005). The carotenoids make the top of the list of natural products isolated from macro- and microalgae. Chronic diseases such as cardiovascular disease, cancer, and several neurological disorders occur mainly due to the presence of free radicals and ROS, and could be prevented by consuming a carotene-rich diet (Gateau et al. 2016).

12.3 Isolation and Purification of Carotenoids from Algae

The isolation of carotenoids in pure form is essential for dietary supplement and commercial applications. The quality of carotenoids depends on the isolation methods, particularly to yield the maximum quantity of carotenoids (Selvameenal et al. 2009; Chan et al. 2013; Gong and Bassi 2016; Flávia Vieira et al. 2017). In commercial production several types of isolation procedures have been developed. These incorporate standard solvent extraction solid–liquid extraction (SLE); supercritical fluid (SCF) extraction using CO_2 (Canela et al. 2002; Valderrama et al. 2003; Montero et al. 2005; Nobre et al. 2006; Reyes et al. 2016; Herrero and Ibañez 2018); ionic liquid extraction such as with 1-ethyl-3-methyl imidazolium acetate, 1-ethyl-3-methyl imidazolium diethylphosphate, 1-ethyl-3-methyl imidazolium tetrafluoroborate, and 1-ethyl-3-methyl imidazolium chloride (Choi et al. 2014); co-solvent assisted SCF extraction; and microwave- and ultrasound assisted extractions (UAEs) (Aryee et al. 2018). The conventional solvent extraction methods have serious setbacks that could be overcome by using SCF extraction and ionic liquid extraction processes. In spite of the environmental issues, volatile organic solvents such as n-hexane, chloroform, methanol, ethyl acetate, and acetone are normally used for extraction. However, greener technologies using supercritical CO_2 ($scCO_2$), co-solvent assisted SCF, and ionic liquids have been developed to achieve maximum extraction as well as techno-economic and environmentally significant techniques (Herrero and Ibañez 2018). SCF extraction techniques have shown feasible recovery of carotenoids from natural sources (Herrero and Ibañez 2018). In addition, the conventional solvent extraction processes promoted by microwave and ultrasound have also been developed to improve the extraction efficiency (Duangkamol et al. 2010; Kim et al. 2016; Jaeschke et al. 2016; Ventura et al. 2017).

Separation methods like centrifugation could be used for the purification of algal biomass on a commercial scale, and after spray drying the algal biomass can be brought to market as tablets or capsules (Chen et al. 2016). The salt-tolerant microalga *D. salina* is an outstanding resource for commercial-scale production of β-carotene (Raja et al. 2007). India represents the greatest producer of carotenoids derived from microalgae, followed by Australia, the United States, and China (Dufossé et al. 2005). Studies have showed that the manufacture of carotenoids by *Botryococcus braunii* is viable, and have confirmed the presence of canthaxanthin, astaxanthin, and β-carotene (Abe et al. 2007). The microalga *Haematococcus* is of great business interest because of the production of astaxanthin, with the largest producers being the United States, Japan, and India (Dufossé et al. 2005).

12.3.1 Conventional Solid-Liquid Extraction (SLE)

Conventional SLE mainly utilizes volatile solvents such as acetone, chloroform, methanol, and ethyl acetate, and in some cases n-hexane. This method could be widely adopted for the isolation of various types of carotenoids; however, the SLE process is not selective for carotenoids only. The crude extract may require a column purification process or another sophisticated method such as preparative high performance liquid chromatography (HPLC) for the elution of the carotenoids. The conventional SLE method includes a soaking or maceration process and has a few downsides; for example, higher amounts of solvent are required, and several extraction steps for the maximum recovery of the target compounds. In some cases, solvent extraction requires saponification of algae by alkali followed by extraction to free carotenoid molecules from the fatty acid esters. Algae species that have a thin cell wall may facilitate easy and efficient extraction of carotenoids without using alkali pretreatment; for instance, *D. salina* and *Dunaliella tertiolecta* (Mäki-Arvela et al. 2014). *Chlorella* species have a thick cell wall that requires alkali pretreatment of algae for the best extraction of carotenoids (Mäki-Arvela et al. 2014). Though the process is simple and widely used, there is always a need for improved approaches that may offer advantages over traditional strategies in terms of efficiency of carotenoid recovery, reduced energy consumption, and the capacity to avoid the use of dangerous substances.

Microalgal species such as *Chlorella* and *Haematococcus* have complex carbohydrate-rich cell walls, which maintain their biological and biomechanical stability. Such cell walls are found to be tough and it is hard to extract the maximum quantity of the biomolecules. Kim et al. (2016) explored the methods for achieving maximum extraction of lipid/astaxanthin from *Chlorella* and *Haematococcus*. The research proved that the cell disruption and extraction strategies are largely dependent on the given microalgal species and cell wall characteristics. Chemical-mediated cell wall rupture has been carried out with chloroform:methanol (1:1, v/v) as well as with 1% H_2SO_4 and yielded the maximum quantity of lipids/astaxanthin from *Chlorella* and *Haematococcus*. Various physico-chemical techniques, namely, microwave and ultrasound promoted cell disruption techniques have been explored and the conventional solvent extraction technique is used to separate the lipids/carotenoids from the algal biomass (Kim et al. 2016). The purification of carotenoids is necessary for the extraction of solid biomass. The disruption of microalgal cell walls is an essential step that should be included in the extraction process to achieve maximum efficiency (Ventura et al. 2017).

The utilization of moderate electrical fields (MEFs) for carotenoid and lipid extraction from the microalgae *Heterochlorella luteoviridis* in ethanol solvent has been investigated (Jaeschke et al. 2016). The study revealed that MEFs combined with ethanol as the solvent allowed 73% of carotenoid extraction and the main carotenoids in the extract were lutein and zeaxanthin.

12.3.2 Microwave and Ultrasound Promoted Extraction

Duangkamol et al. (2010) have explored the recovery of astaxanthin from *H. pluvialis* using various extraction methods including conventional solvent extraction and microwave promoted extraction. The study compared the efficiency of astaxanthin recovery using solvent extraction, UAE and microwave assisted extraction (MAE). Regardless of the extraction method, as compared with other solvents, acetone showed excellent astaxanthin extraction up to 44 and 74.4% using solvent extraction and MAE, respectively. The study suggested that MAE has abundant opportunities for the extraction of valuable compounds, particularly from the microalga *H. pluvialis*. Further, MAE could also be adopted for other algal varieties as well. The microwave and ultrasound techniques have also been used for the interruption of algal biomass with substantial cell walls to enhance the extraction yield.

12.3.3 Super Critical Fluid Extraction

The use of higher temperatures for extraction could possibly destroy the antioxidant functionality of carotenoids. It is a great challenge for any extraction methods that the carotenoids must retain maximum therapeutic value. The nature and abundant availability of CO_2 make it an inexpensive medium for the SCF extraction process. It is a well-known fact that CO_2 is a gas at standard temperature and pressure (STP) and acts as a solid when it is frozen. When the temperature and pressure are both increased over the critical point at 31.10 °C or 304.25 K and pressure 72.9 atm or 7.39 MPa, respectively, it can demonstrate properties in between a gas and a liquid. Thus, CO_2 could act as a greener solvent at normal temperature (304.25 K), which is preferred for temperature- and oxygen-sensitive compounds like carotenoids (Herrero and Ibañez 2018).

Canela Paula et al. (2002) have considered the extraction of fatty acids and carotenoids from the microalga *Spirulina maxima* using $scCO_2$. The effect of pressure and temperature on the extraction yield and chemical composition of the extracts has been thoroughly investigated. The conditions with respect to temperature and pressure have been optimized to obtain the maximum yield of carotenoids and fatty acids. The recovery of astaxanthin from the microalga *H. pluvialis* and of phycocyanin from *S. maxima* have been reported using $scCO_2$ along with ethanol as a co-solvent. The addition of a co-solvent (9.4 mass % of ethanol) enhanced the astaxanthin extraction yield of about 1.7 mass % as compared with the $scCO_2$ alone. By using the SCF technique, a maximum total recovery of astaxantin of up to 97% has been achieved (Valderrama et al. 2003).

Nobre et al. (2006) have investigated the extraction of astaxanthin from algae with various methods using MAE and UAE and also pressurized liquid extraction with $scCO_2$ and ethanol as a co-solvent (Figures 12.3 and 12.4). The investigation was schematically designed to achieve maximum extraction efficiencies of various carotenoids, namely, measuring the effects of solvent, temperature, pressure and mass transfer, extraction kinetics, and modeling. Under the optimized conditions, the highest recovery has been reported for astaxanthin of up to 91.8% using $scCO_2$ under 30 MPa and 60 °C in the presence of 10% ethanol from *H. pluvialis* as compared with other conventional extraction techniques. As ethanol is a polar solvent, its presence could improve the solubility of carotenoids, and it has proved to be the best solvent, giving high yields of astaxanthin while retaining high antioxidative activity.

Similarly, a comparative study explored extraction efficiencies for recovery of carotenoids such as xanthophyll and fucoxanthin from two brown macroalgae, *Fucus serratus* and *Laminaria digitata*, utilizing SLE, $scCO_2$, and ethanol assisted $scCO_2$. The conventional method produced the maximum yield of carotenoid-rich extracts from *F. serratus* using hexane:acetone (70:30) at 50 °C. In $scCO_2$, the maximum carotenoid yield is obtained at 50 °C and at 300 atm pressure (Heffernan et al. 2016). In addition, $scCO_2$ yielded fucoxanthin with higher selectivity, whereas SLE yielded a higher purity of xanthophyll (Heffernan et al. 2016).

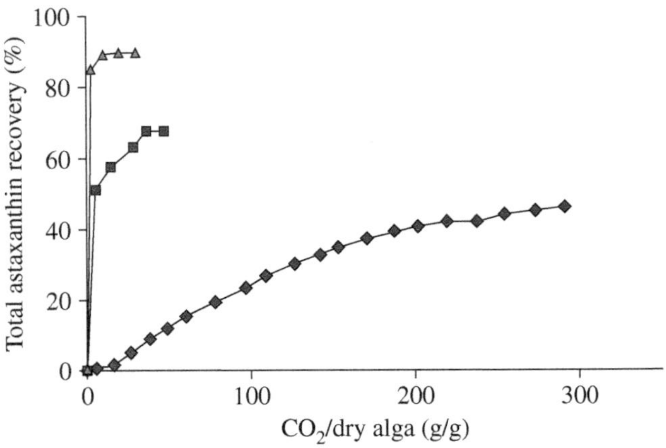

Figure 12.3 Recovery of total astaxanthin (free plus esters) as a function of CO_2 amount with (■) and without (♦) ethanol as a co-solvent at 40 °C, and CO_2 with ethanol at 60 °C and 300 bar (▲). Source Nobre et al. (2006).

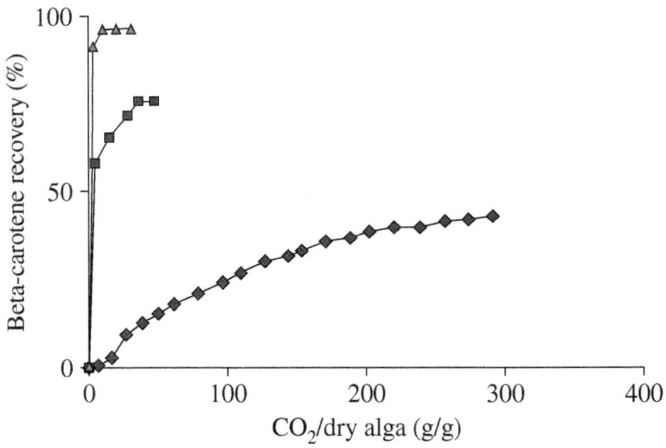

Figure 12.4 Recovery of total β-carotene as a function of CO_2 amount with (■) and without (♦) ethanol as a co-solvent at 40 °C, and CO_2 with ethanol (▲) at 60 °C and 300 bar. Source: Credit: Nobre et al. (2006).

12.3.4 Adsorbent Assisted Carotenoid Extraction

Carotenoid extraction could be improved by converting the algal biomass into a resin paste by mixing it with low-cost adsorbents and subjecting the algal paste to scCO_2 extraction. Microalgal cultures are normally grown in an aqueous medium and supercritical fluid extraction (SFE) in the presence of an aqueous medium requires higher energy. Thus, the addition of a low-cost adsorbent could support extraction from cultures containing higher amounts of a water medium. For example, *Neochloris oleoabundans* is a microalga belonging to the Chlorophyceae family. In addition to carotenoids, due to the presence of high lipid content it is used as an important ingredient in cosmetics and biofuel production as well as a feed for mussels. As previously stated, rupturing of the cell walls plays a major role in extracting maximum biomolecules (Reyes et al. 2016). During their investigation, Reyes et al. (2016) converted *N. oleoabundans* into a paste, oleoresin, using a cryogenic grinding process followed by blending with various adsorbents including activated charcoal and chitosan. As compared with other adsorbents, chitosan adsorbent demonstrated the highest carotenoid recovery of up to 60–140% $g\ g^{-1}$ and the yield is greater than that obtained with acetone. The study revealed that adsorbent assisted extraction obtained extracts with higher amounts of carotenoids from microalgae paste with a high water content. One option is the concurrent extraction procedure of the microalgae paste (containing around 70–80% water), yet there is not much data that investigates this type of extraction. This work investigates the rapid extraction of carotenoids from microalgae paste under supercritical CO_2 and yield of carotenoid extraction using water from *N. oleoabundans* (Reyes et al. 2016).

12.3.5 Ionic Liquid Mediated Carotenoid Extraction

Most of the volatile organic solvents are toxic in nature and the use of volatile solvents should be avoided in the development of greener processes. Ionic liquids are a suitable alternative to the toxic organic solvents since they have low vapor pressure and are less toxic and, in addition, they can be recycled. In general, the ionic liquids contain large organic cations composed of an imidazolium group coupled with smaller inorganic or organic anions. Ionic liquids can play a dual role as catalysts as well as greener solvents for many organic reactions. The utilization of ionic liquids in different industries such as biorefinement and food processing has been explored (Choi et al. 2014). For instance, the ionic liquid derived from substituted imidazolium salts containing acetate, phosphate, and tetrafluoroborate has been used for cell wall disruption, and lipid/astaxanthin extraction has been carried out on *Chlorella* biomass and the efficiency of extraction was found to be dependent on temperature and the type and the dosage of ionic liquid used for the extraction (Choi et al. 2014).

12.3.6 Surfactant Assisted Extraction Methods

There is an absolute necessity for a highly efficient and selective method for the isolation of sensitive biomolecules such as carotenoids that may increase the commercial viability of the algal biomass. Flávia Vieira et al. (2017) explored carotenoid extraction from *Sargassum muticum* and *Sargassum cymosum* using nonionic surfactants in aqueous solution. During this investigation, both dry seaweed and fresh algal biomass were used for the screening of various surfactants with respect to their extraction efficiency. The overall amount of carotenoid obtained from fresh *S. muticum* is $5.28 \pm 2.01\ mg_{carotenoids}\ g_{biomass}^{-1}$ and $1.86 \pm 0.06\ mg_{carotenoids}\ g_{biomass}^{-1}$ when using Tomadol 25-7 and Pluronic P-123 as the surfactants, respectively. In contrast, the conventional extraction method using ethanol as the solvent yielded $6.48 \pm 0.01\ mg_{carotenoids}\ g_{biomass}^{-1}$ of carotenoids (Flávia Vieira et al. 2017). This investigation delineated that fresh algal biomass afforded more carotenoids when compared with the dried counterparts and the use of nonionic surfactants avoids the use of organic solvents like ethanol.

Table 12.2 Summary of astaxanthin extraction methods and yields from *Haematococcus pluvialis* (Mahfuzur et al. 2016)

Astaxanthin extraction/purification method	Astaxanthin yield/ extraction efficiency
$scCO_2$ at 20 MPa, 55 °C, 13% (w/w) ethanol, 120 minutesa	83% recovery
$scCO_2$ expanded ethanol (50% [w/w] ethanol), 7 MPa, 45 °C, 120 minutes	124.2% recovery
$scCO_2$ at 20 MPa, 60 °C, 2 ml of ethanol for 1 hour	2.45 mg g^{-1} dry weight
$scCO_2$, co-solvent 0.154–1% (v/v) ethanol, 7–34 MPa, 30–80 °C, 0–100 minutes	74% recovery
$scCO_2$, co-solvent 1.25–8.75% (v/v) ethanol, 30–50 MPa, 35–75 °C, 210 minutes	87.4% recovery
$scCO_2$, co-solvent 0–12% (v/v) vegetable oils, 30–50 MPa, 50–80 °C, 300 minutes	51% recovery
$scCO_2$, co-solvent, 30–50 MPa, 40–80 °C, 60–240 minutes	84% recovery
$scCO_2$, co-solvent, 1.67–7.5% (v/v) ethanol 20–55 MPa 40–80 °C, 240 minutes	80% recovery
$scCO_2$, co-solvent 0–10% (v/v) ethanol 20–30 MPa, 40–60 °C	90% recovery
$scCO_2$, co-solvent 0-9.4% (w/w) ethanol, 30 MPa, 60 °C	97% recovery
Cell germination (12 hours), ionic liquid (1-ethyl-3-methylimidazolium ethylsulfate), 24 hours	32.5 pg $cell^{-1}$
Direct extraction using liquefied di-methyl ether at 0.59 MPa, 25 °C	1 (mg g^{-1} cell)
HCl : acetone (5:5 v/v%), 70 °C, 20 minutes	19.8 (mg g^{-1} cell)
Ultrasonication in solvent (ethyl acetate and ethanol), 16 minutes, 41 °C, 40 kHz, 200 W, EtOH : ethyl acetate (20:1)	28 (mg g^{-1})
Grinding three repetitions, pressurized hexane (10.3 MPa)	35 (mg g^{-1} cell)
Treating with enzymes (Viscozyme, Alcalase), 50 °C, 2 hours	2649 ± 359 μg g^{-1} cell
Dodecane, 48 hours, saponification with methanolic NaOH (0.02 M), sedimentation in darkness, 4 °C, 12 hours	85% efficiency
2 N HCl, 70 °C, acetone, 1 hour	87% efficiency
NaOH 30 min, acetone, 15 hours	7 (mg g^{-1} cell)
40% (v/v) acetone for 2 minutes at 80 °C, followed by lyophilization or treatment with specific lytic enzymes	70% recovery

[a] $scCO_2$, supercritical carbon dioxide.

As compared with other macro- and microalgae, *H. pluvialis* yielded higher amounts of the commercially important carotenoids such as lutein (75–80%), β-carotene (10–20%), as well as other types of carotenoids such as violaxanthin, neoxanthin, lactucaxanthin, and zeaxanthin at an early stage. The total carotenoid content could be improved, especially astaxanthin content, up to 80–99% of total carotenoids by employing various cultivating conditions (Mahfuzur et al. 2016). Mahfuzur et al. (2016) summarized various extraction techniques and yields of astaxanthin recovery presented in Table 12.2. The discussion indicated that $scCO_2$ along with the presence of 50% ethanol as co-solvent could afford 124.2% recovery of astaxanthin when compared with the extract using $scCO_2$ alone (Table 12.2). As compared with other extraction techniques, SCF seems to be a promising extraction technique that could be adopted for most of the algal species.

Although the separation of carotenoids using conventional SLE is a simple method, it has several limitations, which includes selectivity toward carotenoids due to its structural similarities and high solvent consumption, all of which promote the continuous quest for innovative and economical extraction technologies (Mahesha Poojary et al. 2016).

12.4 Biological Properties of Carotenoids and Possible Health Effects

12.4.1 Cancer Prevention

Carotenoids are additionally utilized in food supplements, cosmetics, and pharmaceuticals (Becker 2004; Guedes et al. 2011; Athreya and Xavier 2017). Numerous *in vitro* and *in vivo* investigations have demonstrated that carotenoids have activity against various types of cancer (Ziegler 1989; Mein et al. 2008; Sathasivam and Ki 2018). The findings from these studies propose that carotenoids may reduce the risk factors for various types of cancer in humans, especially bladder, breast, hepatic, intestinal, leukemic, lung, oral, and prostate cancer (Nishino et al. 2002). The anticancer activity of carotenoids involves varied mechanisms, including induction of cell apoptosis and suppression of cell proliferation. For instance, carotenoids showed anticancer activity against human colorectal adenocarcinoma cell lines such as Caco-2, DLD-1, and HT-29 at a concentration of 15.2 mM (Sathasivam and Ki 2018). β-carotene, astaxanthin, capsanthin, and bixin inhibited the proliferation and decreased the viability of leukemia K562 cells at 8 μM (Zhang et al. 2012).

Astaxanthin has been found to have a role in directing CYP (Cytochrome p450) genes in rat hepatocytes. Additionally, carotenoids are effective inducers of communication between cells at the cell-gap junctions (the water-filled pores in the cell membranes that permit the cell-to-cell communications needed to change tumor cell development and specifically to constrain growth of cancerous cells). In cultured hepatocytes, 100 mg of astaxanthin (3-hydroxy-4-oxo-beta-ionol and 3-hydroxy-4-oxo-beta-ionone) was a significant inducer of the major cytochrome P450 enzyme, CYP3A4, as well as of CYP2B6, but not of other CYPs, including those from CYP1A and CYP2C families (Kistler 2002). Some types of carotenoids have increasingly strong anticarcinogenic activity compared with β-carotene and may be progressively valuable for cancer prevention (Bertram 2001; Vineis et al. 2004; Cardozo et al. 2007). Most of the carotenoids have therapeutic merit, such as β-carotene, astaxanthin, lutein, zeaxanthin, violaxanthin, fucoxanthin, which have anticancer, antitumoral, and anti-inflammatory efficacies, due to their powerful antioxidant effect that is used to defend life forms against oxidative stress (Khan et al. 2009; Milani et al. 2017; Bule et al. 2018). Fucoxanthin has been found to have activity against cancer cells such as Caco-2, DLD-1, and HT-29, which are human colorectal adenocarcinoma cell lines (Hosokawa et al. 2004; Moghadamtousi, et al. 2014). After 72 hours of fucoxanthin treatment (15.2 mM), the viabilities of Caco-2, DLD-1, and HT-29 were reduced to 14.8, 29.4, and 50.8%, respectively (Hosokawa et al. 2004). The impact of various carotenoids such as β-cryptoxanthin, canthaxanthin, fucoxanthin, neoxanthin, phytoene, and zeaxanthin on the prostate cancer cell lines, PL-3, DU 145, and LNCaP has been explored (Kotake Nara et al.

2001). Cells were cultured in a carotenoid-supplemented medium for 72 hours at 20 $\mu M\,l^{-1}$. Neoxanthin from spinach and fucoxanthin from brown algae significantly reduced cell viability to 10.9 and 14.9% for PC-3; 15.0 and 5.0% for DU 145; and nearly zero and 9.8% for LNCaP, respectively. Meanwhile, acyclic carotenoids such as phytofluene, zeta-carotene, and lycopene, all of which are present in tomatos, also considerably reduced cell viability (Kotake Nara et al. 2001).

12.4.2 Antioxidant Activities

The most important biological roles of carotenoids are identified with their antioxidant properties in humans, which occur due to their molecular structure (Abdalla 2003). ROS-induced oxidative stress mechanisms and the methodologies to battle against oxidative stress have been studied in depth (Sharma et al. 2012; Murthy et al. 2002). Astaxanthin (AX) is an important antioxidant as its activity is 10 times greater than that of zeaxanthin, lutein, canthaxanthin, and β-carotene, and 100 times greater than α-tocopherol (Miki 1991; Higuera-Ciapara et al. 2006). Chew et al. (1999) fed mice with a diet containing 0, 0.1%, and 0.4% AX, β-carotene, or canthaxanthin over 3 weeks before inoculating the mammary fat pad with tumor cells. When comparing the antioxidant activities of carotenoid derivatives such as astaxanthin, lutein, lycopene, α-carotene, β-carotene, α-tocopherol, and 6-hydroxy-2,5,7,8-tetramethylchroman-2-carboxylic acid against peroxyl radicals, astaxanthin was the most successful antioxidant (Naguib 2000). Antioxidant activity was assessed using a fluorometric assay based on 4,4-difluoro-3,5-bis(4-phenyl-1,3-butadienyl)-4-bora-3a,4a-diaza-s-indacene (BODIPY 665/676) as an indicator; 2,2′-azobis-2,4-dimethylvaleronitrile (AMVN) as a peroxyl radical generator; and 6-hydroxy-2,5,7,8-tetramethylchroman-2-carboxylic acid (Trolox) as a control in an organic and liposomal media (Naguib 2000). The relative reactivities of astaxanthin, β-carotene, α-tocopherol, and lutein were found to be 1.00, 0.9, 0.6, and 0.6, respectively (Naguib 2000).

Astaxanthin may additionally act as a powerful antioxidant and inhibit free radical chain reactions in a vast array of living organisms (Lorenz and Cysewski 2000; Hussein et al. 2006; Ranga Rao et al. 2010). Free astaxanthin is especially susceptible to oxidation (Hussein et al. 2006). Dietary astaxanthin showed significant reduction in the elastin bands in rat aorta. It also significantly decreased the (wall:lumen) aerial ratio of the coronary arteries. These results suggest that astaxanthin can modulate the oxidative condition and may improve vascular elastin and arterial wall thickness in hypertension. Edge et al. (2010) revealed that β-carotene, lycopene, zeaxanthin, and astaxanthin showed an oxidation ability against guanosine and also helped in minimizing development of guanosine. Moreover, the reaction of carotenoid with the oxidized guanosine produced the radical cation of the carotenoid. Palozza and Krinsk (1992) reported that β-carotene and α-tocopherol can act synergistically as an effective "radical-trapping antioxidant" in biological membranes. The inhibition of lipid peroxidation by a blend of the two fat-soluble antioxidants was shown to be superior to the sum of the individual inhibitions. Carotenoids being antioxidants might prevent lipid peroxidation (Chisté et al. 2014). β-carotene is a strong antioxidant that can protect against cardiovascular diseases (Zhang et al. 2014). Lycopene is able to reduce the danger of cancer and is also involved in the obstruction of different diseases because of its antioxidant properties (Rao and Rao 2007). Oxidative damage to DNA has been significantly reduced by 20% by consumption of lycopene, which possibly prevents cancer, especially prostate cancer (Rao and Rao 2007).

12.4.3 Antidiabetic Activity

Diabetes mellitus is effectively related to oxidative stress, which can be an impact of higher-level production of free radicals, a decrease in the level of antioxidant defenses, or both. Oxidative stress induced by hyperglycemia leads to dysfunction of pancreatic β-cells and different types of tissue damage in patients with diabetes mellitus (Bajaj and Khan 2012). Astaxanthin, shows potential in preventing and treating type II diabetes (Sathsivam and Ki 2018). Nakano et al. (2008) revealed the impact of astaxanthin at approx. $0.1\,g\,kg^{-1}$ in a mixture with antioxidants such as ascorbic acid and α-tocopherol against oxidative damage in streptozotocin-stimulated diabetic osteogenic disorder Shionogi (ODS) rats, and demonstrated that astaxanthin in a blend with α-tocopherol could reduce the effect of oxidative damage through the control of oxidative stress initiated by type II diabetes. The research revealed the promising potential of fucoxanthin isolated from the edible brown algae *Eisenia bicyclis* and *Undaria pinnatifida* as a therapeutic intervention for the management of diabetes as well as diabetes-associated complications. Fucoxanthin showed promising inhibitory activity against advanced glycation end-product (AGE) formation and human recombinant aldose reductase (HRAR) and rat lens aldose reductase (RLAR) activity, which was confirmed with enzyme inhibition in a 3D structure of Tyrosine-protein phosphatase non-receptor type 1 also known as protein-tyrosine phosphatase 1B (PTP1B) using Autodock 4.0 to simulate the binding of fucoxanthin (Jung et al. 2012). Another report supported the hypothesis that fucoxanthin isolated from *U. pinnatifida* suppresses the development of hyperglycemia and hyperinsulinemia by activating the insulin signaling pathway, including glucose transporter type 4 (GLUT4) translocation, and inducing GLUT4 expression in the soleus and extensor digitorum longus muscles, respectively, of diabetic/obese KK-Ay mice with a 0.2% fucoxanthin-containing diet (Nishikawa et al. 2012).

Fucoxanthin has great potential as an antidiabetic agent (Nishikawa et al. 2012). An investigation of fucoxanthin reports that treatment with this carotenoid can restore blood glucose and insulin levels to normal in diabetic/obese mice when the animals are treated with feed containing 0.2% fucoxanthin for 2 weeks (Nishikawa et al. 2012).

Recent research on carotenoids has proved that whether type I or type II, this disease has serious macro- and microvascular complications that constitute the primary cause of morbidity and death. In the past few years, four nonprovitamin A carotenoids, lutein, zeaxanthin, lycopene, and astaxanthin, have been used to prevent the development and progression of diabetic microvascular complications (Murillo and Fernandez 2016)

A few studies have confirmed that levels of dietary carotenoids and concentrations of β-carotene in the blood reduce fasting blood glucose levels and elevated insulin levels in diabetic patients (Ylonen et al. 2003; Sluijs et al. 2015). It has been observed that carotenoid intake is inversely related to HbA1c (hemoglobin A1c) levels (Suzuki et al. 2002; Sluijs et al. 2015). In addition, carotenoids such as lycopene, lutein, and zeaxanthin can act against diabetic retinopathy (Brazionis et al. 2009; Hu et al. 2011). Most of the studies on carotenoids and diabetes report the significance of dietary intake of carotenoids for the prevention and treatment of type II diabetes (Stahl and Sies 2005; Jung et al. 2012; Nishikawa et al. 2012).

Eating a diet rich in carotenoids, especially provitamin A carotenoids, may have helped prevent the development of type II diabetes in Japanese male and female patients aged 30–79 years. The highest tertiles of serum α-carotene, β-cryptoxanthin, and total provitamin A carotenoids against the lowest tertiles supported the hypothesis that they have a vital role in type II diabetes prevention (Sugiura et al. 2015). In addition, studies have demonstrated the connections between serum concentrations of carotenoids, smoking, and the occurrence of diabetes mellitus over time (Hozawa et al. 2006; Brazionis et al. 2009; Sathasivam and Ki 2018; Ramaraj and Ki 2018).

12.4.4 Skin Diseases

Carotenoids may exhibit bioactivity providing photoprotection by means of a photooxidative process in the skin occurring as a reaction to harmful UV light, associated with scavenging of ROS and anti-inflammatory properties (Akyon 2002; Sies and Stahl 2004). Astaxanthin has been described as exerting anti-inflammatory effects while preserving essential lipids and proteins in human lymphocytes when they were treated with 5 μM of astaxanthin, which may be because of superoxide dismutase and catalase enzyme activities (Bolin et al. 2010). The combination of astaxanthin (2 μM) and vitamin C proved to be a powerful antioxidant in human lymphocytes as shown by the marked reduction in superoxide anion, and hydrogen peroxide production as well as increased glutathione (GSH) content, GSH:glutathione disulfide (GSSG) ratio, and glutathione peroxidase (GPx) and glutathione reductase (GR) activities (Bolin et al. 2010).

Other reports have compared the modulation of UVA irradiation by astaxanthin, canthaxanthin, and β-carotene for photoprotection in human dermal fibroblasts, and showed that astaxanthin exhibited a pronounced photoprotective impact and counteracted UVA induced modifications in human dermal fibroblasts (HDF), as detected by MTT assay when treated with 10 μM of astaxanthin (Camera et al. 2009). Uptake of 10 μM of astaxanthin by fibroblasts was greater than that of canthaxanthin and β-carotene, suggesting that astaxanthin may exert a greater preventive effect toward photooxidative changes (Camera et al. 2009). Recently, Suganuma et al. (2010) observed the effect of astaxanthin on the induction of matrix metalloproteinase-1 and skin fibroblast elastase caused by UVA irradiation of cultured human dermal fibroblasts. Among the different cytokines tested they found that astaxanthin only significantly diminished IL-6 secretion (Suganuma et al. 2010). These studies suggest that topical or oral administration of astaxanthin may counteract UVA radiation effects including skin sagging or wrinkling (Lyons and O'Brien 2002). The synthetic carotenoid also prevented DNA damage in both HEMAc and CaCo-2 cells at lower concentrations (10 nM, 100 nM, 10 μM) (Lyons and O'Brien 2002).

12.4.5 Antimicrobial Activities

Carotenoids are an important group of natural pigments with specific applications as colorants, food supplements, and nutraceuticals; they are also used for medical, cosmetic, and biotechnological purposes, especially antimicrobial activity against strains of *Staphylococcus aureus*, and β-lactamase-producing cultures of *Escherichia coli*, *Pseudomonas aeruginosa*, and *Klebsiella* sp. (Kirti et al. 2014). Astaxanthin has also health benefits as an antimicrobial agent, boosting the immune system, exhibiting bioactivity against *Helicobacter pylori*, and preventing cataract because of its high antioxidant activity, which has been examined by *in vitro* studies and preclinical trials (Kirti et al. 2014).

12.4.6 Wound Healing

β-carotene plays a major role within the wound healing process and also the body's immune response (Chow and Barbul 2014). It enhances macrophage influx and activation in skin cell injuries, stimulates fibroblasts to synthesize collagen, and augments cellular proliferation (Patel et al. 2012). Another study reported that the carotenoids may stimulate attacks on foreign cells after the skin has been broken and will facilitate a quick healing of wounds (Rojas et al. 2002). Carotenoids have been shown to significantly enhance the release of interleukin-1α and tumor necrosis factor-α from murine peritoneal adherent cells. Carotenoids such as β-carotene, canthaxanthin, and astaxanthin have possible immuno-modulating activities to enhance the proliferation and functions of murine immune-competent cells (Okai and Higashi-Okai 1996). Researchers showed that vitamin A intensifies the cross-linking as well as tensile strength of wounds (Greenwald et al.1990). Vitamin A, believed to be an antioxidant, increases fibroblast proliferation, collagen, and proteoglycan synthesis, and decreases the matrix metalloproteinase (MMP) levels to prevent degradation of extracellular matrix (ECM) in the healing process (Burgess 2008). Vitamin A increases macrophage influx and activation in wounds, stimulates fibroblasts to synthesize collagen, and increases cellular proliferation (Zaidi et al. 2005).

12.4.7 Miscellaneous Biological Activities

Carotenoids, especially astaxanthin, are efficient for improving muscle tiredness. Astaxanthin can be used as a supplement to improve antioxidant defenses against oxidative damage induced by exhaustive exercise in soleus muscles and plasma. Long-term 1 mg astaxanthin kg^{-1} body weight (BW) supplementation in Wistar rats (for 45 days) significantly delayed time to exhaustion by 29% in a swimming test (Polotow et al. 2014). Remarkably, young men taking natural Astaxanthin showed no increase whatsoever in joint soreness in their knees. It appeared that natural Astaxanthin at a moderate dose of 4 mg day^{-1} completely prevented joint pain after exercise (Fry 2001). Another study also proved that astaxanthin accumulated in gastrocnemius and heart. Astaxanthin can attenuate exercise-induced damage in mouse skeletal muscle and heart, including an associated neutrophil infiltration that induces further damage in C57BL/6 mice (Aoi et al. 2003). The main sources of ROS generation as a result of exercise are the mitochondrial electron transport chain, xanthine oxidase, and phagocytes (Evans 2000). Biological activities ascribed to astaxanthin include anti-inflammatory, immunomodulatory, and neuroprotective effects (Hussein et al. 2006). Humans fed a β-carotene and astaxanthin supplement had enhanced testes weight, sperm count, and sperm head morphology as compared with cyclophosphamide-treated animals, representing the chemoprotective capability of astaxanthin against cyclophosphamide-induced germ cell toxicity in mice (Leon et al. 2003). The administration of β-carotene-rich *Dunaliella* alga inhibited low-density lipoprotein (LDL) oxidation and reduced plasma triglycerides and LDL levels from 140 to 100 mg dl^{-1} and from 1000 to 600 mg dl^{-1}, respectively, and increased high-density lipoprotein (HDL) level from 125 to 140 mg dl^{-1} with 6–10 weeks of treatment in a mouse model (Shaish et al. 2009).

β-carotene-rich *Dunaliella* alga inhibited significantly plasma cholesterol elevation and atherosclerosis progression in $ApoE^{-/-}$ deficient mice fed a high fat diet (Harari et al. 2013). Carotenoids may have preventive and protective effects in various chronic diseases such as diabetes mellitus, metabolic syndrome, cancer, and cardiovascular diseases (Sathsivam and Ki 2018; Sathasivam et al. 2018). It has been reported that a diet rich in carotenoids may decrease the severity of disorders caused by *H. pylori* (Fiedor et al. 2001). Antioxidant and anti-inflammatory properties of astaxanthin and β-carotene may contribute to inhibition of *H. pylori*-induced gastric inflammation. Astaxanthin changes *H. pylori*-induced activation of T helper cell type 1 response toward T helper cell type 2 responses in the infected tissues (Kang and Kim 2017). Astaxanthin can exert preventive actions against atherosclerosis via its potential to improve inflammation, lipid metabolism, and glucose metabolism (Iwamoto et al. 2000; Park et al. 2010; Yoshida et al. 2010; Ursoniu et al. 2015).

12.5 Potential Commercial Applications

According to recent research, carotenoids had a market value of US$1.65 billion in 2018, which was predicted to rise to US$2.16 billion by 2026 at a rate of 3.5% (Globe Newswire 2019). The main sources of carotenoids in the global market include annatto, astaxanthin, β-carotene, β-apo-8-carotenal, β-apo-8-carotenal-ester, canthaxanthin, capsanthin, paprika extract, lutein, lycopene, and zeaxanthin (BCC Research 2018). These carotenoids were mostly used for food, feed, nutraceutical supplements, and cosmetics. Although these carotenoids are obtainable from diverse sources, algal-based carotenoids possess an enormous share of the global market (BCC Research 2018) due to their potential functional properties.

There are various species of microalgae used in the production of carotenoids and its derivatives, which are used as they grow more rapidly than macroalgae (Ishika et al. 2019). Additionally, the global market depends on versatile sources of microalgae to meet the challenges connected with cultivation of specific species, climatic conditions, and cost-effective technology in isolation (Vaz et al. 2016). Some specific Chlorophyta strains such as *D. salina*, *H. pluvialis*, *C. vulgaris*, *Chlorella zofingiensis*, and *Chlorella pyrenoidosa* have been utilized in the large-scale manufacturing of carotenes, astaxanthin, canthaxanthin, lutein, and other carotenoids (Janchot et al. 2019). Recent global market research shows that *Spirulina*, *Chlorella*, and *D. salina* account for the major share of the manufacture of algal-based carotenoids (Persistence Market Research 2018).

12.5.1 Microalgal Carotenoids in Commercial Applications

A recent report shows that Asia, North America, Latin America, and Europe produce an enormous mass of microalgae. The mass production of microalgae such as *Chlorella* and *Spirulina* is mainly from Asia and the United States but these microalgae are grown in various tropical countries like Mexico as well (Lozano-Garcia et al. 2019). Together *Chlorella* and *Spirulina* are the main microalgae worldwide, with 5000 and 2000 t DW year^{-1} produced of each with an estimated value of US$40 million year^{-1} for each (Milledge 2012). This growth rate shows the interest in using microalgae-based products as a source of bioactive food and feed items (Vigani et al. 2015). *Dunaliella salina* is well suited for large-scale production with amounts as much as approx. 14% DW (Sathasivam et al. 2014). This alga tends to grow outside in open lakes under humid conditions, which requires low accessibility of nitrogen, hyper saline, and enormous amounts of UV radiation (Chu 2012). The β-carotene content of *Spirulina* accounts for 140 mg per 100 g wet weight, *Chlorella* consists of 180 mg wet weight, and *H. pluvialis* contains 16.7% (DW). Other carotenoids such as neoxanthin (8.3%), violaxanthin (12.5%), astaxanthin (5%), lutein (56.3%), and zeaxanthin (6.3%) have been found in *H. pluvialis* with some trace amounts of adonixanthin, canthaxanthin, adonirbin, etc. (Borowitzka 2013). The cultivation of *Dunaliella* as a source of β-carotene is increasing with active industrial plants found around the world, including Australia, Israel, the United States, and China with yearly production of dry *Dunaliella* biomass of around 1200 t annually (Milledge 2012).

12.5.2 Commercial Applications of Astaxanthin and Lutein

Astaxanthin is projected to undergo a compound annual growth rate (CAGR) of 4.2% from 2018 to 2024 due to consumer demands for its health benefits (BCC Research 2018). This can be attributed to various benefits; for example, better pigmentation in feed, and better health benefits compared with the petroleum-based synthetic pigments (An et al. 2014). Market research shows that worldwide requirement for astaxanthin is anticipated to rise from US$615.19 million in 2016 to US$1226.14 million by 2023 with a CAGR of 10.3% (James 2017). However, algal astaxanthin adds up to <1% of the worldwide market as compared with the synthetic alternative (Panis et al. 2016). The nutraceutical industries evaluated to have the largest volume of *H. pluvialis* for regular supply of astaxanthin in 2017 represented 54.8% of the global market, and will probably achieve 190 metric t by 2024 (BCC Research 2018). There are a few microalgae strains accounting for the potential production of astaxanthin, such as *Chlorella* sp., *Chlorococcum* sp., and *Scenedesmus* sp. Compared with all these algae, astaxanthin biomass has been accumulated more in *H. pluvialis* in the range of approx. 4% of dry biomass (Wang et al. 2019). The major commercial application of astaxanthin is in aquaculture as a natural substitute for color in feed for salmon, trout, and shrimps (Bishop and Zubeck 2012). It is used as an antioxidant in the cosmetic industry for skin care and antiaging (Hillol et al. 2012). Even astaxanthin-fortified foods and beverages have been used nowadays mainly for sports endurance drinks (Sidari and Tofalo 2019). This color pigment mainly derived from *H. pluvialis* has great natural healing potential as an antiulcerative agent, in immunomodulation, and as a mutant cell inhibitor (Enzing et al. 2014).

The lutein contents (g kg^{-1} biomass) of microalgae include *Chlorella fusca* (4.24), *Chlorococcum citroforme* (7.4), *Coelastrum proboscideum* (3.4–5.0), *Neospondiococcum gelatinosum* (4.4), *Tetracysis aplanosporum* (5.9), *Tetracystis intermedium* (3.5), *Tetracystis tetrasporum* (4.4), and *Chlorella zofingiensis* (2.4–2.8). Approximately 5 g kg^{-1} of DW lutein was recovered from *Scenedesmus* sp. and *Desmodesmus* sp. (Lin et al. 2015). However, high temperature brought about an increase in the lutein content found in some species like *D. salina*, *Scenedesmus almeriensis*, and *Muriellopsis*. As referred to by many researchers the most promising microalgae for the production of lutein are *Muriellopsis* sp., *Scenedesmus* sp., *Chlorella zofingensis*, *Chlorella protothecoides*, *Galdieria sulphuraria*, and *Scenedesmus* sp. (Chan et al. 2013; Wells et al. 2017; Asker et al. 2018), although no lutein extraction plant as of now utilizes microalgal biomass as a source of widespread production. The largest of the extraction plants were under 10 ha and more recently plants of 200 ha have been operational (Acién et al. 2017).

Therefore, the global market mainly focuses on *Spirulina*, *Chlorella*, and *Dunaliella*, broadly utilized in food and pharmaceutical manufacturing for therapeutic purposes (Sidari and Tofalo 2019). The carotenoid derivatives are delivering an assortment of health and nutraceutical supplements in the form of powders, tablets, soft gels, and capsules (Enzing et al. 2014). Further, the food industry uses these three microalgae as a nutrient supplement incorporated into noodles, wholemeal cookies, breads, rolls, confections, desserts, and other nutritional supplements to improve nutritive value and well-being (Liang et al. 2004; Kadam and Prabhasankar 2010; Hossain et al. 2017). The world's largest producers of algal carotenoids are Earthwise *Spirulina*, Neo Algae, Regenurex, BioAstin, Algoma, AstaReal, Nutrex-Hawaii Hawaiian, Astapure®, Bulk Supplements, Taiwan Chlorella Manufacturing Company, Biophyto® Premium Spirulina, Apogen®, and Nutrilite. All these products mainly target potential health problems such as antiviral, antiaging, pigmentation, ocular regeneration, cardiovascular and neurological health, nutritional supplements, etc., and are registered under international associations like the Natural Algae Astaxanthin Association, USA (Sharma and Sharma 2017).

12.5.3 Macroalgal Carotenoids in Commercial Applications

Macroalgae are well known for diverse carotenoids; for example, fucoxanthin, β-carotene, lutein, and siphonaxanthin (Ganesan et al. 2011; Kavalappa et al. 2019). As per a recent report, seaweed (macroalgae) global market shares will increase 11.4% CAGR from 2018 to 2024, and among this 11.8% of human consumption is mostly derived from red seaweed sources (Persistence Market Research 2018). A few species of brown seaweeds such as *Macrocystis pyrifera*, *Hizikia fusiformis*, and *U. pinnatifida* are common in coastal zones of the North Pacific Ocean. However, macroalgae have different carotenoid derivatives, which contain only ~0.05% fucoxanthin (Nunes et al. 2019), owing to low quantification and a tedious process of extraction that increases production costs as compared with microalgae. Some potential producers of seaweed fucoxanthin are TNvitamins, BRI nutrition, Solaray, Best Naturals, Eden Pond, Vitacost, Pure control supplements, Modifilan, Garden of life, Only Natural, and Source Naturals (Grimes 2019). All these producers were using different species of brown seaweed as the principal sources for the production of fucoxanthin in combination with other natural sources like pomegranate and green leaves (Algahealth 2019).

12.5.4 Nutraceutical Supplements

The utilization of algal carotenoids as foodstuffs has been growing due to concerns over comfort and safety measures in terms of side effects. The US Food and Drug Administration (FDA) and European Food Safety Authority (EFSA) have accepted algal-based carotenoids as a nutraceutical supplement under the category GRAS (generally recognized as safe); for example, petroleum-based carotenoid derivatives have been identified to cause lung malignancy and cardiovascular illnesses (Vigani et al. 2015). Therefore, natural-based carotenoid pigments could support various health benefits and these compounds have been included in many food items and blended with sports and energy drinks, bars, soups, pudding, bread, cake mixture, and biscuits (Enzing et al. 2014). For example, *S. platensis* has been added to bread as a substitute for gluten, *H. pluvialis* astaxanthin has been added to sports drinks, etc. (Selmo and Salas-Mellado 2014). As *Spirulina* is commonly known for a high protein content, this also contains carotenoids as a useful compound with the functional properties of antihypercholesterol agent and antihypertensive supplement (Spolaore et al. 2006; Lafarga 2019).

12.5.5 Commercial Application of Algal Carotenoids in Feed

Algal feed is very common in livestock diets, such as feed for poultry and pigs, although no isolated compound is added to the feed (Abdelnour et al. 2019). Approximately 30% of algae harvested and cultivated around the world is utilized in animal diets; for example, *Chlorella* for laying hens (0.5–1% of diet) (Grigorova et al. 2006). Addition of *Sargassum dentifolium* caused a considerable rise in the level of carotenes (22–25 $mg\,kg^{-1}$), lutein plus zeaxanthin (15.5–16.6 $mg\,kg^{-1}$), linoleic acid (0.35–0.51 $mg\,g^{-1}$), and omega 9 fatty acid (6.5–8.2 $mg\,g^{-1}$) contents in the egg yolk (Al-Harthi and El-Deek, 2012). These researchers found that lutein-fortified *Chlorella* improves the lutein absorption in the hen's eggs. Similarly, increasing the quantity of *Chlorella* from 0.5 to 1% in feed increases the egg yolk color from 6.0 to 11.0 (Roche egg color fan); this outcome suggests that the dietary lutein from *Chlorella* is rapidly retained in the serum and liver of laying hens and affects the developing oocyte (An et al. 2014). Predominantly, this diet improves the production of lutein-improved chicken eggs (An et al. 2014).

Fishmeal is usually utilized in fish feed, though, in recent times growth and expansion of the algal industry has led to increased monetary and ecological benefits for the growth of healthy fish to enter into the food chain. Astaxanthin, like alternative carotenoids, is not made by *de novo* synthesis by aquatic heterotrophs. They have to either obtain it through their diet or change the dietary carotenoid precursors through metabolic reactions to increase their supplies (Li and Liu 2019). Macroalgae including *Porphyra dioica* were fed to rainbow trout resulting in a dark orange pigmentation of flesh as compared with the whitish color of control fish. This pigmentation impact on fish muscle by including *P. dioica* in the feed is of substantial interest to the natural salmon-cultivating industry (Soler-Vila et al. 2009).

12.6 Conclusions and Future Recommendations

The commercial utilization of carotenoids seems to be one of the foremost flourishing areas of investigation in blue biotechnology (a branch of biotechnology that utilizes aquatic organisms). The growing market demand for pigments isolated from natural sources has promoted the large-scale cultivation of microalgae for the synthesis of such compounds, thus important decreases in production costs are predicted in coming years. The production of carotenoids by adopting an appropriate biotechnological process, with the added advantage of low cost, high yields, and decreased processing time would be preferred. Information concerning these processes is vital to lead to new technologies within the production of microbial carotenoids.

The significant antioxidant and health-promoting properties of the carotenoids within living organisms have generated enormous interest among behavioral ecologists and researchers. Most of the research completed to date has been based on animal models and *in vitro* models, and the potency of microalgae carotenoids in humans has also been evaluated in some cases.

The recognized therapeutic value of some of the carotenoids in the prevention and treatment of degenerative diseases has therefore opened up new roads for the advancement of large-scale production systems.

Seaweed carotenoids have found several potential biological activities with extensive scope in the supplement and nutraceutical industries. In addition, the molecular mechanisms, actions, and interactions of the anticancer activities of seaweed carotenoids need to be determined through more investigations. Future clinical reviews should center on small and large patient cohorts that are healthy or with chronic disease risk factors. It is still necessary to understand their biological mechanisms of action to determine their efficacy in the potential prevention and treatment of chronic diseases. Although there are several ongoing investigations into the applications of carotenoids to exploit them for healthcare, most of these investigations have used animal models rather than human clinical trials for assessment. It is recommended that the forthcoming areas of analysis should also concentrate on human clinical trials. It is anticipated that such investigations will enable researchers to recognize the potential applications of carotenoids in growing techniques for the prevention, treatment, and management of diseases.

Acknowledgments

The authors would like to thank Dr. N. Shettu, Associate Professor & Head of PG and Research Department of Zoology, Pachaiyappa's College, Chennai, for providing a supportive environment and tireless support while preparing this chapter. In addition, the authors thank Ms. R. Dhanalakshmi and Ms. V.Vinitha for providing documentation support.

References

Abdalla, D.S.P. (2003). *Encyclopedia of Food Sciences and Nutrition*, Coronary Heart Disease | Antioxidant Status, 2e (eds. B.C. Paul and F.F. Toldra), 1654–1663. London: Academic Press.

Abdel-Aal, E.-S.M., Akhtar, H., Zaheer, K., and Ali, R. (2013). Dietary sources of lutein and zeaxanthin carotenoids and their role in eye health. *Nutrients* **13** (5): 1169–1185.

Abdelnour, S., El-Hack, M.A., Arif, M. et al. (2019). The application of the microalgae *Chlorella* spp. as a supplement in broiler feed. *World's Poultry Science Journal* **75** (2): 305–318.

Abe, K., Hattori, H., and Hirano, M. (2007). Accumulation and antioxidant activity of secondary carotenoids in the aerial microalga *Coelastrella striolata* var. multistriata. *Food Chemistry* **100**: 656–661.

Acién, F.G., Molina, E., Fernández-Sevilla, J.M. et al. (2017). Economics of microalgae production. In: *Microalgae-Based Biofuels and Bioproducts* (eds. R. Muñoz and C. Gonzalez-Fernandez), 485–503. Cambridge: Woodhead Publishers.

Akyon, Y. (2002). Effect of antioxidants on the immune response of *Helicobacter pylori*. *Clinical Microbiological Infections* **8**: 438–441.

Algahealth. (2019). Growing microalgal sources of fucoxanthin. AlgaHealth Grant agreement.

Al-Harthi, M.A., and El-Deek, A.A. (2012). Effect of different dietary concentrations of brown marine algae (*Sargassum dentifebium*) prepared by different methods on plasma and yolk lipid profiles, yolk total carotene and lutein plus zeaxanthin of laying hens. *Italian Journal of Animal Science*, 11(4): e64.

An, B.K., Jeon, J.Y., Kang, C.W. et al. (2014). The tissue distribution of lutein in laying hens fed lutein fortified *Chlorella* and production of chicken eggs enriched with lutein. *Korean Journal for Food Science of Animal Resources* **34** (2): 172–177.

Aoi, W., Naito, Y., Sakuma, K., and Kuchide, M. (2003). Astaxanthin limits exercise-induced skeletal and cardiac muscle damage in mice. *Antioxidants & Redox Signaling* **5** (1): 139–144.

Aryee, A.N.A., Agyei, D., and Akanbi, T.O. (2018). Recovery and utilization of seaweed pigments in food processing. *Current Opinion in Food Science* **19**: 113–119.

Asker, D. and Awad, T.S. (2019). Isolation and characterization of a novel lutein-producing marine microalga using high throughput screening. *Food Research International* **116**: 660–667.

Asker, D., Awad, T.S., Beppu, T., and Ueda, K. (2018). Screening and profiling of natural ketocarotenoids from environmental aquatic bacterial isolates. *Food Chemistry* **253**: 247–254.

Athreya, K. and Xavier, M.F. (2017). Antioxidants in the treatment of cancer. *Nutrition and Cancer* **69** (8): 1099–1104.

Aust, O., Stahl, W., Sies, H. et al. (2005). Supplementation with tomato-based products increases lycopene, phytofluene, and phytoene levels in human serum and protects against UV-light-induced erythema. *International Journal for Vitamin and Nutrition Research* **1**: 54–60.

Bajaj, S. and Khan, A. (2012). Antioxidants and diabetes. *Indian Journal of Endocrinology and Metabolism* **16**: S267–S271.

BCC Research. (2018). The global market for carotenoids. www.bccresearch.com/market-research/food-and-beverage/carotenoids-globalmarket-fod025d.html (accessed September 14, 2020).

Becker, E.W. (2004). Microalgae in human and animal nutrition. In: *Handbook of Microalgal Culture* (ed. A. Richmond), 312–351. Oxford: Blackwell.

Bertram, J.S. (2001). The molecular biology of cancer. *Molecular Aspects of Medicine* **21**: 167–223.

Bishop, W.M. and Zubeck, H.M. (2012). Evaluation of microalgae for use as nutraceuticals and nutritional supplements. *Journal of Nutrition and Food Sciences* **2** (5): 1–6.

Bocanegra, A.R.D., Legarreta, I.G., Jeronimo, F.M., and Campocosio, A.T. (2004). Influence of environmental and nutritional factors in the production of astaxanthin from *Haematococcus pluvialis*. *Bioresource Technology* **92** (2): 209–214.

Bolin, A.P., Macedo, R.C., Marin, D.P. et al. (2010). Astaxanthin prevents *in vitro* auto-oxidative injury in human lymphocytes. *Cell Biology and Toxicology* **26** (5): 457–467.

Borowitzka, M.A. (2013). High-value products from microalgae – their development and commercialization. *Journal of Applied Phycology* **25**: 743–756.

Brazionis, L., Rowley, K., Itsiopoulos, C., and O'Dea, K. (2009). Plasma carotenoids and diabetic retinopathy. *British Journal of Nutrition* **101**: 270–277.

Bule, M.H., Ahmed, I., Maqbool, F. et al. (2018). Microalgae as a source of high-value bioactive compounds. *Frontiers in Bioscience* **10**: 197–216.

Burgess, C. (2008). Topical vitamins. *Journal of Drugs in Dermatology* **7**: s2–s6.

Buyuklu, M., Kandemir, F., Ozkaraca, M. et al. (2014). Beneficial effects of lycopene against contrast medium-induced oxidative stress, inflammation, autophagy, and apoptosis in rat kidney. *Human & Experimental Toxicology* **8**: 11–15.

Camera, E., Mastrofrancesco, A., Fabbri, C., and Daubrawa, F. (2009). Astaxanthin, canthaxanthin and β-carotene differently affect UVA-induced oxidative damage and expression of oxidative stress-responsive enzymes. *Experimental Dermatology* **18**: 222–231.

Canela, A.P.R.F., Rosa, P.T.V., Marques, M.O.M., and Meireles, M.A.A. (2002). Supercritical fluid extraction of fatty acids and carotenoids from the microalgae *Spirulina maxima*. *Industrial and Engineering Chemistry Research* **41** (12): 3012–3018.

Canela Paula, A.R., Rosa Paulo, T.V., Marques Marcia, O.M., and Meireles Angela, M.A. (2002). Supercritical fluid extraction of fatty acids and carotenoids from the microalgae *Spirulina maxima*. *Industrial Engineering & Chemical Research* **41**: 3012–3018.

Cardozo, K.H., Guaratini, T., Barros, M.P. et al. (2007). Metabolites from algae with economical impact. *Comparative Biochemistry and Physiology – Part C: Toxicology & Pharmacology* **146**: 60–78.

Cerón, M.C., García-Malea, M.C., Rivas, J. et al. (2007). Antioxidant activity of *Haematococcus pluvialis* cells grown in continuous culture as a function of their carotenoid and fatty acid content. *Applied Microbiology and Biotechnology* **74** (5): 1112–1119.

Cha, K.H., Koo, S.Y., and Lee, D.U. (2008). Antiproliferative effects of carotenoids extracted from *Chlorella ellipsoidea* and *Chlorella vulgaris* on human colon cancer cells. *Journal of Agricultural and Food Chemistry* **56** (22): 10521–10526.

Chan, M.C., Ho, S.H., Lee, D.J. et al. (2013). Characterization, extraction and purification of lutein produced by an indigenous microalga *Scenedesmus obliquus* CNW-N. *Biochemical engineering Journal* **78**: 24–31.

Chen, J., Wang, Y., Benemann, J.R. et al. (2016). Microalgal industry in China: challenges and prospects. *Journal of Applied Phycology* **28**: 715–725.

Chew, B.P., Park, J.S., Wong, M.W., and Wong, T.S. (1999). A comparison of the anticancer activities of dietary beta-carotene, canthaxanthin and astaxanthin in mice in vivo. *Anticancer Research* **19**: 1849–1853.

Chisté, R.C., Freitas, M., Mercadante, A.Z., and Fernandes, E. (2014). Carotenoids are effective inhibitors of in vitro hemolysis of human erythrocytes, as determined by a practical and optimized cellular antioxidant assay. *Journal of Food Science* **79**: H1841–H1847. https://doi.org/10.1111/1750-3841.12580.

Choi, S.-A., Oh, Y.-K., Jeong, M.-J. et al. (2014). Effects of ionic liquid mixtures on lipid extraction from *Chlorella vulgaris*. *Renewable Energy* **65**: 169–174.

Chow, O. and Barbul, A. (2014). Immunonutrition: role in wound healing and tissue regeneration. *Advances in Wound Care (New Rochelle)* **3** (1): 46–53.

Chu, W.L. (2012). Biotechnological applications of microalgae. *International e-Journal of Science and Medicinal Education* **6**: 24–37.

Corol, D., Dorobantu, I.I., Toma, N., and Nitu, R. (2002). Diversity of biological functions of carotenoids. *Romanian Biotechnological Letters* **8** (1): 1067–1074.

Crupi, P., Toci, A.T., Mangini, S. et al. (2013). Determination of fucoxanthin isomers in microalgae (*Isochrysis* sp.) by high-performance liquid chromatography coupled with diode-array detector multistage mass spectrometry coupled with positive electro spray ionization. *Rapid Communication Mass Spectrometry* **27** (9): 1027–1035.

Cysewski, G.R. and Lorenz, R.T. (2004). Industrial production of microalgal cell-mass and secondary products – species of high potential. *Haematococcus*. In: *Handbook of Microalgal Culture: Biotechnology and Applied Phycology* (ed. A. Richmond), 281–288. Oxford: Blackwell Publisher.

D'Alessandro, E.B. and Filho, N.R.A. (2016). Concepts and studies on lipid and pigments of microalgae: a review. *Renewable & Sustainable Energy Reviews* **58**: 832–841.

Dambek, M., Eilers, U., Breitenbach, J. et al. (2012). Biosynthesis of fucoxanthin and diadinoxanthin and function of initial pathway genes in *Phaeodactylum tricornutum*. *Journal of Experimental Botany* **63** (15): 5607–5612.

Dayananda, C., Kumudha, A., Sarada, R., and Ravishankar, G.A. (2010). Isolation, characterization and outdoor cultivation of green microalgae *Botryococcus* sp. *Scientific Research and Essays* **5** (17): 2497–2505.

Duangkamol, R., Shotipruk, A., and Pavasant, P. (2010). Comparison of extraction methods for recovery of astaxanthin from *Haematococcus pluvialis*. *Separation Science and Technology* **46** (1): 64–70.

Dufossé, C.L., Feron, G., Mauvais, G. et al. (2005). Microorganisms and microalgae as sources of pigments for food use: a scientific oddity or an industrial reality? *Trends in Food Science & Technology* **16**: 389–406.

Edge, R., Gaikwad, P., Navaratnam, S. et al. (2010). Reduction of oxidized guanosine by dietary carotenoids: a pulse radiolysis study. *Archives of Biochemistry and Biophysics* **504**: 100–103.

Enzing, C., Ploeg, M., Barbosa, M., and Sijtsma, L. (2014). Microalgae-based products for the food and feed sector: an outlook for Europe. *JRC Scientific and policy reports*: 19–37.

Erdoğan, A., Demirel, Z., Conk Dalay, M., and Eroğlu, A.E. (2016). Fucoxanthin content of *Cylindrotheca closterium* and its oxidative stress mediated enhancement. *Turkish Journal of Fisheries and Aquatic Sciences* **16**: 499–506.

Evans, W.J. (2000). Vitamin E, vitamin C, and exercise. *American Journal of Clinical Nutrition* **72**: 647S–652S.

Fazeli, M.R., Tofighi, H., Samadi, N., and Jamalifar, H. (2006). Effects of salinity on beta-carotene production by *Dunaliella tertiolecta* DCCBC2629 isolated from the Urmia salt lake, north of Iran. *Bioresource Technology* **97**: 2453–2456.

Fiedor, J., Fiedor, L., Winkler, J. et al. (2001). Photodynamics of the bacteriochlorophyll-carotenoid system. 1. Bacteriochlorophyll-photosensitized oxygenation of β-carotene in acetone. *Photochemistry and Photobiology* **74** (1): 64–71.

Flávia Vieira, F., Ricardo Guilherme, J.R., Márcia Neves, C. et al. (2017). Single-step extraction of carotenoids from brown macroalgae using non-ionic surfactants. *Separation and Purification Technology* **172**: 268–276.

Fry, A. (2001). Astaxanthin clinical trial for delayed onset muscular soreness. Human Performance Laboratories. The University of Memphis. Report 1 August 16, 2001. https://www.cyanotech.com/pdfs/bioastin/batl26.pdf (accessed September 14, 2020).

Ganesan, P., Noda, K., Manabe, Y. et al. (2011). Siphonaxanthin, a marine carotenoid from green algae, effectively induces apoptosis in human leukemia (HL-60) cells. *Biochimica et Biophysica Acta (BBA) – General Subjects* **1810** (5): 497–503.

Gateau, H., Solymosi, K., Marchand, J., and Shoefs, B. (2016). Carotenoids of microalgae used in food industry and medicine. *Mini-Reviews in Medicinal Chemistry* **16** (999): 1–1.

Globe Newswire. (2019). carotenoids market to reach USD 2.19 billion by 2026. | Reports and data. https://www.globenewswire.com/news-release/2019/04/11/1802980/0/en/Carotenoids-Market-To-Reach-USD-2-19-Billion-By-2026-Reports-And-Data.html (accessed September 14, 2020).

Gong, M. and Bassi, A. (2016). Carotenoids from microalgae: a review of recent developments. *Biotechnology Advances* **34** (8): 1396–1412.

Goodwin, T.W. (1992). Biosynthesis of carotenoids: an overview. *Methods in Enzymology* **214**: 330–340.

Goodwin, T.W. and Britton, G. (1988). Distribution and analysis of carotenoids. In: *Plant Pigments* (ed. T.W. Goodwin), 62–132. London: Academic Press.

Goss, R. (2003). Substrate specificity of the violaxanthin de-epoxidase of the primitive green alga *Mantoniella squamata* (Prasinophyceae). *Planta* **217**: 801–812.

Grasa-López, A., Miliar-García, A., Quevedo-Corona, L. et al. (2016). *Undaria pinnatifida* and fucoxanthin ameliorate lipogenesis and markers of both inflammation and cardiovascular dysfunction in an animal model of diet-induced obesity. *Marine Drugs* **14**: 148. https://doi.org/10.3390/md14080148.

Graydon, R., Gilchrist, S.E., Young, I.S. et al. (2007). Effect of lycopene supplementation on insulin-like growth factor-1 and insulin-like growth factor binding protein-3: a double-blind, placebo-controlled trial. *European Journal of Clinical Nutrition* **61** (10): 1196–1200.

Graziani, G., Schiavo, S., Nicolai, M.A. et al. (2013). Microalgae as human food: chemical and nutritional characteristics of the thermo-acidophilic microalga *Galdieria sulphuraria*. *Food & Function* **4**: 144–152.

Greenwald, D.P., Sharzer, L.A., Padawer, J. et al. (1990). Zone II flexor tendon repair: effects of vitamins A, E, beta-carotene. *Journal of Surgical Research* **9**: 98–102.

Griendling, K.K., Touyz, R.M., Zweier, J.L. et al. (2016). Measurement of reactive oxygen species, reactive nitrogen species, and redox-dependent signaling in the cardiovascular system: a scientific statement from the American Heart Association. *Circulation Research* **119** (5): e39–e75.

Grigorova, S., Surdjiiska, S., Banskalieva, V., and Dimitrov, G. (2006). The effect of biomass from green algae of *Chlorella* genus on the biochemical characteristics of table eggs. *Journal of Central European Agriculture* **7** (1): 111–116.

Grimes, R. (2019). Best fucoxanthin supplements – top 10 brands reviewed for 2019. https://top10supps.com/best-fucoxanthin-supplements (accessed September 14, 2020).

Guedes, A.C., Amaro, H.M., and Malcata, F.X. (2011). Microalgae as sources of carotenoids. *Marine Drugs* **9** (4): 625–644.

Guerin, M., Huntley, M.E., and Olaizola, M. (2003). *Haematococcus* astaxanthin: applications for human health and nutrition. *Trends in Biotechnology* **21** (5): 210–226.

Harari, A., Abecassis, R., Relevi, N. et al. (2013). Prevention of atherosclerosis progression by 9-cis-β-carotene rich alga *Dunaliella* in apoE-deficient mice. *BioMed Research International*: 169517.

Heffernan, N., Smyth, T.J., FitzGerald, R.J. et al. (2016). Comparison of extraction methods for selected carotenoids from macroalgae and the assessment of their seasonal/spatial variation. *Innovative Food Science & Emerging Technologies* **37B**: 221–228.

Henríquez, V., Escobar, C., Galarza, J., and Gimpel, J. (2016). Carotenoids in microalgae. In: *Carotenoids in Nature* (ed. C. Stange), 219–237. Cham: Springer International Publishing.

Herrero, M. and Ibañez, E. (2018). Green extraction processes, biorefineries and sustainability: recovery of high added-value products from natural sources. *The Journal of Supercritical Fluids* **134**: 252–259.

Higuera-Ciapara, I., Félix-Valenzuela, L., and Goycoolea, F.M. (2006). Astaxanthin: a review of its chemistry and applications. *Critical Reviews in Food Science and Nutrition* **46** (2): 185–196.

Hillol, C., Shrikrishna, D.J., Dolly, W.D., and Sunil, P. (2012). Potential applications of blue green algae. *Journal of Scientific & Industrial Research* **71**: 13–20.

Hosokawa, M., Kudo, M., Maeda, H. et al. (2004). Fucoxanthin induces apoptosis and enhances the antiproliferative effect of the PPAR c-ligand, troglitazone, on colon cancer cells. *Biochimica et Biophysica Acta (BBA) – General Subjects* **1675**: 113–119.

Hossain, A.K.M., Brennan, M.A., Mason, S.L. et al. (2017). The effect of astaxanthin-rich microalgae "*Haematococcus pluvialis*" and wholemeal flours incorporation in improving the physical and functional properties of cookies. *Foods* **6** (8): 57.

Hozawa, A., Jacobs, D.R. Jr., and Steffes, M.W. (2006). Associations of serum carotenoid concentrations with the development of diabetes and with insulin concentration: interaction with smoking: the Coronary Artery Risk Development in Young Adults (CARDIA) Study. *American Journal of Epidemiology* **163**: 929–937.

Hu, B.J., Hu, Y.N., Lin, S. et al. (2011). Application of lutein and zeaxanthin in non-proliferative diabetic retinopathy. *International Journal of Ophthalmology* **4** (3): 303–306.

Hussein, G., Goto, H., Oda, S. et al. (2006). Antihypertensive potential and mechanism of action of astaxanthin: III. Antioxidant and histopathological effects in spontaneously hypertensive rats. *Biological and Pharmaceutical Bulletin* **29**: 684–688.

Inbaraj, B., Chien, J.T., and Chen, B.-H. (2006). Improved high performance liquid chromatographic method for determination of carotenoids in the microalga *Chlorella pyrenoidosa*. *Journal of Chromatography A* **1102** (1–2): 193–199.

Ishika, T., Laird, D.W., Bahri, P.A., and Moheimani, N.R. (2019). Co-cultivation and stepwise cultivation of *Chaetoceros muelleri* and *Amphora* sp. for fucoxanthin production under gradual salinity increase. *Journal of Applied Phycology* **31** (3): 1535–1544.

Iwamoto, T., Hosoda, K., Hirano, R. et al. (2000). Inhibition of low-density lipoprotein oxidation by astaxanthin. *Journal of Atherosclerosis and Thrombosis* **7**: 216–222.

James, L. (2017). Astaxanthin market report, size, share, analysis 2017 and forecast to 2023. Reuters. https://www.reuters.com/brandfeatures/venture-capital/article?id=15886 (accessed September 14, 2020).

Janchot, K., Rauytanapanit, M., Honda, M. et al. (2019). Effects of potassium chloride-induced stress on the carotenoids canthaxanthin, astaxanthin, and lipid accumulations in the green *Chlorococcal microalga* strain TISTR 9500. *Journal of Eukaryotic Microbiology* **66** (5): 778–787.

Jaswir, D., Noviendri, R., Hasrini, F., and Octavianti, F. (2011). Carotenoids: sources, medicinal properties and their application in food and nutraceutical industry. *Journal of Medicinal Plants Research* **5** (33): 7119–7131.

Jung, A.H., Nurul Islam, M., Mee Lee, C. et al. (2012). Promising antidiabetic potential of fucoxanthin isolated from the edible brown algae *Eisenia bicyclis* and *Undaria pinnatifida*. *Fisheries Science* **78** (6): 1321–1329.

Kadam, S.U. and Prabhasankar, P. (2010). Marine foods as functional ingredients in bakery and pasta products. *Food Research International* **43** (8): 1975–1980.

Kang, H. and Kim, J. (2017). Astaxanthin and β-carotene in *Helicobacter pylori*-induced gastric inflammation: a mini-review on action mechanism. *Journal of Cancer Prevention* **22** (2): 57–61.

Kavalappa, Y.P., Rudresh, D.U., Gopal, S.S. et al. (2019). β-Carotene isolated from the marine red alga, *Gracillaria* sp. potently attenuates the growth of human hepatocellular carcinoma (HepG2) cells by modulating multiple molecular pathways. *Journal of Functional Foods* **52**: 165–176.

Khan, Q.A., Lu, J., and Hecht, S.M. (2009). Calothrixins, a new class of human DNA topoisomerase I poisons. *Journal of Natural Products* **72**: 438–442.

Kim, J.H., Kim, S.M., Cha, K.H. et al. (2016). Evaluation of the anti-obesity effect of the microalga *Pheodactylum tricornutum*. *Applied Biological Chemistry* **59**: 283–290.

Kim, S.M., Shang, Y.F., and Um, B.H. (2011). A preparative method for isolation of fucoxanthin from *Eisenia bicyclis* by centrifugal partition chromatography. *Phytochemical Analysis* **22** (4): 322–329. https://doi.org/10.1002/pca.1283.

Kim, S.M., Jung, Y.J., Kwon, O.N. et al. (2012). A potential commercial source of fucoxanthin extracted from the microalga *Phaeodactylum tricornutum*. *Applied Biochemistry and Biotechnology* **166** (7): 1843–1855.

Kirti, K., Amita, S., Priti, S. et al. (2014). Colorful world of microbes: carotenoids and their applications. *Advances in Biology*: 837891.

Kistler, A. (2002). Metabolism and CYP-inducer properties of astaxanthin in man and primary human hepatocytes. *Archives of Toxicolology* **75**: 665–675.

Koka, P. and Song, P.-.S. (1978). Protection of chlorophyll *a* by carotenoid from photodynamic decomposition. *Photochemistry and Photophysiology* **29**: 509–514.

Kotake Nara, E., Kushiro, M., Zhang, H. et al. (2001). Carotenoids affect proliferation of human prostate cancer cells. *Journal of Nutrition* **131**: 3303–3306.

Koyande, A.K., Chew, K.W., Rambabu, K. et al. (2019). Microalgae: a potential alternative to health supplementation for humans. *Food Science and Human Wellness* **8**: 16–24.

Lafarga, T. (2019). Effect of microalgal biomass incorporation into foods: nutritional and sensorial attributes of the end products. *Algal Research* **41**: 101566.

Le, M. and Xiao-Ming, L. (2010). Effects of lutein and zeaxanthin on aspects of eye health. *Journal of the Science of Food and Agriculture* **90** (1): 2–12.

Lemoine, Y. and Schoefs, B. (2010). Secondary ketocarotenoid astaxanthin biosynthesis in algae: a multifunctional response to stress. *Photosynthesis Research* **106** (1–2): 155–177.

Leon, R., Martin, M., Vigara, J. et al. (2003). Microalgae mediated photoproduction of β-carotene in aqueous–organic two phase systems. *Biomolecular Engineering* **20**: 177–182.

Li, H. and Liu, J. (2019). Effects of defatted *Haematococcus pluvialis* meal (DHPM) supplementation on the growth performance, and the carotenoid content and composition in the rotifer (*Brachionus plicatilis*). *Aquaculture* **505**: 34–40.

Liang, S., Liu, X., Chen, F., and Chen, Z. (2004). Current microalgal health food R & D activities in China. In: *Asian Pacific Phycology in the 21st Century: Prospects and Challenges*, 45–48. Dordrecht: Springer.

Lidebjer, C., Leanderson, P., Ernerudh, J., and Jonasson, L. (2007). Low plasma levels of oxygenated carotenoids in patients with coronary artery disease. *Nutrition Metabolism and Cardiovascular Diseases* **17**: 448–456.

Lin, J.H., Lee, D.J., and Chang, J.S. (2015). Lutein production from biomass: marigold flowers versus microalgae. *Bioresource technology* **184**: 421–428.

Long, H., Ting, H., Shabnam, F. et al. (2017). Antioxidants maintain cellular redox homeostasis by elimination of reactive oxygen species. *Cell Physiology and Biochemistry* **44**: 532–553.

Lozano-Garcia, D.F., Cuellar-Bermudez, S.P., del Rio-Hinojosa, E. et al. (2019). Potential land microalgae cultivation in Mexico: from food production to biofuels. *Algal research* **39**: 101459.

Lu, Y.M., Xiang, W.Z., and Wen, Y.H. (2011). *Spirulina* (*Arthrospira*) industry in Inner Mongolia of China: current and prospects. *Journal of Applied Phycology* **23**: 265–269.

Lyons, N.M. and O'Brien, N. (2002). Modulatory effects of analgal extract containing astaxanthin on UVA-irradiated cells in culture. *Journal of Dermatological Science* **30**: 73–84.

Mahesha Poojary, M., Francisco Barba, J., Aliakbarian, B. et al. (2016). Innovative alternative technologies to extract carotenoids from microalgae and seaweeds. *Marine Drugs* **14**: 214.

Mahfuzur, R.S., Yuanmei, L., Cheng, J.J., and Daroch, M. (2016). Astaxanthin-producing green microalga *Haematococcus pluvialis*: from single cell to high value commercial products. *Frontiers in Plant Science* **7**: 531.

Mäki-Arvela, P., Hachemi, I., and Murzin, D.Y. (2014). Comparative study of the extraction methods for recovery of carotenoids from algae: extraction kinetics and effect of different extraction parameters. *Journal of Chemical Technology and Biotechnology* **89**: 1607–1626.

Mein, J.R., Lian, F., and Wang, X.D. (2008). Biological activity of lycopene metabolites: implications for cancer prevention. *Nutrition Reviews* **66**: 667–683.

Meléndez-Martínez, A.J. (2019). An overview of carotenoids, apocarotenoids, and vitamin A in agro-food, nutrition, health, and disease. *Molecular Nutrition and Food Research* **63**: 1801045.

Jaeschke, D.P., Menegol, T., Rech, R. et al. (2016). Carotenoid and lipid extraction from *Heterochlorella luteoviridis* using moderate electric field and ethanol. *Process Biochemistry* **51** (10): 1636–1643.

Miki, W. (1991). Biological functions and activities of animal carotenoids. *Pure & Applied Chemistry* **63**: 141–146.

Milani, A., Basirnejad, M., Shahbazi, S., and Bolhassani, A. (2017). Carotenoids: biochemistry, pharmacology and treatment. *British Journal of Pharmacology* **174**: 1290–1324.

Milledge, J.J. (2012). Microalgae-commercial potential for fuel, food and feed. *Food Science & Technology* **26** (1): 28–30.

Minhas, A.K., Hodgson, P., Barrow, C.J. et al. (2016). The isolation and identification of new microalgal strains producing oil and carotenoid simultaneously with biofuel potential. *Bioresource Technology* **211**: 556–565.

Moghadamtousi, S.Z., Karimian, H., Khanabdali, R. et al. (2014). Anticancer and antitumor potential of fucoidan and fucoxanthin, two main metabolites isolated from brown algae. *The Scientific World Journal*: 768323. https://doi.org/10.1155/2014/768323.

Montero, O., Macías-Sánchez, M.D., Lama, C.M. et al. (2005). Supercritical CO_2 extraction of beta-carotene from a marine strain of the cyanobacterium *Synechococcus* species. *Journal of Agricultural and Food Chemistry* **53** (25): 9701–9707.

Murillo, A.G. and Fernandez, M.L. (2016). Potential of dietary non-provitamin A carotenoids in the prevention and treatment of diabetic microvascular complications. *Advances in Nutrition* **7** (1): 14–24.

Murthy, K.N.C., Singh, R.P., and Jayaprakasha, G.K. (2002). Antioxidant activities of grape (*Vitis vinifera*) Pomaceae extracts. *Toxicology* **40**: 941–947.

Naguib, M.A. (2000). Antioxidant activities of astaxanthin and related carotenoids. *Journal of Agricultural and Food Chemistry* **48** (4): 1150–1154.

Nakano, M., Onodera, A., Saito, E., and Tanabe, M. (2008). Effect of astaxanthin in combination with alpha-tocopherol or ascorbic acid against oxidative damage in diabetic ODS rats. *Journal of Nutritional Science and Vitaminology (Tokyo)* **54**: 329–334.

Nishikawa, S., Hosokawa, M., and Miyashita, K. (2012). Fucoxanthin promotes translocation and induction of glucose transporter 4 in skeletal muscles of diabetic/obese KK-A (y) mice. *Phytomedicine* **19**: 389–394.

Nishino, H., Murakoshi, M., Li, T. et al. (2002). Carotenoids in cancer chemoprevention. *Cancer Metastasis Reviews* **21**: 257–264.

Nobre, B., Marcelo, F., Passos, R. et al. (2006). Supercritical carbon dioxide extraction of astaxanthin and other carotenoids from the microalga *Haematococcus pluvialis*. *European Food Research Technology* **223**: 787–790.

Nunes, N., Leça, J.M., Pereira, A.C. et al. (2019). Evaluation of fucoxanthin contents in seaweed biomass by vortex-assisted solid-liquid microextraction using high-performance liquid chromatography with photodiode array detection. *Algal Research* **42**: 101603.

Okai, Y. and Higashi-Okai, K. (1996). Possible immunomodulating activities of carotenoids in *in vitro* cell culture experiments. *International Journal of Immunopharmacology* **18** (12): 753–758.

Olmedilla, B., Granado, F., Southon, S. et al. (2001). Serum concentrations of carotenoids and vitamins A, E, and C in control subjects from five European countries. *British Journal of Nutrition* **85** (2): 227–238.

Othman, R., Noh, N., Nurrulhidayah, A.F. et al. (2017). Determination of natural carotenoid pigments from freshwater green algae as potential halal food colorants. *International Food Research Journal* **24** (Suppl): S468–S471.

Palozza, P. and Krinsky, N.I. (1992). Astaxanthin and canthaxanthin are potent antioxidants in a membrane model. *Archives of Biochemistry and Biophysics* **297**: 291–295.

Panis, G. and Rosales Carreon, J. (2016). Commercial astaxanthin production derived by green alga *Haematococcus pluvialis*: a microalgae process model and a techno-economic assessment all through production line. *Algal Research* **18**: 175–190.

Park, J.S., Chyun, J.H., Kim, Y.K. et al. (2010). Astaxanthin decreased oxidative stress and inflammation and enhanced immune response in humans. *Nutrition & Metabolism* **7**: 18.

Patel, N.R., Bole, M., Chen, C. et al. (2012). Cell elasticity determines macrophage function. *PLoS One* **2012**: e41024.

Peng, J., Yuan, J.P., Wu, C.F., and Wang, J.H. (2011). Fucoxanthin, a marine carotenoid present in brown seaweeds and diatoms: metabolism and bioactivities relevant to human health. *Marine Drugs* **9**: 1806–1828.

Persistence Market Research (2018). Global crustacean market to reach US$ 147 Bn by 2025. New York: Persistence Market Research Pvt. Ltd.

Polotow, T.G., Vardaris, C.V., Mihaliuc, A.R. et al. (2014). Astaxanthin supplementation delays physical exhaustion and prevents redox imbalances in plasma and soleus muscles of Wistar rats. *Nutrients* **6** (12): 5819–5838.

Pushpa, H. and Purushothama, K.B. (2010). Antimicrobial activity of *Lyophyllum decastes* an edible wild mushroom. *World Journal of Agricultural Sciences* **6** (5): 506–509.

Qian, C., Decker, E.A., Xiao, H., and McClements, D.J. (2012). Physical and chemical stability of β-carotene-enriched nanoemulsions: influence of pH, ionic strength, temperature, and emulsifier type. *Food Chemistry* **132**: 1221–1229.

Raja, R., Haemaiswarya, S., and Rengasamy, R. (2007). Exploitation of *Dunaliella* for β-carotene production. *Applied Microbiology and Biotechnology* **74**: 517–523.

Rajauria, G. and Abu-Ghannam, N. (2013). Isolation and partial characterization of bioactive fucoxanthin from *Himanthalia elongata* brown seaweed: a TLC-based approach. *International Journal of Analytical Chemistry* **2013**: 802573. https://doi.org/10.1155/2013/802573.

Ramaraj, S. and Ki, J.-S. (2018). A review of the biological activities of microalgal carotenoids and their potential use in healthcare and cosmetic industries. *Marine Drugs* **16** (1): 26.

Ranga Rao, A., Raghunath Reddy, R.L., Baskaran, V. et al. (2010). Characterization of microalgal carotenoids by mass spectrometry and their bioavailability and antioxidant properties elucidated in rat model. *Journal of Agriculture and Food Chemistry* **58**: 8553–8559.

Rao, A.V. and Rao, L.G. (2007). Carotenoids and human health. *Pharmacological Research* **55**: 207–216.

Raposo, M.F., de Morais, A.M., and de Morais, R.M. (2015). Carotenoids from marine microalgae: a valuable natural source for the prevention of chronic diseases. *Marine Drugs* **13**: 5128–5155.

Renju, G.L., Muraleedhara Kurup, G., and Bandugula, V.R. (2014). Effect of lycopene isolated from *Chlorella marina* on proliferation and apoptosis in human prostate cancer cell line PC-3. *Tumor Biology* **35** (11): 10747–10758. https://doi.org/10.1007/s13277-014-2339-5.

Reyes, F.A., Mendiola, J.A., Suarez-Alvarez, S. et al. (2016). Adsorbent-assisted supercritical CO_2 extraction of carotenoids from *Neochloris oleoabundans* paste. *The Journal of Supercritical Fluids* **112**: 7–13.

Rojas, I., Padgett, D.A., Sheridan, J.F., and Marucha, P.T. (2002). Stress-induced susceptibility to bacterial infection during cutaneous wound healing. *Brain, Behavior, and Immunity* **16**: 74–84.

Sánchez, J.F., Fernández-Sevilla, J.M., Acién, F.G. et al. (2008). Biomass and lutein productivity of *Scenedesmus almeriensis*: influence of irradiance, dilution rate and temperature. *Applied Microbiology and Biotechnology* **79** (5): 719–729.

Sathasivam, R. and Juntawong, N. (2013). Modified medium for enhanced growth of *Dunaliella* strains. *International Journal of Current Science* **5**: 67–73.

Sathasivam, R. and Ki, J.S. (2018). A review of the biological activities of microalgal carotenoids and their potential use in healthcare and cosmetics industries. *Marine Drugs* **16** (1): 26.

Sathasivam, R., Praiboon, J., Chirapart, A. et al. (2014). Screening, phenotypic and genotypic identification of b-carotene producing strains of *Dunaliella salina* from Thailand. *Indian Journal of Geo-Marine Science* **43** (12): 2198–2216.

Sathasivam, R., Radhakrishnan, R., Hashem, A., and Abd_Allahd, E.F. (2018). Microalgae metabolites: a rich source for food and medicine. *Saudi Journal of Biological Sciences* **26**: 709–722.

Schwarz, S., Obermüller-Jevic, U.C., Hellmis, E. et al. (2008). Lycopene inhibits disease progression in patients with benign prostate hyperplasia. *Journal of Nutrition* **138** (1): 49–53.

Selmo, M.S. and Salas-Mellado, M.M. (2014). Technological quality of bread from rice flour with *Spirulina*. *International Food Research Journal* **21** (4): 1523–1528.

Selvameenal, L., Radhakrishnan, M., and Balagurunathan, R. (2009). Antibiotic pigment from desert soil actinomycetes; biological activity, purification and chemical screening. *Indian Journal of Pharmaceutical Sciences* **71** (5): 499–504.

Shaish, A., Harari, A., Kamari, Y. et al. (2009). Application of *Dunaliella* in atherosclerosis. In: *The Alga Dunaliella: Biodiversity, Physiology, Genomics and Biotechnology* (eds. A. Ben-Amotz, J.E.W. Polle and D.V.S. Rao), 475–494. Jersey Science Publishers.

Sharma, P. and Sharma, N. (2017). Industrial and biotechnological applications of algae: a review. *Journal of Advances in Plant Biology* **1** (1): 01.

Sharma, P., Ambuj Bhushan, J., Rama Shanker, D., and Mohammad, P. (2012). Reactive oxygen species, oxidative damage, and antioxidative defense mechanism in plants under stressful conditions. *Journal of Botany*: 217037.

Shen, H.M. and Mizushima, N. (2014). At the end of the autophagic road: an emerging understanding of lysosomal functions in autophagy. *Trends in Biochemical Sciences* **39**: 61–71.

Shinichi, T. (2011). Carotenoids in algae: distributions, biosyntheses and functions. *Marine Drugs* **9**: 1101–1118. https://doi.org/10.3390/md9061101.

Sidari, R. and Tofalo, R. (2019). A comprehensive overview on microalgal-fortified/based food and beverages. *Food Reviews International*: 1–28.

Sies, H. and Stahl, W. (2004). Nutritional protection against skin damage from sunlight. *Annual Review of Nutrition* **24**: 173–200.

Sluijs, I., Cadier, E., Beulens, J.W. et al. (2015). Dietary intake of carotenoids and risk of type 2 diabetes. *Nutrition, Metabolism & Cardiovascular Diseases* **25**: 376–381.

Soler-Vila, A., Coughlan, S., Guiry, M.D., and Kraan, S. (2009). The red alga *Porphyra dioica* as a fish-feed ingredient for rainbow trout (*Oncorhynchus mykiss*): effects on growth, feed efficiency, and carcass composition. *Journal of Applied Phycology* **21** (5): 617–624.

Soontornchaiboon, W., Joo, S.S., and Kim, S.M. (2012). Anti-inflammatory effects of violaxanthin isolated from microalga *Chlorella ellipsoidea* in RAW 264.7 macrophages. *Biological and Pharmaceutical Bulletin* **35** (7): 1137–1144.

Spolaore, P., Joannis-Cassan, C., Duran, E., and Isambert, A. (2006). Commercial applications of microalgae. *Journal of Bioscience and Bioengineering* **101** (2): 87–96.

Stafsnes, M.H., Josefsen, K.D., Andersen, G.K. et al. (2010). Isolation and characterization of marine pigmented bacteria from norwegian coastal waters and screening for carotenoids with UVA-blue light absorbing properties. *Journal of Microbiolology* **48** (1): 16–23.

Stahl, W. and Sies, H. (2005). Bioactivity and protective effects of natural carotenoids. *Biochimica Biophysica Acta* **1740**: 101–107.

Suganuma, K., Nakajima, H., Ohtsuki, M., and Imokawa, G. (2010). Astaxanthin attenuates the UVA-induced up-regulation of matrix metalloproteinase-1 and skin fibroblast elastase in human dermal fibroblasts. *Journal of Dermatological Science* **58** (2): 136–142.

Sugiura, M., Mieko, N., Kazunori, O. et al. (2015). High-serum carotenoids associated with lower risk for developing type 2 diabetes among Japanese subjects: Mikkabi cohort study. *BMJ Open Diabetes Research and Care* **3**: e000147. https://doi.org/10.1136/bmjdrc-2015-000147.1-8.

Suzuki, K., Ito, Y., Nakamura, S. et al. (2002). Relationship between serum carotenoids and hyperglycemia: a population-based cross-sectional study. *Journal of Epidemiolology* **12**: 357–366.

Todd Lorenz, R. and Cysewski, G.R. (2000). Commercial potential for *Haematococcus* microalgae as a natural source of astaxanthin. *Trends in Biotechnology* **18** (4): 160–167.

Uchiyama, A. and Okada, Y. (2008). Clinical efficacy of astaxanthin-containing *Haematococcus pluvialis* extract for the volunteers at risk of metabolic syndrome. *Journal of Clinical Biochemistry and Nutrition* **43** (Suppl. 1): 38–43.

Uchiyama, K., Naito, Y., Hasegawa, G. et al. (2002). Astaxanthin protects beta-cells against glucose toxicity in diabetic db/db mice. *Redox Reports* **7** (5): 290–293.

Ursoniu, S., Sahebkar, A., Serban, M.C., and Banach, M. (2015). Lipid profile and glucose changes after supplementation with astaxanthin: a systematic review and meta-analysis of randomized controlled trials. *Archives of Medical Science* **11**: 253–266.

Valderrama, J.O., Perrut, M., and Majewski, W. (2003). Extraction of astaxantine and phycocyanine from microalgae with supercritical carbon dioxide. *Journal of Chemical and Engineering Data* **48**: 827–830.

Vaz, B.S., Moreira, J.B., Morais, M.G., and Vieira Costa, J.A. (2016). Microalgae as a new source of bioactive compounds in food supplements. *Current Opinion in Food Science* **7**: 73–77.

Ventura, S.P.M., Nobre, B.P., Ertekin, F. et al. (2017). Extraction of value-added compounds from microalgae. In: *Microalgae-Based Biofuels and Bioproducts* (eds. C. Gonzalez-Fernandez and R. Munoz), 461–483. Cambridge: Woodhead Publishing.

Vigani, M., Parisi, C., Rodríguez-Cerezo, E. et al. (2015). Food and feed products from micro-algae: market opportunities and challenges for the EU. *Trends in Food Science & Technology* **42** (1): 81–92.

Vineis, M., Alavanja, P., Buffler, E. et al. (2004). Doll tobacco and cancer: recent epidemiological evidence. *Journal of the National Cancer Institute* **96**: 99–106.

Wang, W.J., Wang, G.C., Zhang, M., and Teng, C.K. (2005). Isolation of fucoxanthin from the rhizoid of *Laminaria japonica* Aresch. *Journal of Integrative Plant Biology* **47**: 1009–1015.

Wang, F., Gao, B., Wu, M. et al. (2019). A novel strategy for the hyper-production of astaxanthin from the newly isolated microalga *Haematococcus pluvialis* JNU35. *Algal Research* **39**: 101466.

Wells, M.L., Potin, P., Craigie, J.S. et al. (2017). Algae as nutritional and functional food sources: revisiting our understanding. *Journal of Applied Phycology* **29** (2): 949–982.

Xia, S., Wang, K., Wan, L.L. et al. (2013). Production, characterization, and antioxidant activity of fucoxanthin from the marine diatom *Odontella aurita. Marine Drugs* **11** (7): 2667–2681.

Xu, Y., Ibrahim, I.M., and Harvey, P.J. (2016). The influence of photoperiod and light intensity on the growth and photosynthesis of *Dunaliella salina* (Chlorophyta) CCAP 19/30. *Plant Physiology and Biochemistry* **106**, 305e315.

Ylonen, K., Alfthan, G., Groop, L. et al. (2003). Dietary intakes and plasma concentrations of carotenoids and tocopherols in relation to glucose metabolism in subjects at high risk of type 2 diabetes: the Botnia dietary study. *American Journal of Clinical Nutrition* **77**: 1434–1441.

Yoshida, H., Yanai, H., Ito, K. et al. (2010). Administration of natural astaxanthin increases serum HDl-cholesterol and adiponectin in subjects with mild hyperlipidemia. *Atherosclerosis* **209**: 520–523.

Zaidi, S., Patel, A., Mehta, N. et al. (2005). Early biochemical alterations in manganese toxicity: ameliorating effects of magnesium nitrate and vitamins. *Industrial Health* **43**: 663–668.

Zhang, J., Sun, Z., Sun, P. et al. (2014). Microalgal carotenoids: beneficial effects and potential in human health. *Food & Function* **5**: 413–425.

Zhang, X., Zhao, W.E., Hu, L. et al. (2012). Carotenoids inhibit proliferation and regulate expression of peroxisome proliferators-activated receptor gamma (PPARγ) in K562 cancer cells. *Journal of Current Pharmaceutical Biotechnology* **13** (1): 180–190.

Zhao, D., Kwon, S.H., Chun, Y.S. et al. (2017). Anti-neuroinflammatory effects of fucoxanthin via inhibition of Akt/NF-κB and MAPKs/AP-1 pathways and activation of PKA/CREB pathway in lipopolysaccharide-activated BV-2 microglial cells. *Neurochemical Research* **42** (2): 667–677.

Ziegler, R.G. (1989). A review of epidemiologic evidence that carotenoids reduce the risk of cancer. *Journal of Nutrition* **119** (1): 116–122.

13

Algal Derived Functional Lipids and their Role in Promoting Health

Nolwenn Terme[1], Benoît Chénais[2,3], Mathilde Fournière[1,4], Nathalie Bourgougnon[1], and Gilles Bedoux[1]

[1] *Laboratoire de Biotechnologie et Chimie Marines EA 3884, Université Bretagne Sud, IUEM,, Vannes, France*
[2] *Mer Molécules Santé EA2160, Le Mans Université,, Le Mans, France*
[3] *IUML FR3473 CNRS,, Le Mans, France*
[4] *Université Catholique de l'Ouest Bretagne Nord,, Guingamp, France*

13.1 Introduction

Lipids are fatty or waxy organic compounds soluble in nonpolar solvents and include fats, waxes, sterols, fat-soluble vitamins, glycerolipids, phospholipids, or glycolipids among others (Holdt and Kraan 2011). The main roles of lipids comprise energy storage (Reeds et al. 1999), cell signaling, and the structural composition of intracellular and cellular membranes (Thompson 1996). Study of the lipidome consists generally of total lipid content determination and fatty acid (FA) profiling. Eukaryotic algae comprise more than 50 000 species (Guiry and Guiry 2019) and include microalgae (phytoplankton) and macroalgae (seaweeds) separated according to genomic and phenotypic classification. This chapter reviews both microalgae and macroalgae including, but not limited to, Chlorophyta, Rhodophyta, Ochrophyta, Chrysophyta, Dinophyta, Prymnesiophyta, and Bacillariophyceae (diatoms).

Algal FAs account for a wide molecular variety and are studied for their potential nutritional benefits and their capacity to act as chemotaxonomic markers. Moreover, the algal FA content and profile can be affected or even controlled by external parameters such as light, nutrient availability, osmotic stress, temperature, or presence of pollutants (Bhaskar et al. 2004b; Colombo et al. 2006; Floreto et al. 1994a, b; Floreto et al. 1996; Hotimchenko 2002; Khotimchenko and Levchenko 1997; McCauley et al. 2016; Mishra et al. 1993; Schmid et al. 2014).

Recent Advances in Micro- and Macroalgal Processing: Food and Health Perspectives, First Edition.
Edited by Gaurav Rajauria and Yvonne V. Yuan.

This chapter reviews data dealing with FA composition, isolation and purification of FAs, health properties of FAs, and potential commercial applications of FAs whether they are from microalgae or macroalgae.

13.2 Types and Structures of Fatty Acids from Algae

FAs possess a carboxylic group linked to an aliphatic chain that may be straight or branched, saturated or unsaturated, and with a length ranging from 4–28 carbons whether with an odd or even number of carbons. FAs are divided into families according to the degree of unsaturation: saturated fatty acids (SFAs; Figure 13.1) with no double bonds, monounsaturated fatty acids (MUFAs; Figure 13.1) with one double bond, and polyunsaturated fatty acids (PUFAs; Figure 13.1) with two or more double bonds. For MUFAs and PUFAs, the location of the first double bond

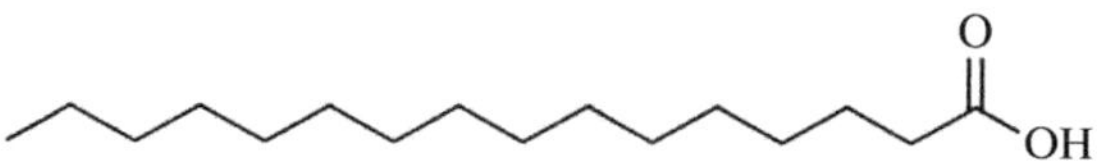

Palmitic acid
SFA
C16:0

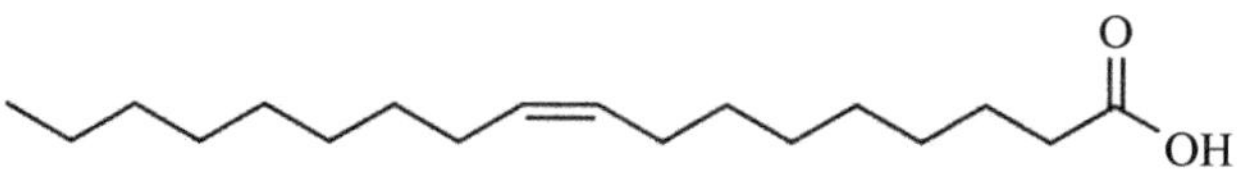

Oleic acid
MUFA
C18:1n-9

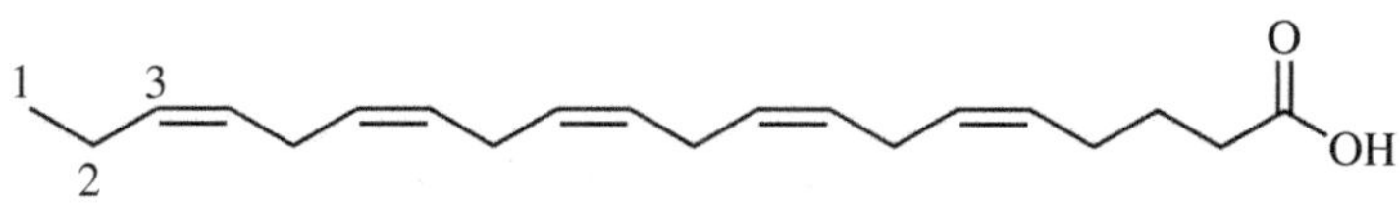

Eicosapentaenoic acid (EPA)
PUFA
C20:5n-3

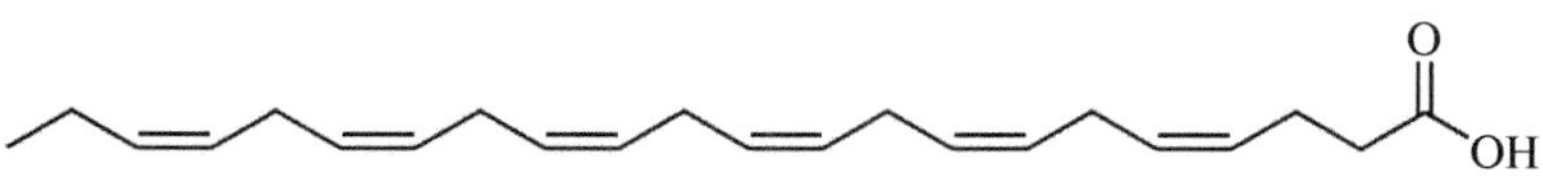

Docosahexaenoic acid (DHA)
PUFA
C22:6n-3

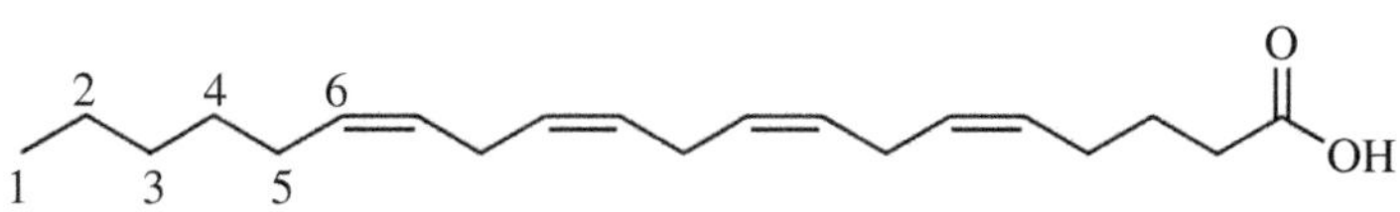

Arachidonic acid (ARA)
PUFA
C20:4n-6

Figure 13.1 Chemical structure examples of saturated fatty acid (SFA), monounsaturated fatty acid (MUFA), and polyunsaturated fatty acid (PUFA)

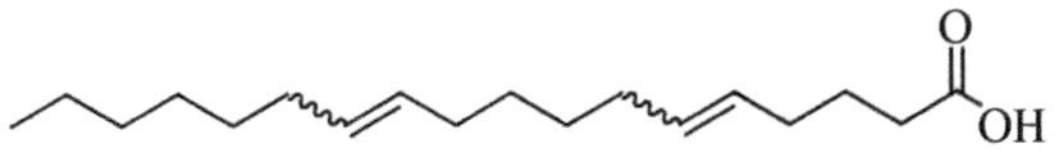

Octadeca-5, 11-dienoic acid
NMI
C18:2n-7,13

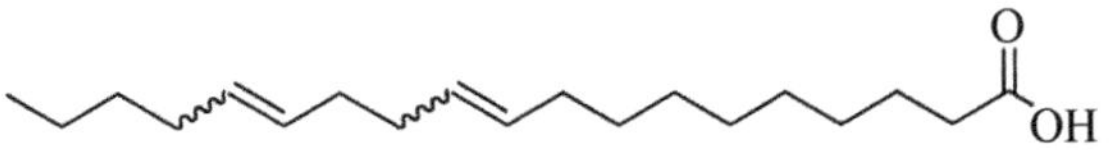

Nonadeca-10, 14-dienoic acid
NMI
C19:2n-5,9

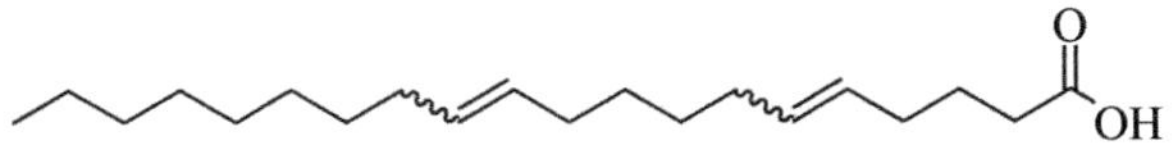

Eicosa-5,11,dienoic acid
NMI
C20:2n-9,15

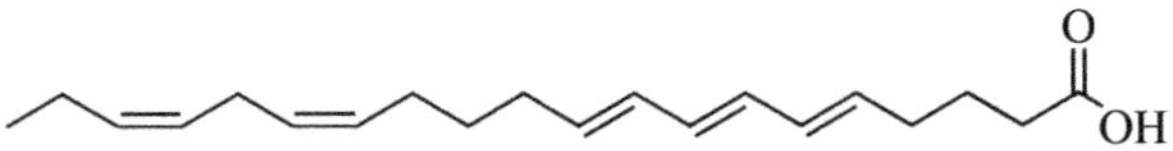

(5E, 7E, 9E, 14Z, 17Z)-eicosa-5,7,9,14,17-pentaenoic acid
Conjugated Fatty Acid

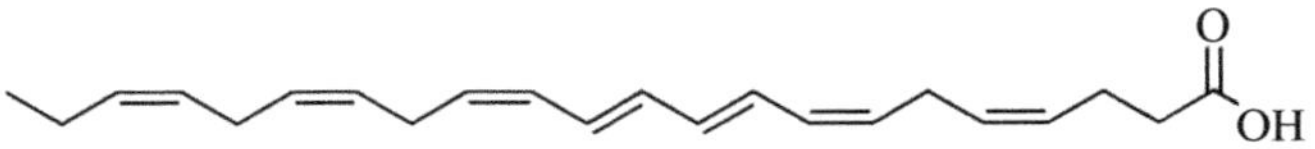

(4Z, 7Z, 9E, 11E, 13Z, 16Z, 19Z)-docosa-4,7,9,11,13,16,19-heptaenoic acid
Conjugated Fatty Acid

Figure 13.2 Chemical structure of nonmethylene-interrupted fatty acids and conjugated fatty acid identified in algae. C18:2n-7,13 is identified in *Cladophora rupestris* (Chlorophyta, *Chladophorales*) (Ratnayake and Ackman 1979); C19:2n-5,9 in *Grateloupia turuturu* (Rhodophyta, *Halymeniales*) (Kendel et al. 2013), and C20:2n-9,15 in *Sargassum* species (Ochrophyta, *Fucales*) (Khotimchenko 1991). The conjugated fatty acid (5E,7E,9E,14Z,17Z)-eicosa-5,7,9,14,17-pentaenoic acid is found in *Acanthophora spicifera* (Rhodophyta, *Ceramiales*) (Bhaskar et al. 2004) and (4Z,7Z,9E,11E,13Z,16Z,19Z)-docosa-4,7,9,11,13,16,19-heptaenoic acid in *Anadyomene stellata* (Chlorophyta, *Chladophorales*) (Mikhailova et al. 1995)

(X) from the methyl end is indicated with the n-X or ω-X number (Figure 13.1). This numbering defines the n-6 (or ω-6) and n-3 (or ω-3) well-known classes of FAs (Figure 13.1). For example, eicosapentaenoic acid (EPA), also called C20:4n-3, indicates that this acid is a 20-carbon-long FA with four double bonds and the first one is located at three carbons from the methyl end (Figure 13.1).

Most of the double bonds of PUFAs are nonconjugated with a methylene group between double bonds. However, non-methylene-interrupted (NMI) FAs with more than one methylene group between double bonds (Figure 13.2) are detected in macroalgae (Jamieson and Reid 1972; Khotimchenko 1991; Ratnayake and Ackman 1979). FAs with conjugated double bonds are also found in the FA profiles of algae (Figure 13.2) (Bhaskar et al. 2004a; Mikhailova et al. 1995).

FAs can also be branched (Kendel et al. 2015; Lang et al. 2011) or contain functional groups such as hydroxyl (Gelin et al. 1997; Kendel et al. 2013; Kendel et al. 2015),

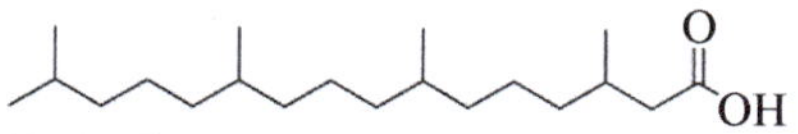

3,7,11,15-tetramethylhexadecanoic acid
Branched Fatty Acid

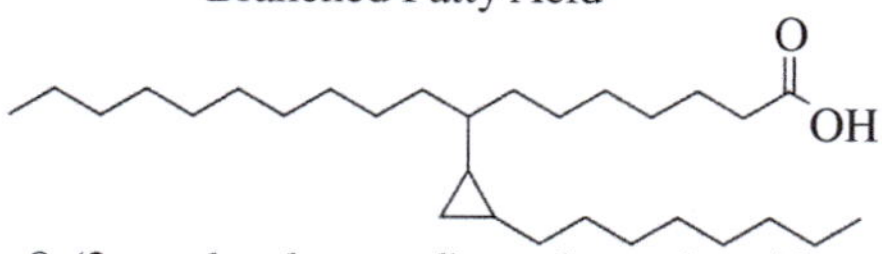

8-(2-octylcyclopropyl)octadecanoic acid
Branched Fatty Acid

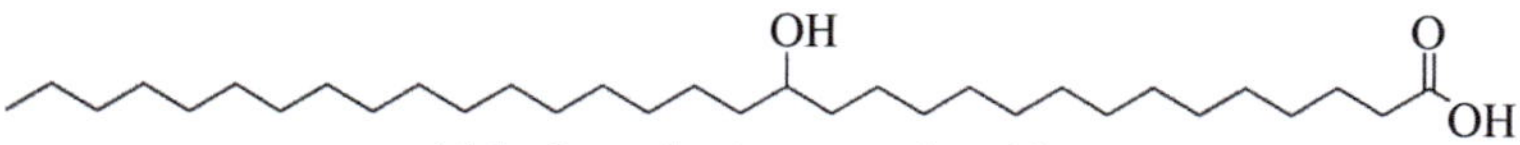

15-hydroxydotriacontanoic acid
C32:0 15-hydroxy

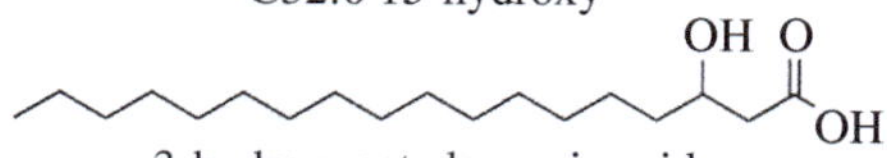

3-hydroxyoctadecanoic acid
C18 3-hydroxy

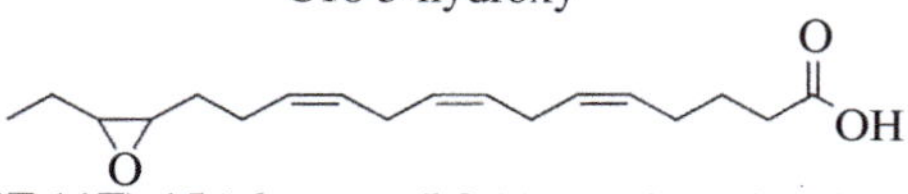

(5Z,8Z,11Z)-15,16-epoxy-5,8,11-octadecatrienoic acid
Fatty acid with epoxy group

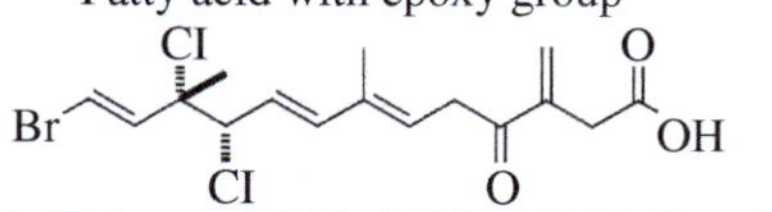

(6E,8E,10S,11S,12E)-13-bromo-10,11-dichloro-7,11-dimethyl-3-methylene-4-oxotrideca-6,8,12-trienoic acid
Fatty acid with keto and halogen group

Figure 13.3 Branched and functionalized fatty acids. 3,7,11,15-tetramethylhexadecanoic acid is identified in *Heterococcus fuornensis* (Ochrophyta, *Tribonematales*) (Lang et al. 2011); 8-(2-octylcyclopropyl)octadecanoic acid in *Chlamydomonas zebra* (Chlorophyta, *Chlamydomonadales*) (Lang et al. 2011); 15-hydroxydotriacontanoic acid in *Nannochloropsis* sp. (Ochrophyta, *Eustigmatales*) (Gelin et al. 1997); 3-hydroxyoctadecanoic acid in *Solieria chordalis* (Rhodophyta, *Gigartinales*) (Kendel et al. 2015); (5Z,8Z,11Z)-15,16-epoxy-5,8,11-octadecatrienoic acid in *Chlamydomyxa montana* (Ochrophyta, *Chlamydomyxales*) (Lang et al. 2011); and (6E,8E,10S,11S,12E)-13-bromo-10,11-dichloro-7,11-dimethyl-3-methylene-4-oxotrideca-6,8,12-trienoic acid in *Plocamium cartilagineum* (Rhodophyta, *Plocamiales*) (Dembitsky and Srebnik 2002)

halogen (Dembitsky and Srebnik 2002; Kornprobst 2014), keto (Eltgroth et al. 2005), or epoxy groups (Lang et al. 2011) (Figure 13.3).

Oxylipins have also been identified in algae (Figure 13.4). They are oxidized FAs formed by enzyme or chemical oxidation (Kumari et al. 2013b).

This family contains hydroxyl, oxo, epoxy FAs, polyunsaturated aldehydes, prostaglandins, leukotriene, or polycyclic FAs (Barofsky and Pohnert 2007; Bernart et al. 1993; Bouarab 2004; D'Ippolito et al. 2004, 2005; Fontana et al. 2007).

FAs are rarely free in the biological matrix. They are linked by an ester bond to a glycerol moiety forming an acylglycerol (mono-, di-, or tri- depending on the quantity of FAs bound to each glycerol), to a sugar (simple, complex, or sulfated) forming a

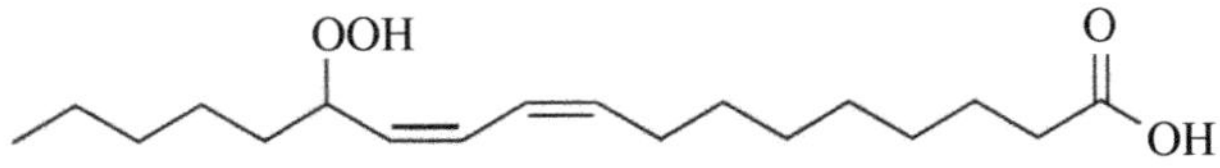

(9Z,11Z)-13-hydroperoxyoctadeca-9,11-dienoic acid
13-HpODE

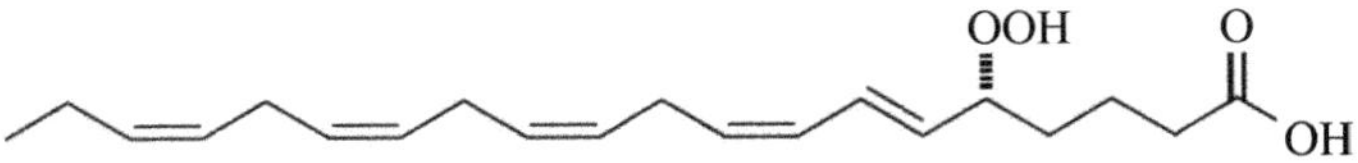

(R,6E,8Z,11Z,14Z,17Z)-5-hydroperoxyicosa-6,8,11,14,17-pentaenoic acid
5R-HpEPE

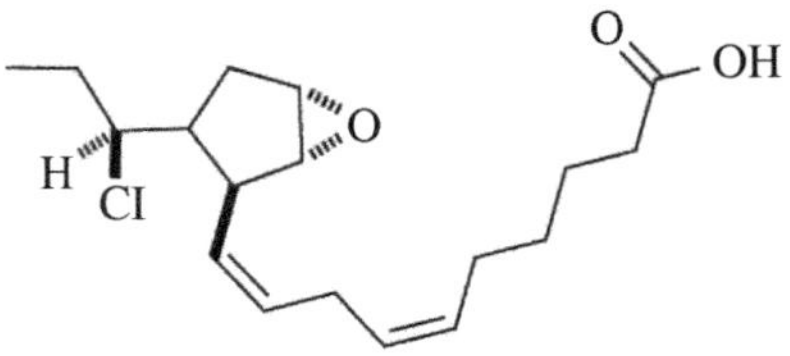

Chlorinated oxylipin

Figure 13.4 Oxylipins in algae. 13-HpODE is identified in *Chondrus crispus* (Rhodophyta, *Gigartinales*) (Fontana et al. 2007); 5R-HpEPE in *Skeletonema marinoi* (Bacillariophyta, *Thalassiosirales*) (D'Ippolito et al. 2005); and the chlorinated oxylipin in *Egregia menziesii* (Ochrophyta, *Laminariales*) (Dembitsky and Srebnik 2002)

glycolipid, or to a phosphatidylglycerol group then forming a phospholipid. Thus, FAs are present in the three lipid classes, i.e. neutral lipids, glycolipids, and phospholipids. Triacylglycerols (TAGs) have storage and energy functions in algal cells (Khotimchenko and Yakovleva 2004; MacDougall et al. 2011; Thompson 1996). Glycolipids play an important role in energy supply and cell protection against stresses by stabilizing the membrane bilayer and acting as markers for cellular recognition (Boudière et al. 2014; Holdt and Kraan 2011). Phospholipids act as transport materials for membrane structure preservation (Holdt and Kraan 2011).

Several species of freshwater and marine microalgae produce high quantities of lipids, generally about 10–25% of dry weight and up to about 50–60% in some diatoms or *Chlorella* species (Chlorophyta), for example (Table 13.1; Mata et al. 2010; Mimouni et al. 2012, 2015). The C16 and C18 SFAs and MUFAs are present in all microalgal groups but in variable amounts ranging from 5– 40% and 1.8–40% of total FAs, respectively (Hu et al. 2008; Mimouni et al. 2018). However, the n-3 and n-6 long-chain polyunsaturated fatty acids (LC-PUFAs) arachidonic acid (C20:4n-6, ARA), α-linolenic acid (C18:3n-3, ALA), γ-linolenic acid (C18:3n-6, GLA), docosahexaenoic acid (C22:6n-3, DHA), and EPA (C20:5n-3), which are of interest for human health applications, are mainly present in marine species (De Jesus Raposo et al. 2013; Mimouni et al. 2012) while also available from freshwater species such as *Dunaliella* sp. (Chlorophyta, *Chlamydomonadales*) (Bhosale et al. 2010; Chen et al. 2011; Sheffer et al. 1986) or *Chlorella* sp. (Chlorophyta, *Chlorellales*) (Buono et al. 2014; Petkov and Garcia 2007) under specific conditions of culture.

Table 13.1 Approximate amount of total lipids, docosahexaenoic acid (DHA), and eicosapentaenoic acid (EPA) in some marine and freshwater microalgae

Classes	Species	Total lipid content (% of dry weight)[a,b]	DHA (molar %)[b]	EPA (molar %)[b]
Bacillariophytes (diatoms)	*Nitzschia* sp.	16–47[a]	<1	25–30
	Odontella aurita	7–13[b]	1–2	>25
	Phaeodactylum tricornutum	18–57[a]	2	26
	Skeletonema costatum	13–51[a]	1–5	10–20
	Thalassiosira pseudonana	20–24[a,b]	1	15
Chlorophytes	*Chlorella vulgaris*	5–58[a]	<1	1–5
	Dunaliella salina	6–25[a]		
	Dunaliella primolecta	23[a,b]	<1	<1
	Tetraselmis suecica	8–23[a]	<1	1–5
Dinophytes	*Crypthecodinium cohnii*	20–51[a]	<1	45
Prymnesiophytes	*Diacronema lutheri*	20–35[a,b]	10–20	>20
	Isochrysis sp.	7–40[a]	10–20	<1
Rhodophytes	*Porphyridium cruentum*	9–19[a]	<1	21

[a] Data from Mata et al. (2010).
[b] Data from Mimouni et al. (2012).

Species rich in EPA include diatoms (Bacillariophyceae) such as *Phaeodactylum tricornutum* (Bacillariophyta), *Odontella aurita* (Bacillariophyta, *Eupodiscales*), *Nitzschia* sp. (Ochrophyta, *Bacillariales*), *Thalassiosira pseudonana* (Bacillariophyta, *Thalassiosirales*), and *Skeletonema costatum* (Bacillariophyta, *Thalassiosirales*) (Mata et al. 2010; Mimouni et al. 2012), and also the rhodophyte *Porphyridium cruentum* (Rhodophyta, *Porphyridiales*), the dinophyte *Crypthecodinium cohnii* (Miozoa, *Peridiniales*), and the prymnesiophyte *Isochrysis* sp. (Haptophyta, *Isochrysidales*) (including the species *Tisochrysis lutea*) (Table 13.1; Mata et al. 2010; Mimouni et al. 2012). Interestingly, the prymnesiophyte *Diacronema lutheri* (previously *Pavlova lutheri*, Haptophyta, *Pavlovales*) displays high contents of both DHA and EPA (De Jesus Raposo et al. 2013) (Table 13.1). The LC-PUFAs of marine microalgae are incorporated into TAGs (neutral lipids) as storage and into polar lipids such as phospholipids and galactolipids as membrane constituents (Ulmann et al. 2017).

The lipid content of microalgae can be modulated by culture conditions and several stresses (Sayanova et al. 2017). For example, the addition of sodium salts of organic acids, i.e. sodium acetate, pyruvate, citrate, and malate, to the culture medium of the marine microalgae *Thraustochytrium* sp. T01 (Labyrinthulomycetes, *Thraustochytriaceae*) increases DHA production by 40–46% (Chandrasekaran et al. 2018). As another example, fermentation strategies using heterotrophic microalgae such as *Schizochytrium mangrovei* (*Thraustochytriaceae*) can influence the production of lipids and especially of DHA (Hoang et al. 2018). However, most of the studies aim to increase lipid production, which could be achieved by modifying the light spectrum exposure of *Dunaliella salina* and *Nannochloropsis oculata* (Ochrophyta, *Eustigmatophyceae*) cultures (Gilbert et al. 2013), under osmotic stress in *Chlamydomonas reinhardtii* (Chlorophyta, *Chlamydomonadales*) (Yang et al. 2018), by nutrient stress such as nitrogen limitation in *Chlorella vulgaris* and *Chaetoceros muelleri* (Ochrophyta) (Adamakis et al. 2018; Lin et al. 2018), or phosphate limitation in *Thalassiosira weissflogii* (Lin et al. 2018). However, the increase in the overall amount of FAs is not sufficient and particular attention must also be paid to their nature; nutrient limitation, for example, leads to a lower proportion of PUFAs (Lin et al. 2018), which could be interesting for biodiesel production but not for human or animal health/feeding purposes. In addition, the effects of stress or culture conditions are also species-specific (Pavón-Suriano et al. 2018). Environmental contaminants such as ethinylestradiol (among several other chemicals) could also have an impact on lipid metabolism; in this case, ethinylestradiol impairs the production of LC-PUFAs, affects the galactolipid versus phospholipid balance, and triggers the recycling of FAs from membrane lipids to TAGs in *Phaeodactylum tricornutum* (Conte et al. 2018).

Unlike microalgae, macroalgae produce a low quantity of lipids generally about 1–6% DW (Rodrigues et al. 2015). Chain length and degree of unsaturation are higher than those of terrestrial plants (Kumari et al. 2013b). Palmitic acid is the most common SFA (Gressler et al. 2010). A high content of PUFAs is typical for seaweeds, especially ALA, EPA, ARA, and stearidonic acid (C18:4n-3, STA) (Dawczynski et al. 2007; Murata and Nakazoe 2001). FA distribution can be linked to the phylum and some FAs can serve as taxonomic markers (Table 13.2; Galloway et al. 2012; Kumari et al. 2013a). LC-PUFAs are more abundant in red and brown seaweeds than in green (Schmid et al. 2014). Phaeophyta demonstrate a higher total lipid content than other phyla and SFAs and PUFAs are the main classes of FA representing up to 80% of FAs (Table 13.2; Wielgosz-Collin et al. 2016). C18 and C20 are the major PUFAs present in similar quantities and DHA is rarely isolated from brown seaweeds except in Fucales and Scytosiphonales (Wielgosz-Collin et al. 2016). High proportions of ARA (13% of total FAs), EPA (13% of total FAs), and linoleic acid (C18:2n-6, LA), and lower content of palmitic and stearic acids than Rhodophyta are typical for Phaeophyta (Table 13.2; Galloway et al. 2012; Schmid et al. 2014).

Rhodophyta are characterized by a high quantity of C20 PUFAs with four or five double bonds (around 11% of ARA and 17% EPA) (Dawczynski et al. 2007; Galloway et al. 2012; Schmid et al. 2014; Wielgosz-Collin et al. 2016). Abundant quantities of palmitic and oleic acids are found in red seaweeds, whereas DHA is absent or present at low concentrations (Table 13.2; Dawczynski et al. 2007; Schmid et al. 2014). Halogenated FAs such as short-chain chlorinated, brominated, or iodinated FAs have been identified specifically in *Asparagopsis* (Rhodophyta, *Bonnemaisoniales*) red seaweeds (Dembitsky and Srebnik 2002). The Chlorophyta phylum is characterized by a high content of C18 PUFAs (LA and ALA) (Khotimchenko et al. 2002; Li et al. 2002) but the C20 content (ARA and EPA) is significantly lower than in the Phaeophyta and Rhodophyta (Table 13.2; Schmid et al. 2014). Contents around 5% of LA, 7% of STA, and presence of ALA are markers for Chlorophyta seaweeds (Galloway et al. 2012). C16 PUFAs have chemotaxonomic value for green seaweeds (Khotimchenko 1993). Indeed, hexadecatrienoic acid C16:3n-3 is specific to the *Codium* green seaweed genus (Chlorophyta, *Bryopsidales*) (Goecke et al. 2010).

Table 13.2 Fatty acid distribution characteristics of macroalgal phyla

Phylum	Specificity	References
Phaeophyta	• High content of C18 and C20 polyunsaturated fatty acids (PUFAs) (13% of arachidonic acid [ARA] and 13% eicosapentaenoic acid [EPA]) • High content of linoleic acid (LA) • Lower content of palmitic and stearic acids than Rhodophyta • Very low content of docosahexaenoic acid (DHA) except for Fucales and Scytosiphonales	(Galloway et al. 2012; Schmid et al. 2014; Wielgosz-Collin et al. 2016)
Rhodophyta	• High content in C20 PUFAs (11% of ARA and 17% of EPA) • High content of palmitic and oleic acids • Absence or very low content of DHA • Halogenated fatty acids specific for *Asparagopsis*	(Dawczynski et al. 2007; Dembitsky and Srebnik 2002; Galloway et al. 2012; Schmid et al. 2014; Wielgosz-Collin et al. 2016)
Chlorophyta	• High content of C18 PUFAs • Lower content of C20 PUFAs • 5% of LA • 7% of stearidonic acid (STA) • Presence of ALA • C16:3n-3 specific for *Codium*	(Galloway et al. 2012; Goecke et al. 2010; Khotimchenko 1993; Khotimchenko et al. 2002; Li et al. 2002; Schmid et al. 2014)

As with microalgae, lipid content and FA distribution of macroalgae are modulated by external parameters (Bhaskar et al. 2004b; Colombo et al. 2006; Denis et al. 2010; Floreto et al. 1994a, [b], 1996; Khotimchenko and Levchenko 1997; Kim et al. 1996; McCauley et al. 2016; Mishra et al. 1993; Tasende 2000). Cold conditions of growth such as cold or deep water increase the total lipid content of red and brown seaweeds (Bhaskar et al. 2004b; Colombo et al. 2006; Denis et al. 2010; Kim et al. 1996; Mishra et al. 1993). FAs are longer and more unsaturated for cold species than for tropical or temperate water species (Bhaskar et al. 2004b; Colombo et al. 2006). For example, the PUFA content of seaweeds from the Canadian coasts is twice as large as in those from the south China coast (52.1 vs. 22.3%, respectively) and the mean chain length is 17.8 carbons for the cold water species, whereas it is 16.3 carbons for the temperate water species (Colombo et al. 2006). In culture conditions, nitrogen starvation leads to a lower total lipid content, a higher SFA and low unsaturated (one or two double bonds) content, and a lower PUFA content (McCauley et al. 2016; Mishra et al. 1993). Phosphorus deprivation has no significant impact on the total lipid content. However, the starvation of phosphorus decreased the storage FA content such as palmitic acid, and increased the PUFA content such as hexadecatetraenoic acid C16:4n-3 (Floreto et al. 1996). Light intensity does not affect the total lipid content. However, light is necessary for efficient lipid production (Floreto et al. 1994b). Seaweed FAs are not affected by anchoring on the seabed, whereas total lipid content is reduced if seaweeds are attached on the seabed (Khotimchenko and Levchenko 1997). The stage of development of the seaweeds also influences the FA content and distribution. Gametophytes of the Rhodophyta *Chondrus crispus* (Rhodophyta, *Gigartinales*) exhibit more MUFAs such as palmitoleic C16:1n-7 and oleic C18:1n-9 acids than sporophytes, whereas sporophytes are richer in SFAs such as palmitic and stearic acids and in ALA (Tasende 2000). For the red seaweed *Gracilaria verrucosa* (Rhodophyta, *Gracilariales*), a difference in ARA content is also noticed between cystocarps and branches (Khotimchenko and Levchenko 1997).

13.3 Isolation and Purification of FAs from Algae

13.3.1 Isolation of FAs from Algae

Isolation of FAs can be done just after the extraction of lipids from algae (see Chapter 10 for lipid extraction). Chemical saponification is the most commonly used method to release FAs from glycerol or sugar moieties. For chemical saponification, an alkali hydro-alcoholic solution is refluxed over a short time period (generally 1–2 hours) or stirred at room temperature over a longer time (17–24 hours) for the hydrolysis of the ester linkages. These parameters do not significantly influence the FA profile (Cartens et al. 1996). Then, after acidification, FAs can be recovered directly (Zhang et al. 2018) or by liquid–liquid extraction (Kendel et al. 2015). The saponification can also take place during the extraction of FAs. Alkali is directly added to the solvent extraction system and FAs are recovered after acidification and liquid–liquid partition (Cartens et al. 1996; Guil-Guerrero et al. 2001; Paul et al. 2014). This direct saponification of biomass increases the yield of FAs extracted, and reduces operating time and possible degradation (Cartens et al. 1996; Molina Grima et al. 1994). It should be noted that as a lot of studies are based on the identification and quantification of FAs, the saponification is often replaced by a transesterification to fatty acid methyl esters (FAMEs), which can be injected directly in a gas chromatography system for analysis or used for further purification (Mansour 2005; Nagappan and Kumar Verma 2018).

Supercritical fluid extraction is an eco-friendly alternative method to isolate lipids from seaweeds. Until now, supercritical carbon dioxide ($scCO_2$) has been the most commonly used supercritical fluid, due to its low critical pressure and temperature (73.9 bar and 31.1 °C). $scCO_2$ is currently used for the extraction of microalgae but it is little used for seaweed lipid extraction (Grosso et al. 2015; Terme et al. 2017; Terme et al. 2018).

13.3.2 Purification of FAs from Algae

Purification of FAs can be done from the free fatty acids (FFAs) or esters (glycerides or FAME) and is generally conducted to obtain FAs with a high added value, i.e. PUFAs, in a multistep process for high purity (Namal Senanayake 2013; Robles Medina et al. 1998; Shahidi and Wanasundara 1998). The separation techniques reviewed here include physicochemical methods such as crystallization by urea inclusion compounds or use of low temperatures and distillation, chromatographic methods such as reverse phase chromatography, silver nitrate adsorption, centrifugal partition chromatography (CPC), and supercritical fluid chromatography and enzymatic methods.

13.3.2.1 Urea Crystallization Urea fractionation is widely used both for analytical and preparative purposes for FA concentration of marine oils, but is not often used for algal oils. It is based on the formation of hexagonal crystals enclosing straight-chain molecules during crystallization (Smith 1952). The affinity of FAs and esters with urea decreases when unsaturated bonds are present in the chain. Thus, SFAs and MUFAs are first precipitated from the solution while PUFAs remain in solution (Iverson and Weik 1967; Strocchi and Bonaga 1975). The parameters governing the crystallization have been extensively studied in the form of the urea adductability values (binding properties between urea and FAs) (Iverson and Weik 1967), the stability constants, and the heats of formation of crystals (Schlenk 1954; Swern 1964). To form complexes, the urea concentration should be near saturation; the fractionation is greatly influenced by urea:FA ratio and temperature can be adjusted according to the desired concentration of FAs.

An algal oil from the dinoflagellate *Crypthecodinium cohnii* was enriched in DHA from 47.7 to 97.1% of the total FA fraction by using a urea:FA ratio of 3:1 at 4 °C in methanol (Namal Senanayake and Shahidi 2000). The soluble fraction comprised 98.2% of PUFAs whereas the urea complexing fraction comprised 66.9% of SFAs and MUFAs. When the urea:FA ratio increases, more DHA is complexed and a lower recovery yield of DHA is obtained (Namal Senanayake and Shahidi 2000). For the Rhodophyta *Porphyridium cruentum*, an EPA- and ARA-enriched fraction is targeted (Guil-Guerrero et al. 2001). The urea:FA ratio of 4:1 was tested in methanol at 4 and 28 °C (Guil-Guerrero et al. 2001). Both temperatures resulted in a similar lipid concentrate composition with 57% ARA and 34% EPA but 28 °C led to a better recovery yield because it is the optimal crystallization temperature for EPA. This enriched fraction also contained interesting FAs such as LA (8.2%) and homo-GLA (1.3%). All the SFAs were eliminated with 0.2% palmitoleic acid remaining (Guil-Guerrero et al. 2001). Extraction of the diatom *Phaeodactylum tricornutum* produced an oil enriched in EPA by urea fractionation with a urea:FA ratio of 4:1 at 28 °C (Cartens et al. 1996). Methanol and ethanol were both tested for dissolving urea. SFA and MUFA are effectively removed with both solvents (Cartens et al. 1996). Methanol leads to a more concentrated fraction in EPA, DHA, and ARA (55.2, 1.5, and 5.9%, respectively) but ethanol recovers more EPA than methanol; 84% of the total EPA amount was recovered by an ethanolic solution of urea compared with 79% for the methanolic urea solution. However, overall yields (45% for methanol and 53% for ethanol) are acceptable in comparison with other purification processes (Cartens et al. 1996). When a second urea crystallization was used to purify EPA from the diatom *Phaeodactylum tricornutum*, the EPA content reached 80.7% of total FAs but with a very low yield (23%; Zhang et al. 2018). This fraction also comprised 12.2% ARA, 1.1% LA, and approx. 2% MUFAs and SFAs (Zhang et al. 2018). For *Isochrysis galbana*, purification with a 4:1 urea:FA ratio at 4 °C in methanol was efficient to produce an STA-, EPA-, and DHA-enriched fraction representing 85.4% of the urea concentrate FAs. It was noticed that the recovery yield of DHA in the urea concentrate is 100% (Robles Medina et al. 1995a, [b]). The purification can also be conducted on FAME obtained by transmethylation of lipids from *Porphyridium cruentum* (Cohen and Cohen 1991). The EPA methyl ester proportion increased from 47.5 to 81.9% of the fraction, whereas the SFA methyl ester content decreased from 35.6 to 3.1% of the fraction (Cohen and Cohen 1991). The fraction was also enriched in ARA (5.4 to 6.6%). The previous FA profile seems to be an important factor for enrichment. By using a strain of *Porphyridium cruentum* identified as a rich source of ARA (41.7%), the urea purification in the same conditions led to an 80% ARA-enriched fraction (Cohen and Cohen 1991).

13.3.2.2 Low-Temperature Crystallization Low-temperature crystallization is based on the melting points of FAs. Using different temperatures and successive filtrations, it is possible to purify PUFAs from algae, as SFAs and MUFAs have higher melting points than PUFAs. Fatty acid esters or FAs can be purified by low-temperature crystallization depending on the solvent (Privett 1971; Wang et al. 2018; Zhang et al. 2018). Acetone is used for methyl esters while hydrocarbons are used for acids (Privett 1971). A docosapentaenoic acid (C22:5, DPA) rich fraction was obtained from *Schizochytrium* sp. oil (Wang et al. 2018). A crystallization at −80 °C over 8 hours in acetone enriched the fraction in DPA from 35.8 to 51.2% and decreased the content of SFAs and MUFAs from 41.7 to 15.1% (Wang et al. 2018). Low-temperature crystallization of *Phaeodactylum tricornutum* lipids led to an EPA-rich fraction (Zhang et al. 2018). After 24 hours at −80 °C in hexane, EPA represented 40.7% of the total FAs of the fraction, whereas SFAs and MUFAs are reduced from 61.9 to 17.9% (Zhang et al. 2018).

13.3.2.3 Distillation Distillation is based on the boiling points of FAME. The longer the FAME carbon chain, the higher the boiling point, with straight chains having higher boiling points than their branched chain analogues (Cason et al. 1951). Industrial application of fractional distillation is possible as apparatus and techniques have been developed to accommodate up to 20 kg of esters with a high-performance column (Privett 1971). The main drawback of this technique is the use of heating that can lead to degradation of FA by loss of unsaturation, formation of cyclic compounds, or isomerization (Privett 1971). To avoid degradation, the distillation temperature must be below 200 °C. However, temperatures greater than 200 °C are necessary for LC-PUFA distillation. However, a decrease in pressure can lead to a decreased boiling point allowing lower distillation temperature use (Namal Senanayake 2013). On the other hand, decreased pressure results in a loss of distillation column efficiency. This method, called molecular distillation, is applied to fish and aquatic organism oil enrichment in some n-3 PUFAs but is poorly applied to algae (Namal Senanayake 2013).

13.3.2.4 Chromatography FAs can be separated according to the carbon chain length and degree of unsaturation using reverse phase, silver nitrate adsorption, centrifugal partition chromatography (CPC), or supercritical fluid chromatography at analytical or preparative scales. The separation can be conducted whether on FFAs or on fatty esters.

For chromatography, the choice of detector is a key point. The mass spectrometer is the most suitable and most used detector for identification. As it is a destructive method, it cannot be used for purification of FAs. However, the analytical and separation methodology can be optimized using this detector, and subsequently used for purification without the detector. The differential refractometer (refractive index detector) needs a sufficient concentration of FAs in the sample and an elution gradient is not feasible with this detector (Robles Medina et al. 1998). Most FAs do not absorb ultraviolet (UV) radiation or interfere with the solvent absorption. Therefore, their conversion to UV-visible sensitive derivatives is necessary for detection (Robles Medina et al. 1998). A multiple wavelength detection can help with the identification of PUFAs. The wavelength of 192 nm is quite PUFA selective with sensitivity increasing with the number of double bonds. The wavelength of 217 nm can be used for EPA and DHA detection (Robles Medina et al. 1995a) and 220 nm for TAG detection because of the specific absorbance due to the carbonyl (C=O) group (Shukla 1988).

Reverse phase chromatography of FAs is based on the adsorption of hydrophobic soluble molecules from a polar solvent to a nonpolar sorbent under pressure such as in high-pressure liquid chromatography. Octadecylsilyl (C18) and Octasilyl (C8) stationary phases are used (Aveldano et al. 1983; Cartens et al. 1996; Cohen and Cohen 1991; Mansour 2005; Molina Grima et al. 1994, 1995; Robles Medina et al. 1995a; Robles Medina et al. 1998). C18 columns lead to a better separation of FAs whereas C8 allows a faster separation of very long FAs (Aveldano et al. 1983). The separation depends on chain length, degree, and configuration of unsaturation. Elution time increases with chain length and decreases with the amount of unsaturation for the same chain length (Robles Medina et al. 1998). FFAs separate faster than the corresponding esters because they are more polar. The most commonly used mobile phases are 60–100% methanol or acetonitrile in water (Aveldano et al. 1983). Acetonitrile seems to be more selective probably due to its lower viscosity, but this solvent cannot dissolve all the FAs and separations are longer than with methanol. For biocompatible (i.e. non-toxic and/or food-grade) separations, methanol can be replaced by ethanol but the flow rate must be decreased and the resolution is lower (Robles Medina et al. 1995a). Reverse phase chromatography was used to obtain three fractions rich in STA, EPA, and DHA, respectively, from an *I. galbana* urea concentrate at the semi-preparative scale with a good purity (Molina Grima et al. 1994, 1995). *Phaeodactylum tricornutum* led to a 93.6% EPA fraction after high-performance liquid chromatography (HPLC) (Cartens et al. 1996). At the semi-preparative scale, 98% of the EPA contained in the diatom was recovered with a 94% purity. An EPA concentrate was also obtained from *Porphyridium cruentum* (Cohen and Cohen 1991). The reverse phase chromatography enriched the EPA fraction from 81.9 to 97.3% and decreased the ARA content from 6.6 to 1.4%. LC-PUFA methyl esters from *Scrippsiella* sp. CS-295/c (Haptophyta, *Coccolithophyceae*) were isolated with repeated injections using preparative HPLC with a high purity (Mansour 2005).

Silver nitrate silicic acid HPLC is a quick semi-preparative fractionation methodology for highly unsaturated fatty esters with three to six double bonds (Robles Medina et al. 1998). The fractionation is based on the formation of a complex between the column silver ions and double bonds by charge transfer (Guil-Guerrero et al. 2001). Elution time increases with the number of double bonds because sample–column interactions are stronger. Therefore, SFAs are eluted first followed by unsaturated FAs. The order of elution for unsaturated esters is determined by the number, the position, and the geometric configuration of double bonds (Scholfield 1979). For a good purification, the ratio of the fatty esters and stationary phase should be 4% (w/w) (Belarbi et al. 2000). Various concentrations of acetone in hexane as the mobile phase allowed the separation of fatty esters from *Porphyridium cruentum* urea concentrate (Belarbi et al. 2000). Five percent acetone in hexane enriched the fraction in ARA while 10% enriched the fraction in EPA (Belarbi et al. 2000). This method was also applied to *Monodus subterraneus* (Ochrophyta, *Xanthophyceae*) oil and led to an EPA-rich fraction with more than 92% of purity. The scale-up of this process was conducted with *Porphyridium cruentum* by increasing the column diameter and demonstrated the possibility of EPA and ARA large-scale production using this method (Belarbi et al. 2000).

The use of supercritical fluids for nontoxic and food-safe production of high-value natural bioactives has been reviewed recently (Catchpole et al. 2012). $scCO_2$ is generally used for extraction of nonpolar lipophilic compounds and a wide range of polar co-solvents can be used to improve the extraction of polar compounds (Catchpole et al. 2012). Combining $scCO_2$ and chromatography principles led to a separation of FAs on the basis of the chain length ($scCO_2$ properties) and the degree of unsaturation (chromatography solid phase properties) (Montañés et al. 2013). Supercritical fluid chromatography has been used for the isolation of EPA ethyl esters from an algal oil (Montañés et al. 2013). The particle size, the stationary phase, sample loading, and temperature/pressure are the most important parameters for achieving separation of PUFAs (Montañés et al. 2013). Under optimized conditions ($scCO_2$, 7.5 ml minute^{-1}, 170 bar, 333 K, GreenSep Nitro column), EPA with greater than 95% purity is obtained in a single pass from an algal oil (Montañés et al. 2013).

CPC is a liquid–liquid chromatography without sorbent using two immiscible solvent systems (Becerra et al. 2015; Boulho et al. 2017; Namal Senanayake 2013; Wanasundara and Fedec 2002; Yoon et al. 2010). CPC is derived from counter-current chromatography and relies on the partition of compounds between the two solvent systems (Becerra et al. 2015). In a CPC system, the liquid stationary phase remains in the partition cells thanks to the centrifugal force created by the spinning rotor (800–1000 rpm) while the liquid mobile phase passes from cell to cell by ducts (Wanasundara and Fedec 2002). This technique is particularly suitable for the isolation of molecules from complex natural matrices on a large scale (Becerra et al. 2015; Yoon et al. 2010). CPC has been used for the purification of fucosterol from the brown alga *Lessonia vadosa* (Ochrophyta, *Laminariales*) and recovered between 70 and 93% of fucosterol present in the extracted fraction with a high purity (more than 97%) (Becerra et al. 2015). CPC has also been used for the isolation and purification of PUFAs from microalgae. The purification of an oil extract from *Skeletonema costatum* led to a fraction rich in essential FAs (45% of C20:5, 43% of C16:4, 7.5% of C18:4, and 4.5% of C22:6) with a 42% yield (Bousquet and Le Goffic 1995). After purification by CPC of a microalgal oil containing 39.7% DHA and 15.2% DPA n-6, samples at 84.6% DHA and 84.9% DPA n-6 were prepared using a solvent system composed of heptane/methanol/water (Wanasundara and Fedec 2002).

13.3.2.5 Enzymatic Purification of FAs Highly PUFA-enriched triglycerides can be obtained by lipase-catalyzed reactions (Ishihara et al. 2000; Namal Senanayake and Shahidi 2002; Robles Medina et al. 1998). Lipases are enzymes that can catalyze the synthesis or hydrolysis of an ester linkage in acylglycerols in a reversible way depending on the water content in the reaction media (Robles Medina et al. 1998). Therefore, lipases can catalyze exchanges of FAs in acylglycerols (Marangoni and Rousseau 1995). The type of enzymes, concentration and ratios of surfactants, initial composition of FA mixtures, solvents, water content, elimination method (i.e. evaporation or freeze drying), temperature, pH, agitation method and speed, and type of reactor are all parameters that affect the enzymatic ratio rate and the type of product (Robles Medina et al. 1998). However, mild temperature and pH conditions are typically used for lipases (Gandhi 1997), allowing their use for oils enriched in PUFAs. As the acylglycerol form of FAs is preferred for improved nutrition applications, this method can be taken in account for obtaining PUFAs for medical or dietetic purposes (Namal Senanayake 2013).

Lipase-catalyzed esterification of glycerol and PUFAs from microalgae leads to a triglyceride-rich fraction (Robles Medina et al. 1999). The lipase Novozyme 435 isolated from *Candida antarctica*, and immobilized on acrylic resin, is used in hexane without water, at 50 °C, with 1 g of molecular sieves added at the beginning of the reaction, with a glycerol:PUFA molar ratio of 1.2:3, an agitation rate of 200 rpm, and a concentration of 100 mg of lipase for 9 ml of hexane (Robles Medina et al. 1999). With these conditions, a triglyceride yield of 96.5% was obtained from *Phaeodactylum tricornutum* after 72 h (Robles Medina et al. 1999). The triglyceride fraction comprised 42.5% of EPA (Robles Medina et al. 1999). With another microalga, *Porphyridium cruentum*, the triglyceride yield was lower, i.e. 89.3% after 96 hours of reaction and the fraction comprised 45.6% of EPA and 43.4% of ARA (Robles Medina et al. 1999). The same enzyme was used in a one-pot process of extraction and purification of triglycerides from *Chlorella* sp. KR-1 (Lee et al. 2013). Almost all the total lipids were extracted and the FAME production was 293 mg per biomass gram in 6 hours at 60 °C. The triglyceride fraction comprised 25% palmitic acid, 17% oleic acid, and 15% LA (Lee et al. 2013). The total PUFA content represented 21% of the total FAs. Twelve lipases derived from *Penicillium camemberti* (lipase G), *Candida rugosa* (lipase AY), *Penicillium roqueforti* (lipase R), *Rhizopus oryzae* (lipase F-AP), *Aspergillus niger* (lipase A), *Mucor javanicus* (lipase M), *Rhizopus* sp. (lipase Ta), *Alcaligenes* sp. (lipases PL and QL), *Candida cylindracea* (lipase QF and MY), and *Rhizomucor miehei* lipozyme-IM were tested for STA and hexadecatetraenoic acid (C16:4n-3) purifications from *Undaria pinnatifida* (Phaeophyta, *Laminariales*) and *Ulva pertusa* (Chlorophyta, *Ulvales*) (Ishihara et al. 2000). For *U. pinnatifida*, all the enzymes except R, PL, and QL enriched the fraction in STA. The best results were obtained with lipase M with 61.6% of free STA in the fraction with 75.7% of recovery. For *U. pertusa*, all the enzymes except QL enriched the fraction in C16:4n-3 up to 30.6% of total FA content. For STA, the best results were obtained with the lipozyme-IM. Thus, STA represented 42.6% of the total FA content. The lipase M led to a fraction with 35.5% of STA and 30.6% of C16:4n-3. The recovery was 79.5% for C16:4n-3 and 69% for STA from *U. pertusa* with this lipase (Ishihara et al. 2000). Lipase AK from *Pseudomonas fluorescens* led to an enriched fraction in EPA up to 75.9% from *Phaeodactylum tricornutum* cells (Ramírez Fajardo et al. 2006). This study demonstrated that the initial concentration of EPA did not influence the final concentration or the recovery yield of EPA. Lipase-catalyzed reactions were used for DHA incorporation in borage oil (*Borago officinalis* L.; Namal Senanayake and Shahidi 2002). Here, the source of DHA was an algal oil. From an algal oil with 47.5% of DHA, a borage oil with 35.6% of DHA was obtained with 165 *C. antarctica* lipase units, at 50 °C for 25 hours (Namal Senanayake and Shahidi 2002).

As can be seen from the above discussion, applications of lipases are well established and proven. Industrial lipase reaction systems are also available. Further development of lipase and lipase-catalyzed reactions can lead to the production of novel oils enriched in essential FAs from natural sources and to the production of nonnatural esters for use as bioactive compounds.

13.3.2.6 Highly Pure PUFAs For purification of FAs, two or more procedures are required to obtain highly purified molecules from algae (Ishihara et al. 2000; Mendes et al. 2007; Robles Medina et al. 1995a; Shinde et al. 2018). A sequential procedure developed for concentration of DHA from the dinoflagellate *C. cohnii* biomass (Mendes et al. 2007) using a low-temperature crystallization followed by urea crystallization, purified DHA up to 99% of the FA fraction. The combination of lipase M from *M. javanicus* and medium pressure liquid chromatography was used to purify STA and hexadecatetraenoic acid (C16:4n-3) from the brown seaweed *U. pinnatifida* and the green seaweed *U. pertusa* (Ishihara et al. 2000). Highly pure fractions (more than 95% purity) were obtained and the overall yields are over 60% for *U. pertusa* and 52.9% for *U. pinnatifida.* The key step for improving purity and yield is the optimization of the lipase reactions (Ishihara et al. 2000). A two-step process combining urea crystallization and HPLC led to three fractions enriched in STA, EPA, and DHA from the Prymnesiophyte *I. galbana* with high yields and high purity (Robles Medina et al. 1995a). A multistep process combining urea crystallization, distillation, and silver ion chromatography was used to purify n-7 FA like palmitoleic acid (C16:1n-7) from algal oils (Shinde et al. 2018). In this process, fractions enriched in n-3, n-6, and n-9 FA were also obtained from microalgae from genera such as *Nannochloropsis*, *Nitzschia*, *Thalassiosira*, and *Phaeodactylum* (Shinde et al. 2018).

13.4 Health Properties of FAs

Dietary lipids have a vast array of activities that can impact human health. Here, we describe the activities of lipids and FAs from microalgae and macroalgae related to cosmetics, antivirals, cardiovascular diseases (CVDs), metabolic syndrome (MetS), and cancer prevention and/or therapy.

13.4.1 Lipids, FAs from Seaweeds and Cosmetic or Cosmeceutical Uses

Lipids and FAs from macroalgae may demonstrate four biological activities linked with cosmetics or cosmeceutical applications. They demonstrate skin hydration and skin elasticity enhancement efficacy and antimicrobial, anti-inflammatory, and antioxidant activities (Al-Fadhli et al. 2006; Banskota et al. 2014a, [b]; Choi et al. 2012; Fabrowska et al. 2017; Ishihara et al. 1998; Mendes et al. 2013; Park et al. 2013; Plaza et al. 2010; Santos et al. 2017; Terme et al. 2018).

13.4.1.1 Skin Care Lipids and FAs in cosmetics are used for their ability to protect the skin barrier and maintain the hydration level of the skin (Coderch et al. 2002). In our skin, they may incorporate themselves into cell membranes and a lack of cutaneous lipids may exacerbate scratches and discomfort (Bonnet 2018). Lipids and their derivatives are commonly used in cosmetic emulsions as emollients or surfactants. Bio-based lipids are of primary interest in this field. The lipid structure (FA chain length, saturation level, and branching) defines the functionality of the ingredient. For example, short-chain FAs (fewer than 8 carbons) exhibit solubilizing and detergent properties, intermediate chains (between 8 and 12 carbons) have foaming properties, and for long chains (more than 12 carbons) have emulsifying properties. Emulsion fluidity is expected from short chains and stability provided by long chains in fatty alcohols (Duprat-de-Paule et al. 2018). Lipids in cosmetics can be used directly as active ingredients to improve skin appearance (Rabasco Alvarez et al. 2000). Emulsions in cosmetic products contain a large variety of oils (Duprat-de-Paule et al. 2018). From seaweed sources, few studies show their direct use in cosmetics (Fabrowska et al. 2017).

$scCO_2$ extracts from the green seaweed *Cladophora glomerata* (Chlorophyta, *Chladophorales*), enriched in nonpolar compounds such as FAs improved *in vivo* skin hydration and *stratum corneum* water retention (Fabrowska et al. 2017). The skin hydration measured by corneometer increased up to +42–45% after 4 weeks of application by a group of women of 20+ and 40+ years of age (Fabrowska et al. 2017). FAs were observed to act as complementary occlusive compounds forming a barrier or seal that contributed to skin hydration (Fabrowska et al. 2017). An improvement in skin elasticity was also observed from an emulsion containing the *C. glomerata* algae extract (Fabrowska et al. 2017).

13.4.1.2 Antimicrobial Activity Glycoglycerolipids from the red seaweed *Chondria armata* (Rhodophyta, *Ceramiales*) were isolated from the chloroform-soluble fraction of a crude methanolic extract (Al-Fadhli et al. 2006). Glycoglycerolipids are compounds with one or more sugar residues glycosidically linked to a lipid containing a glycerol residue. Fractions PF_2 and PF_3, (PF refers to the polarity of the fraction isolated from the chloroform-soluble fraction) containing the two major glycoglycerolipids ((2R)-2-*O*-(5,8,11,14-eicosatetranoyl)-3-*O*-α-D-galactopyranosyl-*sn*-glycerol and 2R-1-*O*-(palmitoyl)-2-*O*-(5,8,11,14,17-eicosapentanoyl)-3-*O*-β-D-galactopyranosyl-*sn*-glycerol) were assessed for their antimicrobial properties (Al-Fadhli et al. 2006). Antibacterial and antifungal activities were measured using the paper disk assay method and using as positive control streptomycin for antibacterial assay and nystatin for antifungal assay (Al-Fadhli et al. 2006). The diameter of the growth inhibition halos induced by the sample was evaluated. PF_2 and PF_3 showed mild antibacterial activity against *Shigella flexneri* and *Vibrio cholerae*, respectively (Al-Fadhli et al. 2006). PF_2 (130 μg $disk^{-1}$) exhibited antimicrobial activity against *Escherichia coli*, *Staphylococcus aureus*, and *Salmonella typhi*, and antifungal activity against *Aspergillus fumigatus* and *niger*, *Cryptococcus neoformans*, and *Rhodotorula* sp. PF_3 was effective against the bacteria *Klebsiella* sp. and yeasts *Candida albicans*, *A. fumigatus*, and *C. neoformans* (Al-Fadhli et al. 2006). Ethyl acetate extracts from two red seaweeds *C. crispus* and *Gracilaria vermiculophylla* from an integrated multi-trophic aquaculture (IMTA) system exhibited higher antimicrobial activity when compared with other extraction solvents (methanol and diethyl ether) and cultivation regimes (IMTA or wild) (M. Mendes et al. 2013). All ethyl acetate extracts exhibited greater amounts of SFAs (mean of 69% of total FA) than MUFAs and PUFAs (means of 8 and 22%, respectively). The antimicrobial properties by the agar diffusion method assessed against *S. aureus* and *Enterococcus faecalis* were higher than those of the positive control (lactic acid 30%). The antimicrobial activity appeared to be more effective against Gram-positive bacteria (Mendes et al. 2013). Thus, ethyl acetate was determined in this study to be the best solvent for isolation of antimicrobial compounds. Further studies should be performed in order to identify, isolate, and characterize the specific compounds with antimicrobial activities (Mendes et al. 2013). STA and GLA from *Ulva linza* (previously the Chlorophyta *Enteromorpha linza*) have been identified as active compounds against Gram-negative oral pathogenic bacteria *Porphyromonas gingivalis* with a greater activity than the reference drug, triclosan (Choi et al. 2012; Park et al. 2013). The minimal inhibitory concentrations (MICs) of STA and GLA were established at 9.76 against 78.12 $\mu g \cdot ml^{-1}$ for triclosan. This seaweed could provide 500 mg of STA and 140 mg of GLA from 100 g of powder (Choi et al. 2012; Park et al. 2013). Plaza et al. (2010) reported that pressurized liquid ethanol extracts of the brown seaweed *Himanthalia elongata* (Ochrophyta, *Fucales*) were more effective for antimicrobial activity (minimal bactericidal concentration (MBC) and minimal fungicidal concentration (MFC) between 6 and 12 mg·ml^{-1}) than water (MBC and MFC between 12.25 and 14 mg·ml^{-1}) or hexane (MBC and MFC between 7 and 14 mg·ml^{-1}) extracts against *S. aureus*, *E. coli*, *C. albicans*, and *A. niger*. These extracts contained greater amounts of FAs compared with water and hexane extracts. In addition, ethanol extracts contained large amounts of palmitoleic and oleic acid (2.5 and 17.9%, respectively) that could be related to the antimicrobial activity (Plaza et al. 2010). According to Zheng et al. (2005), LC-PUFAs were selective inhibitors of FabI, an enoyl-acyl carrier protein reductase involved in the synthesis of FAs in bacteria and so inhibited the FA biosynthesis of the tested microorganisms (Zheng et al. 2005). The brown seaweed *Bifurcaria bifurcata* (Ochrophyta, *Fucales*) is well known for its composition of diterpenes (Santos et al. 2017). Lipophilic extracts of *B. bifurcata*, enriched in FAs exhibited antioxidant activity, anti-inflammatory potential with inhibition of nitric oxide production, and antibacterial activity *in vitro* (Santos et al. 2017). The dichloromethane extract was mainly composed of diterpenes (1892.8 ± 134.0 mg·kg^{-1} DW), free SFAs (550.4 ± 15.7 mg·kg^{-1} DW), free unsaturated FAs (397.1 ± 18.4 mg·kg^{-1} DW), which represented 42% of the total FAs, long-chain aliphatic alcohols (C14–C28), and sterols (406.5 ± 26.2 mg·kg^{-1} DW). FAs were the second most abundant compounds detected in the lipophilic extract (947.9 ± 21.9 mg·kg^{-1} DW) with palmitic acid predominant for the saturated FAs and octadec-9-enoic acid (C18:1n-9) for the unsaturated FAs (Santos et al. 2017). Antibacterial activity of the lipophilic extract was assessed against *S. aureus*, *E. coli*, *Staphylococcus epidermidis*, and *Pseudomonas aeruginosa* with MIC determination. Inhibition against both Gram-negative and Gram-positive bacteria was observed (against *S. aureus* and *E. coli* with MIC of 1024 and 2048 µg·ml^{-1}, respectively) but no growth inhibition against *S. epidermidis* and *Pseudomonas aeruginosa* in the range of the tested concentrations (MIC >2048 µg·ml^{-1}) (Santos et al. 2017).

Taken together, the above evidence suggests that macroalgal FAs with antimicrobial activity could be potentially used as preservatives in cosmetic products or to maintain the stability of the skin microbiome.

13.4.1.3 Anti-Inflammatory Activity PUFAs isolated from *U. pinnatifida* and *Ulva australis* inhibited the production of metabolites involved in the lipoxygenase pathway (Ishihara et al. 1998). Indeed, C16:4n-3 and STA significantly suppressed the production of B_4 and C_4 leukotrienes and 5-hydroxyeicosatetraenoic acid in MC/9 mouse mast cells (Ishihara et al. 1998). The anti-inflammatory activity of these seaweeds is of interest against skin inflammation, common in cutaneous diseases such as atopic dermatitis (Banskota et al. 2014b). A lipophilic extract of *B. bifurcata* inhibited lipopolysaccharide (LPS) induced nitric oxide production to 6 and 40% at 50 and 25 µg·ml^{-1} in murine RAW264.7 cells (Santos et al. 2017). EPA and ARA isolated from *C. crispus* also inhibited nitric oxide production in murine LPS-induced macrophages RAW264.7 to 50 and 62% at 100 µM, respectively (Banskota et al. 2014a). These results are limited to mouse macrophages and more research must be done with cell lines from human skin for anti-inflammatory assessment.

13.4.1.4 Antioxidant Activity Free radicals and reactive oxygen species (ROS) may induce skin damage associated with aging and inflammatory disorders (Oresajo et al. 2012; Pillai et al. 2005). Lipid-based antioxidant compounds that may help to prevent and control oxidative damage are therefore of huge interest in cosmetics and cosmeceuticals. Ethanol extracts of the brown seaweed *H. elongata* exhibited antioxidant activity according to Trolox equivalent antioxidant capacity (TEAC) assay (radical cation inhibition) (Plaza et al. 2010). These activities could be linked to lipid content but deeper study should be done (Plaza et al. 2010). A lipophilic fraction of *B. bifurcata* exhibited strong antioxidant activity evaluated by 2,2-diphenyl-1-picrylhydrazyl (DPPH) and 2,2′-azino-bis(3-ethylbenzothiazoline)-6-sulfonic acid (ABTS) *in vitro* assays. For DPPH, the antioxidant activity of the lipophilic fraction was expressed by a half maximal inhibitory concentration (IC_{50}) of $365.6 \pm 10.0\,\mu g{\cdot}ml^{-1}$ compared with ascorbic acid (IC_{50} of $4.08 \pm 0.05\,\mu g{\cdot}ml^{-1}$) and butylated hydroxytoluene (BHT) (IC_{50} of $14.32 \pm 0.69\,\mu g{\cdot}ml^{-1}$). For ABTS assay, the lipophilic fraction exhibited an IC_{50} of $116.3 \pm 2.5\,\mu g{\cdot}ml^{-1}$ compared with Trolox (IC_{50} of $365.6 \pm 10.0\,\mu g{\cdot}ml^{-1}$) (Santos et al. 2017). Neutral lipids, glycolipids, and phospholipids extracted by solvent extraction (chloroform/methanol) and $scCO_2$ ($scCO_2$, $scCO_2$ + ethanol 2%, $scCO_2$ + ethanol 8%) from two seaweeds, the red macroalga *Solieria chordalis* (Rhodophyta, *Gigartinales*) and the brown *Sargassum muticum* (Ochrophyta, *Fucales*) demonstrated free radical scavenging activity with DPPH from 16 to 86.6% after a 30-minute incubation at 37 °C (Terme et al. 2018). All lipid classes from *S. chordalis* and *S. muticum* demonstrated DPPH free radical scavenging activities at $1\,mg{\cdot}ml^{-1}$. The antioxidant activity of the phospholipid class of *S. chordalis* $scCO_2$ + ethanol 8% and *S. muticum* $scCO_2$ was greater than the chloroform/methanol solvent, respectively (half maximal effective concentration [EC_{50}] of 1.1 ± 0.1 and $1.0 \pm 0.1\,mg{\cdot}ml^{-1}$ against 4.9 ± 0.5 and $4.8 \pm 0.1\,mg{\cdot}ml^{-1}$) (Terme et al. 2018). Phospholipids with PUFAs were likely extracted selectively and exhibited antioxidant properties *in vitro* (Terme et al. 2018). The glycolipid and phospholipid fractions represented up to 90% of the lipid fraction from *S. muticum*. $scCO_2$ appears to be a good eco-responsible technique for the extraction of antioxidant lipids since antioxidant activity of glycolipids and phospholipids from *S. muticum* $scCO_2$ are twice that of the chloroform/methanol solvent system (Terme et al. 2018). More research needs to be done on macroalgal lipids to assess their *in vitro* activity on skin cells (keratinocytes and fibroblasts) for anti-aging and skin hydration assessment and potential relationships to antioxidant activity for example.

13.4.2 Preventive Effects of n-3 PUFAs on CVD and Metabolic Syndrome

Numerous investigations have been carried out in an attempt to examine the effect of n-3 PUFA intake for the management of CVDs and CVD risk factors, and there is a large body of evidence supporting their cardioprotective effects (AbuMweis et al. 2018; Bird et al. 2018; Innes and Calder 2018; Manuelli et al. 2017; O'Mahoney et al. 2018). CVDs are the leading cause of mortality among developed countries, even in apparently healthy individuals. In addition to genetic predisposition and a few nonmodifiable factors including age, gender, and ethnic origin, the development of CVDs is strongly associated with the presence of MetS (also referred to as Syndrome X, insulin resistance syndrome, or dysmetabolic syndrome) and the deregulation of clinical parameters such as increased very low density lipoprotein (VLDL) and triglyceride levels, decreased high density lipoprotein (HDL) levels, obesity, diabetes, and hypertension (Gonzalez-Chávez et al. 2018). Lifestyle and diet alterations, especially an n-3 LC-PUFA-enriched diet, could help to modulate these factors and reduce MetS and CVD risk.

13.4.2.1 Cardioprotective Effects of n-3 PUFAs Cardioprotective effects of n-3 LC-PUFAs were initially reported in a landmark study comparing the diets and CVD rates of Greenland Inuit to the Danish population (Bang et al. 1980). These benefits of n-3 LC-PUFAs were further supported by epidemiological studies associating fish consumption with a reduced CVD mortality in different populations (Daviglus et al. 1997; Kagawa et al. 1982; Kromhout et al. 1985; Newman et al. 1993). Various mechanisms have been proposed to explain the reduction in cardiovascular risk by n-3 PUFAs, including prevention of cardiac arrhythmias, decreased plasma triglycerides, reduction of blood pressure, decreased platelet aggregation, and reduction of inflammation (Calder 2004). Interestingly, the effects of DHA and EPA are not identical as suggested by a recent systematic review (Innes and Calder 2018), which discussed that DHA has a greater triglyceride-lowering effect, a greater effect on vascular function improvement and lowering of heart rate and blood pressure, and finally that only DHA increased HDL- and low density lipoprotein (LDL-) cholesterol concentration and LDL particle size (Innes and Calder 2018). Consumption of n-3 PUFAs has also been related to the regulation of eicosanoid concentrations, influencing several physiological functions in relation to the increase of plasma LDL-cholesterol levels, protection against cardiovascular, coronary heart diseases, atherosclerosis, diabetes, hypertension, and metabolic diseases (Jung et al. 2008; Kaur et al. 2012; Zárate et al. 2017).

Nutrition feeding studies in healthy animal models showed that ALA, the metabolic precursor of EPA and DHA, could reduce myocardial damage during cardiomyopathic disease in hamsters fed a high-fat diet with ALA representing 52% of total lipids (Fiaccavento et al. 2006). Reduced atherosclerosis, antithrombotic, and anti-inflammatory effects have also been reported in C57/B16 mice either wild-type or deficient for LDL-receptor, or deficient for APOE gene and fed diets rich in ALA (Bassett et al. 2011; Holy et al. 2011; Winnik et al. 2011). In addition, a diet enriched in n-3 LC-PUFAs, when fed after the onset of the ischemia/reperfusion period, reduced apoptosis in the limbic system of the brain, reduced circulating pro-inflammatory cytokines and attenuated post-myocardial infarction depression in a rat model of ischemia/reperfusion (Gilbert et al. 2013). However, a protective effect of n-3 PUFAs against CVD was not always detected in normal animals, although present in diabetic animals, as shown in a myocardial ischemia/reperfusion injury rat model (Xie et al. 2011). At the cellular level, recent studies reported the involvement of the peroxisome proliferator activated receptor (PPAR)-δ signaling pathway and enhanced ceramide levels in the cytotoxicity of DHA toward rat cardiomyocytes (Samokhvalov et al. 2015). In addition to an impact on PPAR-α and -γ signaling, n-3 PUFAs may act through inhibition of cyclic adenosine monophosphate-dependent protein kinase C (PKC) activation and calcium release at the intracellular level, and through inhibition of both Na^+-H^+ and Na^+-Ca^{2+} ion exchange as well as by reducing ligand availability for angiotensin-II, endothelin-1, and thromboxane receptors (Poudyal et al. 2011).

Early randomized controlled trials showed a reduction in risk of cardiovascular mortality after increasing consumption of fatty fish or n-3 LC-PUFA dietary supplements

(Burr et al. 1989; Gissi-Prevenzione Investigators 1999; Singh et al. 1997). However, more recent studies do not show significant effects of EPA and/or DHA supplementation (Aung et al. 2018; Kromhout et al. 2012; Maki et al. 2017; Manson et al. 2019). This lack of effect of n-3 PUFAs in recent prevention studies may have several explanations, among which is the frequent use of statin therapy in study patients (Maki et al. 2017; Sethi et al. 2016). Indeed, the mechanisms of action of n-3 PUFAs overlap with the pleiotropic effects of statins, such as antithrombotic and antioxidant effects, and improving endothelial function (Bird et al. 2018; Sethi et al. 2016). In addition, statins may interfere with cytochrome P450 enzymes and PPAR to affect PUFA concentration and eicosanoid production (Bird et al. 2018). Interestingly, DHA from algal oil reduced blood TAGs and increased HDL- but also LDL-cholesterol in patients without coronary disease, demonstrating a positive effect in the risk of initiation of factors involved in CVD (Bernstein et al. 2012).

13.4.2.2 Prevention of CVD Risk Associated with MetS and Diabetes Numerous nutrition studies have been conducted in animals with an enhanced risk of CVD, namely obesity, dyslipidemia and/or diabetes models, which highlighted the preventive effects of n-3 PUFAs (Mimouni et al. 2015; Ulmann et al. 2017). The efficacy of n-3 PUFAs to reduce the risk of CVD is linked to a reduction of factors involved in MetS development, mainly through modification of the serum lipid profile (Manuelli et al. 2017). The main effects of n-3 LC-PUFAs, mainly EPA and DHA, on plasma lipids were a reduction of adiposity, a diminution of TAG synthesis, and a decrease in the concentration of plasma TAG in obese patients (Micallef et al. 2009; Ulmann et al. 2017). In hypercholesterolemic rats, DHA supplementation reduced total weight gain, adiposity index, plasma HDL-cholesterol, and glucose concentrations regardless of the dose and form (i.e. DHA ethyl esters and DHA re-esterified TAG) of supplementation (Tabernero et al. 2013). Reductions in serum cholesterol and TAG levels, and a decrease in platelet aggregation were also observed in hypercholesterolemic rats fed EPA and DHA (Adan et al. 1999). Consumption of n-3 PUFAs had beneficial effects on obesity with increased β-oxidation or adiponectin levels in obese rats (Shirouchi et al. 2007). Moreover, the body mass index and waist circumference of obese patients were inversely correlated with EPA and DHA intakes (Micallef et al. 2009) owing to increased lipolysis and decreased lipogenesis in the liver (Harris and Bulchandani 2006). In the same way, a significant decrease in blood TAG and increase in HDL-cholesterol were observed in patients with dyslipidemia after consumption of 3 g PUFAs per day in a proportion of 0.9:1.5 for EPA and DHA, respectively, during 3 and 6 months (Derosa et al. 2009). A decrease in TAG and increase in HDL-cholesterol in blood were also reported in Type II diabetes patients receiving 460 mg of EPA and 380 mg of DHA ethyl esters per day for 8 weeks (Valdivielso et al. 2009) and similar conclusions have been drawn from a meta-analysis of Type II diabetes randomized controlled trials (O'Mahoney et al. 2018).

Concerning the use of microalgal n-3 PUFAs as dietary source of PUFAs in human or animal nutrition protocols, several studies highlighted the benefits of microalgae (Mimouni et al. 2015; Ulmann et al. 2014, 2017). In hypertriglyceridemic men, the concentration of fasting TAG and the number of small dense LDL particles were decreased after 45 days of a diet containing 7.5 g per day of DHA oil from *C. cohnii*, corresponding to about 3 g of DHA per day (Kelley et al. 2007). The use of the EPA-rich diatom *O. aurita* as a diet supplement reduced the risk factors for high-fat-diet induced MetS including hyperlipidemia, platelet aggregation, and oxidative stress in high-fat fed rats (Haimeur et al. 2012). Moreover, the ability of *O. aurita* to reduce CVD risk factors in high-fat-fed rats was similar or even greater than that of fish oil, potentially due to a synergistic interaction of n-3 PUFAs with other bioactive components of the microalga such as pigments or phytosterols (Haimeur et al. 2016). In alloxan-induced diabetic rats, diets supplemented with either *N. oculata* or *I. galbana* at $50\,mg\,d^{-1}$ decreased blood levels of glucose, TAG, and cholesterol (Nuño et al. 2013). Additionally, *Chlorella*, a freshwater microalgal genus rich in GLA, was demonstrated to prevent dyslipidemia in rat and hamster models fed with high-fat diets and subsequently prevented hyperlipidemia as well as atherosclerosis (Cherng and Shih 2005; Yamagishi et al. 2005). Consumption of *Chlorella pyrenoidosa* in the diet enhanced the hypoglycemic effects of exogenous insulin in streptozotocin-induced diabetic mice (Cherng and Shih 2006; Jong-Yuh and Mei-Fen 2005). Our current studies are investigating the potential of the two diatoms *Phaeodactylum tricornutum*, *T. lutea*, and the haptophyte *D. lutheri*, to reduce MetS-related risk factors in high-fat-fed rats (Mayer et al. 2018a, [b]). *Phaeodactylum tricornutum* supplementation has a real impact on MetS (Mayer et al. 2019). Nevertheless, caution in the interpretation of the above results is mandatory since they were obtained using whole microalgal cells that provide a variety of bioactive molecules with potential synergistic effects.

13.4.3 Contribution of n-3 PUFAs in Cancer Risk Factor Prevention and/or Therapy

13.4.3.1 Epidemiological Studies Highlight the Benefit of n-3 PUFA-Rich Diet

Increasing evidence suggests that n-3 PUFAs have anticancer activity and improve the effect of conventional cancer therapy (Chénais and Blanckaert 2012; de Lorgeril and Salen 2012; Ulmann et al. 2014, 2017; Vaughan et al. 2013).

High fat consumption is commonly associated with increased risk for several types of diet-related cancers such as breast, colonic, or pancreatic tumors (Chénais and Blanckaert 2012; de Lorgeril and Salen 2012; Ulmann et al. 2014, 2017; Vaughan et al. 2013). Furthermore, epidemiological studies highlight a 4- to 5-fold greater rate of breast cancer in Western countries than in Japan, associated, at least in part, with a diet low in fatty fish rich in PUFAs (Holmes and Willett 2004; Hursting et al. 1990; Kaizer et al. 1989; Kinlen 1991; Sasaki et al. 1993). These observations suggested that diets rich in n-3 and n-6 LC-PUFAs may help to reduce the risk of cancers (de Lorgeril and Salen 2012; Vaughan et al. 2013). However, while dietary n-3 PUFAs appear to possess a preventive effect on cancer (Hursting et al. 1990; Kaizer et al. 1989; Sasaki et al. 1993), n-6 PUFAs have been related to a higher risk of inducing tumor formation and inflammatory processes (Chénais and Blanckaert 2012; Weisburger 1997). On the other hand, SFAs and MUFAs have been shown to have either no effect on tumor formation or a moderate tumor-promoting effect (de Lorgeril and Salen 2012; Weisburger 1997). Recent population studies have shown that n-3 PUFA consumption reduced the risk of hepatocellular carcinoma (Gao et al. 2015) and enhanced survival after breast cancer (Khankari et al. 2015). Population studies show that intake of n-3 PUFAs is not associated with an overall increased incidence of colorectal cancer (Song et al. 2015) but may have a protective role against colorectal cancer, by reducing the risk of tumor initiation (Hodge et al. 2015; Song et al. 2015). Nevertheless, different n-3 PUFA exposures may exhibit different associations with cancer risk, and observational studies on colorectal, prostate, and breast cancers provide only limited evidence of a possible role of n-3 PUFAs in cancer prevention because of insufficient homogeneity of the observations (Gerber 2012; Hodge et al. 2015; Holmes et al. 2004; Khankari et al. 2015; MacLean et al. 2006; Shen et al. 2012; Song et al. 2015).

13.4.3.2 Antiproliferative and Pro-apoptotic Effects of n-3 PUFAs Understanding the cellular and molecular mechanisms of the anticancer effect of n-3 PUFAs remains an important area of current research. An increasing number of investigations have been performed in diverse human cancer cell lines using purified n-3 PUFAs, mainly DHA, and highlighting their antiproliferative and pro-apoptotic effects (D'Eliseo and Velotti 2016; Moloudizargari et al. 2018; Song and Kim 2016; Ulmann et al. 2017; VanderSluis et al. 2017). It is noteworthy that n-3 PUFAs had no pro-apoptotic effects on nontumoral cells including the human MCF-10A and H184-A1N4 mammary epithelial cell lines (Rovito et al. 2015; Tsai et al. 2017), embryonic kidney HEK-293 cells, and human hepatocyte-like WRL-68 cells, as well as Sprague Dawley rat primary cortical neuronal cells and murine peritoneal macrophages (So et al. 2015). Cell proliferation was reduced by DHA whether it originated from fish oil or microalgae (Judé et al. 2006; van Beelen et al. 2009). DHA acted as an antiproliferative agent by lengthening the cell cycle at the G_2/M transition (Newell et al. 2017) such as in the MDA-MB-231 breast cancer cell line (Barascu et al. 2006), or mainly by G_0/G_1 cell cycle arrest (Newell et al. 2017) such as in LA-N-1 neuroblastoma cells (So et al. 2015). The antiproliferative effects of DHA also involved increased cell sensitivity to ROS (Siddiqui et al. 2008; Song and Kim 2016) through the downregulation of superoxide dismutase 1 (SOD1) (Ding et al. 2004) and glutathione peroxidase 1 (GPX1) (Vibet et al. 2008). In addition, DHA was recently reported to induce the expression and nuclear translocation of the oxidative stress sensitive transcription factor nuclear factor erythroid 2 like 2/nuclear factor (erythroid derived 2)-like 2 (NFE2L2/Nrf2) (Pettersen et al. 2016; Tsai et al. 2017) and to increase the expression of oxidative stress-induced growth inhibitor 1 (OSGIN1) in MCF-7 and Hs578T breast cancer cells (Tsai et al. 2017). However, DHA also increased the activity of antioxidant enzymes (SOD, CAT, and GPX) in breast cancer tissues (Geng et al. 2018), suggesting that the anti-/pro-oxidant effects of DHA may be dependent of the cell type and concentration used.

Apoptosis was induced by DHA and, to a lesser extent by EPA (Sam et al. 2016; Sun et al. 2017; Wan et al. 2016), but not by ALA (Mason et al. 2015). Apoptosis was enhanced in DHA-treated cells through impairment of the activity of protein kinase Akt/PKB, p53 activation and increased caspase-3, caspase-9, and Bax pro-apoptotic enzyme levels or activity and decreased survival and Bcl-X_L in various cancer cell lines and with DHA concentration ranging from 10 to 200 μM (Ahangar et al. 2016; Chamras et al. 2002; Han et al. 2016; Liu et al. 2016; Mason et al. 2015; Park et al. 2018; Sam et al. 2017; Sam et al. 2018; So et al. 2015; Sun et al. 2017; Tasaki et al. 2017; Wan et al. 2016; Xue et al. 2017; Yin et al. 2017; Table 13.3).

The inactivation of the PI3K/Akt pathway is the main apoptosis pathway mentioned in the literature (see Table 13.3 for references). However, some other apoptotic pathways such as the Bax-independent pathway could be also involved in HL-60 promyelocytic leukemia (Miura et al. 2004). In the breast cancer cell line MCF-7, DHA-induced apoptosis was linked to both increased death receptors (DR-4 [death receptor 4], TRAIL [tumor necrosis factor-related apoptosis inducing ligand], and Fas) expression and mitochondrial release of the caspase activator SMAC (second mitochondria

Table 13.3 Examples of cell death signaling pathways triggered by n-3 polyunsaturated fatty acids (PUFAs) in human cancer cells

Type of cancer	Cell lines	n-3 PUFAs	Antiproliferative effect	Signaling pathway elements	References
Acute lymphoblastic leukemia	Molt-4	DHA	Apoptosis	↑p53, ↓survivin	(Sam et al. 2017)
Adrenocortical carcinoma	SW13, H295R[a]	DHA	Apoptosis, G_0/G_1 arrest	↓Akt, ↓mTor	(Liu et al. 2016)
Breast cancer	Human breast cancer tissue	DHA	Apoptosis	↑PPAR-α, TLR-4, ↑cAMP, GMPc, oxidative stress enzyme	(Geng et al. 2018)
	MCF-7	DHA	Apoptosis	↑p53 (PI3K), ↑NFE2L2, ↑ROS, ↑OSGIN1	(Tsai et al. 2017)
	MCF-7	DHA	Apoptosis	↑Fas, DR-4, TRAIL	(Xue et al. 2017)
	BT-474	DHA	Apoptosis	↓Akt, ↓Erk-1/2	(Mason et al. 2015)
	MCF-7, SKBR3, MDA-MB-231	DHA, EPA[b]	Apoptosis, autophagy	↑PPAR-γ	(Rovito et al. 2015)
Colorectal cancer	HCT116	DHA	Apoptosis	↑p53, ↓survivin, miR-1G1	(Sam et al. 2018)
	HCT116[a]	DHA	Apoptosis	↓survivin, β-catenin blockage	(Han et al. 2016)
	HCT116, HCT8[a]	DHA	Apoptosis	↑TNF-α, ↓miR-21, ↓AMPK, ↓RIP1 kinase	(Fluckiger et al. 2016)
	LS174T	DHA, EPA	Apoptosis	↓survivin	(Ahangar et al. 2016; Sam et al. 2016)
Glioblastoma	D54-MG, U-87-MG, U-251-MG	DHA	Apoptosis, autophagy, G_0/G_1 arrest	↓Akt, ↓mTor, ↑AMPK	(Kim et al. 2017)

(*continued*)

Table 13.3 *(continued)*

Type of cancer	Cell lines	n-3 PUFAs	Antiproliferative effect	Signaling pathway elements	References
Lung cancer (nonsmall cell)	A549	DHA	Apoptosis	↓Akt, PI3K, ↑ROS	(Yin et al. 2017)
	A549	DHA, EPA	Apoptosis, autophagy	↑ROS	(Zajdel et al. 2015)
Multiple myeloma	RPMI-8226, OPM-2	DHA	Apoptosis, autophagy	↓STAT3	(D'Eliseo et al. 2017)
Ovarian cancer	KF-28, HAC-2	DHA, GLA	Apoptosis	↑MAPK (JNK, p38), ↑ROS	(Tanaka et al. 2017)
	TOV-21G	DHA, EPA	Apoptosis	↑p53, ↑PPAR-γ	(Wan et al. 2016)
Pancreatic cancer	PANC-1	DHA	Apoptosis	↓survivin, ↓STAT3, ↓EGFR, ↓NF-κB	(M. Park et al. 2018)
Prostate cancer	DU-145	DHA, EPA	Apoptosis	↑p53, PI3K/Akt, ↑MAPK (JNK, p38), ↑TNF-α, ↑NF-κB	(Sun et al. 2017)
Renal cancer	Caki-1, 786-O	DHA	Apoptosis, G_0/G_1 arrest, G_2/M arrest	↓Akt, ↓STAT3, ↑EGFR	(Tasaki et al. 2017)

[a] Publication including animal model.

[b] dopamine-conjugated DHA or EPA.

Akt, protein kinase B; AMPK, adenosine monophosphate activated protein kinase; cAMP, cyclic adenosine monophosphate; DHA, docosahexaenoic acid; DR-4, death receptor 4; EGFR, epidermal growth factor; EPA, eicosapentaenoic acid; Erk, extracellular signal-regulated kinase; GLA, γ-linolenic acid; GMPc, guanosine monophosphate c; JNK, c-Jun N-terminal kinase; MAPK, mitogen-activated protein kinase; miR, microRNA; mTor, mammalian target of rapamycin; NFE2L2, nuclear factor erythroid 2 like 2; NF-κB, nuclear factor κ B; OSGIN, oxidative stress-induced growth inhibitor; PI3K, phosphoinositide 3-kinase; PPAR, peroxisome proliferator activated receptor; RIP, receptor-interacting protein; ROS, reactive oxygen species; TLR-4, Toll like receptor 4; TNF-α, tumor necrosis factor-α; TRAIL, tumor necrosis factor-related apoptosis inducing ligand.

derived activator of caspases)/Diablo (Xue et al. 2017). The inhibition of the STAT3 survival pathway has been reported for several cell types, including pancreatic and renal cancer cells and multiple myeloma (D'Eliseo et al. 2012, 2017, 2012; Park et al. 2018; Tasaki et al. 2017). The activation of the MAP kinase pathway, especially that of p38 and JNK (c-Jun N-terminal kinase), was also reported a few times to activate apoptosis and/or autophagy in the human prostate cancer cell line DU145 and KF-28 ovarian cancer cells (Sun et al. 2017; Tanaka et al. 2017). In addition, DHA and EPA are natural ligands of PPAR-α and PPAR-γ, thereby DHA-induced apoptosis may be linked to PPAR-γ overexpression in an epithelial ovarian cancer cell line (Wan et al. 2016), and to PPAR-α overexpression in breast cancer tissue (Table 13.3; Geng et al. 2018). Dopamine-conjugates of DHA and EPA induced breast cancer cell death through recruitment of PPAR-γ (Rovito et al. 2015). However, the role of PPAR-α and PPAR-γ in controlling cancer cell proliferation and apoptosis is controversial (Yousefnia et al. 2018). Besides apoptosis, recent studies have also highlighted that DHA may also induce pyroptosis, a form of programmed cell death mediated by inflammatory caspases (i.e. caspase-1, -4, and -5 in humans) and leading to pore formation in cell membrane by the N-terminal region of GasderminD in breast cancer cells (Pizato et al. 2018), and autophagy in breast, colon, and lung cancer cells as well as in glioblastoma cell lines (Kim et al. 2017; Pettersen et al. 2016; Rovito et al. 2015; Zajdel et al. 2015). Distinctive features of immunogenic apoptosis include the cell surface exposure of calreticulin and/or HSP90 in pre- or early-apoptotic stages and the release of nonhistone chromatin protein high mobility group box 1 in late-apoptosis, which will stimulate antitumor immune responses through antigen-presenting cells (Serrano-del Valle et al. 2019). DHA has been reported to promote immunogenic apoptosis and activated autophagy in multiple myeloma cells and inhibited the STAT3 survival pathway (Table 13.3; D'Eliseo et al. 2017). This study also reported the activation of autophagy by DHA in peripheral blood macrophages and dendritic cells, suggesting DHA acted as an immune stimulator, enhancing the presentation of tumor antigens by phagocytic cells (D'Eliseo et al. 2017).

Studies have been conducted in animal models of chemically induced tumors or tumor xenografts that reported antiproliferative and pro-apoptotic effects of DHA (Fluckiger et al. 2016; Liu et al. 2016), its metabolic precursor GLA (Das et al. 1995), or dietary fats (Han et al. 2016; Ramesh and Das 1995). Moreover, animal studies that demonstrated the potential preventive effects of n-3 PUFAs against several types of cancer have been reported using the *fat*-1 transgenic mouse that expresses n-3 desaturase missing in mammalian cells. These studies focused on colorectal cancer and colitis-associated cancer (Algamas-Dimantov et al. 2014; Han et al. 2016; Jia et al. 2008; Lim et al. 2009; Liu et al. 2016; Nowak et al. 2007; Weylandt et al. 2011), but have also targeted breast (Zou et al. 2013), liver (Lim et al. 2009; Weylandt et al. 2011), lung (Xia et al. 2005), pancreatic (Mohammed et al. 2012), and prostate (Lu et al. 2008) cancers as well as melanoma (Xia et al. 2006) and adrenocortical carcinoma (Liu et al. 2016).

13.4.3.3 Anti-Invasive and Antimetastatic Effects of n-3 PUFAs A few studies have shown that the diet can affect the metastatic potential of cancer cells known to have a high metastatic phenotype such as breast cancer (Bougnoux et al. 2009; Bougnoux et al. 2010). The antimetastatic effect of DHA was highlighted in several cancer cell lines (Chénais and Blanckaert 2012; Ulmann et al. 2014, 2017). DHA, at a concentration ranging from 10–100 μM, reduced the invasive potential of the MDA-MB-231 breast cancer cell line (Blanckaert et al. 2010, 2015; Yun et al. 2016) as well as 0.1% (v/v) fish oil with the tamoxifen-resistant (TamR) MCF-7 cells (Davison et al. 2018). DHA also suppressed the invasiveness of A549 lung adenocarcinoma (Yin et al. 2017) and renal cancer cell lines Caki-1 and 786-O (Tasaki et al. 2017). This anti-invasive effect of DHA was also demonstrated in several human colorectal cancer cell lines and may be linked to inhibition of granzyme B, a serine protease most commonly found in the granules of cytotoxic lymphocytes (CTLs), natural killer (NK) cells, and cytotoxic T cells (D'Eliseo et al. 2016). The mechanisms and signaling pathways involved in the antimetastatic effects of DHA remain to be understood and the current data are insufficient. However, this antimetastatic effect is corroborated by *in vivo* animal studies using *fat*-1 transgenic mice capable of producing n-3 FAs from the n-6 type, leading to abundant n-3 FAs with reduced levels of n-6 FAs in their organs and tissues, without the need for a dietary n-3 supply (Kang 2007). The use of *fat*-1 transgenic mice has shown a decrease of tumor growth and diminution of lung metastasis of syngeneic breast cancer cells in this DHA-rich environment (Yun et al. 2016).

13.4.3.4 n-3 PUFAs as Adjuvant of Chemotherapy Several studies have highlighted the potential of n-3 PUFAs, either fish oil or purified EPA/DHA, as an adjuvant in the treatment of cancer (Corsetto et al. 2017; Murphy et al. 2012; Siddiqui et al. 2011; Volpato and Hull 2018). Indeed, DHA enhanced the cytotoxic effects of docetaxel in prostate (LNCaP, PC3, and DU145) and mammary (MDA-MB-231) cancer cell lines through increased apoptosis (Chauvin et al. 2016; Shaikh et al. 2008). A similar enhancement of apoptosis was observed *in vitro* when combining DHA with diverse chemotherapeutic drugs, including lomustine with glioblastoma cell lines (Harvey et al. 2015), all-*trans* retinoic acid with the breast cancer cell line MCF-7 (Abdolahi et al. 2016), cisplatin with gastric cancer cells (Sheng et al. 2016); or with other traditional adjuvants such as dexamethasone in multiple myeloma cells (Dai et al. 2017) or curcumin in breast cancer cell lines or an *in vivo* mouse model of 7,12-dimethylbenz[a]anthracene (DMBA) induced mammary tumorigenesis (Altenburg et al. 2011; Siddiqui et al. 2013). Combining DHA-rich fish oil with 5-fluorouracil, irinotecan, or oxaliplatin also enhanced apoptosis in the colorectal cell line HT-29 by 120, 43, and 55%, respectively (Granci et al. 2013). Even radiation therapy such as single X-ray radiotherapy (up to 4 Gy) may be improved by n-3 PUFA exposure of colorectal HT-29 and LST174T cell lines (Cai et al. 2014). *In vivo* experiments using a model of N-methylnitrosurea-induced mammary tumor showed that the reduction of the tumor size induced by epirubicin was 40% greater when approx. 0.7 g DHA was provided daily in the diet (Colas et al. 2006). Furthermore, this effect of DHA was linked to a selective increase of oxidative damage as demonstrated by elevated lipid hydroperoxide level in tumors (Hajjaji et al. 2012). In addition, a clinical phase-II trial showed that the addition of DHA to anthracycline-based treatment targeting metastatic breast cancer improved the outcome of chemotherapy (Bougnoux et al. 2009). Moreover, DHA has the potential to specifically sensitize tumoral cells to chemotherapy or radiotherapy while protecting nontumor cells (Bougnoux et al. 2010; Hajjaji and Bougnoux 2013). Indeed, high incorporation of DHA during chemotherapy was devoid of adverse side effects and can improve the outcome of chemotherapy or radiotherapy (Bougnoux et al. 2010; Hajjaji and Bougnoux 2013).

Taking the evidence discussed above, DHA is a safe, natural compound that can greatly improve the anticancer properties of anticancer drugs by additive or synergistic interactions (Corsetto et al. 2017; Siddiqui et al. 2011; Volpato and Hull 2018). In addition, n-3 PUFAs reduced the risk of obesity-related breast cancer (Manni et al. 2017) and had protective effects toward the cardiotoxicity of anthracyclines, the most extensively used chemotherapeutics (Serini et al. 2017; Xue et al. 2016). Thus, current results of cohort studies and investigations in cell lines or animal models demonstrated that DHA could reduce tumor cell number by acting as soon as the cell begins its neoplastic transformation through a decrease in proliferation and an increase in apoptosis; this might explain the low level of breast cancer in populations with a high intake of DHA such as Japanese, Scandinavians, and people from Greenland and Nunavut (Bougnoux et al. 2010). According to Stark et al. (2016), regions with high EPA + DHA blood levels (>6%) included the Sea of Japan, Scandinavia, Greenland, Nunavut, Mongolia, and some other areas with indigenous population or populations not fully adapted to Westernized food habits (Stark et al. 2016). More importantly, DHA may also reduce the invasive potential of certain cancers, which is one of the main complications with advanced cancers.

13.4.4 Antiviral Activities

Sulfolipids like 1,2-di-*O*-acyl-3-*O*-(α-D-sulphoquinovosyl)-glyceride with two palmitic acids seemed to be responsible for the antiviral activities of extracts from the green seaweed, *Ulva fasciata*, the red seaweed *Laurencia papillosa* (Rhodophyta, *Ceramiales*), and the brown seaweed *Sargassum vulgare* against herpes simplex virus 1 and 2 *in vitro* (El Baz et al. 2014; Plouguerné et al. 2013). Palmitic acid extracted from *Sargassum fusiforme* also demonstrated antiviral activity against human immunodeficiency virus 1 (HIV-1) blocking virus entry and infection *in vitro* (Lee et al. 2009).

13.5 Potential Commercial Applications

Algal use by local populations across the globe is an old tradition in China, Japan, and Korea. In recent decades, progress in biotechnology has increased the development of commercial and industrial scale of algal bioactives. Macroalgae are mainly used for the production of phycocolloids, particularly, the Rhodophyta and Phaeophyta. However, their richness in the essential n-3 and n-6 PUFAs and their long-chain metabolites and derivatives EPA and DHA (Banskota et al. 2014a; Khotimchenko 2002) have strengthened their importance for human and animal diets.

IMTA systems are based on the use of organisms from different trophic levels where the excretion of upper-level organisms becomes a resource utilized by the lower levels (Pliego-Cortés et al. 2019). The use of aquaculture wastewater as a nutrient feed for seaweeds is recognized as a way to obtain algal biomass (Chopin et al. 2001; Neori et al. 2004). Recently, Peñuela et al. (2018) showed that the PUFA content was doubled in the biomass of the carragenophyte *Solieria filiformis* cultured in an IMTA system (Peñuela et al. 2018). Coupling ecological aquaculture or bioextraction to obtain algal biomass with the use of environmentally friendly food-safe techniques and the biorefinery concept could be a research strategy focus into the "Blue Economy" that highlights the sustainable use of oceanic resources by providing economic and ecological benefits.

The successful use of microalgae in biotechnology relies on the choice of the algal strain in accordance with their specific culture conditions to obtain the desired products with desirable properties (Pulz and Gross 2004). Currently, only a small number of microalgal species are produced on an industrial scale for their lipid content (Gouveia et al. 2008). They are mainly produced as human nutritional supplements and additives for animal feed (Kovač et al. 2013). The most important species in terms of annual world production are the Chlorophytes *Chlorella* sp. (2000 t year^{-1}), *D. salina* (1200 t year^{-1}), and *Haematococcus pluvialis* (Chlorophyta, *Chlamydomonadales*, 300 t year^{-1}), the dinoflagellate *C. cohnii* (240 t year^{-1} for DHA oil), and *Schizochytrium* sp. (10 t year^{-1} for DHA oil production) (Van der Voort et al. 2017).

For human nutrition, microalgae are sold in different forms including tablets, capsules, and liquids, or incorporated into snack foods, pasta, candies, or beverages (Liang et al. 2004). In our diet, PUFAs are generally supplied by fish and fish oils. However, fish oil as a food additive has drawbacks including an unpleasant taste and fishy smell. When one considers that PUFAs in fish are derived from their diet and especially from microalgae consumption, it makes sense to consider microalgae as a direct source of essential PUFAs (Jiang et al. 1999). The rhodophyte *Porphyridium cruentum* has been cultivated in artificial seawater and used for ARA production (Pulz and Gross 2004). Bacillariophytes including *Phaeodactylum tricornutum* can accumulate lipid up to 60% DW under nitrogen starvation making them a good source of PUFAs, especially EPA (Borowitzka 1997).

The global value for n-3 oils was around €320 million in 2014 (Van der Voort et al. 2017). Infant formula and dietary supplements are the most important applications for DHA-rich oils (Van der Voort et al. 2017). TAGs obtained from *Isochrysis* sp. and *I. galbana* 2307 exhibited FA composition and positional distribution in TAGs, crystallization, and melting properties similar to those of human milk fats (He et al. 2019). Therefore, they are promising sources of TAGs for infant formulas. Algal oils accounted for 3% of the EPA and DHA volume and 18% of the market value in recent years and the demand is growing related to the demand of nutrition and food labeling with terms such as "vegetarian" or "natural" (Van der Voort et al. 2017).

The economic value of algal cultivation is not the only parameter to consider in commercial applications of algae. The sustainable development of algae cultivation must also be taken into account to meet the needs of the present without compromising the ability of future generations to meet their own needs (World Commission on Environment and Development 1987). DHA can be produced by green strategies related to waste consumption. Indeed, *Schizochytrium* sp. grown on cane molasses as a carbon source and algal residue (*Schizochytrium* residue after a first FA extraction) as a nitrogen source has been used to produce DHA (Yin et al. 2019). The technical feasibility and sustainability of *Nannochloropsis gaditana* cultivation was demonstrated in the circular economy framework at the semi-industrial scale (López et al. 2019). The use of flue gases from a coal fired power plant produced a biomass in accordance with regulations for animal feed (López et al. 2019).

13.6 Conclusion and Future Trends

Very few algal species are used for their FA content for commercial purposes, despite a wide range of biological activities potentially impacting human health and wellness.

The cultivation conditions whether *in vitro* or at sea must be controlled for a high lipid quantity and purity. Molecular biology and genetic engineering could be promising approaches to increase the lipid content or FA profile of a specific interest by strain selection or gene overexpression. In the context of climate change, the biorefinery approach allows the global valorization of biomass by making successive extractions of compounds of interest. Improvement of processes for extraction and purification of FAs will extend the development of new markets with high added value without the drawback of the costs of cultivation.

Acknowledgments

The authors want to thank Newonat (Arzal, France) for the production of $scCO_2$ extracts. M. Fournière thanks the Conseil départemental des Côtes d'Armor (CD22) and Université Catholique de l'Ouest for PhD financial support. This work is a part of research conducted by N. Terme in a temporary lecturer position at Université Bretagne Sud and at the LBCM laboratory.

References

Abdolahi, M., Shokri, F., Hosseini, M. et al. (2016). The combined effects of all-*trans*-retinoic acid and docosahexaenoic acid on the induction of apoptosis in human breast cancer MCF-7 cells. *Journal of Cancer Research and Therapeutics* **12** (1): 204–208. https://doi.org/10.4103/0973-1482.154071.

AbuMweis, S., Jew, S., Tayyem, R., and Agraib, L. (2018). Eicosapentaenoic acid and docosahexaenoic acid containing supplements modulate risk factors for cardiovascular disease: a meta-analysis of randomised placebo-control human clinical trials. *Journal of Human Nutrition and Dietetics* **31** (1): 67–84. https://doi.org/10.1111/jhn.12493.

Adamakis, I.D., Lazaridis, P.A., Terzopoulou, E. et al. (2018). Cultivation, characterization, and properties of *Chlorella vulgaris* microalgae with different lipid contents and effect on fast pyrolysis oil composition. *Environmental Science and Pollution Research* **25** (23): 23018–23032. https://doi.org/10.1007/s11356-018-2368-5.

Adan, Y., Shibata, K., Sato, M. et al. (1999). Effects of docosahexaenoic and eicosapentaenoic acid on lipid metabolism, eicosanoid production, platelet aggregation and atherosclerosis in Hypercholesterolemic rats. *Bioscience, Biotechnology, and Biochemistry* **63** (1): 111–119. https://doi.org/10.1271/bbb.63.111.

Ahangar, P., Sam, M.R., Nejati, V., and Habibian, R. (2016). Treatment of undifferentiated colorectal cancer cells with fish-oil derived docosahexaenoic acid triggers caspase-3 activation and apoptosis. *Journal of Cancer Research and Therapeutics* **12** (2): 798–804. https://doi.org/10.4103/0973-1482.157326.

Al-Fadhli, A., Wahidulla, S., and D'Souza, L. (2006). Glycolipids from the red alga *Chondria armata* (Kütz.) Okamura. *Glycobiology* **16** (10): 902–915. https://doi.org/10.1093/glycob/cwl018.

Algamas-Dimantov, A., Yehuda-Shnaidman, E., Hertz, R. et al. (2014). Prevention of diabetes-promoted colorectal cancer by (n-3) polyunsaturated fatty acids and (n-3) PUFA mimetic. *Oncotarget* **5** (20): 9851–9863. https://doi.org/10.18632/oncotarget.2453.

Altenburg, J.D., Bieberich, A.A., Terry, C. et al. (2011). A synergistic antiproliferation effect of curcumin and docosahexaenoic acid in SK-BR-3 breast cancer cells: unique signaling not explained by the effects of either compound alone. *BMC Cancer* **11**: 149. https://doi.org/10.1186/1471-2407-11-149.

Aung, T., Halsey, J., Kromhout, D. et al. (2018). Associations of omega-3 fatty acid supplement use with cardiovascular disease risks meta-analysis of 10 trials involving 77 917 individuals. *JAMA Cardiology* **3** (3): 225–234. https://doi.org/10.1001/jamacardio.2017.5205.

Aveldano, M.I., VanRollins, M., and Horrocks, L.A. (1983). Separation and quantitation of free fatty acids and fatty acid methyl esters by RP HPLC. *Journal of Lipid Research* **24** (1): 83–93.

Bang, H.O., Dyerberg, J., and Sinclair, H.M. (1980). The composition of the Eskimo food in North Western Greenland. *American Journal of Clinical Nutrition* **33** (12): 2657–2661. https://doi.org/10.1093/ajcn/33.12.2657.

Banskota, A.H., Stefanova, R., Sperker, S. et al. (2014a). Lipids isolated from the cultivated red alga *Chondrus crispus* inhibit nitric oxide production. *Journal of Applied Phycology* **26** (3): 1565–1571. https://doi.org/10.1007/s10811-013-0174-5.

Banskota, A.H., Stefanova, R., Sperker, S. et al. (2014b). Polar lipids from the marine macroalga *Palmaria palmata* inhibit lipopolysaccharide-induced nitric oxide production in RAW264.7 macrophage cells. *Phytochemistry* **101**: 101–108. https://doi.org/10.1016/j.phytochem.2014.02.004.

Barascu, A., Besson, P., Le Floch, O. et al. (2006). CDK1-cyclin B1 mediates the inhibition of proliferation induced by omega-3 fatty acids in MDA-MB-231 breast cancer cells. *International Journal of Biochemistry and Cell Biology* **38** (2): 196–208. https://doi.org/10.1016/j.biocel.2005.08.015.

Barofsky, A. and Pohnert, G. (2007). Biosynthesis of polyunsaturated short chain aldehydes in the diatom *Thalassiosira rotula*. *Organic Letters* **9** (6): 1017–1020. https://doi.org/10.1021/ol063051v.

Bassett, C.M.C., McCullough, R.S., Edel, A.L. et al. (2011). The α-linolenic acid content of flaxseed can prevent the atherogenic effects of dietary trans fat. *AJP: Heart and Circulatory Physiology* **301** (6): H2220–H2226. https://doi.org/10.1152/ajpheart.00958.2010.

Becerra, M., Boutefnouchet, S., Córdoba, O. et al. (2015). Antileishmanial activity of fucosterol recovered from *Lessonia vadosa* Searles (Lessoniaceae) by SFE, PSE and CPC. *Phytochemistry Letters* **11**: 418–423. https://doi.org/10.1016/j.phytol.2014.12.019.

van Beelen, V.A., Spenkelink, B., Mooibroek, H. et al. (2009). An n-3 PUFA-rich microalgal oil diet protects to a similar extent as a fish oil-rich diet against AOM-induced colonic aberrant crypt foci in F344 rats. *Food and Chemical Toxicology* **47** (2): 316–320. https://doi.org/10.1016/j.fct.2008.11.014.

Belarbi, E.-H., Molina Grima, E., and Chisti, Y. (2000). A process for high yield and scaleable recovery of high purity eicosapentaenoic acid esters from microalgae and fish oil. *Enzyme and Microbial Technology* **26** (7): 516–529. https://doi.org/10.1016/S0141-0229(99)00191-X.

Bernart, M.W., Whatley, G.G., and Gerwick, W.H. (1993). Unprecedented oxylipins from the marine green alga *Acrosiphonia coalita*. *Journal of Natural Products* **56** (2): 245–259. https://doi.org/10.1021/np50092a010.

Bernstein, A.M., Ding, E.L., Willett, W.C., and Rimm, E.B. (2012). A meta-analysis shows that docosahexaenoic acid from algal oil reduces serum triglycerides and increases HDL-cholesterol and LDL-cholesterol in persons without coronary heart disease. *Journal of Nutrition* **142** (1): 99–104. https://doi.org/10.3945/jn.111.148973.

Bhaskar, N., Kinami, T., Miyashita, K. et al. (2004a). Occurrence of conjugated polyenoic fatty acids in seaweeds from the Indian Ocean. *Zeitschrift Für Naturforschung C* **59** (5–6): 310–314. https://doi.org/10.1515/znc-2004-5-602.

Bhaskar, N., Miyashita, K., and Hosokawa, M. (2004b). Comparative evaluation of fatty acid composition of different *Sargassum* (Fucales, Phaeophyta) species harvested from temperate and tropical waters. *Journal of Aquatic Food Product Technology* **13** (4): 53–70. https://doi.org/10.1300/J030v13n04.

Bhosale, R.A., Rajabhoj, M.P., and Chaugule, B.B. (2010). *Dunaliella salina* Teod. As a prominent source of eicosapentaenoic acid. *International Journal on Algae* **12** (2): 185–189. https://doi.org/10.1615/InterJAlgae.v12.i2.70.

Bird, J., Calder, P., and Eggersdorfer, M. (2018). The role of n-3 long chain polyunsaturated fatty acids in cardiovascular disease prevention, and interactions with statins. *Nutrients* **10** (6): 775. https://doi.org/10.3390/nu10060775.

Blanckaert, V., Ulmann, L., Mimouni, V. et al. (2010). Docosahexaenoic acid intake decreases proliferation, increases apoptosis and decreases the invasive potential of the human breast carcinoma cell line MDA-MB-231. *International Journal of Oncology* **36** (3): 737–742. https://doi.org/10.3892/ijo-00000549.

Blanckaert, V., Kerviel, V., Lépinay, A. et al. (2015). Docosahexaenoic acid inhibits the invasion of MDA-MB-231 breast cancer cells through upregulation of cytokeratin-1. *International Journal of Oncology* **46** (6): 2649–2655. https://doi.org/10.3892/ijo.2015.2936.

Bonnet, C. (2018). Lipids, a natural raw material at the heart of cosmetics innovation. *OCL* **25** (5): D501. https://doi.org/10.1051/ocl/2018055.

Borowitzka, M.A. (1997). Microalgae for aquaculture: opportunities and constraints. *Journal of Applied Phycology* **9** (5): 393–401. https://doi.org/10.1023/A:1007921728300.

Bouarab, K. (2004). The innate immunity of a marine red alga involves oxylipins from both the eicosanoid and octadecanoid pathways. *Plant Physiology* **135** (3): 1838–1848. https://doi.org/10.1104/pp.103.037622.

Boudière, L., Michaud, M., Petroutsos, D. et al. (2014). Glycerolipids in photosynthesis: composition, synthesis and trafficking. *Biochimica et Biophysica Acta (BBA) – Bioenergetics* **1837** (4): 470–480. https://doi.org/10.1016/j.bbabio.2013.09.007.

Bougnoux, P., Hajjaji, N., Ferrasson, M.N. et al. (2009). Improving outcome of chemotherapy of metastatic breast cancer by docosahexaenoic acid: a phase II trial. *British Journal of Cancer* **101** (12): 1978–1985. https://doi.org/10.1038/sj.bjc.6605441.

Bougnoux, P., Hajjaji, N., Maheo, K. et al. (2010). Fatty acids and breast cancer: sensitization to treatments and prevention of metastatic re-growth. *Progress in Lipid Research* **49** (1): 76–86. https://doi.org/10.1016/j.plipres.2009.08.003.

Boulho, R., Le Roux, J., Le Quémener, C. et al. (2017). Fractionation of UV-B absorbing molecules and of free radical scavenging compounds from *Solieria chordalis* by using centrifugal partition chromatography. *Phytochemistry Letters* **20**: 410–414. https://doi.org/10.1016/j.phytol.2017.03.010.

Bousquet, O. and Le Goffic, F. (1995). Counter-current chromatographic separation of polyunsaturated fatty acids. *Journal of Chromatography A* **704** (1): 211–216. https://doi.org/10.1016/0021-9673(94)01233-5.

Buono, S., Langellotti, A.L., Martello, A. et al. (2014). Functional ingredients from microalgae. *Food & Function* **5** (8): 1669–1685. https://doi.org/10.1039/c4fo00125g.

Burr, M.L., Gilbert, J.F., Holliday, R.M. et al. (1989). Effects of changes in fat, fish, and fibre intakes on death and myocardial reinfarction: diet and reinfarction trial (dart). *The Lancet* **334** (8666): 757–761. https://doi.org/10.1016/S0140-6736(89)90828-3.

Cai, F., Sorg, O., Granci, V. et al. (2014). Interaction of ω-3 polyunsaturated fatty acids with radiation therapy in two different colorectal cancer cell lines. *Clinical Nutrition* **33** (1): 164–170. https://doi.org/10.1016/j.clnu.2013.04.005.

Calder, P. (2004). N-3 fatty acids and cardiovascular disease: evidence explained and mechanisms explored. *Clinical Science* **107** (1): 1–11. https://doi.org/10.1042/CS20040119.

Cartens, M., Molina Grima, E., Robles Medina, A. et al. (1996). Eicosapentaenoic acid (20,5n-3) from the marine microalga *Phaeodactylum tricornutum*. *Journal of the American Oil Chemists' Society* **73** (8): 1025–1031. https://doi.org/10.1007/BF02523411.

Cason, J., Allinger, N.L., Sumrell, G., and Williams, D.E. (1951). Branched-chain fatty acids. XVII. Synthesis of two trimethylalkanoic acids. Certain relationships of boiling point and index of refraction to structure. *Journal of Organic Chemistry* **16** (7): 1170–1176. https://doi.org/10.1021/jo50001a023.

Catchpole, O.J., Tallon, S., Dyer, P. et al. (2012). Integrated supercritical fluid extraction and bioprocessing. *American Journal of Biochemistry and Biotechnology* **8** (4): 263–287. https://doi.org/10.3844/ajbbsp.2012.263.287.

Chamras, H., Ardashian, A., Heber, D., and Glaspy, J.A. (2002). Fatty acid modulation of MCF-7 human breast cancer cell proliferation, apoptosis and differentiation. *Journal of Nutritional Biochemistry* **13** (12): 711–716. https://doi.org/10.1016/S0955-2863(02)00230-9.

Chandrasekaran, K., Dhanraj, M., and Chadha, A. (2018). Effects of organic and inorganic salts on docosahexaenoic acid (DHA) production by a locally isolated strain of *Thraustochytrium* sp. T01. *Preparative Biochemistry and Biotechnology* **5**: 1–6. https://doi.org/10.1080/10826068.2018.1476882.

Chauvin, L., Goupille, C., Blanc, C. et al. (2016). Long chain n-3 polyunsaturated fatty acids increase the efficacy of docetaxel in mammary cancer cells by downregulating Akt and PKCε/δ-induced ERK pathways. *Biochimica et Biophysica Acta (BBA) – Molecular and Cell Biology of Lipids* **1861** (4): 380–390. https://doi.org/10.1016/j.bbalip.2016.01.012.

Chen, M., Tang, H., Ma, H. et al. (2011). Effect of nutrients on growth and lipid accumulation in the green algae *Dunaliella tertiolecta*. *Bioresource Technology* **102** (2): 1649–1655. https://doi.org/10.1016/j.biortech.2010.09.062.

Chénais, B. and Blanckaert, V. (2012). The Janus face of lipids in human breast cancer: how polyunsaturated fatty acids affect tumor cell hallmarks. *International Journal of Breast Cancer* **2012**: 712536. https://doi.org/10.1155/2012/712536.

Cherng, J.Y. and Shih, M.F. (2005). Preventing dyslipidemia by *Chlorella pyrenoidosa* in rats and hamsters after chronic high fat diet treatment. *Life Sciences* **76** (26): 3001–3013. https://doi.org/10.1016/j.lfs.2004.10.055.

Cherng, J.-Y. and Shih, M.-F. (2006). Improving glycogenesis in streptozocin (STZ) diabetic mice after administration of green algae *Chlorella*. *Life Sciences* **78** (11): 1181–1186. https://doi.org/10.1016/j.lfs.2005.06.050.

Choi, J.-S., Ha, Y.-M., Joo, C.-U. et al. (2012). Inhibition of oral pathogens and collagenase activity by seaweed extracts. *Journal of Environmental Biology* **33** (1): 115–121.

Chopin, T., Buschmann, A.H., Halling, C. et al. (2001). Integrating seaweeds into marine aquaculture systems: a key toward sustainability. *Journal of Phycology* **37** (6): 975–986. https://doi.org/10.1046/j.1529-8817.2001.01137.x.

Coderch, L., De Pera, M., Fonollosa, J. et al. (2002). Efficacy of *stratum corneum* lipid supplementation on human skin. *Contact Dermatitis* **47** (3): 139–146. https://doi.org/10.1034/j.1600-0536.2002.470303.x.

Cohen, Z. and Cohen, S. (1991). Preparation of eicosapentaenoic acid (EPA) concentrate from *Porphyridium cruentum*. *Journal of the American Oil Chemists' Society* **68** (1): 16–19. https://doi.org/10.1007/BF02660301.

Colas, S., Mahéo, K., Denis, F. et al. (2006). Sensitization by dietary docosahexaenoic acid of rat mammary carcinoma to anthracycline: a role for tumor vascularization. *Clinical Cancer Research* **12** (19): 5879–5886. https://doi.org/10.1158/1078-0432.CCR-06-0386.

Colombo, M.L., Risè, P., Giavarini, F. et al. (2006). Marine macroalgae as sources of polyunsaturated fatty acids. *Plant Foods for Human Nutrition* **61** (2): 67–72. https://doi.org/10.1007/s11130-006-0015-7.

Conte, M., Lupette, J., Seddiki, K. et al. (2018). Screening for biologically annotated drugs that trigger triacylglycerol accumulation in the diatom *Phaeodactylum*. *Plant Physiology* **177** (2): 532–552. https://doi.org/10.1104/pp.17.01804.

Corsetto, P., Colombo, I., Kopecka, J. et al. (2017). ω-3 long chain polyunsaturated fatty acids as sensitizing agents and multidrug resistance Revertants in cancer therapy. *International Journal of Molecular Sciences* **18** (12): 2770. https://doi.org/10.3390/ijms18122770.

Dai, X., Li, M., and Geng, F. (2017). Omega-3 polyunsaturated fatty acids eicosapentaenoic acid and docosahexaenoic acid enhance dexamethasone sensitivity in multiple myeloma cells by the p53/miR-34a/Bcl-2 axis. *Biochemistry (Moscow)* **82** (7): 826–833. https://doi.org/10.1134/S0006297917070082.

Das, U.N., Prasad, V.V.S.K., and Reddy, D.R. (1995). Local application of γ-linolenic acid in the treatment of human gliomas. *Cancer Letters* **94** (2): 147–155. https://doi.org/10.1016/0304-3835(95)03844-M.

Daviglus, M.L., Stamler, J., Orencia, A.J. et al. (1997). Fish consumption and the 30-year risk of fatal myocardial infarction. *New England Journal of Medicine* **336** (15): 1046–1053. https://doi.org/10.1056/NEJM199704103361502.

Davison, Z., Nicholson, R.I., Hiscox, S., and Heard, C.M. (2018). Co-administration of fish oil with signal transduction inhibitors has anti-migration effects in breast cancer cell lines. *The Open Biochemistry Journal* **12** (1): 130–148. https://doi.org/10.2174/1874091X01812010130.

Dawczynski, C., Schubert, R., and Jahreis, G. (2007). Amino acids, fatty acids, and dietary fibre in edible seaweed products. *Food Chemistry* **103** (3): 891–899. https://doi.org/10.1016/j.foodchem.2006.09.041.

De Jesus Raposo, M.F., de Morais, R.M.S.C., and de Morais, A.M.M.B. (2013). Health applications of bioactive compounds from marine microalgae. *Life Sciences* **93** (15): 479–486. https://doi.org/10.1016/j.lfs.2013.08.002.

D'Eliseo, D. and Velotti, F. (2016). Omega-3 fatty acids and cancer cell cytotoxicity: implications for multi-targeted cancer therapy. *Journal of Clinical Medicine* **5** (2): 15. https://doi.org/10.3390/jcm5020015.

D'Eliseo, D., Manzi, L., Merendino, N., and Velotti, F. (2012). Docosahexaenoic acid inhibits invasion of human RT112 urinary bladder and PT45 pancreatic carcinoma cells via down-modulation of granzyme B expression. *The Journal of Nutritional Biochemistry* **23** (5): 452–457. https://doi.org/10.1016/j.jnutbio.2011.01.010.

D'Eliseo, D., Di Rocco, G., Loria, R. et al. (2016). Epitelial-to-mesenchimal transition and invasion are upmodulated by tumor-expressed granzyme B and inhibited by docosahexaenoic acid in human colorectal cancer cells. *Journal of Experimental & Clinical Cancer Research* **35** (1): 24. https://doi.org/10.1186/s13046-016-0302-6.

D'Eliseo, D., Di Renzo, L., Santoni, A., and Velotti, F. (2017). Docosahexaenoic acid (DHA) promotes immunogenic apoptosis in human multiple myeloma cells, induces autophagy and inhibits STAT3 in both tumor and dendritic cells. *Genes & Cancer* **8**: 426–437. https://doi.org/10.1016/j.mechmat.2013.11.011.

Dembitsky, V.M. and Srebnik, M. (2002). Natural halogenated fatty acids: their analogues and derivatives. *Progress in Lipid Research* **41** (4): 315–367. https://doi.org/10.1016/S0163-7827(02)00003-6.

Denis, C., Morançais, M., Li, M. et al. (2010). Study of the chemical composition of edible red macroalgae *Grateloupia turuturu* from Brittany (France). *Food Chemistry* **119** (3): 913–917. https://doi.org/10.1016/j.foodchem.2009.07.047.

Derosa, G., Maffioli, P., D'Angelo, A. et al. (2009). Effects of long chain ω-3 fatty acids on metalloproteinases and their inhibitors in combined dyslipidemia patients. *Expert Opinion on Pharmacotherapy* **10** (8): 1239–1247. https://doi.org/10.1517/14656560902865601.

Ding, W.-Q., Vaught, J.L., Yamauchi, H., and Lind, S.E. (2004). Differential sensitivity of cancer cells to docosahexaenoic acid-induced cytotoxicity: the potential importance of down-regulation of superoxide dismutase 1 expression. *Molecular Cancer Therapeutics* **3** (9): 1109–1117.

D'Ippolito, G., Tucci, S., Cutignano, A. et al. (2004). The role of complex lipids in the synthesis of bioactive aldehydes of the marine diatom *Skeletonema costatum*. *Biochimica et Biophysica Acta (BBA) – Molecular and Cell Biology of Lipids* **1686** (1–2): 100–107. https://doi.org/10.1016/j.bbalip.2004.09.002.

D'Ippolito, G., Cutignano, A., Briante, R. et al. (2005). New C16 fatty-acid-based oxylipin pathway in the marine diatom *Thalassiosira rotula*. *Organic and Biomolecular Chemistry* **3** (22): 4065–4070. https://doi.org/10.1039/b510640k.

Duprat-de-Paule, S., Guilbot, J., Roso, A. et al. (2018). Augmented bio-based lipids for cosmetics. *OCL* **25** (5): D503. https://doi.org/10.1051/ocl/2018036.

El Baz, F.K., El Baroty, G.S., Ibrahim, E.A., and Abd El Baky, H.H. (2014). Cytotoxicity, antioxidants and antimicrobial activities of lipids extracted from some marine algae. *Journal of Aquaculture Research & Development* **05** (07): 1–5. https://doi.org/10.4172/2155-9546.1000284.

Eltgroth, M.L., Watwood, R.L., and Wolfe, G.V. (2005). Production and cellular localization of neutral long-chain lipids in the haptophyte algae *Isochrysis galbana* and *Emiliania huxleyi*. *Journal of Phycology* **41** (5): 1000–1009. https://doi.org/10.1111/j.1529-8817.2005.00128.x.

Fabrowska, J., Kapuścińska, A., Łęska, B. et al. (2017). *In vivo* studies and stability study of *Cladophora glomerata* extract as a cosmetic active ingredient. *Acta Poloniae Pharmaceutica. Drug Research* **74** (2): 633–641.

Fiaccavento, R., Carotenuto, F., Minieri, M. et al. (2006). α-Linolenic acid-enriched diet prevents myocardial damage and expands longevity in cardiomyopathic hamsters. *American Journal of Pathology* **169** (6): 1913–1924. https://doi.org/10.2353/ajpath.2006.051320.

Floreto, E.A.T., Hirata, H., Yamasaki, S., and Castro, S.C. (1994a). Effect of salinity on the growth and fatty acid composition of *Ulva pertusa* Kjellman (Chlorophyta). *Botanica Marina* **37** (2): 151–156. https://doi.org/10.1515/botm.1994.37.2.151.

Floreto, E.A.T., Hirata, H., Yamasaki, S., and Castro, S.C. (1994b). Influence of light intensity on the fatty acid composition of *Ulva pertusa* Kjellman (Chlorophyta). *Botanica Marina* **37** (2): 143–150. https://doi.org/10.1515/botm.1994.37.2.143.

Floreto, E.A.T., Teshima, S., and Ishikawa, M. (1996). Effects of nitrogen and phosphorus on the growth and fatty acid composition of *Ulva pertusa* Kjellman (Chlorophyta). *Botanica Marina* **39** (1–6): 69–74. https://doi.org/10.1515/botm.1996.39.1-6.69.

Fluckiger, A., Dumont, A., Derangère, V. et al. (2016). Inhibition of colon cancer growth by docosahexaenoic acid involves autocrine production of TNFα. *Oncogene* **35** (35): 4611–4622. https://doi.org/10.1038/onc.2015.523.

Fontana, A., D'Ippolito, G., Cutignano, A. et al. (2007). LOX-induced lipid peroxidation mechanism responsible for the detrimental effect of marine diatoms on zooplankton grazers. *ChemBioChem* **8** (15): 1810–1818. https://doi.org/10.1002/cbic.200700269.

Galloway, A.W.E., Britton-Simmons, K.H., Duggins, D.O. et al. (2012). Fatty acid signatures differentiate marine macrophytes at ordinal and family ranks. *Journal of Phycology* **48** (4): 956–965. https://doi.org/10.1111/j.1529-8817.2012.01173.x.

Gandhi, N.N. (1997). Applications of lipase. *Journal of the American Oil Chemists' Society* **74** (6): 621–634. https://doi.org/10.1007/s11746-997-0194-x.

Gao, M., Sun, K., Guo, M. et al. (2015). Fish consumption and n-3 polyunsaturated fatty acids, and risk of hepatocellular carcinoma: systematic review and meta-analysis. *Cancer Causes and Control* **26** (3): 367–376. https://doi.org/10.1007/s10552-014-0512-1.

Gelin, F., Volkman, J.K., De Leeuw, J.W., and Sinninghe Damsté, J.S. (1997). Mid-chain hydroxy long-chain fatty acids in microalgae from the genus *Nannochloropsis*. *Phytochemistry* **45** (4): 641–646. https://doi.org/10.1016/S0031-9422(97)00068-X.

Geng, L., Zhou, W., Liu, B. et al. (2018). DHA induces apoptosis of human malignant breast cancer tissues by the TLR-4/PPAR-α pathways. *Oncology Letters* **15** (3): 2967–2977. https://doi.org/10.3892/ol.2017.7702.

Gerber, M. (2012). Omega-3 fatty acids and cancers: a systematic update review of epidemiological studies. *British Journal of Nutrition* **107** (Suppl. 2): S228–S239. https://doi.org/10.1017/S0007114512001614.

Gilbert, K., Arseneault-Bréard, J., Flores Monaco, F. et al. (2013). Attenuation of post-myocardial infarction depression in rats by n-3 fatty acids or probiotics starting after the onset of reperfusion. *British Journal of Nutrition* **109** (1): 50–56. https://doi.org/10.1017/S0007114512003807.

Goecke, F., Hernández, V., Bittner, M. et al. (2010). Fatty acid composition of three species of *Codium* (Bryopsidales, Chlorophyta) in Chile. *Revista de Biología Marina y Oceanografía* **45** (2): 325–330. https://doi.org/10.4067/S0718-19572010000200014.

Gonzalez-Chávez, A., Chávez-Fernández, J.A., Elizondo-Argueta, S. et al. (2018). Metabolic syndrome and cardiovascular disease: a health challenge. *Archives of Medical Research* **49** (8): 516–521. https://doi.org/10.1016/j.arcmed.2018.10.003.

Gouveia, L., Batista, A.P., Sousa, I. et al. (2008). Microalgae in novel food product. In: *Food Chemistry Research Developments* (ed. K.N. Papadopoulos), 75–112. New York: Nova Science Publishers.

Granci, V., Cai, F., Lecumberri, E. et al. (2013). Colon cancer cell chemosensitisation by fish oil emulsion involves apoptotic mitochondria pathway. *British Journal of Nutrition* **109** (7): 1188–1195. https://doi.org/10.1017/S000711451200308X.

Gressler, V., Yokoya, N.S., Fujii, M.T. et al. (2010). Lipid, fatty acid, protein, amino acid and ash contents in four Brazilian red algae species. *Food Chemistry* **120** (2): 585–590. https://doi.org/10.1016/j.foodchem.2009.10.028.

Grosso, C., Valentão, P., Ferreres, F., and Andrade, P.B. (2015). Alternative and efficient extraction methods for marine-derived compounds. *Marine Drugs* **13** (5): 3182–3230. https://doi.org/10.3390/md13053182.

Guil-Guerrero, J.L., Belarbi, E.-H., and Rebelloso-Fuentes, M.M. (2001). Eicosapentanoic and arachinodic acids purification from the red microalga *Porphyridium cruentum*. *Bioseparation* **9**: 299–306. https://doi.org/10.1023/A:1011124624001.

Guiry, M.D. and Guiry, G.M. (2019). AlgaeBase. World-wide electronic publication. www.algaebase.org (accessed January 21, 2019).

Haimeur, A., Ulmann, L., Mimouni, V. et al. (2012). The role of *Odontella aurita*, a marine diatom rich in EPA, as a dietary supplement in dyslipidemia, platelet function and oxidative stress in high-fat fed rats. *Lipids in Health and Disease* **11**: 147. https://doi.org/10.1186/1476-511X-11-147.

Haimeur, A., Mimouni, V., Ulmann, L. et al. (2016). Fish oil and microalga omega-3 as dietary supplements: a comparative study on cardiovascular risk factors in high-fat fed rats. *Lipids* **51** (9): 1037–1049. https://doi.org/10.1007/s11745-016-4177-2.

Hajjaji, N. and Bougnoux, P. (2013). Selective sensitization of tumors to chemotherapy by marine-derived lipids: a review. *Cancer Treatment Reviews* **39** (5): 473–488. https://doi.org/10.1016/j.ctrv.2012.07.001.

Hajjaji, N., Besson, P., and Bougnoux, P. (2012). Tumor and non-tumor tissues differential oxidative stress response to supplemental DHA and chemotherapy in rats. *Cancer Chemotherapy and Pharmacology* **70** (1): 17–23. https://doi.org/10.1007/s00280-012-1884-0.

Han, Y.-M., Jeong, M., Park, J.-M. et al. (2016). The ω-3 polyunsaturated fatty acids prevented colitis-associated carcinogenesis through blocking dissociation of β-catenin complex, inhibiting COX-2 through repressing NF-κB, and inducing 15-prostaglandin dehydrogenase. *Oncotarget* **7** (39): 63583–63595. https://doi.org/10.18632/oncotarget.11544.

Harris, W.S. and Bulchandani, D. (2006). Why do omega-3 fatty acids lower serum triglycerides? *Current Opinion in Lipidology* **17** (4): 387–393. https://doi.org/10.1097/01.mol.0000236363.63840.16.

Harvey, K.A., Xu, Z., Saaddatzadeh, M.R. et al. (2015). Enhanced anticancer properties of lomustine in conjunction with docosahexaenoic acid in glioblastoma cell lines. *Journal of Neurosurgery* **122** (3): 547–556. https://doi.org/10.3171/2014.10.JNS14759.

He, Y., Wu, T., Sun, H. et al. (2019). Comparison of fatty acid composition and positional distribution of microalgae triacylglycerols for human milk fat substitutes. *Algal Research* **37**: 40–50. https://doi.org/10.1016/j.algal.2018.11.004.

Hoang, L.A.T., Nguyen, H.C., Le, T.T. et al. (2018). Different fermentation strategies by *Schizochytrium mangrovei* strain pq6 to produce feedstock for exploitation of squalene and omega-3 fatty acids. *Journal of Phycology* **54** (4): 550–556. https://doi.org/10.1111/jpy.12757.

Hodge, A.M., Williamson, E.J., Bassett, J.K. et al. (2015). Dietary and biomarker estimates of fatty acids and risk of colorectal cancer. *International Journal of Cancer* **137** (5): 1224–1234. https://doi.org/10.1002/ijc.29479.

Holdt, S.L. and Kraan, S. (2011). Bioactive compounds in seaweed: functional food applications and legislation. *Journal of Applied Phycology* **23** (3): 543–597. https://doi.org/10.1007/s10811-010-9632-5.

Holmes, M.D. and Willett, W.C. (2004). Does diet affect breast cancer risk? *Breast Cancer Research* **6** (4): 170–178. https://doi.org/10.1186/bcr909.

Holmes, M.D., Liu, S., Hankinson, S.E. et al. (2004). Dietary carbohydrates, fiber, and breast cancer risk. *American Journal of Epidemiology* **159** (8): 732–739. https://doi.org/10.1093/aje/kwh112.

Holy, E.W., Forestier, M., Richter, E.K. et al. (2011). Dietary α-linolenic acid inhibits arterial thrombus formation, tissue factor expression, and platelet activation. *Arteriosclerosis, Thrombosis, and Vascular Biology* **31** (8): 1772–1780. https://doi.org/10.1161/ATVBAHA.111.226118.

Hotimchenko, S.V. (2002). Fatty acid composition of algae from habitats with varying amounts of illumination. *Russian Journal of Marine Biology* **28** (3): 218–220. https://doi.org/10.1023/A:1016861807103.

Hu, Q., Sommerfeld, M., Jarvis, E. et al. (2008). Microalgal triacylglycerols as feedstocks for biofuel production: perspectives and advances. *The Plant Journal* **54** (4): 621–639. https://doi.org/10.1111/j.1365-313X.2008.03492.x.

Hursting, S.D., Thornquist, M., and Henderson, M.M. (1990). Types of dietary fat and the incidence of cancer at five sites. *Preventive Medicine* **19** (3): 242–253. https://doi.org/10.1016/0091-7435(90)90025-F.

Innes, J. and Calder, P. (2018). The differential effects of eicosapentaenoic acid and docosahexaenoic acid on cardiometabolic risk factors: a systematic review. *International Journal of Molecular Sciences* **19** (2): 532. https://doi.org/10.3390/ijms19020532.

Gissi-Prevenzione Investigators (1999). Prevenzione Investigators – dietary supplementation with n-3 polyunsaturated fatty acids and vitamin E after myocardial infarction: results of the Gissi-Prevenzione trial. *Lancet* **354**: 447–455. https://doi.org/10.1016/S0140-6736(99)07072-5.

Ishihara, K., Murata, M., Kaneniwa, M. et al. (1998). Inhibition of icosanoid production in MC/9 mouse mast cells by n-3 polyunsaturated fatty acids isolated from edible marine algae. *Bioscience, Biotechnology, and Biochemistry* **62** (7): 1412–1415. https://doi.org/10.1271/bbb.62.1412.

Ishihara, K., Murata, M., Kaneniwa, M. et al. (2000). Purification of stearidonic acid (18:4(n-3)) and hexadecatetraenoic acid (16:4(n-3)) from algal fatty acid with lipase and medium pressure liquid chromatography. *Bioscience, Biotechnology, and Biochemistry* **64** (11): 2454–2457. https://doi.org/10.1271/bbb.64.2454.

Iverson, J.L. and Weik, R.W. (1967). Correlation of fatty acid structure with preferential order of urea complexac formation. *Journal – Association of Official Analytical Chemists* **50** (5): 1111–1118.

Jamieson, G.R. and Reid, E.H. (1972). The component fatty acids of some marine algal lipids. *Phytochemistry* **11** (4): 1423–1432. https://doi.org/10.1016/S0031-9422(00)90096-7.

Jia, Q., Lupton, J.R., Smith, R. et al. (2008). Reduced colitis-associated colon cancer in *Fat*-1 (n-3 fatty desaturase) transgenic mice. *Cancer Research* **68**: 3985–3991.

Jiang, Y., Chen, F., and Liang, S.Z. (1999). Production potential of docosahexaenoic acid by the heterotrophic marine dinoflagellate *Crypthecodinium cohnii*. *Process Biochemistry* **34** ((6–7), 637): 633. https://doi.org/10.1016/S0032-9592(98)00134-4.

Jong-Yuh, C. and Mei-Fen, S. (2005). Potential hypoglycemic effects of *Chlorella* in streptozotocin-induced diabetic mice. *Life Sciences* **77** (9): 980–990. https://doi.org/10.1016/j.lfs.2004.12.036.

Judé, S., Roger, S., Martel, E. et al. (2006). Dietary long-chain omega-3 fatty acids of marine origin: a comparison of their protective effects on coronary heart disease and breast cancers. *Progress in Biophysics and Molecular Biology* **90** (1–3): 299–325. https://doi.org/10.1016/j.pbiomolbio.2005.05.006.

Jung, U.J., Torrejon, C., Tighe, A.P., and Deckelbaum, R.J. (2008). n-33 Fatty acids and cardiovascular disease: mechanisms underlying beneficial effects. *The American Journal of Clinical Nutrition* **87** (6): 2003S–2009S. https://doi.org/10.1093/ajcn/87.6.2003S.

Kagawa, Y., Nishizawa, M., Suzuki, M. et al. (1982). Eicosapolyenoic acids of serum lipids of Japanese islanders with low incidence of cardiovascular diseases. *Journal of Nutritional Science and Vitaminology* **28** (4): 441–453. https://doi.org/10.3177/jnsv.28.441.

Kaizer, L., Boyd, N.F., Kriukov, V., and Tritchler, D. (1989). Fish consumption and breast cancer risk: an ecological study. *Nutrition and Cancer* **12** (1): 61–68. https://doi.org/10.1080/01635588909514002.

Kang, J.X. (2007). *Fat*-1 transgenic mice: a new model for omega-3 research. *Prostaglandins, Leukotrienes and Essential Fatty Acids* **77** (5–6): 263–267. https://doi.org/10.1016/J.PLEFA.2007.10.010.

Kaur, N., Chugh, V., and Gupta, A.K. (2012). Essential fatty acids as functional components of foods-a review. *Journal of Food Science and Technology* **51** (10): 2289–2303. https://doi.org/10.1007/s13197-012-0677-0.

Kelley, N.S., Hubbard, N.E., and Erickson, K.L. (2007). Conjugated linoleic acid isomers and cancer. *The Journal of Nutrition* **137** (12): 2599–2607. https://doi.org/10.1093/jn/137.12.2599.

Kendel, M., Barnathan, G., Fleurence, J. et al. (2013). Non-methylene interrupted and hydroxy fatty acids in polar lipids of the alga *Grateloupia turuturu* over the four seasons. *Lipids* **48** (5): 535–545. https://doi.org/10.1007/s11745-013-3783-5.

Kendel, M., Wielgosz-Collin, G., Bertrand, S. et al. (2015). Lipid composition, fatty acids and sterols in the seaweeds *Ulva armoricana*, and *Solieria chordalis* from Brittany (France): an analysis from nutritional, chemotaxonomic, and antiproliferative activity perspectives. *Marine Drugs* **13** (9): 5606–5628. https://doi.org/10.3390/md13095606.

Khankari, N.K., Bradshaw, P.T., Steck, S.E. et al. (2015). Dietary intake of fish, polyunsaturated fatty acids and survival after breast cancer: a population-based follow-up study on

Long Island, New York: fish, PUFAs, and breast cancer survival. *Cancer* **121**: 2244–2252. https://doi.org/10.1007/s10549-015-3663-1.Progestin.

Khotimchenko, S.V. (1991). Fatty acid composition of seven *Sargassum* species. *Phytochemistry* **30** (8): 2639–2641. https://doi.org/10.1016/0031-9422(91)85113-E.

Khotimchenko, S.V. (1993). Fatty acids of green macrophytic algae from the sea of Japan. *Phytochemistry* **32** (5): 1203–1207. https://doi.org/10.1016/S0031-9422(00)95092-1.

Khotimchenko, S.V. (2002). Distribution of glyceroglycolipids in marine algae and grasses. *Chemistry of Natural Compounds* **38** (3): 223–229. https://doi.org/10.1023/A:1020471709232.

Khotimchenko, S.V. and Levchenko, E.V. (1997). Lipids of the red alga *Gracilaria verrucosa* (Huds.) Papenf. *Botanica Marina* **40** (1–6): 541–545. https://doi.org/10.1515/botm.1997.40.1-6.541.

Khotimchenko, S.V. and Yakovleva, I.M. (2004). Effect of solar irradiance on lipids of the green alga *Ulva fenestrata* Postels et Ruprecht. *Botanica Marina* **47** (5): 395–401. https://doi.org/10.1515/BOT.2004.050.

Khotimchenko, S.V., Vaskovsky, V.E., and Titlyanova, T.V. (2002). Fatty acids of marine algae from the Pacific Coast of North California. *Botanica Marina* **45** (1): 17–22. https://doi.org/10.1515/BOT.2002.003.

Kim, M.K., Dubacq, J.-P., Thomas, J.-C., and Giraud, G. (1996). Seasonal variations of triacylglycerols and fatty acids in *Fucus serratus*. *Phytochemistry* **43** (1): 49–55. https://doi.org/10.1016/0031-9422(96)00243-9.

Kim, S., Jing, K., Shin, S. et al. (2017). ω3-polyunsaturated fatty acids induce cell death through apoptosis and autophagy in glioblastoma cells: *in vitro* and *in vivo*. *Oncology Reports* **39** (1): 239–246. https://doi.org/10.3892/or.2017.6101.

Kinlen, L.J. (1991). Diet and breast cancer. *British Medical Bulletin* **47** (2): 462–469. https://doi.org/10.1093/oxfordjournals.bmb.a072484.

Kornprobst, J.-M. (2014). *Encyclopedia of Marine Natural Products*. Weinheim: Wiley-VCH Verlag GmbH & Co. KGaA https://doi.org/10.1002/9783527335855.

Kovač, D.J., Simeunović, J.B., Babić, O.B. et al. (2013). Algae in food and feed. *Food and Feed Research* **40** (1): 21–31.

Kromhout, D., Bosschieter, E.B., and de Lezenne Coulander, C. (1985). The inverse relation between fish consumption and 20-year mortality from coronary heart disease. *New England Journal of Medicine* **312** (19): 1205–1209. https://doi.org/10.1056/NEJM198505093121901.

Kromhout, D., Yasuda, S., Geleijnse, J.M., and Shimokawa, H. (2012). Fish oil and omega-3 fatty acids in cardiovascular disease: do they really work? *European Heart Journal* **33** (4): 436–443. https://doi.org/10.1093/eurheartj/ehr362.

Kumari, P., Bijo, A.J., Mantri, V.A. et al. (2013a). Fatty acid profiling of tropical marine macroalgae: an analysis from chemotaxonomic and nutritional perspectives. *Phytochemistry* **86**: 44–56. https://doi.org/10.1016/j.phytochem.2012.10.015.

Kumari, P., Kumar, M., Reddy, C.R.K., and Jha, B. (2013b). Algal lipids, fatty acids and sterols. In: *Functional Ingredients from Algae for Foods and Nutraceuticals* (ed. H. Domínguez), 87–134. Cambridge: Woodhead Publishing https://doi.org/10.1533/9780857098689.1.87.

Lang, I., Hodac, L., Friedl, T., and Feussner, I. (2011). Fatty acid profiles and their distribution patterns in microalgae: a comprehensive analysis of more than 2000 strains from the SAG culture collection. *BMC Plant Biology* **11** (1): 124. https://doi.org/10.1186/1471-2229-11-124.

Lee, D.Y.W., Lin, X., Paskaleva, E.E. et al. (2009). Palmitic acid is a novel CD4 fusion inhibitor that blocks HIV entry and infection. *AIDS Research and Human Retroviruses* **25** (12): 1231–1241. https://doi.org/10.1089/aid.2009.0019.

Lee, O.K., Kim, Y.H., Na, J.G. et al. (2013). Highly efficient extraction and lipase-catalyzed transesterification of triglycerides from *Chlorella* sp. KR-1 for production of biodiesel. *Bioresource Technology* **147**: 240–245. https://doi.org/10.1016/j.biortech.2013.08.037.

Li, X., Fan, X., Han, L., and Lou, Q. (2002). Fatty acids of some algae from the Bohai Sea. *Phytochemistry* **59** (2): 157–161. https://doi.org/10.1016/S0031-9422(01)00437-X.

Liang, S.Z., Liu, X., Chen, F., and Chen, Z. (2004). Current microalgal health food R&D activities in China. *Hydrobiologia* **512**: 45–48. https://doi.org/10.1023/B:HYDR.0000020366.65760.98.

Lim, K., Han, C., Dai, Y. et al. (2009). Omega-3 polyunsaturated fatty acids inhibit hepatocellular carcinoma cell growth through blocking β-catenin and cyclooxygenase-2. *Molecular Cancer Therapeutics* **8** (11): 3046–3055. https://doi.org/10.1158/1535-7163.MCT-09-0551.

Lin, Q., Zhuo, W.H., Wang, X.W. et al. (2018). Effects of fundamental nutrient stresses on the lipid accumulation profiles in two diatom species *Thalassiosira weissflogii* and *Chaetoceros muelleri*. *Bioprocess and Biosystems Engineering* **41** (8): 1213–1224. https://doi.org/10.1007/s00449-018-1950-z.

Liu, J., Xu, M., Zhao, Y. et al. (2016). N-3 polyunsaturated fatty acids abrogate mTORC1/2 signaling and inhibit adrenocortical carcinoma growth *in vitro* and *in vivo*. *Oncology Reports* **35** (6): 3514–3522. https://doi.org/10.3892/or.2016.4720.

López, A.R., Rodríguez, S.B., Vallejo, R.A. et al. (2019). Sustainable cultivation of *Nannochloropsis gaditana* microalgae in outdoor raceways using flue gases for a complete 2-year cycle: a circular economy challenge. *Journal of Applied Phycology* **31** (3): 1515–1523. https://doi.org/10.1007/s10811-018-1710-0.

de Lorgeril, M. and Salen, P. (2012). New insights into the health effects of dietary saturated and omega-6 and omega-3 polyunsaturated fatty acids. *BMC Medicine* **10** (1): 50. https://doi.org/10.1186/1741-7015-10-50.

Lu, Y., Nie, D., Witt, W.T. et al. (2008). Expression of the *fat*-1 gene diminishes prostate cancer growth in vivo through enhancing apoptosis and inhibiting GSK-3 phosphorylation. *Molecular Cancer Therapeutics* **7** (10): 3203–3211. https://doi.org/10.1158/1535-7163.MCT-08-0494.

MacDougall, K.M., McNichol, J., McGinn, P.J. et al. (2011). Triacylglycerol profiling of microalgae strains for biofuel feedstock by liquid chromatography-high-resolution mass spectrometry. *Analytical and Bioanalytical Chemistry* **401** (8): 2609–2616. https://doi.org/10.1007/s00216-011-5376-6.

MacLean, C.H., Newberry, S.J., Mojica, W.A. et al. (2006). Effects of omega-3 fatty acids on cancer risk:a systematic review. *JAMA* **295** (4): 403. https://doi.org/10.1001/jama.295.4.403.

Maki, K.C., Palacios, O.M., Bell, M., and Toth, P.P. (2017). Use of supplemental long-chain omega-3 fatty acids and risk for cardiac death: an updated meta-analysis and review of research gaps. *Journal of Clinical Lipidology* **11** (5): 1152–1160. https://doi.org/10.1016/j.jacl.2017.07.010.

Manni, A., El-Bayoumy, K., and Thompson, H. (2017). Docosahexaenoic acid in combination with dietary energy restriction for reducing the risk of obesity related breast cancer. *International Journal of Molecular Sciences* **19** (1): 28. https://doi.org/10.3390/ijms19010028.

Manson, J.E., Cook, N.R., Lee, I.-M. et al. (2019). Marine n-3 fatty acids and prevention of cardiovascular disease and cancer. *New England Journal of Medicine* **380** (1): 23–32. https://doi.org/10.1056/NEJMoa1811403.

Mansour, M.P. (2005). Reversed-phase high-performance liquid chromatography purification of methyl esters of C16–C28 polyunsaturated fatty acids in microalgae, including octacosaoctaenoic acid [28:8(n-3)]. *Journal of Chromatography A* **1097** (1–2): 54–58. https://doi.org/10.1016/j.chroma.2005.08.011.

Manuelli, M., Della Guardia, L., and Cena, H. (2017). Enriching diet with n-3 PUFAs to help prevent cardiovascular diseases in healthy adults: results from clinical trials. *International Journal of Molecular Sciences* **18** (7): 1552. https://doi.org/10.3390/ijms18071552.

Marangoni, A.G. and Rousseau, D. (1995). Engineering triacylglycerols: the role of interesterification. *Trends in Food Science and Technology* **6** (10): 329–335. https://doi.org/10.1016/S0924-2244(00)89167-0.

Mason, J.K., Klaire, S., Kharotia, S. et al. (2015). α-Linolenic acid and docosahexaenoic acid, alone and combined with trastuzumab, reduce HER2-overexpressing breast cancer cell growth but differentially regulate HER2 signaling pathways. *Lipids in Health and Disease* **14** (1): 91. https://doi.org/10.1186/s12944-015-0090-6.

Mata, T.M., Martins, A.A., and Caetano, N.S. (2010). Microalgae for biodiesel production and other applications: a review. *Renewable and Sustainable Energy Reviews* **14** (1): 217–232. https://doi.org/10.1016/j.rser.2009.07.020.

Mayer, C., Côme, M., Guéno, F. et al. (2018a). Effets bénéfiques de la micro-algue *Phaeodactylum tricornutum* dans la prévention du syndrome métabolique et de l'obésité chez le rat Wistar. *Nutrition Clinique et Métabolisme* **32** (4): 305. https://doi.org/10.1016/j.nupar.2018.09.155.

Mayer, C., Côme, M., Ulmann, L., Nazih, H., Ouguerram, K., Chénais, B., & Mimouni, V. (2018b). Comparative effects of *Phaeodactylum tricornatum* and *Diacronema lutheri* on risk factors associated with metabolic syndrome (MS) and obesity in Wistar rat. Paper for Lipids in the Ocean: Structure, Function, Ecological Role and Applications, Brest, November 20–22. https://marinelipids.sciencesconf.org/data/pages/Lipids_in_the_Ocean_2018_abstract_book.pdf (accessed September 25, 2020).

Mayer, C., Côme, M., Ulmann, L. et al. (2019). Preventive effects of the marine microalga *Phaeodactylum tricornutum*, used as a food supplement, on risk factors associated with metabolic syndrome in Wistar rats. *Nutrients* **11** (5): 1069. https://doi.org/10.3390/nu11051069.

McCauley, J.I., Meyer, B.J., Winberg, P.C., and Skropeta, D. (2016). Parameters affecting the analytical profile of fatty acids in the macroalgal genus *Ulva*. *Food Chemistry* **209**: 332–340. https://doi.org/10.1016/j.foodchem.2016.04.039.

Mendes, A., Da Silva, T.L., and Reis, A.D. (2007). DHA concentration and purification from the marine heterotrophic microalga *Crypthecodinium cohnii* CCMP 316 by winterization and urea complexation. *Food Technology and Biotechnology* **45** (1): 38–44. https://doi.org/10.4152/pea.201106445.

Mendes, M., Pereira, R.C., Sousa Pinto, I. et al. (2013). Antimicrobial activity and lipid profile of seaweed extracts from the north Portuguese coast. *International Food Research Journal* **20** (6): 3337–3345.

Micallef, M., Munro, I., Phang, M., and Garg, M. (2009). Plasma n-3 polyunsaturated fatty acids are negatively associated with obesity. *British Journal of Nutrition* **102** (9): 1370–1374. https://doi.org/10.1017/S0007114509382173.

Mikhailova, M.V., Bemis, D.L., Wise, M.L. et al. (1995). Structure and biosynthesis of novel conjugated polyene fatty acids from the marine green alga *Anadyomene stellata*. *Lipids* **30** (7): 583–589. https://doi.org/10.1007/BF02536993.

Mimouni, V., Ulmann, L., Pasquet, V. et al. (2012). The potential of microalgae for the production of bioactive molecules of pharmaceutical interest. *Current Pharmaceutical Biotechnology* **13** (15): 2733–2750. https://doi.org/10.2174/138920112804724828.

Mimouni, V., Ulmann, L., Haimeur, A. et al. (2015). Marine microalgae used as food supplements and their implication in preventing cardiovascular diseases. *OCL* **22** (4): D409. https://doi.org/10.1051/ocl/2015015.

Mimouni, V., Couzinet-Mossion, A., Ulmann, L., and Wielgosz-Collin, G. (2018). Lipids from microalgae. In: *Microalgae in Health and Disease Prevention* (eds. I. Levine and J. Fleurence), 109–131. Cambridge: Academic Press https://doi.org/10.1016/B978-0-12-811405-6.00005-0.

Mishra, V.K., Temelli, F., Ooraikul, B. et al. (1993). Lipids of the red alga, *Palmaria palmata*. *Botanica Marina* **36** (2): 169–174. https://doi.org/10.1515/botm.1993.36.2.169.

Miura, Y., Takahashi, K., Murata, Y. et al. (2004). Docosahexaenoic acid induces apoptosis *via* the Bax-independent pathway in HL-60 cells. *Bioscience, Biotechnology, and Biochemistry* **68** (11): 2415–2417. https://doi.org/10.1271/bbb.68.2415.

Mohammed, A., Janakiram, N.B., Brewer, M. et al. (2012). Endogenous n-3 polyunsaturated fatty acids delay progression of pancreatic ductal adenocarcinoma in Fat-1-p48$^{Cre/+}$-LSL-Kras$^{G12D/+}$ mice. *Neoplasia* **14** (12): 1249–1259. https://doi.org/10.1593/neo.121508.

Molina Grima, E., Robles Medina, A., Giménez Giménez, A. et al. (1994). Comparison between extraction of lipids and fatty acids from microalgal biomass. *Journal of the American Oil Chemists' Society* **71** (9): 955–959. https://doi.org/10.1007/BF02542261.

Molina Grima, E., Sanchez Pérez, J.A., Garcia Camacho, F. et al. (1995). The production of polyunsaturated fatty acids by microalgae: from strain selection to product purification. *Process Biochemistry* **30** (8): 711–719. https://doi.org/10.1016/0032-9592(94)00047-6.

Moloudizargari, M., Mortaz, E., Asghari, M.H. et al. (2018). Effects of the polyunsaturated fatty acids, EPA and DHA, on hematological malignancies: a systematic review. *Oncotarget* **9** (14): 11858–11875. https://doi.org/10.18632/oncotarget.24405.

Montañés, F., Catchpole, O.J., Tallon, S. et al. (2013). Semi-preparative supercritical chromatography scale plant for polyunsaturated fatty acids purification. *The Journal of Supercritical Fluids* **79**: 46–54. https://doi.org/10.1016/j.supflu.2012.11.018.

Murata, M. and Nakazoe, J. (2001). Production and use of marine algae in Japan. *Japan Agricultural Research Quarterly: JARQ* **35** (4): 281–290. https://doi.org/10.6090/jarq.35.281.

Murphy, R.A., Mourtzakis, M., and Mazurak, V.C. (2012). n-3 Polyunsaturated fatty acids: the potential role for supplementation in cancer. *Current Opinion in Clinical Nutrition and Metabolic Care* **15** (3): 246–251. https://doi.org/10.1097/MCO.0b013e328351c32f.

Nagappan, S. and Kumar Verma, S. (2018). Co-production of biodiesel and alpha-linolenic acid (omega-3 fatty acid) from microalgae, *Desmodesmus* sp. MCC34. *Energy Sources, Part A: Recovery, Utilization, and Environmental Effects* **40** (24): 2933–2940. https://doi.org/10.1080/15567036.2018.1514434.

Namal Senanayake, S.P.J. (2013). Methods of concentration and purification of omega-3 fatty acids. In: *Separation, Extraction and Concentration Processes in the Food, Beverage and Nutraceutical Industries* (ed. S.S.H. Rizvi), 483–505. Cambridge: Woodhead Publishing https://doi.org/10.1533/9780857090751.2.483.

Namal Senanayake, S.P.J. and Shahidi, F. (2000). Concentration of docosahexaenoic acid (DHA) from algal oil via urea complexation. *Journal of Food Lipids* **7** (1): 51–61. https://doi.org/10.1111/j.1745-4522.2000.tb00160.x.

Namal Senanayake, S.P.J. and Shahidi, F. (2002). Lipase-catalyzed incorporation of docosahexaenoic acid (DHA) into borage oil: optimization using response surface methodology. *Food Chemistry* **77** (1): 115–123. https://doi.org/10.1016/S0308-8146(01)00311-9.

Neori, A., Chopin, T., Troell, M. et al. (2004). Integrated aquaculture: rationale, evolution and state of the art emphasizing seaweed biofiltration in modern mariculture. *Aquaculture* **231**: 361–391. https://doi.org/10.1016/j.aquaculture.2003.11.015.

Newell, M., Baker, K., Postovit, L., and Field, C. (2017). A critical review on the effect of docosahexaenoic acid (DHA) on cancer cell cycle progression. *International Journal of Molecular Sciences* **18** (8): 1784. https://doi.org/10.3390/ijms18081784.

Newman, W.P., Middaugh, J.P., Propst, M.T., and Rogers, D.R. (1993). Atherosclerosis in Alaska natives and non-natives. *The Lancet* **341** (8852): 1056–1057. https://doi.org/10.1016/0140-6736(93)92413-N.

Nowak, J., Weylandt, K.H., Habbel, P. et al. (2007). Colitis-associated colon tumorigenesis is suppressed in transgenic mice rich in endogenous n-3 fatty acids. *Carcinogenesis* **28** (9): 1991–1995. https://doi.org/10.1093/carcin/bgm166.

Nuño, K., Villarruel-López, A., Puebla-Pérez, A.M. et al. (2013). Effects of the marine microalgae *Isochrysis galbana* and *Nannochloropsis oculata* in diabetic rats. *Journal of Functional Foods* **5** (1): 106–115. https://doi.org/10.1016/j.jff.2012.08.011.

O'Mahoney, L.L., Matu, J., Price, O.J. et al. (2018). Omega-3 polyunsaturated fatty acids favourably modulate cardiometabolic biomarkers in type 2 diabetes: a meta-analysis and meta-regression of randomized controlled trials. *Cardiovascular Diabetology* **17** (1): 98. https://doi.org/10.1186/s12933-018-0740-x.

Oresajo, C., Pillai, S., Manco, M. et al. (2012). Antioxidants and the skin: understanding formulation and efficacy. *Dermatologic Therapy* **25** (3): 252–259. https://doi.org/10.1111/j.1529-8019.2012.01505.x.

Park, N.-H., Choi, J.-S., Hwang, S.-Y. et al. (2013). Antimicrobial activities of stearidonic and gamma-linolenic acids from the green seaweed *Enteromorpha linza* against several oral pathogenic bacteria. *Botanical Studies* **54** (1): 1–9. https://doi.org/10.1186/1999-3110-54-39.

Park, M., Lim, J., and Kim, H. (2018). Docoxahexaenoic acid induces apoptosis of pancreatic cancer cells by suppressing activation of STAT3 and NF-κB. *Nutrients* **10** (11): 1621. https://doi.org/10.3390/nu10111621.

Paul, N.A., Neveux, N., Magnusson, M., and de Nys, R. (2014). Comparative production and nutritional value of "sea grapes" – the tropical green seaweeds *Caulerpa lentillifera* and *C. racemosa*. *Journal of Applied Phycology* **26** (4): 1833–1844. https://doi.org/10.1007/s10811-013-0227-9.

Pavón-Suriano, S.G., Ortega-Clemente, L.A., Curiel-Ramírez, S. et al. (2018). Evaluation of colour temperatures in the cultivation of *Dunaliella salina* and *Nannochloropsis oculata* in the production of lipids and carbohydrates. *Environmental Science and Pollution Research* **25** (22): 21332–21340. https://doi.org/10.1007/s11356-017-9764-0.

Peñuela, A., Robledo, D., Bourgougnon, N. et al. (2018). Environmentally friendly valorization of *Solieria filiformis* (Gigartinales, Rhodophyta) from IMTA using a biorefinery concept. *Marine Drugs* **16** (12): 487. https://doi.org/10.3390/md16120487.

Petkov, G. and Garcia, G. (2007). Which are fatty acids of the green alga *Chlorella*? *Biochemical Systematics and Ecology* **35** (5): 281–285. https://doi.org/10.1016/j.bse.2006.10.017.

Pettersen, K., Talstad, V., Hild, C. et al. (2016). Free radical biology and medicine DHA-induced stress response in human colon cancer cells – focus on oxidative stress and autophagy. *Free Radical Biology and Medicine* **90**: 158–172. https://doi.org/10.1016/j.freeradbiomed.2015.11.018.

Pillai, S., Oresajo, C., and Hayward, J. (2005). Ultraviolet radiation and skin aging: roles of reactive oxygen species, inflammation and protease activation, and strategies for prevention of inflammation-induced matrix degradation – a review. *International Journal of Cosmetic Science* **27** (1): 17–34. https://doi.org/10.1111/j.1467-2494.2004.00241.x.

Pizato, N., Luzete, B.C., Kiffer, L.F.M.V. et al. (2018). Omega-3 docosahexaenoic acid induces pyroptosis cell death in triple-negative breast cancer cells. *Scientific Reports* **8** (1): 9775. https://doi.org/10.1038/s41598-018-27850-y.

Plaza, M., Santoyo, S., Jaime, L. et al. (2010). Screening for bioactive compounds from algae. *Journal of Pharmaceutical and Biomedical Analysis* **51** (2): 450–455. https://doi.org/10.1016/j.jpba.2009.03.016.

Pliego-Cortés, H., Bedoux, G., Boulho, R. et al. (2019). Stress tolerance and photoadaptation to solar radiation in *Rhodymenia pseudopalmata* (Rhodophyta) through mycosporine-like amino acids, phenolic compounds, and pigments in an integrated multi-trophic aquaculture system. *Algal Research* **41**: 101542. https://doi.org/10.1016/j.algal.2019.101542.

Plouguerné, E., de Souza, L.M., Sassaki, G.L. et al. (2013). Antiviral sulfoquinovosyldiacylglycerols (SQDGs) from the Brazilian brown seaweed *Sargassum vulgare*. *Marine Drugs* **11** (11): 4628–4640. https://doi.org/10.3390/md11114628.

Poudyal, H., Panchal, S.K., Diwan, V., and Brown, L. (2011). Omega-3 fatty acids and metabolic syndrome: effects and emerging mechanisms of action. *Progress in Lipid Research* **50** (4): 372–387. https://doi.org/10.1016/j.plipres.2011.06.003.

Privett, O.S. (1971). Preparation of polyunsaturated fatty acids from natural sources. *Progress in the Chemistry of Fats and Other Lipids* **9** (C): 407–452. https://doi.org/10.1016/0079-6832(71)90033-4.

Pulz, O. and Gross, W. (2004). Valuable products from biotechnology of microalgae. *Applied Microbiology and Biotechnology* **65** (6): 635–648. https://doi.org/10.1007/s00253-004-1647-x.

Rabasco Alvarez, A.M., González Rodríguez, M.L., and Rodríguez, M.L.G. (2000). Lipids in pharmaceutical and cosmetic preparations. *Grasas y Aceites* **51** (1–2): 74–96. https://doi.org/10.3989/gya.2000.v51.i1-2.409.

Ramesh, G. and Das, U.N. (1995). Effect of dietary fat on diethylnitrosamine induced hepatocarcinogenesis in Wistar rats. *Cancer Letters* **95** (1–2): 237–245. https://doi.org/10.1016/0304-3835(95)03896-5.

Ramírez Fajardo, A., Esteban Cerdán, L., Robles Medina, A. et al. (2006). Concentration of eicosapentaenoic acid by selective esterification using lipases. *Journal of the American Oil Chemists' Society* **83** (3): 215–221. https://doi.org/10.1007/s11746-006-1196-9.

Ratnayake, W.M.N. and Ackman, R.G. (1979). Identification of novel octadecadienoic fatty acids in the seaweed *Cladophora rupestris* through oxidative ozonolysis of the alcohols prepared from the acids. *Lipids* **14** (6): 580–584. https://doi.org/10.1007/BF02533536.

Reeds, D.N., Brzezinski, M.A., Coury, D.A. et al. (1999). Neutral lipids in macroalgal spores and their role in swimming. *Marine Biology* **133** (4): 737–744. https://doi.org/10.1007/s002270050515.

Robles Medina, A., Giménez Giménez, A., Garcia Camacho, F. et al. (1995a). Concentration and purification of stearidonic, eicosapentaenoic, and docosahexaenoic acids from cod liver oil and the marine microalga *Isochrysis galbana*. *Journal of the American Oil Chemists' Society* **72** (5): 575–583. https://doi.org/10.1007/BF02638859.

Robles Medina, A., Molina Grima, E., and García Sánchez, J.L. (1995b). Obtaining of polyunsaturated fatty acids concentrates by the urea complexes method. *Grasas y Aceites* **46** (3): 174–182. https://doi.org/10.3989/gya.1995.v46.i3.922.

Robles Medina, A., Molina Grima, E., Giménez Giménez, A., and Ibáñez González, M.J. (1998). Downstream processing of algal polyunsaturated fatty acids. *Biotechnology Advances* **16** (3): 517–580. https://doi.org/10.1016/S0734-9750(97)00083-9.

Robles Medina, A., Esteban Cerdán, L., Giménez Giménez, A. et al. (1999). Lipase-catalyzed esterification of glycerol and polyunsaturated fatty acids from fish and microalgae oils. *Progress in Industrial Microbiology* **35** (70): 379–391. https://doi.org/10.1016/S0079-6352(99)80131-3.

Rodrigues, D., Freitas, A.C., Pereira, L. et al. (2015). Chemical composition of red, brown and green macroalgae from Buarcos Bay in central west coast of Portugal. *Food Chemistry* **183**: 197–207. https://doi.org/10.1016/j.foodchem.2015.03.057.

Rovito, D., Giordano, C., Plastina, P. et al. (2015). Omega-3 DHA- and EPA-dopamine conjugates induce PPARγ-dependent breast cancer cell death through autophagy and apoptosis. *Biochimica et Biophysica Acta (BBA) – General Subjects* **1850** (11): 2185–2195. https://doi.org/10.1016/j.bbagen.2015.08.004.

Sam, M.R., Ahangar, P., Nejati, V., and Habibian, R. (2016). Treatment of LS174T colorectal cancer stem-like cells with n-3 PUFAs induces growth suppression through inhibition of survivin expression and induction of caspase-3 activation. *Cellular Oncology* **39** (1): 69–77. https://doi.org/10.1007/s13402-015-0254-4.

Sam, M.R., Esmaeillou, M., and Shokrgozar, M.A. (2017). Fish-oil-derived DHA-mediated enhancement of apoptosis in acute lymphoblastic leukemia cells is associated with accumulation of p53, downregulation of survivin, and caspase-3 activation. *Nutrition and Cancer* **69** (1): 64–73. https://doi.org/10.1080/01635581.2017.1247884.

Sam, M.R., Tavakoli-Mehr, M., and Safaralizadeh, R. (2018). Omega-3 fatty acid DHA modulates p53, survivin, and microRNA-16-1 expression in KRAS-mutant colorectal cancer stem-like cells. *Genes & Nutrition* **13** (1): 8. https://doi.org/10.1186/s12263-018-0596-4.

Samokhvalov, V., Zlobine, I., Jamieson, K.L. et al. (2015). PPARδ signaling mediates the cytotoxicity of DHA in H9c2 cells. *Toxicology Letters* **232** (1): 10–20. https://doi.org/10.1016/j.toxlet.2014.09.029.

Santos, S.A.O., Trindade, S.S., Oliveira, C.S.D. et al. (2017). Lipophilic fraction of cultivated *Bifurcaria bifurcata* R. Ross: detailed composition and in vitro prospection of current challenging bioactive properties. *Marine Drugs* **15** (11): 1–17. https://doi.org/10.3390/md15110340.

Sasaki, S., Horacsek, M., and Kesteloot, H. (1993). An ecological study of the relationship between dietary fat intake and breast cancer mortality. *Preventive Medicine* **22** (2): 187–202. https://doi.org/10.1006/pmed.1993.1016.

Sayanova, O., Mimouni, V., Ulmann, L. et al. (2017). Modulation of lipid biosynthesis by stress in diatoms. *Philosophical Transactions of the Royal Society, B: Biological Sciences* **372** (1728): 20160407. https://doi.org/10.1098/rstb.2016.0407.

Schlenk, H. (1954). Urea inclusion compounds of fatty acids. *Progress in the Chemistry of Fats and Other Lipids* **2**: 243–267. https://doi.org/10.1016/0079-6832(54)90007-5.

Schmid, M., Guihéneuf, F., and Stengel, D.B. (2014). Fatty acid contents and profiles of 16 macroalgae collected from the Irish coast at two seasons. *Journal of Applied Phycology* **26** (1): 451–463. https://doi.org/10.1007/s10811-013-0132-2.

Scholfield, C.R. (1979). Silver nitrate-high performance liquid chromatography of fatty methyl esters. *Journal of the American Oil Chemists' Society* **56** (4): 510–511. https://doi.org/10.1007/BF02680190.

Serini, S., Ottes Vasconcelos, R., Nascimento Gomes, R., and Calviello, G. (2017). Protective effects of ω-3 PUFA in anthracycline-induced cardiotoxicity: a critical review. *International Journal of Molecular Sciences* **18** (12): 2689. https://doi.org/10.3390/ijms18122689.

Serrano-del Valle, A., Anel, A., Naval, J., and Marzo, I. (2019). Immunogenic cell death and immunotherapy of multiple myeloma. *Frontiers in Cell and Development Biology* **7**: 50. https://doi.org/10.3389/fcell.2019.00050.

Sethi, A., Bajaj, A., Khosla, S., and Arora, R.R. (2016). Statin use mitigate the benefit of omega-3 fatty acids supplementation-a meta-regression of randomized trials. *American Journal of Therapeutics* **23** (3): e737–e748. https://doi.org/10.1097/MJT.0000000000000048.

Shahidi, F. and Wanasundara, U.N. (1998). Omega-3 fatty acid concentrates: nutritional aspects and production technologies. *Trends in Food Science and Technology* **9** (6): 230–240. https://doi.org/10.1016/S0924-2244(98)00044-2.

Shaikh, I.A.A., Brown, I., Schofield, A.C. et al. (2008). Docosahexaenoic acid enhances the efficacy of docetaxel in prostate cancer cells by modulation of apoptosis: the role of genes associated with the NF-κB pathway. *The Prostate* **68** (15): 1635–1646. https://doi.org/10.1002/pros.20830.

Sheffer, M., Fried, A., Gottlieb, H.E. et al. (1986). Lipid composition of the plasma-membrane of the halotolerant alga, *Dunaliella salina*. *Biochimica et Biophysica Acta (BBA) – Biomembranes* **857** (2): 165–172. https://doi.org/10.1016/0005-2736(86)90344-5.

Shen, X.J., Zhou, J.D., Dong, J.Y. et al. (2012). Dietary intake of n-3 fatty acids and colorectal cancer risk: a meta-analysis of data from 489000 individuals. *British Journal of Nutrition* **108** (9): 1550–1556. https://doi.org/10.1017/S0007114512003546.

Sheng, H., Chen, X., Liu, B. et al. (2016). Omega-3 polyunsaturated fatty acids enhance cisplatin efficacy in gastric cancer cells by inducing apoptosis via ADORA1. *Anti-Cancer Agents in Medicinal Chemistry* **16** (9): 1085–1092. https://doi.org/10.2174/1871520616666160330104413.

Shinde, S., Ventre, S., Lloyd-Randolfi, J., and Lamont, M. (2018). Isolation of omega-7 fatty acid ethyl esters from natural oils. US 9895403 B2. https://patents.google.com/patent/US9895403B2/en (accessed September 15, 2020)

Shirouchi, B., Nagao, K., Inoue, N. et al. (2007). Effect of dietary omega 3 phosphatidylcholine on obesity-related disorders in obese Otsuka Long-Evans Tokushima fatty rats. *Journal of Agricultural and Food Chemistry* **55** (17): 7170–7176. https://doi.org/10.1021/jf071225x.

Shukla, V.K.S. (1988). Recent advances in the high performance liquid chromatography of lipids. *Progress in Lipid Research* **27** (1): 5–38. https://doi.org/10.1016/0163-7827(88)90003-3.

Siddiquí, R.A., Harvey, K.A., and Stillwell, W. (2008). Anticancer properties of oxidation products of docosahexaenoic acid. *Chemistry and Physics of Lipids* **153** (1): 47–56. https://doi.org/10.1016/j.chemphyslip.2008.02.009.

Siddiqui, R.A., Harvey, K.A., Xu, Z. et al. (2011). Docosahexaenoic acid: a natural powerful adjuvant that improves efficacy for anticancer treatment with no adverse effects. *BioFactors* **37** (6): 399–412. https://doi.org/10.1002/biof.181.

Siddiqui, R.A., Harvey, K.A., Walker, C. et al. (2013). Characterization of synergistic anti-cancer effects of docosahexaenoic acid and curcumin on DMBA-induced mammary tumorigenesis in mice. *BMC Cancer* **13**: 418. https://doi.org/10.1186/1471-2407-13-418.

Singh, R.B., Niaz, M.A., Sharma, J.P. et al. (1997). Randomized, double-blind, placebo-controlled trial of fish oil and mustard oil in patients with suspected acute myocardial infarction: the Indian experiment of infarct survival-4. *Cardiovascular Drugs and Therapy* **11** (3): 485–491. https://doi.org/10.1023/A:1007757724505.

Smith, A.E. (1952). The crystal structure of the urea–hydrocarbon complexes. *Acta Crystallographica* **5** (2): 224–235. https://doi.org/10.1107/S0365110X52000629.

So, W.W., Liu, W.N., and Leung, K.N. (2015). Omega-3 polyunsaturated fatty acids trigger cell cycle arrest and induce apoptosis in human neuroblastoma LA-N-1 cells. *Nutrients* **7** (8): 6956–6973. https://doi.org/10.3390/nu7085319.

Song, E. and Kim, H. (2016). Docosahexaenoic acid induces oxidative DNA damage and apoptosis, and enhances the chemosensitivity of cancer cells. *International Journal of Molecular Sciences* **17** (8): 1257. https://doi.org/10.3390/ijms17081257.

Song, M., Nishihara, R., Wu, K. et al. (2015). Marine ω-3 polyunsaturated fatty acids and risk for colorectal cancer according to microsatellite instability. *JNCI: Journal of the National Cancer Institute* **107** (4): 1879–1879. https://doi.org/10.1093/jnci/djv007.

Stark, K.D., Van Elswyk, M.E., Higgins, M.R. et al. (2016). Global survey of the omega-3 fatty acids, docosahexaenoic acid and eicosapentaenoic acid in the blood stream of healthy adults. *Progress in Lipid Research* **63**: 132–152. https://doi.org/10.1016/j.plipres.2016.05.001.

Strocchi, A. and Bonaga, G. (1975). Correlation between urea inclusion compounds and conformational structure of unsaturated C18 fatty acid methyl esters. *Chemistry and Physics of Lipids* **15** (2): 87–94. https://doi.org/10.1016/0009-3084(75)90033-X.

Sun, Y., Jia, X., Hou, L. et al. (2017). Involvement of apoptotic pathways in docosahexaenoic acid-induced benefit in prostate cancer: pathway-focused gene expression analysis using RT2 profile PCR array system. *Lipids in Health and Disease* **16** (1): 59. https://doi.org/10.1186/s12944-017-0442-5.

Swern, D. (1964). Techniques of separation. Urea complexes. In: *Fatty Acids. Their Chemistry, Properties, Production and Uses* (ed. K.S. Markley), 2309–2358. New York: Interscience Publishers.

Tabernero, M., Bermejo, L.M., Elvira, M. et al. (2013). Metabolic effect of docosahexaenoic acid supplementation in different doses and formulations (ethyl- and glyceryl-) in hypercholesterolemic rats. *Journal of Functional Foods* **5** (2): 755–762. https://doi.org/10.1016/j.jff.2013.01.021.

Tanaka, A., Yamamoto, A., Murota, K. et al. (2017). Polyunsaturated fatty acids induce ovarian cancer cell death through ROS-dependent MAP kinase activation. *Biochemical and Biophysical Research Communications* **493** (1): 468–473. https://doi.org/10.1016/j.bbrc.2017.08.168.

Tasaki, S., Horiguchi, A., Asano, T. et al. (2017). Docosahexaenoic acid inhibits the phosphorylation of STAT3 and the growth and invasion of renal cancer cells. *Experimental and Therapeutic Medicine* **14** (2): 1146–1152. https://doi.org/10.3892/etm.2017.4616.

Tasende, M.G. (2000). Fatty acid and sterol composition of gametophytes and sporophytes of *Chondrus crispus* (Gigartinaceae, Rhodophyta). *Scientia Marina* **64** (4): 421–426. https://doi.org/10.3989/scimar.2000.64n4421.

Terme, N., Boulho, R., Kendel, M. et al. (2017). Selective extraction of lipid classes from *Solieria chordalis* and *Sargassum muticum* using supercritical carbon dioxide and conventional solid–liquid methods. *Journal of Applied Phycology* **29** (5): 2513–2519. https://doi.org/10.1007/s10811-017-1084-8.

Terme, N., Boulho, R., Kucma, J.-P. et al. (2018). Radical scavenging activity of lipids from seaweeds isolated by solid-liquid extraction and supercritical fluids. *OCL* **25** (5): D505. https://doi.org/10.1051/ocl/2018054.

Thompson, G.A. (1996). Lipids and membrane function in green algae. *Biochimica et Biophysica Acta (BBA) – Lipids and Lipid Metabolism* **1302** (1): 17–45. https://doi.org/10.1016/0005-2760(96)00045-8.

Tsai, C.H., Shen, Y.C., Chen, H.W. et al. (2017). Docosahexaenoic acid increases the expression of oxidative stress-induced growth inhibitor 1 through the PI3K/Akt/Nrf2 signaling pathway in breast cancer cells. *Food and Chemical Toxicology* **108**: 276–288. https://doi.org/10.1016/j.fct.2017.08.010.

Ulmann, L., Mimouni, V., Blanckaert, V. et al. (2014). The polyunsaturated fatty acids from microalgae as potential sources for health and disease. In: *Polyunsaturated Fatty Acids* (ed. A. Catala), 23–43. New York: Nova Science Publishers.

Ulmann, L., Blanckaert, V., Mimouni, V. et al. (2017). Microalgal fatty acids and their implication in health and disease. *Mini-Reviews in Medicinal Chemistry* **17** (12): 1112–1123. https://doi.org/10.2174/1389557516666160722132736.

Valdivielso, P., Rioja, J., García-Arias, C. et al. (2009). Omega 3 fatty acids induce a marked reduction of apolipoprotein B48 when added to fluvastatin in patients with type 2 diabetes and mixed hyperlipidemia: a preliminary report. *Cardiovascular Diabetology* **8**: 1. https://doi.org/10.1186/1475-2840-8-1.

Van der Voort, M., Spruijt, J., Potters, J., De Wolf, P., and Elissen, H. (2017). Socio-economic assessment of Algae-based PUFA production. Public output report of the PUFAChain project, Göttingen, December 2017. www.pufachain.eu. https://doi.org/10.18174/440229 (accessed September 15, 2020).

VanderSluis, L., Mazurak, V., Damaraju, S., and Field, C. (2017). Determination of the relative efficacy of eicosapentaenoic acid and docosahexaenoic acid for anti-cancer effects in human breast cancer models. *International Journal of Molecular Sciences* **18** (12): 2607. https://doi.org/10.3390/ijms18122607.

Vaughan, V.C., Hassing, M.R., and Lewandowski, P.A. (2013). Marine polyunsaturated fatty acids and cancer therapy. *British Journal of Cancer* **108** (3): 486–492. https://doi.org/10.1038/bjc.2012.586.

Vibet, S., Goupille, C., Bougnoux, P. et al. (2008). Sensitization by docosahexaenoic acid (DHA) of breast cancer cells to anthracyclines through loss of glutathione peroxidase (GPx1) response. *Free Radical Biology and Medicine* **44** (7): 1483–1491. https://doi.org/10.1016/j.freeradbiomed.2008.01.009.

Volpato, M. and Hull, M.A. (2018). Omega-3 polyunsaturated fatty acids as adjuvant therapy of colorectal cancer. *Cancer and Metastasis Reviews* **37** (2–3): 545–555. https://doi.org/10.1007/s10555-018-9744-y.

Wan, X.H., Fu, X., and Ababaikeli, G. (2016). Docosahexaenoic acid induces growth suppression on epithelial ovarian cancer cells more effectively than eicosapentaenoic acid. *Nutrition and Cancer* **68** (2): 320–327. https://doi.org/10.1080/01635581.2016.1142581.

Wanasundara, U. and Fedec, P. (2002). Centrifugal partition chromatography (CPC): emerging separation and purification technique for lipid and related compounds. *INFORM – International News on Fats, Oils and Related Materials* **13** (9): 726–730.

Wang, X., Wang, X., Wang, W. et al. (2018). Synthesis of docosapentaenoic acid-enriched diacylglycerols by enzymatic glycerolysis of *Schizochytrium* sp. oil. *Bioresource Technology* **262**: 278–283. https://doi.org/10.1016/j.biortech.2018.04.061.

Weisburger, J.H. (1997). Dietary fat and risk of chronic disease. *Journal of the American Dietetic Association* **97** (7): S16–S23. https://doi.org/10.1016/S0002-8223(97)00725-6.

Weylandt, K.H., Krause, L.F., Gomolka, B. et al. (2011). Suppressed liver tumorigenesis in *fat*-1 mice with elevated omega-3 fatty acids is associated with increased omega-3 derived lipid mediators and reduced TNF-α. *Carcinogenesis* **32** (6): 897–903. https://doi.org/10.1093/carcin/bgr049.

Wielgosz-Collin, G., Kendel, M., and Couzinet-Mossion, A. (2016). Lipids, fatty acids, glycolipids, and phospholipids. In: *Seaweed in Health and Disease Prevention*, 185–221. San Diego, CA: Academic Press https://doi.org/10.1016/B978-0-12-802772-1.00007-5.

Winnik, S., Lohmann, C., Richter, E.K. et al. (2011). Dietary α-linolenic acid diminishes experimental atherogenesis and restricts T cell-driven inflammation. *European Heart Journal* **32** (20): 2573–2584. https://doi.org/10.1093/eurheartj/ehq501.

World Commission on Environment and Development (1987). *Our Common Future*, 27. Oxford: Oxford Unviersity Press.

Xia, S.H., Wang, J., and Kang, J.X. (2005). Decreased n-6/n-3 fatty acid ratio reduces the invasive potential of human lung cancer cells by downregulation of cell adhesion/invasion-related genes. *Carcinogenesis* **26** (4): 779–784. https://doi.org/10.1093/carcin/bgi019.

Xia, S.H., Lu, Y., Wang, J. et al. (2006). Melanoma growth is reduced in *fat*-1 transgenic mice: impact of omega-6/omega-3 essential fatty acids. *Proceedings of the National Academy of Sciences* **103** (33): 12499–12504. https://doi.org/10.1073/pnas.0605394103.

Xie, N., Zhang, W., Li, J. et al. (2011). α-Linolenic acid intake attenuates myocardial ischemia/reperfusion injury through anti-inflammatory and anti-oxidative stress effects in diabetic but not Normal rats. *Archives of Medical Research* **42** (3): 171–181. https://doi.org/10.1016/j.arcmed.2011.04.008.

Xue, H., Ren, W., Denkinger, M. et al. (2016). Nutrition modulation of cardiotoxicity and anticancer efficacy related to doxorubicin chemotherapy by glutamine and ω-3 polyunsaturated fatty acids. *Journal of Parenteral and Enteral Nutrition* **40** (1): 52–66. https://doi.org/10.1177/0148607115581838.

Xue, M., Ge, Y., Yu, C. et al. (2017). Apoptosis is induced by docosahexaenoic acid in breast cancer cells via death receptor and mitochondria-mediated pathways. *Molecular Medicine Reports* **16** (1): 978–982. https://doi.org/10.3892/mmr.2017.6678.

Yamagishi, S., Nakamura, K., and Inoue, H. (2005). Therapeutic potentials of unicellular green alga *Chlorella* in advanced glycation end product (AGE)-related disorders. *Medical Hypotheses* **65** (5): 953–955. https://doi.org/10.1016/j.mehy.2005.05.006.

Yang, A., Suh, W.I., Kang, N.K. et al. (2018). MAPK/ERK and JNK pathways regulate lipid synthesis and cell growth of *Chlamydomonas reinhardtii* under osmotic stress, respectively. *Scientific Reports* **8** (1): 13857. https://doi.org/10.1038/s41598-018-32216-5.

Yin, Y., Sui, C., Meng, F. et al. (2017). The omega-3 polyunsaturated fatty acid docosahexaenoic acid inhibits proliferation and progression of non-small cell lung cancer cells through the reactive oxygen species-mediated inactivation of the PI3K/Akt pathway. *Lipids in Health and Disease* **16** (1): 87. https://doi.org/10.1186/s12944-017-0474-x.

Yin, F.W., Zhu, S.Y., Guo, D.S. et al. (2019). Development of a strategy for the production of docosahexaenoic acid by *Schizochytrium* sp. from cane molasses and algae-residue. *Bioresource Technology* **271**: 118–124. https://doi.org/10.1016/j.biortech.2018.09.114.

Yoon, K.D., Chin, Y.W., and Kim, J. (2010). Centrifugal partition chromatography: application to natural products in 1994-2009. *Journal of Liquid Chromatography and Related Technologies* **33** (9–12): 1208–1254. https://doi.org/10.1080/10826076.2010.484374.

Yousefnia, S., Momenzadeh, S., Seyed Forootan, F. et al. (2018). The influence of peroxisome proliferator-activated receptor γ (PPARγ) ligands on cancer cell tumorigenicity. *Gene* **649**: 14–22. https://doi.org/10.1016/j.gene.2018.01.018.

Yun, E.-J., Song, K.-S., Shin, S. et al. (2016). Docosahexaenoic acid suppresses breast cancer cell metastasis by targeting matrix-metalloproteinases. *Oncotarget* **7** (31): 49961–49971. https://doi.org/10.18632/oncotarget.10266.

Zajdel, A., Wilczok, A., and Tarkowski, M. (2015). Toxic effects of n-3 polyunsaturated fatty acids in human lung A549 cells. *Toxicology in Vitro* **30** (1): 486–491. https://doi.org/10.1016/j.tiv.2015.09.013.

Zárate, R., el Jaber-Vazdekis, N., Tejera, N. et al. (2017). Significance of long chain polyunsaturated fatty acids in human health. *Clinical and Translational Medicine* **6** (1): 25. https://doi.org/10.1186/s40169-017-0153-6.

Zhang, W., Wang, F., Gao, B. et al. (2018). An integrated biorefinery process: stepwise extraction of fucoxanthin, eicosapentaenoic acid and chrysolaminarin from the same *Phaeodactylum tricornutum* biomass. *Algal Research* **32**: 193–200. https://doi.org/10.1016/j.algal.2018.04.002.

Zheng, C.J., Yoo, J.S., Lee, T.G. et al. (2005). Fatty acid synthesis is a target for antibacterial activity of unsaturated fatty acids. *FEBS Letters* **579** (23): 5157–5162. https://doi.org/10.1016/j.febslet.2005.08.028.

Zou, Z., Bellenger, S., Massey, K.A. et al. (2013). Inhibition of the HER2 pathway by n-3 polyunsaturated fatty acids prevents breast cancer in *fat*-1 transgenic mice. *Journal of Lipid Research* **54** (12): 3453–3463. https://doi.org/10.1194/jlr.M042754.

14

Algal Proteins and Peptides: Current Trends and Future Prospects

Abirami Ramu Ganesan[1], Shanmugam Munisamy[2], Rajeev Bhat[3], Palaniappan Seedevi[4], Kannan Mohan[5], and Shingo Matsukawa[6]

[1]*Department of Food Science and Home Economics, College of Engineering, Science and Technology, Fiji National University, Suva, Fiji Islands*
[2]*Research and Development Division (DSIR-Lab), Aquagri Processing Private Limited, Manamadurai, India*
[3]*ERA-Chair in VALORTECH, Estonia University of Life Sciences, Tartu, Estonia*
[4]*Department of Environmental Science, Periyar University, Salem, India*
[5]*Postgraduate and Research Department of Zoology, Sri Vasavi College, Erode, India*
[6]*Department of Food Science and Technology, Tokyo University of Marine Science and Technology, Tokyo, Japan*

14.1 Introduction

The investigation of complex protein structures is progressively growing and is an important field of research in recent times. Basic characterization of proteins and peptides is complicated due to the complexity and presence of polypeptides in quaternary structures, especially in the case of lower plants; for example, proteins from macroalgae (seaweeds) are bound to other nonprotein structures such as polysaccharides and polyphenols (Abirami and Kowsalya, 2017) that require extra effort to disintegrate the cell wall materials by physical or chemical methods (Kadam et al. 2017). There are several rapid methods of protein extraction that have been used in the literature such as microwave assisted extraction (MAE) (Chew et al. 2019), supercritical fluid extraction (SFE) (Herrero et al. 2006), ultrahigh pressure extraction (UPE), pressurized liquid extraction (PLE) (Tran et al. 2019), and ultrasound assisted extraction (UAE) (Kadam et al. 2017). Extraction of protein from algal sources requires hydrolysis processes to release peptides for specific functional bioactivities (Kumar 2019). Enzymatic hydrolyzes include proteases, cellulases, amylases, glucanases, and

Recent Advances in Micro- and Macroalgal Processing: Food and Health Perspectives, First Edition.
Edited by Gaurav Rajauria and Yvonne V. Yuan.

endoproteases used for the degradation of extracellular matrices in macroalgae like *Ascophyllum nodosum* to release proteins and peptides (Kadam et al. 2017).

Among the diverse hydrolysis strategies, enzymatic hydrolysis is commonly used in nutraceutical applications including antihypertensive (Sheih et al. 2009) and antidiabetic (Fan et al. 2018) effects and gives reliable results as compared with other methods such as SFE (Herrero et al. 2006). Other techniques including fermentation using microorganisms have also been effectively used for protein extraction in which macromolecules are separated using yeast, molds, and bacteria. For example, *Candida lipolytica*, *Candida rugopelliculosa*, and *Rhizopus oligosporus* have been used in the extraction of small peptide chains from microalgae like *Pavlova lutheri* under anaerobic conditions (Ryu et al. 2012). Fermentation-induced proteolysis is one of the major biochemical steps chiefly used for the production of polypeptides, smaller peptides, amino acids, and amines (Oh et al. 2015). Some methanol-utilizing yeast species such as *Candida boidinii*, *Pichia pastoris*, *Pichia methanolica*, *Candida rugopelliculosa*, and *Hansenula polymorpha* (thermotolerant) have been used for the fermentation and production of peptide from algae like *P. lutheri* (Oh et al. 2015). Therefore, proteolytic hydrolysis has been reported to assist in releasing peptides, which may be useful bioactive ingredients in reducing the risk of specific diseases related to radical scavenging and α-glucosidase inhibition (Rodrigues et al. 2015). This chapter is focused on the structure, extraction, and function of micro- and macroalgal proteins and peptides as biologically active molecules and their potential applications in improving human health or reducing the risk of chronic diseases such as diabetes, cancer, hypertension, and immunomodulation (Figure 14.1).

14.2 Isolation and Purification of Proteins from Algae

The extraction of proteins from micro- and macroalgae is inadequately reported in contrast to proteins from different terrestrial plant sources such as chickpea, soybean, pea, lentil, and mung bean (Apone et al. 2019). In general, algal proteins have been extracted using aqueous, acidic, and/or alkaline media using various methodologies (Zhang et al. 2019a, 2019b). Details of the extraction and isolation of proteins from micro- and macroalgae using different techniques and their recovery levels are given in Table 14.1.

Some effective methods of protein separation from algae such as *A. nodosum*, *Ulva* spp., and *Laminaria digitata* require acid and alkali hydrolysis (Yang et al., 2019). Rhodophyta and Ochraphyta algae contain insoluble cell wall polysaccharides including carrageenans, agar, alginates, and fucoidans, which require additional efforts to extract protein from these algae (Suwal et al. 2019). Harnedy and FitzGerald (2013) reported that mechanical grinding, osmotic shock, and enzymatic treatment of *Palmaria palmata* showed better protein yield compared with other polysaccharidase treatments yielding 11.57 g 100 g^{-1} of protein. More sophisticated methods including UAE, MAE, and pulse electric fields (PEFs) have also been used to separate proteins from macroalgae such as *P. palmata*, *A. nodosum*, and *L. digitata* (Bleakley and Hayes 2017). Seyfabadi et al. (2011) reported recovery of 46.0% protein from *Chlorella vul-*

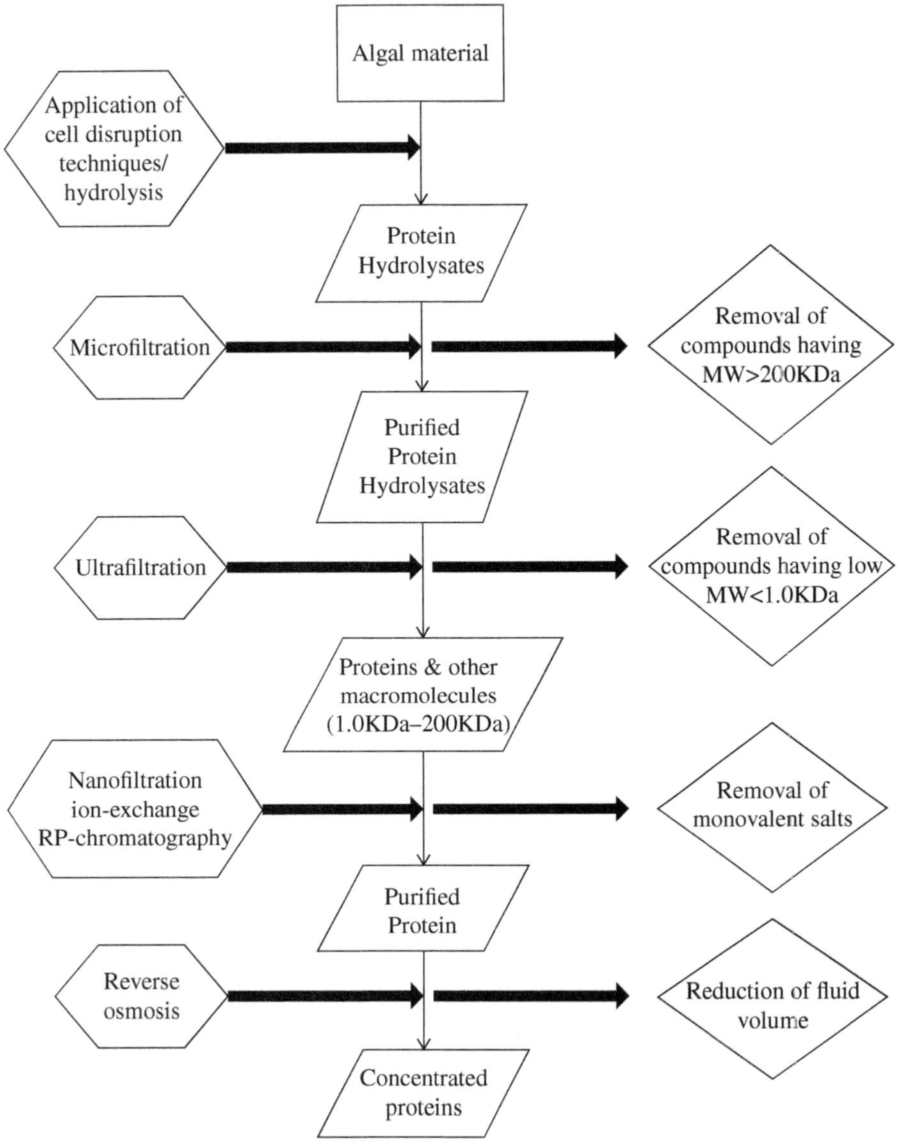

Figure 14.1 Application of membrane technologies in isolating and enriching protein fractions from micro- and macroalgae. Source: Bleakley and Hayes (2017).

garis through combined PEF–temperature treatment sonic disruption, whereas it was 8.40% with enzymatic treatment (Alzahrani et al. 2018). It was reported that fresh samples also showed better total protein yield quantitatively in comparison with dried samples; for example, *Spirulina platensis* fresh alga yield was 67.18% protein, whereas the dried sample yielded 72.85% (Agustini et al. 2015).

Table 14.1 Extraction and isolation of protein from macroalgae using different methods.

Species	Extraction method	Extraction and isolation methods	Protein yield g 100 g^{-1} dry weight	References
Palmaria palmata	Enzymatic hydrolysis	Polysaccharidase degradation	3.3	Joubert and Fleurence 2008
			6.7	Harnedy and FitzGerald 2013
	Physical process	Osmotic stress	6.77	Harnedy and FitzGerald 2013
		High shear force	6.92	
	Chemical extraction	Alkaline and aqueous	4.16	
Acanthophora spicifera	Physical process	Aqueous treatment in combination with Potter homogenization	8.9	Barbarino and Lourenço (2005)
Sargassum vulgare			6.9	
Ulva fasciata			7.3	
Ulva rigida	Physical process	Osmotic shock	9.7	Fleurence et al. 1995
	Enzymatic incubation	Cellulase treatment	18.5	
Ulva rotundata	Physical process	Osmotic shock	14.0	
	Enzymatic incubation	Cellulase treatment	18.5	
Ulva lactuca	Physical process	Pulsed electric field	< 1.0	Polikovsky et al. 2016

14.3 Structural Characteristics of Micro- and Macroalgae Peptides

14.3.1 Structures of Peptides from Microalgae

Some of the peptides isolated from microalgae and their biological activities reported in the literature are provided in Table 14.2. Peptides of microalgae derived from enzymatic hydrolyzes have been reported to exhibit a variety of biological activities including cell proliferation, carbohydrate enzyme inhibition, and antioxidant activity (Heo et al. 2017). The peptide sequences vary from a few amino acids to more than 10 amino acid residues (Kang et al. 2012). A peptide with the sequence of Val-Glu-Cys-Lyr-Gly-Pro-Asn-Arg-Pro-Glu-Phe was isolated from *C. vulgaris* through pepsin hydrolysis and was reported to have angiotensin I-converting enzyme (ACE) inhibitory action *in vitro* with a half maximal inhibitory concentration (IC_{50}) value of 29.6 μM (Sheih et al. 2009).

Table 14.2 Peptides from microalgae and their potential bioactivities.

Microalgae	Peptide sequences	Extraction method	Bioactivity	References
Tetradesmus obliquus	Trp-Pro-Arg-Gly-Tyr-Phe-Leu Gly-Pro-Asp-Arg-Pro-Lys-Phe-Leu-Gly-Pro-Phe Try-Tyr-Gly-Pro-Asp-Arg-Pro-Lys-Phe-Leu Ser-Asp-Try-Asp-Arg-Phe	Alcalase®	ACE inhibition; antioxidant ABTS and DPPH activity	Montone et al. 2018
Pavlova lutheri	Glu-Pro-Gln-Trp-Phe-Leu	Fermentation by *Hansenula polymorpha*	Osteoblastic differentiation and bone health in MG-63 cells	Qian et al. 2018
Pavlova lutheri	Met-Gly-Arg-Tyr	Fermentation by *Hansenula polymorpha*	Antioxidant, Inhibitory against α-MSH	Oh et al. 2015
Pavlova lutheri	Met-Pro-Gly-Pro-Leu-Ser-Pro-Leu	Fermentation by *Candida rugopelliculosa*	Myofibroblast differentiation	Ryu et al. 2012
Nannochloropsis oculata	Leu-Glu-Gln Gly-Met-Asn-Asn-Leu-Thr-Pro	Pepsin	ACE inhibitory activity	Samarakoon et al. 2013
Navicula incerta	Pro-Gly-Trp-Asn-Gln-Trp-Phe-Leu Val-Glu-Val-Leu-Pro-Pro-Ala-Glu-Leu	Pepsin	Hepatic fibrosis inhibitory effect in gamma-glutamyl transpeptidase assay	Kang et al. 2012
Navicula incerta	Glu-Asp-Lys-Arg	Pepsin	Antioxidative *in vitro* assay	Kang et al. 2012
Navicula incerta	Pro-Gly-Trp-Asn-Gln-Trp-Phe-Leu, Val-Glu-Val-Leu-Pro-Pro-Ala-Glu-Leu	Alcalase®, neutrase, papain, pepsin, pronase, E trypsin, and α-chymotrypsin	Inhibitory effects on collagen release in hepatic fibrosis in hepatic stellate cells LX-2	Kang et al. 2013
Spirulina maxima	Leu-Asp-Ala-Val-Asn-Arg Met-Met-Leu-Asp-Phe	Pepsin, trypsin, and chymotrypsin	Anti-inflammatory peptides in RBL-2H3 mast cells	Vo et al. 2013
Spirulina platensis	Ile-Ala-Glu Phe-Ala-Leu Ala-Glu-Leu Ile-Ala-Pro-Gly Val-Ala-Phe	Pepsin	ACE inhibitory activity in rat model	Suetsuna and Nakano, 2000

(*continued*)

Table 14.2 (*continued*)

Microalgae	Peptide sequences	Extraction method	Bioactivity	References
Spirulina sp.	Thr-Met-Glu-Pro-Gly-Lys-Pro	Gastrointestinal enzymes	ACE inhibitory activity *in vitro* assay	Heo et al. 2017
Chlorella ellipsoidea	Val-Glu-Gly-Tyr	Alcalase	ACE inhibitory activity in rat model	Ko et al. 2012
Chlorella vulgaris	Ile-Val-Val-Glu Ala-Phe-Leu Phe-Ala-Leu Ala-Glu-Leu Val-Val-Pro-Pro-Ala	Pepsin	ACE inhibitory activity in rat model	Suetsuna and Nakano 2000
Chlorella vulgaris	Val-Glu-Cys-Lyr-Gly-Pro-Asn-Arg-Pro-Glu-Phe	Pepsin	Antiproliferation *in vitro* ACE assay ACE-inhibitory, antioxidative superoxide radical	Sheih et al. 2009

α-MSH, melanocyte stimulating hormone; ABTS, 2,2′-azino-bis(3-ethylbenzothiazoline-6-sulfonic acid); ACE, angiotensin I-converting enzyme; DPPH, 2,2-diphenyl-1-picrylhydrazyl.

Five peptides, Ile-Ala-Glu, Phe-Ala-Leu, Ala-Glu-Leu, Ile-Ala-Pro-Gly, and Val-Ala-Phe, obtained through pepsin hydrolysis of protein from *S. platensis* (Suetsuna and Nakano 2000), and heptameric peptide Thr-Met-Glu-Pro-Gly-Lys-Pro from an unknown species of *Spirulina*, tested using an *in vitro* ACE assay exhibited ACE inhibition with an IC_{50} value of 0.98 mg ml^{-1} (Heo et al. 2017) and thereby have potential to reduce hypertension in cardiovascular diseases. Peptides with amino acid sequences Met-Met-Leu-Asp-Phe isolated from *S. maxima* following hydrolysis with pepsin, trypsin, and chymotrypsin have been reported to have anti-inflammatory activity against histamine release from RBL-2H3 mast cells (Vo et al. 2013). Kang et al. (2012) isolated longer-chain peptides from *Navicula incerta*, such as Pro-Gly-Trp-Asn-Gln-Trp-Phe-Leu-NIPP1 (Nuclear inhibitor of protein phosphatase-1) and Val-Glu-Val-Leu-Pro-Pro-Ala-Glu-Leu-NIPP2 (Nuclear inhibitor of protein phosphatase-2), through hydrolysis using selective enzymes like trypsin and then α-chymotrypsin to isolate peptides NIPP1 and NIPP2, which decreased gamma-glutamyl transferase activity in HepG2 cells. Further, NIPP1 showed better activity than NIPP2 in the cytotoxicity of liver cells and lowered cytokine levels. Therefore, the structure of peptides derived from microalgae would be a potential nutraceutical ingredient to treat specific diseases.

14.3.2 Structure of Protein and Peptides from Macroalgae

Macroalgae (seaweeds) are rich sources of bioactive protein hydrolysates and peptides (Harnedy et al. 2017). To date, potential functional food applications of seaweeds such as *Gracilariopsis lemaneiformis* and *P. palmata* have been screened, with wide varieties of peptides showing bioactive properties like immunomodulation, antihypertensive action, and cell proliferation (see Table 14.3) (Fitzgerald et al. 2014; Vásquez et al. 2019). The proteins extracted from seaweeds are hydrolyzed with enzymes including pepsin, trypsin, chymotrypsin, and Alcalase® in order to obtain bioactive protein hydrolysates and peptides (Vásquez et al. 2019). These protein hydrolysates and peptides have different amino acid sequences with interesting biological activities (Table 14.3) such as antioxidant properties against 2,2-diphenyl-1-picrylhydrazyl (DPPH) and 2,2′-azino-bis(3-ethylbenzothiazoline-6-sulfonic acid) (ABTS) (Zhang et al. 2019b), and ACE inhibitory activity (Furuta et al. 2016; de Marco Castro et al. 2019), antihypertensive (Chen et al. 2016), and anticancer activities (Chaves et al. 2018) with *in vitro* models.

When the proteins of *G. lemaneiformis* were hydrolyzed by different protease enzymes including trypsin, pepsin, papain, α-chymotrypsin, and Alcalase®, an isolated peptide Glu-Leu-Trp-Lys-Thr-Phe exhibited DPPH scavenging activity at a half maximal effective concentration (EC_{50}) of 1.541 mg ml^{-1} (Zhang et al. 2019a, 2019b). Deng et al. (2018) isolated peptides from *G. lemaneiformis* that exhibited strong ACE inhibitory activity with an IC_{50} value of 9.64 μM; these peptides were administered to rats at a dose level of 10 mg ml^{-1}, which reduced systolic blood pressure to normal (Table 14.3). A peptide (Ile-Arg-Leu-Ile-Val-Leu-Met-Pro-Ile-Leu-Met-Ala) isolated from *P. palmata* by alkaline hydrolysis exhibited dipeptidyl peptidase (DPP) IV inhibitory activity with an IC_{50} value of 1.65 mg ml^{-1} (Harnedy et al. 2015). As compared with these values *P. palmata* peptides (Ile-Leu-Ala-Pro, Leu-Leu-Ala-Pro, Met-Ala-Gly-Val-Asp-His-Ile) isolated using enzyme Corolase® protease for protein hydrolysis exhibited better DPP-IV inhibitory activity with an IC_{50} value of 1.42 mg ml^{-1} under porcine kidney DPP-IV assay (Harnedy et al. 2015).

14.4 Protein and Peptide Extraction Methods from Algae

14.4.1 Physical Processes

Physical grinding, osmotic stress, and pressurized cell disruption using chemical reagents have been reported to yield better recoveries of algal proteins (Bleakley and Hayes 2017). High-pressure cell disruption using ultrasonication at a pressure of 2700 bar exhibited algal proteins in the range between 41 and 90% (dry weight, DW) from *H. pluvialis* and *Porphyridium cruentum*, respectively; the lowest yields of 7.4% were obtained from manual grinding (ground using a mortar and pestle for 5 minutes), followed by ultrasonication (30 minutes), which yielded 8.5% from *H. pluvialis* (Safi et al. 2014). Marrion et al. (2003) estimated that osmotic shock coupled with ultrasonication for 1 hour enhanced extraction of algal proteins from 0.5 to 1.35% in *P. palmata*. Similarly, osmotic shock in the aqueous protein extraction method slightly increased the protein yield from *P. palmata*, i.e. 1.02 g 100 g^{-1} DW compared with high shear force using a homogenizer at 24 000 rpm, which yielded 0.74 g 100 g^{-1} DW. Further, enzymes like polysaccharidase used in hydrolysis yielded the greatest recovery of protein from *P. palmata* (11.57 g 100 g^{-1} DW) (Harnedy and FitzGerald 2013).

Table 14.3 Peptides from macroalgae and their potential bioactivities.

Macroalgae	Peptide sequence	Extraction and digestion methods	Bioactivity	References
Gracilariopsis lemaneiformis	Glu-Leu-Trp-Lys-Thr-Phe	Pepsin	DPPH radical scavenging activity	Zhang et al. 2019a, 2019b
Gracilariopsis lemaneiformis	Phe-Leu-Ile-Met and Lys-Gln-Glu-Glu-His-Tyr-Arg	Trypsin	ACE inhibition *in vitro* assay	Deng et al. 2018
Solieria filiformis	*Solieria filiformis* hydrolysate	Phosphate buffer precipitation	Anticancer activity against human breast adenocarci-noma cell line (MCF-7)	Chaves et al. 2018
Ulva spp.	Protein hydrolysates and Peptide fractions	Purazyme® + Flavourzyme®	Regulate cytokine activity in cytokine interleukin-10 spleen cells	Cian et al. 2018
Ulva rigida	IP, AFL	Pepsin bromelain	ACE inhibitory *in vitro* assay	Paiva et al. 2016
Palmaria palmata	Ile-Arg-Leu-Ile-Val-Leu-Met-Pro-Ile-Leu-Met-Ala	Papain	ACE and rennin inhibitory *in vitro* assay	Fitzgerald et al. 2012
Palmaria palmata	Alkaline protein extract hydrolysate	Alcalase®,Corolase®, and Flavourzyme hydrolysis	ACE and rennin inhibitory *in vitro* assay	Harnedy and FitzGerald 2013
Palmaria palmata	Ile-Leu-Ala-Pro Leu-Leu-Ala-Pro Met-Ala-Gly-Val-Asp-His-Ile	Corolase hydrolysis	Antidiabetic, dipeptidyl peptidase-IV inhibitory activity *in vitro* assay	Harnedy et al. 2015
Palmaria palmata	Tyr-Arg-Asp Ala-Gly-Gly-Glu-Tyr Val-Tyr-Arg-The Val-Asp-His-Tyr Ile-Lys-Gly-His-Tyr Leu-Lys-Asn-Pro-Gly Leu-Asp-Tyr Leu-Arg-Tyr Phe-Glu-Gln-Asp-Try-Ala-Ser	Thermolysin hydrolysis	ACE inhibitory and antihyper-tensive *in vitro* assay	Furuta et al. 2016

(*continued*)

Table 14.3 (*continued*)

Macroalgae	Peptide sequence	Extraction and digestion methods	Bioactivity	References
Palmaria palmata	Protein hydrolysate fraction	Chymotrypsin hydrolysis	Antioxidant activity	Beaulieu et al. 2016
Porphyra columbina	Residual seaweed cake hydrolysate	Fungal protease and Flavourzyme hydrolysis	ACE and rennin inhibitory *in vitro* assay	Cian et al. 2012a
Porphyra yezoensis	Ala-Lys-Tyr-Ser-Tyr	Pepsin	Antihypertensive in rat model	Saito and Hagino 2005
Pyropia colombina	*Pyropia colombina* hydrolysates	Alcalase®, Flavourzyme	ACE and rennin inhibitory *in vitro* assay	Cian et al. 2012b
Undaria pinnatifida	Tyr-His Lys-Trp Lys-Tyr Lys-Phe Phe-Tyr Val-Trp Val-Phe Lie-Tyr Lie-Trp Val-Tyr	Hot water extract	Antihypertensive in rat model	Suetsuna and Nakano 2000
Undaria pinnatifida	Val-Tyr Ile-Tyr Ala-Trp Phe-Tyr Val-Trp Ile-Trp Leu-Trp	Alginate lyase followed by protease	ACE inhibitory *in vitro* assay	Minoru et al. 2005
Undaria pinnatifida	Val-Tyr Ile-Tyr Ala-Trp Phe-Tyr Val-Trp Ile-Trp Leu-Trp	Protease S	Antihypertensive *in vitro* assay	Sato et al. (2002)
Undaria pinnatifida	Ala-Ile-Tyr-Lys Tyr-Lys-Tyr-Tyr Lys-Phe-Tyr-Gly Tyr-Asn-Lys-Leu	Pepsin	ACE inhibitory activity *in vitro* assay	Suetsuna and Nakano 2000
Porphyra yezoensis	Ile-Tyr, Met-Lys-Tyr Ala-Lys-Tyr-Ser-Tyr Leu-Arg-Tyr	Pepsin	ACE-1 inhibitory activity *in vitro* assay	Lin et al. 2018
Porphyra yezoensis	Protein hydrolysates	Hot water extract	Chemoprotective effect in MTS assay	Lee et al. 2018

(*continued*)

Table 14.3 (*continued*)

Macroalgae	Peptide sequence	Extraction and digestion methods	Bioactivity	References
Pyropia yezoensis	Protein hydrolysates	Water extract followed by methanol and chloroform precipitation	Antioxidant	Kim et al. 2018
Pyropia yezoensis	Crude protein	Dialysis	Protein prevents dexamethasone-induced myotube atrophy in rats	Lee et al. 2018
Laminaria japonica	Lys-Tyr, Gly-Lys-Tyr, Ser-Lys-Thr-Tyr, Ala-Lys-Tyr Ala-Lys-Tyr-Ser-Tyr, Lys-Lys-Phe-Tyr, Phe-Tyr, Lys-Phe-Lys-Tyr	Papain, Alcalase®, and trypsin	Antihypertensive *in vitro* assay	Chen et al. 2016

ACE, angiotensin I-converting enzyme; DPPH, 2,2-diphenyl-1-picrylhydrazyl; IP, Ile-Pro; AFL, Ala-Phe-Leu; MCF-7, Michigan Cancer Foundation-7; MTS, 3-(4,5-dimethylthiazol-2-yl)-5-(3-carboxymethoxy-phenyl)-2-(4-sulfophenyl)-2H-tetrazolium.

14.4.2 Enzymatic Hydrolysis

A portion of the peptide sections of microalgae proteins, for example, in *C. vulgaris*, *Dunaliella salina*, and *S. plantesis*, can be released from native proteins by enzymatic hydrolysis, particularly pepsin, trypsin, and chymotrypsin using gastrointestinal digestion (Sedighi et al. 2019). Joubert and Fleurence, (2008) reported that the protein yield increased by 10-fold in *Chondrus crispus* when algal tissue was hydrolyzed with a combination of cellulase and carrageenase (1.5 to 2 mg g^{-1} wet weight) as compared with the enzyme-free method (0.7 mg g^{-1} wet weight). A similar result was obtained with *P. palmata*, which yielded 10-fold more phycoerythrin pigment protein (4.36 g kg^{-1} wet ground algae) upon treatment with xylanase and cellulase compared with nonenzymatic extraction (0.11 g kg^{-1} dry ground algae; Dumay et al. 2013). In other work, Mæhre et al. (2016) reported that the essential amino acid yield increased from 38.9 to 42.5% after enzymatic treatment of xylase and cellulase in a concentration of 10 U in *Trichoderma longibrachiatum*. Similarly, the protein extraction without enzyme delivered a yield of 4.40% (w/w) in *Chlorella sorokiniana* in contrast with when an enzyme like thermolysin was used in the extraction, which gave the highest protein yield of 65.08%. This result reported that thermolysin hydrolysates have the greatest degree of hydrolysis (18.8%) after 4 hours of hydrolysis (Tejano et al. 2019).

14.4.3 Enzyme Assisted Extraction (EAE)

EAE methods of extracting micro- and macroalgal proteins involve hydrolytic activity using cellulase, polysaccharidases, and α-amylase to disrupt the cell wall structure and liberate intracellular materials including polysaccharides, peptides, or amino acids (Vásquez et al. 2019). In general, micro- and macroalgal cell walls are composites of microfibrillar polysaccharides made up of xylan and proteoglycans (Dumay et al. 2013). Rodrigues et al. (2015) compared the protein yields and functionality of EAE and UAE: EAE in the presence of Alcalase® (pH 8.0) yielded 29.6 mg $g_{lyoph}{}^{-1}$ of protein/nitrogen from *Sargassum muticum*, but UAE under 400 W, 50/60 Hz for 60 minutes at 50 °C extracted 24.4%. In other species such as *Undaria pinnatifida*, EAE alone using Alcalase® yielded 15.56%, and UAE alone yielded 10.36% from *U. pinnatifida*, whereas UAE yielded 19.06% and EAE 22.26% from *Codium tomentosum*. This work showed that EAE seems to be a promising adjunct to protein extraction protocols. Vásquez et al. (2019) reported that EAE was an effective method of extracting protein, even though macroalgae have a high percentage of polysaccharides in the outer cell matrix. These researchers isolated 74.6 and 36.1% protein from polysaccharide-rich seaweeds such as *Macrocystis pyrifera* and *Chondracanthus chamissoi* through EAE using cellulases.

14.4.4 Ultrasound Assisted Extraction

Ultrasound assisted extraction (UAE) using soundwaves has also been applied to extract protein from micro- and macroalgae (Kadam et al. 2015). UAE techniques have been used to increase the protein yield from microalgae including *Chlorella* and *Scenedesmus* species (El-Chaghaby et al. 2019). Ultrasonic energy using forces from 0.1 kWh l^{-1} up to 0.4 kWh l^{-1} has been used to extract microalgal proteins; for example, the protein estimated in the supernatants of aqueous microalgal solutions produced from *Chlorella* spp. and *Scenedesmus* spp. increased from 35 to 80% when increasing the sonication power up to 0.4 kWh;$^{-1}$ compared with low intensity at 0.1 kWh l^{-1} (Keris-Sen et al. 2014). However, at a higher intensity of 0.5 kWh l^{-1} the cell disintegration was observed to be decreased with a low protein content of 50% compared with 0.4 kWh l^{-1} (Keris-Sen et al. 2014).

It has also been reported that using two ultrasonic frequencies 15 kHz and 20 kHz together in extraction is a viable method for macroalgal protein extraction; for example, the protein yield was increased from 18.42 to 24.35% in *Porphyra yezoensis*; this value was 50% higher and extraction time was reduced by 18% compared with using a single frequency during the extraction process because the soundwaves caused implosion of cavitation bubbles resulting in a high protein yield (Qu et al. 2013). There are several advantages to using UAE including rapid processing (10–60 minutes), nonthermal treatment, and lower consumption of solvents (50–200 ml) (Chemat and Khan 2011). Kadam et al. (2017) have reported that ultrasound pretreated *A. nodosum* in an aqueous suspension with hydrochloric acid and alkaline treatments (NaOH, 0.1–0.4 M) exhibited increased protein yields from 18.94 to 57.23%, as compared with untreated material (7.97%) and reduced processing times from 60 to 10 minutes.

14.4.5 Pulsed Electric Field

Pulsed electric field extraction (PEF) involves applying high electric currents of 15 kV to perforate cell walls or membranes resulting in enhanced extraction of intracellular components including proteins (Töpfl 2006). PEF is a destructive technique generally used for extraction of lipids from microalgae such as *Chlorella* species for biofuel purposes (Vanthoor-Koopmans et al. 2013); it has also been used to extract multiple intracellular components including carbohydrates, proteins, and lipids from microalgae like *C. vulgaris* (Goettel et al. 2013). The untreated biomass consists of 163 μg g^{-1} DW; however, PEF at the highest electric strength with 25 kV cm^{-1} for 75 μs at 40 °C increased the lutein concentration 4.5-fold, i.e. 753 μg g^{-1} DW in *C. vulgaris* (Luengo et al. 2015). Pulse electric strength of 10.42 kWh kg^{-1} in an aqueous medium gave 10% of protein (w/w) from *Nannochloropsis* sp.; this proteins yield is found to be low compared with other studies using similar electric strength directed on *Nannochloropsis* sp., which acquired higher yields of proteins, i.e. 30% (Coustets et al. 2013), yet the PEF treatments in these examinations were conducted with a blend of ethanol and dimethyl sulfoxide, which enhanced the release of proteins (Parniakov et al. 2015). Protein extracted from *Ulva* species through PEF under conditions of field strength 2.964 kV cm^{-1}, pulse duration 5.70 μs, at 0.5 Hz, exhibited a yield of 59.13 μg protein ml^{-1} of algal extract compared with the control samples with a yield of 23.80 μg protein ml^{-1} of algal extract as determined by the Bradford assay (Polikovsky et al. 2016). It is noteworthy that this treatment protocol does not result in a thermic effect on the proteins as the highest temperature examined was 35.50 °C (Polikovsky et al. 2016). Postma et al. (2017) compared the effects of various modes of PEF with bead milling and mechanical beating for protein extraction: PEF variables from 0.03 up to 150 kWh kg^{-1} DW resulted in protein yields of 2.5 and 3.2% for *C. vulgaris* and 1.9–2.5% for *Neochloris oleoabundans*. However, continuous flow of PEF (0.4 and 0.6 kWh kg^{-1} DW) yielded up to 2.3 and 10.5% protein for *C. vulgaris* and *N. oleoabundans*, respectively; it was noted that no protein release resulted at 0 kWh kg^{-1} DW in an aqueous medium (Postma et al. 2017).

14.4.6 Microwave Assisted Extraction

Microwave assisted extraction (MAE) involves heating material such as micro- and macroalgae using radio waves, causing moisture to vaporize, thus creating localized high pressure, which can then rupture and disrupt cell contents (Barba et al. 2015). Increased yields of soluble proteins (193 mg l^{-1} protein) were extracted from microalgal biomass of *Stigeoclonium* sp. and *Monoraphidium* sp. and diatoms, namely, *Nitzschia* sp. and *Navicula* sp., using microwave pretreatment of cell suspensions compared with UAE, which yielded protein recoveries of 135 mg l^{-1} protein (Passos et al. 2015). Low energy input and costs are the primary advantages of MAE; however, the application of MAE in micro- and macroalgae is limited due to its impaired function with dried samples (Chemat and Khan 2011). Chew et al. (2019) reported that the yield of protein from *C. vulgaris* through MAE was 2.54-fold increased from 24.9 to 63.2%; MAE along with three-phase partitioning (TPP) using ammonium sulfate at 30% concentration recovered 63.2% protein, whereas 24.9% protein was obtained from TPP alone. They reported that MAE resulted in cell degradation in microalgae, which helped to extract protein and different biomolecules out of the microalgal tissues (Chew et al. 2019).

14.4.7 Membrane Filtration

Membrane technologies have the advantage of being nonthermal and environmentally friendly due to fewer solvents consumed in the extraction (Kumar et al. 2013). Microfiltration (MF), ultrafiltration (UF), nano-filtration (NF), and reverse osmosis (RO) are the most commonly used membrane technologies to separate macromolecules from supernatants (Bleakley and Hayes 2017). Membrane technologies can be used as one of the strategies for improving micro- and macroalgal protein yields when used in combination with cell disruption techniques such as polysaccharidases, UAE, or PEF (Bleakley and Hayes 2017). MF can be used to remove micro- and macroalgal cell wall components such as cellulose, homogalacturonan (HG), xyloglucan, mannans, and xylans from suspensions of disrupted cells (Herburger et al. 2019), whereas UF would be used to isolate proteins and different macromolecules like polysaccharide from 1–200 kDa molecular weight (Denis et al. 2009). On the other hand, NF has been used to remove salts to minimize osmolality, followed by RO to reduce the fluid volume of algal extracts (Kumar et al. 2013; Morales et al. 2019).

Denis et al. (2009) used UF at 20 °C with a pressure of 4 bar to isolate phycoerythrin from *Grateloupia turuturu* followed by tissue homogenization. Alternatively, algal protein enrichment can be achieved through two-stage UF as demonstrated by the separation of cell wall components from *Tetraselmis suecica* using different-sized pore membranes with molecular cutoff 10 and 100 kDa following high-pressure homogenization at 200 and 1000 bar, which gave a better yield of protein 0.70 g l^{-1} at high pressure and its counterpart was 0.23 g l^{-1} (200 bar) at 100 kDa membrane of the aqueous phase after cell disruption (Safi et al. 2014). UF in combination with gel filtration chromatography assay resulted in a greater protein yield from *G. lemaneiformis* of 58.02% total protein of <3 kDa compared with a UF fraction of 3–10 kDa in the extraction process (Zhang et al. 2019a, 2019b).

14.4.8 High Hydrostatic Pressure (HHP)

HHP using pressure up to 1000 MPa and ultrahigh pressure (100–300 MPa) have been investigated for their impacts on proteins and extractability of bioactive peptides and nutrients from micro- and macroalgal sources like *Parachlorella kessleri* (Zhang et al. 2019a). According to Suwal et al. (2019), HHP at 400 MPa for 20 minutes with enzymes cellulase and hemicellulase at a pH of 4.5 increased protein yield from 30 to 34 mg g^{-1} in *P. palmata*. They also examined the effect of HHP alone without the addition of enzymes, which yielded 8.4% of protein, which confirms that HHP along with enzymes in the extraction system gives a better quantity of protein. However, Tran et al. (2019) reported contrary effects of HHP treatment on the extraction of β-phycoerythrin from *P. cruentum*. They reported that HHP at 500 MPa for 5 minutes had no impact on cell integrity, while HHP treatment at low and high levels in the range of between 50 and 500 MPa failed to separate β-phycoerythrin from a *P. cruentum* cell suspension. Interestingly, HHP at 400 MPa decreased the β-phycoerythrin yield to 66.6 mg g^{-1} DW as compared with the untreated sample yield of 73.8 mg g^{-1} DW. Therefore, HHP is not recommended for the extraction of β-phycoerythrin from *P. cruentum* biomass or suspensions but can be used up to 300 MPa, which yielded 78.1 mg g^{-1} DW with no structural damage to β-phycoerythrin (Tran et al. 2019).

14.5 Biological Properties of Micro- and Macroalgal Peptides and Possible Health Effects

14.5.1 Antihypertensive Peptides

Cermeno et al. (2019) extracted a peptide from *Porphyra dioica* protein extract using enzymatic hydrolysis and then fractionated it using semi-preparative reverse-phase high-performance chromatography, which gave Tyr-Leu-Val-Ala peptide, which exhibited DPP-IV inhibitory activity against *in vitro* simulated gastrointestinal digestion, with an IC_{50} of 439 μM. A similar report is also available for another green microalga *Chlorella ellipsoidea* hydrolysates consisting of Val-Glu-Gly-Tyr that had the ability to reduce systolic blood pressure (a reduction of 22.8 mmHg during rest 189.5 mmHg) and had a higher ACE activity of IC_{50} 128.4 μM in rats injected at a dose of 10 mg kg^{-1} body weight (Ko et al. 2012). This research also showed that peptides consisting of fewer than 20 amino acids with low molecular weight were more effective than high molecular weight peptide 10 kDa tuna fish protein hydrolysates (Ko et al. 2012). Further, enzymatic hydrolysis using proteases on *Ulva intestinalis* led to amino acid sequences of ACE inhibitory peptides such as Phe-Gly-Met-Pro-Leu-Asp-Arg and Met-Glu-Leu-Val-Leu-Arg using the ultra-performance liquid chromatography-tandem mass spectrometry technique (Sun et al. 2019). These two peptides showed IC_{50} values of 219.35 and 236.85 μM, respectively; however, trypsin hydrolysates displayed the highest ACE inhibitory action compared with these two peptides from *U. intestinalis*. Similarly, a genomic study on plastid proteins of *Palmaria* species (Japan) showed amino acids with a sequence of large core-membrane linker protein (apcE) in phycobilisomes, which were responsible for ACE inhibitory action in the majority of species from *Palmaria*. They compared ACE inhibitory peptides between protein sequences and a database *in silico* analysis, and they identified that photosystems consisting of 177 ACE inhibitory peptides are the most predominant source of ACE inhibitory action in *Palmaria* sp. (Kumagai et al. 2019).

14.5.2 Anticancer Peptides and Proteins

Peptides with anticancer bioactivities such as those from micro- and macroalgae have received attention in recent times due to their multifunctionality and *in vivo* digestion (Stack et al. 2018). There is extensive research in this field to study the impact of micro- and macroalgal-based proteins and peptides against cancer cells both *in vitro* and *in vivo* (Nongonierma and FitzGerald 2019). Nutraceutical and pharmaceutical functionalities of micro- and macroalgal proteins and peptides have been recently reported (Stack et al. 2018; Nongonierma and FitzGerald 2019). For example, peptides from red seaweed *Solieria filiformis* (Sf) were described as two types of isolectins, SfL-1 and SfL-2, with molecular weights of 27 552 and 27 985 Da each with 67 amino acids. Both peptides showed inhibition of tumor cell viability at doses 62.5, 250, and 500 μg ml^{-1} against human breast cancer cells (MCF-7 cells) with a significant loss of cells from 43.4, 58.27, and 61.2% (Chaves et al. 2018). Sheih et al. (2009) reported that an 11-amino acid peptide from *C. vulgaris* exerted anticancer activity against the human gastric cancer cell line AGS at a dose of 36 μg ml^{-1}. After 24 hours of peptide administration, the cells in the G1 stage decreased, and cell growth was arrested in post-G1 phase by the peptide fraction. Fernández-Acero et al. (2018) isolated a prohibitin protein (known to inhibit DNA synthesis and thereby influence proliferation) from *Nannochloropsis gaditana* microalga for potential use in the treatment of diseases influenced by cell replication such as carcinogenesis. This alga also yielded more than 7500 peptides and 655 proteins with potential biomedical applications including treatment for cancer, and cell proliferation using prohibitin (Fernández-Acero et al. 2018). However, as compared with fresh or intact microalgae such as *Spirulina* sp., fermented micro- or macroalgal peptides have been reported to exhibit greater efficacies in both antioxidant and anticancer bioactivities; for example, a purified peptide, Met-Gly-Arg-Tyr, from fermented *P. lutheri* extracted by quadrupole time-of-flight mass spectrometry protected genomic DNA of B16F10 melanoma cells against hydroxyl radicals produced by Fe (II)/H_2O_2 (Oh et al. 2015). Moreover, this peptide from *P. lutheri* decreased the production of melanin and tyrosinase activity through an α-melanocyte-stimulating hormone (α-MSH) in B16F10 melanoma cells in a dose-dependent manner (25–200 μM concentration) (Oh et al. 2015).

14.5.3 Antioxidant Micro- and Macroalgal Peptides

Flavourzyme®, Alcalase®, and trypsin enzymes were used for the hydrolysis of *Nitzschia*, *Spirulina*, and *Chlorella* algae, which yielded the highest protein from *Spirulina* (42.46%), then *Nitzschia* (23.42%), and then *Chlorella* (8.4%). The protein extracted from endopeptidase Alcalase® showed effective scavenging action of 66.77% against ABTS+• assay *in vitro* as compared with other enzymes like Flavourzyme® (55%) and trypsin (45%) used in protein extraction (Alzahrani et al. 2018). Similar results are available from enzymatic hydrolysis of marine microalgae *Isochrysis zhanjiangensis*. Peptide Asn-Asp-Ala-Glu-Tyr-Gly-Ile-Cys-Gly-Phe with molecular weight 1088.16 Da inhibited the production of intracellular reactive oxygen species (ROS) by dichloro-dihydro-fluorescein diacetate (DCFH-DA) assay (Chen et al. 2019). Among various enzymes used in the hydrolysis process like chymotrypsin, trypsin, pepsin, and *in vitro* gastrointestinal digestion, the peptide extracted from gastrointestinal hydrolysate showed relatively high free radical scavenging ability (Chen et al. 2019). Further, phycobiliprotein (PBP) from *P. yezoensis* showed potent inhibition of ROS. Specifically, PBP 1-2 peptides and PBP 7-9 peptides showed potential antioxidant action against HepG2 cells (Kim et al. 2018). They reported that PBP1, 2, and 7-9 peptides increased the number of viable cells by 23–32%, whereas the control sample was reduced to 47% by 5 mM H_2O_2, and PBP 1-13 decreased dead cells by 30–143%. This result shows PBP 1, 2, and 7-9 protected cells from oxidative stress by H_2O_2, thereby acting as effective antioxidants (Kim et al. 2018).

14.5.4 Anti-Inflammatory Peptides

Protein hydrolysate obtained from green seaweed *Ulva* sp. showed pro-anti-inflammatory activity against cytokines tumor necrosis factor (TNF), interferon gamma (IFN-γ), and interleukin 10 (IL-10) in rat spleen cells (Cian et al. 2018). Hydrolysis by two different mixtures of enzymes, namely Purazyme/Flavourzyme (PF) and alkaline protease Protex 6 L/Flavourzyme (AF) resulted in a large number of peptides using the PF system (3150 kDa) as compared with AF used in the extraction

(2160 kDa; Cian et al. 2018). The protein obtained from *Ulva* by PF hydrolysate was 16.7–23.6%, which found to be similar to that of the crude protein content of *Ulva fasciata* in the range of 22.7% DW (Abirami, 2012). A protein hydrolysate from *Porphyra columbina* digested with Flavourzyme exhibited inhibition against the proinflammatory cytokines of IL-10 and TNF in a study of splenocyte cell viability at a dose of 1 g l^{-1} (Cian et al. 2012a, b). Further, the two dipeptides, namely histidine–glutamic acid (HE) and glycine–proline (GP), isolated from *Porphyridium purpureum* with a total protein of 29.9% DW and purified phycoerythrin of 2.98% DW were evaluated for atherogenic foam cell prevention capacity against RAW 264.7 cell line. They showed IC_{50} values of 91.2 µg/ml (GP) and 103.3 µg/ml (HE) in MTT assay, which reduces foam cell formation, and secretion of TNF-α and IL-6 in the RAW 264.7 cell line. They found that molecular interaction of GP and HE peptides targeted protein mediators such as CD36, SRA1, and MAP kinase p38 as a scavenging receptor (Kavitha et al. 2019). Thus, hydrolysates of micro- and macroalgal food protein sources may have immunomodulatory impacts, which may be of interest to be used as a functional food or nutraceutical.

14.5.5 Algal Proteins and Peptides on Immunomodulation

Peptide-based medications for hormonal treatment have been used for hormones (e.g. insulin, insulin-like growth factors) and neurotransmitters since the early 1950s (Gokhale and Satyanarayanajois 2014). A few proteins from *Spirulina* and *Scenedesmus obliquus* are connected with cell wall polysaccharide, which show an effective immunological response (Perez Espitia et al. 2012). In a human trial, elder adults of 60–87 years who consumed 8 g day^{-1} of *Spirulina* for 16 continuous weeks showed significant increases in plasma IL-2 and decreases in IL-6, which was found to be a significant immune modulation reaction (Park et al. 2008). Similarly, *Spirulina* protein was also effective in modulating the immune system of HIV patients in a human trial discussed below (Azabji-Kenfack et al. 2011). In other work, the efficiency of *S. platensis* protein was compared with soybean protein isolate in HIV-infected adults (both males and females) of 18–35 years with severe immune deficiency of CD4 count 96 cells mm^{-3} through regular supplementation of *S. platensis* of 0.20–0.37 g kg^{-1} day^{-1} for 12 weeks. The experimental group receiving *S. platensis* showed significantly increased CD4 cells (195 cells mm^{-3}) and decreases in HIV viral load (4.45 $\log_{10}$ copies mm^{-3}) in contrast to the soybean-fed group with CD4 levels of 143 cells mm^{-3} and HIV viral load of 4.75 $\log_{10}$ copies mm^{-3} (Azabji-Kenfack et al. 2011). Afify et al. (2018) identified an effective protein hydrolysate (Sd1pa, Sd2pa, Sd1pep, and Sd1Try) from green microalgae *S. obliquus*, which inhibited Coxsackie B_3 virus (CVB_3) cell replication in the range of 57.6–66.2%, at a concentration of 100 µg ml^{-1}. In addition, the antiviral effect of these peptides depends on direct interaction with viral glycoproteins like gB, gC, and gD. Some peptides have a binding capacity on gp120 glycoprotein, which plays a role in the adsorption and penetration of HIV in the host cells (Perez Espitia et al. 2012); thus, *S. obliquus*-based peptides directly interact with the virus envelope and inhibit the growth of viral cells. A recent study conducted with Polish consumers (online survey) showed that regular consumption of *Spirulina*, *Chlorella*, and *Aphanizomenon* supplements can act as an immunity boost in 60.7% of the population surveyed (Rzymski and Jaśkiewicz 2017).

14.5.6 Antiobesity Peptides

Spirulina platensis protein was hydrolyzed using papain, pepsin, trypsin, Alcalase®, and protamex individually in the extraction process, yielding four peptides: Asn-Ala-Leu-Lys-Cys-Cys-His-Ser-Cys-Pro-Asn-Lys (NALKCCHSCPA), Leu-Asn-Asn-Pro-Ser-Val-Cys-Asp-Cys-Asp-Cys-Met-Met-Lys-Ala-Ala-Arg (LNNPSVCD-CDCMMKAAR), Asn-Pro-Val-Try-Lys-Arg-Lys (NPVWKRK), and Cys-Ala-Asn-Pro-His-Glu-Leu-Pro-Asn-Lys (CANPHELPNK) (Fan et al. 2018). These peptides were tested for preadipocyte 3T3-L1 cell proliferation; the pepsin hydrolysate peptide (CANPHELPNK) exhibited better antiproliferation activity (77.37%) at a concentration of 0.125–2 mg ml^{-1} than Simvastatin (70.32%), however other peptides showed inhibition in the range of 37.86–60.08%. A molecular docking study demonstrated that decreased apoptosis-based adipocytes led to the loss of body fat, which was seen in CANPHELPNK peptides (Fan et al. 2018). Similarly, whole *S. platensis* (WSP-2 g kg^{-1} day^{-1}), *S. platensis* protein (SPP-2 g kg^{-1} day^{-1}), and *S. platensis* protein hydrolysate (SPPH-2 g kg^{-1} day^{-1}) were given to mice along with a high-fat diet. The results showed that SPPH exhibited good antiobesity effects (reducing body weight by 39.8%); WSP and SPP reduced it by 33.5 and 33.1%, respectively (Zhao et al. 2019).

14.5.7 Antidiabetic Proteins and Peptides

The current technologies for the treatment of diabetes mellitus depend on incretin analogues, i.e. agents that act like incretin hormones such as glucagon-like peptide-1 (GLP-1) and dipeptidyl peptidase 4 (DPP-IV) inhibitors (Zhang et al., 2018). In general GLP-1 and glucose-dependent insulinotropic polypeptide (GIP) were responsible for DPP- IV inhibitory activation (Nongonierma and FitzGerald 2019). Hydrolysates from the red seaweed *Porphyra* sp. yielded two novel peptides, Gly-Gly-Ser-Lys and Glu-Leu-Ser, which exhibited inhibition of α-amylase action *in vitro*, whereas low molecular weight <3 KDa peptides exhibited strong *in vitro* α-amylase activity with an IC_{50} of 0.96 mg ml^{-1} compared with synthetic peptides, which had an IC_{50} value of 2.58 mM (Admassu et al. 2018). Moreover, *U. fasciata* crude extract containing 22.37% protein significantly upregulated carbohydrate metabolism enzymes uch as hexokinase, glucokinase, and glucose-6-phosphostase in the liver in alloxan-induced diabetic rats at a dose of 200 mg kg^{-1} day^{-1} for 28 days (Abirami and Kowsalya 2013). Similarly, active peptides were extracted from *S. platensis* crude protein using ultrasound power 220 W with pressure 10 MPa for 60 minutes. Using an *in silico* method it was found that Gly-Val-Pro-Met-Pro-Asp-Asn-Lys (GVPMPNK), Arg-Asn-Pro-Phe-Val-Phe-Ala-Pro-Thr-Leu-Leu-Thr-Val-Ala-Ala-Arg (RNPFV-FAPTLLTVAAR), and Leu-Arg-Ser-Glu-Leu-Ala-Ala-Try-Ser-Arg (LRSE-LAAWSR) peptides exhibited antidiabetic action. Among them, LRSELAAWSR showed good action against α-amylase, with an IC_{50} of 313.6 μg ml^{-1}, but the strongest action on α-glucosidase with an IC_{50} of 134.2 μg ml^{-1} and DPP-IV with an IC_{50} of 167.3 μg ml^{-1} (Hu et al. 2019).

14.5.8 Antimicrobial Algal Peptides

Various secondary metabolites from microalgae like *D. salina* and *S. platensis*, and macroalgae like *Codium* spp., have been reported to exhibit antimicrobial activities against various Gram-positive species like *Staphylococcus*, *Streptococcus*, and Gram-negative bacteria including *E. coli* (Sun et al. 2016; Darvish et al. 2018). The protein hydrolysate from macroalga *Saccharina longicruris* exhibited significant antibacterial action against *Staphylococcus aureus*. The fraction composed of molecular weight >10 kDa showed the maximum reduction of 40% μ_{max} bacterial growth rate at a concentration of 2.5 mg ml^{-1}; this acts as an antibacterial defensin-like peptide (Beaulieu et al. 2015). Other macroalgae such as *Saccharina latissima*, *Codium* spp., and *Mastocarpus stellatus* Pérez-Míguez et al. (2019) also showed defensin-like peptides that were found to be 100% similar to a ubiquitin-protein sequence commonly found in Pacific oysters. In addition, *S. platensis* protein hydrolysates showed less bactericidal activities against *S. aureus* and *E.coli* at a higher concentration of 16 and 8 mg ml^{-1} with a zone of inhibition of 12 and 16 mm, respectively (Sun et al. 2016). Further, they identified an 18-amino acid sequence from *S. platensis* of Lys-Leu-Val-Asp-Ala-Ser-His-Arg-Leu-Ala-Thr-Gly-Asp-Val-Ala-Val-Arg-Ala (KLVDASHRLATGDVAVRA) with molecular weight of 1878.97 Da responsible for antibacterial action. The molecular weight of proteins/peptides has been reported to be an important attribute in terms of antibacterial activities; for example, a protein fraction from *D. salina* with a molecular weight of 63 kDa exhibited stronger antibacterial effects against *E. coli* and *S. aureus* at 59.4 and 42.9% inhibition as compared with its peptide fraction from trypsin and chymotrypsin of 3–10 kDa and >10 kDa, whereas, <3 kDa demonstrated 16.8, 7.8, and 10.3% inhibition against *E.coli* at a concentration of 50 µl (Darvish et al. 2018). The peptide fraction <3 kDa from *D. salina* exhibited bactericidal action against *Helicobacter pylori*, which is considered as one of the antibiotic-resistant species, with minimum inhibition concentration (MIC) of 0.175 mg *in vitro*. This proves that low molecular weight peptide from *D. salina* exhibits action against gastric bacteria and is potentially a promising naturally derived peptide (Darvish et al. 2018).

14.5.9 Biological Value of Algal Proteins in Human Nutrition

The most popularly consumed seaweeds include *Porphyra tenera* (nori) and *P. palmata* (dulse) (Urbano and Goñi 2002). *Ulva* species are among the most noteworthy consumed types in Asia, and Western nations, in the form of sushi wrapping and alone, respectively, because of their higher protein contents and flavors (Kazir et al. 2019). The biological value of *P. tenera*, *Laminaria japonica*, and *U. pinnatifida* proteins was evaluated through an *in vivo* study with Wistar rats, which reported that that the fiber in the dietary seaweeds negatively affected protein efficiency ratio (PER) (Janczyk et al. 2005). This reveals that phlorotannins and high insoluble polysaccharide (10–76%) contents in these algae were principal factors that negatively impacted PERs of these algal proteins (Bleakley and Hayes 2017). Another *in vitro* digestion study demonstrated that proteins from wild and cultivated macroalgae exhibited moderately similar amino acid scores to regularly consumed plant-based proteins such as grains (69– 84%), pulses (72– 92%), fruits and vegetables (68–92%) via *in vitro* digestibility using multienzyme hydrolysis (Tibbetts et al. 2016). *Palmaria palmata* displayed all the essential amino acids in its protein sequence (Dawczynski et al. 2007). Bjarnadóttir et al. (2018) reported an enzymatic hydrolysis method to the rigid cell wall β-D-xylans in *P. palmata*; a pretreatment with xylanase enabled improved protein yield of 33.3%, while umamizyme (commercial protease enzyme) brought about 37% protein compared with untreated *P. palmata* 19.4% protein (Bjarnadóttir et al. 2018). Further, no reduction in any of the essential amino acids was found in the solid phase of these two hydrolysates, with loss of tryptophan occurring in the extraction process. Therefore, enzymatic hydrolysis is recommended to obtain improved protein biological value and digestibility from algal sources (Obata et al. 2015).

14.6 Potential Commercial Applications of Micro- and Macroalgal Peptides and Proteins

Algal protein in the global market has an increasing number of producers worldwide, and the key players are Nutrex Hawaii Inc., Cyanotech Corporation, Heliae Development LLC, Allma, Far East Bio-Tech Co., Rainbow Light Nutritional System, TerraVia Holdings Inc., etc. (Persistence Market Research 2018). This rising demand is anticipated to develop at a compound annual growth rate of 7.03% to achieve an aggregate market size of US$838 billion by 2023, expanding from US$596 billion in 2018 (Wood 2018).

14.6.1 Microalgae Peptides and Proteins in Commercial Applications

Among the microalgal species, *S. platensis* protein is one of the most studied and tested proteins so far. It is equivalent to meat protein (710–760 g kg^{-1} dry matter base) and soybeans (~400 g kg^{-1} dry matter base), and also contains methionine, which is not present in any other microalgae (Neumann et al. 2017). *Spirulina* is legally approved for human consumption as a supplement in Europe Regulation (EC) No. 396/2005 by the European Food Safety Authority (EFSA), Japan Codex Alimentarius, and in the United States by the Food and Drug Administration, because of its nondetrimental effects (de Sécurité Sanitaire 2017). In Brazil, despite the fact that Agencia Nacional de Vigilancia Sanitaria (ANVISA), a National Health Surveillance Agency, permits the promotion of *Spirulina* as a supplement (Huynh-Ba and Sassi 2018), products where this microalga is blended with other ingredients are required to be registered. For transparency and informational purposes, the microalgal species and harvesting or cultivation locations should be displayed on labels of nutritional supplements or nutraceutical products as required by the French agency for food (ANSES, 2017), environmental and occupational health and safety (de Sécurité Sanitaire 2017).

The protein pigments (PBPs) from cyanobacterium *Arthrospira* sp. and microalga *Porphyridium* sp., as well as Rhodophyta macroalgae, have potential market demand as a nutraceutical supplement. They already do as fluorescent indicators in biomedical and immunological research (Román et al. 2002). These pigments have an expanding number of applications related to their natural dyes and wide scope in pharmaceutical applications (Becker 2004); for example, the most common use of phycocyanin derived from *Spirulina* (11–27% phycocyanin) is as a natural color in foods and in biomedical research laboratories as a fluorescent reagent (Spolaore et al. 2006). Pure synergy organics (https://synergynatural.com/pages/spirulina), Natural Blue-green algae (https://www.thesynergycompany.com/blue-green-algae-capsules), Super algae (https://www.naturessunshine.com/us/product/super-algae-100-caps/1056), Antenna (http://www.spirufoundation.org/products.php), BioChlorella (https://www.biochlorella.com), Microingredients (https://microingredients.com/products/organic-spirulina-tablets), Fairvital (https://www.fairvital.com/en/index), Super Spirulina® (www.naturesway.com.au/product/nw-super-spirulina-tabs-150s), and AlgaVia® (http://algavia.com) represent commercial brands marketing microalgae protein and peptides in the form of tablets, pills, and powders. All these products are approved by the US FDA and are recognized as GRAS (Valensa International 2012). These products are considered as vegan in nature, free from gluten and other allergens (product nutritional label), and as a source of essential amino acids. The products tend to be utilized as nutraceutical supplements, and additives in food for pastry, bakery, and confectionaries (Finamore et al. 2017).

14.6.2 Macroalgal Peptides and Proteins in Commercial Applications

Some commercially available macroalgal peptides marketed for antihypertensive properties are wakame jelly from *U. pinnatifida*, and Peptide Nori from *P. yezoensis* and *P. tenera*. (https://emeraldisleseaweed.com/). All of these peptides were approved by the US FDA and are considered as GRAS for consumption exclusively for antihypertensive cases (Seca and Pinto 2018). Although these peptides were obtained through proteolytic hydrolysis, they showed specific resistance to gastrointestinal proteases (Seca and Pinto 2018).

14.7 Conclusion and Future Recommendations

Algal proteins/peptides undergo a succession of steps involved in the isolation of algal peptides as the proteins are intact with rigid cell wall polysaccharides. There are a few proteolytic enzymes used to cleave specific sites of protein chains, and this cleavage could be facilitated by bioassays or peptidomics devices. Similarly, other strategies including precipitation, maceration, dialysis, and chromatographic techniques have been applied in the separation of peptides. However, these techniques have a few disadvantages including high cost, tedious processing, and low yield. In order to scale up effectiveness in the isolation of peptides, the latest techniques are involved like "flow chemistry," which accelerates the extraction time and elution of peptides, and some other technologies like UF, the phase separation method, EAE, and US have also been utilized effectively. All these methods signify future chances to produce algal peptides in specific sizes, with C- or N-terminal, for better functionalities. Algal peptides have demonstrated different functional properties in disease prevention. Antihypertensive, anticancer, antiviral, and immunomodulation activities etc. have been reported frequently. Thus, promoting the use of these peptides as a food supplement would be beneficial. Further study of algal peptides for pharmacokinetics is essential to perform phase IV clinical trials before human applications. Further, some algal proteins and peptides are as of now legitimately approved; however, undiscovered varieties of proteins/peptides from seaweeds might be a significant source of novel peptides for future health applications in the commercial market.

Acknowledgments

ARG thanks Fiji National University for the facilities provided. RB thanks EU Horizon's 2020 Research and Innovation program funding (VALORTECH Grant Agreement No. 810630).

References

Abirami, R.G. (2012). Nutritional and safety evaluation of underexploited seaweeds and nutraceutical potentials of *Ulva fasciata*. Doctoral dissertation. Avinashilingam Deemed University for Women, Coimbatore, Tamilnadu, India. http://hdl.handle.net/10603/13460 (accessed September 16, 2020).

Abirami, R.G. and Kowsalya, S. (2013). Antidiabetic activity of *Ulva fasciata* and its impact on carbohydrate metabolism enzymes in alloxan induced diabetic rats. *International Journal of Research in Phytochemistry & Pharmacology* **3** (3): 136–141.

Abirami, R.G. and Kowsalya, S. (2017). Quantification and correlation study on derived phenols and antioxidant activity of seaweeds from Gulf of Mannar. *Journal of Herbs, Spices & Medicinal Plants* **23** (1): 9–17.

Admassu, H., Gasmalla, M.A., Yang, R., and Zhao, W. (2018). Identification of bioactive peptides with α-amylase inhibitory potential from enzymatic protein hydrolysates of red seaweed (*Porphyra* spp). *Journal of Agricultural and Food Chemistry* **66** (19): 4872–4882.

Afify, A.E.M.M., El Baroty, G.S., El Baz, F.K. et al. (2018). *Scenedesmus obliquus*: antioxidant and antiviral activity of proteins hydrolyzed by three enzymes. *Journal, Genetic Engineering & Biotechnology* **16** (2): 399–408.

Agustini, T.W., Suzery, M., Sutrisnanto, D., and Ma'ruf, W.F. (2015). Comparative study of bioactive substances extracted from fresh and dried *Spirulina* sp. *Procedia Environmental Sciences* **23**: 282–289.

Alzahrani, M.A.J., Perera, C.O., and Hemar, Y. (2018). Production of bioactive proteins and peptides from the diatom *Nitzschia laevis* and comparison of their *in vitro* antioxidant activities with those from *Spirulina platensis* and *Chlorella vulgaris*. *International Journal of Food Science & Technology* **53** (3): 676–682.

ANSES. (2017). OPINION of the French Agency for Food, Environmental and Occupational Health & Safety on the risks associated with the consumption of food supplements containing spirulina. ANSES. https://www.anses.fr/en/system/files/NUT2014SA0096EN.pdf (accessed September 16, 2020).

Apone, F., Barbulova, A., and Colucci, G. (2019). Plant and microalgae derived peptides are advantageously employed as bioactive compounds in cosmetics. *Frontiers in Plant Science* **10**: 756.

Azabji-Kenfack, M., Dikosso, S.E., Loni, E.G. et al. (2011). Potential of *Spirulina platensis* as a nutritional supplement in malnourished HIV-infected adults in sub-Saharan Africa: a randomised, single-blind study. *Nutrition and Metabolic Insights* **4**: 29–37.

Barba, F.J., Grimi, N., and Vorobiev, E. (2015). New approaches for the use of non-conventional cell disruption technologies to extract potential food additives and nutraceuticals from microalgae. *Food Engineering Reviews* **7** (1): 45–62.

Barbarino, E. and Lourenço, S.O. (2005). An evaluation of methods for extraction and quantification of protein from marine macro-and microalgae. *Journal of Applied Phycology* **17** (5): 447–460.

Beaulieu, L., Bondu, S., Doiron, K. et al. (2015). Characterization of antibacterial activity from protein hydrolysates of the macroalga *Saccharina longicruris* and identification of peptides implied in bioactivity. *Journal of Functional Foods* **17**: 685–697.

Beaulieu, L., Sirois, M., and Tamigneaux, É. (2016). Evaluation of the in vitro biological activity of protein hydrolysates of the edible red alga, *Palmaria palmata* (dulse) harvested from the Gaspe coast and cultivated in tanks. *Journal of Applied Phycology* **28** (5): 3101–3115.

Becker, W. (2004). Microalgae in human and animal nutrition. In: *In Handbook of Microalgal Culture: Biotechnology and Applied Phycology*, vol. **312** (ed. A. Richmond), 312–325. Oxford: Blackwell Science.

Bjarnadóttir, M., Aðalbjörnsson, B.V., Nilsson, A. et al. (2018). *Palmaria palmata* as an alternative protein source: enzymatic protein extraction, amino acid composition, and nitrogen-to-protein conversion factor. *Journal of Applied Phycology* **30** (3): 2061–2070.

Bleakley, S. and Hayes, M. (2017). Algal proteins: extraction, application, and challenges concerning production. *Food* **6** (5): 1–34.

Cermeno, M., Stack, J., Tobin, P. et al. (2019). Peptide identification from a *Porphyra dioica* protein hydrolysate with antioxidant, angiotensin converting enzyme and dipeptidyl peptidase IV inhibitory activities. *Food & Function* **10** (6): 3421–3429.

Chaves, R.P., da Silva, S.R., Neto, L.G.N. et al. (2018). Structural characterization of two isolectins from the marine red alga *Solieria filiformis* (Kützing) PW Gabrielson and their anticancer effect on MCF-7 breast cancer cells. *International Journal of Biological Macromolecules* **107** (part A): 1320–1329.

Chemat, F. and Khan, M.K. (2011). Applications of ultrasound in food technology: processing, preservation and extraction. *Ultrasonics Sonochemistry* **18** (4): 813–835.

Chen, J.C., Wang, J., Zheng, B.D. et al. (2016). Simultaneous determination of 8 small antihypertensive peptides with tyrosine at the C-terminal in *Laminaria japonica* hydrolysates by RP-HPLC method. *Journal of Food Processing and Preservation* **40** (3): 492–501.

Chen, M.F., Zhang, Y.Y., Di He, M. et al. (2019). Antioxidant peptide purified from enzymatic hydrolysates of *Isochrysis Zhanjiangensis* and its protective effect against ethanol induced oxidative stress of HepG2 cells. *Biotechnology and Bioprocess Engineering* **24** (2): 308–317.

Chew, K.W., Chia, S.R., Lee, S.Y. et al. (2019). Enhanced microalgal protein extraction and purification using sustainable microwave-assisted multiphase partitioning technique. *Chemical Engineering Journal* **367**: 1–8.

Cian, R.E., López-Posadas, R., Drago, S.R. et al. (2012a). Immunomodulatory properties of the protein fraction from *Porphyra columbina*. *Journal of Agricultural and Food Chemistry* **60** (33): 8146–8154.

Cian, R.E., Martínez-Augustin, O., and Drago, S.R. (2012b). Bioactive properties of peptides obtained by enzymatic hydrolysis from protein byproducts of *Porphyra columbina*. *Food Research International* **49** (1): 364–372.

Cian, R., Hernández-Chirlaque, C., Gámez-Belmonte, R. et al. (2018). Green alga *Ulva* spp. hydrolysates and their peptide fractions regulate cytokine production in splenic macrophages and lymphocytes involving the TLR4-NFκB/MAPK pathways. *Marine Drugs* **16** (7): 235.

Coustets, M., Al-Karablieh, N., Thomsen, C., and Teissié, J. (2013). Flow process for electroextraction of total proteins from microalgae. *The Journal of Membrane Biology* **246** (10): 751–760.

Darvish, M., Jalili, H., Ranaei-Siadat, S.O., and Sedighi, M. (2018). Potential cytotoxic effects of peptide fractions from *Dunaliella salina* protein hydrolyzed by gastric proteases. *Journal of Aquatic Food Product Technology* **27** (2): 165–175.

Dawczynski, C., Schubert, R., and Jahreis, G. (2007). Amino acids, fatty acids, and dietary fibre in edible seaweed products. *Food Chemistry* **103** (3): 891–899.

Deng, Z., Liu, Y., Wang, J. et al. (2018). Antihypertensive effects of two novel angiotensin I-converting enzyme (ACE) inhibitory peptides from *Gracilariopsis lemaneiformis* (Rhodophyta) in spontaneously hypertensive rats (SHRs). *Marine Drugs* **16** (9): 299.

Denis, C., Massé, A., Fleurence, J., and Jaouen, P. (2009). Concentration and pre-purification with ultrafiltration of a R-phycoerythrin solution extracted from macro-algae *Grateloupia turuturu*: process definition and up-scaling. *Separation and Purification Technology* **69** (1): 37–42.

Dumay, J., Clément, N., Morançais, M., and Fleurence, J. (2013). Optimization of hydrolysis conditions of *Palmaria palmata* to enhance R-phycoerythrin extraction. *Bioresource Technology* **131**: 21–27.

El-Chaghaby, G., Rashad, S., Abdel-Kader, S. et al. (2019). Assessment of phytochemical components, proximate composition and antioxidant properties of *Scenedesmus obliquus*, *Chlorella vulgaris* and *Spirulina platensis* algae extracts. *Egyptian Journal of Aquatic Biology and Fisheries* **23** (4): 521–526.

Fan, X., Cui, Y., Zhang, R., and Zhang, X. (2018). Purification and identification of anti-obesity peptides derived from *Spirulina platensis*. *Journal of Functional Foods* **47**: 350–360.

Fernández-Acero, F.J., Amil-Ruiz, F., Durán-Peña, M.J. et al. (2018). Valorisation of the microalgae *Nannochloropsis gaditana* biomass by proteomic approach in the context of circular economy. *Journal of Proteomics* **193**: 239–242.

Finamore, A., Palmery, M., Bensehaila, S., and Peluso, I. (2017). Antioxidant, immunomodulating, and microbial-modulating activities of the sustainable and ecofriendly *Spirulina*. *Oxidative Medicine and Cellular Longevity* **2017**.

Fitzgerald, C., Mora-Soler, L., Gallagher, E. et al. (2012). Isolation and characterization of bioactive pro-peptides with *in vitro* renin inhibitory activities from the macroalga *Palmaria palmata*. *Journal of Agricultural and Food Chemistry* **60** (30): 7421–7427.

Fitzgerald, C., Aluko, R.E., Hossain, M. et al. (2014). Potential of a renin inhibitory peptide from the red seaweed *Palmaria palmata* as a functional food ingredient following confirmation and characterization of a hypotensive effect in spontaneously hypertensive rats. *Journal of Agricultural and Food Chemistry* **62** (33): 8352–8356.

Fleurence, J., Le Coeur, C., Mabeau, S. et al. (1995). Comparison of different extractive procedures for proteins from the edible seaweeds *Ulva rigida* and *Ulva rotundata*. *Journal of Applied Phycology* **7** (6): 577–582.

Furuta, T., Miyabe, Y., Yasui, H. et al. (2016). Angiotensin I converting enzyme inhibitory peptides derived from phycobiliproteins of dulse *Palmaria palmata*. *Marine Drugs* **14** (2): 1–10.

Goettel, M., Eing, C., Gusbeth, C. et al. (2013). Pulsed electric field assisted extraction of intracellular valuables from microalgae. *Algal Research* **2** (4): 401–408.

Gokhale, A.S. and Satyanarayanajois, S. (2014). Peptides and peptidomimetics as immunomodulators. *Immunotherapy* **6** (6): 755–774.

Harnedy, P.A. and FitzGerald, R.J. (2013). Extraction of protein from the macroalga *Palmaria palmata*. *LWT – Food Science and Technology* **51** (1): 375–382.

Harnedy, P.A., O'Keeffe, M.B., and FitzGerald, R.J. (2015). Purification and identification of dipeptidyl peptidase (DPP) IV inhibitory peptides from the macroalga *Palmaria palmata*. *Food Chemistry* **172**: 400–406.

Harnedy, P.A., O'Keeffe, M.B., and FitzGerald, R.J. (2017). Fractionation and identification of antioxidant peptides from an enzymatically hydrolysed *Palmaria palmata* protein isolate. *Food Research International* **100**: 416–422.

Heo, S.Y., Ko, S.C., Kim, C.S. et al. (2017). A heptameric peptide purified from *Spirulina sp.* gastrointestinal hydrolysate inhibits angiotensin I-converting enzyme- and angiotensin II-induced vascular dysfunction in human endothelial cells. *International Journal of Molecular Medicine* **39** (5): 1072–1082.

Herburger, K., Xin, A., and Holzinger, A. (2019). Homogalacturonan accumulation in cell walls of the green alga *Zygnema* sp.(Charophyta) increases desiccation resistance. *Frontiers in Plant Science* **10**: 1–13.

Herrero, M., Cifuentes, A., and Ibañez, E. (2006). Sub-and supercritical fluid extraction of functional ingredients from different natural sources: plants, food-by-products, algae and microalgae: a review. *Food Chemistry* **98** (1): 136–148.

Hu, S., Fan, X., Qi, P., and Zhang, X. (2019). Identification of anti-diabetes peptides from *Spirulina platensis*. *Journal of Functional Foods* **56**: 333–341.

Huynh-Ba, K. and Sassi, A.B. (2018). ANVISA: an introduction to a new regulatory agency with many challenges. *AAPS Open* **4** (1): 9.

Janczyk, P., Wolf, C., and Souffrant, W.B. (2005). Evaluation of nutritional value and safety of the green microalgae *Chlorella vulgaris* treated with novel processing methods. *Arch Zootech* **8**: 132–147.

Joubert, Y. and Fleurence, J. (2008). Simultaneous extraction of proteins and DNA by an enzymatic treatment of the cell wall of *Palmaria palmata* (Rhodophyta). *Journal of Applied Phycology* **20** (1): 55–61.

Kadam, S.U., Tiwari, B.K., and O'Donnell, C.P. (2015). Effect of ultrasound pre-treatment on the drying kinetics of brown seaweed *Ascophyllum nodosum*. *Ultrasonics Sonochemistry* **23**: 302–307.

Kadam, S.U., Álvarez, C., Tiwari, B.K., and O'Donnell, C.P. (2017). Extraction and characterization of protein from Irish brown seaweed *Ascophyllum nodosum*. *Food Research International* **99**: 1021–1027.

Kang, K.H., Qian, Z.J., Ryu, B. et al. (2012). Antioxidant peptides from protein hydrolysate of microalgae *Navicula incerta* and their protective effects in HepG2/CYP2E1 cells induced by ethanol. *Phytotherapy Research* **26** (10): 1555–1563.

Kang, K.H., Qian, Z.J., Ryu, B. et al. (2013). Hepatic fibrosis inhibitory effect of peptides isolated from *Navicula incerta* on TGF-β1 induced activation of LX-2 human hepatic stellate cells. *Preventive Nutrition and Food Science* **18** (2): 124–132.

Kavitha, M.D., Gouda, K.G.M., Rao, S.J.A. et al. (2019). Atheroprotective effect of novel peptides from *Porphyridium purpureum* in RAW 264.7 macrophage cell line and its molecular docking study. *Biotechnology Letters* **41** (1): 91–106.

Kazir, M., Abuhassira, Y., Robin, A. et al. (2019). Extraction of proteins from two marine macroalgae, *Ulva* sp. and *Gracilaria* sp., for food application, and evaluating digestibility, amino acid composition and antioxidant properties of the protein concentrates. *Food Hydrocolloids* **87**: 194–203.

Keris-Sen, U.D., Sen, U., Soydemir, G., and Gurol, M.D. (2014). An investigation of ultrasound effect on microalgal cell integrity and lipid extraction efficiency. *Bioresource Technology* **152**: 407–413.

Kim, E.Y., Choi, Y.H., and Nam, T.J. (2018). Identification and antioxidant activity of synthetic peptides from phycobiliproteins of *Pyropia yezoensis*. *International Journal of Molecular Medicine* **42** (2): 789–798.

Ko, S.C., Kang, N., Kim, E.A. et al. (2012). A novel angiotensin I-converting enzyme (ACE) inhibitory peptide from a marine *Chlorella ellipsoidea* and its antihypertensive effect in spontaneously hypertensive rats. *Process Biochemistry* **47** (12): 2005–2011.

Kumagai, Y., Miyabe, Y., Takeda, T. et al. (2019). In silico analysis of relationship between proteins from plastid genome of red alga *Palmaria* sp. (Japan) and angiotensin I converting enzyme inhibitory peptides. *Marine Drugs* **17** (3): 1–11.

Kumar, M.S. (2019). Peptides and peptidomimetics as potential Antiobesity agents: overview of current status. *Frontiers in Nutrition* **6** (11): 1–12.

Kumar, P., Sharma, N., Ranjan, R. et al. (2013). Perspective of membrane technology in dairy industry: a review. *Asian-Australasian Journal of Animal Sciences* **26** (9): 1347–1358.

Lee, M.K., Choi, J.W., Choi, Y., and Nam, T.J. (2018). *Pyropia yezoensis* protein prevents dexamethasone-induced myotube atrophy in C2C12 myotubes. *Marine Drugs* **16** (12): 497.

Lin, Y.H., Chen, G.W., Yeh, C. et al. (2018). Purification and identification of angiotensin I-converting enzyme inhibitory peptides and the antihypertensive effect of *Chlorella sorokiniana* protein hydrolysates. *Nutrients* **10** (10): 1–12.

Luengo, E., Martínez, J.M., Bordetas, A. et al. (2015). Influence of the treatment medium temperature on lutein extraction assisted by pulsed electric fields from *Chlorella vulgaris*. *Innovative Food Science & Emerging Technologies* **29**: 15–22.

Mæhre, H., Jensen, I.J., and Eilertsen, K.E. (2016). Enzymatic pre-treatment increases the protein bioaccessibility and extractability in dulse (*Palmaria palmata*). *Marine Drugs* **14** (11): 196.

de Marco Castro, E., Shannon, E., and Abu-Ghannam, N. (2019). Effect of fermentation on enhancing the nutraceutical properties of *Arthrospira platensis* (*Spirulina*). *Fermentation* **5** (1): 1–16.

Marrion, O., Schwertz, A., Fleurence, J. et al. (2003). Improvement of the digestibility of the proteins of the red alga *Palmaria palmata* by physical processes and fermentation. *Food/Nahrung* **47** (5): 339–344.

Minoru, S., Takashi, O., Takao, H. et al. (2005). Production of the blood pressure lowing peptides from brown alga (*Undaria pinnatifida*). *Journal of Ocean University of China* **4** (3): 209–213.

Montone, C.M., Capriotti, A.L., Cavaliere, C. et al. (2018). Peptidomic strategy for purification and identification of potential ACE-inhibitory and antioxidant peptides in *Tetradesmus obliquus* microalgae. *Analytical and Bioanalytical Chemistry* **410** (15): 3573–3586.

Morales, D., Smiderle, F.R., Villalva, M. et al. (2019). Testing the effect of combining innovative extraction technologies on the biological activities of obtained β-glucan-enriched fractions from *Lentinula edodes*. *Journal of Functional Foods* **60**: 103446.

Neumann, C., Velten, S., and Liebert, F. (2017). Improving the dietary protein quality by amino acid fortification with a high inclusion level of micro algae (*Spirulina platensis*) or insect meal (*Hermetia illucens*) in meat type chicken diets. *Open Journal of Animal Sciences* **8** (1): 12–26.

Nongonierma, A.B. and FitzGerald, R.J. (2019). Features of dipeptidyl peptidase IV (DPP-IV) inhibitory peptides from dietary proteins. *Journal of Food Biochemistry* **43** (1): e12451.

Obata, O., Akunna, J.C., and Walker, G. (2015). Hydrolytic effects of acid and enzymatic pre-treatment on the anaerobic biodegradability of *Ascophyllum nodosum* and *Laminaria digitata* species of brown seaweed. *Biomass and Bioenergy* **80**: 140–146.

Oh, G.W., Ko, S.C., Heo, S.Y. et al. (2015). A novel peptide purified from the fermented microalga *Pavlova lutheri* attenuates oxidative stress and melanogenesis in B16F10 melanoma cells. *Process Biochemistry* **50** (8): 1318–1326.

Paiva, L., Lima, E., Neto, A.I., and Baptista, J. (2016). Isolation and characterization of angiotensin I-converting enzyme (ACE) inhibitory peptides from *Ulva rigida* C Agardh protein hydrolysate. *Journal of Functional Foods* **26**: 65–76.

Park, H.J., Lee, Y.J., Ryu, H.K. et al. (2008). A randomized double-blind, placebo-controlled study to establish the effects of spirulina in elderly Koreans. *Annals of Nutrition and Metabolism* **52** (4): 322–328.

Parniakov, O., Barba, F.J., Grimi, N. et al. (2015). Pulsed electric field and pH assisted selective extraction of intracellular components from microalgae *Nannochloropsis*. *Algal Research* **8**: 128–134.

Passos, F., Carretero, J., and Ferrer, I. (2015). Comparing pretreatment methods for improving microalgae anaerobic digestion: thermal, hydrothermal, microwave and ultrasound. *Chemical Engineering Journal* **279**: 667–672.

Perez Espitia, P.J., de Fátima Ferreira Soares, N., dos Reis Coimbra, J.S. et al. (2012). Bioactive peptides: synthesis, properties, and applications in the packaging and preservation of food. *Comprehensive Reviews in Food Science and Food Safety* **11** (2): 187–204.

Pérez-Míguez, R., Plaza, M., Castro-Puyana, M., and Marina, M.L. (2019). Separation and identification of peptides in hydrolysed protein extracts from edible macroalgae by HPLC-ESI-QTOF/MS. *Algal Research* **39**: 101465.

Persistence Market Research. (2018). Algal protein market: global industry trend analysis 2012 to 2017 and forecast 2017–2025. https://www.persistencemarketresearch.com/market-research/algal-protein-market.asp (accessed December 21, 2018)

Polikovsky, M., Fernand, F., Sack, M. et al. (2016). Towards marine biorefineries: selective proteins extractions from marine macroalgae *Ulva* with pulsed electric fields. *Innovative Food Science & Emerging Technologies* **37**: 194–200.

Postma, P.R., Fernandes, D.A., Timmermans, R.A.H. et al. (2017). Pulsed electric field for protein release of the microalgae *Chlorella vulgaris* and *Neochloris oleoabundans*. *Algal Research* **24**: 181–187.

Qian, Z.J., Ryu, B., Kang, K.H. et al. (2018). Cellular properties of the fermented microalgae *Pavlova lutheri* and its isolated active peptide in osteoblastic differentiation of MG-63 cells. *Molecular Medicine Reports* **17** (1): 2044–2050.

Qu, W., Ma, H., Wang, T., and Zheng, H. (2013). Alternating two-frequency countercurrent ultrasonic-assisted extraction of protein and polysaccharide from *Porphyra yezoensis*. *Transactions of the Chinese Society of Agricultural Engineering* **29** (1): 285–292.

Rodrigues, D., Sousa, S., Silva, A. et al. (2015). Impact of enzyme- and ultrasound-assisted extraction methods on biological properties of red, brown, and green seaweeds from the central west coast of Portugal. *Journal of Agricultural and Food Chemistry* **63** (12): 3177–3188.

Román, R.B., Álvarez-Pez, J.M., Fernández, F.A., and Grima, E.M. (2002). Recovery of pure B-phycoerythrin from the microalga *Porphyridium cruentum*. *Journal of Biotechnology* **93** (1): 73–85.

Ryu, B., Kang, K.H., Ngo, D.H. et al. (2012). Statistical optimization of microalgae *Pavlova lutheri* cultivation conditions and its fermentation conditions by yeast, *Candida rugopelliculosa*. *Bioresource Technology* **107**: 307–313.

Rzymski, P. and Jaśkiewicz, M. (2017). Microalgal food supplements from the perspective of Polish consumers: patterns of use, adverse events, and beneficial effects. *Journal of Applied Phycology* **29** (4): 1841–1850.

Safi, C., Ursu, A.V., Laroche, C. et al. (2014). Aqueous extraction of proteins from microalgae: effect of different cell disruption methods. *Algal Research* **3**: 61–65.

Sato, M., Hosokawa, T., Yamaguchi, T. et al. (2002). Angiotensin I-converting enzyme inhibitory peptides derived from wakame (*Undaria pinnatifida*) and their antihypertensive effect in spontaneously hypertensive rats. *Journal of Agricultural and Food Chemistry* **50** (21): 6245–6252.

Saito, M. and Hagino, H. (2005). Antihypertensive effect of oligopeptides derived from nori (*Porphyra yezoensis*) and Ala-Lys-Tyr-Ser-Tyr in rats. *Journal of Japanese Society of Nutrition and Food Science (Japan)* **58** (12): 177–184.

Samarakoon, K.W., Kwon, O.N., Ko, J.Y. et al. (2013). Purification and identification of novel angiotensin-I converting enzyme (ACE) inhibitory peptides from cultured marine microalgae (*Nannochloropsis oculata*) protein hydrolysate. *Journal of Applied Phycology* **25** (5): 1595–1606.

Seca, A. and Pinto, D. (2018). Overview on the antihypertensive and anti-obesity effects of secondary metabolites from seaweeds. *Marine Drugs* **16** (7): 237.

Sedighi, M., Jalili, H., Darvish, M. et al. (2019). Enzymatic hydrolysis of microalgae proteins using serine proteases: a study to characterize kinetic parameters. *Food Chemistry* **284**: 334–339.

Seyfabadi, J., Ramezanpour, Z., and Khoeyi, Z.A. (2011). Protein, fatty acid, and pigment content of *Chlorella vulgaris* under different light regimes. *Journal of Applied Phycology* **23** (4): 721–726.

Sheih, I.C., Fang, T.J., and Wu, T.K. (2009). Isolation and characterisation of a novel angiotensin I-converting enzyme (ACE) inhibitory peptide from the algae protein waste. *Food Chemistry* **115** (1): 279–284.

Spolaore, P., Joannis-Cassan, C., Duran, E., and Isambert, A. (2006). Commercial applications of microalgae. *Journal of Bioscience and Bioengineering* **101** (2): 87–96.

Stack, J., Le Gouic, A.V., Tobin, P.R. et al. (2018). Protein extraction and bioactive hydrolysate generation from two microalgae, *Porphyridium purpureum* and *Phaeodactylum tricornutum*. *Journal of Food Bioactives* **1**: 153–165.

Suetsuna, K. and Nakano, T. (2000). Identification of an antihypertensive peptide from peptic digest of wakame (*Undaria pinnatifida*). *The Journal of Nutritional Biochemistry* **11** (9): 450–454.

Sun, Y., Chang, R., Li, Q., and Li, B. (2016). Isolation and characterization of an antibacterial peptide from protein hydrolysates of *Spirulina platensis*. *European Food Research and Technology* **242** (5): 685–692.

Sun, S., Xu, X., Sun, X. et al. (2019). Preparation and identification of ACE inhibitory peptides from the marine macroalga *Ulva intestinalis*. *Marine Drugs* **17** (3): 179.

Suwal, S., Perreault, V., Marciniak, A. et al. (2019). Effects of high hydrostatic pressure and polysaccharidases on the extraction of antioxidant compounds from red macroalgae, *Palmaria palmata* and *Solieria chordalis*. *Journal of Food Engineering* **252**: 53–59.

Tejano, L.A., Peralta, J.P., Yap, E.E.S., and Chang, Y.W. (2019). Bioactivities of enzymatic protein hydrolysates derived from *Chlorella sorokiniana*. *Food Science & Nutrition* **7**: 2381–2390.

Tibbetts, S.M., Milley, J.E., and Lall, S.P. (2016). Nutritional quality of some wild and cultivated seaweeds: nutrient composition, total phenolic content and in vitro digestibility. *Journal of Applied Phycology* **28** (6): 3575–3585.

Töpfl, S. (2006). Pulsed electric fields (PEF) for permeabilization of cell membranes in food- and bioprocessing–applications, process and equipment design and cost analysis. Technische Universität Berlin. http://dx.doi.org/10.14279/depositonce-1441 (accessed September 16, 2020).

Tran, T., Denimal, E., Lafarge, C. et al. (2019). Effect of high hydrostatic pressure on extraction of B-phycoerythrin from *Porphyridium cruentum:* use of confocal microscopy and image processing. *Algal Research* **38**: 101394.

Urbano, M.G. and Goñi, I. (2002). Bioavailability of nutrients in rats fed on edible seaweeds, nori (*Porphyra tenera*) and wakame (*Undaria pinnatifida*), as a source of dietary fibre. *Food Chemistry* **76** (3): 281–286.

Valensa International. (2012). Parry organic spirulina first to receive FDA GRAS status for organic spirulina ingredient. https://www.prnewswire.com/news-releases/parry-organic-spirulina-first-to-receive-fda-gras-status-for-organic-spirulina-ingredient-177461581.html (accessed September 16, 2020).

Vanthoor-Koopmans, M., Wijffels, R.H., Barbosa, M.J., and Eppink, M.H. (2013). Biorefinery of microalgae for food and fuel. *Bioresource Technology* **135**: 142–149.

Vásquez, V., Martínez, R., and Bernal, C. (2019). Enzyme-assisted extraction of proteins from the seaweeds *Macrocystis pyrifera* and *Chondracanthus chamissoi*: characterization of the extracts and their bioactive potential. *Journal of Applied Phycology* **31**: 1999–2010.

Vo, T.S., Ryu, B., and Kim, S.K. (2013). Purification of novel anti-inflammatory peptides from enzymatic hydrolysate of the edible microalgal *Spirulina maxima*. *Journal of Functional Foods* **5** (3): 1336–1346.

Wood, L. (2018). Global algae protein market 2017–2023 – $800+ million industry trends, opportunities and forecasts. https://www.businesswire.com/news/home/20180209005673/en/Global-Algae-Protein-Market-2017-2023---800 (accessed December 21, 2018).

Yang, H.S., Haj, F.G., Lee, M. et al. (2019). *Laminaria japonica* extract enhances intestinal barrier function by altering inflammatory response and tight junction-related protein in lipopolysaccharide-stimulated Caco-2 cells. *Nutrients* **11** (5): 1001.

Zhang, L., Zhang, S.T., Yin, Y.C. et al. (2018). Hypoglycemic effect and mechanism of isoquercitrin as an inhibitor of dipeptidyl peptidase-4 in type 2 diabetic mice. *RSC Advances* **8** (27): 14967–14974.

Zhang, R., Grimi, N., Marchal, L., and Vorobiev, E. (2019a). Application of high-voltage electrical discharges and high-pressure homogenization for recovery of intracellular compounds from microalgae *Parachlorella kessleri*. *Bioprocess and Biosystems Engineering* **42** (1): 29–36.

Zhang, X., Cao, D., Sun, X. et al. (2019b). Preparation and identification of antioxidant peptides from protein hydrolysate of marine alga *Gracilariopsis lemaneiformis*. *Journal of Applied Phycology*: 1–12.

Zhao, B., Cui, Y., Fan, X. et al. (2019). Anti-obesity effects of *Spirulina platensis* protein hydrolysate by modulating brain-liver axis in high-fat diet fed mice. *PLoS One* **14** (6): e0218543.

15
Algal Dietary Fiber and its Health Benefits

Shakeel Ramzan[1], Muhammad Mushtaq[1], Sumia Akram[2], and Ahmad Adnan[1]
[1]*Department of Chemistry, GC University, Lahore, Pakistan*
[2]*Division of Science and Technology, University of Education, Lahore, Pakistan*

15.1 Introduction

Macroalgae or marine algae are the eukaryotic organisms that contain chlorophyll for photosynthesis but lack other membranes or organs like leaves, roots, stem, cell walls, and sterile coverings around the reproductive cells of the plant. These organisms commonly grow underwater or in shaded areas with plenty of water including river rocks, buildings in contact with water, and tree stems or roots. The literature lacks a universally accepted definition or classification of algal biomass and these may fall into different divisions depending upon their various attributes like the organization of photosynthesis membranes, their pigments, the chemical composition of photosynthesis storage products, and other morphological attributes. Overall, algal biomass has been categorized into four main groups based on their colors such as brown algae comprising more than 1750 species of class Phaeophyceae and Ochrophyta phylum. The red algae cover the most abundant class of algal species (more than 6000 members) of the Rhodophyta phylum. The green and blue or blue-green algae comprise between approx. 1200 and 1500 species of phylum Chlorophyta and Cyanophyta, respectively. The algal biomass of the blue-green algae is mainly spread over temperate sands, trees, and rocky shores (Kılınç et al. 2013).

Algal biomass is found growing throughout the world's seas and oceans but none of them has been found to be poisonous or detrimental to humans (Guiry 2009; Wynne and Bold 1985). The utilization of macroalgae as human food has been reported since ancient times, but their commercial utilization began after World War II. Meanwhile, research regarding the nutritional potential of algae revealed that algae could work as a good source of carbohydrates and protein to fulfill the protein requirements of the rapidly growing world population. Nowadays, marine macroalgae are the major coastal resource in many countries for human consumption. Figure 15.1 compares the total production in thousands of metric tons ($X \times 10^3$) of wild and cultivated seaweeds. According to the plotted data, China covers the highest fraction (698 000 metric tons) followed by France (616 000 metric tons), and the UK (205 000 metric tons).

Recent Advances in Micro- and Macroalgal Processing: Food and Health Perspectives, First Edition.
Edited by Gaurav Rajauria and Yvonne V. Yuan.

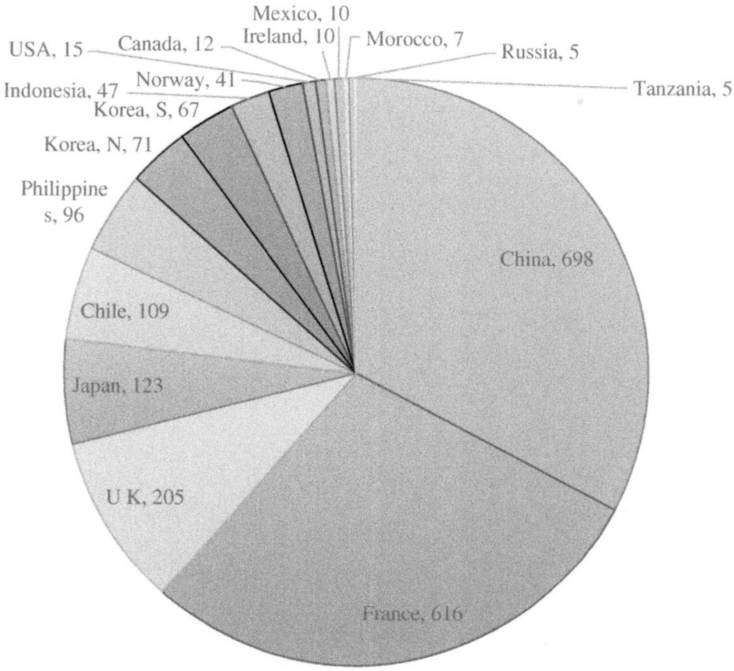

Figure 15.1 Distribution of total seaweed production (wild + cultivated) in x × 10^3 metrictons

Awareness regarding the fiber content and nutritional value of seaweeds has initiated cultivation of algal species in various parts of the world. Figure 15.2 gives an estimation of hundreds of metric tons of algae cultivated across the map. China ranks top with annual cultivation of 67 500 metric tons of algae followed by Japan and the Philippines with an annual production of 10 700 and 9000 metric tons, respectively.

The macroalgae occupy a major portion of the producers in the food chain or food web. Although these organisms follow the same photosynthetic mechanism as land-based plants, the macroalgae, can capture sunlight, carbon dioxide, and water more efficiently. Likewise, algal structures occupy more surface area when present in the form of colonies and algal blooms so become more efficient in converting sunlight energy into biomass. In general, algal biomass represents autotrophic producers in the food chain, particularly for marine animals, but algae may develop a symbiotic relationship with various hosts to supply them with energy or nutrients. The algal biomass is not only a primary producer in the food web but also provides proteins, polysaccharides, lipids, minerals, enzymes, and vitamins. Nowadays, algae have become a potential food source, particularly in Asia, and algae intake not only provides fiber but also vitamins, iodine, niacin, and calcium (Kılınç et al. 2013).

15.2 Dietary Fiber

The term dietary fiber was first used for digestible fiber in 1973 as opposed to crude fiber, which may refer to nondigestible components of foods (Potty 1996).

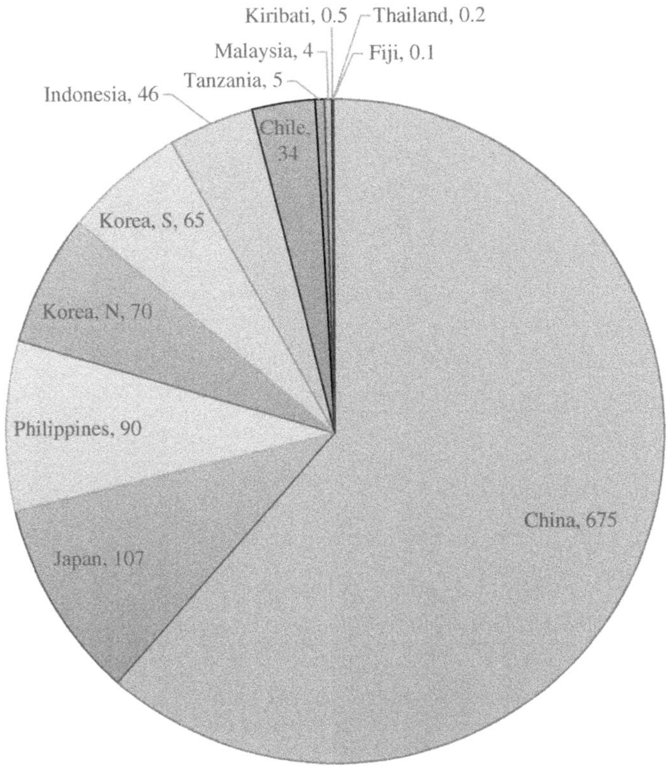

Figure 15.2 Worldwide production volume (x × 100 metricton) of cultivated algae

The next year Trowell (1974) defined dietary fiber as the part of plant cell-based food that resists hydrolysis (digestion) by the human enzyme systems. It mainly consists of particular oligosaccharides, celluloses, hemicelluloses, lignins, pectins, waxes, and gums. From an analytical point of view, dietary fibers cover nonstarchy polysaccharides of plant origin. Most researchers label nonstarchy polysaccharides of plant cell wall materials as dietary fiber (Schweizer 1991); however, lignin and the majority of modified starches produced during the course of food manufacturing or processing are often nondigestible by a human being, and therefore must be considered as dietary fiber (Potty 1996). Nowadays, dietary fiber covers the fraction of food containing modified starches, oligosaccharides, hydrolysis-resistant proteins, and many other bioactives with complex structures like polyphenols (Calixto 1997; Jiménez-Escrig and Sánchez-Muniz 2000).

Dietary fiber comprises the macromolecules similar to plant cell wall components that normally resist hydrolysis by human endogenous enzymes like amylases and maltases. The majority of these biomolecules are polymers of glucose, such as pectin substances, cellulose and hemicellulose, inulin, starch, and modified moieties like phytates, gums, polyphenols, saponins, waxes, and cutin (Lahaye 1991; Trowell 1974). Many of these biomolecules do not dissolve or withstand digestion in the human digestion system. The digestible carbohydrates like starch and lactose may become indigestible after certain modifications. Starch has been also categorized according to whether it is physically accessible, gelatinized, retrograded, or chemically modified (Elleuch et al. 2011).

Dietary fiber consists of a complex and bulky arrangement of elements like carbon, hydrogen, oxygen, nitrogen, and elements whose concentration and composition in different sources are neither uniform nor constant (Potty 1996). These chemical and physical variables explain the number and complexity of physiological principles associated with dietary fiber. With respect to polysaccharides, each and every type of dietary fiber is characterized by the nature of the bonds between them and their sugar residues.

15.2.1 Algae as a Source of Dietary Fiber

The edible seaweeds or marine macroalgae are the sea vegetables that can be taken directly or added to human foods. These algal strains might be from any class but broadly have been grouped as brown (Phaeophyceae), green (Chlorophyceae), and red (Rhodophyceae) algae (Renn 1990). These edible sea vegetables are rich in fiber and cell wall polysaccharides whose concentration may vary from species to species. The most well known species of algae used in cuisines include *Undaria* sp. (wakame), *Laminaria* sp. (kombu), and *Hizikia* sp. (hiziki) from brown seaweeds; laverbread, grape stones, *Carola*, and *Porphyra* sp. (nori) of the red group (McHugh 1991); and *Chlorella*, gutweed (*Ulva intestinalis*), sea grapes and sea lettuce of the green algae. Each group of algae varies in polysaccharides present in the form of cellulose, laminarans, alginates, and fucans. For example, the main cell walls of brown algae contain alginates, cellulose, and fucans, whereas those of red may be composed of sulfated galactans like carrageenans and agar, xylans, mannans, and cellulose. Similarly, uronic acids, rhamnose, xylose, or galactose, cellulose, mannans, and sulfate ionic polysaccharides have been found in the cell walls of green algae (Lahaye 1991).

The relative amounts of dietary fiber in algal biomass are considerably higher than in fruits and vegetables or their by-products. Table 15.1 compares the percentage amounts (g/100 g^{-1}) of dietary fibers reported in various species of brown, green, and red algae. It is obvious from the collected data that a few algal species like *Sargassum hemiphyllum*, *Ulva reticulata*, *Eisenia bicyclis*, *Gracilaria changii*, and *Sargassum henslowianum* contain about 61.3, 65.7, 10–75, 64.7, and 61.1% total dietary fiber (TDF). It is interesting to note that the majority of algal strains screened for their fiber content contain more than 30% TDF, which is significantly higher than well-known fruits like avocado, banana, guava, jackfruit, longan, mango, and pomegranate.

The dietary fibers of algal biomass and of plant origin are classified into soluble and insoluble fiber. The soluble fiber includes agars, furan, alginic acid, laminaran or laminarin, porphyran pectic substances, algal polysaccharides, and some of the hemicelluloses are soluble dietary fiber, while mannans, cellulose, xylan, hemicellulose, and lignin are insoluble dietary fiber (Lahaye 1991; Roehrig 1988). The TDF contents are 50% dry weight for *Fucus*, 58% for *Undaria*, 29% for *Saccharina*, and 30% for *Porphyra* (Lahaye 1991; Murata and Nakazoe 2001). According to Fleury and Lahaye

Table 15.1 A comparison of percentage of dietary fiber of various algal species

Brown seaweeds	Total dietary fiber (TDF) (%)	References	Green algae	TDF %	References	Red algae	TDF (%)	References
Sargassum hemiphyllum	61.3	Chan et al. (1997)	*Caulerapa racemosa*	33–40	Patara et al. (2011)	*Gracilaria changii*	22.7	Marinho-Soriano et al. (2006)
Eisenia bicyclis	10–75	Patara et al. (2011)	*Ulva compressa*	41.1–55.4	Parthiban et al. (2013)	*Gracilaria changii*	64.7	Chan and Matanjun (2017)
Sargassum horneri	42–55	Murakami et al. (2011)	*Ulva pertusa*	52.1	Yoshie et al. (1997)	*Euchema cottonii*	25.5	Msuya and Neori (2002)
Sargassum wightii	48.0	Prosky et al. (1988)	*Ulva reticulata*	65.7	Yoshie et al. (1997)	*Gracilaria crassa*	22.7	MacArtain et al. (2007)
Laminaria sp.	36.0	Kılınç et al. (2013)	*Ulva rigida*	38–40	Yoshie et al. (1997)	*Pterocladiella. capillacea*	52.0	Mišurcová et al. (2010)
Sargassum fusiforme	35–45.9	Burtin (2003)	*Ulva* sp.	38.0	Patara et al. (2011)	*Porphyra umbilicalis*	33.7	Mišurcová et al. (2010)
S. henslowianum	61.1	Wong and Cheung (2001)	*Ulva lactuca*	38.1–43	Burtin (2003)	*Palmaria palmata*	33.7	Matanjun et al. (2009)
Sargassum mangarevense	42.8	Zubia et al. (2003)				*Porphyra* sp.	48.6	Matanjun et al. (2009)
Sargassum patens	54.8	Wong and Cheung (2001)				*Gracilaria verrucosa*	52.0	Wong and Cheung (2000)
Sargassum polycytum	39.6	Zubia et al. (2003)				*Hypnea charoides*	50.3	Wong and Cheung (2000)
Sargassum wightii	44–53	Zubia et al. (2003)				*Hypnea japonica*	53.2	Norziah and Ching (2000)
Undaria pinnatifida	16–51	Dawczynski et al. (2007)				*Gracilaria verrucosa*	50–56	Zubia et al. (2003)

(1991) *Undaria pinnatifida* (wakame), *Porphyra*, and *Chondrus* contain 15–22% soluble dietary fiber while *Laminaria* and *Fucus* may contain 27–40% insoluble dietary fiber.

15.2.2 Marine Algal Polysaccharides

Marine macroalgae or seaweeds are rich in bioactive compounds like polysaccharides called dietary fiber. Dietary fiber has a potential prebiotic effect on human health. Out of the TDF content (25–70%) present in seaweeds, the soluble dietary fiber accounts for 50–80% (de Jesus Raposo et al. 2016). Dietary fiber of macroalgae possesses several biological properties like antioxidant activity (Chandini et al. 2008), anti-inflammatory activity (Kang et al. 2008; Suleria et al. 2016), antiviral activity (Lozano et al. 2016; Sinha et al. 2010), and anticoagulant potency (Jin et al. 2013). Terrestrial plants and marine seaweeds are natural sources of dietary fiber. Due to their physiology, marine seaweeds contain more dietary fiber (de Jesus Raposo et al. 2016). For example, laminarin, mainly present in brown algae, is a linear polysaccharide made of β (1→3) glucan with β (1→6) branches at a 3:1 ratio. Its reducing ends are often replaced with 2–3% D-mannitol and it works as a carbohydrate reserve. It can be hydrolyzed into sugars by an enzyme laminarinase, namely EC 3.2.1.6. Polyuronide, the main matrix part of brown algae, is known as a gelling alginate and is mainly composed of alternating units of two hexaronic acids, i.e. β-D-mannuronic acid (β-(1→4)-D-mannuronic acid [M]) and its C_5 epimer α-(1→4)-L-guluronic acid (L). Polyuronide may consist of homo, hetero, or alternating M and L units depending upon the maturity of the seaweed and area of cultivation. In general, the distribution of guluronic blocks affects the gel-forming capacity of polyuronides.

Fucans or sulfur-containing heterogeneous polysaccharides may fall into three categories. The first class of fucans, i.e. fucoidans contains 1→3 and (1→4) linked α-L-fucopyranose residues with small amounts of D-xylose, D-mannose, D-galactose, and uronic acids. Fucoidans comprise 20–30% on a dry weight basis of brown seaweed and have been found to be antioxidant, cognitive protective, anticancer, antiangiogenic, anti-inflammatory, and antiviral in preclinical trials (Burtin 2003).

Members of the second class of fucans, namely glycuronogalactofucans, contain linear chains of (1,4)- D-galactose having a branch at C5 with L-fucosyl-3-sulfate or sometimes uronic acid. Ascophyllans or xylofucoglycuronans comprise a backbone of polyuronide, mostly of poly-β-(1,4)-D-mannuronic acid having a branch with 3-O-D-sylosyl-L-fucose-4-sulfate or sometimes with uronic acid (Fleury and Lahaye 1991). The sulfated galactans (agar and carrageenans), mannans, xylans, and cellulose are present in the cell walls of red algae, while starch constitutes the reserve polysaccharide of red algae (Lahaye 1991).

The term carrageenans has been used for the family of complex red algae polysaccharides and they contain linear galactans, namely β-(1,4,3,6)-anhydro-D-galactose alternating with α-(1,3)-galactose. However, these polysaccharides may differ in the position and degree of sulfate substituents. The commercial carrageenans also vary in sulfate distribution and the ratio of 3,6-anhydro galactose content. The agars are another important class of polysaccharides present in red algae like *Gelidium* sp. (known as tengusa) and *Gracilaria* sp. (ogonori). The commercial production of agar for jellies, custards, and other culinary uses is mainly from *Gracilaria*. Chemically, agar consists of about 70% agarose and agaropectin. The former is basically a polymer of agarbiose: (3,6)-anhydro-L-galactopyranose and D-galactose (Renn 1990), whereas the latter is made up of alternating units of L-galactose and D-galactose with extensive sulfate-based acidic groups.

Green algae contain cellulose, arabinogalactan proteins, β-xylans, sulfated polysaccharides, and β-mannans. Moreover, rhamnogalacturonan, 2-keto sugars, and mixed linkage glucans have also been reported in green algae (Jiménez-Escrig and Sánchez-Muniz 2000; Lahaye 1991).

15.3 Physical Properties of Dietary Fiber (Dispersibility, Viscosity, Binding Capacity, Fermentability)

Although seaweeds or cultivated algae contain fibrous carbohydrates, their dispersal, dissolution, or digestion in the human gut system or intestines depends upon the chemical composition of the fiber. It is therefore important to discuss the physical properties of algal fiber to understand its characteristic responses in the human gut and potential health benefits or risks. The physical properties that can control the physiological functions of dietary fiber include but are not limited to its viscosity, dispersibility, or water-holding capacity (WHC), and fermentability or fecal bulking or swelling capacity (Schneeman 1999). Actually, the basic definition of dietary fiber, i.e. cell wall constituents resistant to human gut and intestine secretions, is more physiological in nature (Jiménez-Escrig and Sánchez-Muniz 2000; Lahaye 1991).

15.3.1 Dispersibility

Dietary fiber falls into two categories, i.e. water-soluble or insoluble on the basis of ability to form a homogeneous mixture when mixed with water. In general, the polysaccharide polymers bearing polar substituents like SO_4^{2-}, COOH, or terminal OH groups are soluble in water and their solubility further increases with an increase in temperature and ionic strength or polarity (Bertin et al. 1988; Fleury and Lahaye 1991; Manas et al. 1994). In this context, polysaccharides like fucans, laminarans, pectin, and alginates form gelatinous masses when mixed with water, whereas cellulose, lignin, resistant starch, and a few β-glucans are insoluble when exposed to water. The algal biomasses, in general, was found to be rich in soluble type fibers as compared with fruits, vegetables, and cereal grain (Elleuch et al. 2011).

The key health benefits of dietary fiberd have been associated with their ability to bulk, ferment, or increase the viscosity of ingested foods. All of these properties in one way or other depend on water absorption, swelling, or WHC. The hydrolysis of dietary fiber also depends upon fiber particle size, gut pH, temperature, and porosity of ingested fiber in addition to the chemical structure (Elleuch et al. 2011). The hydrolysis or WHC of fiber has been extensively studied and was found to be temperature-, pH-, and electrolyte-dependent. Moreover, cooking and chewing of dietary fiber may affect their molecular entanglement or extent of crosslinking to affect the solubility and WHC of fiber (Fleury and Lahaye 1991).

The WHC of dietary fiber, in general, depends upon the structure and composition of the component polysaccharides. The simplest approach to determine WHC involves centrifugation of precisely weighed fiber. Water may become entrapped in fiber depending upon its polysaccharide structure. Moreover, WHC may vary with soaking time, temperature, agitation speed, and centrifugation time. So WHC is generally measured as the amount of water retained by 1.0 g of the fiber under specific conditions of temperature and agitation (Guillon and Champ 2000). Moreover, the dissolution of fiber during the experimental course of time may ultimately affect the WHC of the final product (Fleury and Lahaye 1991). The swelling ability of dietary fiber, like WHC, can be easily estimated by swelling the fiber in an excess of water or other solvent of interest in a graduated volumetric cylinder, overnight at 37 °C (Kuniak and Marchessault 1972). Another similar physiological parameter to assess the ability of dietary fiber to retain lipids is its oil holding capacity (OHC), which is denoted by the number of grams of oil retained (g oil per g of dietary fiber) during sufficient interaction with corn oil. Out of these parameters, the WHC in general increases with an increase in pH and temperature of dietary fiber or digestion media (Wong and Cheung 2000).

It is interesting to note that WHC of algal fiber from wakame (19.0–44.0 g g^{-1}) on a dry mass basis is much higher than that of dietary fiber of whole foods such as wheat bran (2.8–3.6 g g^{-1}), rice bran (4.89 g g^{-1}), orange (7.3 g g^{-1}), peach (12.9 g g^{-1}), and sugarbeet (34.5 g g^{-1}) (Mehta et al. 2015). Likewise, the OHC of dietary fiber from *Lminaria digitata* was found to be higher than that of fruit fiber obtained from the fruit juice industry (Elleuch et al. 2011). The higher OHC and WHC of algal fiber have been attributed to composition, charge density, hydrophilic behavior, and surface characteristics of algae fiber constituents like fucans and alginates (Caprez et al. 1986; Elleuch et al. 2011; Fleury and Lahaye 1991).

The WHC and OHC and swellability of algal fiber may vary from species to species, maturity/harvesting stage, and marine environment. In general, the dried algal matrix can swell up to 20 times its dry matter volume once exposed to water (Kuda et al. 1997). Alginate, a gelling polyuronide and a major part of algal fiber in brown algae, forms tough jelly-like viscous materials due to calcium cations (Fleury and Lahaye 1991). As a gelling agent, cationic alginate containing guluronic acid has much greater solubility in water than alginate with mannuronic acid, which is responsible for gel production in the stomach after dietary intake of alginate-rich food. Carrageenan also produces robust and thick jelly materials when it binds with calcium and potassium, respectively. Similarly, the gelling behavior of alginic acid in stomach varies widely with composition. In general, the solubility of sodium alginate containing guluronic acid is more than in alginate bearing more mannuronic acid. Moreover, *in vivo* investigation has revealed that animals fed with feed containing guluronic acid-rich alginates take less food and face growth retardation compared with those fed with fibers mainly consisting of mannuronic acid-rich alginates (Kimura et al. 1996). According to Torsdottir et al. (1991) sodium alginate also retards gastric evacuation in humans.

15.3.2 Viscosity (η)

From a health point of view, dietary fiber falls into two categories, namely, dietary fiber and functional fiber. The viscosity plays an important role regarding flow behavior and dietary applications of fiber; however, discrepancies exist regarding definitions and principles of viscosity. Therefore, before we turn to the viscosity of dietary fiber, it is important to make a brief overview of viscosity. Sir Isaac Newton was the first scientist who defined viscosity as "the ratio flow of fluid in response to force applied on the fluid." The method used to calculate viscosity compares force applied tangentially to a fluid plane "shear stress" (Γ Nm^{-2}) with flow rate "shear rate" (γ; S^{-1}). The majority of liquid foods and biological matrixes like concentrated orange juice, apple sauce concentrates, intestinal fluid, mayonnaise, and honey do not follow Newtonian fluid principles and their viscosities change with a change in shear rate, concentration, particle size, temperature, and, above all, size of undigested particles. However, the available literature indicates that many instruments intended to determine the viscosity of Newtonian fluids are erroneously used to monitor the viscosity of non-Newtonian fluids (Elleuch et al. 2011).

The characterization of soluble dietary fiber depends upon their capacity to enhance the viscosity of the solution and to decrease plasma cholesterol and glycemic responses, while the characterization of insoluble dietary fibers is made according to their low density, their porosity, their capability to increase fecal bulk, and to limit the intestinal transit time. In food processing, soluble dietary fiber exhibits greater ability to impart viscosity, produce gels, or act as emulsifiers without giving any bad taste or texture as compared with insoluble dietary fibers and also can be utilized more easily in processed drinks and foods. The ability of dietary fiber to form a gel or thicken when brought into contact with a solution mainly depends upon its chemical composition, nevertheless fluidic behavior of dietary fiber and other biological material changes with a change in shear rates, moisture level, temperature, particle size, and pH. In addition, the chemical composition and physicochemical characteristics of dietary fiber play a strategic role in enhancing the viscosity of a diet and reducing its intestinal transit time (Abdul-Hamid and Luan 2000; Olson et al. 1987; Roehrig 1988; Schneeman 1987). An increase in the intestinal viscosity of the diet with the incorporation of dietary fiber inhibits the glycemic response (availability of glucose), cholesterol, and many other toxins present in the diet from penetrating into the bloodstream. Finally, on viscosity: the physicochemical characteristics of soluble dietary fiber may help us to predict the thickening of polysaccharide fibers like pectins, alginates, gums, and β-glucans, changes in intestinal enzyme activities, glycemic response, blood cholesterol and lipid attenuation, laxation, and digestibility.

15.3.3 Binding Capacity

The hypocholesterolemic effect, anticancer behavior, and ability of dietary fiber to check obesity have been mainly linked to its binding capacity with bile acids. In addition, the binding of dietary fiber with bile acids and salts also controls or often reduces the availability of certain metals, minerals, nutrients, and vitamins. The literature contains a plethora of research reports regarding the binding of dietary fibers with bile acids. The bile materials are mainly composed of amphiphilic (both hydrophilic and phobic) steroids, namely cholic and deoxycholic acids (acids synthesized in the liver), which are conjugated with glycine or taurine to become hydrophilic, whereas in the colon these biomolecules deconjugate and/or dehydroxylate into hydrophobic deoxycholic and lithocholic acid. In general, a decrease in bile pH and an increase in hydrophobicity of dietary fibers and bile acids enhance their binding capacity. The attachment of bile acids/salts to the fiber molecules reduces their concentration in the colon, which eventually reduces the risk of colon cancer. Moreover, the retention of fecapentaenes and heterocyclic amines also guards against various toxicities (Potty 1996). Suzuki et al. (1996) had investigated fibers of brown, green, and red algae for their ability to bind bile acids and observed that nori and cholate species of red algae can bind 12.6–15.5% of bile acids, followed by green alga (aonori) (9.7%), and other seaweeds. The lowest bile acid-binding capacity was shown by species kombu and hiziki of brown algae, which could not adsorb cholic acid or sodium cholate. As stated above, the binding capacity of algal fibers decreases with an increase in pH and polarity of bile acids (Suzuki et al. 1996).

Besides the benefits associated with the intake of dietary fiber, its intake may reduce the availability of minerals and vitamins. In this context, pectins exhibit the highest mineral-binding capacity, while methoxy derivatives of pectin do not bind mineral cations (Jiménez-Escrig and Sánchez-Muniz 2000). It is interesting to note that brown seaweed fiber, when tested in *in vitro* models studies, scavenged sodium from the environment containing sodium and potassium cations. Likewise, 1 g of fiber from brown algae may adsorb 59 mg of sodium and offer good sodium–potassium exchange capacity (Krotkiewski and Aurell 1997). In contrast, seaweed alginates can bind barium, strontium, and calcium cations via conformational transformation of polyuronide chains in eggshells where aggregation of alginates leads to the formation of gels (Fleury and Lahaye 1991; Jiménez-Escrig and Sánchez-Muniz 2000).

15.3.4 Fermentability

When food enters the large bowel (colon) along with various enzymes and biomolecules from the liver and small intestine, it undergoes bacterial fermentation. The exact site and rate of fermentation depend upon the chemical structure, composition, solubility, microflora, and bioavailability of a few more readily fermentable substrates. In general, food fermentation in the colon produces a large amount of short-chain fatty acids (acetic, propanoic, and butyric acids), methane (CH_4), hydrogen (H_2), and carbon dioxide (CO_2). As a result of the fermentation reaction, the physiochemical environment of the large intestine changes. Likewise, the presence of carbohydrates may boost bacterial growth or metabolism of particular organisms at the expense of other ones (Guillon and Champ 2000). The research data available related to algal dietary fiber indicate sulfate and fucose concentration and their arrangement play a key role during the bacterial degradation of these products. According to Michell et al. (1996), alginates of algal fiber take 6 hours for their latency phase while following a particular fermentation pattern. The authors report that about 65% of algal alginates degrade and ferment to produce short-chain fatty acids, which contradicts the general perception that water-soluble fibers are highly fermentable (Topping 1991). Overall, the ability of algal dietary fibers to resist bacterial fermentation at least retains a few of their physicochemical characteristics that may impart a variety of benefits in the colon (Michell et al. 1996). Another report regarding the behavior of water-soluble algal polysaccharides (brown algae) suggests that bacterial flora present in the human intestine can only ferment laminarin and alginates (Fujii 1992).

15.4 Therapeutic Effect of Algal Dietary Fibers

A great deal of research has been focused on demonstrating the chemical composition and nutritional profile of dietary fibers after 1974 when Burkitt, Paninter, and Walker suggested an inverse relationship between the intake of dietary fiber and prevalence of colon cancer, diabetes, and cardiovascular diseases (Jiménez-Escrig and Sánchez-Muniz 2000). Later on, Burkitt also found that many metabolic and digestive disorders can be linked to reduced consumption of dietary fiber (Lahaye 1991). At present, a general perception prevails that diets rich in dietary fiber can significantly reduce the risks of noncommunicable diseases (NCD) particularly obesity, diabetes, coronary heart diseases, and colon cancer (Elleuch et al. 2011; Mann and Cummings 2009).

In addition to the potential health benefits, dietary fiber improves digestion, hydrolysis, colon fermentation, fecal bulk, stool volume, and changes the absorption kinetics of nutrients like glucose and minerals (Elleuch et al. 2011). The incorporation of algal fiber into the human diet can offer a diversity of benefits against NCD. Other important benefits associated with diets rich in fiber include the protection and growth of intestinal flora responsible for proper function and maintenance of gut health (Fujii 1992; Goni et al. 2001). The following sections contain examples of various *in vitro* and *in vivo* studies undertaken to establish key health benefits and activities of dietary fiber from algal biomasses.

15.4.1 Antihypertensive Effects

Ren et al. (1994) evaluated the polysaccharides of 26 fractions of algal strains (green, red, and brown) for their antihypertensive and antihyperlipidemic activities. The researchers fed Wistar strain male rats with high salts, cholesterol, seaweed powder, and polysaccharide fractions like fucoidan, funoran, porphyran, and alginate for 28 days and noticed a significant drop in systolic blood pressure of rats fed with diets containing polyanionic polysaccharides like fucoidan, funoran, porphyran, and alginate. It was astonishing to note that male Wistar rats fed on algal powder often faced a rise in systolic blood pressure. From this perspective, it would be reasonable to conclude that not all algal polysaccharides or powders will offer the same extent of benefits against hypertension-related disorders. In another report, Ren et al. (1994) found that the algal polysaccharide funoran caused a significant fall in the systolic blood pressure of animals during supplementation of a sodium diet with algal polysaccharide for 26 days. The intake of algal polysaccharides may cause about a 39% increase in urinary excretion rate and a 14% fall in systolic blood pressure level. The serum electrolytes of the funoran group of animals contained relatively higher potassium (sodium:potassium ratio 13% lower) as compared with the control. But the levels of sodium in both of the groups were almost identical. In this way, this study showed a positive relationship between blood pressure and urine sodium:potassium ratio, and between urinary sodium excretion and systolic blood pressure in rats fed funoran. A similar study was conducted by Krotkiewski and Aurell (1997), who evaluated the antihypertensive effect of brown alga (*Ascophyllum nodosum*) fiber in slightly hypertensive patients. The brown algae fiber was mixed with a suitable amount of potassium and, by the end of the experiment, the systolic blood pressure had dropped from 111.50 to 101.40 mmHg. Like the previous report, urinary excretion of potassium was increased in the treatment group as compared with the control so an antihypertensive effect can be correlated with enhanced intestinal absorption of potassium. It can also be hypothesized that the digestion of algal fiber reduces the intestinal absorption of sodium, as fiber can bind with sodium more efficiently than potassium (Jiménez-Escrig and Sánchez-Muniz 2000).

15.4.2 Antiobesity Attributes

Obesity is the foremost epidemic, which has a great effect on human health and it renders the obese subject more susceptible to other NCD like diabetes, colon and liver cancers, metabolic syndrome, osteoarthritis, and cardiovascular diseases. The medical solution to obesity involves the inhibition of pancreatic lipase via synthetic inhibitors like orlistat. The administration of such drugs may cause severe adverse effects on human health. The incorporation of an algal dietary fiber component offers a safer and more benign solution to obesity. In this context, algal polysaccharides like fucoidans, alginates, and phlorotannins and the carotenoid fucoxanthin are the four major bioactive compounds found in macroalgae that act as antiobesity agents through different mechanisms. Fucoidans and fucoxanthin control or inhibit lipid absorption and metabolism, alginates influence feelings of satiety, and fucoxanthin also manages the inhibition of adipocyte differentiation (Wan-Loy and Siew-Moi 2016).

15.4.3 Diabetes Control

Diabetes mellitus is a set of metabolic disorders of the endocrine system marked by the term hyperglycemia. The majority of diabetes patients all around the world have type II diabetes mellitus (TIIDM), for reasons such as sedentary lifestyle, the upsurge of obesity in the population, as well as unhealthy lifestyle. In this regard, macroalgae demonstrate potential benefits in managing TIIDM as they contain a significant amount of dietary fiber, polyphenolic compounds, and unsaturated fatty acids. Edible species especially have myriad compounds with various modes of action to interact with crucial proteins, control anti-inflammatory responses, as well as upregulating of antioxidant enzymes, and all of these can be applied in the treatment strategies of TIIDM. Macroalgae contain dietary fiber and polysaccharides that increase post-prandial satiety, assist in improving insulin sensitivity, and reducing blood glucose levels. Dietary fibers, monounsaturated fatty acids, and polyunsaturated fatty acids also reduce the inflammatory response associated with adiposity and hyperglycemia. The phenolic and nonphenolic compounds obtained from seaweeds show a positive influence on symptoms of TIIDM (such as hyperlipidemia and hyperglycemia). These bioactive compounds show modes of action similar to those of known antidiabetic medicines. The bioactive compounds and extracts from macroalgae can also exertheir antidiabetic attributes through increasing cellular uptake of glucose, inhibition of enzymes like protein tyrosine phosphatase 1B (PTP1B), dipeptidyl peptidase-4 (DPP-4) and aldose reductase, β-cell cytoprotection, diminution of advanced glycation end-products (AGE) formation, and action against obesity. Hence, algal bioactive compounds hold the potential to manage TIIDM either as purified pharmacological agents and supplements or as part of dietary ingestion (Sharifuddin et al. 2015).

15.5 Potential Commercial Applications

According to the recommendations of nutritionists and diet experts (Institute of Medicine (US) Panel on the Definition of Dietary Fiber and the Standing Committee on the Scientific Evaluation of Dietary Reference 2001), the average daily requirement of dietary fiber for women younger than 50 years is 25 g day^{-1} and about 21 g day^{-1} for women older than 50 years. Similarly, the requirement for a man up to 50 years is 38 g day^{-1} and a man above 50 years requires 30 g day^{-1}. And from these amounts, 20–30% of daily fiber intake should be taken from soluble fiber (Elleuch et al. 2011).

Dietary fiber gives some functional attributes to foods; for example, enhancing OHC, WHC, emulsification, or gel formation. In fact, dietary fiber used in foods like dairy products, baked goods, jams, soups, and meats can change the textural properties, stabilize high-fat food and emulsions, avoid syneresis (separation of liquid from gel), and improve shelf-life as well. It illustrates that the food industry can take advantage of these physicochemical properties of dietary fiber to improve the quality of their products in terms of viscosity, sensory characteristics, texture, and shelf-life. However, it can cause unwanted and undesirable changes in the texture and color of foods so the percentage of fiber that may be added to the food product is finite (Elleuch et al. 2011).

Fiber can be incorporated into fish products. According to (Borderías et al. 2005), the use of soluble fibers like carrageenan in fish products improves their functional properties like water-binding, emulsion capacity, thickening, and gelling properties of products prepared with minced fish muscle, particularly when the raw material utilized is of poor functionality. On the other hand, it may cause extensive loss of rigidity and elasticity in muscle protein gels (Elleuch et al. 2011).

The total volume of marine algae used in food products is significantly greater than its use in industrial applications especially in terms of monetary value. According to Jiménez-Escrig and Sánchez-Muniz (2000) the food product value is more than six times that of industrial products (Jensen 1993).

Macroalgae, which are traditionally used in the Western food industry due to their polysaccharide extractives like agar, alginate, and carrageenan, also contain particular compounds that have potential nutritional benefits. They are also used as an ingredient in cosmetics and global food industries, and moreover seaweeds are also used as animal feed additives and as fertilizer (Kılınç et al. 2013).

The use of chemical preservatives can be reduced by replacing them with seaweeds or their extracts in food (Gupta and Abu-Ghannam 2011; Kılınç et al. 2013).

Owing to gelling properties and high viscosity, the food industry uses some types of algal fiber as texture modifiers. Carrageenan has a positive influence on sausage attributes like pH, lipid oxidation, weight loss as well as sensory attributes; levels up to 2% show a positive influence on microbiological and physicochemical characteristics of fermented low-fat sausages. However, a level of 3% shows a negative effect on the firmness of sausages (Koutsopoulos et al. 2008).

Researchers prepared breads by utilizing *Ulva rigida* and *Lemna minor*, and evaluated their shelf-lives. According to them, the shelf-life of *U. rigida*-containing bread was found unacceptable on day 10 at 4 °C and on day 5 at room temperature, which was longer when compared with the shelf-life of control groups and extended for 2 days in both storage periods. *Lemna minor* also extended the shelf-life of the breads compared with the control and extended the limit of acceptance on day 12 at 4 °C and on day 8 at room temperature, while the control could extend the acceptable limit on day 8 at 4 °C and on day 3 at room temperature (Kılınç et al. 2013). This means algal fibers can be utilized to increase the shelf-life of our edible products.

Seaweed can be used as a fertilizer for organic agriculture and energy-rich methane from seaweed can be utilized by anaerobic digestion, but the high content of heavy metals in it and its digestates are a reason to limit their utilization as fertilizers. However, the production of biogas from seaweed and mobilization of heavy metals allow removal of metals for better-quality fertilizers (Nkemka and Murto 2012).

The OHC, WHC, swelling capacity, and high antioxidant activities of algal dietary fibers pose some possibilities for its use as functional ingredients in the food industry. Dietary fiber with high OHC stabilizes fatty food products and emulsions, while dietary fiber with high WHC can be utilized to control or modify the viscosity, avoid synaeresis, and to improve the texture of some formulated food items (Elleuch et al. 2011; Grigelmo-Miguel et al. 1999). Dietary fiber with high antioxidant activities stabilizes high-fat food while improving the oxidative stability of that food and extending shelf-life. So, myriad technological attributes like water swelling capacity, WHC, water solubility, viscosity, fat/oil-binding capacity, and antioxidant properties warrant the use of algal dietary fiber as ingredients in the food industry (Elleuch et al. 2011).

15.6 Conclusions and Future Recommendations

Marine macroalgae are an important source of a plethora of various bioactive polysaccharides with potential ranging from novel food applications to industrial applications and these interesting and exotic polysaccharides are currently utilized for their functional properties in biomedicine and food. Moreover, myriad applications for use of macroalgae cultivation for alternative fuel sources may be possible. However, the community has to make a transition from a hydrocarbon to a carbohydrate economy for the enlarged benefits of carbon-neutral biofuel, medicine, and plastics (Kraan 2012). Nowadays, macroalgae are being continuously investigated for their use in many industrial applications like cosmetics, food, chemistry, medicine, paint, etc. In addition to this, biologically active compounds (such as carotenoids, phlorotannins, fucoidans, alginic acid, and peptides) present in macroalgae have proven their important role in the prevention of some degenerative ailments such as inflammation, cancer, hypertension, arthritis, and diabetes. Hence, macroalgae derived active components have novel chemical components as functional ingredients in a number of industrial applications (Wijesinghe and Jeon 2012). Nowadays, about 15–20 edible algae strains are being marketed for consumption purposes in Europe, which are significantly different in quality, consistency, color, and nutrient contents. Hence, for these reasons the studies of algology compare and evaluate the chemical and nutrient content of various commercially available marine macroalgae products at food stores and specialty shops (Dawczynski et al. 2007; Herbreteau et al. 1997). The algal biomass can convert solar energy very efficiently and produce huge amounts of biomass in a short period of time; therefore, these microorganisms potentially represent a significant and overlooked source of polysaccharides and a renewable energy source (Kraan 2012). The establishment of new pharmacological products and algal bioactive-enriched functional food requires more extensive and molecular-level design for structure–activity relationships for antiobesity drugs, particularly inhibitors of pancreatic lipase (Wan-Loy and Siew-Moi 2016). Further studies are also necessary for the complete capitalization on the benefits of algal bioactive components for the prevention and management of diabetes and gastrointestinal disorders (Sharifuddin et al. 2015).

References

Abdul-Hamid, A. and Luan, Y.S. (2000). Functional properties of dietary fibre prepared from defatted rice bran. *Food Chemistry* **68** (1): 15–19.

Bertin, C., Rouau, X., and Thibault, J.F. (1988). Structure and properties of sugar beet fibres. *Journal of the Science of Food and Agriculture* **44** (1): 15–29.

Borderías, A.J., Sánchez-Alonso, I., and Pérez-Mateos, M. (2005). New applications of fibres in foods: addition to fishery products. *Trends in Food Science & Technology* **16** (10): 458–465.

Burtin, P. (2003). Nutritional value of seaweeds. *Electronic Journal of Environmental, Agricultural and Food Chemistry* **2** (4): 498–503.

Calixto, F.S. (1997). La fibra dietética en nutrición y salud. *Alimentación, nutrición y salud* **4** (1): 17–21.

Caprez, A., Arrigoni, E., Amadò, R., and Neukom, H. (1986). Influence of different types of thermal treatment on the chemical composition and physical properties of wheat bran. *Journal of Cereal Science* **4** (3): 233–239.

Chan, P.T. and Matanjun, P. (2017). Chemical composition and physicochemical properties of tropical red seaweed, *Gracilaria changii*. *Food Chemistry* **221**: 302–310.

Chan, J.C.-C., Cheung, P.C.-K., and Ang, P.O. (1997). Comparative studies on the effect of three drying methods on the nutritional composition of seaweed *Sargassum hemiphyllum* (Turn.) C. Ag. *Journal of Agricultural and Food Chemistry* **45** (8): 3056–3059.

Chandini, S.K., Ganesan, P., and Bhaskar, N. (2008). In vitro antioxidant activities of three selected brown seaweeds of India. *Food Chemistry* **107** (2): 707–713.

Dawczynski, C., Schubert, R., and Jahreis, G. (2007). Amino acids, fatty acids, and dietary fibre in edible seaweed products. *Food Chemistry* **103** (3): 891–899.

Elleuch, M., Bedigian, D., Roiseux, O. et al. (2011). Dietary fibre and fibre-rich by-products of food processing: characterisation, technological functionality and commercial applications: a review. *Food Chemistry* **124** (2): 411–421. https://doi.org/10.1016/j.foodchem.2010.06.077.

Fleury, N. and Lahaye, M. (1991). Chemical and physico-chemical characterisation of fibres from *Laminaria digitata* (kombu breton): a physiological approach. *Journal of the Science of Food and Agriculture* **55** (3): 389–400.

Fujii, T. (1992). Fermentation of water-soluble polysaccharides of brown algae by human intestinal bacteria in vitro. *Nippon Suisan Gakkaishi* **58**: 147–152.

Goni, I., Gudiel-Urbano, M., Bravo, L., and Saura-Calixto, F. (2001). Dietary modulation of bacterial fermentative capacity by edible seaweeds in rats. *Journal of Agricultural and Food Chemistry* **49** (5): 2663–2668.

Grigelmo-Miguel, N., Carreras-Boladeras, E., and Martín-Belloso, O. (1999). Development of high-fruit-dietary-fibre muffins. *European Food Research and Technology* **210** (2): 123–128.

Guillon, F. and Champ, M. (2000). Structural and physical properties of dietary fibres, and consequences of processing on human physiology. *Food Research International* **33** (3–4): 233–245.

Guiry, M. (2009). Seaweeds. National University of Ireland, Galway. www.seaweed.ie (accessed September 22, 2020).

Gupta, S. and Abu-Ghannam, N. (2011). Recent developments in the application of seaweeds or seaweed extracts as a means for enhancing the safety and quality attributes of foods. *Innovative Food Science & Emerging Technologies* **12** (4): 600–609.

Herbreteau, F., Coiffard, L., Derrien, A., and De Roeck-Holtzhauer, Y. (1997). The fatty acid composition of five species of macroalgae. *Botanica Marina* **40** (1–6): 25–28.

Institute of Medicine (US) Panel on the Definition of Dietary Fiber and the Standing Committee on the Scientific Evaluation of Dietary Reference Intakes (2001). *Dietary Reference Intakes: Proposed Definition of Dietary Fiber: a Report of the Panel on the Definition of Dietary Fiber and the Standing Committee on the Scientific Evaluation of Dietary Reference Intakes*. National Academy Press.

Jensen, A. (1993). Present and future needs for algae and algal products. In: *Fourteenth International Seaweed Symposium. Developments in Hydrobiology*, vol. **85** (eds. A.R.O. Chapman, M.T. Brown and M. Lahaye). Dordrecht: Springer https://doi.org/10.1007/978-94-011-1998-6_2.

de Jesus Raposo, M.F., De Morais, A.M.M.B., and De Morais, R.M.S.C. (2016). Emergent sources of prebiotics: seaweeds and microalgae. *Marine Drugs* **14** (2): 27.

Jiménez-Escrig, A. and Sánchez-Muniz, F. (2000). Dietary fibre from edible seaweeds: chemical structure, physicochemical properties and effects on cholesterol metabolism. *Nutrition Research* **20** (4): 585–598.

Jin, W., Zhang, Q., Wang, J., and Zhang, W. (2013). A comparative study of the anticoagulant activities of eleven fucoidans. *Carbohydrate Polymers* **91** (1): 1–6.

Kang, J., Khan, M., Park, N. et al. (2008). Antipyretic, analgesic, and anti-inflammatory activities of the seaweed *Sargassum fulvellum* and *Sargassum thunbergii* in mice. *Journal of Ethnopharmacology* **116** (1): 187–190.

Kılınç, B., Cirik, S., Turan, G. et al. (2013). Seaweeds for food and industrial applications. In: *Food Industry* (ed. I. Muzzalupo), 736–745. London: IntechOpen.

Kimura, Y., Watanabe, K., and Okuda, H. (1996). Effects of soluble sodium alginate on cholesterol excretion and glucose tolerance in rats. *Journal of Ethnopharmacology* **54** (1): 47–54.

Koutsopoulos, D., Koutsimanis, G., and Bloukas, J. (2008). Effect of carrageenan level and packaging during ripening on processing and quality characteristics of low-fat fermented sausages produced with olive oil. *Meat Science* **79** (1): 188–197.

Kraan, S. (2012). Algal polysaccharides, novel applications and outlook. In: *Carbohydrates – Comprehensive Studies on Glycobiology and Glycotechnology* (ed. C.-F. Chang), 490–518. London: IntechOpen.

Krotkiewski, M. and Aurell, M. (1997). Hipertensión leve tratada con un preparado de algas marinas intercambiador de iones sodio-potasio. *Cardiovascular* **1**: 6–11.

Kuda, T., Yokoyama, M., and Fujii, T. (1997). Effects of marine algal diets hijiki, aonori, and nori on levels of serum lipid and cecal microflora in rats. *Fisheries Science* **63** (3): 428–432.

Kuniak, L. and Marchessault, R. (1972). Study of the crosslinking reaction between epichlorohydrin and starch. *Starch-Stärke* **24** (4): 110–116.

Lahaye, M. (1991). Marine algae as sources of fibres: determination of soluble and insoluble dietary fibre contents in some 'sea vegetables'. *Journal of the Science of Food and Agriculture* **54** (4): 587–594. https://doi.org/10.1002/jsfa.2740540410.

Lozano, I., Wacyk, J.M., Carrasco, J., and Cortez-San Martín, M.A. (2016). Red macroalgae *Pyropia columbina* and *Gracilaria chilensis*: sustainable feed additive in the *Salmo salar* diet and the evaluation of potential antiviral activity against infectious salmon anemia virus. *Journal of Applied Phycology* **28** (2): 1343–1351.

MacArtain, P., Gill, C.I., Brooks, M. et al. (2007). Nutritional value of edible seaweeds. *Nutrition Reviews* **65** (12): 535–543.

Manas, E., Bravo, L., and Saura-Calixto, F. (1994). Sources of error in dietary fibre analysis. *Food Chemistry* **50** (4): 331–342.

Mann, J. and Cummings, J. (2009). Possible implications for health of the different definitions of dietary fibre. *Nutrition, Metabolism, and Cardiovascular Diseases* **19** (3): 226–229.

Marinho-Soriano, E., Fonseca, P., Carneiro, M., and Moreira, W. (2006). Seasonal variation in the chemical composition of two tropical seaweeds. *Bioresource Technology* **97** (18): 2402–2406.

Matanjun, P., Mohamed, S., Mustapha, N.M., and Muhammad, K. (2009). Nutrient content of tropical edible seaweeds, *Eucheuma cottonii, Caulerpa lentillifera* and *Sargassum polycystum. Journal of Applied Phycology* **21** (1): 75–80.

McHugh, D.J. (1991). Worldwide distribution of commercial resources of seaweeds including Gelidium. In: *International Workshop on Gelidium. Developments in Hydrobiology*, vol. **68** (eds. J.A. Juanes, B. Santelices and J.L. McLachlan). Dordrecht: Springer https://doi.org/10.1007/978-94-011-3610-5_2.

Mehta, N., Ahlawat, S., Sharma, D., and Dabur, R. (2015). Novel trends in development of dietary fiber rich meat products – a critical review. *Journal of Food Science and Technology* **52** (2): 633–647.

Michell, C., Lahaye, M., Bonnet, C. et al. (1996). In vitro fermentation by human faecal bacteria of total and purified dietary fibres from brown seaweeds. *British Journal of Nutrition* **75** (2): 263–280.

Mišurcová, L., Kráčmar, S., Klejdus, B., and Vacek, J. (2010). Nitrogen content, dietary fiber, and digestibility in algal food products. *Czech Journal of Food Sciences* **28**: 27–35.

Msuya, F.E. and Neori, A. (2002). *Ulva reticulata* and *Gracilaria crassa*: macroalgae that can biofilter effluent from tidal fishponds in Tanzania. *Western Indian Ocean Journal of Marine Science* **1**: 117–126.

Murakami, K., Yamaguchi, Y., Noda, K. et al. (2011). Seasonal variation in the chemical composition of a marine brown alga, *Sargassum horneri* (Turner) C Agardh. *Journal of Food Composition and Analysis* **24** (2): 231–236.

Murata, M. and Nakazoe, J.-I. (2001). Production and use of marine Algae in Japan. *Japan Agricultural Research Quarterly: JARQ* **35** (4): 281–290. https://doi.org/10.6090/jarq.35.281.

Nkemka, V. and Murto, M. (2012). Exploring strategies for seaweed hydrolysis: effect on methane potential and heavy metal mobilisation. *Process Biochemistry* **47** (12): 2523–2526.

Norziah, M.H. and Ching, C.Y. (2000). Nutritional composition of edible seaweed *Gracilaria changgi. Food Chemistry* **68** (1): 69–76.

Olson, A., Gray, G., and Chiu, M.-C. (1987). Chemistry and analysis of soluble dietary fiber. *Food Technology (Chicago)* **41** (2): 71–80.

Parthiban, C., Saranya, C., Girija, K. et al. (2013). Biochemical composition of some selected seaweeds from Tuticorin coast. *Advances in Applied Science Research* **4** (3): 362–366.

Patara, L., Visbeck, M., Masina, S. et al. (2011). Marine biogeochemical responses to the North Atlantic Oscillation in a coupled climate model. *Journal of Geophysical Research, Oceans* **116** (C7): C07023. https://doi.org/10.1029/2010JC006785, 2011C07023.

Potty, V. (1996). Physio-chemical [physico-chemical] aspects, physiological functions, nutritional importance and technological significance of dietary fibres: a critical appraisial. *Journal of Food Science and Technology* **33** (1): 1–18.

Prosky, L., Asp, N.-G., Schweizer, T. et al. (1988). Determination of insoluble, soluble, and total dietary fiber in foods and food products: interlaboratory study. *Journal of the Association of Official Analytical Chemists* **71** (5): 1017–1023.

Ren, D., Noda, H., Amano, H. et al. (1994). Study on antihypertensive and antihyperlipidemic effects of marine algae. *Fisheries Science* **60** (1): 83–88.

Ren, D., Noda, H., Amano, H., and Nisizawa, K. (1994). Antihypertensive and antihyperlipidemic effects of funoran. *Fisheries Science* **60** (4): 423–427.

Renn, D.W. (1990). Seaweeds and biotechnology—inseparable companions. In: *Thirteenth International Seaweed Symposium. Developments in Hydrobiology*, vol. **58** (eds. S.C. Lindstrom and P.W. Gabrielson). Dordrecht: Springer https://doi.org/10.1007/978-94-009-2049-1_2.

Roehrig, K.L. (1988). The physiological effects of dietary fiber—a review. *Food Hydrocolloids* **2** (1): 1–18.

Schneeman, B.O. (1987). Soluble vs insoluble fiber: different physiological responses. *Food Technology* **41**: 81–82.

Schneeman, B.O. (1999). *Building Scientific Consensus: The Importance of Dietary Fiber*. Oxford: Oxford University Press.

Schweizer, T.F. (1991). What is dietary fibre? *Trends in Food Science & Technology* **2**: 254–255.

Sharifuddin, Y., Chin, Y.-X., Lim, P.-E., and Phang, S.-M. (2015). Potential bioactive compounds from seaweed for diabetes management. *Marine Drugs* **13** (8): 5447–5491. https://doi.org/10.3390/md13085447.

Sinha, S., Astani, A., Ghosh, T. et al. (2010). Polysaccharides from *Sargassum tenerrimum*: structural features, chemical modification and anti-viral activity. *Phytochemistry* **71** (2–3): 235–242.

Suleria, H.A.R., Gobe, G., Masci, P., and Osborne, S.A. (2016). Marine bioactive compounds and health promoting perspectives; innovation pathways for drug discovery. *Trends in Food Science & Technology* **50**: 44–55.

Suzuki, T., Ohsugi, Y., Yoshie, Y. et al. (1996). Dietary fiber content, water-holding capacity and binding capacity of seaweeds. *Fisheries Science* **62** (3): 454–461.

Topping, D.L. (1991). Soluble fiber polysaccharides: effects on plasma cholesterol and colonic fermentation. *Nutrition Reviews* **49** (7): 195–203.

Torsdottir, I., Alpsten, M., Holm, G. et al. (1991). A small dose of soluble alginate-fiber affects postprandial glycemia and gastric emptying in humans with diabetes. *The Journal of Nutrition* **121** (6): 795–799.

Trowell, H. (1974). Definitions of fibre. *The Lancet* **303** (7856): 503.

Wan-Loy, C. and Siew-Moi, P. (2016). Marine algae as a potential source for anti-obesity agents. *Marine Drugs* **14** (12): 222. https://doi.org/10.3390/md14120222.

Wijesinghe, W. and Jeon, Y.-J. (2012). Enzyme-assistant extraction (EAE) of bioactive components: a useful approach for recovery of industrially important metabolites from seaweeds: a review. *Fitoterapia* **83** (1): 6–12.

Wong, K. and Cheung, P.C. (2000). Nutritional evaluation of some subtropical red and green seaweeds: part I – proximate composition, amino acid profiles and some physico-chemical properties. *Food Chemistry* **71** (4): 475–482. https://doi.org/10.1016/S0308-8146(00)00175-8.

Wong, K. and Cheung, P.C. (2001). Influence of drying treatment on three *Sargassum* species. *Journal of Applied Phycology* **13** (1): 43–50.

Wynne, M.J. and Bold, H. (1985). *Introduction to the Algae: Structure and Reproduction*. Upper Saddle River, NJ: Prentice-Hall.

Yoshie, Y., Suzuki, T., Shirai, T., and Hirano, T. (1997). Analytical procedure and distribution of soluble and insoluble dietary fibers in seaweed foods. *Journal of the Tokyo University of Fisheries (Japan)* **83**: 1–12.

Zubia, M., Payri, C.E., Deslandes, E., and Guezennec, J. (2003). Chemical composition of attached and drift specimens of *Sargassum mangarevense* and *Turbinaria ornata* (Phaeophyta: Fucales) from Tahiti, French Polynesia. *Botanica Marina* **46** (6): 562–571.

Section III

Application of Algae and Algal Components

16

Applications of Algae and Algae Extracts in Human Food and Feed

Sara Amiri Samani[1], Maryam Jafari[1,2], Sayed Mohammad Sahafi[3], and Shahin Roohinejad[4]

[1]*Department of Food Science and Technology, Shahrekord Branch, Islamic Azad University, Shahrekord, Iran*
[2]*Research Center of Nutrition and Organic Products, Shahrekord Branch, Islamic Azad University, Shahrekord, Iran*
[3]*Department of Food Science and Technology, Isfahan University of Technology, Isfahan, Iran*
[4]*Burn and Wound Healing Research Center, Division of Food and Nutrition, Shiraz University of Medical Sciences, Shiraz, Iran*

16.1 Introduction

Interest in using algae products has increased over the past few decades. Currently, global demand is increasing for consumption of algae as an interesting source of food and feed. The reason for the growing attention for algae consumption is that they are a rich source of physiologically active substances such as proteins, carbohydrates, essential fatty acids (e.g. docosahexaenoic acid [DHA], eicosapentaenoic acid [EPA], arachidonic acid [ARA], and alpha-linolenic acid [ALA]), pigments (carotenoids, chlorophyll, phycocyanin), enzymes (catalases, superoxide dismutase), polyphenols, and fiber as well as many vitamins and minerals (e.g. vitamins A, C, B_1, B_2, B_6, niacin, potassium, iodine, iron, calcium, and magnesium) (Priyadarshani and Rath 2012). Some species of macro algae such as *Himanthalia elongata*, *Undaria pinnatifida*, *Chondrus crispus*, and *Porphyra* sp. are more in demand due to their low calories and high vitamin and mineral contents (Plaza et al. 2008). Algae are used in human diets and as animal feed in the poultry and aquarium industries (Hasan and Chakrabarti 2009). According to the Food and Agriculture Organization of the United Nations (FAO) 2014, 38% of the 23.8 million t of harvested seaweed in the world are consumed by humans. This does not include the hydrocolloids that are extracted from marine algae (agar, carrageen, and alginate) and used as thickening, gelling,

Recent Advances in Micro- and Macroalgal Processing: Food and Health Perspectives, First Edition.
Edited by Gaurav Rajauria and Yvonne V. Yuan.

and emulsifying agents in food products. In this chapter, the nutritional compounds of algae as well as their potential applications in food and feed are highlighted.

16.2 Nutritional Composition of Algae

Algae are considered as a good source of protein and amino acids compared with other food sources (Becker 2007). For instance, dried *Spirulina* contains 68% proteins, which is three times higher than beef. *Chlorella* contains 50–60% protein, which is comparable with yeast, flour, milk powder, and soy (Blazencic 2007). Besides protein, algae are a good source of fiber (Plaza et al. 2008). The main products from algae, which are mainly used in the food industry as thickening agents, are polysaccharides like carrageenan, agar, and alginates that are used in marmalade, jellies, ice cream, etc. Algae are a good source of polyunsaturated fatty acids (PUFAs) such as ω-3 and gamma linolenic acid (GLA). Moreover, algae are a rich source of minerals and vitamins and they are widely used in food supplements (Kovac et al. 2013). For example, Mohammad et al. (2011) reported that the amount of β-carotene in *Spirulina* was 10 times higher than carrots. Since the global preference has changed from artificial colors to natural colors, algae would be a good alternative that can respond to this demand. Other kinds of pigments like carotenoids and phycobiliproteins can be found in addition to chlorophylls in algae (Kovac et al. 2013). Phycobiliproteins are a group of pigments that are used as a food colorant in chewing gums, jellies, dairy products, and soft drinks, etc. (Gouveia et al. 2008a, b). Phycobiliproteins, polyphenols, and vitamins are the most potent antioxidants in algae (Plaza et al. 2008).

16.3 Application of Whole Algae in Food Products

16.3.1 Muscle-Based Foods

Algal species can be used for development of muscle-based foods. For instance, sea lettuce (*Ulva lactuca*) is one of the commonly consumed marine vegetables, which is a rich source of dietary fiber and essential vitamins, especially vitamin B_{12} and vitamin C. This type of algae is consumed in different ways such as juices after boiling (in Cuba), in salad or soup (in the Philippines), or as toasted sea lettuce (in the UK) (Kim et al. 2011). Kumarathunge et al. (2016) investigated the potential of adding sea lettuce powder to fish burgers at four different levels (0.5, 1.0, 1.5, and 2.0% w/w). Incorporation of 0.5% (w/w) algae powder resulted in a higher amount of protein and fiber compared with the control.

Several studies have evaluated the feasibility of adding wakame/sea mustard (*U. pinnatifida*) to meat products (up to 5.6% w/w) such as patties (Lopez-Lopez et al. 2010, 2011; Jeon and Choi 2012) and gel/emulsion meat systems (Cofrades et al. 2008; Lopez-Lopez et al. 2009) with the aim of producing low-fat and low-salt products. Addition of wakame powder increased the polyphenol and mineral content of products, improved the water and fat-binding properties, created harder and chewier structures, and solved the problems related to low salt content.

Sea spaghetti (*H. elongata*) is known for high total dietary fiber and mineral content (especially K, Mg, and Ca) (Cofrades et al. 2008, 2011). The potential for using sea spaghetti as a functional ingredient in beef patties (Cox and Abu-Ghannam 2013), gel/emulsion meat systems (Cofrades et al. 2008; Lopez-Lopez et al.

2009), low-fat/low-salt frankfurters (Jimenez-Colmenero et al. 2010), low-fat/low-salt restructured poultry steaks (Cofrades et al. 2011), and pork meat batter (Fernandez-Martin et al. 2009) has been previously reported. Addition of *H. elongata* (10–40% w/w) as a source of antioxidants and dietary fiber to beef patties resulted in an increase in the nutritional and technological quality (reduced cooking losses and improved texture, mouth feel, and tenderness nearly 50% compared with the patties prepared without algae powder) (Cox and Abu-Ghannam 2013). In gel/emulsion meat systems, in the presence of seaweed, it is possible to achieve desirable rheological properties only by adding 0.5% NaCl, which is a much smaller amount than those commonly used in meat products (Cofrades et al. 2008).

Sea tangle, especially genus *Laminaria* such as *Laminaria japonica*, is a rich source of dietary fiber (mainly laminaran, fucoidan, and alginic acid), vitamins, minerals, and proteins, and is used in many Asian countries as seafood (Kim et al. 2008, 2010). Incorporation of *L. japonica* (1–5%) into pork patties as a fat replacer did not have an effect on the quality characteristics (textural and sensory properties) of the final product containing 10% fat compared with control patties with 20% fat (Choi et al. 2012). Lee et al. (2018) examined the possibility of using sea tangle powder (1.5 and 3%) and/or its combination with high pressure as substitutes for phosphate in emulsion-type sausages. They reported satisfactory results in terms of cooking quality and overall acceptability and suggested this method could be applied directly in the industry. Oh and Lim (2011) reported that incorporation of sea tangle (2.5%) into the patties resulted in a healthier product with improved fat- and water-binding properties and oxidation stability without any adverse effect on sensory perception.

Sargassum species are a rich source of bioactive compounds such as polyphenols, vitamins, dietary fiber, carotenoids, and proteins. Hence, they have great potential to be used in nutraceutical and pharmaceutical areas (Yende et al. 2014). Addition of *Sargassum thunbergii* (known as hede) up to 5% w/w in hamburger patties has been reported to increase the cooking yield (Chun et al. 1999).

Cofrades et al. (2008) evaluated the potential of adding nori (*Porphyra umbilicalis*) (2.5% and 5% w/w), a rich source of protein and phenolic content, to a meat emulsion model system. In addition to improving nutritional value, the emulsion stability of the meat system was also affected depending on the concentration of alga (Cofrades et al. 2008).

Eucheuma (*Kappaphycus alverezii*), as an important source of various carrageenans, was used in the formulation of fish cutlets at various concentrations (5, 7.5, 10, 12.5, and 15% w/w). Sensory evaluation of fish cutlets revealed that incorporation of eucheuma up to 10% influenced the texture of fish cutlets without any adverse effects on their acceptability and appearance (Senthil et al. 2005). In another study, *Gelidium amansii* was added to hamburger patties at a concentration of 1–5% w/w and the sensory evaluation for color and overall acceptability in patties containing 3% *G. amansii* were found to be comparable with regular patties (Chun et al. 1999).

16.3.2 Dairy Products

The potential for adding algal biomass into dairy products such as yogurts and cheeses to increase their nutritional and functional properties along with enhancing the viability of probiotics has been previously reported (Table 16.1). Nuñez and Picon (2016) investigated the supplementation of yogurt and quark with five dehydrated edible seaweeds. *Porphyra umbilicalis*, *U. lactuca*, and *U. pinnatifida* had the most intense effect

Table 16.1 Examples of algae incorporation in dairy products

Product	Algae incorporation	Addition (% w/w)	Parameter	References
Yogurt and quark	*Himanthalia elongata*, *Porphyra umbilicalis*, *Saccharina latissima*, *Ulva lactuca*, and *Undaria pinnatifida*	0.5–1.0	Sensory characteristics	Nuñez and Picon (2016)
Probiotic yogurt	*Spirulina platensis*	0.25–1.0	Techno-functional properties	Beheshtipour et al. (2012)
Yogurt	*Spirulina platensis*	0.5–1.0	Techno-functional properties	Mocanu et al. (2013)
Yogurt and acidophilus milk	*Spirulina platensis*	0.5–1.0	Techno-functional properties	Guldas and Irkin (2010)
Natural and probiotic yogurt	*Spirulina platensis*	0.1–0.8	Techno-functional and nutritional properties	Molnar et al. (2005)
Appenzeller cheese	*Chlorella sp.*	0–2.0	Techno-functional and nutritional properties	Heo et al. (2006)
Processed cheese	*Chlorella sp.*	0.5–1.0	Techno-functional and nutritional properties	Jeon (2006)
Cottage cheese	*Undaria pinnatifida* and *Laminaria japonica*	3–15	Techno-functional and nutritional properties	Lalic and Berkovic (2005)

on the yogurt and quark flavor at 0.50% w/w concentration, while yogurt and quark supplemented with *Saccharina latissima* at the same concentration received the highest odor and flavor quality scores. Beheshtipour et al. (2012) investigated the impact of different concentrations (0.25, 0.50, and 1.00% w/w) of *Arthospira platensis* on the physicochemical properties and viability of different probiotic bacteria in probiotic yogurt. Samples containing 1% of algal biomass showed higher counts for *Lactobacillus acidophilus* and bifidobacteria than two other concentrations at the end of fermentation and during the storage period, while the 0.5% addition of microalgae biomass gave more satisfactory organoleptic evaluation results than the concentration of 1%. According to results reported by Mocanu et al. (2013) and Molnar et al. (2005), *Spirulina platensis* biomass was effective on the growth of coccus-shaped starter bacteria. Guldas and Irkin (2010) showed that viable counts in 1% *Spirulina*-enriched yogurts were similar to that of the 0.5% addition but sensory scores of 0.5% *Spirulina* were better than 1% ones. They suggested that fruit yogurt or fruit-flavored yogurts might be a good choice for the addition of 1% of *S. platensis* powder without a negative effect on the organoleptic properties of the final products. Also, Heo et al. (2006) reported that lactic acid bacteria counts in Appenzeller cheese containing *Chlorella sp.* powder (up to 2% w/w) were higher than in the control cheese. The optimum addition level of *Chlorella sp.* powder was 0.5%, which produced Appenzeller cheese of acceptable quality. In a study conducted by Jeon (2006), *Chlorella sp.* was added to processed cheese at a concentration of 0.5–1% and the physical and sensory properties of the final product were investigated. Despite some differences in color and texture, the protein, fat, and moisture contents, and the degree of oiling off, were similar to the control. Lalic and Berkovic (2005) incorporated *L. japonica* and *U. pinnatifida* at three concentrations (3, 9, and 15%) in cottage cheeses. The samples containing 15% algae presented higher mineral content, while consistency and firmness were optimum at concentrations of 9% of *L. japonica* or *U. pinnatifida*.

16.3.3 Cereal-Based Food Products

Algal powders can be added into cereal-based products for different reasons (Table 16.2). For example, *Chlorella vulgaris* was incorporated into cookies as a coloring agent and as a potential antioxidant and nutritional supplement (Gouveia et al. 2007). In other studies, *Isochrysis galbana* was added as a source of ω-3 PUFAs (Gouveia et al. 2008a, b) and whole *Arthospira platensis* was incorporated to enhance the protein and fiber content in biscuits (Singh et al. 2015). Pasta is another widely accepted product with low protein and essential amino acid contents. Therefore, a number of studies have focused on pasta supplementation with high-protein sources such as soy isolates and flours, whey proteins, etc. (Prabhasankar et al. 2007). El-Baz et al. (2017) studied the effect of mixing *Dunaliella salina* algae powder (1–3%) with semolina on the quality of pasta (cooking, sensory, and nutritional properties). The results showed that increasing levels of algae resulted in increasing the nutritional value of pasta including protein, fat, ash, and carbohydrate contents. Also, phytochemical content and cooking properties (weight and volume) were improved compared with the control. Prabhasankar et al. (2009) evaluated the effect of different concentrations (0–30%) of *U. pinnatifida* on the cooking, sensory, nutritional, and bio-functional quality of pasta. Addition of algae up to 20% did not negatively affect the sensory characteristics. The incorporation of *U. pinnatifida* resulted in production of pasta with a higher amount of total phenolics, fucosterol, and fucoxanthin, and better antioxidant activity, fatty acids, and amino acids profiles.

Table 16.2 Examples of algae incorporation in cereal-based products

Product	Algae incorporation	Addition (% w/w)	Parameters	References
Cookies	*Chlorella vulgaris*	0.5–3.0	Coloring and antioxidant properties	Gouveia et al. (2007)
Biscuits	*Isochrysis galbana*	1 and 3	Techno-functional and nutritional properties (ω-3 polyunsaturated fatty acids)	Gouveia et al. (2008a, b)
	Arthospira platensis	1.63–8.36	Techno-functional and nutritional properties	Singh et al. (2015)
Pasta	*Dunaliella salina*	1–3	Techno-functional and nutritional properties	El-Baz et al. (2017)
	Undaria pinnatifida	0–30	Cooking, sensory, nutritional, and bio-functional properties	Prabhasankar et al. (2009)
	Isochrysis galbana and *Diacronema vlkianum*	0.5–2.0	Techno-functional and nutritional properties (ω-3 polyunsaturated fatty acids)	Fradique et al. (2013)
	Arthospira platensis	5–20	Techno-functional and nutritional properties	Rodríguez De Marco et al. (2014)
	Dunaliella salina	1–3	Techno-functional and nutritional properties	El-Baz et al. (2017)
Bread	*Dunaliella* sp.	10	Nutritional properties	Finney et al. (1984)
	Ascophyllum nodosum	1–4	Nutritional properties	Hall et al. (2012)
	Arthospira platensis	11	Techno-functional and nutritional properties	Ak et al. (2016)
Gluten-free bread	*Arthospira platensis*	2–5	Nutritional properties	Figueira et al. (2011)

Several studies have reported the incorporation of algae to enhance the nutritional properties of bread. For instance, some algae species such as *Dunaliella sp.* and *Arthrospira sp.* were incorporated into bread to increase its protein and essential amino acid contents (Finney et al. 1984; Ak et al. 2016; Figueira et al. 2011). Addition of other microalgae species to bread resulted in changing the color, crust, and crumb (an increase in browning and evolution to more green-yellow tonalities), but did not affect hardness, chewiness, and resilience (Garcia-Segovia et al. 2017). According to Hall et al. (2012), the incorporation of *Ascophyllum nodosum* (1–4%) into bread significantly reduced subsequent energy intake, while no significant differences were observed in the area under the curve for glycemia or cholesterolemia.

16.3.4 Beverages

Along with increasing consumer awareness of food health and increasing demand for natural ingredients, functional botanical ingredients are more popular on the beverage market. In this regard, the addition of algae to beverages to supply nutrients like vitamins (A, B_1, B_2, and C), proteins, minerals, and antioxidants, with proven health benefits, has been the subject of several studies. Formulation of beverages using different species of algae such as wakame, *Ulva pertusa* (sea lettuce), *Hizikia sp.*, and *Ecklonia cava* (sea trumpet), and assessment of functional properties of products have been targeted in several studies (Nagai et al. 2006; Nagai and Yukimoto 2003). They reported that beverages prepared from free algae, except for sea lettuce, possessed high radical and superoxide scavenging activities. Therefore, they suggested these types of beverages for patients suffering chronic diseases, such as cancer, cardiovascular problems, and diabetes. Sharoba et al. (2017) incorporated *Spirulina sp.* into kiwifruit and cantaloupe nectar blends at different concentrations (2.5–15% w/w) to improve the nutritional values. According to their results, all nectar blends prepared and supported by *Spirulina sp.* were highly accepted. Ratanaburee et al. (2011) studied the preparation of fermented red seaweed (*Gracilaria fisheri*) beverage by a selected strain of lactic acid bacteria (*Lactobacillus plantarum* DW12) for the enrichment of the gamma-aminobutyric acid (GABA) content in the beverage. They concluded that enrichment of the GABA content in fermented red seaweed beverage could be possible by adding monosodium glutamate (MSG) and the suitable GABA-producing strain. However, the appropriate amount of MSG to add should be further investigated due to the creation of an unsatisfactory salty taste. Prachyakij et al. (2008) formulated a fermented beverage from the same red algae using *Lactobacillus plantarum* DW3 as a starter inoculum to supply more minerals without disturbing the sensory characteristics of the beverage. Several patents have also been registered based on enrichment of beverage formulation with algae and preparation methods (Matsuzaki and Yoshida 2007; Kuhara 2006) for use in healthy or functional foods.

16.4 Application of Whole Algae in Feed

The use of algae for animal feed and aquaculture is of particular interest. Algal biomass is full of primary and secondary metabolites such as essential vitamins and minerals, but they are considered as an ideal candidate for feed supplementation because of their protein content and fatty acid profiles. For example, protein accounts for about 60% of the *Chlorella* sp. and *Spirulina* sp. biomass.

Different strains of micro- and macroalgae can be used directly as live cultures or as value-added feed supplements for both aquaculture species, especially fish and penaeid prawn larvae, and terrestrial livestock (Khatoon et al. 2010).

Algal genera such as *Chlorella*, *Spirulina*, *Scenedesmus*, *Dunaliella*, and *Nannochloropsis* are popularly used as aquaculture feed for their high nutritious value (Avron and Ben-Amotz 1992; Lee 1997; Yamaguchi 1997). Also, some other algal genera such as *Skeletonema*, *Phaeodactylum*, *Pavlova*, *Chaetoceros*, *Tetraselmis*, and *Isochrysis* are used in aquaculture due to their high PUFA, DHA, and EPA content (Benemann 1992; Wang, 2003; Knuckey et al. 2005). In addition to essential fatty acids, the extracted pigments from algae (such as fucoxanthin and astaxanthin) provide attractive color to the flesh of aquatic animals, which enhances their economic value and consumer acceptability (Spolaore et al. 2006). In addition, microalgae are used directly as a feed source for filter-feeding aquaculture species such as bivalve mollusks, polychaete worms, or gastropod mollusks and echinoderms. In other cases, they are indirectly given as food to the zooplanktonic live prey fed to small fish larvae (Conceição et al. 2010; Muller-Feuga 2000).

Subsequently, in terrestrial animals, algae-supplemented diets significantly affect the physiology and metabolic pathways, improve immune response, microbial counts in the gut, and overall performance of the targeted animals (Doherty et al. 2010). For example, supplementation of broiler chickens' diet with organic forms of selenium (Se) using Se-enriched alga increased the Se concentration in the muscle and improved the oxidative stability of meat compared to inorganic Se addition (sodium selenite) (Ševčíková et al. 2006; Dlouhá et al. 2008). Also, supplementation of laying hens' and broilers' diets with Se-enriched *Chlorella sp.* and Se-enriched yeast (organic dietary Se sources) enhanced the nutritional value of meat and eggs for human consumption (Skřivan et al. 2008).

Some reports suggest that algae such as *Spirulina sp.* not only contain digestible amino acids and available minerals for poultry but also decrease pellet mill production rate and increase pellet durability. Algae have potential as a pellet binder (up to 16%) and improve the pelleting process without being detrimental to performance or amino acid digestibility (Evans et al. 2015).

Addition of ω-3 fatty acids to dairy cattle diets using fish oil, which is a common additive, has been found to improve reproductive efficiency, reduce prostaglandin secretion, and improve fertility and embryo survival in dairy cattle (Staples et al. 1998; Mattos et al. 2000; Mattos et al. 2004; Santos et al. 2008). New technology allows for heterotrophic production of algal biomass, which is a high-quality source of DHA (C22:6 n-3) and could be used as a ration supplement for dairy cattle. Previous studies have shown that feeding ruminants with algal biomass causes a significant increase in the level of ω-3 fatty acids in milk and modulates the fatty acid composition of meats (Stamey et al. 2012). Šefer et al. (2011) reported that supplementation of hens' diets with above 0.5% *Schizochytrium* sp. led to a higher amount of ω-3 PUFAs and ω-6/ω-3 PUFA ratio in egg yolks. The addition of microalgae rich in DHA (C22:6n-3) to lambs' diets and its effect on the fatty acid composition of different fat deposits and muscles was investigated by Díaz et al. (2017). Their findings showed that dietary supplementation with microalgae improved the PUFA/saturated fatty acid and ω-6/ω-3 ratios in conjunction with increased levels of DHA and total ω-3 fatty acids in lamb muscle. Despite the beneficial effects of algae in animal feeds, some undesirable effects such as deteriorative impact of prolonged feeding of algae on color of chicken and the quality of eggs and meat (Becker 2004) or perception of off-flavor in meat originated from algae or lipid oxidation (owing to an increase in PUFAs in muscles) should not be underestimated (Norcross 2015). Also, high cultivation costs, and difficulty in production and application in fuel production should be considered as the other challenges for the usage of algae in the feed sector.

16.5 Algal Extracts as Ingredients in Food Products

Certain strains of algae offer a host of advantages that could considerably improve the quality of food. Commercialization of algal species is underway with the aim of introducing algal biomass into the food market as a high-value ingredient. In most cases, these high-value ingredients are free from contaminants or undesirable by-products, which can improve taste and stability of the product, in addition to health and nutrition claims. They are also free of heavy metals, harmful microbes, and toxins. These extracts could serve as potential ingredients in dry mixes, veggie smoothies, protein replacements, fruit/vegetable mixes, and dozens of other foods and beverages. Broadly, the versatility of algae points to their prospective role as food ingredients. Studies show that some algal strains can produce considerable amounts of ingredients in comparison with routine sources and even compete with them in this regard. Seaweeds contain substances such as polysaccharides, proteins, lipids, pigments, and polyphenols with antibacterial, antiviral, and antifungal activities, as well as many other benefits. This gives seaweeds great potential as a supplement in functional foods or for the extraction of compounds (Holdt and Kraan 2011). The following is a list of the most important compounds that can be extracted from algae and used as ingredients in food.

16.5.1 Proteins

Protein content is widely differentiated among algal groups. The filamentous cyanobacterium *Arthrospira platensis* (*Spirulina*) and various commercial species of the unicellular green alga *Chlorella* contain high amounts of protein (up to 70% based on dry weight). These microalgae notably contain all of the essential amino acids that must be obtained from foods and their amino acid profile is often on par with other protein sources (such as soybean and egg) (Bleakley and Hayes 2017; Wells et al. 2017). From ancient times to now, *Spirulina sp.* and *Chlorella sp.* have been harvested on a large scale as protein-rich foodstuffs in many cultures (Wells et al. 2017).

Macroalgae contain relatively high protein levels ranging from 10 to 47% (based on dry weight) (Bocanegra et al. 2009; Lordan et al. 2011; Stengel et al. 2011). Among them, red and green algae such as *Porphyra* spp. (laver), *Pyropia* spp. (nori) (up to 44%), *Palmaria palmata* (dulse) (up to 35%), and *Ulva* spp. (sea lettuce) (up to 44%) often contain higher protein content in comparison with most brown algae (3–16% dry weight) (Bocanegra et al. 2009; Holdt and Kraan 2011; Lordan et al. 2011; Wells et al. 2017). As shown in Table 16.3, the amount of protein in algae is comparable with high-protein plant sources such as soybeans (40%). Their proteins are also good in terms of quality; for example, the amino acid composition of *Porphyra tenera* protein is close to that of ovalbumin (Holdt and Kraan 2011). However, similar to plants, the

Table 16.3 Comparison of total protein content (% of dry weight) in seaweed and foods

Algal genera/food	Protein content (% w/w)	References
Laminaria saccharina	3–21	Harnedy and FitzGerald (2011); Holdt and Kraan (2011)
Fucus	5–57	Holdt and Kraan (2011)
Ascophyllum	1.2–12	Holdt and Kraan (2011)
Undaria	11–24	Harnedy and FitzGerald (2011); Holdt and Kraan (2011)
Sargassum	9–20	Holdt and Kraan (2011)
Ulva	7–74	Holdt and Kraan (2011); Mac Artain et al. (2007)
Chondrus	6–29	Holdt and Kraan (2011)
Porphyra	15–47	Mac Artain et al. (2007)
Gracilaria	5–23	Holdt and Kraan (2011)
Palmaria	8–35	Harnedy and FitzGerald (2011); Holdt and Kraan (2011)
Konbu	8.1–15	Bocanegra et al. (2009)
Chlorella sp. and *Spirulina*	50	Andrade et al. (2018)
Soybean (white)	40.3	Bocanegra et al. (2009)
Pea (green)	28.8	Bocanegra et al. (2009)
Carrot	11	Bocanegra et al. (2009)
Tomato	14.5	Bocanegra et al. (2009)
Egg	49.80	Bocanegra et al. (2009)

protein content in marine algae varies depending on genus, species, phylum, season, environment, and life cycle (Bocanegra et al. 2009; Holdt and Kraan 2011; Lordan et al. 2011; Stengel et al. 2011; Wells et al. 2017).

Marine algae species are rich in essential amino acids (Stengel et al. 2011; Wells et al. 2017). Most of the amino acids found in algal proteins are acidic amino acids such as glutamic and aspartic acids (Holdt and Kraan 2011; Wells et al. 2017). Although, lysine, threonine, tryptophan, histidine, and sulfur amino acids such as methionine and cysteine have been reported as limiting amino acids in algal proteins (Bleakley and Hayes 2017; Holdt and Kraan 2011; Mac Artain et al., 2007), their total amount are higher than those found in plants (Holdt and Kraan 2011). Taurine (a nonproteinaceous amino acid) is abundant in red algae. It is not an essential amino acid, but as a component of bile acids it can complex with cholesterol and reduce its levels in the blood of humans (Holdt and Kraan 2011).

In a number of previous studies, it has been reported that the peptides extracted from algae have hormonal effects on the physiological stages of the human body. These peptides showed antioxidant, anti-HIV, antimutagenic, antihypertensive, anticoagulant, antimicrobial, immunomodulatory, and blood sugar and cholesterol-lowering functions (Andrade et al. 2018; Harnedy and FitzGerald 2011; Lordan et al. 2011; Stengel et al. 2011).

As well as the nutritional value and health benefits associated with the consumption of seaweed proteins, they are also used as natural dyes (phycobiliproteins) in different food products, such as desserts, milkshakes, fermented milk, and ice creams (Rioux and Turgeon 2015).

16.5.2 Polysaccharides

Polysaccharides (polymers composed of simple monosaccharides) are widely used by industries, especially the food industry (Andrade et al. 2018; Holdt and Kraan 2011). Algal polysaccharide content is relatively high (33–75% dry matter), but due to low digestibility, algae cannot be considered as a potential energy-rich food (Bocanegra et al. 2009; Lordan et al. 2011). The total polysaccharide contents in algal species ranges from 4 to 76%. *Ascophyllum*, *Palmaria*, and *Porphyra* are the most important algae genera in terms of polysaccharide content. However, green seaweed species such as *Ulva* also have a high amount of polysaccharide (up to 65% of dry weight) (Holdt and Kraan 2011). Direct comparisons show that algae have similar or slightly elevated levels of total polysaccharides compared with terrestrial plants (Mac Artain et al., 2007). Algal polysaccharides differ from those of conventional plants as they contain uncommon polysaccharides that may be acetylated, methylated, sulfated, or pyruvylated (Bocanegra et al. 2009; Mac Artain et al., 2007). Most algal carbohydrates are considered as dietary fiber because of their resistance to digestion by intestinal enzymes in the human gastrointestinal tract, so they can be partially fermented by colonic bacteria (Bocanegra et al. 2009; Lordan et al. 2011; Mac Artain et al., 2007). The total dietary fiber content of seaweeds (29.3–62.3%) is higher than the fiber content of most fruits and vegetables (Lordan et al. 2011). Algal polysaccharides are widely used in the food industry (including functional foods) as valuable bioactive ingredients because they are easy to extract and have numerous health benefits (Lordan et al. 2011).

Storage polysaccharides, such as carrageenans, agar, and alginates are the most commercially extracted components from algae. These polysaccharides are used as thickening, gelling, stabilizing, and packaging agents in various food products (Lordan et al. 2011; Stengel et al. 2011). Agar, a soluble polysaccharide extracted from red algae genera *Gelidium* and *Gracilaria*, forms a gel at low concentrations (0.5–2%) over a wide range of pH values (Bocanegra et al. 2009; Holdt and Kraan 2011). Therefore, it is widely used as a gelling and stabilizing agent in confectionery, bakery products, dairy products, canned meat and fish, water gels, beverages, and various other food products (Rioux and Turgeon 2015).

Carrageenans are used as thickeners and stabilizers in food products such as canned foods, bakery fillings, salad dressings, dessert mousses, ice cream, and instant desserts (Holdt and Kraan 2011). Carrageenans form gels upon cooling at a temperature around 40–60 °C and the resulting gel is thermally reversible by heating above its gelation temperature. In combination with an antibrowning agent, carrageenan can extend the shelf-life of fresh-cut fruits such as apples and bananas (Rioux and Turgeon 2015).

Brown algae are a potential source of alginate, which accounts for 17–35% of *Sargassum* sp. and about 28% of *Laminaria gurjanovae* (Bocanegra et al. 2009; Wells et al. 2017). Alginate is used as a stabilizer, emulsifier, gelling, and thickening agent in various food systems such as margarine, mayonnaise, ice creams, ready-to-eat soups, ketchup, Alfredo sauces, caramels, dehydrated soups, frozen meals, desserts, and purées. Alginate is also used to facilitate heat exchange during sterilization in canned meat meals. It could reduce the size of ice crystals, improve texture, and prevent syneresis in ice creams. In addition, alginate is suitable to use as an encapsulating agent in pharmaceutical products (Rioux and Turgeon 2015).

Fucan, which is abundant in the cell walls of brown algae (about 3.6–20% based on dry matter) such as *Fucus*, *Chordaria*, and several members of the *Laminariaceae* family, is a complex of sulfated polysaccharides (Lordan et al. 2011; Bocanegra et al. 2009). Numerous physiological and health properties including anticoagulant, antiviral, anti-liver failure, antithrombotic, antitumor, anti-inflammatory, and antioxidant activities have been reported for fucan (Garcia-Vaquero et al. 2019; Holdt and Kraan 2011; Lordan et al. 2011; Stengel et al. 2011).

Porphyran is another sulfated polysaccharide found in the cell walls of red macroalgae (main portion of *Porphyra*) (Bocanegra et al. 2009; Lordan et al., 2011). However, porphyran isolated from different species has shown great variations in the chemical and structural components (Bocanegra et al. 2009).

Neutral glucans, such as laminaran and mannitol, are the other storage polysaccharides in brown algae. Mannitol is the primary end-product of photosynthesis in brown algae and constitutes up to 30% of them. Laminaran can be found abundantly in all *Laminaria* species (22% based on dry matter). Several physiological functions have been reported for laminaran including modulation of intestinal metabolism through its effects on mucus composition, promotion of cell adhesion, immune-stimulatory, antimicrobial, antioxidant, and antitumor activities (Garcia-Vaquero et al. 2018; Lordan et al. 2011; Stengel et al. 2011).

Ulvan is the major water-soluble sulfated heteropolysaccharide (about 8–29% based on dry matter) of green seaweeds, *Ulva* and *Enteromorpha* species (Bocanegra et al. 2009). A semi-dilute solution of ulvan showed a rod-climbing effect and the gel formed on cooling without cation addition, which suggests ulvan could be a new source of water-soluble gelling polysaccharide (Rioux and Turgeon 2015).

Oligosaccharides can be obtained from algal sources either naturally or by physical, chemical, or biochemical degradation of algal polysaccharides. According to previous studies, oligosaccharides have also shown different physiological effects such as immunostimulation activities, and antioxidant and antitumor properties. Moreover, oligosaccharides can promote the growth of probiotic bacteria when they are added to the diet (Holdt and Kraan 2011; Lordan et al. 2011). In this case, digestion-resistant oligomers are used as a specific substrate for the growth of health-beneficial bacteria such as bifidobacteria and lactobacilli (Lordan et al. 2011).

16.5.3 Lipids

The lipid content of macroalgae represents up to 1–5% (dry weight), which is lower than that of other marine sources and their contribution as a food energy source appears to be low (Bocanegra et al. 2009; Holdt and Kraan 2011; Lordan et al. 2011; Mac Artain et al., 2007; Wells et al. 2017). The algal fatty acid profile differs from that of plants as algae have a higher proportion of PUFAs (almost half of lipid content), most of them are omega-3 (ω-6) and omega-6 (ω-6) fatty acids (Bocanegra et al. 2009; Lordan et al. 2011; Mac Artain et al., 2007). These fatty acids are of particular interest with respect to functional foods because they provide a wide range of functions in the body including antioxidant, antimicrobial, and anti-inflammatory activities, blood pressure regulatory and blood clotting inhibitory effects, rheumatoid arthritis and heart disease risk reduction, and roles in development and functioning of the brain and nervous systems (Lordan et al. 2011; Stengel et al. 2011). Both ω-3 and ω-6 fatty acids are essential for humans and should be consumed in a balanced proportion with an ideal ratio of ω-6:ω-3 ranging from 3:1 to 5:1. The predominant fatty acid in various seaweed products is EPA (C20:5,n-3), which accounts for 50% of the total fatty acid content (Holdt and Kraan 2011). The triglyceride composition in brown and red algae mainly consists of ω-3 and ω-6 fatty acids such as EPA, α-linolenic acid, and arachidonic and linoleic acids, respectively, along with relatively high levels of oleic and palmitic acids, while green seaweeds are characterized by the presence of hexadecatetraenoic, oleic, and palmitic acids (Bocanegra et al. 2009; Holdt and Kraan 2011; Lordan et al. 2011).

Like macroalgae, microalgae are rich sources of long-chain PUFAs, especially γ-linolenic acid, arachidonic acid, EPA, and DHA (Andrade et al. 2018). The lipid fraction of *C. vulgaris* is mainly composed of oleic, palmitic, and linolenic acids accounting for 72% of total fatty acids. In *D. salina*, palmitic, linolenic, and oleic acid contents are more than 85% of the total fatty acids. On the other hand, short-chain fatty acids have been detected in the lipid fraction of the green microalga, *Haematococcus* sp. (Lordan et al. 2011).

16.5.4 Pigments

According to the color of the pigment, algae can be classified as Rhodophyceae (red algae), Phaeophyceae (brown algae), or Chlorophyceae (green algae). Green macroalgae are abundant in coastal waters, where sunlight can easily penetrate, while brown and red macroalgae are found at greater depths (Lordan et al. 2011). Some of the possible microalgal sources of chlorophylls include *Spirulina* sp., such as *S. platensis*, and *Aphanizomenon flos-aquae* (Rasmussen and Morrissey 2007). Chlorophylls are primarily used as natural dyes in the food and beverage industries. Additionally, these pigments and their derivatives have shown anticancer activity because of their ability to bind carcinogenic hydrophobic compounds such as heterocyclic amines, polycyclic aromatic hydrocarbons, and aflatoxin (Rasmussen and Morrissey 2007).

Green seaweed species contain β-carotene, lutein, neoxanthin, zeaxanthin, and violaxanthin, while brown seaweed species contain β-carotene, fucoxanthin, and violaxanthin, and red seaweed species contain mainly α- and β-carotene, zeaxanthin, and lutein (Rajauria et al. 2017; Holdt and Kraan 2011). A number of algal strains investigated as natural producers of commercial carotenoids include *Spirulina (Arthrospira) maxima*, *D. salina*, *Chlorella protothecoides*, *C. vulgaris*, and *Haematococcus pluvialis* (Rasmussen and Morrissey 2007). The carotene levels in algae show seasonal variations, with the highest content in summer (420 ppm) and the lowest in winter (37 ppm) (Holdt and Kraan 2011). Various species of the green microalgae such as *D. salina* and *H. pluvialis* can accumulate about 8% β-carotene based on their dry weight (Wells et al. 2017).

Astaxanthin, the major carotenoid pigment with an orange-red color, can be derived from marine algae. Astaxanthin supplements from algae have been available to the public since 2000 onwards, and astaxanthin in commercial form (Zanthin) was approved by the US Food and Drug Administration (FDA) in 2005 as a dietary supplement. Zanthin derived from *H. pluvialis* is the richest source of natural astaxanthin (more than 3% of dry weight at an industrial scale) (Guerin et al. 2003). In addition to its use in dietary supplements, *H. pluvialis* can be added to aquaculture feed for enhanced pigmentation of salmon flesh (Rasmussen and Morrissey 2007).

Phycobiliproteins are a group of protein-pigment complexes with linear tetrapyrrole groups (bilins) such as phycoerythrobilin (red) and phycocyanobilin (blue) (Andrade et al. 2018; Holdt and Kraan 2011). Generally, phycobiliproteins are produced by algae at 10% dry mass; therefore, they have a high market value (Skulberg 2004). Phycobiliproteins play an important role in the photosynthetic process of Rhodophyta, Cyanophyta, and Cryptophyta. They include a major proportion of the red algae cellular proteins (e.g.1.2 and 0.5% of dry weight for *P. palmata* and *Gracilaria tikvahiae*, respectively; Holdt and Kraan 2011). In recent years, phycobiliproteins have been used as natural colorants in various food products such as soft drinks, fermented milk products, milkshakes, ice creams, chewing gum, jellies, ice sherbets, and for sweet cake decoration (Andrade et al. 2018; Sekar and Chandramohan 2008).

16.5.5 Phenolic Compounds

Phenolic compounds as secondary metabolites are not directly involved in algal primary processes such as cell division, photosynthesis, etc. However, some phenolic compounds, such as phlorotannins in brown algae, exhibit primary functions in growth and cell wall development (Stengel et al. 2011). Phlorotannins exist at concentrations of 20–250 (mg g^{-1} of dry mass) in *A. nodosum*, *Fucus vesiculosus*, *Sargassum spinuligerum*, and *Cystophora retroflexa* (Bocanegra et al. 2009). Phenolic compounds are present in most algae, but unlike plants, anthocyanins have not been found in algae (Stengel et al. 2011). The amount of phenolic compounds in green and red algae is lower than in brown algae species (Holdt and Kraan 2011). Bromophenol as a major phenolic compound is found at high levels in seaweeds such as *Polysiphonia urceolata* (Li et al. 2007). Phenolic content in seaweed varies from 1 to 14% of dry weight and species of the *Ascophyllum* and *Fucus* genera contain the highest phenolic contents (14 and 12%, respectively). Brown algae such as *Fucus*, *Sargassum*, and *A. nodosum* contain high levels of polyphenols (fucophlorethol, fucol, fucodiphloroethol G, and ergosterol) and the phenolic compound phlorotannin, which give them strong antioxidant activities (Rajauria et al. 2016). Like algal pigments, the amount of polyphenols depends on seasonal variations (Holdt and Kraan 2011). Besides phloroglucinol, many other flavonoids and their glycosides such as catechin and epicatechin, rutin, and hesperidin are present in brown, red, and green seaweeds (Holdt and Kraan 2011). A number of other nontypical phenolic compounds have been reported in different brown, red, and green algae; for example colpol in *Colpomenia sinuosa* (brown seaweed), tichocarpols as phenylpropanoid derivatives in *Tichocarpus crinitus* (red algae), coumarins in *Dasycladus vermicularis* (green algae), and some vanillic acid derivatives in *Cladophora socialis* (green algae) (Stengel et al. 2011). Previous investigations of extracted polyphenols have revealed that the antioxidant activity of some seaweed species such as *Kappaphycus*, *Eucheuma*, and *Turbinaria conoides* are stronger than α-tocopherol as a standard antioxidant (Ganesan et al. 2008).

16.6 Conclusion and Future Recommendations

Considering the fact that algae are good sources of nutritional compounds, they are promising sources of ingredients in both food and feed industries. However, the safety issues of the products such as allergens, toxins, heavy metals, or other harmful compounds potentially produced/transferred by the algae should be further evaluated before application in food products and feed.

References

Ak, B., Avsaroglu, E., Isik, O. et al. (2016). Nutritional and physicochemical characteristics of bread enriched with microalgae *Spirulina platensis*. *International Journal of Engineering Research and Applications* **6**: 30–38.

Andrade, L.M., Andrade, C.J., Dias, M. et al. (2018). *Chlorella* and *Spirulina* microalgae as sources of functional foods, nutraceuticals, and food supplements; an overview. *MOJ Food Process Technology* **6** (1): 45–58.

Avron, M. and Ben-Amotz, A. (1992). *Dunaliella; Physiology, Biochemistry and Biotechnology*. Boca Raton, FL: CRC Press.

Becker, W. (2004). Microalgae in human and animal nutrition. In: *Handbook of Microalgal Culture* (ed. A. Richmond), 312–351. Oxford: Blackwell Publishing Ltd.

Becker, E.W. (2007). Micro algae as a source of protein. *Biotechnology Advances* **25** (2): 207–210.

Beheshtipour, H., Mortazavian, A.M., Haratian, P., and Darani, K.K. (2012). Erratum to: effects of *Chlorella vulgaris* and *Arthrospira platensis* addition on viability of probiotic bacteria in yogurt and its biochemical properties. *European Food Research and Technology* **235**: 1213–1213.

Benemann, J.R. (1992). Microalgae aquaculture feeds. *Journal of Applied Phycology* **4**: 23.

Blazencic, J. (2007). *Sistematika algi*. Belgrade: NNK Internacional.

Bleakley, S. and Hayes, M. (2017). Algal proteins: extraction, application, and challenges concerning production. *Food* **6** (5): 1–33.

Bocanegra, A., Bastida, S., Benedi, J. et al. (2009). Characteristics and nutritional and cardiovascular-health properties of seaweeds. *Journal of Medicinal Food* **12** (2): 236–258.

Choi, Y.S., Choi, J.H., Han, D.J. et al. (2012). Effects of *Laminaria japonica* on the physico-chemical and sensory characteristics of reduced-fat pork patties. *Meat Science* **91**: 1–7.

Chun, S.S., Park, J.R., Park, J.C. et al. (1999). Quality characteristics of hamburger patties added with seaweed powder. *Journal of the Korean Society of Food Science and Nutrition* **28**: 140–144.

Cofrades, S., Lopez-Lopez, I., Solas, M.T. et al. (2008). Influence of different types and proportions of added edible seaweeds on characteristics of low-salt gel/emulsion meat systems. *Meat Science* **79**: 767–776.

Cofrades, S., Lopez-Lopez, I., Ruiz-Capillas, C. et al. (2011). Quality characteristics of low-salt restructured poultry with microbial transglutaminase and seaweed. *Meat Science* **87**: 373–380.

Conceição, L.E.C., Yúfera, M., Makridis, P. et al. (2010). Live feeds for early stages of fish rearing. *Aquaculture Research* **41**: 613–640.

Cox, S. and Abu-Ghannam, N. (2013). Enhancement of the phytochemical and fibre content of beef-patties with *Himanthalia elongata* seaweed. *International Journal of Food Science and Technology* **48** (11): 2239–2249.

Díaz, M.T., Perez, C., Sanchez, C.I. et al. (2017). Feeding microalgae increases omega 3 fatty acids of fat deposits and muscles in light lambs. *Journal of Food Composition and Analysis* **56**: 115–123.

Dlouhá, G., Ševčíková, S., Dokoupilová, A. et al. (2008). Effect of dietary selenium sources on growth performance, breast muscle selenium, glutathione peroxidase activity and oxidative stability in broilers. *Czech Journal of Animal Science* **53**: 265–269.

Doherty, O., Dillon, J.V., Figat, S. et al. (2010). The effects of lactose inclusion and seaweed extract derived from *Laminaria* spp. On performance, digestibility of diet components and microbial populations in newly weaned pigs. *Animal Feed Science and Technology* **157** (3–4): 173–180.

El-Baz, F.K., Abdo, S.M., and Hussein, A.M.S. (2017). Microalgae *Dunaliella salina* for use as food supplement to improve pasta quality. *International Journal of Pharmaceutical Sciences and Research* **46**: 45–51.

Evans, A.M., Smith, D.L., and Moritz, J.S. (2015). Effects of algae incorporation intobroiler starter diet formulations on nutrient digestibility and 3 to 21d bird performance. *Journal of Applied Poultry Research* **24**: 206–214.

FAO (2014). *The State of the World Fisheries and Aquaculture 2014.* Rome: FAO.

Fernandez-Martin, F., Lopez-Lopez, I., Cofrades, S., and Jimenez-Colmenero, F. (2009). Influence of adding sea spaghetti seaweed and replacing the animal fat with olive oil or a konjac gel on porkmeat batter gelation. Potential protein/alginate association. *Meat Science* **83**: 209–217.

Figueira, F.D.S., Crizel, T.D.M., Silva, C.R., and Sallas-Mellado, M.D.L.M.S. (2011). Elaboration of gluten-free bread enriched with the microalgae *Spirulina platensis*. *Brazilian Journal of Food Technology* **14**: 308–316.

Finney, K.F., Pomeranz, Y., and Bruinsma, B.L. (1984). Use of algae *Dunaliella* as a protein supplement in bread. *Cereal Chemistry* **61**: 402–406.

Fradique, M., Batista, A.P., Nunes, M.C. et al. (2013). *Isochrysis galbana* and *Diacronema vlkianum* biomass incorporation in pasta products as PUFA's source. *LWT Journal of Food and Science Technology* **50**: 312–319.

Ganesan, P., Kumar, C.S., and Bhaskar, N. (2008). Antioxidant properties of methanol extract and its solvent fractions obtained from selected Indian red seaweeds. *Bioresource Technology* **99**: 2717–2723.

Garcia-Segovia, P., Pagan-Moreno, M.J., Lara, I.F., and Martinez-Monzo, J. (2017). Effect of microalgae incorporation on physicochemical and textural propertiesin wheat bread formulation. *Food Science and Technology International* **23**: 437–447.

Garcia-Vaquero, M., Rajauria, G., Tiwari, B. et al. (2018). Extraction and yield optimisation of fucose, glucans and associated antioxidant activities from *Laminaria digitata* by applying response surface methodology to high intensity ultrasound-assisted extraction. *Marine Drugs* **16** (8): 257.

Garcia-Vaquero, M., O'Doherty, J.V., Tiwari, B.K. et al. (2019). Enhancing the extraction of polysaccharides and antioxidants from macroalgae using sequential hydrothermal-assisted extraction followed by ultrasound and thermal technologies. *Marine Drugs* **17** (8): 457.

Gouveia, L., Batista, A.P., Miranda, A. et al. (2007). *Chlorella vulgaris* biomass used as coloring source in traditional butter cookies. *Innovative Food Science & Emerging Technologies* **8**: 433–436.

Gouveia, L., Batista, A.P., Sousa, I. et al. (2008a). Microalgae in novel food products. In: *Papadoupoulos, K*, 75–112. Food Chemistry Research Developments, Hauppauge, NY: Nova Science Publishers.

Gouveia, L., Coutinho, C., Mendonça, E. et al. (2008b). Functional biscuits with PUFA-ω3 from *Isochrysis galbana*. *Journal of the Science of Food and Agriculture* **88**: 891–896.

Guldas, M. and Irkin, R. (2010). Influence of *Spirulina platensis* powder on the microflora of yoghurt and acidophilus milk. *Mljekarstvo.* **60**: 237–243.

Guerin, M., Huntley, M.E., and Olaizola, M. (2003). *Haematococcus astaxanthin*: applications for human health and nutrition. *Trends in Biotechnology* **21**: 210–216.

Hall, A.C., Fairclough, A.C., Mahadevan, K., and Paxman, J.R. (2012). *Ascophyllum nodosum* enriched bread reduces subsequent energy intake with no effect on postprandial glucose and cholesterol in healthy, overweight males. A pilot study. *Appetite* **58**: 379–386.

Harnedy, P.A. and FitzGerald, R.J. (2011). Bioactive proteins, peptides, and amino acids from macroalgae. *Journal of Phycology* **47**: 218–232.

Hasan, M.R. and Chakrabarti, R. (2009). Use of algae and aquatic macrophytes as feed in small scale aquaculture: a review. Bulletin: FAO Fisheries and Aquaculture Technical Paper, No. 531. Rome: FAO.

Heo, J.Y., Shin, H.J., Oh, D.H. et al. (2006). Quality properties of Appenzeller cheese added with *Chlorella*. *Korean Journal for Food Science of Animal Resources* **26**: 525–531.

Holdt, S.L. and Kraan, S. (2011). Bioactive compounds in seaweeds: functional food application and legislation. *Journal of Applied Phycology* **23**: 543–597.

Jeon, H. (2006). Effect of *Chlorella* addition on the quality of processed cheese. *Journal of the Korean Society of Food Science and Nutrition* **35**: 373–377.

Jeon, M.R. and Choi, S.H. (2012). Quality characteristics of pork patties added with seaweed powder. *Korean Journal for Food Science of Animal Resources* **32**: 77–83.

Jimenez-Colmenero, F., Cofrades, S., Lopez-Lopez, I. et al. (2010). Technological and sensory characteristics of reduced/low fat, low-salt frankfurters as affected by the addition of konjac and seaweed. *Meat Science* **84**: 356–363.

Khatoon, N., Sengupta, P., Homechaudhuri, S., and Pal, R. (2010). Evaluation of algae based feed in goldfish (*Carassius auratus*) nutrition. *Proceedings of the Zoological Society (Calcutta)* **63** (2): 109–114.

Kim, J.H., Kim, J.H., and Yoo, S.S. (2008). Impacts of the proportion of sea-tangle on quality characteristics of muffin. *Korean Journal of Food and Cookery Science* **24**: 565–572.

Kim, H.W., Choi, J.H., Choi, Y.S. et al. (2010). Effects of sea tangle (*Laminaria japonica*) powder on quality characteristics of breakfast sausages. *Korean Journal for Food Science of Animal Resources* **30**: 55–61.

Kim, S.K., Pangestuti, R., and Rahmadi, P. (2011). Sea lettuces: culinary uses and nutritional value. *Advances in Food and Nutrition Research* **64**: 57–70.

Knuckey, R.M., Semmens, G.L., Mayer, R.J., and Rimmer, M.A. (2005). Development of an optimal micro algal diet for the culture of the calanoid copepod *Acartia sinjiensis*: effect of algal species and feed concentration on copepod development. *Aquaculture* **249** (1–4): 339–351.

Kovac, D., Simeunovic, J., Babic, O. et al. (2013). Algae in food and feed. *Food and Feed Research* **40** (1): 21–31.

Kuhara, T. (2006). Liquidized seaweed, method for producing the same, and raw material. Japanese Patent Application JP 2006254899 A.

Kumarathunge, N.C., Jayasinghe, J.M.P., and Abeyrathne, E.D.N.S. (2016). Development of sea lettuce (*Ulva lactuca*) and Catla (*Catla catla*) incorporated protein and fiber rich fish burger. *International Journal of Agricultural Science and Research* **3** (4): 229–233.

Lalic, L.M. and Berkovic, K. (2005). The influence of algae addition on physicochemical properties of cottage cheese. *Milchwissenschaft* **60**: 151–154.

Lee, H., Choe, J., Yong, H.I. et al. (2018). Combination of sea tangle powder and high-pressure treatment as an alternative to phosphate in emulsion-type sausage. *Journal of Food Processing & Preservation* **42** (9): 1–9.

Lee, Y.K. (1997). Commercial production of micro algae in the Asia Pacific rim. *Journal of Applied Phycology* **9**: 403–411.

Li, K., Li, X.M., Ji, N.Y., and Wang, B.G. (2007). Natural bromophenols from the marine red alga *Polysiphonia urceolata* (Rhodomelaceae): structural elucidation and DPPH radical-scavenging activity. *Bioorganic & Medicinal Chemistry* **15**: 6627–6631.

Lopez-Lopez, I., Bastida, S., Ruiz-Capillas, C. et al. (2009). Composition and antioxidant capacity of low-salt meat emulsion model systems containing edible seaweeds. *Meat Science* **83**: 492–498.

Lopez-Lopez, I., Cofrades, S., Yakan, A. et al. (2010). Frozen storage characteristics of low-salt and low-fat beef patties as affected by wakame addition and replacing pork backfat with olive oil-in-water emulsion. *Food Research International* **43**: 1244–1254.

Lopez-Lopez, I., Cofrades, S., Caneque, V. et al. (2011). Effect of cooking on the chemical composition of low-salt, low-fat wakame/olive oil added beef patties with special reference to fatty acid content. *Meat Science* **89**: 27–34.

Lordan, S., Ross, R.P., and Stanton, C. (2011). Marine bioactives as functional food ingredients: potential to reduce the incidence of chronic diseases. *Marine Drugs* **9**: 1056–1100.

Mac Artain, P., Gill, C.I.R., Brooks, M. et al. (2007). Nutritional value of edible seaweeds. *Nutrition Reviews* **65**: 535–543.

Matsuzaki, T. and Yoshida, K. (2007). Seasoning liquid containing *Undaria pinnatifida* and *Chlorella*, and a method for producing the same. Japanese Patent Application JP 2007319105 A.

Mattos, R., Staples, C.R., and Thatcher, W.W. (2000). Effects of dietary fatty acids on reproduction in ruminants. *Reviews of Reproduction* **5**: 38–45.

Mattos, R., Staples, C.R., Arteche, A. et al. (2004). The effects of feeding fish oil on uterine secretion of PGF2α, milk composition, and metabolic status of periparturient Holstein cows. *Journal of Dairy Science* **87**: 921–932.

Mocanu, D.G., Botez, E., Nistor, V.O. et al. (2013). Influence of *Spirulina platensis* biomass over some starter culture of lactic bacteria. *Journal of Agroalimentary Processes and Technologies* **19**: 474–479.

Mohammed, M.K. and Mohd, M.K. (2011). Production of carotenoids (antioxidants/colourant) in Spirulina platensis in response to indole acetic acid (IAA). *International Journal of Engineering Science and Technology (IJEST)* **3**(6): 4973–4979.

Molnar, N., Gyenis, B., and Varga, L. (2005). Influence of a powdered *Spirulina platensis* biomass on acid production of lactococci in milk. *Milchwissenschaft* **60**: 380–382.

Muller-Feuga, A. (2000). The role of microalgae in aquaculture: situation and trends. *Journal of Applied Phycology* **12**: 527–534.

Nagai, T. and Yukimoto, T. (2003). Preparation and functional properties of beverages made from sea algae. *Food Chemistry* **81**: 327–332.

Nagai, T., Suzuki, N., and Nagashima, T. (2006). Angiotensin I-converting enzyme inhibitory activities of beverages made from sea algae and commercially available tea extracts. *Journal of Food, Agriculture and Environment* **4**: 17–19.

Norcross, R.G. (2015). Impact of algae supplemented diets combined with antioxidants on the nutritional profile, quality attributes and storage stability of chicken breast meat. MSc thesis. College of Agriculture, Food and Environment. University of Kentucky.

Nuñez, M. and Picon, A. (2016). Seaweeds in yogurt and quark supplementation: influence of five dehydrated edible seaweeds on sensory characteristics. *International Journal of Food Science and Technology* **52** (2): 1–8.

Oh, H.K. and Lim, H.S. (2011). Quality characteristics of the hamburger patties with sea tangle (*Laminaria japonica*) powder and/or cooked rice. *Korean Journal for Food Science of Animal Resources* **31**: 570–579.

Plaza, M., Cifuentes, A., and Ibanez, E. (2008). In the search of new functional food ingredients from algae. *Trends in Food Science & Technology* **19** (1): 31–39.

Prabhasankar, P., Jyotsna, R., Indrani, D., and Rao, G.V. (2007). Influence of whey protein concentrate, additives, their combination on the quality and microstructure of vermicelli made from Indian *T. durum* wheat variety. *Journal of Food Engineering* **80**: 1239–1245.

Prabhasankar, P., Ganesan, P., Bhaskar, N. et al. (2009). Edible Japanese seaweed, wakame (*Undaria pinnatifida*) as an ingredient in pasta: chemical, functional and structural evaluation. *Food Chemistry* **115**: 501–508.

Prachyakij, P., Charernjirakul, W., and Kantachote, D. (2008). Improvement in the quality of a fermented seaweed beverage using an antiyeast starter of *Lactobacillus plantarum* DW3 and partial sterilization. *World Journal of Microbiology and Biotechnology* **24**: 1713–1720.

Priyadarshani, I. and Rath, B. (2012). Commercial and industrial applications of micro algae – a review. *Journal of Algal Biomass Utilization* **3** (4): 89–100.

Rajauria, G., Foley, B., and Abu-Ghannam, N. (2016). Identification and characterization of phenolic antioxidant compounds from brown Irish seaweed *Himanthalia elongata* using LC-DAD–ESI-MS/MS. *Innovative Food Science & Emerging Technologies* **37**: 261–268.

Rajauria, G., Foley, B., and Abu-Ghannam, N. (2017). Characterization of dietary fucoxanthin from *Himanthalia elongata* brown seaweed. *Food Research International* **99**: 995–1001.

Rasmussen, R.S. and Morrissey, M.T. (2007). Marine biotechnology for production of food ingredients. In: *Advances in Food and Nutrition Research*, vol. **52** (ed. S.L. Taylor), 237–292. New York: Elsevier.

Ratanaburee, A., Kantachote, D., Charernjiratrakul, W. et al. (2011). Enhancement of γ-aminobutyric acid in a fermented red seaweed beverage by starter culture *Lactobacillus plantarum* DW12. *Electronic Journal of Biotechnology* **14** (3): 1–13.

Rioux, L.-E. and Turgeon, S. (2015). Seaweed carbohydrates. In: *Seaweed Sustainability: Food and Non-food Applications* (eds. B. Tiwari and D. Troy), 141–192. Amsterdam: Elsevier.

Rodríguez De Marco, E., Steffolani, M.E., Martínez, C.S., and León, A.E. (2014). Effects of *Spirulina* biomass on the technological and nutritional quality of bread wheat pasta. *LWT Journal of Food and Science Technology* **58**: 102–108.

Santos, J.E., Bilby, T.R., Thatcher, W.W. et al. (2008). Long-chain fatty acids of diet as factors influencing reproduction in cattle. *Reproduction in Domestic Animals* **43** (Suppl. 2): 23–30.

Šefer, D., Andonov, A., Sobajic, S. et al. (2011). Effect of feeding laying hens diets supplemented with omega 3 fatty acids on the egg fatty acid profile. *Biotechnology in Animal Husbandry* **27** (3): 679–686.

Sekar, S. and Chandramohan, M. (2008). Phycobiliproteins as a commodity: trends in applied research, patents and commercialization. *Journal of Applied Phycology* **20**: 113–136.

Senthil, A., Mama, B.S., and Mahadevaswamy, M. (2005). Effect of using seaweed (*Eucheuma*) powder on the quality of fish cutlet. *Journal of Food Science and Nutrition* **56**: 327–335.

Ševčíková, S., Skřivan, M., Dlouhá, G., and Koucký, M. (2006). The effect of selenium source on the performance and meat quality of broiler chickens. *Czech Journal of Animal Science* **51**: 449–457.

Sharoba, A.M., Morsy, O.M., El-Desouky, A. I., Bahlol, H.E.M., Abd El Mawla, E.M. (2017). Utilization of *Spirulina* algae to improve the nutritional value of kiwifruits and cantaloupe nectar blends. 2nd International Sino-Egyptian Congress on Agriculture, Veterinary Sciences and Engineering (2nd ISEC-AVE), October 7–10, 2017, Benha, Egypt.

Singh, P., Singh, R., Jha, A. et al. (2015). Optimization of a process for high fibre and high protein biscuit. *Journal of Food Science and Technology* **52**: 1394–1403.

Skřivan, M., Marounek, M., Dlouhá, G., and Ševčíková, S. (2008). Dietary selenium increases vitamin E contents of egg yolk and chicken meat. *British Poultry Science* **49**: 482–486.

Skulberg, O.M. (2004). Bioactive chemicals in microalgae. In: *Handbook of Microalgal Culture: Biotechnology and Applied Phycology* (ed. A. Richmond), 485–512. Oxford: Blackwell Publishing.

Spolaore, P., Joannis Cassan, C., Duran, E., and Isambert, A. (2006). Commercial applications of microalgae. *Journal of Bioscience and Bioengineering* **101** (2): 87–96.

Stamey, J.A., Shepherd, D.M., de Veth, M.J., and Corl, B.A. (2012). Influence of high-oil algae biomass as a feed intake and growth-performance enhancer in feedlot cattle during period of high ambient temperature. *Journal of Dairy Science* **95**: 5269–5275.

Staples, C.R., Burke, J.M., and Thatcher, W.W. (1998). Influence of supplemental fats on reproductive tissues and performance of lactating cows. *Journal of Dairy Science* **81**: 856–871.

Stengel, D.B., Connan, S., and Popper, Z.A. (2011). Algal chemodiversity and bioactivity: sources of natural variability and implications for commercial application. *Biotechnology Advances* **29**: 483–501.

Wang, J.K. (2003). Conceptual design of a microalgae-based recirculating oyster and shrimp system. *Aquacultural Engineering* **28**: 37–46.

Wells, M.L., Potin, P., Craigie, J.S. et al. (2017). Algae as nutritional and functional food sources: revisiting our understanding. *Journal of Applied Phycology* **29** (2): 949–982.

Yamaguchi, K. (1997). Recent advances in micro algal bioscience in Japan, with special reference to utilization of biomass and metabolites: a review. *Journal of Applied Phycology* **8**: 227–233.

Yende, S.R., Harle, U.N., and Chaugule, B.B. (2014). Therapeutic potential and health benefits of *Sargassum* species. *Pharmacognosy Reviews* **8** (15): 1–7.

17
Role of Algal Compounds for Human Health

Sidra Ehsan[1], Sumia Akram[2], Zohaib Saeed[1], Muhammad Pervaiz[1], and Muhammad Mushtaq[1]

[1]*Department of Chemistry, GC University, Lahore, Pakistan*
[2]*Division of Science and Technology, University of Education, Lahore, Pakistan*

17.1 Introduction

The massive increase in the global population over the past couple of decades has led to concerns regarding the depletion of agricultural and pharmaceutical resources, particularly food and medicine-related products. In the same context, malnutrition has continued to be a prevalent global problem. In such a situation, alternative food sources like seaweeds and their derived products can provide hope of solutions to malnutrition and food security-related issues. Based on archeological evidence, it can be seen that algae have been used as foods and medicines under certain conditions throughout human history. In 2013 the worldwide cultivation and production of algae using aquaculture methods was up to 21 million tons with an estimated value of US$6.7 billion, and more than 38% of the total algal production (23.8 million tons) was meant for human and animal consumption. Macroalgae have been used as foods worldwide and their therapeutic and medicinal applications have been frequently reported from various geographical locations. Increased awareness regarding its nutritional profile, bioactive composition, and potential health attributes has increased the demand for algal biomass and derived products globally (Wells et al. 2017).

At this time, China stands at the top among algae producing nations and perhaps it will remain in the same position, as a number of focused efforts have been made in China to improve the production of macro- and microalgae. In the same region, Japan has become the largest consumer of algae, where the use of algae as a foodstuff may range up to 1.6 kg per person per annum. The presence of phenolic compounds, vitamins, polysaccharides, carotenes, proteins, and minerals in algal biomass may offer a variety of health benefits to consumers in addition to dietary and essential energy requirements. However, a great deal of research is required regarding the bioavailability and accumulation of algal bioactive compounds. The presence of naturally occurring antioxidants and other bioactive compounds in the macroalgae is gaining the

Recent Advances in Micro- and Macroalgal Processing: Food and Health Perspectives, First Edition. Edited by Gaurav Rajauria and Yvonne V. Yuan.

attention of scientists for *in vitro* and *in vivo* clinical trials to promote the usage of algae as a food additive in beverages, nutraceuticals, food supplements, and processed meat (Cornish and Garbary 2010). In turn, the algal industry is realizing the potential therapeutic and medicinal uses of algae as a food additive. Various species of algae provide iodine (*Laminaria*), phycocyanin (*Spirulina platensis*), β-carotene (*Dunaliella salina*), anthelmintic, kainic acid (*Caloglossa leprieurii*), etc. used for goiter, inflammation, vision problems, and intestinal worms, respectively (Tseng 2001). The present chapter highlights the importance of various bioactive compounds synthesized by algal weeds and some microalgae species cultivated worldwide.

More than 25 000 species of algae have been reported in the world with particular algal species varying from a single cell (microalgae) up to 150 ft long giant structures (macroalgae). Likewise, the algal biomass may bear blue, green, red, or brown coloration depending upon the bioactive compounds, especially terpenoids, it synthesizes. Algae are present everywhere, on plants, rocks, soils, oceans, and nearby wetlands. In addition to their nutritional profile and potential as industrial products, macroalgae and microalgae are responsible for the consumption of CO_2 and in return produce oxygen that keeps us alive. In any food chain, they act as primary producers; approx. 70 algal species are used for food, fertilizers, animal feed, biochemical processes, and pharmaceuticals (Edwards 2008).

17.2 Classification of Algae

Algae have been classified on the basis of their morphology, cell walls, the biochemistry of their pigments, energy storage compounds, and photosynthetic pigments because they contain a combination of one or more of chlorophyll and other necessary pigments called accessory pigments (Davis et al. 2003).

17.2.1 Euglenophyta

The euglenoids contain around 800 species of unicellular algae that normally live in freshwater, especially when it contains plenty of organic matter. These species do not have a true cell wall; instead, a proteinaceous-bound covering called a pellicle keeps the cell structure together. These microalgae migrate via flagella and most of these species produce carbohydrates via photosynthesis and store them as paramylon, a carbohydrate similar to starch. Chlorophyll *a* and *b* are considered to be the primary photosynthetic pigments, while some species rely on organic matter suspended in water for their survival. A few euglenoid species can survive even kept in the dark if these are provided with organic matter. The blue-green algae of the Euglenophyta division are often considered a rich source of protein, minerals, and carotenoids that provide immunity to the living cells. Once digested, these algal species work as a detoxifier to clean and strengthen the human digestive system, which in turn improves energy levels, helps in the proper functioning of the liver and kidneys, improves the working of the cardiovascular system, and lowers inflammation (Sahoo and Kumar 2015).

17.2.2 Chrysophyta

The Chrysophyta division covers 1100 species of golden-brown algae and about half a million diatoms. The majority of these algal species grow in the marine system but many can survive both in fresh and marine waters. Structurally, cellulose and pectin materials mainly constitute the cell wall of both divisions. However, in the case of diatoms, the cell wall polymers are extensively crosslinked with silicon and are therefore rigid and resistant to decay. These species, like other algal biomass, produce carbohydrates via photosynthesis and store them in the form of leucosin. The photosynthetic pigments include chlorophyll *a* and *c*, and carotenoids and xanthophylls are the accessory pigments, with a special pigment known as fucoxanthin. The diatom species are mainly made of silica, have a double-shelled structure that can stack into each other like a pillbox, and are distinguished on the basis of their shell shape. The other class of golden-brown algae is less diverse than diatoms, and most species lack cell walls, while others have pectin material in the cell wall. The cells of golden-brown algae are smaller than 0.05 mm in diameter and they are known as nanoplankton (Caron and Brown 1987).

17.2.3 Pyrrophyta

These are flame or fire algae and dinoflagellates, and account for 1100 species of unicellular algae. Some species of fire algae live in freshwater, while most live in marine water. The cell wall of dinoflagellates is made of cellulose; they have two flagella for locomotion and store energy in the form of starch. Chlorophyll *a* and *c* are the photosynthetic pigments of pyrrophyta, while carotenoids, xanthophyll, and fucoxanthin are the accessory pigments. Some dinoflagellates result in the production of red tides, which are harmful to marine life due to the presence of toxic chemicals produced by the dinoflagellates, while some species of dinoflagellates can produce bioluminescence that can be seen in clearly in the dark (Burkholder 1973).

17.2.4 Chlorophyta (Green Algae)

Chlorophyta, known as green algae, comprise more than 7000 species and are mostly found in freshwater with some in marine water. Green algae of both unicellular and multicellular types mostly have cell walls made of cellulose with hemicellulose and calcium carbonate. Like other algal species, they contain photosynthetic pigments chlorophyll *a* and *b* to synthesize carbohydrates, which are subsequently stored in the form of starch. A flagellum-like structure helps the algal species with migration. The green algae known as *Gonium sp.* form small spherical colonies of 4–32 cells, while other species such as *Volvox* form large, hollow, spherical colonies of ten to thousands of cells. *Chlorella sp.* is considered a food supplement in the form of a tablet, acts as a detoxifier, and contains a high content of minerals, proteins, and vitamins (Mohammed et al. 2019).

17.2.5 Rhodophyta (Red Algae)

More than 4000 species including both micro- and macroscopic sizes of Rhodophyta or red algae have been identified, mainly from the marine ecosystem. The cell wall of Rhodophyta comprises cellulose and other polysaccharides in addition to accessory pigments of carotenoids, xanthophylls, and phycobilin derivatives. This class of algae lacks a flagellum-like structure for their migration but contains photosynthetic pigments chlorophyll *a* and *d*, and stores the photosynthetic products as Floridian starch. These algal species may contain substantial amounts of minerals, vitamins, and antioxidants useful for human growth and health (Woelkerling et al. 1993).

17.2.6 Phaeophyta (Brown Algae)

Around 1500 species of Phaeophyta or brown algae have been identified in the marine ecosystem. The brown algae are macroscopic in size and often form large kelps that may cover tens of meters. The members of this algal division bear a cell wall made of cellulose and polysaccharides called alginic acid; some algae have a complex tissue system. The brown algae have two flagella for locomotion, and store energy in the form of carbohydrate polymers called laminarin. Chlorophyll *a* and *c* are the photosynthetic pigments, while carotenoids and xanthophylls are the accessory pigments (Li et al. 2011).

17.2.7 Xanthophyta

The Xanthophyta, also known as yellow-green algae, comprise about 750 species living in the freshwater ecosystem. These are unicellular species that form small colonies and their cell wall is usually made up of cellulose, pectin material, and to some extent silica is present. These species store energy in the form of a carbohydrate called leucosin, and have two flagella for locomotion. Chlorophyll *a* is the photosynthetic pigment, while carotenoids and xanthophylls act as accessory pigments (Khataee et al. 2011).

17.3 Proximate Composition of Algae

The algal biomass generally comprises carbohydrates, proteins, vitamins, fats, fiber, minerals, nucleic acids, and pigments. The exact composition of various elements, biomolecules, minerals, and nutrients differs from species to species, and with geological territory, growth level, and growth conditions (Wang et al. 2010). A similar trend has been observed regarding the proximate composition of some frequently investigated seaweeds (Table 17.1).

17.3.1 Algal Carbohydrates

Carbohydrates or hydrates of carbon are considered to be a quick and major source of energy for heterotrophs like humans. In plants, and likewise in algae, carbohydrates are mainly present in the form of sugars, starches, cellulose, hemicellulose, chitin, and

Table 17.1 Proximate composition of some frequently investigated algae species.

Algal species	Proteins	Carbohydrates	Lipids	Moisture	Ash	Fiber	References
Caulerpa serrulata	14.48 ± 0.006	45.6 ± 0.003	4.24 ± 0.003	10.6 ± 0.025	17.05 ± 0.003	18.6 ± 0.007	Osman et al. (2011)
Padina tetrastromatica	3.873 ± 0.009	15.54 ± 0.003	3.920 ± 0.009	13.37 ± 0.11	21.20 ± 0.009	55.41 ± 0.003	
Turbinaria triquatra	4.133 ± 0.009	16.30 ± 0.006	1.62 ± 0.003	23.62 ± 0.42	29.57 ± 0.007	48.30 ± 0.007	
Sargassum subrepandum	4.22 ± 0.006	17.21 ± 0.008	3.83 ± 0.006	13.02 ± 0.027	26.75 ± 0.003	47.94 ± 0.006	
Acanthophora spicifera	5.07 ± 0.01	44.76 ± 0.01	0.55 ± 0.01	18.84 ± 0.13	28.38 ± 0.39	2.42 ± 0.24	D'Armas et al. (2019)
Centroceras clavulatum	4.78 ± 0.02	32.24 ± 0.12	0.75 ± 0.02	23.54 ± 0.22	36.69 ± 0.22	2.02 ± 0.11	
Hypnea spinella	8.02 ± 0.01	34.46 ± 0.18	1.44 ± 0.01	18.61 ± 0.11	33.07 ± 0.12	4.41 ± 0.19	
Kappaphycus alvarezii	4.86 ± 0.01	41.15 ± 0.11	0.57 ± 0.01	22.77 ± 0.15	27.49 ± 0.15	3.18 ± 0.11	
Padina pavonica	5.53 ± 0.01	43.39 ± 0.16	0.83 ± 0.01	20.47 ± 0.26	24.85 ± 0.26	4.94 ± 0.16	
Spatoglossum schroederi	5.21 ± 0.02	40.04 ± 0.21	3.07 ± 0.02	12.84 ± 0.18	34.58 ± 0.20	4.28 ± 0.20	
Ulva lactuca	5.54 ± 0.02	45.52 ± 0.04	0.33 ± 0.01	20.67 ± 0.27	26.99 ± 0.26	0.96 ± 0.03	
Grateloupia turuturu	22.9 ± 2.0	nd	2.6 ± 0.1	nd	18.5 ± 0.6	60.4 ± 2.3	Denis et al. (2010)
Padina pavonia	35.40 ± 0.56	nd	5.89 ± 0.24	nd	44.92 ± 1.60	13.64 ± 0.75	
Laurencia papillosa	34.65 ± 0.48	nd	6.73 ± 0.33	nd	44.05 ± 1.10	13.55 ± 1.36	
Jania rubens	7.20 ± 0.19	nd	0.12 ± 0.01	nd	80.73 ± 3.16	11.62 ± 1.40	
Heterosiphonia japonica	19.0 ± 0.36	4.28 ± 1.52	1.42 ± 0.35	9.95 ± 0.27	22.1 ± 0.72	53.2 ± 0.56	Wong and Cheung (2000)
Hypnea charoides	18.4 ± 0.30	7.02 ± 4.06	1.48 ± 0.15	10.9 ± 0.62	22.8 ± 2.23	50.3	

(continued)

Table 17.1 (*continued*)

Algal species		Proteins	Carbohydrates	Lipids	Moisture	Ash	Fiber	References
Ulva lactuca		7.06 ± 0.06	14.6 ± 4.94	1.64 ± 0.10	10.6 ± 1.14	21.3 ± 2.78	55.4	
Caulerpa lentillifera		19.38 ± 1.48	44.02 ± 2.01	2.87 ± 0.03	87.05 ± 0.50*	29.61 ± 1.50	4.12 ± 0.16	Nagappan and Vairappan (2014)
Caulerpa racemosa	*Var. CM*	17.36 ± 0.72	52.81 ± 1.89	2.21 ± 0.05	91.36 ± 1.09*	23.81 ± 1.35	3.11 ± 0.32	
	Var. LV	17.28 ± 0.63	50.19 ± 1.35	2.11 ± 0.04	93.20 ± 0.81*	26.74 ± 2.17	3.18 ± 0.38	
Cymbula compressa		28.97 ± 3.73	12.25 ± 1.60	nd	nd	1.66 ± 0.29	nd	Ozgun et al. (2015)
Dactyladenia dichotoma		40.44 ± 3.27	47.92 ± 5.66	nd	nd	7.60 ± 1.614	nd	
Padina pavonia		31.91 ± 4.59	14.74 ± 3.08	nd	nd	18.19 ± 2.66	nd	
Sargassum vulgare		35.09 ± 2.49	31.03 ± 6.59	nd	nd	16.07 ± 2.92	nd	
Stypopodium schimperi		65.19 ± 4.32	41.92 ± 2.32	nd	nd	4.66 ± 1.72	nd	
Cystoseira corniculata		43.72 ± 3.22	20.74 ± 1.37	nd	nd	8.67 ± 2.02	nd	
Cystoseira barbata		53.18 ± 9.00	19.71 ± 3.40	nd	nd	14.13 ± 1.19	nd	
Stypocaulon scoparium		35.88 ± 2.88	13.43 ± 1.07	nd	nd	7.43 ± 2.43	nd	

All the values are mean ± SD of g 100 g^{-1} of dry mass except *, which indicates g 100 g^{-1} of fresh weight; nd indicates no data available.

certain fibers. Carbohydrates are the macronutrients, present in different food items like maize, corn, milk, fruits, grains, and cereals, which provide sufficient energy for the proper functioning of muscles and the central nervous system of our body (Sarwar et al. 2015). The algal carbohydrates may compete with other carbohydrates sources used as food for living organisms. Algal biomass has been reported (Table 17.1) as an abundant source of polysaccharides of various origins, states, and classes like starch, fiber, agar, alginates, carrageenans, and agarose depending upon the class of algae. For example, the Chlorophyta contain polysaccharides in the form of amylopectin and ulvans, while the Rhodophyta and Phaeophyta store these biomolecules in the form of agar, carrageenans, and alginates and homofucans, respectively (Priyadarshani and Rath 2012).

Ulvans are sulfated polysaccharide bioactive compounds with antitumor, immunomodulation, antihyperlipidemic, and anticoagulant characteristics. Mannitol present in brown algae is reported to have antioxidant properties and is used in the cosmetic and pharmaceutical industries. Alginates from red alga being polymeric acids in nature, act as a carrier to deliver zinc, silver, and other bioactive substances for multiple biological actions. Zhang et al. (2010) extracted the polysaccharides from biomass of different algal species *Ulva pertusa*, *Laminaria japonica*, *Enteromorpha linza*, and *Bryopsis plumosa*, which comprised 33.4, 66.7, 47.9, 41.8, and 78.9% of the total sugar, respectively. Arabinose contributed the major fraction of total sugars in *B. plumosa* species, whereas *B. plumosa* species were high in fucose. Likewise, galactose was the main sugar present in *B. plumosa*, *U. pertusa*, and *L. japonica.* Wang et al. (2014) have observed that the polysaccharides of these algal species have good reducing power, and hydroxyl radical or superoxide scavenging capacity.

Additionally, Lewin (1956) explained the chemical composition of a marine algae *Rhizoclonium* sp., which act as a substituent for wood fiber and comprise 57.4% of total carbohydrates, containing glucose as a major constituent (78.4%); mannose 1.3%, galactose 12.5%, and xylose 19.8% are also present.

Leyton et al. (2016) extracted polysaccharides and phlorotannins from the brown algae *Macrocystis pyrifera* and observed that 62.14% of dry matter was sugars along with $191.7 \pm 3.4\,mg\,g^{-1}$ dry weight (DW) of mannitol, and $138.1 \pm 2.3\,mg\,g^{-1}$ DW of phlorotannins. The relative concentrations of these biomolecules however changed with changes in extraction conditions particularly the liquid to solid (S/L) ratio, extraction time, particle size, and extractant composition. Optimum conditions for maximum extraction enlist a pretreatment with hexane, with a drying temperature of 40 °C, extraction carried out with water, size of the particles should below 1.4 mm, and S/L ratio should be 1:15. At the end, two phlorotannins, phloroeckol and phloroglucinol tetramer, were found in the extract of water which have an antidiabetic effect and preventative effect on Alzheimer's disease in the case of phloroeckol, and an antiallergic effect, with the ability to scavenge free radicals in the case of phloroglucinol tetramer. Thus, macroalgae can be exploited for human consumption due to the presence of a variety of carbohydrates with clinically proven therapeutic and pharmacological effects. Results showed that all the collected samples possess potential antioxidant activities, especially radical scavenging effects, and have potential use as food and for many pharmacological applications. Overall, phlorotannin extracts have a wide potential for functional foods and for various applications of human health.

17.3.2 Proteinaceous Biomolecules in Algae

Proteins play a vital role in the development and functioning of key body organs and control material transportation across the membranes. Moreover, a few proteins or their derivatives such as amino acids and enzymes work as building blocks and catalysts for the synthesis of other biomolecules (Hicke and Dunn 2003). The human body needs particular enzymes and amino acids for proper growth and function and algal protein may compete with other traditional protein sources like egg, meat, milk, and soybeans, in both quantitative and qualitative aspects. For example, *Chlorella vulgaris*, a species of the Chlorophyta family, has been reported to contain 51–58% DW of protein. Table 17.2 compares a variety of amino acids present in macroalgae; predominantly, aspartic acid and glutamic acid constituted a higher proportion among all the amino acids present in algae (Chronakis and Madsen 2011). Another study (Ursu et al. 2014) indicates that *C. vulgaris* can contain 76% protein on a dry mass basis, which mainly comprises alanine, glutamic acid, and aspartic acid.

A highly consumed alga, *Spirulina sp.*, became popular mainly for its higher levels of proteins and other beneficial nutrients. This species has been labeled as a "superfood" by the World Health Organization (WHO) due to its nutrient profile. *Spirulina sp.* contains 180% more calcium than milk, 670% more protein than tofu, 3100% more β-carotene than carrots, along with 5100% more iron than spinach. *Chlorella sp.* is also reported as a species with 48% DW of protein. Pharmacological applications of *Spirulina sp.* include renal protection, antihypertension, antihyperlipidemia, and antihyperglycemic activities. Tchorbanov and Bozhkova (1988) recovered protein of 60–70% of dry mass from *Chlorella* and *Scenedesmus* sp. containing about 12.2% of alanine. Phycobilins and lectins are bioactive algal proteins exploited for many industrial and pharmaceutical applications (Jiang et al. 2015). Some green microalgal species such as *Chlorella sp.* result in a reduction in the extraction yield of intracellular proteins and as a result all biomass applications result in lowering digestibility in humans. The protein content in microalgae is determined by a total nitrogen to protein conversion factor (Ramanna et al. 2014).

Ursu et al. (2014) extracted proteins from melted biomass of *C. vulgaris* indigenous to France, under various extraction conditions of temperature, pH, and centrifugation speed or tangential ultrafiltration. Under optimal conditions, the researchers isolated more than 50 g of protein from 100 g of biomass, which mainly comprised amino acids like alanine, glutamic acid, and aspartic acid. It was observed that *C. vulgaris* microalgae biomass works as a good source of valuable amino acids. Moreover, mechanical treatment or alkaline hydrolysis prior to isoelectric precipitation may provide better process efficiency. Overall, proteins from *C. vulgaris* biomass can be used as a food complement or as techno-functional ingredients in the food industry or cosmetics for their enhanced emulsifying properties and neutral conditions. Thus, microalgae contain a significant amount of high-value proteinaceous biomolecules and should be further exploited as alternative food and medicine for human beings.

Mæhre et al. (2014) also extracted protein from different micro- and macroalgal species of the marine ecosystem and quantified the protein contents extracted from different algal species using Lowry and Bradford's method with the help of two standard proteins bovine serum albumin (BSA) and casein. The highest protein contents were measured in *Aglaothamnion uruguayense* belonging to the kingdom Prymnesiophyta: $15.6 \pm 0.3\%$ of the dry biomass and the major constituent found was

Table 17.2 Amino acid profile of some selected brown, red, and green algae harvested from the coast of Norway (Mæhre et al. 2014).

	Alaria esculenta	*Laminaria digitata*	*Laminaria hyperborea*	*Fucus vesiculosus*	*Pelvetia canaliculata*	*Cladophora rupestris*	*Enteromorpha intestinalis*	*Ulva lactuca*	*Palmaria palmata*	*Vertebrata lanosa*
Essential amino acids										
Threonine	5.1 ± 0.4c	3.8 ± 0.3b	3.5 ± 0.3b	3.4 ± 0.4b	3.5 ± 0.1b	2.2 ± 0.3a	8.0 ± 0.8def	6.2 ± 0.3d	7.1 ± 0.2e	7.8 ± 0.3f
Valine	5.5 ± 0.3c	3.6 ± 0.3b	3.5 ± 0.2b	3.7 ± 0.6ab	3.9 ± 0.2b	2.4 ± 0.3a	8.4 ± 1.3 cde	7.1 ± 0.1d	9.6 ± 0.4e	7.6 ± 0.3d
Methionine	2.4 ± 0.3 cde	1.8 ± 0.1bc	1.6 ± 0.1b	1.5 ± 0.2b	1.4 ± 0.1b	0.9 ± 0.1a	2.3 ± 0.4bcde	2.2 ± 0.1d	3.1 ± 0.2e	1.8 ± 0.2bcd
Isoleucine	3.8 ± 0.5bc	2.7 ± 0.1b	2.2 ± 0.2a	2.7 ± 0.3ab	3.0 ± a0b	1.6 ± 0.4a	5.9 ± 1.0 cde	4.4 ± 0.2c	6.5 ± 0.1d	7.2 ± 0.2e
Leucine	7.5 ± 0.9c	5.2 ± 0.1b	4.5 ± 0.5b	5.0 ± 0.7b	5.2 ± 0.3b	2.7 ± 0.5a	9.5 ± 1.2 cde	8.5 ± 0.3c	11.3 ± 0.3e	9.9 ± 0.2d
Phenylalanine	4.8 ± 0.5c	3.4 ± 0.3b	3.1 ± 0.1b	3.3 ± 0.4b	3.4 ± 0.1b	2.1 ± 0.3a	7.4 ± 1.1 cdef	6.0 ± 0.2d	7.1 ± 0.2e	8.2 ± 0.2f
Lysine	5.3 ± 0.5c	3.7 ± 0.2b	3.4 ± 0.3b	4.3 ± 0.6bcd	3.7 ± 0.2b	2.1 ± 0.4a	6.4 ± 0.9c	5.1 ± 0.2c	8.9 ± 0.4d	12.6 ± 0.3e
Histidine	1.6 ± 0.2bcde	1.2 ± 0.1b	1.2 ± 0.1bc	1.1 ± 0.1b	1.0 ± 0.1ab	0.7 ± 0.2a	2.1 ± 0.4bcde	1.6 ± 0.1 cd	1.8 ± 0.1de	2.0 ± 0.0e
Tryptophan	na	na	na	na	na	na	na	na	na	na
Nonessential amino acids										
Aspartic acid*	8.4 ± 0.7c	6.2 ± 0.2b	5.9 ± 0.4b	8.3 ± 1.1bc	5.9 ± 0.3b	3.5 ± 0.4a	14.6 ± 1.8de	9.0 ± 0.3c	13.1 ± 0.3e	12.3 ± 0.2d
Serine	5.2 ± 0.4c	3.6 ± 0.1b	3.5 ± 0.3b	3.5 ± 0.5ab	3.6 ± 0.1b	2.2 ± 0.3a	7.8 ± 1.1 cde	5.9 ± 0.3c	8.4 ± 0.2e	7.7 ± 0.3d
Glutamic acid*	20.1 ± 1.1e	8.5 ± 0.6b	8.6 ± 0.6b	17.9 ± 2.2 cde	15.0 ± 1.2 cd	5.7 ± 0.8a	18.2 ± 2.0de	12.2 ± 0.5c	21.3 ± 0.5e	16.3 ± 0.4d
Proline	5.1 ± 0.8abc	3.9 ± 02b	3.5 ± 0.5ab	3.1 ± 0.5ab	3.2 ± 0.2a	2.9 ± 0.3a	6.6 ± 1.0c	5.8 ± 05c	9.7 ± 0.3d	10.8 ± 0.5d
Glycine	5.7 ± 0.6b	4.1 ± 0.2a	3.8 ± 0.2a	3.8 ± 0.5a	4.1 ± 0.2a	3.3 ± 0.4a	8.5 ± 0.9 cd	7.3 ± 0.2c	9.6 ± 0.4d	8.9 ± 0.2d
Alanine	18.9 ± 1.1 g	5.2 ± 3.0abcef	6.2 ± 0.5b	5.0 ± 0.7b	5.5 ± 0.3b	3.1 ± 0.5a	14.7 ± 1.8dg	10.1 ± 0.3de	12.2 ± 0.5df	7.6 ± 0.5c
Cysteine	n	n	n	n	n	0.5 ± 0.2bd	1.4 ± 0.4cef	1.0 ± 0.2de	0.5 ± 0.1bc	2.1 ± 0.1f
Tyrosine	2.9 ± 0.4c	1.8 ± 0.2b	1.6 ± 0.1ab	1.5 ± 0.2ab	1.4 ± 0.1a	1.5 ± 0.3ab	3.8 ± 0.5 cd	3.4 ± 0.4c	4.7 ± 0.2de	5.4 ± 0.4e
Arginine	4.8 ± 0.6 cd	3.4 ± 0.2bc	3.0 ± 0.1ab	3.2 ± 0.4ab	3.2 ± 0.2ab	25 ± 0.3a	7.4 ± 1.2def	6.0 ± 0.3d	8.6 ± 0.3f	7.0 ± 0.4e
Sum TAA	107.2 ± 6.6c	62.2 ± 4.2b	58.9 ± 3.3b	71.2 ± 8.4b	66.8 ± 3.2b	40.1 ± 5.0a	132.9 ± 17.1 cd	101.5 ± 3.9c	143.6 ± 3.7d	135.1 ± 2.7d
Relative amount essential amino acids (%)	33.5 ± 1.4a	40.9 ± 2.2 cdefg	38.9 ± 0.3 cd	35.0 ± 1.1ab	37.7 ± 0.6bc	36.7 ± 0.9abcd	37.5 ± 0.4be	40.3 ± 0.4 g	38.6 ± 0.2c	42.3 ± 0.1f
Chemical score	0.84	1.00	0.89	0.80	0.82	0.96	0.91	0.92	0.75	0.87

na, Not analyzed.

Values are expressed as mean ± SD and in g kg^{-1} dry weight. Different letters in each row indicate significant differences ($P < 0.05$) between species.

[a] Values for aspartic acid and glutamic acid represent the sums of aspartic acid + asparagine and glutamic acid + glutamine, respectively, as asparagine and glutamine are present in their acid forms after acidic hydrolysis.

glutamic acid (14.9 ± 1.5). The experimenters, in this case, suggested that the results are more reliable with Lowry's method using (BSA) standard as compared with Bradford's method with casein standard. Fleurence (1999) recovered 47% protein (dry mass basis) from red algal species *Porphyra tenera* belonging to the Rhodophyta from Europe containing aspartic acid (8.5–18.5), compared with different algal species and nutritious traditional foods *Ulva armoricana* (green seaweed), *U. pertusa* (green seaweed), *Porphyra tenera* (red seaweed), a leguminous plant, and ovalbumin under the influence of strong alkaline conditions. Among all the seaweeds, the red seaweed *P. tenera* the Rhodophyceae has potential application for nutritional food that is beneficial for human health, animal feed, and *in vitro* protein digestibility. Fleurence et al. (1995) found that the edible algae *Ulva rigida Agardh* and *Ulva rotundata*, when macerated with different enzymatic formulations or using classical methods under reductive conditions using NaOH or with a two-phase system (polyethylene glycol PEG/K_2CO_3), offered good quantity and quality of protein normally rich in aspartic and glutamic acids.

Tchorbanov and Bozhkova (1988) used organic solvents to wash unicellular algae *Chlorella* and *Scenedesmus sp.* before the enzymatic hydrolysis of proteins. Both the species were found to comprise approx. 60–70% total dry biomass containing alanine as a major constituent. The composition of amino acids extracted from protein hydrolysates meets the requirements for balanced and effective protein products for human health. Results obtained from experiments showed that cell proteins were effectively hydrolyzed after extraction with different organic solvents in the above-mentioned algal species. This makes the enzymatic hydrolysate process a very effective, efficient, and economically beneficial process for the extraction of proteins. Galland-Irmouli et al. (1999) observed that the protein content of algal biomass varies according to season as well as the algal species and maturity state. Moreover, *Palmaria palmata*, a red seaweed, contained 21.9 ± 3.5% of protein on a dry mass basis comprising mainly acidic amino acids (28.5 ± 8.7% of total amino acids) particularly aspartic acid (27.9%). Similar algal species when processed after de-fatting produced 40–50% protein on a dry mass basis (Gerde et al. 2013). The major component found was proline with 14.6% of the total proteineic mass. A sufficient amount of nonprotein nitrogen was present in the biomass, which divided into different fractions. The protein-rich product that is extracted through the isolation process has functional properties due to the presence of a high degree of glycosylation. Moreover, the recovery of protein is relatively low, compared with soybean and yeast sources. The protein contents, amino acid composition, and digestibility of protein were studied with different algal species. The digestibility of *P. palmata* protein is often reduced due to the presence of the nonprotein fraction in these algae. Table 17.3 provides an idea about the bioactivities of various enzyme hydrolysates present in algal biomass.

17.3.3 Algal Lipids

As well as proteins and carbohydrates, algae may contain substantial amounts of fats and organoleptic bioactives. The data assembled in Table 17.1 indicate that lipid content may vary from species to species and with geographical conditions. In general, algae contain lipids up to 10% of their dry mass, except some variants of *C. vulgaris*, which may contain lipids up to 19% of their dry mass. From an economic and health point of view these lipids compete with the carbohydrates and proteins. The

Table 17.3 Some selected proteinaceous enzyme atic hydrolysates and their algal sources and bioactivities.

Marine algae	Bioactivity	Type of enzymes	Origin (country)	References
Navicula incerta	Antioxidative	Pepsin α-chymotrypsin	South Korea	Kang et al. (2011)
Navicula incerta	Hepatic fibrosis inhibitory effect	Papain	South Korea	Kang et al. (2012)
Chlorella vulgaris	Antioxidative superoxide radical	Pepsin	Taiwan	Sheih et al. (2009)
Chlorella vulgaris	Angiotensin-converting enzyme (ACE) inhibitory	Pepsin	Taiwan	Sheih et al. (2010)
Chlorella vulgaris	Antiproliferation	Pepsin	Taiwan	Sheih et al. (2010)
Spirulina platensis	ACE-I inhibitory	Pepsin	Japan	Suetsuna and Chen (2001)
Undaria pinnatifida	Antihypertensive	Protease	Japan	Suetsuna et al. (2004)

oleaginous bioactives most frequently reported in algae have been classified into three groups, e.g. glycerolipids (nonpolar; neutral), phospholipids, and glycolipids or glycosylglycerides. Although algal lipids resemble those in higher plants in most cases their chain length and degree of unsaturation has been found to be higher than lipids present in land plants (Table 17.4).

The phospholipids are among the most abundant and useful lipids. The most abundant algal phospholipids include phosphatidyl glycerol, phosphatidyl choline, phosphatidyl ethanolamine, phosphatidyl inositol, and phoshatidic acid or their esters with glycerol, serine, myo-inositol, choline, and ethanolamine. The phospholipids normally represent 10–20% of algal fats, but dinophytes like *Kraenia*, *Karlodinium*, and *Takayama* species, and *Polarella glacialis* may contain phospholipids up to 90% of their total lipids. Phosphatidylglycerol and phosphatidylcholine mainly present in green (40%) and red (62%) algae, respectively, and help to maintain the photosynthetic assembly (Kumari et al. 2013) .

Algal glycolipids often comprise monogalactosyl diacylglycerol, digalactosyl diacylglycerol, and sulfolipids. The neutral glycerolipids may contain esters of various fatty acids with glycerol, and betaine lipids contain links with glycerol and fatty acids via an ether linkage. The latter class of algal lipids works as a zwitterion at a neutral pH. Some species of red algae like *Chondrus crispus*, *Polysiphonia lanosa*, *Ceratodictyon spongiosum*, and *Halymenia* sp. also contain sphingolipids. Overall, macroalgae are considered to be a low-calorie food with a high content of polyunsaturated fatty acids along with C_{28} and C_{29} sterols that have been found to exhibit antihypertensive, anti-inflammatory, antifungal, anticancer, antidiabetic, and antibacterial activities. Lipids in algae are a better alternative to fish oil with higher resistance to oxidation and enhanced bioavailability (Ibañez and Cifuentes 2013).

Paiva et al. (2014) observed that edible species of *Porphyra sp.*, *Osmundea pinnatifida*, and *Fucus spiralis* may contain lipids at values of 8.88 ± 0.05, 7.53 ± 0.07, and 5.23 ± 0.03 of their body weight, respectively. The fatty acids extracted from these

Table 17.4 Fatty acid profiles of some selected brown, red, and green algae harvested from the coast of Norway (Mæhre et al. 2014).

	Alaria esculenta	*Laminaria digitata*	*Laminaria hyperborea*	*Fucus vesiculosus*	*Pelvetia canaliculata*	*Cladophora rupestris*	*Enteromorpha intestinalis*	*Ulva lactuca*	*Palmaria palmata*	*Vertebrata lanosa*
C14:0	8.9 ± 0.2b	9.1 ± 0.1b	9.0 ± 0.8bcd	12.4 ± 0.0d	9.5 ± 0.2bc	9.0 ± 3.2abcd	1.8 ± 0.5a	0.9 ± 0.1a	10.2 ± 02c	2.2 ± 0.2a
C16:0	26.9 ± 0.4d	21.7 ± 0.3c	23.3 ± 0.4c	11.4 ± 0.2b	9.8 ± 0.1a	31.8 ± 2.8 cde	23.2 ± 1.2 cd	26.0 ± 0.4d	31.9 ± 0.5e	25.6 ± 0.1d
C18:0	1.7 ± 0.0c	0.8 ± 0.1ab	1.3 ± 0.5abcd	0.6 ± 0.0b	1.9 ± 0.0d	nda	nda	nda	1.6 ± 01 cd	0.9 ± 0.1b
Sum saturated acids	37.4 ± 0.6e	31.5 ± 0.3d	33.7 ± 0.7d	24.3 ± 0.2b	21.2 ± 0.3a	40.8 ± 0.5f	25.0 ± 0.7bc	26.9 ± 0.4c	43.7 ± 0.6 g	28.6 ± 0.2c
C16:1, n-7	1.5 ± 0.0 cd	0.9 ± 0.0b	nda	1.1 ± 0.1bc	1.4 ± 0.0 cd	8.3 ± 1.1ef	1.8 ± 0.1de	0.9 ± 0.0b	1.4 ± 0.1bcd	8.0 ± 0.0f
C18:1, n-9	23.9 ± 0.5bd	17.8 ± 0.5ce	26.5 ± 4.2acdfg	46.0 ± 0.4 g	40.8 ± 0.3f	10.5 ± 2.1abc	5.4 ± 3.3be	0.8 ± 0.0ab	5.1 ± 1.1ab	5.6 ± 1.0ab
C18:1, n-7	nda	nda	nda	nda	nda	$8.6 \pm 2.$abcd	15.2 ± 0.9d	14.6 ± 0.0d	2.2 ± 0.0b	9.0 ± 0.2c
Sum monounsaturated fatty acids	25.4 ± 0.5d	18.7 ± 0.5bc	26.5 ± 4.2abcdef	47.1 ± 0.3f	42.2 ± 0.3e	27.3 ± 1.0d	22.4 ± 2.3bd	16.3 ± 0.0b	8.7 ± 1.1a	22.6 ± 0.8 cd
C16:3, n-3	nda	nda	nda	nda	nda	nda	1.2 ± 0.1b	2.6 ± 0.0c	nda	nda
C16:4, n-3	nda	nda	nda	nda	nda	2.1 ± 0.8ab	7.6 ± 0.4C	7.1 ± 0.0bc	nda	nda
C18:2, n-6	8.2 ± 0.2e	9.5 ± 0.0d	5.0 ± 0.2c	8.0 ± 0.0e	13.4 ± 0.1 g	7.4 ± 0.8bcdef	5.8 ± 0.6bcde	10.5 ± 0.0f	0.6 ± 0.0a	4.1 ± 0.1b
C18.3, n-3	5.1 ± 0.0e	7.5 ± 0.1f	3.8 ± 0.4cde	2.7 ± 0.0c	3.4 ± 0.0d	5.2 ± 1.7abcdefg	14.4 ± 0.8 h	15.2 ± 0.1 gh	nda	0.8 ± 0.1b
C18:4, n-3	8.1 ± 0.2e	10.2 ± 0.1f	8.1 ± 0.8def	2.2 ± 0.1c	1.9 ± 0.1c	4.3 ± 1.4abcdef	6.1 ± 0.2d	6.3 ± 0.1d	nda	1.0 ± 0.1b
C20:2, n-6	nda	nda	nda	0.9 ± 0.0b	1.0 ± 0.0c	nda	nda	nda	nda	0.7 ± 0.0b
C20:3, n-6	nda	nda	nda	1.0 ± 0.0b	2.1 ± 0.0d	nda	nda	nda	nda	1.5 ± 0.0c
C20:4, n-6	4.6 ± 0.0c	7.0 ± 0.1e	7.6 ± 0.8 cde	7.4 ± 0.1e	8.2 ± 0.3e	nda	nda	nda	0.7 ± 0.0b	5.6 ± 0.2d
C20:5, n-3	7.1 ± 0.1d	11.4 ± 0.1e	9.5 ± 1.0 cde	3.7 ± 0.0bc	4.0 ± 0.1bc	2.5 ± 0.6ab	0.8 ± 0.1a	0.9 ± 0.2a	34.3 ± 0.1f	32.1 ± 1.0f
C22:5, n-3	nda	nda	nda	nda	nda	nda	1.2 ± 0.0b	1.2 ± 0.0b	n.d.a	n.d.a
Sum polyunsaturated fatty acids	33.2 ± 0.2b	45.6 ± 0.2d	34.2 ± 3.2abcd	25.8 ± 0.1a	34.0 ± 0.3b	21.5 ± 3.1b	37.1 ± 0.8ab	42.6 ± 0.1c	35.4 ± 0.5b	45.8 ± 0.9 cd
n-3	20.4 ± 0.3b	29.1 ± 0.2 cde	21.5 ± 2.2abcdfh	8.6 ± 0.1a	9.3 ± 0.2b	14.1 ± 2.3ab	31.3 ± 1.4defgh	32.1 ± 0.1 fg	34.3 ± 0.1 hi	33.8 ± 0.9egi
n-6	12.8 ± 0.1 g	16.5 ± 0.1 h	12.7 ± 1.0efghi	17.2 ± 0.1i	24.6 ± 0.3j	7.4 ± 0.8bcd	5.8 ± 0.6b	10.5 ± 0.0cf	1.1 ± 04a	11.9 ± 0.0de
n-6/n-3	0.6 ± 0.8d	0.6 ± 0.0d	0.6 ± 0.0d	2.0 ± 0.0e	2.6 ± 0.1f	0.5 ± 0.0 cd	0.2 ± 0.0ab	0.3 ± 0.0b	0.0 ± 0.0a	0.4 ± 0.0bc
ni	4.0 ± 0.9ab	4.2 ± 0.5ab	5.6 ± 0.3b	2.8 ± 0.1a	2.6 ± 0.0a	10.3 ± 1.9abc	15.5 ± 1.0c	14.2 ± 0.4c	12.2 ± 0.5c	3.0 ± 0.2a

nd, Not detected; ni, not identified.
Values are given as mean ± SD and in percentage of total fatty acid content. Different letters indicate significant difference ($P < 0.05$) between species.

species can be used in food supplements and in various pharmaceutical products for a balanced diet. The lipids of *Porphyra* species can be used in fish feed as food additives to increase body weight and levels of triglyceride deposited in the muscles of fish, which also support the fish in stress conditions. These researchers ranked the above algal species as among the most beneficial for human health if these are regularly consumed and they have protective and effective effects against degenerative diseases. Similarly, Gressler et al. (2010) extracted lipids and fatty acids from four algal species belonging to the Rhodophyta, with values of 1.1–6.2% and 16:0 (5.3 ± 0.00), 16:0 (5.8 ± 0.2), 16:0 (4.1 ± 0.1), and 16:0 (3.1 ± 0.2), respectively. The algal species *Gracilaria domingensis* and *Gracilaria birdiae* have the same amount of lipid content, but slightly differ in fatty acid contents.

Baghel et al. (2014) extracted the total fatty acid contents from a red algal species (*Gracilaria crassa*) and found palmitic acid (52.89 ± 0.59) and stearic acid (32.56 ± 0.9) as major components in the chemical composition. This nutritional composition of algal species can be used as a human diet source and for pharmacological activities. (Kim et al. 2012) extracted lipids from biomass of alga *C. vulgaris* using Bligh and Dyer's method and ionic liquid mixtures using methanol. The lipid content extracted with the first method was 10.6 and 11.1%, respectively, and 12.5 and 19.0% of lipid content were extracted using a mixture of ionic liquids [Bmim] [CF_3SO_3]. They also found that lipid content extracted from ionic liquid mixtures had higher efficiencies compared with the Bligh and Dyers' method. The experiments showed that wide ranges of fatty acids can extracted using ionic liquid methanol mixtures, in which C16:0, C16:1, and C18:2 fatty acids were dominantly extracted. Moreover, imidazolium-based ionic liquids have some disadvantages since they are expensive and toxic aquatically. However, the ionic liquid mixture with methanol produces an efficient and environmentally friendly system to extract the lipids from different algal species due to the green solvent properties of ionic liquids. Hence, due to the habitat diversity of algae and the presence of heterogeneous forms of lipids, utilization of lipids as food and nutraceuticals has been immensely enhanced. The presence of lipids in algae illustrate the importance of its use as food additives and as nutraceuticals.

17.3.4 Algal Minerals

Algae are considered to be one of the richest sources of minerals. The most common minerals found in algae are potassium, iron, copper, calcium, sodium, iodine, magnesium, and phosphorus. All these minerals are required for the proper functioning of different catabolic and anabolic processes in human beings and other living organisms. For example, calcium, phosphorus, and magnesium are used to build bones and teeth, while sodium and potassium are used to maintain water balance, maintain acid–base levels, and for transfer of nutrients in and outside of an individual cell. Deficiencies of these minerals may cause severe impairments to human health. For example, osteoporosis in females may occur because of lack of calcium and deficiency of iron may lead to anemia. Baghel et al. (2014) extracted the total mineral content from red algal species *G. crassa*, which was16 027.4 ± 344.08 mg $(100\,g)^{-1}$ DW, containing sodium (4105 ± 682.0 mg) and potassium (11 170 ± 686.94 mg) as the main fractions in their chemical composition. Table 17.5 provides a typical comparison of mineral macronutrients, and heavy metal contents of brown, green, and red algae. The results showed that macroalgae can work as a potential source of various macro- and micronutrients, especially potassium followed by sodium. The high level of K > Na is beneficial for the health of humans and helps in the reduction of obesity and blood lipid concentrations, and reduces the coronary heart disease risk. It has been found that intake of algae can overcome calcium (Ca) and Iron (Fe) deficiency; the latter is particularly important for growing children and women at pre- and post-menopausal stages (Cofrades et al. 2010). Their intake has been found to be associated with maintenance of proper sugar levels, maintenance of cholesterol level, etc. Microalgae are also rich in calcium and magnesium.

17.3.5 Algal Vitamins

Vitamins play a vital role in many chemical processes in the human body and are considered as micronutrients. Vitamins are required in small quantities but the deficiency of vitamins in the human body may lead to some diverse effects such as loss of vision, rickets, scurvy, beriberi, etc. Thus, vitamins are among the most important nutrients for the proper growth and function of the human body and health of an individual. Algae are reported to contain some essential vitamins. Vitamins (A, B^1, B^2, B^6, B^{12}, C, E) are present in various species of algae. Marine algae have been used for the treatment of goiter and scurvy, which is an indication of the presence of vitamin C in algae. Cyanobacteria have also been reported to contain vitamin B^{12}. Therefore, macroalgae can be a potential source of vitamins for human beings (Priyadarshani and Rath 2012).

17.4 Commercial Importance of Macroalgae in Human Nutrition

There are many species of macro- and microalgae that have been used by humans to meet nutritional requirements or health benefits. For example, algal species of *Nostoc*, *Arthrospira*, and *Aphanizomenon*, also known as blue-green algae, have been used in the human diet for thousands of years. As stated above, Japan was the first to cultivate *Chlorella sp.* at commercial levels for food and pharmaceutical use. This genus covers the unicellular algae of the Chlorophyta division or simply green algae. The most interesting features of these algae include their higher photosynthetic efficiency (may exceed that of several land crops such as sugarcane) and the ability to store food/energy. These algal species are usually considered to be a rich source of protein (amino acids), dietary fiber, minerals, and vitamins. Following Japan, the United States, China, Taiwan, and Indonesia also produce *Chlorella sp.* on a commercial scale. There are many companies across the globe, like Prime Chlorella™, Taiwan Chlorella, Sun Chlorella, Lucky Vitamin™, and HerbMark, which produce and market *Chlorella sp.* for its potential health benefits. Taiwan Chlorella Manufacturing Co. Ltd. is considered as the largest producer of this microalga, with 400 tons of dry biomass produced per year, followed by Klotz, Germany, with 130–150 tons of dried mass per year. The worldwide annual business of *Chlorella*-based products ranges up to US$38 billion. The microalgae of genus *Chlorella* contain almost all essential amino acids and a substantial level of vitamin B_{12}, magnesium, lutein, and other

Table 17.5 Mineral profile and heavy metal content of some selected brown, red, and green algae harvested from the coast of Norway (Mæhre et al. 2014).

	Alaria esculenta	*Laminaria digitata*	*Laminaria hyperborea*	*Fucus vesiculosus*	*Pelvetia canaliculata*	*Cladophora rupestris*	*Enteromorpha intestinalis*	*Ulva lactuca*	*Palmaria palmata*	*Vertebrata lanosa*
Macrominerals										
Calcium	8000	10 000	8000	12 000	8300	29 000	5500	3500	3600	6400
Magnesium	8700	8400	6400	7400	9600	12 000	15 000	26 000	5300	6000
Phosphorus	2300	1200	1600	840	730	870	1200	500	2700	1100
Microminerals										
Copper	2.4	1.6	1.7	1.8	2.6	17	4.9	6	4.9	8
Iron	87	58	120	92	130	10 000	6000	210	100	480
Iodine	220	3100	3500	130	210	63	130	21	260	1300
Manganese	5.6	3.1	6.5	34	8.6	240	130	11	11	20
Selenium	0.041	0.021	0.033	0.03	0.035	0.066	0.028	0.049	0.14	0.53
Zinc	49	24	22	26	31	30	25	6	29	81
Heavy metals										
Arsenic	48	64	55	41	28	9.4	4.9	7.9	10	93
Cadmium	3.4	0.1	0.48	1.2	0.48	0.091	0.12	0.092	0.48	3.8
Mercury	<0.005	0.006	0.007	0.011	0.047	0.006	0.014	0.005	0.005	0.01

Values are expressed as mean of two parallels and in mg kg^{-1} dry weight.

carotenoids. The extracts of these microalgae are thought to be effective against macular degeneration and cataracts. Other health-promoting attributes associated with *Chlorella* include atherosclerosis and hypercholesterolemia and antitumor activity. Meanwhile, β-1,3-glucan present in *Chlorella* is an immunostimulator, free radical scavenger, and blood lipid reducer.

Subsequent to *Chlorella*, *Spirulina sp.*, a prokaryotic cyanobacterium, has been frequently produced during the past couple of decades for fish and poultry feed, dyes and pigmentation, vitamins and pharmaceutical supplementation. More than 5000 t of these algal species are produced worldwide, mainly in the United States, China, Taiwan, India, Japan, and Thailand. Many companies are producing and selling nutraceuticals based on *Spirulina sp.*, but Hainan Simai Enterprising Ltd. is the world's largest producer, located in China. Likewise, Yangon (Myanmar) Spirulina factory sells various products like chips, tablets, pasta made up of *Spirulina* and a liquid extract containing *Spirulina*. Another corporation, Cyanotech (Hawaii, USA), offers a variety of products under the brand name Spirulina. *Spirulina* species mainly consist of protein but they contain β-carotene in quantities about 10 times larger than in carrots. These algal species have been found to be useful for persons fighting obesity, diabetes, high cholesterol, and hypertension. *Spirulina* (*Arthrospira*) *sp.* also works well to remedy hyperlipidemia and renal failure and can be used for growth promotion of intestinal *Lactobacilli* and to control elevated serum glucose levels.

Dunaliella or its most dominant species *Dunaliella salina* (*D. salina*) has also become a good source of dietary protein and carbohydrates. The interesting features of this algal species include their very thin cell wall, which favors its application in the pharmaceutical and functional food industries. Moreover, this algal division is much more halotolerant. The world's largest producer of *D. salina* is Cognis Nutrition and Health, Australia. This strain of microalga is famous due to the presence of β-carotene (14% DW). *Dunaliella* is used in the form of powder in dietary supplements and functional foods. Another major commercial microalga is called *Aphanizomenon flos-aquae*, which is used as a health promoter alone or in combination with other nutraceuticals. All the pharmacological and biological properties associated with micro- and macroalgae are down to the presence of potentially bioactive compounds. These bioactives have been clinically exploited using many *in vitro* and *in vivo* studies (Hashemian et al. 2019).

Macroalgae are nature's most potent source of bioactive compounds. Algae are being used as a source of food, food additives, animal feed, and for pharmacological purposes in different regions across the world. The high content of polysaccharides and amino acids, and low content of lipids with higher polyunsaturated fatty acids, variety of vitamins, β-carotene, antioxidants, dietary fiber, and richness in minerals all add to the health benefits and render macroalgae an important source of food. Moreover, due to the nutritional attributes of the macroalgae, countries like China, Japan, Korea, and now many European countries have developed industries for the production of macroalgae to use in bakery products, meats, and other processed foods. Thus, more research is required to explore the potential of algae for the presence of novel bioactive compounds to benefit humans and other living organisms.

References

Baghel, R.S., Kumari, P., Reddy, C.R.K., and Jha, B. (2014). Growth, pigments, and biochemical composition of marine red alga *Gracilaria crassa*. *Journal of Applied Phycology* **26** (5): 2143–2150. https://doi.org/10.1007/s10811-014-0250-5.

Burkholder, P.R. (1973). The ecology of marine antibiotics and coral reefs. *Biology and Geology of Coral Reefs* **2**: 117–182.

Caron, L. and Brown, J. (1987). Chlorophyll-carotenoid protein complexes from the diatom, Phaeodactylum tricornutum: spectrophotometric, pigment and polypeptide analyses. *Plant and Cell Physiology* **28** (5): 775–785.

Chronakis, I.S. and Madsen, M. (2011). Algal proteins. In: *Handbook of Food Proteins*, 353–394. London: Elsevier.

Cofrades, S., López-Lopez, I., Bravo, L. et al. (2010). Nutritional and antioxidant properties of different brown and red Spanish edible seaweeds. *Food Science and Technology International* **16**: 361–371.

Cornish, M.L. and Garbary, D.J. (2010). Antioxidants from macroalgae: potential applications in human health and nutrition. *Algae* **25** (4): 155–171.

D'Armas, H., Jaramillo, C., D'Armas, M. et al. (2019). Proximate composition of several macroalgae from the coast of Salinas Bay, Ecuador. *Revista de Biología Tropical* **67** (1): 61–68.

Davis, T.A., Volesky, B., and Mucci, A. (2003). A review of the biochemistry of heavy metal biosorption by brown algae. *Water Research* **37** (18): 4311–4330.

Denis, C., Morançais, M., Li, M. et al. (2010). Study of the chemical composition of edible red macroalgae *Grateloupia turuturu* from Brittany (France). *Food Chemistry* **119** (3): 913–917. https://doi.org/10.1016/j.foodchem.2009.07.047.

Edwards, M.R. (2008). *Green Algae Strategy: End Biowar I and Engineer Sustainable Food and Biofuel*. Lulu. com.

Fleurence, J. (1999). Seaweed proteins: biochemical, nutritional aspects and potential uses. *Trends in Food Science & Technology* **10** (1): 25–28.

Fleurence, J., Le Coeur, C., Mabeau, S. et al. (1995). Comparison of different extractive procedures for proteins from the edible seaweeds *Ulva rigida* and *Ulva rotundata*. *Journal of Applied Phycology* **7** (6): 577–582.

Galland-Irmouli, A.-V., Fleurence, J., Lamghari, R. et al. (1999). Nutritional value of proteins from edible seaweed *Palmaria palmata* (dulse). *The Journal of Nutritional Biochemistry* **10** (6): 353–359.

Gerde, J.A., Wang, T., Yao, L. et al. (2013). Optimizing protein isolation from defatted and non-defatted *Nannochloropsis* microalgae biomass. *Algal Research* **2** (2): 145–153.

Gressler, V., Yokoya, N.S., Fujii, M.T. et al. (2010). Lipid, fatty acid, protein, amino acid and ash contents in four Brazilian red algae species. *Food Chemistry* **120** (2): 585–590.

Hashemian, M., Ahmadzadeh, H., Hosseini, M. et al. (2019). Production of microalgae-derived high-protein biomass to enhance food for animal feedstock and human consumption. In: *Advanced Bioprocessing for Alternative Fuels, Biobased Chemicals, and Bioproducts*, 393–405. London: Elsevier.

Hicke, L. and Dunn, R. (2003). Regulation of membrane protein transport by ubiquitin and ubiquitin-binding proteins. *Annual Review of Cell and Developmental Biology* **19** (1): 141–172.

Ibañez, E. and Cifuentes, A. (2013). Benefits of using algae as natural sources of functional ingredients. *Journal of the Science of Food and Agriculture* **93** (4): 703–709.

Jiang, L., Pei, H., Hu, W. et al. (2015). The feasibility of using complex wastewater from a monosodium glutamate factory to cultivate *Spirulina subsalsa* and accumulate biochemical composition. *Bioresource Technology* **180**: 304–310.

Kang, E.-H., Choi, S.-W., Chung, S.E. et al. (2011). Photoluminescence characteristics of Sr3SiO5: Eu2+ yellow phosphors synthesized by solid-state method and pechini process. *Journal of The Electrochemical Society* **158** (11): J330.

Kang, K.-H., Qian, Z.-J., Ryu, B. et al. (2012). Protective effects of protein hydrolysate from marine microalgae *Navicula incerta* on ethanol-induced toxicity in HepG2/CYP2E1 cells. *Food Chemistry* **132** (2): 677–685.

Khataee, A., Zarei, M., Dehghan, G. et al. (2011). Biotreatment of a triphenylmethane dye solution using a Xanthophyta alga: modeling of key factors by neural network. *Journal of the Taiwan Institute of Chemical Engineers* **42** (3): 380–386.

Kim, Y.H., Choi, Y.K., Park, J. et al. (2012). Ionic liquid-mediated extraction of lipids from algal biomass. *Bioresource Technology* **109**: 312–315. https://doi.org/10.1016/j.biortech.2011.04.064.

Kumari, P., Kumar, M., Reddy, C., and Jha, B. (2013). Algal lipids, fatty acids and sterols. In: *Functional Ingredients from Algae for Foods and Nutraceuticals*, 87–134. London: Elsevier.

Lewin, R.A. (1956). Extracellular polysaccharides of green algae. *Canadian Journal of Microbiology* **2** (7): 665–672.

Leyton, A., Pezoa-Conte, R., Barriga, A. et al. (2016). Identification and efficient extraction method of phlorotannins from the brown seaweed *Macrocystis pyrifera* using an orthogonal experimental design. *Algal Research* **16**: 201–208.

Li, Y.-X., Wijesekara, I., Li, Y., and Kim, S.-K. (2011). Phlorotannins as bioactive agents from brown algae. *Process Biochemistry* **46** (12): 2219–2224.

Mæhre, H.K., Malde, M.K., Eilertsen, K.E., and Elvevoll, E.O. (2014). Characterization of protein, lipid and mineral contents in common Norwegian seaweeds and evaluation of their potential as food and feed. *Journal of the Science of Food and Agriculture* **94** (15): 3281–3290.

Mohammed, H., Abdelgeliel, A.S., Cochis, A. et al. (2019). Bioactivity of Red Sea algae for industrial application and biomedical engineering. In: *Marine-Derived Biomaterials for Tissue Engineering Applications*, 491–522. Springer.

Nagappan, T. and Vairappan, C.S. (2014). Nutritional and bioactive properties of three edible species of green algae, genus *Caulerpa* (*Caulerpaceae*). *Journal of Applied Phycology* **26** (2): 1019–1027. https://doi.org/10.1007/s10811-013-0147-8.

Osman, N., El-Manawy, I., and Amin, A. (2011). Nutritional composition and mineral content of five macroalgae from Red Sea. *Egyptian Journal of Phycology* **12** (90): 89–102.

Ozgun, S., Turan, F., Çinar, M.E. et al. (2015). Biochemical composition of some brown algae from Iskenderun Bay, the northeastern Mediterranean coast of Turkey. *Journal of Black Sea/Mediterranean Environment* **21** (2): 125–134.

Paiva, L., Lima, E., Patarra, R.F. et al. (2014). Edible Azorean macroalgae as source of rich nutrients with impact on human health. *Food Chemistry* **164**: 128–135.

Polat, S. and Ozogul, Y. (2009). Fatty acid, mineral and proximate composition of some seaweeds from the northeastern Mediterranean coast. *Italian Journal of Food Science* **21** (3).

Priyadarshani, I. and Rath, B. (2012). Commercial and industrial applications of micro algae – a review. *Journal of Algal Biomass Utilization* **3** (4): 89–100.

Ramanna, L., Guldhe, A., Rawat, I., and Bux, F. (2014). The optimization of biomass and lipid yields of *Chlorella sorokiniana* when using wastewater supplemented with different nitrogen sources. *Bioresource Technology* **168**: 127–135.

Sahoo, D. and Kumar, S. (2015). Xanthophyceae, Euglenophyceae and Dinophyceae. In: *The Algae World*, 259–305. Springer.

Sarwar, M.H., Sarwar, M.F., Khalid, M.T., and Sarwar, M. (2015). Effects of eating the balance food and diet to protect human health and prevent diseases. *American Journal of Circuits, Systems and Signal Processing* **1** (3): 99–104.

Sheih, I.-C., Wu, T.-K., and Fang, T.J. (2009). Antioxidant properties of a new antioxidative peptide from algae protein waste hydrolysate in different oxidation systems. *Bioresource Technology* **100** (13): 3419–3425.

Sheih, I.-C., Fang, T.J., Wu, T.-K., and Lin, P.-H. (2010). Anticancer and antioxidant activities of the peptide fraction from algae protein waste. *Journal of Agricultural and Food Chemistry* **58** (2): 1202–1207.

Suetsuna, K. and Chen, J.-R. (2001). Identification of antihypertensive peptides from peptic digest of two microalgae, *Chlorella vulgaris* and *Spirulina platensis*. *Marine Biotechnology* **3** (4): 305–309.

Suetsuna, K., Maekawa, K., and Chen, J.-R. (2004). Antihypertensive effects of *Undaria pinnatifida* (wakame) peptide on blood pressure in spontaneously hypertensive rats. *The Journal of Nutritional Biochemistry* **15** (5): 267–272.

Tchorbanov, B. and Bozhkova, M. (1988). Enzymatic hydrolysis of cell proteins in green algae *Chlorella* and *Scenedesmus* after extraction with organic solvents. *Enzyme and Microbial Technology* **10** (4): 233–238.

Tseng, C. (2001). Algal biotechnology industries and research activities in China. *Journal of Applied Phycology* **13** (4): 375–380.

Ursu, A.-V., Marcati, A., Sayd, T. et al. (2014). Extraction, fractionation and functional properties of proteins from the microalgae *Chlorella vulgaris*. *Bioresource Technology* **157**: 134–139. https://doi.org/10.1016/j.biortech.2014.01.071.

Wang, L., Min, M., Li, Y. et al. (2010). Cultivation of green algae *Chlorella* sp. in different wastewaters from municipal wastewater treatment plant. *Applied Biochemistry and Biotechnology* **162** (4): 1174–1186.

Wang, L., Wang, X., Wu, H., and Liu, R. (2014). Overview on biological activities and molecular characteristics of sulfated polysaccharides from marine green algae in recent years. *Marine Drugs* **12** (9): 4984–5020.

Wells, M.L., Potin, P., Craigie, J.S. et al. (2017). Algae as nutritional and functional food sources: revisiting our understanding. *Journal of Applied Phycology* **29** (2): 949–982.

Woelkerling, W.J., Irvine, L., and Harvey, A.S. (1993). Growth-forms in non-geniculate coralline red algae (Coralliinales, Rhodophyta). *Australian Systematic Botany* **6** (4): 277–293.

Wong, K.H. and Cheung, P.C.K. (2000). Nutritional evaluation of some subtropical red and green seaweeds: part I – proximate composition, amino acid profiles and some physico-chemical properties. *Food Chemistry* **71** (4): 475–482. https://doi.org/10.1016/S0308-8146(00)00175-8.

Zhang, Z., Wang, F., Wang, X. et al. (2010). Extraction of the polysaccharides from five algae and their potential antioxidant activity in vitro. *Carbohydrate Polymers* **82** (1): 118–121.

18
Advancements in Algae in Nutraceutical and Functional Food

Froylán M.E. Escalante and Daniel A. Pérez-Rico
Department of Chemistry, Autonomous University of Guadalajara, Zapopan, Mexico

18.1 Introduction

Algae, namely seaweeds (macroalgae), microalgae, and cyanobacteria, are the oldest members of the plant kingdom, dating back 3 billion years and distributed from the polar region to tropical areas and from nutrient-rich coastal seas to oligotrophic open oceans. Marine algae range in size from microalgae, microscopic individual cells, to macroalgae, pluricellular organisms reaching up to 30 m in size (Qin et al. 2012; Sathasivam et al. 2017). These plants have been consumed by humans for thousands of years, as proven by archeological evidence from 14 000 BCE, being used for food and medicinal purposes (Wells et al. 2017).

The medicinal value of cyanobacteria was appreciated as early as 1500 BCE (other authors date it back even further to 2000 years ago) in China when *Nostoc* strains were used to treat gout, fistula, and several forms of cancer, while *Spirulina* (*Arthrospira*) from Lake Texcoco was already collected by the Aztec population c. 1300 CE. The very high incidence of the novel, biologically active compounds isolated so far indicates that cyanobacteria and microalgae are a rich source of potentially useful natural products. On the other hand, the first report referring to seaweeds use dealt with "nori" (*Porphyra*), which has been collected since the year 530 CE (García et al. 2017; Priyadarshani and Rath 2012; Pulz and Gross 2004; Singh et al. 2002).

Traditionally, both seaweeds and microalgae, have been especially used as food in Asian countries like China, Japan, and Korea, while in Western countries, seaweeds are mainly used in the pharmaceutical, food, and cosmetic industries as a source of hydrocolloids (Jiménez-Escrig et al. 2011). Moreover, they are a component of the bait sources for animal aquaculture and produce abundant valuable compounds for the chemical industry and human health, including lipids (e.g. fatty acids), polysaccharides (e.g. alginate, agar, carrageenan, laminarin, and sulfated carbohydrates), proteins and

Recent Advances in Micro- and Macroalgal Processing: Food and Health Perspectives, First Edition.
Edited by Gaurav Rajauria and Yvonne V. Yuan.

amino acids, pigments (e.g. chlorophylls, carotenoids, and phycobiliproteins), and also potential new pharmaceuticals (e.g. peptides, oral vaccines), leading to their use as nutraceuticals.

The term nutraceutical derives from joining the terms "nutrition" and "pharmaceutical." It refers to foods or food ingredients with medical or health benefits. Through food-based approaches, active substances with pharmaceutical properties are given to humans to prevent or treat certain diseases linked to food. Several active compounds produced by different marine organisms have a wide role in nutraceutical applications. These marine derived active ingredients (including polyunsaturated fatty acids [PUFAs], polysaccharides, polyphenols, bioactive peptides, and carotenoids) are known for their anticancer, anti-inflammatory, antioxidant, and antimicrobial activities. They are applied as nutraceuticals, for example, to combat obesity (Ruocco et al. 2016). However, the terms "nutraceutical" or "functional food" have no legal status in many nations. The path from algal research to the launching of new food products or dietary supplements is strongly affected by industrial, regulatory, and nutritional considerations. For instance, the European regulations on novel food and its safety affect the marketing of microalgae products if the toxins, allergens, or other harmful compounds potentially produced by algae are not assessed (Vigani et al. 2015; Wells et al. 2017).

Even though many studies report the potential nutritional or bioactive content of different algae, far fewer studies quantify the nutrient bioavailability and phytochemicals from algal-enriched foods (Wells et al. 2017). Therefore, the purpose of this chapter is to give the first glance to the most relevant reports in the past decade referring to the use of algae as a source of valuable food and nutraceutical products. The structure of the chapter depicts four main groups of molecules: carbohydrates, lipids, proteins, and pigments from seaweeds and microalgae. After a general description of each group, the most representative molecule subclasses in each group are analyzed. Culture conditions, extraction, and purification, as well as a deeper understanding of the physiological effects of the most important molecules, are discussed in detail.

18.2 Algal Derived Molecules

18.2.1 Carbohydrates

In the biosphere, carbohydrates are the major organic compounds produced by photosynthetic, aquatic, and terrestrials organisms used as a source of energy for heterotrophic organisms. They are also important because of their participation in the cellular structure, immune system, fertilization, and food storage (Ruocco et al. 2016).

18.2.1.1 Carbohydrates in Seaweed Seaweeds have been studied for a long time owing to their importance in the production of carbohydrates, mainly polysaccharides, such as cellulose, fucoidans, laminarin, alginic acid from brown seaweeds (Figure 18.1), carrageenan and agar mainly from red seaweeds, and sulfated polysaccharides such as ulvan from green seaweeds. In comparison with cultivated vegetables, edible seaweeds are potentially good sources of nonstarch polysaccharides, minerals, trace elements, and certain vitamins (Burtin 2003; Gupta and Abu-Ghannam 2011; Kumar et al. 2008). The total carbohydrate content ranges from 20 to 76% on a dry weight

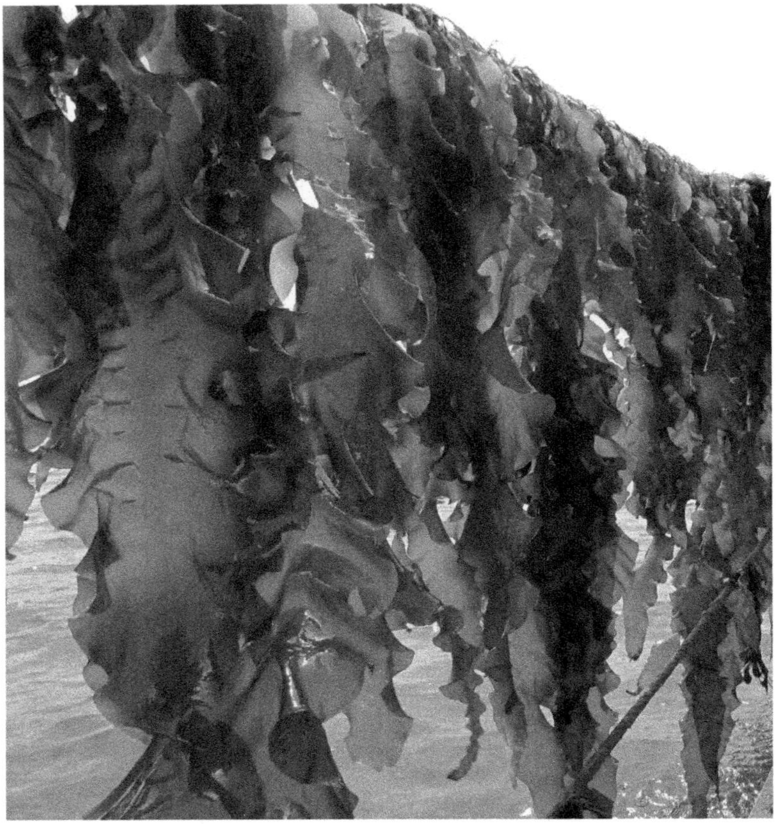

Figure 18.1 Sweet kelp (*Saccharina lattisima*) previously known as *Laminaria saccharina*. Source: Courtesy of Merinov Québec Fisheries and Aquaculture Innovation Centre.

basis, mainly dietary fiber; therefore, seaweeds are not a good source of carbohydrates in terms of bioavailability (Rajapakse and Kim 2011).

In general, the carbohydrate content in seaweeds varies depending on the group to which they belong, i.e. brown seaweed (Phaeophyta), red seaweed (Rhodophyta), or green seaweed (Chlorophyta). Brown seaweeds like *Sargassum* and *Macrocystis* are industrially important mainly for their alginic acid content; red seaweeds, mainly *Kappaphycus* and *Beaphycus*, are commercially exploited for agar and carrageenan production for foods; meanwhile, green seaweeds, mainly from the Ulvaceae family, are able to accumulate up to 65% carbohydrates on a dry weight basis, being a rich source of ulvan and glucuronic acid (Dawczynski et al. 2007; Holdt and Kraan 2011; Kumar et al. 2008; Tanna and Mishra 2018).

Among the main polysaccharides from seaweeds, alginate, carrageenan, fucoidan, and ulvan are widely applied in the biological and biochemical areas owing to their biocompatibility and availability (Wijesekara and Karunarathna 2017). Some of these molecules have been related to immunomodulatory and anticarcinogenic activities (Burtin 2003; Gupta and Abu-Ghannam 2011).

18.2.1.2 Carbohydrates in Microalgae Microalgae are an unrecognized and unexploited source of carbohydrates. Compared with higher plants, they use sunlight energy more efficiently (Priyadarshani and Rath 2012) and are responsible for almost 50% of the photosynthetic activity on Earth (Milledge 2011). Most of the carbohydrates in nature are found as polysaccharides, which is itself a very complex group of molecules due to the variety of its monomers, linkages, polymerization levels, and conjugation with other molecules (Hayes 2012). With more than 30 000 species documented, microalgae provide an immense diversity of polysaccharides (Foley et al. 2011; Tomaselli 2003).

Glucose, galactose, and xylose are the predominant carbohydrates in microalgae, while mannose, rhamnose, and fucose are notably present as well (Cesário et al. 2018; De Jesus Raposo et al. 2015; Delattre et al. 2016). Most of their polysaccharides are conformed heterogeneously of such monomers. The most abundant polysaccharides are cellulose and starch, accumulating in the cell wall and intracellularly as reserve material, respectively (Chew et al. 2017). Carbohydrates can constitute up to 64% of microalgal biomass on a dry weight basis, with *Porphyridium cruentum* and *Spirogyra* sp. being two of the higher producers with ranges from 40–57% and 33–64%, respectively (Priyadarshani and Rath 2012).

Microalgal carbohydrates appear to have good overall digestibility. The lack of lignin in microalgal biomass facilitates its transformation processes (Khan et al. 2018). Still, the presence of complex polysaccharides makes microalgae a considerable source of dietary fiber, which is an important ingredient of a functional food (Dhingra et al. 2012). Digestibility of microalgae has been poorly studied and is an issue that should be clarified along with a proper understanding of the interactions with human metabolism (Wells et al. 2017).

Microalgae have not been associated long with commercial carbohydrate production; however, *Chlorella* sp. has dominated the microalgal market next to *Spirulina*, and the largest amounts of polysaccharides produced are associated with it (Milledge 2011). Despite not having the highest carbohydrate concentrations, *Chlorella* sp. is widely produced as a health food due to its carbohydrate active substances (Barka and Blecker 2016). Polysaccharide extracts from it have proven antioxidant, immunomodulating, and anticancer activities (Kwak et al. 2012; Sheng et al. 2007; Song et al. 2018), although the structures and mechanisms responsible for such physiological functions are poorly understood.

18.2.1.3 Dietary Fiber Fiber is a well-established ingredient in the nutraceutical and functional food industry. Its diverse beneficial effects are known (Dhingra et al. 2012), but the complexity of interactions (Kostic et al. 2013) and the differences in microbiome competencies (Hehemann et al. 2010) keep us far from completely understanding the activity of dietary fiber in our body.

As mentioned above, most of the seaweed polysaccharides are not degraded by human endogenous enzymes. Seaweeds contain an important amount of dietary fiber, varying from 36–60% on a dry weight basis (Holdt and Kraan 2011; Rajapakse and Kim 2011). Nearly 55–70% of its total dietary fiber is soluble including agar, alginates, and carrageenan; the insoluble fiber includes cellulose, mannans, and xylan. The soluble fiber in seaweed added to the diet can enhance water binding to the food pellet in the gut facilitating stool bulking and decrease transit in the colon, which in turn is a positive factor in preventing cancer. The inclusion of seaweed dietary fiber has been reported to aid in the reduction of obesity, suppression of gastrointestinal inflammation, and encourage the action of probiotics (Rajapakse and Kim 2011). Seaweeds like *Fucus* and *Laminaria* have the highest insoluble dietary fiber content (40–27%), while *Undaria pinnatifida*, *Condrus* sp., and *Porphyra* sp. have the highest soluble dietary fiber content (Holdt and Kraan 2011).

Some of the most notable polysaccharides in this group include: ulvan, from green seaweed like the "sea lettuce" (*Ulva lactuca*), which is found in amounts from 8–29%; laminarin, mainly isolated from the brown seaweed *Laminaria digitata*, which is also a sulfated polysaccharide; alginate from brown seaweeds like *Laminaria hyperborean*, *L. digitata*, *Laminaria japonica*, *Ascophyllum* sp., and *Macrocystis pyrifera*; and carrageenan, mainly extracted from red algae *Kappaphycus* sp. and *Betaphycus* sp., which have been extensively studied. They have many health applications, including: strong antioxidant, antitumoral, immunostimulant, anti-inflammatory, anticoagulant/antithrombotic, lipid-lowering, antiviral, antibacterial, and antiprotozoal properties among many others. They have great potential for use in food, pharmaceutical, agricultural, and chemical applications (Kumar et al. 2008; Lahaye and Robic 2007; Moroney et al. 2015; Tanna and Mishra 2018; Venkatesan et al. 2015; Wijesekara and Karunarathna 2017).

Another group of dietary fiber polysaccharides is β-glucans, a heterogeneous group consisting of D-glucose monomers linked by β-glycosidic bonds (Zeković et al. 2005). They can be found in the cell wall of yeast, fungi, plants, bacteria, and algae (Du et al. 2014). They are a form of soluble fiber, as the β-linkages make them nondigestible for humans. Such resistant material can make it almost intact to the colon where it is fermented by our microbial co-metabolism, shaping the microbiome and chemical environment (Wells et al. 2017).

Owing to their multiple functional and bioactive properties, β-glucans are increasingly used in the food industry (Zhu et al. 2016). These include immunomodulating effects, anticancer, antimicrobial, antiviral, and hematopoietic activities, as well as reducing lipid and sugar levels (Kim et al. 2006; Yaakob et al. 2014). β-glucans' most remarkable activity is as potent immunomodulators (Kankkunen et al. 2010). The immunomodulatory functions of β-glucans explain many of their other activities, such as their anticancer, antimicrobial, antiviral, and hematopoietic effects (Chan et al. 2009; Cramer et al. 2006; Medina-Gali et al. 2018; Samuelsen et al. 2014).

The main sources of β-glucans are yeast, fungi, and cereals (Ahmad et al. 2012b), but, as with other applications, microalgae present themselves as a novel alternative with lots of advantages regarding production. The possibility of producing β-glucans in microalgae is recent and promising. Some species have up to 24% in dry weight (Schulze et al. 2016), while the most important bioactive compounds in *Chlorella* sp. are β-glucans (Sathasivam et al. 2017). Seaweeds also contain β-glucans, for example, in the form of laminarin in brown seaweeds (Kumar et al. 2008).

18.2.1.4 Sulfated Polysaccharides Sulfated polysaccharides are those in which some hydroxyl groups are replaced by sulfate groups (Korzeniowska et al. 2018). The presence of glucuronic acid and half-ester sulfate groups give them acidic character and, along with the carboxyl groups, anionic nature (Eteshola et al. 1998; Geresh and Arad 1991). They contain up to 15% of sulfate residues (De Jesus Raposo et al. 2015). Several biological activities make sulfated polysaccharides an attractive functional ingredient for the food industry.

The antiviral activity of the sulfated polysaccharides is their most remarkable attribute. The sulfate content is proportional to antiviral activity (Arad and

Levy-Ontman 2010). Such an effect has been demonstrated on several viruses, including herpes simplex virus (HSV), HIV, respiratory syncytial virus (RSV), influenza, measles, mumps, and polio, and it is associated with the anionic nature of the polymers, which blocks internalization into the host (Ahmadi et al. 2015). In addition, sulfated polysaccharides have immunostimulant, antiadhesive, antioxidant, anticancer, anticoagulant, antiarteriosclerosis, and hypolipidemic properties (Chen et al. 2010; Dvir et al. 2009; Gardeva et al. 2009; Guzman-Murillo and Ascencio 2000; Jiménez-Escrig et al. 2011; Khan et al. 2005; Namikoshi et al. 1996).

Among the most recurrent sulfated polysaccharides in literature are: ulvan and laminarin (mentioned above as dietary fiber), fucoidan carbohydrates mainly composed of L-fucose, which appears in brown seaweeds in amounts of around 2–10%, especially in the cell walls of seaweed species in the Fucaceae and Laminariaceae families. They have been reported with several biological properties including anticoagulant capacity, which in turn has resulted in their use as possible substitutes for heparin; for their antithrombotic activity, since they act on inflammation and the immune system; and as protection against viral infection, as well as for their interference in mammalian fertilization mechanisms (Berteau and Mulloy 2003; Jiménez-Escrig et al. 2011).

Though microalgae are not an especially rich source of these kinds of carbohydrates, the red microalgae are the most relevant group in the production of sulfated carbohydrates, especially *Porphyridium* sp. It is among the microalgae gaining acceptance in the health food industry owing to the polysaccharides it produces (Chacón-Lee and González-Mariño 2010; Mobin and Alam 2017). Their cells are encapsulated within a sulfated polysaccharide gel, which provides a variety of functions such as protection, mechanical support, and biorecognition (Arad and Levy-Ontman, 2010; Shimona Geresh et al. 2002; Ngo and Kim 2013). Another sulfated carbohydrate from microalgae is spirulan from *Spirulina platensis*, which also shows antithrombogenic properties (Ruocco et al. 2016). Little is known about the relationship between the biochemical structure and the physiological properties of these compounds, but their potential to be included in food for health benefits is clear.

18.2.2 Lipids

Lipids are a broad group of naturally occurring molecules that include fats, waxes, sterols, fat-soluble vitamins (such as A, D, E, and K), mono-, di-, and triacylglycerols, diglycerides, phospholipids, and other related molecules. Lipids account for about 40% of the total calories in most industrialized countries. Vegetable oils contribute 70% of the dietary lipids, while marine oils contribute about 2% of the global oil production, with the remainder coming from fats from land animals. Particularly, marine oils consist primarily of C14–C22 fatty acids (Holdt and Kraan 2011).

Long-chain omega-3 fatty acids, mainly eicosapentaenoic acid (EPA) and docosahexaenoic acid (DHA), are essential in human nutrition since they cannot be synthesized by human or animals; these are constituents of higher vertebrate membranes, particularly neuronal cells in humans, infant nutrition, retinal development, and ongoing visual, cognitive, as well as important acids in human breast milk. Based on their health benefits, global demand for omega-3 fatty acids has significantly increased over the past two decades, but there is mounting concern about the sustainability of sourcing these compounds from wild fish (Adarme-Vega et al. 2012; Christaki et al. 2011; Gouveia et al. 2008).

Traditionally, the main sources of this group of long-chain fatty acids are fish and fish oils, but a long list of disadvantages including fish odor, heavy metal contamination, toxins, etc., led to the search for other alternatives. The biotechnological production of long-chain fatty acids has been considered a feasible alternative using marine plants as the main source. In general, microalgae show higher lipid contents varying from 20–50%, but as with other metabolites, the environmental and culture conditions could increase these values up to 70% on a dry weight basis (Bellou et al. 2014; Christaki et al. 2011). In contrast, seaweed lipid content has been consistently reported as low, ranging from 1–5% on a dry weight basis (Holdt and Kraan 2011; Mohamed et al. 2012; Rajapakse and Kim 2011; Tanna and Mishra 2018). However, their valuable fatty acid content is considerable.

18.2.2.1 Fatty Acids from Seaweeds The predominant fatty acid in various seaweeds products is EPA, which is at concentrations as high as 50% of the total fatty acid content, and $\omega6$ fatty acids such as arachidonic acid (AA). In addition, marine algae also contain octadecatetraenoic acid (C18:3ω6), which is not present in other organisms; this fatty acid was suggested to affect the immune system in humans (Holdt and Kraan 2011; Rajapakse and Kim 2011). Gosch et al. (2012) studied brown, green, and red seaweeds from different sites in Australia and reported that brown seaweeds typically showed the highest lipid content. Sánchez-Machado et al. (2004) analyzed seven seaweed samples (two red and four brown) from the northwest Iberian coast and found that brown species have a higher content of unsaturated fatty acids while red ones showed a higher content of saturated fatty acids.

18.2.2.2 Fatty Acids from Microalgae Recently, there has been an increased interest in the use of microalgal lipids in numerous commercial applications, such as in the food, chemical, cosmetic, and pharmaceutical industries (Bellou et al. 2014), since they are a good source of valuable nutritional ingredients as described above (Figure 18.2). Nevertheless, microalgae have long been seen as a potential source of fatty acids, especially the long-chain PUFAs such as γ-linolenic acid (GLA, 18:3ω6), AA (20:4ω6), EPA (20:5ω3), and DHA (22:6ω3). They have been associated with prevention and treatment of several diseases including cardiovascular disorders, cancer, type II diabetes, inflammatory bowel disorders, asthma, arthritis, kidney and skin disorders, depression, and schizophrenia (Ravishankar and Ambati 2019). In addition, they contribute to the production of prostaglandins, prostacyclins, leucotrienes, and thromboxanes (Borowitzka 2013; Christaki et al. 2011; Gouveia et al. 2008; Khozin-Goldberg 2016; Priyadarshani and Rath 2012; Chandini et al. 2008). These long-chain fatty acids cannot be synthesized by higher plants and animals; only microalgae can supply the whole food chains with these components. The main advantage of microalgae as a PUFA source is the lack of unpleasant odor, reduced risk of chemical contamination, and better purification potential (Pulz and Gross 2004).

The most exploited microalgae for PUFAs have been *Nannochloropsis*, *Phaeodactylum*, *Schizochytrium*, *Thraustochytrium*, *Arthrospira*, *Porphyridium*, *Isochrysys*, *Diacronema*, and *Crypthecodinium* sp. (Adarme-Vega et al. 2014). However, this list is not as extensive as research in this field. The fatty acid composition of cyanobacteria is generally limited to C16 and C18 fatty acids; among the most common are linoleic acid (LA, 18:2ω6), α-linoleic acid (ALA, 18:3ω3), and GLA, while marine planktonic species of *Bacillariophyta*, *Dinophyta*, *Eustigmatophyta*, *Haptophyta*, and *Rhodophyta* produce the long-chain PUFAs of the ω3 family EPA and/or

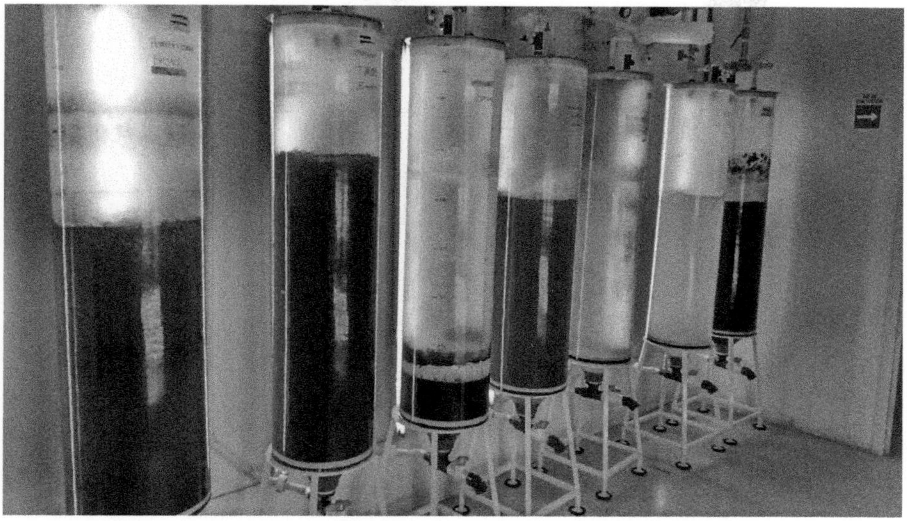

Figure 18.2 Pilot-scale cultivation of several microalgae for lipid production. Source: Courtesy of Biotecnología Mexicana de Microalgas, SA de CV (BIOMEX).

DHA (Khozin-Goldberg 2016). Particularly, *Phaeodactylum* and *Nanochloropsis* are suitable for EPA, while *Isochrysis* and *Schizochytrium* are right for DHA production (Ryckebosch et al. 2012). Some of the abovementioned microalgal species can be cultivated under heterotrophic conditions including *Chlorella*, *Nitzschia*, *Cyclotella*, *Tetraselmis*, *Schizochytrium*, and *Crypthecodinium* (Ryckebosch et al. 2012), representing a strong productive potential given their ease of handling compared with phototrophic cultures.

18.2.3 Proteins

Proteins are fundamental components and nutrients for the human body. They are the most versatile group of macromolecules and have the widest range of activities. Microalgae are an extraordinary source of protein and it is the main reason why they have been consumed for centuries. They have bioactive compounds with several uses in the food and health industry. Their potential for novel applications and to supply the protein demand efficiently has increased over the years, emphasizing the need for this to be explored.

Since the early 1950s, intense efforts have been made to explore new alternative protein sources as food supplements, primarily in anticipation of insufficient protein supply. The investigations conducted so far confirm that algal biomass shows promising qualities as a novel source of protein: the average quality of most of the algae examined is equal, sometimes even superior to conventional plant proteins (Becker 2007).

18.2.3.1 Proteins from Seaweeds Among seaweeds, red and green seaweeds contain higher amounts of proteins, varying from 10–47% on a dry weight basis, compared

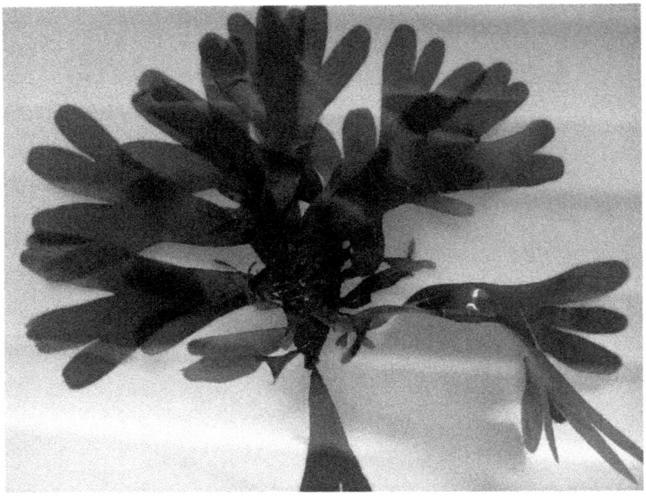

Figure 18.3 *Palmaria palmata* (dulse seaweed). Source: Courtesy of Merinov Québec Fisheries and Aquaculture Innovation Centre.

with brown seaweeds which contain 3–15%. In some red seaweeds, such as *Palmaria palmata* (dulse, Figure 18.3) and *Porphyra tenera* (nori), proteins can represent up to 35 and 47% of dry matter, respectively. These levels are comparable with those found in high-protein vegetables; for example, soybeans (in which proteins represent 35% of dry mass). As with other molecules, the amount of protein in seaweeds varies according to the species, environmental conditions, habitats, maturity, and applied methods used for protein and amino acid determination (Burtin 2003; Černá 2011; Tanna and Mishra 2018).

Most seaweeds contain all essential amino acids and are also a rich source of acidic amino acids such as glutamic acid and aspartic acid. Although cysteine, methionine, threonine, tryptophan, lysine, and histidine are limited in seaweed proteins, they are still present in higher amounts than in terrestrial plants. The final amino acid composition depends on the seasonal period. Generally, the highest protein value has been found during the period of winter–early spring and the lowest during summer–early autumn (Černá 2011; Dawczynski et al. 2007; Tanna and Mishra 2018). Despite this, in comparison with the standard proteins, seaweed proteins (as well as other plant proteins) are not full-valued proteins because of their low amounts of some amino acids. Nevertheless, the presence of all essential amino acids in considerable quantities indicates that seaweed proteins are nutritionally superior to terrestrial plant proteins (Černá 2011).

18.2.3.2 Proteins from Microalgae Microalgae protein contents are among the best in nature. Animal food is the traditional source of protein, having great protein levels, but animal diets have negative effects on human health (Ekmekcioglu et al. 2018) and their production is unsustainable (Henchion et al. 2017). Plants as a protein source are a viable alternative (Tuso 2013), but their protein content and quality are not as good as animal protein, given that the quality of proteins depends on their digestibility; proteins from plants are typically harder to digest (due to the high fiber content of the cell wall) than those coming from animals (Bleakley and Hayes 2017). Several species of microalgae have higher protein content (dry weight basis) than all of the traditional sources, e.g. *Anabaena cylindrica*, 43–56%; *Arthrospira maxima*, 60–71%; *Scenedesmus obliquus*, 50–56%; and *S.* (*Arthrospira*) *platensis*, 60–71% on a dry weight basis. In particular, *Arthrospira* sp. are the most consumed microalgae and one of the most nutritious food known in nature (Capelli and Cysewski 2010). Their biomass is commercialized under the name *Spirulina* and it is exploited mainly because of its high protein content (Priyadarshani and Rath 2012). *Arthrospira* sp. are also important for their various health-promoting effects and ability to produce phycobiliproteins, which can represent up to 20% of their total protein content (Barka and Blecker 2016) (see pigments in Section 18.2.4).

In general, the amino acid profile of microalgae also makes them a great source of protein. Similar to animal-sourced protein, algae are considered a complete source of proteins as they are rich in all the essential amino acids that humans must obtain from food (Hoffman and Falvo 2004; Wells et al. 2017). Most plants are incomplete protein sources (Tien Lea et al. 2016), although some of them like soybean have all of the essential amino acids; however, microalgae have an amino acid profile comparable with the best animal and plant sources of protein (Becker 2007).

Despite the potential of microalgae as a source of proteins with good overall digestibility, they have been ignored and poorly examined, which may be down to factors such as the powder-like consistency of dried biomass and its dark-green color, which limits the incorporation of the algal material into conventional foodstuff. The socio-ethnological barriers and very conservative food restrictions in developing countries present a great challenge as well (Becker 2007; Kose et al. 2017; Lonnie et al. 2018).

18.2.3.3 Bioactive Peptides Bioactive peptides are sequences between 2 and 30 amino acids long, generally encrypted within the sequence of the parent protein, which only become active after being released (Harnedy and Fitzgerald 2011; Hayes 2013). The activation can be done chemically or enzymatically during digestion or food processing, providing diverse opportunities to include them in food (Sánchez and Vázquez 2017). Owing to their various health benefits, e.g. properties such as opioid, immunomodulatory, antibacterial, antithrombotic, and hypertensive activity, the commercial interest in them has increased considerably in recent years, although industrial production has been limited by the lack of technology (Bleakley and Hayes 2017; Fan et al. 2014; Harnedy and Fitzgerald 2011; Holdt and Kraan 2011; Jiménez-Escrig et al. 2011; Kim and Kang 2011; Rico et al. 2017; Sheih et al. 2010; Suetsuna and Chen 2001). Most of these activities have been only demonstrated *in vitro*; however, more *in vivo* studies are required as the environment there is much more complicated. Additionally, production on a large scale, isolation methods, and understanding their bioactivity remain as challenges (Fan et al. 2014). Yet, the increasing interest in these compounds will develop our knowledge and technologies.

Animal foods are the main source of bioactive peptides (Albenzio et al. 2017), but they can also be obtained from agroindustrial residues (Lemes et al. 2016). Seaweeds and microalgae are an important alternative to produce bioactive peptides, as many of their health benefits are caused by these compounds, especially in cyanobacteria (Sigamani et al. 2016). However, peptides isolation from seaweeds is a difficult task owing to the link between polysaccharides and protein within the seaweed matrix. Some peptides from seaweeds have been reported to present a antihypertensive effect, namely angiotensin-converting enzyme (ACE) inhibitory activity, e.g. protein hydrolysates from *U. pinnatifida*, which has been reported by Sato et al. (2002). In any case, there is not much information related to peptides from algae with biological activity.

18.2.3.4 Recombinant Proteins The development of genetic engineering has provided the capacity to change organisms and food at a constitutional level. They can be modified to produce molecules for any purpose, including enhancing their nutritional and health properties. Despite having a considerable image problem, genetically modified food has been commercialized and consumed for many years (Wunderlich and Gatto 2015). The debate regarding its use is still ongoing, but considering all the advantages and current global conditions, it seems unlikable that its development will ever stop. Genetic modification provides many benefits to food by enhancing productivity, nutritional value, and by generating new therapeutic applications for traditional food. In order to deal with the expansion of the population, the demand for more food in some regions and healthier food in others, the decrease of resources, health challenges, and ecological concerns, genetically modified food stands, not as an absolute solution, but as an important tool to help diminish such problems (Bawa and Anilakumar 2013; Zhang et al. 2016).

Scarce information is available about recombinant protein production with macroalgae. On the other hand, the enormous potential in microalgae is better established (Yan et al. 2016). They present numerous advantages over all the other organisms, especially when the final objective is for human consumption, which include rapid growth, safety, scalability, simple growth requirements, no risk of contamination or harm to humans, metabolic diversity, and transformation stability (Rasala and Mayfield 2015).

The three microalgae genomes, nuclear, mitochondrial, and chloroplast can be transformed, and each with distinct attributes. The nuclear genome can perform all post-translational modifications, including glycosylation, and can secrete proteins (Specht et al. 2010). The chloroplast cannot glycosylate proteins, but it can accumulate them at much higher levels owing to the lack of silencing mechanisms, reaching levels as high as 21% of the recombinant protein (Gong et al. 2011). Both genomes have the ability to express complex proteins, including therapeutic ones. Proteins such as erythropoietin, antibodies, and vaccines have successfully been produced in microalgae (Eichler-Stahlberg et al. 2009; Rasala et al. 2010; Tran et al. 2009). These organisms generate the possibility to produce all types of nutritional, gut regulatory, therapeutic, and immunomodulating proteins, and deliver them directly into the body without purification. The ultimate goal of functional food and nutraceuticals is human health, and expressing recombinant proteins in microalgae provides a resourceful and adaptable alternative to achieve it.

18.2.3.5 Oral Vaccines Microalgae are ideal organisms to deliver vaccines orally. It is among the most promising applications of expressing recombinant proteins in food. Oral vaccines present several advantages over traditional ones, such as eliminating the need for trained personnel, equipment for administration and storage; inducing mucosal and systemic immunity; increased safety; reduced costs: and higher compliance from patients (Specht and Mayfield 2014). Microalgae are of great interest for this application as they are safe to eat, they have the ability to express complex proteins, they can be grown on a large scale, and their rigid cell walls provide antigen protection during their storage and digestion (Kwon and Daniell 2016). Plants also present such benefits, but microalgae grow faster and with more control in bioreactors; they are easier to transform, and their entire biomass can be consumed, making them a more suitable organism for oral vaccine production.

The idea of edible vaccines is not new – it has been around for decades (Jan et al. 2016). The first reported vaccine antigen expressed in a microalga dates back to 2003 (Sun et al. 2003). It is clear that microalgae have the potential to deliver oral vaccines as immunization has been shown to be effective (Dreesen et al. 2010; Gregory et al. 2012). A relevant success is a vaccine effective against malaria (Dauvillée et al. 2010), although the production of vaccines for noninfectious diseases, such as diabetes and cancer, is encouraging as well (Demurtas et al. 2013; Wang et al. 2008). Diseases are still a global problem, and producing edible vaccines in microalgae could contribute substantially to solving it by increasing their safety and reducing costs, which is especially important in developing countries.

18.2.4 Pigments

Pigments are high-value molecules in the industrial sector including food, cosmetics, and pharmaceutics, which have been widely used mostly to enhance the product appearance. Over the past few decades, the tendency for more natural products, especially in food, has led to the substitution of synthetic dyes for natural pigments. The latter, apart from enhancing color and improving the sensorial experience of the consumer, include the added value of nutraceutical properties such as antioxidant, anticarcinogenic, and anti-inflammatory activity.

Plants and microorganisms are the two major sources of natural pigments. The natural pigments from plants have drawbacks such as instability against light, heat, or adverse pH, and low water solubility, and are often unavailable throughout the year. Hence, the microbial pigments are of great interest owing to the stability of the pigments produced and the availability of cultivation technology (Kumar et al. 2015).

18.2.4.1 Pigments from Seaweeds Algae represent a promising source of natural pigments with potential nutraceutical activity. The major carotenoids that occur in algae include β-carotene, lutein, violaxanthin, neoxanthin, and zeaxanthin in green seaweed; α- and β-carotene, lutein, and zeaxanthin in red seaweed; and β-carotene, violaxanthin, and fucoxanthin in brown seaweed (Kumar et al. 2008), with fucoxanthin being probably the most exploited pigment from brown seaweed.

18.2.4.2 Pigments from Microalgae Among the most promising microorganisms for pigment production are microalgae. However, as with many other biotechnological processes, microbial pigment production still faces a considerable technology gap. Nonetheless, this gap is now closing every day. Among the advantages of microalgae as pigment producers are the ease of growth and cultivation in bioreactors, as well as the capacity to produce a wide range of natural and safe colorants (Figure 18.4).

18.2.4.3 Chlorophyll The most abundant light-harvesting pigments in nature are chlorophylls. They are greenish in color, fat-soluble pigments with polycyclic planar structures esterified by a long phytol side-chain where Mg^{2+} occupies the central position, in green leafy plants. The other pigments are often masked by chlorophyll and are often shown in autumn in senescence, where chlorophyll degrades and the

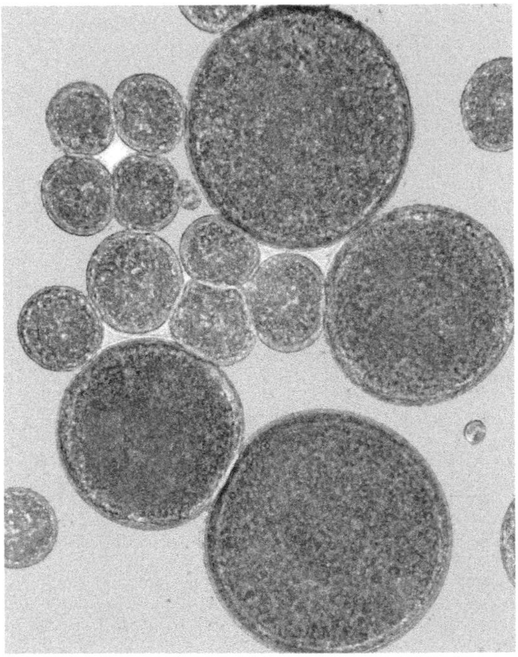

Figure 18.4 *Haematoccocus pluvialis* growing under standard conditions producing chlorophyll.

synthesis of other pigments is induced (Ferruzzi and Blakeslee 2007; Lev-Yadun and Gould 2007). There are two main types of chlorophyll, chlorophyll *a* being a blue/green pigment and chlorophyll *b*, a green/yellow pigment. These are differentiated by a simple change of substituent groups on ring B from methyl to formyl. These two forms of chlorophyll coexist together in plants in the approximate ratio of 3:1 with the methyl variant (chlorophyll *a*) predominating. The *a* variant with the methyl substituent is less stable and has a bluer green character than the *b* variant with the formyl substituent (Humphrey 2004). Other chlorophylls include chlorophyll *c* yellow/green, chlorophyll *d* brilliant/forest green, and chlorophyll *f* emerald green (Mulders et al. 2014).

Chlorophylls and their various derivatives have a long-established history of use in traditional medicine and for therapeutic purposes. Both natural chlorophyll and commercial-grade derivatives, such as sodium copper chlorophyllin (SCC), have been widely investigated for a range of beneficial biological activities including speeding up wound healing, tissue growth stimulation, anti-inflammatory properties, control of calcium oxalate crystals, treatment of ulcers and oral sepsis, antioxidant and antimutagenic properties, and internal deodorization. Furthermore, the ability of both natural and commercial chlorophyll derivatives to act as photosensitizers has enabled their utilization as effective agents in photodynamic therapy for cancer (Ferruzzi and Blakeslee 2007; Halim et al. 2010). However, exposure of chlorophyll molecules to weak acids, oxygen, or light accelerates their oxidation and results in the formation of numerous degradation products (Halim et al. 2010). Natural chlorophyll is highly unstable and, additionally, it is more expensive than artificial colorings, requiring it to undergo a chemical modification by replacing the magnesium center with a copper ion in order to improve its stability as a food coloring agent (Halim et al. 2010; Humphrey 2004).

Manifold applications of chlorophylls are found in the kitchen as the greater part of industrially prepared chlorophyll derivatives are destined for the increasing demand of natural colorants for food and beverages. These pigments are approved as a food additive (E140) for coloration. Famous *chefs de cuisine* use chlorophyll to provide a green coloring for a variety of foodstuffs and beverages, such as pasta, pesto, or absinthe. In addition, wasabi surrogates consisting of "simple" horseradish colorized with *Spirulina* chlorophyll are found in retail. Some of the industrial production is also destined for the cosmetic, toiletry, and pharmaceutical market. Owing to its high deodorant capacity, chlorophyll *a* is also used as an ingredient in items of personal hygiene, such as deodorants, or, as pastilles, it is commercialized in formulations against bad breath (Begum et al. 2016; Gouveia et al. 2008; Koller et al. 2014).

Given the commercial importance of chlorophylls and their derivates, most of the commercial chlorophyll is obtained from vegetable sources. Nevertheless, there is a growing interest in the biotechnology field for obtaining nonvegetable sources of colors (Rangel-Yagui et al. 2004). A good source of natural chlorophyll is microalgae; these are an abundant source material but can be difficult to extract and often contain a high level of undesirable metallic contaminants (Humphrey 2004). Chlorophyll *a* is the primary photosynthetic pigment in all algae and it is the only chlorophyll in cyanobacteria (blue-green algae) and Rhodophyta. Like all higher plants, Chlorophyta and Euglenophyta contain chlorophyll *b* as well; chlorophylls *c*, *d*, and *e* can be found in several marine algae and freshwater diatoms. These chlorophylls differ according to the substituents on their porphyrin ring (D'Alessandro and Antoniosi Filho 2016; Gouveia et al. 2008; Hu et al. 2018; Mulders et al. 2014; Pignolet et al. 2013). The most used microalgae for chlorophyll production on a large scale have been reported to be *Dunaliella* sp., *Spirulina* sp., and *Chlorella sorokiniana* (Begum et al. 2016; Harun et al. 2010; Mulders et al. 2014).

18.2.4.4 Carotenoids Carotenoids are the second most abundant pigments on Earth. These pigments are responsible for the different colors of fruits, vegetables, and other plants (Gouveia et al. 2010). Chemically, they are lipophilic isoprenoid compounds composed of a C40 backbone of isoprene units, usually colored yellow, orange, and red. The structural diversity for the various carotenoids is provided by the number and position of the conjugate double bonds, cyclization at one or both ends and oxygenation of the backbone. Carotenes are the hydrocarbon carotenoids, while xanthophylls are the oxygenated version (Gong and Bassi 2016; Hu et al. 2018; Sathasivam et al. 2017). There are over 400 carotenoids identified, but β-carotene and astaxanthin are the most commercialized, followed by lutein, zeaxanthin, and lycopene (Gouveia et al. 2010; Sathasivam et al. 2017). Microalgae are recognized as an excellent source of carotenoids, mainly β-carotene; its hydroxyl derivate, zeaxanthin; its keto derivates, echinenone and canthaxanthin; and the carotenoid glycosides, myxoxanthophyll (Rodrigues et al. 2014).

18.2.4.4.1 β-Carotene β-carotene is mainly produced by *Dunaliella salina*, which can accumulate up to 14% w/w on a dry weight basis, especially if the microalgae are cultured under nitrogen-deficient media, with high salt concentration and intense solar radiation. This pigment is readily used in cosmetics and food industry – in the latter for the production of cheese, butter, margarine, soft drinks, etc. (Christaki et al. 2011; Mobin and Alam 2017).

Among the important carotenoids for humans, β-carotene is a major source of vitamin A, which is necessary for retina functions and has an effect on many tissue types through its action as a regulator of gene expression. In addition, β-carotene helps protect the skin against photoaging by its antioxidant activity. The natural form of this pigment has a stronger effect and can be easily absorbed by the body when compared with the synthetic form (Fu et al. 2013; Mary Leema et al. 2010; Sathasivam et al. 2017). The consumption of carotenoids in the diet has been epidemiologically correlated with a lower risk for several diseases, particularly those in which free radicals are thought to play a role in the initiation, such as arteriosclerosis, cataracts, night blindness, age-related macular degeneration (AMD), multiple sclerosis, and cancer. In addition, it has been suggested that β-carotene is responsible for the prevention of toxin build-up in the liver and potentially improves the immune system. However, some long-term studies with β-carotene suggest that the threshold between the beneficial and adverse effects of some carotenoids is low and provides a strong stimulus to further understanding the functional effects of specific carotenoids, e.g. long-term β-carotene intake increases the risk of cancer as well as the cancer death rate (Gong and Bassi 2016; Gouveia et al. 2008).

18.2.4.4.2 Astaxanthin *Haematococcus pluvialis* (Figure 18.5) could be considered the main commercial producing organism of astaxanthin and the best natural source of this high-value carotenoid. It has been stated that it can accumulate astaxanthin up to 1–8% dry weight, but a more conservative quantity is around 1–3% dry weight

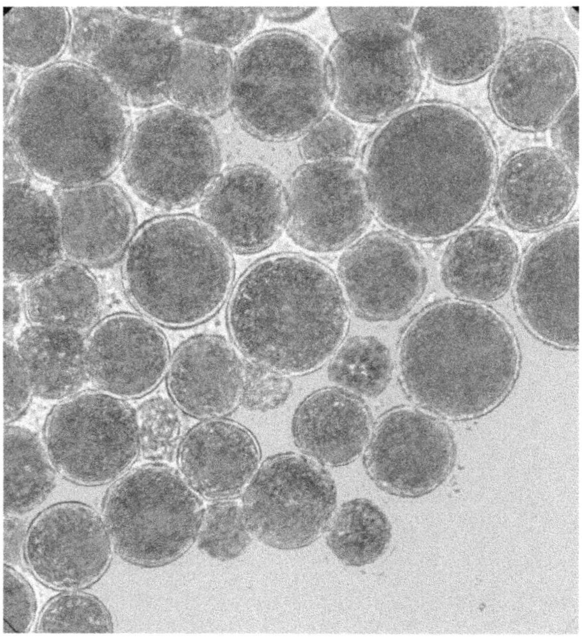

Figure 18.5 *Haematoccocus pluvialis* growing under stress conditions producing asthaxanthin.

(D'Alessandro and Antoniosi Filho 2016; Gouveia et al. 2008; Mobin and Alam 2017). Another natural source is *Phaffia rhodozyma* yeast, although it requires a large amount of feed for sufficient pigmentation (Gouveia et al. 2008).

Astaxanthin is best recognized for the pinkish color it produces in aquatic fish and shrimp. It is insoluble in water and a by-product of β-carotene, since under stress β-carotene is converted into astaxanthin through β-carotene oxygenase and β-carotene hydroxylase. There are three stereoisomers of astaxanthin: (3R, 3′R), (3R, 3′S), and (3S, 3′S) are reported; the synthetic astaxanthin contains an approximately 1:2:1 mixture of these stereoisomers. *Haematococcus pluvialis* produces only the (3S, 3′S) stereoisomers in free and esterified conditions (Christaki et al. 2011; D'Alessandro and Antoniosi Filho 2016; Gong and Bassi 2016; Gouveia et al. 2008; Sathasivam et al. 2017).

Astaxanthin is the strongest antioxidant of all the carotenoids and exhibits several-fold stronger antioxidant activity than vitamin E, vitamin C, and β-carotene. It sequesters free radicals by removing reactive oxygen. Despite this, these antioxidants are weaker than synthetic antioxidants such as butylated hydroxytoluene or butylated hydroxyanisole, but natural antioxidants have higher bioavailability and, therefore, exert a better protective effect than synthetic ones (Christaki et al. 2011; D'Alessandro and Antoniosi Filho 2016; Gong and Bassi 2016; Gouveia et al. 2008).

Given its natural origin, astaxanthin, like other carotenoids, is preferred for functional foods, especially in beverages. Some reports support the assumption that daily ingestion of astaxanthin may protect body tissues from oxidative damage, which might be a practical and beneficial strategy in health management (Gouveia et al. 2008). But the most promising commercial application is in pharmaceuticals and cosmetics: astaxanthin has the potential to enhance antibody production, antiaging, and sunproofing, and it also demonstrates anti-inflammatory effects when administered with aspirin. Because of this, it is used in disease treatment such as atherosclerosis and heart disease, diabetes, skin conditions, chronic inflammatory diseases, and prevention of some cancers (Christaki et al. 2011; D'Alessandro and Antoniosi Filho 2016; Gong and Bassi 2016).

18.2.4.4.3 Lutein Lutein is yellowish at low concentrations and red-orangish at high concentrations. It is a primary xanthophyll pigment, mainly lipophilic but with polar hydroxyl groups at both ends of the conjugated polyisoprenoid chain (Gouveia et al. 2008; Hu et al. 2018). Lutein and its stereo isomer zeaxanthin are xanthophyll carotenoids abundant in egg yolks and dark-green leafy vegetables such as spinach and kale. Although these carotenoids are similar in structure to α- and β-carotene, they do not have provitamin A activity. Like other carotenoids, it is involved in light-harvesting during photosynthesis and protection of the photosystems from photo-oxidative damage (Hu et al. 2018; Ma and Lin 2010).

Lutein is exclusively found in the Chlorophyta and in some green Dinophyta. In some of the Chlorophyta, this yellow pigment can be converted into loroxanthin (Mulders et al. 2014). The most studied microalgae for lutein production are *Muriellopsis* sp. and *Scenedesmus almeriensis*, surpassing lutein production from marigold (D'Alessandro and Antoniosi Filho 2016; Fernández-Sevilla et al. 2010). Nonetheless, other strains such as *S. almeriensis, Chlorella protothecoides, Chlorella zofingiensis, Chlorococcum citriforme*, and *Neospongiococcus gelatinosum* have been used. The most important environmental factors for lutein productions seem to be temperature, irradiance, pH and availability, and source of nitrogen, salinity, and the presence of oxidizing substances (Fernández-Sevilla et al. 2010; Guedes et al. 2011). The lutein productivity varies among strains, but for *Muriellopsis* sp. it has been reported as ranging from 1 mg m^{-2} day^{-1} to 180 mg m^{-2} day^{-1} (Fernández-Sevilla et al. 2010).

Lutein is one of the most important carotenoids in food and human serum. It is an essential component present in the macula lutea (or yellow spot) in the retina and eyes lens, as well as in almost all the structures of the definitive human eye: retinal pigment epithelium, choroid, iris, ciliary body, and the matrix of the subretinal space, with the exception of the vitreous body, which lacks carotenoids (Panova et al. 2017; Sathasivam et al. 2017). The macular pigment, as it is called, protects the eyes from oxidative damage by blue light, improves visual acuity, and increased lutein intake was shown to protect against AMD (Hu et al. 2018).

Together with zeaxanthin, lutein has garnered increasing attention on the grounds of recent studies that show how an adequate intake of this product might help prevent or ameliorate the effects of degenerative human diseases, such as AMD or cataracts, as well as skin health (Fernández-Sevilla et al. 2010). In addition, recent findings have confirmed that, along with carotenoids such as lycopene and zeaxanthin, lutein can protect against diabetic retinopathy. Besides, it has been found that lutein can lower streptozotocin (STZ)-induced hyperglycemia and shows significant antioxidant effects in kidneys of diabetic rats. In the epidermal and dermal skin layers, the carotenoid lutein has been shown to protect against UV-induced oxidative damage, especially in combination with other antioxidant systems and immunoprotective substances (Sathasivam and Ki 2018).

Although lutein and zeaxanthin are not essential nutrients for human health, they can be incorporated into the human diet with the consumption of green leafy vegetables and even cultivars, but this has several disadvantages. It requires a discipline hard to maintain for practical reasons, the amount of lutein varies in the different vegetables and even cultivars, and the most important difficulty is that the effective dose of lutein derived to the bloodstream (bioavailability) depends on the preparation, the presence of other foods (particularly fats or fiber), and even the patient's physiology (Fernández-Sevilla et al. 2010; Ma and Lin 2010). Although lutein and zeaxanthin are considered to be major carotenoids in the normal Western diet, data available from population-based studies showed that lutein intake tended to decline in both the US and Europe, particularly from dark-green leafy vegetables. Therefore, it is worth noting that increasing intake of food sources rich in xanthophylls is warranted (Ma and Lin 2010).

18.2.4.4.4 Fucoxanthin Fucoxanthin is a major marine brown carotenoid, occurs abundantly in some macro- and microalgae, and contributes more than 10% of the estimated total production of carotenoids in nature. Fucoxanthin has an unusual allenic bond and some oxygenic functional groups such as epoxy, hydroxyl, carbonyl, and carboxyl moieties in its molecule that contribute to its unique structure. The allenic bond is found mainly in carotenoids such as fucoxanthin, which was the first allenic carotenoid found in brown seaweeds. It is responsible for higher antioxidant activity (Maeda et al. 2008; Peng et al. 2011).

Fucoxanthin was first isolated from the marine brown seaweeds *Fucus*, *Dictyota*, and *Laminaria* by Willstätter and Page in 1914 (Peng et al. 2011). In some Southeast Asian countries, some seaweeds containing fucoxanthin are often used as a food source including *Undaria*, *Laminaria*, *Hizikia*, and *Sargassum* (Maeda et al. 2008; Yan et al. 1999). Fucoxanthin is also found in microalgae, particularly in the Haptophyta, the fucoxanthin-containing Dinophyta, the Chrysophyta, and the Bacillariophyta; the latter two classes belong to a group referred to as the Heterokontophyta (Mulders et al. 2014). Diatoms exhibit a characteristic golden-brown color owing to a high amount of the xanthophyll fucoxanthin that plays a major role in the light-harvesting complex of their photosystems. The diatom *Phaeodactylum tricornutum* has been proposed as a commercial source for fucoxanthin, with production higher than 1.5% dry weight. A similar amount of fucoxanthin was produced by the Haptophyta *Isochrysis* sp. (Talero et al. 2015).

Fucoxanthin is bound to several proteins and, together with chlorophyll *a*, it forms fucoxanthin–Chl *a*–protein complexes in the thylakoids, where it acts as a primary carotenoid to harvest light and transfer energy. This protein has been extensively investigated in microalgae. However, it is not known whether this pigment functions as a secondary carotenoid relating to photo-oxidative protection. Fucoxanthin has been found to have several therapeutic activities, including anticancer, antihypertensive, anti-inflammatory, and antiobesity effects. However, most of these studies were conducted with fucoxanthin isolated from macroalgae; no studies have reported on the commercial production of fucoxanthin derived from microalgae (Gong and Bassi 2016; Kim et al. 2012; Mikami and Hosokawa 2013; Peng et al. 2011; Talero et al. 2015).

Fucoxanthin has been reported to effectively scavenge chemically generated free radicals, such as 1,1-diphenyl-2-picrylhydrazyl (DPPH) (Rajauria et al., 2017). It acts as an antioxidant under anoxic conditions, whereas other carotenoids, such as β-carotene and lutein, show little or no quenching activity in such chemical assessment systems. This molecule could effectively inhibit intracellular reactive oxygen species formation, DNA damage, and apoptosis induced by H_2O_2, possibly because of the ability of fucoxanthin to increase catalase (Mikami and Hosokawa 2013; Peng et al. 2011; Yan et al. 1999).

Fucoxanthin has also been attributed to antidiabetic and hepatoprotective activity. It has been reported that dietary fucoxanthin can attenuate both body weight and white adipose tissue; the latter is induced through excessive fat accumulation and induces insulin resistance, which leads to type II diabetes (Mikami and Hosokawa 2013; Miyashita et al. 2011). It has been suggested that fucoxanthin improves insulin resistance and decreases blood glucose levels (Miyata et al. 2009; Peng et al. 2011).

18.2.4.5 Phycobiliproteins Phycobiliproteins are brilliantly colored, highly fluorescent, water-soluble protein components of the photosynthetic light-harvesting antenna. Unlike other natural colorants, the phycobilin pigments phycocyanin (blue), phycoerythrin (red), phycoerythrocyanin (orange), and allophycocyanin (green-bluish) are only found in algae. The main source of phycobiliproteins is the cyanobacterium *Spirulina* (*Arthrospira*) for phycocyanin (it may reach up to 20% in dry weight of the cell protein), although *Galdieria sulphuraria* has also been shown to be a candidate for phycocyanin production, while the rhodophyte *Porphyridium* is the main source of phycoerythrin (red). Phycocyanin is formed by α and β subunits and has linear tetrapyrrole phytochromobilin covalently attached to its polypeptides via a thioether linkage to a conserved Cys residue. Phycocyanin exists as a complex interacting mixture of the trimer, hexamer, and decamer aggregates, which has been reported to be a function of pH and ionic strength of the medium, protein concentration, and algal origin. Furthermore, the stage of aggregation affects the molecular weight as well as the position and intensity of the maximum absorbance peak of phycocyanin (Antelo et al. 2008; Dasgupta 2015; Gouveia et al. 2008; Wu et al. 2016).

Cyanobacterial phycobiliproteins have an important role in the commercial and biotechnological sectors. In general, phycocyanin has a wide range of applications including food and cosmetic colors; it can be used as fluorescent tags in flow cytometry and immunology, as possible antioxidants in cosmetics, as a component of functional foods, as photosensitizers in photodynamic therapy for treatment of cancers, and for other therapeutic benefits (Antelo et al. 2008; Borowitzka 2013; D'Alessandro and Antoniosi Filho 2016; Gouveia et al. 2008; Sloth et al. 2006). Phycoerythrins and phycocyanins are the major commercially important phycobiliproteins given their cost and wide application range, with C-phycocyanin (C-PC) being the most important; it is sold for US$500 to 100 000 kg^{-1} depending on its purity (Borowitzka 2013; Kannaujiya and Sinha 2016). Both pigments, phycoerythrin and phycocyanin, are actually used in the industrial sector as colorants for chewing gum, ice cream, beverages, milk products, candies, and cosmetics (Kannaujiya and Sinha 2016; Sarada et al. 1999).

Purified C-PC has nutraceutical and pharmaceutical potential. More attention has been paid to the use of C-PC as a nutraceutical, particularly in health foods in which dried *S. platensis* is the functional component. Beyond their nutritional value, whole cyanobacteria are suggested to stimulate the immune defense system and possess antioxidant, anti-inflammatory, antiviral, anticancer, and cholesterol-lowering effects, partly because of their C-PC contents. The largest route for human intake of C-PC is in the nonpurified form via *S. platensis* health food products. However, cyanobacteria may also contain a range of other biologically active compounds, and it is, therefore, difficult to attribute health effects from consumption of whole cyanobacteria directly to the C-PC component (Dasgupta 2015).

18.3 Perspectives

With global population growth, food production must enhance its productivity both quantitatively and qualitatively. In addition, the rise of collective consciousness in search of health and wellness results in an increased demand for nutraceuticals and functional food. Algae are an unexploited source of compounds with a wide range of biological activities to supply such demand. The immense diversity of species makes their compound reservoir inestimable. Although research has focused on few of them (Wells et al. 2017), especially carbohydrates, they produce compounds well-known for their beneficial effects that are already used in the food industry (Ahmad et al. 2012a; Arad & Levy-Ontman 2010).

Algae are an alternative source for the production of traditional and novel compounds with several advantages over the conventional ones, being completely ecological, renewable, and safe (Korzeniowska et al. 2018). In addition, not having lignin facilitates the separation of highly valuable polysaccharides (Foley et al. 2011). Producing carbohydrates as functional ingredients in algae has enormous potential, especially for the discovery of novel compounds, but several challenges must be tackled before turning it into a reality.

To date, only seaweeds have been studied and exploited significantly for their carbohydrate content. The variety of these molecules in seaweeds is extensive and there is still a long way to go in the search for more functionalities and other health benefits. On the other hand, the main obstacle for producing polysaccharides in microalgae might be the lack of knowledge on the technology to increase their potential as polysaccharide sources. Although they have been consumed for many years and have known benefits, most of the algal structures, interactions, and action mechanisms remain unexplained. Productivity and technological constraints also limit their potential. Under current circumstances, carbohydrates should be produced in microalgae under a biorefinery process in order to be viable (Mehta et al. 2018). The demand for healthier food, the pressure on climate change, as well as technological development will increase the search for high-value compounds, such as polysaccharides, PUFAs, pigments, and proteins in seaweeds and microalgae.

Protein supply, in particular, will be short in the future (Godfray et al. 2010). The potential of algae, especially microalgae, to supply the demand and provide several health benefits at the same time has not been noticed in most of the world. Nearly all its limitations could be overcome through research and technological development, but the lack of algal consumption hinders their progress. The necessity to explore alternative protein sources and the potential of microalgae have been identified since the 1950s (Chacón-Lee and González-Mariño 2010). Although the predictions of those years regarding global food requirements were inaccurate, algae have not become a major source of food either, and the demand for alternative protein sources is present and bigger than ever (Henchion et al. 2017). Increase in population and consciousness for sustainability are the major causes of such demand. Terrestrial agriculture is the traditional protein source, but it requires too much water and arable land, as well as being environmentally expensive (Tanentzap et al. 2015). Microalgae can solve these problems and that is why they have immense market potential.

The microalgae market in the health food industry already exists, and it is mostly because of their protein content. More than 12 000 t of *Spirulina* biomass are produced every year for around US\$30 kg^{-1} (Figure 18.6) (García et al. 2017). The price of phycobiliproteins can reach up to US\$25 mg^{-1} (Milledge 2011). Algae are a relevant ingredient for traditional Asian cuisine, but they are not widely accepted in Western cultures. Enhancement of their sensory properties is still required (Becker 2007). Microalgal proteins might be able to replace conventional proteins someday bringing numerous benefits to the world, but obtaining high-value compounds, such as phycobiliproteins, first; it is imperative to develop technology further in order to make this and other microalgal applications feasible (Vigani et al. 2015). As consumers move toward healthier food, and environmental concerns rise, the importance of microalgae as a source of proteins will increase. Even though seaweeds are considered low-protein organisms, they contain the most essential amino acids. In addition, the potential of seaweeds as source of biopeptides is considered a challenge given the link between polysaccharides and proteins.

Other inestimable molecules from algae are the antioxidants, either in the form of PUFAs or pigments. Both molecules are highly valued for their health benefits. PUFAs are considered nutrients and antioxidants, and their inclusion in the daily diet has been highly recommended. With the increasing interest in healthier foods and dietetic supplements the production of algal PUFAs has also grown, most of them marketed as extracts or powder. According to PUFAChain Project (Marcel van der Voort et al. 2017) the price ranges for algae or fish oil are approx. €400 – €1500 kg^{-1} EPA/DHA and algae DHA supplements are approx. €5500 kg^{-1} DHA. Regarding pigments, the market opportunities are very similar to those for PUFAs as shown above in Section 18.2. Many companies around the world are including natural colorants in their formulations to satisfy global market demands as well as the governmental regulations.

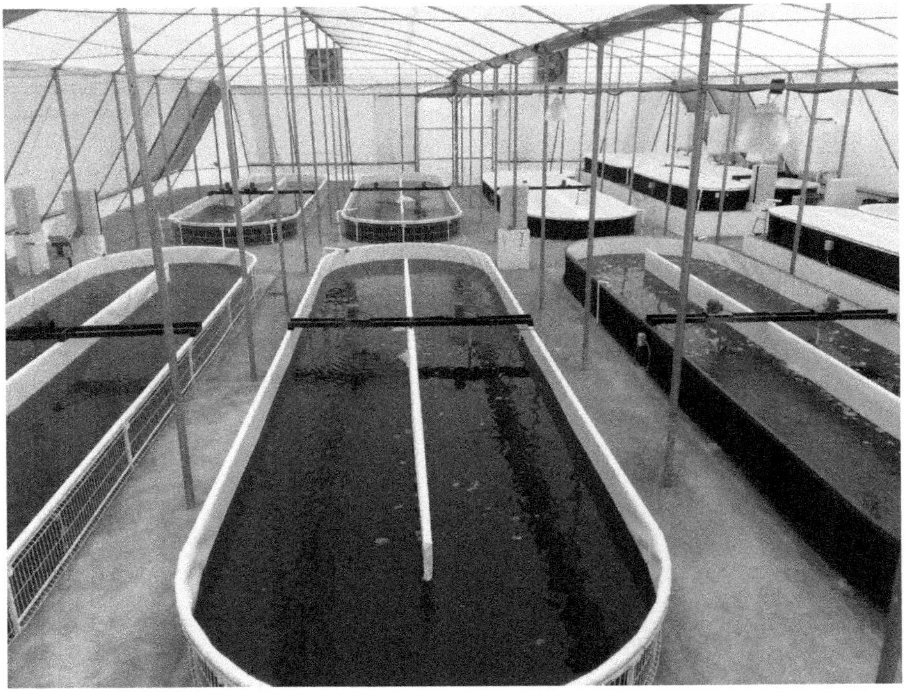

Figure 18.6 Large-scale cultivation of *Spirulina platensis* in raceways for food supplements production. Source: Courtesy of Biotecnología Mexicana de Microalgas, SA de CV (BIOMEX).

Both, micro- and macroalgae (seaweeds) are a rich source of PUFAs and pigments. Their large-scale production is still a challenge as well as a great business opportunity for emerging economies, mostly those with access to the sea.

But perhaps the most significant challenge for micro- and macroalgal production at a commercial scale is the cultural change in the market and consumers regarding the acceptance and use of algae as food and/or nutraceuticals.

References

Adarme-Vega, T., Lim, D.K.Y., Timmins, M. et al. (2012). Microalgal biofactories: a promising approach towards sustainable omega-3 fatty acid production. *Microbial Cell Factories* **11**: 96. https://doi.org/10.1186/1475-2859-11-96.

Adarme-Vega, T.C., Thomas-Hall, S.R., and Schenk, P.M. (2014). Towards sustainable sources for omega-3 fatty acids production. *Current Opinion in Biotechnology* **26**: 14–18. https://doi.org/10.1016/j.copbio.2013.08.003.

Ahmad, A., Anjum, F.M., Zahoor, T. et al. (2012a). Beta glucan: a valuable functional ingredient in foods. *Critical Reviews in Food Science and Nutrition*. https://doi.org/10.1080/10408398.2010.499806.

Ahmad, A., Munir, B., and Abrar, M. (2012b). β-Glucan as functional ingredient for food industry. *Journal of Nutrition & Food Sciences* **02** (02) https://doi.org/10.4172/2155-9600.1000133.

Ahmadi, A., Zorofchian Moghadamtousi, S., Abubakar, S., and Zandi, K. (2015). Antiviral potential of algae polysaccharides isolated from marine sources: a review. *BioMed Research International* **2015**: 1–10. https://doi.org/10.1155/2015/825203.

Albenzio, M., Santillo, A., Caroprese, M., and Malva, A. (2017). Bioactive peptides in animal food products. *Foods* **6** (5): 35. https://doi.org/10.3390/foods6050035.

Antelo, F.S., Costa, J.A.V., and Kalil, S.J. (2008). Thermal degradation kinetics of the phycocyanin from *Spirulina platensis*. *Biochemical Engineering Journal* **41** (1): 43–47. https://doi.org/10.1016/j.bej.2008.03.012.

Arad, S. and Levy-Ontman, O. (2010). Red microalgal cell-wall polysaccharides: biotechnological aspects. *Current Opinion in Biotechnology* **21** (3): 358–364. https://doi.org/10.1016/j.copbio.2010.02.008.

Barka, A. and Blecker, C. (2016). Microalgae as a potential source of single-cell proteins. A review. *Biotechnology, Agronomy and Society and Environment* **20** (3): 427–436.

Bawa, A.S. and Anilakumar, K.R. (2013). Genetically modified foods: safety, risks and public concerns – a review. *Journal of Food Science and Technology*. https://doi.org/10.1007/s13197-012-0899-1.

Becker, E.W. (2007). Micro-algae as a source of protein. *Biotechnology Advances* **25** (2): 207–210. https://doi.org/10.1016/j.biotechadv.2006.11.002.

Begum, H., Yusoff, F.M.D., Banerjee, S. et al. (2016). Availability and utilization of pigments from microalgae. *Critical Reviews in Food Science and Nutrition* **56** (13): 2209–2222. https://doi.org/10.1080/10408398.2013.764841.

Bellou, S., Baeshen, M.N., Elazzazy, A.M. et al. (2014). Microalgal lipids biochemistry and biotechnological perspectives. *Biotechnology Advances* **32** (8): 1476–1493. https://doi.org/10.1016/j.biotechadv.2014.10.003.

Berteau, O. and Mulloy, B. (2003). Sulfated fucans, fresh perspectives: structures, functions, and biological properties of sulfated fucans and an overview of enzymes active toward this class of polysaccharide. *Glycobiology* **13** (6): 29–40. https://doi.org/10.1093/glycob/cwg058.

Bleakley, S. and Hayes, M. (2017). Lgal proteins: extraction, application, and challenges concerning production. *Foods* **6** (5): 33. https://doi.org/10.3390/foods6050033.

Borowitzka, M.A. (2013). High-value products from microalgae-their development and commercialisation. *Journal of Applied Phycology* **25** (3): 743–756. https://doi.org/10.1007/s10811-013-9983-9.

Burtin, P. (2003). Nutritional value of seaweeds. *Journal of Environmental Agriculture and Food Chemistry* **2** (4): 498–503. https://doi.org/ISSN:1579-4377.

Capelli, B. and Cysewski, G.R. (2010). Potential health benefits of spirulina microalgae. A review of the existing literature. *Nutra Food* **9** (2): 19–26. https://doi.org/10.1007/BF03223332.

Černá, M. (2011). *Seaweed Proteins and Amino Acids as Nutraceuticals. Advances in Food and Nutrition Research*, 1e, vol. **64**. Elsevier Inc https://doi.org/10.1016/B978-0-12-387669-0.00024-7.

Cesário, M.T., da Fonseca, M.M.R., Marques, M.M., and de Almeida, M.C.M.D. (2018). Marine algal carbohydrates as carbon sources for the production of biochemicals and biomaterials. *Biotechnology Advances* **36** (3): 798–817. https://doi.org/10.1016/j.biotechadv.2018.02.006.

Chacón-Lee, T.L. and González-Mariño, G.E. (2010). Microalgae for "healthy" foods-possibilities and challenges. *Comprehensive Reviews in Food Science and Food Safety* **9** (6): 655–675. https://doi.org/10.1111/j.1541-4337.2010.00132.x.

Chan, G., Chan, W., and Sze, D. (2009). The effects of β-glucan on human immune and cancer cells. *Journal of Hematology & Oncology* https://doi.org/10.1186/1756-8722-2-25.

Chandini, S.K., Ganesan, P., Suresh, P.V., and Bhaskar, N. (2008). Seaweeds as a source of nutritionally beneficial compounds – a review. *Journal of Food Science and Technology – Mysore* **45** (1): 1–13.

Chen, B., You, W., Huang, J. et al. (2010). Isolation and antioxidant property of the extracellular polysaccharide from *Rhodella reticulata*. *World Journal of Microbiology and Biotechnology*. https://doi.org/10.1007/s11274-009-0240-y.

Chew, K.W., Yap, J.Y., Show, P.L. et al. (2017). Microalgae biorefinery: high value products perspectives. *Bioresource Technology*. https://doi.org/10.1016/j.biortech.2017.01.006.

Christaki, E., Florou-Paneri, P., and Bonos, E. (2011). Microalgae: a novel ingredient in nutrition. *International Journal of Food Sciences and Nutrition* **62** (8): 794–799. https://doi.org/10.3109/09637486.2011.582460.

Cramer, D.E., Allendorf, D.J., Baran, J.T. et al. (2006). β-Glucan enhances complement-mediated hematopoietic recovery after bone marrow injury. *Blood* **107**: 835–840. https://doi.org/10.1182/blood-2005-07-2705.

D'Alessandro, E.B. and Antoniosi Filho, N.R. (2016). Concepts and studies on lipid and pigments of microalgae: a review. *Renewable and Sustainable Energy Reviews* **58**: 832–841. https://doi.org/10.1016/j.rser.2015.12.162.

Dasgupta, C.N. (2015). Algae as a source of phycocyanin and other industrially important pigments. In: *Algal Biorefinery: An Integrated Approach* (ed. D. Das), 253–276. Cham: Springer International Publishing https://doi.org/10.1007/978-3-319-22813-6_12.

Dauvillée, D., Delhaye, S., Gruyer, S. et al. (2010). Engineering the chloroplast targeted malarial vaccine antigens in Chlamydomonas starch granules. *PLoS ONE* **5** (12): e15424.

Dawczynski, C., Schubert, R., and Jahreis, G. (2007). Amino acids, fatty acids, and dietary fibre in edible seaweed products. *Food Chemistry* **103** (3): 891–899. https://doi.org/10.1016/j.foodchem.2006.09.041.

De Jesus Raposo, M.F., De Morais, A.M.B., and De Morais, R.M.S.C. (2015). Marine polysaccharides from algae with potential biomedical applications. *Marine Drugs* **13** (5): 2967–3028. https://doi.org/10.3390/md13052967.

Delattre, C., Pierre, G., Laroche, C., and Michaud, P. (2016). Production, extraction and characterization of microalgal and cyanobacterial exopolysaccharides. *Biotechnology Advances* **34** (7): 1159–1179. https://doi.org/10.1016/j.biotechadv.2016.08.001.

Demurtas, O.C., Massa, S., Ferrante, P. et al. (2013). A *Chlamydomonas*-derived human papillomavirus 16 E7 vaccine induces specific tumor protection. *PLoS One* **8** (4): e61473. https://doi.org/10.1371/journal.pone.0061473.

Dhingra, D., Michael, M., Rajput, H., and Patil, R.T. (2012). Dietary fibre in foods: a review. *Journal of Food Science and Technology* **49**: 255–266. https://doi.org/10.1007/s13197-011-0365-5.

Dreesen, I.A.J., El Hamri, G.C., and Fussenegger, M. (2010). Heat-stable oral alga-based vaccine protects mice from *Staphylococcus aureus* infection. *Journal of Biotechnology* **145**: 273–280. https://doi.org/10.1016/j.jbiotec.2009.12.006.

Du, B., Bian, Z., and Xu, B. (2014). Skin health promotion effects of natural Beta-Glucan derived from cereals and microorganisms: a review. *Phytotherapy Research* **28**: 159–166. https://doi.org/10.1002/ptr.4963.

Dvir, I., Stark, A.H., Chayoth, R. et al. (2009). Hypocholesterolemic effects of nutraceuticals produced from the red microalga *Porphyridium* sp. in rats. *Nutrients*. https://doi.org/10.3390/nu1020156.

Eichler-Stahlberg, A., Weisheit, W., Ruecker, O., and Heitzer, M. (2009). Strategies to facilitate transgene expression in *Chlamydomonas reinhardtii*. *Planta*. https://doi.org/10.1007/s00425-008-0879-x.

Ekmekcioglu, C., Wallner, P., Kundi, M. et al. (2018). Red meat, diseases, and healthy alternatives: a critical review. *Critical Reviews in Food Science and Nutrition*. https://doi.org/10.1080/10408398.2016.1158148.

Eteshola, E., Karpasas, M., Arad, S.M., and Gottlieb, M. (1998). Red microalga exopolysaccharides: 2. Study of the rheology, morphology and thermal gelation of aqueous preparations. *Acta Polymerica* **49** (10–11): 549–556.

Fan, X., Bai, L., Zhu, L. et al. (2014). Marine algae-derived bioactive peptides for human nutrition and health. *Journal of Agricultural and Food Chemistry* **62** (38): 9211–9222. https://doi.org/10.1021/jf502420h.

Fernández-Sevilla, J.M., Acién Fernández, F.G., and Molina Grima, E. (2010). Biotechnological production of lutein and its applications. *Applied Microbiology and Biotechnology* **86** (1): 27–40. https://doi.org/10.1007/s00253-009-2420-y.

Ferruzzi, M.G. and Blakeslee, J. (2007). Digestion, absorption, and cancer preventative activity of dietary chlorophyll derivatives. *Nutrition Research* **27** (1): 1–12. https://doi.org/10.1016/j.nutres.2006.12.003.

Foley, P.M., Beach, E.S., and Zimmerman, J.B. (2011). Algae as a source of renewable chemicals: opportunities and challenges. *Green Chemistry* **13** (6): 1399. https://doi.org/10.1039/c1gc00015b.

Fu, W., Guomundsson, Ó., Paglia, G. et al. (2013). Enhancement of carotenoid biosynthesis in the green microalga Dunaliella salina with light-emitting diodes and adaptive laboratory evolution. *Applied Microbiology and Biotechnology* **97** (6): 2395–2403. https://doi.org/10.1007/s00253-012-4502-5.

García, J.L., de Vicente, M., and Galán, B. (2017). Microalgae, old sustainable food and fashion nutraceuticals. *Microbial Biotechnology* **2783**. https://doi.org/10.1111/1751-7915.12800.

Gardeva, E., Toshkova, R., Minkova, K., and Gigova, L. (2009). Cancer protective action of polysaccharide, derived from red microalga *Porphyridium cruentum* – a biological background. *Biotechnology and Biotechnological Equipment*. https://doi.org/10.1080/13102818.2009.10818540.

Geresh, S. and Arad, S. (1991). The extracellular polysaccharides of the red microalgae: chemistry and rheology. *Bioresource Technology*. https://doi.org/10.1016/0960-8524(91)90154-C.

Geresh, S., Mamontov, A., and Weinstein, J. (2002). Sulfation of extracellular polysaccharides of red microalgae: preparation, characterization and properties. *Journal of Biochemical and Biophysical Methods*. https://doi.org/10.1016/S0165-022X(01)00185-3.

Godfray, H.C.J., Beddington, J.R., Crute, I.R. et al. (2010). Food security: the challenge of feeding 9 billion people. *Science*. https://doi.org/10.1126/science.1185383.

Gong, M. and Bassi, A. (2016). Carotenoids from microalgae: a review of recent developments. *Biotechnology Advances* **34** (8): 1396–1412. https://doi.org/10.1016/j.biotechadv.2016.10.005.

Gong, Y., Hu, H., Gao, Y. et al. (2011). Microalgae as platforms for production of recombinant proteins and valuable compounds: progress and prospects. *Journal of Industrial Microbiology & Biotechnology* **38** (12): 1879–1890. https://doi.org/10.1007/s10295-011-1032-6.

Gosch, B.J., Magnusson, M., Paul, N.A., and de Nys, R. (2012). Total lipid and fatty acid composition of seaweeds for the selection of species for oil-based biofuel and bioproducts. *GCB Bioenergy* **4** (6): 919–930. https://doi.org/10.1111/j.1757-1707.2012.01175.x.

Gouveia, L., Batista, A.P., Sousa, I. et al. (2008). Microalgae in novel food products. In: *Food Chemistry Research Developments* (ed. K.N. Papadopoulos), 75–112. New York: Nova Publishers.

Gouveia, L., Marques, A.E., Sousa, J.M. et al. (2010). Microalgae – source of natural bioactive molecules as functional ingredients. *Food Science & Technology Bulletin: Functional Foods* **7** (2): 21–37. https://doi.org/10.1616/1476-2137.15884.

Gregory, J.A., Li, F., Tomosada, L.M. et al. (2012). Algae-produced pfs25 elicits antibodies that inhibit malaria transmission. *PLoS One*. https://doi.org/10.1371/journal.pone.0037179.

Guedes, A.C., Amaro, H.M., and Malcata, F.X. (2011). Microalgae as sources of carotenoids. *Marine Drugs* **9** (4): 625–644. https://doi.org/10.3390/md9040625.

Gupta, S. and Abu-Ghannam, N. (2011). Bioactive potential and possible health effects of edible brown seaweeds. *Trends in Food Science and Technology* **22** (6): 315–326. https://doi.org/10.1016/j.tifs.2011.03.011.

Guzman-Murillo, M.A. and Ascencio, F. (2000). Anti-adhesive activity of sulphated exopolysaccharides of microalgae on attachment of red sore disease-associated bacteria and *Helicobacter pylori* to tissue culture cells. *Letters in Applied Microbiology*. https://doi.org/10.1046/j.1472-765x.2000.00751.x.

Halim, R., Hosikian, A., Lim, S., and Danquah, M.K. (2010). Chlorophyll extraction from microalgae: a review on the process engineering aspects. *International Journal of Chemical Engineering* **2010**. https://doi.org/10.5268/IW-6.4.874.

Harnedy, P.A. and Fitzgerald, R.J. (2011). Bioactive proteins, peptides, and amino acids from macroalgae. *Journal of Phycology* **47** (2): 218–232. https://doi.org/10.1111/j.1529-8817.2011.00969.x.

Harun, R., Singh, M., Forde, G.M., and Danquah, M.K. (2010). Bioprocess engineering of microalgae to produce a variety of consumer products. *Renewable and Sustainable Energy Reviews* **14** (3): 1037–1047. https://doi.org/10.1016/j.rser.2009.11.004.

Hayes, M. (2012). *Marine bioactive compounds*. In: *Marine Bioactive Compounds: Sources, Characterization and Applications* (ed. M. Hayes). Boston, MA: Springer US https://doi.org/10.1007/978-1-4614-1247-2.

Hayes, M. (2013). Biological activities of proteins and marine-derived peptides from byproducts and seaweeds. In: *Marine Proteins and Peptides: Biological Activities and Applications*, 139–165. Chichester: Wiley https://doi.org/10.1002/9781118375082.ch7.

Hehemann, J.H., Correc, G., Barbeyron, T. et al. (2010). Transfer of carbohydrate-active enzymes from marine bacteria to Japanese gut microbiota. *Nature*. https://doi.org/10.1038/nature08937.

Henchion, M., Hayes, M., Mullen, A. et al. (2017). Future protein supply and demand: strategies and factors influencing a sustainable equilibrium. *Foods* **6** (7): 53. https://doi.org/10.3390/foods6070053.

Hoffman, J.R. and Falvo, M.J. (2004). Protein - Which is best? *Journal of Sports Science and Medicine*. https://doi.org/10.1016/j.compstruct.2011.11.030.

Holdt, S.L. and Kraan, S. (2011). Bioactive compounds in seaweed: functional food applications and legislation. *Journal of Applied Phycology* **23** (3): 543–597. https://doi.org/10.1007/s10811-010-9632-5.

Hu, J., Nagarajan, D., Zhang, Q. et al. (2018). Heterotrophic cultivation of microalgae for pigment production: a review. *Biotechnology Advances* **36** (1): 54–67. https://doi.org/10.1016/j.biotechadv.2017.09.009.

Humphrey, A. (2004). Chlorophyll as a color and functional ingredient. *Journal of Food Science* **69** (5): C422–C425. https://doi.org/10.1111/j.1365-2621.2004.tb10710.x.

Jan, N., Shafi, F., Hameed, O. et al. (2016). An overview on edible vaccines and imunization. *Austin Journal of Nutrition and Food Sciences* **4** (2): 1078.

Jiménez-Escrig, A., Gómez-Ordóñez, E., and Rupérez, P. (2011). Seaweed as a source of novel nutraceuticals: sulfated polysaccharides and peptides. *Advances in Food and Nutrition Research* **64**: 325–337. https://doi.org/10.1016/B978-0-12-387669-0.00026-0.

Kankkunen, P., Teirila, L., Rintahaka, J. et al. (2010). (1,3)-Beta-glucans activate both dectin-1 and NLRP3 inflammasome in human macrophages. *The Journal of Immunology* **184** (11): 6335–6342. https://doi.org/10.4049/jimmunol.0903019.

Kannaujiya, V.K. and Sinha, R.P. (2016). Thermokinetic stability of phycocyanin and phycoerythrin in food-grade preservatives. *Journal of Applied Phycology* **28** (2): 1063–1070. https://doi.org/10.1007/s10811-015-0638-x.

Khan, Z., Bhadouria, P., and Bisen, P. (2005). Nutritional and therapeutic potential of Spirulina. *Current Pharmaceutical Biotechnology* **6** (5): 373–379. https://doi.org/10.2174/138920105774370607.

Khan, M., Shin, J.H., and Kim, J.D. (2018). The promising future of microalgae: current status, challenges, and optimization of a sustainable and renewable industry for biofuels, feed, and other products. *Microbial Cell Factories* **17** (1): 36. https://doi.org/10.1186/s12934-018-0879-x.

Khozin-Goldberg, I. (2016). Lipid metabolism in microalgae. In: *The Physiology of Microalgae* (eds. M.A. Borowitzka, J. Beardall and J.A. Raven), 413–484. Cham: Springer International Publishing https://doi.org/10.1007/978-3-319-24945-2_18.

Kim, S.-K. and Kang, K.-H. (2011). Medicinal effects of peptides from marine microalgae. In: *Advances in Food and Nutrition Research*, 1e, vol. **64**, 313–323. Elsevier Inc. https://doi.org/10.1016/B978-0-12-387669-0.00025-9.

Kim, S.Y., Song, H.J., Lee, Y.Y. et al. (2006). Biomedical issues of dietary fiber beta-glucan. *Journal of Korean Medical Science* **21** (5): 781–789. https://doi.org/10.3346/jkms.2006.21.5.781.

Kim, S.M., Jung, Y.J., Kwon, O.N. et al. (2012). A potential commercial source of fucoxanthin extracted from the microalga *Phaeodactylum tricornutum*. *Applied Biochemistry and Biotechnology* **166** (7): 1843–1855. https://doi.org/10.1007/s12010-012-9602-2.

Koller, M., Muhr, A., and Braunegg, G. (2014). Microalgae as versatile cellular factories for valued products. *Algal Research* **6** (PA): 52–63. https://doi.org/10.1016/j.algal.2014.09.002.

Korzeniowska, K., Górka, B., Lipok, J., and Wieczorek, P.P. (2018). Algae and their extracts in medical treatment. In: *Algae Biomass: Characteristics and Applications*, vol. **8**, 73–87. Cham: Springer International Publishing https://doi.org/10.1007/978-3-319-74703-3_7.

Kose, A., Ozen, M.O., Elibol, M., and Oncel, S.S. (2017). Investigation of in vitro digestibility of dietary microalga *Chlorella vulgaris* and cyanobacterium *Spirulina platensis* as a nutritional supplement. *3 Biotech*. https://doi.org/10.1007/s13205-017-0832-4.

Kostic, A.D., Howitt, M.R., and Garrett, W.S. (2013). Exploring host-microbiota interactions in animal models and humans. *Genes and Development*. https://doi.org/10.1101/gad.212522.112.

Kumar, C.S., Ganesan, P., and Bhaskar, N. (2008). Seaweeds as a source of nutritionally beneficial compounds – a review. *Journal of Food Science and Technology* **45** (1): 1–13.

Kumar, A., Shankar Vishwakarma, H., Singh, J., and Kumar, M. (2015). Microbial pigments: production and their applications in various industries. *International Journal of Pharmaceutical, Chemical and Biological Sciences* **2015** (1): 203–212.

Kwak, J.H., Baek, S.H., Woo, Y. et al. (2012). Beneficial immunostimulatory effect of short-term *Chlorella* supplementation: enhancement of natural killer cell activity and early inflammatory response (randomized, double-blinded, placebo-controlled trial). *Nutrition Journal*. https://doi.org/10.1186/1475-2891-11-53.

Kwon, K.-C. and Daniell, H. (2016). Oral delivery of protein drugs bioencapsulated in plant cells. *Molecular Therapy* **24** (8): 1342–1350. https://doi.org/10.1038/mt.2016.115.

Lahaye, M. and Robic, A. (2007). Structure and function properties of ulvan, a polysaccharide from green seaweeds. *Biomacromolecules* **8** (6): 1765–1774. https://doi.org/10.1021/bm061185q.

Lemes, A.C., Sala, L., Ores, J.D.C. et al. (2016). A review of the latest advances in encrypted bioactive peptides from protein-rich waste. *International Journal of Molecular Sciences*. https://doi.org/10.3390/ijms17060950.

Lev-Yadun, S. and Gould, K.S. (2007). What do red and yellow autumn leaves signal. *The Botanical Review* **73** (4): 279–289. https://doi.org/10.1663/0006-8101(2007)73[279:WDRAYA]2.0.CO;2.

Lonnie, M., Hooker, E., Brunstrom, J.M. et al. (2018). Protein for life: review of optimal protein intake, sustainable dietary sources and the effect on appetite in ageing adults. *Nutrients*. https://doi.org/10.3390/nu10030360.

Ma, L. and Lin, X.M. (2010). Effects of lutein and zeaxanthin on aspects of eye health. *Journal of the Science of Food and Agriculture* **90** (1): 2–12. https://doi.org/10.1002/jsfa.3785.

Maeda, H., Tsukui, T., Sashima, T. et al. (2008). Seaweed carotenoid, fucoxanthin, as a multi-functional nutrient. *Asia Pacific Journal of Clinical Nutrition* **17** (Suppl. 1): 196–199. https://doi.org/10.1186/1475-2891-10-83.

Marcel van der Voort, A., Spruijt, J., Potters, J., de Wolf, P., and Elissen, H. (2017). Socio-economic assessment of algae-based PUFA production. The value chain from microalgae to PUFA ('PUFAChain'). www.pufachain.eu (accessed September 22, 2020).

Mary Leema, J.T., Kirubagaran, R., Vinithkumar, N.V. et al. (2010). High value pigment production from *Arthrospira* (*Spirulina*) *platensis* cultured in seawater. *Bioresource Technology* **101** (23): 9221–9227. https://doi.org/10.1016/j.biortech.2010.06.120.

Medina-Gali, R., Ortega-Villaizan, M.d.M., Mercado, L. et al. (2018). Beta-glucan enhances the response to SVCV infection in zebrafish. *Developmental and Comparative Immunology*. https://doi.org/10.1016/j.dci.2018.02.019.

Mehta, P., Singh, D., Saxena, R. et al. (2018). High-value coproducts from algae – an innovational way to deal with advance algal industry. In: *Waste to Wealth*, 343–363. Singapore: Springer. https://doi.org/10.1007/978-981-10-7431-8_15.

Mikami, K. and Hosokawa, M. (2013). Biosynthetic pathway and health benefits of fucoxanthin, an algae-specific xanthophyll in brown seaweeds. *International Journal of Molecular Sciences* **14** (7): 13763–13781. https://doi.org/10.3390/ijms140713763.

Milledge, J.J. (2011). Commercial application of microalgae other than as biofuels: a brief review. *Reviews in Environmental Science and Bio/Technology* **10** (1): 31–41. https://doi.org/10.1007/s11157-010-9214-7.

Miyashita, K., Nishikawa, S., Beppu, F. et al. (2011). The allenic carotenoid fucoxanthin, a novel marine nutraceutical from brown seaweeds. *Journal of the Science of Food and Agriculture* **91** (7): 1166–1174. https://doi.org/10.1002/jsfa.4353.

Miyata, M., Koyama, T., Kamitani, T. et al. (2009). Anti-obesity effect on rodents of the traditional Japanese food, tororokombu, shaved *Laminaria*. *Bioscience, Biotechnology, and Biochemistry* **73** (10): 2326–2328. https://doi.org/10.1271/bbb.90344.

Mobin, S. and Alam, F. (2017). Some promising microalgal species for commercial applications: a review. *Energy Procedia* **110** (December 2016): 510–517. https://doi.org/10.1016/j.egypro.2017.03.177.

Mohamed, S., Hashim, S.N., and Rahman, H.A. (2012). Seaweeds: a sustainable functional food for complementary and alternative therapy. *Trends in Food Science and Technology* **23** (2): 83–96. https://doi.org/10.1016/j.tifs.2011.09.001.

Moroney, N.C., O'Grady, M.N., Lordan, S. et al. (2015). Seaweed polysaccharides (laminarin and fucoidan) as functional ingredients in pork meat: an evaluation of anti-oxidative potential, thermal stability and bioaccessibility. *Marine Drugs* **13** (4): 2447–2464. https://doi.org/10.3390/md13042447.

Mulders, K.J.M., Lamers, P.P., Martens, D.E., and Wijffels, R.H. (2014). Phototrophic pigment production with microalgae: biological constraints and opportunities. *Journal of Phycology* **50** (2): 229–242. https://doi.org/10.1111/jpy.12173.

Namikoshi, M., Rinehart, K.L., and Ave, S.M. (1996). Bioactive compounds produced by cyanobacteria. *Journal of Industrial Microbiology & Biotechnology*. https://doi.org/10.1007/BF01574768.

Ngo, D.H. and Kim, S.K. (2013). Sulfated polysaccharides as bioactive agents from marine algae. *International Journal of Biological Macromolecules*. https://doi.org/10.1016/j.ijbiomac.2013.08.036.

Panova, I.G., Yakovleva, M.A., Tatikolov, A.S. et al. (2017). Lutein and its oxidized forms in eye structures throughout prenatal human development. *Experimental Eye Research* **160**: 31–37. https://doi.org/10.1016/j.exer.2017.04.008.

Peng, J., Yuan, J.P., Wu, C.F., and Wang, J.H. (2011). Fucoxanthin, a marine carotenoid present in brown seaweeds and diatoms: metabolism and bioactivities relevant to human health. *Marine Drugs* **9** (10): 1806–1828. https://doi.org/10.3390/md9101806.

Pignolet, O., Jubeau, S., Vaca-Garcia, C., and Michaud, P. (2013). Highly valuable microalgae: biochemical and topological aspects. *Journal of Industrial Microbiology and Biotechnology* **40** (8): 781–796. https://doi.org/10.1007/s10295-013-1281-7.

Priyadarshani, I. and Rath, B. (2012). Commercial and industrial applications of micro algae – a review. *Journal of Algal Biomass Utilization* **3** (4): 89–100. https://doi.org/10.1016/j.(73).

Pulz, O. and Gross, W. (2004). Valuable products from biotechnology of microalgae. *Applied Microbiology and Biotechnology* **65** (6): 635–648. https://doi.org/10.1007/s00253-004-1647-x.

Qin, S., Lin, H., and Jiang, P. (2012). Advances in genetic engineering of marine algae. *Biotechnology Advances* **30** (6): 1602–1613. https://doi.org/10.1016/j.biotechadv.2012.05.004.

Rajapakse, N. and Kim, S.K. (2011). *Nutritional and Digestive Health Benefits of Seaweed. Advances in Food and Nutrition Research*, 1e, vol. **64**. Elsevier Inc https://doi.org/10.1016/B978-0-12-387669-0.00002-8.

Rajauria, G., Foley, B. and Abu-Ghannam, N. (2017). Characterization of dietary fucoxanthin from Himanthalia elongata brownseaweed. *Food Research International* **99** (part 3): 995–1001. https://doi.org/10.1016/j.foodres.2016.09.023.

Rangel-Yagui, C.D.O., Danesi, E.D.G., De Carvalho, J.C.M., and Sato, S. (2004). Chlorophyll production from *Spirulina platensis*: cultivation with urea addition by fed-batch process. *Bioresource Technology* **92** (2): 133–141. https://doi.org/10.1016/j.biortech.2003.09.002.

Rasala, B.A. and Mayfield, S.P. (2015). Photosynthetic biomanufacturing in green algae; production of recombinant proteins for industrial, nutritional, and medical uses. *Photosynthesis Research* **123** (3): 227–239. https://doi.org/10.1007/s11120-014-9994-7.

Rasala, B.A., Muto, M., Lee, P.A. et al. (2010). Production of therapeutic proteins in algae, analysis of expression of seven human proteins in the chloroplast of *Chlamydomonas reinhardtii. Plant Biotechnology Journal*. https://doi.org/10.1111/j.1467-7652.2010.00503.x.

Ravishankar, G.A. and Ambati, R.R. (2019). *Handbook of Algal Technologies and Phytochemicals* (eds. G. Ravishankar and R.R. Ambati). Boca Raton, FL: CRC Press https://doi.org/10.1201/9780429054242.

Rico, M., González, A.G., Santana-Casiano, M. et al. (2017). Production of primary and secondary metabolites using algae. In: *Prospects and Challenges in Algal Biotechnology* (eds. B.N. Tripathi and D. Kumar), 311–326. Singapore: Springer Singapore https://doi.org/10.1007/978-981-10-1950-0_12.

Rodrigues, D.B., Flores, É.M.M., Barin, J.S. et al. (2014). Production of carotenoids from microalgae cultivated using agroindustrial wastes. *Food Research International* **65** (PB): 144–148. https://doi.org/10.1016/j.foodres.2014.06.037.

Ruocco, N., Costantini, S., Guariniello, S., and Costantini, M. (2016). Polysaccharides from the marine environment with pharmacological, cosmeceutical and nutraceutical potential. *Molecules* **21** (5): 1–16. https://doi.org/10.3390/molecules21050551.

Ryckebosch, E., Bruneel, C., Muylaert, K., and Foubert, I. (2012). Microalgae as an alternative source of omega-3 long chain polyunsaturated fatty acids. *Lipid Technology* **24** (6): 128–130. https://doi.org/10.1002/lite.201200197.

Samuelsen, A.B.C., Schrezenmeir, J., and Knutsen, S.H. (2014). Effects of orally administered yeast-derived beta-glucans: a review. *Molecular Nutrition and Food Research*. https://doi.org/10.1002/mnfr.201300338.

Sánchez, A. and Vázquez, A. (2017). Bioactive peptides: a review. *Food Quality and Safety* **1** (1): 29–46. https://doi.org/10.1093/fqs/fyx006.

Sánchez-Machado, D.I., López-Cervantes, J., López-Hernández, J., and Paseiro-Losada, P. (2004). Fatty acids, total lipid, protein and ash contents of processed edible seaweeds. *Food Chemistry* **85** (3): 439–444. https://doi.org/10.1016/j.foodchem.2003.08.001.

Sarada, R., Pillai, M.G., and Ravishankar, G. (1999). Phycocyanin from *Spirulina* sp: influence of processing of biomass on phycocyanin yield, analysis of efficacy of extraction methods and stability studies on phycocyanin. *Process Biochemistry* **34** (8): 795–801. https://doi.org/10.1016/S0032-9592(98)00153-8.

Sathasivam, R. and Ki, J.S. (2018). A review of the biological activities of microalgal carotenoids and their potential use in healthcare and cosmetic industries. *Marine Drugs* **16** (1) https://doi.org/10.3390/md16010026.

Sathasivam, R., Radhakrishnan, R., Hashem, A., and Abd Allah, E.F. (2017). Microalgae metabolites: a rich source for food and medicine. *Saudi Journal of Biological Sciences*. https://doi.org/10.1016/j.sjbs.2017.11.003.

Sato, M., Hosokawa, T., Yamaguchi, T. et al. (2002). Angiotensin I-converting enzyme inhibitory peptides derived from wakame (*Undaria pinnatifida*) and their antihypertensive effect in spontaneously hypertensive rats. *Journal of Agricultural and Food Chemistry* **50** (21): 6245–6252. https://doi.org/10.1021/jf020482t.

Schulze, C., Wetzel, M., Reinhardt, J. et al. (2016). Screening of microalgae for primary metabolites including β-glucans and the influence of nitrate starvation and irradiance on β-glucan production. *Journal of Applied Phycology* **28** (5): 2719–2725. https://doi.org/10.1007/s10811-016-0812-9.

Sheih, I.C., Fang, T.J., Wu, T.K., and Lin, P.H. (2010). Anticancer and antioxidant activities of the peptide fraction from algae protein waste. *Journal of Agricultural and Food Chemistry*. https://doi.org/10.1021/jf903089m.

Sheng, J., Yu, F., Xin, Z. et al. (2007). Preparation, identification and their antitumor activities in vitro of polysaccharides from *Chlorella pyrenoidosa*. *Food Chemistry*. https://doi.org/10.1016/j.foodchem.2007.04.018.

Sigamani, S., Ramamurthy, D., and Natarajan, H. (2016). A review on potential biotechnological applications of microalgae. *Journal of Applied Pharmaceutical Science*. https://doi.org/10.7324/JAPS.2016.60829.

Singh, S.C., Sinha, R.P., and Häder, D.-P. (2002). Role of lipids and fatty acids in stress tolerance in cyanobacteria. *Acta Protozoologica* **41**: 297–308.

Sloth, J.K., Wiebe, M.G., and Eriksen, N.T. (2006). Accumulation of phycocyanin in heterotrophic and mixotrophic cultures of the acidophilic red alga *Galdieria sulphuraria*. *Enzyme and Microbial Technology* **38** (1–2): 168–175. https://doi.org/10.1016/j.enzmictec.2005.05.010.

Song, H., He, M., Gu, C. et al. (2018). Extraction optimization, purification, antioxidant activity, and preliminary structural characterization of crude polysaccharide from an arctic *Chlorella* sp. *Polymers*. https://doi.org/10.3390/polym10030292.

Specht, E.A. and Mayfield, S.P. (2014). Algae-based oral recombinant vaccines. *Frontiers in Microbiology* **5** (Feb) https://doi.org/10.3389/fmicb.2014.00060.

Specht, E., Miyake-Stoner, S., and Mayfield, S. (2010). Micro-algae come of age as a platform for recombinant protein production. *Biotechnology Letters* **32** (10): 1373–1383. https://doi.org/10.1007/s10529-010-0326-5.

Suetsuna, K. and Chen, J.R. (2001). Identification of antihypertensive peptides from peptic digest of two microalgae, *Chlorella vulgaris* and *Spirulina platensis*. *Marine Biotechnology*. https://doi.org/10.1007/s10126-001-0012-7.

Sun, M., Qian, K., Su, N. et al. (2003). Foot-and-mouth disease virus VP1 protein fused with cholera toxin B subunit expressed in *Chlamydomonas reinhardtii* chloroplast. *Biotechnology Letters*. https://doi.org/10.1023/A:1024140114505.

Talero, E., García-Mauriño, S., Ávila-Román, J. et al. (2015). Bioactive compounds isolated from microalgae in chronic inflammation and cancer. *Marine Drugs* **13** (10): 6152–6209. https://doi.org/10.3390/md13106152.

Tanentzap, A.J., Lamb, A., Walker, S., and Farmer, A. (2015). Resolving conflicts between agriculture and the natural environment. *PLoS Biology* **13** (9): e1002242. https://doi.org/10.1371/journal.pbio.1002242.

Tanna, B. and Mishra, A. (2018). Metabolites unravel nutraceutical potential of edible seaweeds: an emerging source of functional food. *Comprehensive Reviews in Food Science and Food Safety* **17** (6): 1613–1624. https://doi.org/10.1111/1541-4337.12396.

Tien Lea, D., Duc Chua, H., and Quynh Lea, N. (2016). Improving nutritional quality of plant proteins through genetic engineering. *Current Genomics* **17** (3): 220–229. https://doi.org/10.2174/1389202917666160202215934.

Tomaselli, L. (2003). The microalgal cell. In: *Handbook of Microalgal Culture: Biotechnology and Applied Phycology* (ed. A. Richmond). Oxford: Blackwell Publishing Ltd https://doi.org/10.1002/9780470995280.

Tran, M., Zhou, B., Pettersson, P.L. et al. (2009). Synthesis and assembly of a full-length human monoclonal antibody in algal chloroplasts. *Biotechnology and Bioengineering*. https://doi.org/10.1002/bit.22446.

Tuso, P. (2013). Nutritional update for physicians: plant-based diets. *The Permanente Journal* **17** (2): 61–66. https://doi.org/10.7812/TPP/12-085.

Venkatesan, J., Lowe, B., Anil, S. et al. (2015). Seaweed polysaccharides and their potential biomedical applications. *Starch/Staerke* **67** (5–6): 381–390. https://doi.org/10.1002/star.201400127.

Vigani, M., Parisi, C., Rodríguez-Cerezo, E. et al. (2015). Food and feed products from micro-algae: market opportunities and challenges for the EU. *Trends in Food Science and Technology* **42** (1): 81–92. https://doi.org/10.1016/j.tifs.2014.12.004.

Wang, X., Brandsma, M., Tremblay, R. et al. (2008). A novel expression platform for the production of diabetes-associated autoantigen human glutamic acid decarboxylase (hGAD65). *BMC Biotechnology*. https://doi.org/10.1186/1472-6750-8-87.

Wells, M.L., Potin, P., Craigie, J.S. et al. (2017). Algae as nutritional and functional food sources: revisiting our understanding. *Journal of Applied Phycology* **29** (2): 949–982. https://doi.org/10.1007/s10811-016-0974-5.

Wijesekara, I. and Karunarathna, W.K.D.S. (2017). Usage of seaweed polysaccharides as nutraceuticals. In: *Seaweed Polysaccharides: Isolation, Biological and Biomedical Applications* (eds. J. Venkatesan, S. Anil and S.-K. Kim), 341–348. Elsevier https://doi.org/10.1016/B978-0-12-809816-5.00018-9.

Wu, H.L., Wang, G.H., Xiang, W.Z. et al. (2016). Stability and antioxidant activity of food-grade phycocyanin isolated from *Spirulina platensis*. *International Journal of Food Properties* **19** (10): 2349–2362. https://doi.org/10.1080/10942912.2015.1038564.

Wunderlich, S. and Gatto, K.A. (2015). Consumer perception of genetically modified organisms and sources of information. *Advances in Nutrition* **6** (6): 842–851. https://doi.org/10.3945/an.115.008870.

Yaakob, Z., Ali, E., Zainal, A. et al. (2014). An overview: biomolecules from microalgae for animal feed and aquaculture. *Journal of Biological Research (Greece)*. https://doi.org/10.1186/2241-5793-21-6.

Yan, X., Chuda, Y., Suzuki, M., and Nagata, T. (1999). Fucoxanthin as the major antioxidant in *Hijikia fusiformis*, a common edible seaweed. *Bioscience, Biotechnology, and Biochemistry* **63** (3): 605–607. https://doi.org/10.1271/bbb.63.605.

Yan, N., Fan, C., Chen, Y., and Hu, Z. (2016). The potential for microalgae as bioreactors to produce pharmaceuticals. *International Journal of Molecular Sciences*. https://doi.org/10.3390/ijms17060962.

Zeković, D.B., Kwiatkowski, S., Vrvić, M.M. et al. (2005). Natural and modified (1→3)-β-D-glucans in health promotion and disease alleviation. *Critical Reviews in Biotechnology*. https://doi.org/10.1080/07388550500376166.

Zhang, C., Wohlhueter, R., and Zhang, H. (2016). Genetically modified foods: a critical review of their promise and problems. *Food Science and Human Wellness*. https://doi.org/10.1016/j.fshw.2016.04.002.

Zhu, F., Du, B., and Xu, B. (2016). A critical review on production and industrial applications of beta-glucans. *Food Hydrocolloids* **52**: 275–288. https://doi.org/10.1016/j.foodhyd.2015.07.003.

19
Role of Algal Derived Compounds in Pharmaceuticals and Cosmetics

María Lourdes Mourelle, Carmen P. Gómez, and José L. Legido
Applied Physics Department, Faculty of Sea Sciences, University of Vigo, Vigo, Spain

19.1 Introduction

Algae, like other sessile organisms such as sponges, corals, and other invertebrates, need to adapt to a very competitive and sometimes hostile environment (Alves et al. 2018). They therefore synthesize substances to protect themselves from ultraviolet A (UVA) (320–400 nm) and -B (280–320 nm) irradiation as well as predation from marine organisms. Hence, algae produce primary and secondary metabolites; the former are directly related to their growth, development, and reproduction, while the latter are produced as an adaptive response to stress conditions to which they are subjected (changes in temperature, salinity, UV radiation, water depth, etc.) (Alves et al. 2018). Primary metabolites are mainly proteins, polysaccharides, and fatty acids, while secondary metabolites are polyphenols, pigments, vitamins, sterols, and other bioactive compounds (Alves et al. 2018; Pereira 2018a), which are of great interest in the functional food and nutraceutical, pharmacological, and cosmetic industries.

More than 3000 algal compounds have been discovered in the past five decades, such as peptides, polyacetylenes, alkaloids, and halogenated compounds (Leal et al. 2013; Blunt et al. 2017), even though in the 1990s attention was mainly focused on marine microorganisms such as fungus, microalgae, and cyanobacteria, etc. (Smit 2004). New screening programs based on the ecology of marine organisms (i.e. benthic, littoral, eulittoral, sublittoral), the development of new molecular biology tools (i.e. DNA extraction, DNA sequencing, gene expression, and bioinformatic analysis), the interest in studying toxins produced by marine organisms, and the growing industrial demand for the application of natural compounds extracted from algae and their metabolites with potential economic impact (e.g. asthaxantin, sulfated

Recent Advances in Micro- and Macroalgal Processing: Food and Health Perspectives, First Edition.
Edited by Gaurav Rajauria and Yvonne V. Yuan.

polysaccharides [SPs], etc.) have led to the discovery of a wide variety of biologically active compounds (Alves et al. 2018).

This growth in discovery is also linked to new research techniques from metabolomics, genomics, and proteomics, which have facilitated breakthroughs in macroalgae and microalgae cultivation methods, as well as in the study of their primary and secondary metabolites (Beetul et al. 2016).

19.2 Algae as a Source of Active Ingredients for Pharmaceutical Products

Interest in studying algae for food has been around for a while now; in many countries, the food industries utilize a wide range of algae, which are well known to have high contents of fiber, minerals, vitamins, and different antioxidants (Cardozo et al. 2007), principally marine macroalgae (Beetul et al. 2016), however attention is now moving toward microalgae (both of marine and freshwater origin) (Mourelle et al. 2017). Recent decades have seen increasing research into the extraction of their bioactive compounds for pharmacological use (Beetul et al. 2016). The increased research is facilitated by the ready availability and ease of exploitation (currently obtained by cultivation), as well as their biochemical properties and high nutritional value of macro- and microalgae (Alves et al. 2018; Bule et al. 2018). Added to this is the demand for new natural sources of biologically active compounds that are free of side effects and help treat diseases such as allergies, cardiovascular diseases, cancer, obesity, diabetes, high blood pressure, atopic dermatitis, or Alzheimer's disease (Alves et al. 2018). Therefore, the pharmaceutical, cosmetic, and food industries are seeking new bioactive compounds of marine origin and from macro- and microalgae, in particular. There continues to be a need to provide more scientific evidence through *in vitro*, *in vivo* studies, and especially clinical studies, on the beneficial health effects of algal bioactive compounds (Beetul et al. 2016).

Even though the chemical composition of macro- and microalgae varies depending on the species, location grown, weather conditions, and harvesting season (Gómez-Ordoñez et al. 2010), in general, as photosynthetic organisms subjected to oxidative stress, they will contain several bioactive compounds depending on their classification as Ochraphyta, Rhodophyta, Chlorophyta for macroalgae, and Dinoflagellata, Cryptophyta, or Raphidophyceae for microalgae. These include: polysaccharides; phenolic compounds such as phlorotannins; diverse pigments such as the chlorophylls and carotenoids, including fucoxanthin; mycosporine-like amino acids (MAAs); halogenated compounds; proteins, peptides, and amino acids; essential and long-chain marine polyunsaturated fatty acids (PUFAs); sterols; and other lipids, vitamins, and minerals (Cardozo et al. 2007; Chandini et al. 2008; Gómez-Ordoñez et al. 2010; Fitzgerald et al. 2011; Mohamed et al. 2012; Wijesinghe and Jeon 2012; Mikalak and Chojnacka 2015; Blunt et al. 2017; Alves et al. 2018).

Of all the macroalgal and microalgal bioactive compounds, only a small group such as SPs, sterols, phlorotannins, carotenoids and other pigments, PUFAs, and proteins may have applications in the pharmaceutical industry. The scientific literature contains a great number of *in vitro* and *in vivo* studies on the pharmacological activities of these bioactive compounds; however, due to space limitations, only a few of the most recent ones are reviewed here and a summary of their mechanisms of action is provided.

19.2.1 Sulfated Polysaccharides and Other Phycocolloids

Polysaccharides and, in particular, the sulfated ones are the most studied of all algal bioactive compounds (Pereira 2018a). Many species of macroalgae are rich in polysaccharides, which are mainly found in the cell wall of brown algae (*Phaeophyceae*) and red algae (*Rhodophyceae*), and to a lesser extent in the green algae (*Chlorophyceae*) (Pereira 2018a). The most abundant SPs found in brown algae are fucans (generic term used to define sulfated polysaccharides found in the cell walls of brown algae), fucoidans, ascophyllan, glucuronxylofucan, and sargassan (Ngo and Kim, 2013), while those that abound in red algae are the agars and carrageenans (Ngo and Kim, 2013). On the other hand, the SPs from green algae are usually sulfated heteropolysaccharides containing xylose, arabinose, mannose, glucuronic acid, or glucose (Ngo and Kim, 2013).

A large number of SPs (mainly carrageenans) are used in the food industry as hydrocolloid thickeners (Pereira 2018a), but in recent years, special attention has been paid to other biological activities such as anticoagulant, antioxidant, antiviral, and immunoinflammatory activities of fucoidans, carrageenans, and fucans (Table 19.1) (Jiao et al. 2011, Ngo and Kim, 2013; Vo et al. 2012; Raguraman et al. 2019; Mezdour et al. 2017). The biological activity of fucans and carrageenans has been studied for years now due to their anti-inflammatory and antiviral properties *in vitro* and *in vivo* (Boisson-Vidal et al. 1995). Fucans are obtained mainly from the genera *Fucus* and *Laminaria*, and also from other species such as *A. nodosum* (Boisson-Vidal et al. 1995). These authors studied the activity of low molecular weight fucans *in vitro* and observed that they were potent inhibitors of the human complement activation *in vitro* (40× more active than heparin on a molar basis). In addition to fucans, polysaccharides of the genera *Codium* and *Ulva* (Jiao et al. 2011), such as galactan sulfates and ulvans, also have anticoagulant properties. Recently, Adrien et al. (2019) demonstrated the anticoagulant activities of ulvan. The potential anticoagulant activity of both ulvan fractions was then assessed using different assays, targeting the intrinsic and/or common (activated partial thromboplastin time, APTT), extrinsic (prothrombin time, PT), and common (thrombin time, TT) pathways, and the specific antithrombin-dependent pathway (anti-Xa and anti-IIa) of the coagulation cascade. Furthermore, their anticoagulant properties were compared with those of commercial anticoagulants: heparin and Lovenox®. The results showed that the anticoagulant activity of the chemically sulfated ulvan fraction was stronger than that of Lovenox® against both the intrinsic and extrinsic coagulation pathways (Adrien et al. 2019).

The same is also true for other galactan sulfates obtained from red algae (Farias et al. 2000). These authors obtained a sulfated D-galactan from the red algae *Botryocladia occidentalis* and studied the anticoagulant activities by different assays (APTT, inactivation of thrombin and factor Xa, inactivation of thrombin by antithrombin, inactivation of thrombin by heparin cofactor II, and inactivation of factor Xa by antithrombin); the results showed that algal sulfated D-galactan had a potent anticoagulant activity (similar potency to unfractionated heparin) (Farias et al. 2000). Attention is now being paid to low molecular weight polysaccharides (LMWPs) from species of the genus *Sargassum* (Sun et al. 2018). The authors prepared LMWPs from *Sargassum fusiforme* via H_2O_2 oxidative degradation and investigated *in vitro* the relationship between LMWPs and anticoagulant activity, and studied the anticoagulant activities by APTT, PT, and TT assays, showing that these LMWPs possessed anticoagulant activity in the intrinsic, extrinsic, and common coagulation pathways (Sun et al. 2018).

Table 19.1 Biological activities and potential pharmaceutical uses of micro- and macroalgal bioactive compounds.

Biological activity/potential pharmaceutical use	Bioactive compounds/specific compound	Mechanism	References
Antitumor, cytotoxic, antiproliferative activity	Polysaccharides - Fucoidans	Activation of apoptosis (in human lymphoma HS-Sultan cell line) Suppression of angiogenesis (in human uterine carcinoma HeLa cells) Increase in the immune response in mice Reduction in the adhesion of tumor cells to human platelets	Kwon and Nam (2006); Koyanagi et al. (2003); Li et al. (2008); Wijesekara et al. (2011); Vo and Kim (2013); Moghadamtousi et al. (2014); Bae et al. (2015); Kalimuthu and Kim (2015); Alves et al., (2017); Pereira et al. (2018a); Rahnasto-Rilla et al. (2017)
	Oligosaccharides (from alginates)	Inhibition of TGF-β1/Smad signaling activation in osteosarcoma cells	Chen et al. (2017)
	- Exopolysaccharide	Immunomodulatory activity (inducing B cell proliferation and decreasing the formation of IL-6 and INF-γ)	Park et al. (2017a)
	- Porphyran	Activation caspase-1 and caspase-6 AGS human gastric cancer cells Decreasing the IGF-IR phosphorylation and downregulated a serine/threonine kinase (Akt) phosphorylation AGS human gastric cancer cells	Kwon and Nam (2006)
	- Laminaran	Induction of apoptosis in HT-29 colon cancer cells	Park et al. (2013)
	- Carrageenan	Induction of apoptosis in human intestine (Caco-2) and hepatic (HepG2) Inhibition of angiogenesis in mice Enhance the antitumor activity of 5-fluorouracile on S180 xenograft in mice	Zhou et al. (2005)

(*continued*)

Table 19.1 (*continued*)

Biological activity/potential pharmaceutical use	Bioactive compounds/ specific compound	Mechanism	References
	Carotenoids - Fucoxanthin	Induction of apoptosis in different cancer cells (HL-60, PC3, DU145, LNCaP, HT29) Inhibition of angiogenesis in HUVEC cells	Hosokawa (2004); Peng (2011), Mori (2004); Moghadamtousi et al. (2014); Yousefi et al. (2018); Rocha et al. (2018); Jin et al. (2018)
	- Fucoxanthinol	Induction of anoikis (programmed cell death that occurs in anchorage-dependent cells when they detach from the surrounding ECM)	Terasaki et al. (2017)
	Phlorotannins	Induction of apoptosis MCF-7 human breast cancer cells, HeLa, HT1080, A549, and HT-29 cells	Kong et al. (2009); Li et al., (2011a); Namvar et al. (2013), Narasimham et al. (2013)
	- Phloroglucinol	Inhibits metastatic ability of breast cancer cells, decreased the expression of SLUG, EMT master regulator through inhibition of PI3K/Akt and Ras/Raf-1/ERK signaling pathways	Kim et al. (2015a,b,c,d)
	- Dieckol	Modulation of the expression of key molecules that regulate apoptosis, inflammation, invasion, and angiogenesis	Sadeeshkumar et al. (2017)
	Bromophenols	Induction of apoptosis in several cell lines (DLD-1, HCT-116, etc.)	Rocha et al. (2018)
	Terpenes - Halomon (monoterpene)	Inhibited activity DNA methyltransferase-1 in colon cancer cell lines (HCT-116)	Rocha et al. (2018)
	- Laurinterol (sesquiterpene)	Inhibit melanoma cells via activation of p-53 transcription factor	Rocha et al. (2018)
	- Dactilone (sesquiterpenoid)	Inhibit epidermal growth factor-induced transformation in JB6P + Cl41 cells, induces G_1–S cell progression arrest and apoptosis of tumor cells	Rocha et al. (2018)

(*continued*)

Table 19.1 *(continued)*

Biological activity/potential pharmaceutical use	Bioactive compounds/ specific compound	Mechanism	References
Antithrombotic and antihypertensive activity (cardiovascular health)	Peptides (from digestion of wakame proteins)	Inhibition of ACE in spontaneously hypertensive rats	Sato et al. (2002)
	Phlorotannins	Inhibition of ACE *in vitro*	Jung et al. (2006); Li et al. (2011a)
	Sulfated polysaccharides	Anticoagulant activity (*in vitro* studies)	Wijesekara et al. (2011); Costa et al. (2010); Sun et al. (2018)
	Fucoidans	Antithrombotic: increases secretion of PGI_2 in healthy volunteers	Ren et al. (2013)
Antilipidemic and anticholesterolemic activity	Sulfated polysaccharides - Ulvan	Upregulate mRNA expression of FXR and PPARγ and downregulate the expression of LXR in hypercholesterolemic rats	Penzhang et al. (2003a,b)
	- Porphyran	Improved ratio of low-density lipoprotein cholesterol/high-density lipoprotein cholesterol in mice	Cao et al. (2016) Wang et al. (2017)
	Phytosterols	Decreased plasma total cholesterol levels (mechanism not mentioned) in humans and rats	Lopes et al. (2013)
Antiobesity and antidiabetic activity	Fucoidans	Increased serum concentrations of adiponectin in mice	Jeong et al. (2013)
		Stimulated the release of pancreatic insulin in diabetic rats	Wang et al. (2014)
		α-glucosidase inhibition in mice	Shan et al. (2016)
		Decreased blood pressure Increased insulin secretion Increased insulin resistance in obese or overweight humans	Hernández-Corona et al. (2014)

(continued)

Table 19.1 (*continued*)

Biological activity/potential pharmaceutical use	Bioactive compounds/specific compound	Mechanism	References
	Alginates	Inhibited the activity of pancreatic lipase *in vitro*	Wilcox et al. (2014)
	Fucoxanthin	Improved insulin resistance Reduced lipogenesis (activation of AMPK and ACC in epididymal adipose tissue) in mice	Maeda et al. (2009), Fumiaki et al. (2012) Kang et al. (2012)
	Fucosterol	Inhibition of adipogenesis (modulation of FoxO signaling pathway) in 3T3-L1 adipocytes	Lee et al. (2017)
	Phlorotannins	Inhibition of α-glucosidase and α-amylase Glucose absorption inhibition Protection of β-cells in rats	Lopes et al. (2016)
	Indole derivatives	Inhibition of adipogenesis (activation of AMPK signal pathway) in 3T3-L1 preadipocytes	Kang et al. (2017)
	Methanolic extracts (*Derbesia marina* and *Symphycladia latiscula*)	Inhibitory activity of protein tyrosine phosphatase 1B *in vitro*	Lee et al. (2007)
	Extracts rich in flavonoids (*Enteromorpha prolifera*)	Modulation of hyperglycemia via activation of IRS1 and PI3K/AKT and inhibition of the JNK1/2 insulin pathway in liver of type II diabetic mice	Yan et al. (2019)
Antibacterial, antiviral, and antifungal activity	Ethanolic extracts (several macroalgae, e.g. *Turbinaria ornata*, *E. cava*, *Bifurcaria bifurcata*)	Antibacterial against Gram + and Gram – (e.g. *Enterococcus faecalis*, *Streptococcus iniae*, *Vibrio harveyi*, *Staphylococcus aureus*, *Escherichia coli*)	Vijayabaskar and Shiyamala (2011) Kim et al. (2015d); Lee et al. (2016) Santos et al. (2017)
	Fucoidans	Anti-HIV *in vitro*	Wijesekara et al. (2011); Dinesh et al. (2016)

(*continued*)

Table 19.1 (*continued*)

Biological activity/potential pharmaceutical use	Bioactive compounds/ specific compound	Mechanism	References
	Galactan sulfate (*Agardhiella tenera*)	Anti-HIV (*in vitro*, blocking the viral adhesion to cells)	Yasuhara and Lu (2010)
	Galactofucan (*Adenocystis utricularis*)	Anti-HIV (inhibition of virus replication) in human PBMC primary cell culture	Trinchero et al. (2009)
	Several sulfated polysaccharides from macroalgae (carrageenan, galatan, alginate, fucan, and laminaran) and microalgae (naviculan, calcium spirulan, and nostaflan)	Anti-HIV *in vitro*	Ahmadi et al. (2015) Bule et al. (2018)
	Iota-carrageenan (carragelose)	Antiviral (ability to block viral attachment to the host cells) (in cold virus, in clinical trials)	Ludwig et al. (2013); Calado et al. (2018); http://marinomed.com
	Phlorotannin: 8,4‴-dieckol	Anti-HIV (inhibit the activity of HIV-1 reverse transcriptase) *in vitro*	Karadeniz et al. (2014)
	Lectins: cyanovirin-N	Anti-HIV (inhibit the penetration of the virus in the target cells *in vitro*)	Zappe et al. (2008)
		Inhibition of Ebola virus (*in vitro*)	Matei et al. (2016)
	Dipterpenes, sesquiterpenes (e.g. elatol), fucoidans	Antiprotozoal (against *Leishmania donovani* strains) in BALB/c mice	Torres et al. (2014)
Immunomodulatory and anti-inflammatory activities	Sulfated polysaccharides and lectins (*Ulva lactuca*)	Inhibition of TNF-α cytokine release and downregulation of NO production in Wistar rats	Mezdour et al. (2017)

(*continued*)

Table 19.1 (*continued*)

Biological activity/potential pharmaceutical use	Bioactive compounds/specific compound	Mechanism	References
	Several sulfated polysaccharides (fucoidan, sulfated galactan) from *Gelidium crinale* and *Cytoseira sedoides*	Stimulation of macrophages and potentiation of cytokine production (TNF-α, IL-1β, IL-6, and IL-10) in paw edema rat model	Xu et al. (2017)
	Fucoidans	Activation of natural killer cells in RAW264.7 macrophages	Xu et al. (2017)
	Astaxanthin	Inhibition of IL-1β, IL-6, and TNF-α secretion Inhibition of production NO and PGE_2 (on endotoxin-induced uveitis in rats and in RAW264.7 macrophages)	Ohgami et al. (2003); Shiratori et al. (2005); Lee et al. (2003)
	Sargaquinone	Inhibition of the biosynthesis of leukotrienes (*in vitro* assay with pork leukocytes)	Tziveleka et al. (2005)
	Aryl polyketide lactones	5-lipoxygenase inhibitory activity *in vitro*	Maneesh and Chakraborty (2017)
	Isoprenoid (3-hydroxy-4,7-megastigmadien-9-one)	Inhibition of proinflammatory cytokines by downregulating TLR9-dependent AP-1 and NF-κB activation in BMDCs	Ali et al. (2017)
	Aqueous extracts of *Codium fragile*	Alleviation of osteoarthritis progression Reduction of proteoglycan loss and lower OARSI scores in IL-1β-induced rat primary chondrocytes and a rat osteoarthritis (rat model)	Moon et al. (2018)
	Malyngamides (dicarboximide) from microalgae and cyanobacteria	Inhibition of NO production in RAW264.7 macrophages	Villa et al. (2010)

(*continued*)

Table 19.1 (*continued*)

Biological activity/potential pharmaceutical use	Bioactive compounds/ specific compound	Mechanism	References
Neuroprotective activity (nervous system health)	Fucoxanthin	Neuroprotective activity (in rat hippocampal neurons in both hypoxia-induced oxidative stress and normoxic conditions)	Mohibbullah et al. (2018)
	Pheophytin	Promotes neuronal development in embryogenesis in PC12 cells	Pangestuti and Kim (2011)
	Fucosterol	Inhibition of acetylcholinesterase and butyryl cholinesterase in amyloid-induced microglial cells	Wong et al. (2018)
	Alkaloids: racemosin A and B	Protective effects against Aβ-mediated neuroinflammation in SH-SY5Y cells	Liu et al. (2013)
	Homotaurine (3-amino-1-propanesulfonic acid)	Prevention of the neurotoxicity of A*β* peptide by reducing amyloid aggregation in humans	Kocis et al. (2017) Ricciardi et al. (2015); Bossù et al. (2018)
		Increased memory in Parkinson's disease in clinical study (100 mg homotaurine)	
	Eckol and dieckol	Inhibition of peroxisome proliferator-activated receptor c (protection against Parkinson's disease neurodegeneration) in *in vitro* and *in vivo* Parkinson's disease models	Carta (2013)
		Inhibition of monoamine oxidases in enzyme-based chemiluminiscent immunoassay	Jung et al. (2017)
Other activities	Polysaccharides (*A. nodosum, L. digitata, L. hyperborea,* etc.)	Prebiotic *in vitro*, in mice and weaned pig	Brown et al. (2014); Hamed et al. (2015); Gómez-Guzmán et al. (2018); Kearney et al. (2018)

(*continued*)

Table 19.1 (*continued*)

Biological activity/potential pharmaceutical use	Bioactive compounds/specific compound	Mechanism	References
	Fucoidans	Enhancement of intestinal epithelial barrier function by upregulating the expression of claudin-1 in Caco-2 cell monolayer model	Iraha et al. (2013)
		Relief of the symptoms of non-ulcer dyspepsia in experimental models on oral administration in clinical study	Nagaoka et al. (2000)
		Prevention of gastric ulcer (preventing adhesion of *Helicobacter pylori* to gastric cells in experimental models)	
		Induction of human osteoblast differentiation and inhibition of osteoclast differentiation in human mesenchymal stem cells	Kim et al. (2015d)
	Fucoxanthin	Induction of osteoclast apoptosis in RAW264.7 cells	Das et al. (2010)

Aβ, β-amyloid; ACC, acetyl-CoA carboxylase; ACE, angiotensin I-converting enzyme; Akt, protein kinase; AMPK, AMP-activated protein kinase; AP, activator protein; BALB, albino mouse; BMDC, bone marrow-derived dendritic cell; ECM, extracellular matrix; ERK, extracellular signal-regulated kinase; EMT, epithelial–mesenchymal transition; FXR, farnesoid X receptor; HUVEC, human umbilical vein endothelial cell; IGF-IR, insulin-like growth factor-I receptor; IL, interleukin; INF, interferon; IRS, insulin receptor substrate; JNK, c-Jun N-terminal kinase; LXR, liver X receptor; NF-κB, nuclear factor kappa B; OARSI, osteoarthritis cartilage histopathology assessment system; PBMC, peripheral blood mononuclear cell; PC, human prostate cancer cell; PGE_2, prostaglandin E_2; PI3K, phosphatidylinositol-4,5-bisphosphate 3-kinase; PPARγ, peroxisome proliferator-activated receptor γ; Raf, rapidly accelerated fibrosarcoma; Ras, rat sarcoma; TGF, transforming growth factor; TLR, toll-like receptor.

Another aspect of pharmacological interest is the antiviral properties of fucans and carrageenans, since they have been reported to inhibit the first phase of the HIV-1 replication cycle (Table 19.1; Boisson-Vidal et al. 1995; Girond et al. 1991; Damonte et al. 2004). Carrageenans have likewise been reported as effective against herpes simplex virus (HSV)-1 and HSV-2, possibly due to their *in vitro* interaction with the positive charges in the viral envelope regions that are rich in amino acids (Damonte et al. 2004). Mohsen et al. (2007) investigated the antiviral activity of crude water-soluble SPs and three ethanol fractions; antiviral capacity has been observed to increase with an increase in the degree of sulfation (dose 10 μg μl^{-1} in plaque reduction assay) (Mohsen et al. 2007).

Other studies have confirmed this observation (Jiao et al. 2011), and it has been shown that the activity of fucans against the dengue virus depends on sulfation and that their antiviral capacity increases with molecular weight (Jiao et al. 2011). Peng et al. (2013) demonstrated the antiviral capacity against HSV-1 *in vitro* with the half maximal effective concentration (EC_{50}) of 8.92 μg ml^{-1} of polysaccharides (identified as alginates and fucoidans) obtained from the species *Sargassum naozhouense*.

The SPs fucoidan and laminarin have recently aroused more interest because of their potential pharmaceutical applications. They have been shown to have a wide range of biological properties such as anti-inflammatory, anticoagulant, antioxidant, antiviral, antitumoral, antiapoptosis, antiproliferative, and immunostimulant activities (Collins et al. 2016). Garcia-Vaquero et al. (2017) discussed methods for extraction and purification of fucoidan and laminarin from macroalgae. They reviewed the biological properties of these polysaccharides from *in vivo* and *in vitro* studies to confirm their biological properties and discussed their antioxidant, antitumoral, anticoagulant, and anti-inflammatory properties. For example, laminarin exhibited an anti-inflammatory function *in vivo* by reducing inflammatory cytokines in the colon and liver, and by downregulating interleukin (IL)-6, IL-17A, IL-1b, and IL-10 in the colon of post-weaning pigs. They also discussed antitumoral activity of fucoidans against A20 mouse leukemia cells, among others (Garcia-Vaquero et al. 2017). A recent review by Weelden et al. (2019) provided details on the anticancer mechanisms of action of fucoidan, mainly associated with the phosphatidylinositol-4,5-bisphosphate 3-kinase/protein kinase B (PI3K/Akt), mitogen-activated protein kinase (MAPK), and caspase pathways. The PI3K/Akt signaling pathway is a central player in diverse cellular functions. This pathway is often upregulated in tumor cells and is often targeted in cancer treatment (Weelden et al. 2019).

There is *in vitro* evidence that fucoidan and carrageenans increase the cytotoxicity of natural killer cells against lymphocytes and mast cells; Costa et al. (2010) investigated the cytotoxic activity of SPs from 11 species of seaweeds (*Caulerpa prolifera*, *Sargassum filipendula*, *Dictyopteris delicatula*, and *Dictyota menstrualis* among others) on HeLa cells (doses <2 mg ml^{-1}) and found that all SPs showed antiproliferative activity in a dose-dependent manner (Costa et al. 2010). Kalimuthu and Kim (2015) described the principal antitumoral actions of fucoidans that can be summarized as growth inhibition of cancer cells and in metastasis by prevention of matrigel invasion *in vitro*, and induction of apoptosis through cell cycle arrest or caspases.

With regard to the anti-inflammatory and immunomodulatory activities of fucoidans, there are numerous studies on their potential use in stimulating an immune response and in controlling immune cell activity to mitigate negative effects such as inflammation (Mezdour et al. 2017; Xu et al. 2017, Chen et al. 2008). Therefore, the interest in their use as anti-inflammatory agents has grown from year to year, since there is evidence that they interfere with leukocyte migration to inflammation sites; for example, in a rabbit model of bacterial meningitis, leukocyte rolling was markedly reduced by intravenous infusion of fucoidan (Granert et al. 1994) and also reduced synthesis and expression of nitric oxide and proinflammatory cytokines (IL1β, tumor necrosis factor [TNF]α) in RAW 264.7 cells (dose between 50 and 500 μg ml^{-1}) (Lee et al. 2018).

The antioxidant activities of SPs have been known for years, but they are now receiving more attention (Rocha de Souza et al. 2007; Raguraman et al. 2019; Jin et al. 2018). Research is ongoing into their isolation and purification from different macroalgal genera, mainly *Fucus* and *Laminaria* because of evidence that fucans have a considerable ferric reduction/antioxidant power and superoxide radical scavenging ability *in vitro*. For example, with respect to the inhibition of superoxide radical formation, fucoidan had a half maximal inhibitory concentration (IC_{50}) of 0.058 mg ml^{-1}, while the IC_{50} values for the kappa, iota, and lambda carrageenans were 0.112, 0.332, and 0.046 mg ml^{-1}, respectively (Rocha de Souza et al. 2007); and also *in vitro* and *in vivo* assays showed scavenging activity (Raguraman et al. 2019). Moreover, the antioxidant capacities of carrageenans (kappa, iota, and lambda) and ulvans have also been determined, and they likewise seem to be related to sulfate content (Rocha de Souza et al. 2007). Jin et al. (2018) observed that their antioxidant capacity depended on the degree of polymerization. They studied glucuronomannan oligosaccharides derived from fucoidan, which was extracted from the brown alga *Sargassum thunbergii*, and evaluated the antioxidant activities (hydroxyl radical scavenging activity, superoxide radical scavenging activity, reducing power, and 2,2-diphenyl-1-picrylhydrazyl [DPPH] radical scavenging activity); the findings showed that the higher the degree of polymerization, the better the activity, except for the hydroxyl radical scavenging activity. In addition, the higher the sulfate content, the lower the activities for the reducing power and DPPH radical scavenging activity (Jin et al. 2018). These studies have important applications in pharmaceuticals because it is very well known that oxidative stress and reactive oxygen species (ROS) are involved in several diseases. Elevated levels of ROS result in generation of free radicals, which can cause deleterious effects on protein, lipids, and DNA (Schieber and Chandel 2014). Free radical-induced oxidative stress has emerged as a critical player in the pathophysiology of various conditions like neurodegenerative disorders, cancer, cardiovascular, inflammatory diseases, and aging (Raguraman et al. 2019).

Another highly interesting biological activity of polysaccharides is their ability to reduce blood lipid levels (Pengzhan et al., 2003a, b; Korukanti et al. 2013). Extracts of *Fucus vesiculosus* have been found to reduce triglyceride and cholesterol levels in a dose-dependent manner in Wistar albino hyperlipemic rats (fed with cafeteria diet for 42 days) (Korukanti et al. 2013). Other studies in Triton-induced-hyperlipemic rats fed a high cholesterol diet for 21 days, showed that supplementation of the diet with ulvan from *Ulva pertusa* led to reductions in serum total cholesterol and low-density lipoprotein cholesterol (LDL-C) with no significant alteration in serum triglycerides (Pengzhan et al. 2003a, b). The mechanisms involved in this process are yet to be discovered. Likewise, supplementation (intragastric administration) with extracts of SPs from *Ulva lactuca* in the diet of hypercholesterolemic rats (fed with cholesterol powder, bile salt, and animal lard) lowered oxidative stress and hypercholesterolemia (serum total lipids, triglycerides, total cholesterol, LDL-C, and very low-density lipoprotein cholesterol [VLDL-C] levels, whereas, high-density lipoprotein cholesterol [HDL-C] concentration was markedly increased by 180%) and ameliorated hepatic enzymatic (catalase, glutathione peroxidase, and superoxide dismutase [SOD]), non-enzymatic (reduced glutathione and total thiol) antioxidant defenses and thiobarbituric acid reactive substances (TBARS) (Hassan et al. 2011).

19.2.2 Phlorotannins and Other Polyphenols

Polyphenols such as phlorotannins have been known for years for their *in vitro* and *in vivo* antioxidant, anticoagulant, antibacterial, anti-inflammatory, and anticancer properties (Nwosu et al. 2011; Lee and Jeon 2013; Agregán et al. 2017; Kim et al.

2015c; Li et al. 2011b). Marine algae are particularly rich in polyphenolic compounds such as catechins, flavan-3-ols, flavonols, and the phloroglucinol polymers known as phlorotannins (Gómez-Guzman et al. 2018). The most abundant polyphenols in red and green algae are bromophenols, phenolic acids, and flavonoids (Gómez-Guzman et al. 2018). However, phlorotannins are the predominant polyphenolic secondary metabolites in brown algae such as *Laminaria ochroleuca*, *Eisenia bicyclis*, *Ecklonia maxima*, *A. nodosum*, etc. (Gómez-Guzman et al. 2018) which comprise phloroglucinol units (1,3,5-trihydroxybenzene). They are especially abundant in brown algae and the most studied are *Ecklonia cava*, *F. vesiculosus*, *A. nodosum*, and *Himanthalia elongata* (Gómez-Guzman et al. 2018). Scientific literature also reports on polyphenol-rich extracts (expressed as gallic acid equivalents) obtained from other algae such as *Palmaria palmata*, *Laminaria setchellii*, *Macrocystis integrifolia*, and *Nereocystis luetkeana* (Yuan and Walsh 2006). Different types of phlorotannins such as eckol, dieckol, phlorofucofuroeckol, and dioxinodehydroeckol among others have been researched and identified in brown algae such as *E. cava* and *Ishige okamurae* (Lee and Jeon 2013; Agregán et al. 2017). Dieckol and 6,6′-bieckol phlorofucofuroeckol-A from these algae have be shown to have antidiabetic effects, both *in vivo* and *in vitro*, through a variety of mechanisms, by inhibiting the activity of intestinal α-glucosidase, lowering postprandial hyperglycemia levels, reducing glucose uptake by muscle cells reducing production of hepatic glucose in type II diabetes mellitus, or by protecting against diabetes complications by preventing oxidative stress (Table 19.1) (Lee and Jeon 2013; Kang et al. 2013).

In other studies, phlorotannins extracted from *E. cava*, *Ecklonia stolonifera*, *E. bicyclis*, and *Eisenia arborea* have shown antiallergy activity by preventing binding between IgE and FcεRI (a high-affinity IgE receptor), and a methanolic extract of *E. cava* caused a concentration-dependent reduction in the cell surface expression of FcεRI in the human basophilic KU812F cells (Li et al. 2011a). Other researchers have confirmed phlorotannins to be potent inhibitors of hyaluronidase, phospholipase A2, cyclooxygenase, and lipoxygenase, linked to the suppression of synthesis and release of leukotrienes and prostaglandins in rat basophilic leukemia RBL cells used *in vitro* in allergy studies; for example, among phlorotannins obtained from *E. arborea*, phlorofucofuroeckol-B exhibited the strongest activity against histamine and β-hexosaminidase release with an IC_{50} value of 7.8 μM (Shibata et al. 2002; Li et al. 2011a; Vo et al. 2012). Moreover, two bioactive phlorotannin derivatives, 6,6′-bieckol (3) and 1-(3′,5′-dihydroxyphenoxy)-7-(2″,4″,6-trihydroxyphenoxy)-2,4,9-trihydroxydibenzo-1,4-dioxin, have been reported to be potent inhibitors of histamine release by human basophilic leukemia (KU812) and RBL-2H3 cultured cell lines with IC_{50} values ranging between 38 and 98 μM (corresponding to approx. 23–32 μg ml^{-1}) (Le et al. 2009).

A review by Li et al. 2011a refers to several studies which have shown that phlorotannins have strong antioxidant activities against free radical-mediated oxidation damage (DPPH, hydroxyl, superoxide, and peroxyl radicals) *in vitro*, using an electron spin resonance (ESR) technique (Li et al. 2011a), and that the phlorotannins derived from *Hizikia fusiformis* are potential free radical scavengers (Li et al. 2011a; Siriwardhana et al. 2005). Likewise, several purified phlorotannins from *E. cava*, *Ecklonia kurome*, *E. bicyclis*, and *H. fusiformis* are potent antioxidants and protected against hydrogen peroxide-induced damage in lung fibroblast cells (at 30 μM) (Kang et al. 2006). Recently, ethanolic extracts thought to contain phlorotannins from

E. cava acted as hepatic protectors through two mechanisms: elevation of antioxidant enzymes and normalization of the cytochrome P4502E1 enzyme in carbon tetrachloride (CCl_4)-induced liver injury (Byun et al. 2018).

Antioxidant activities were also observed with alcoholic extracts rich in polyphenols (as gallic acid equivalents) obtained from *P. palmata* (Yuan et al. 2005), where they scavenged hydroxyl ion (•OH) radicals. Moreover, purified eckol, phlorofucofuroeckol-A, dieckol, and 8,8′-bieckol exhibited inhibition of lipid peroxidation *in vitro* and scavenging of superoxide (O_2^-) and DPPH• radicals compared with ascorbic acid and α-tocopherol at 1 μM in a liposome system (Shibata et al. 2008). Likewise, ethanol extracts rich in oligomeric and polymeric phlorotannins obtained from *F. vesiculosus* showed powerful DPPH• scavenging activities comparable with or even greater than those of commercial antioxidants such as ascorbic acid, butylated hydroxytoluene, and α-tocopherol (Wang et al. 2012a). Other research by Yotsu-Yamasita et al. (2013) into *E. kurome* extracts has led to the identification of two new phlorotannins (of molecular weight 974 kDa) that have DPPH• radical scavenging activities and are as potent as dieckol and phlorofucofuroeckol-A, and more potent than phlorofucofuroeckol-B, phloroglucinol, α-tocopherol, and ascorbic acid. They also showed significantly higher intracellular radical scavenging activities than phlorofucofuroeckol-A, phlorofucofuroeckol-B, and quercetin using the cell-permeable and oxidation-sensitive dye dichloro-dihydro-fluorescein diacetate (DCFH-DA) (Yotsu-Yamasita et al. 2013). In addition to phloroglucinol, other polyphenols extracted from *H. elongata* including gallic acid, chlorogenic acid, caffeic acid, ferulic acid, myricetin, and quercetin have shown antioxidant activities using DPPH and ferric reducing antioxidant power (FRAP) assays (Rajauria et al. 2017; Rajauria 2018).

Other studies have focused on the bactericidal activity of phlorotannins, showing that phlorofucofuroeckol-A extracted from *E. kurome* had a higher bactericidal activity than the catechins (Nagayama et al. 2002) on bacteria such as *Campylobacter* spp. or *Staphylococcus aureus*, and that the phlorotannins in *A. nodosum* kill *E. coli* (it is bacteriostatic at concentrations of 25 μg ml^{-1} or higher and at ≥50 μg ml^{-1} is bacteriocidal) (Wang et al. 2009). The antiviral activities of phlorotannins such as 8,8′-bieckol′ and 8,4′-bieckol obtained from *E. cava* have also been studied against HIV-1 by inhibiting activity of the polymerase and ribonuclease in HIV-1 reverse transcriptase (IC_{50} 0.51 μM) (Ahn et al. 2004) and against HIV-1 induced syncytia formation (EC_{50} 1.72 μM) (Artan et al. 2008). A derivative of the phlorotannins, dioxinodehydroeckol, obtained from *E. cava*, reduced the growth of breast cancer MCF-7 cells, via induction of apoptosis (Kong et al. 2009). Moreover, other phlorotannin derivatives such as fucodiphloroethol-G, eckol, dieckol, and phlorofucofuroeckol have shown potent cytotoxic effects on diverse human cancer cell lines such as HeLa, HT1080, A549, and HT-29 (Li et al. 2011a).

The potential effects on enzymatic activities of phlorotannins have been cited by several authors (Li et al. 2011a). Lee et al. (2010b) highlighted the inhibition of α-glucosidase and α-amylase by dieckol with IC_{50} values of 10.8 (α-glucoidase) and 124.9 μmol l^{-1} (α-amylase), respectively, and its possible application in slowing the digestion of oligosaccharides and disaccharides, and, therefore, of glucose absorption in the small intestine in management of diabetes mellitus. The inhibition of angiotensin-I converting enzyme, which plays an important role in blood pressure regulation, has been demonstrated *in vitro* using ethanolic extracts from 10 algal species from Korea (*E. cava*, *E. stolonifera*, *Pelvetia siliquosa*, *H. fusiforme*, and

Undaria pinnatifida) at more than 50% inhibition at a concentration of 163.93 $\mu g\,ml^{-1}$ (Jung et al. 2006). A recent review by Gómez-Guzman et al. (2018) points out that even though more clinical studies are needed, algal polyphenols such as catechins, flavonols, and phlorotannins may exert an antihypertensive effect, to intervene in cardiovascular health, by acting as inhibitors of angiotensin-converting enzyme (ACE) (Gómez-Guzman et al. 2018).

Other actions of phlorotannins include inhibition of matrix metalloproteinases involved in the degradation of extracellular components of the extracellular matrices closely associated with chronic inflammation, arthritis, osteoporosis, metastasis, skin firmness, and aging etc. Kim et al. (2006), in a gelatin digestion assay, showed that phlorotannins derived from *E. cava* could result in complete inhibition of bacterial collagenase-1 activity at 20 $\mu g\,ml^{-1}$ of *E. cava* extract. In addition, artificially induced activities of matrix metalloproteinase (MMP)-2 and MMP-9 in human dermal fibroblast and HT 1080 cells have been inhibited by *E. cava* extract (at 10 $\mu g\,ml^{-1}$) in a more or less similar manner to the positive control doxycycline (Kim et al. 2006; Thomas and Kim 2011).

Bromophenols also have been widely studied and a recent review by Rocha et al. (2018) discussed 10 compounds from different algae (*Vertebrata lanosa*, *Neorhodomela larix*, *Odonthalia corymbifera*, *Osmundaria serrata*, *Rhodomela confervoides*, and *Leathesia marina*) with cytotoxic activities with $IC_{50} \leq 15\,\mu M$ against cancer cell lines of the lung (A549), gastric (BGC-823), breast (MCF-7), and colon (DLD-1), although not all studies used positive controls (only Shoeib et al. 2004 reported such data). Bromophenol (bis(2,3-dibromo-4,5-dihydroxybenzyl) ether, BDDE) obtained by synthesis (in order to obtain sufficient quantities of pure BDDE) has also been found to have antifungal activity. The authors tested BDDE (100 $\mu g\,ml^{-1}$) against *Botrytis cinerea* and they found an inhibition rate of $83.3 \pm 6.8\%$ (Liu et al. 2014). And BDDE isolated from the methanolic extract of the marine alga *Rhodomela confervoides* was found to have antibacterial activity against four strains of bacteria (*S. aureus*, *S. epidermidis*, *E. coli*, and *P. aeruginosa*) with the minimal inhibitory concentration (MIC) $<70\,mg\,ml^{-1}$ (Xu et al. 2003).

Antioxidant activities have also been seen with bromophenols derived from algae such as *R. confervoides* (Li et al. 2012a) using the DPPH assay with IC_{50} values ranging from 5.22 to 23.60 μM and *Symphyocladia latiuscula* by DPPH radical with the IC_{50} value of $\leq 20.5\,\mu g\,ml^{-1}$, (Xu et al. 2013). Another biological activity of bromophenols worth highlighting is that bromophenol derivatives from the red alga *R. confervoides* that contain one or two 2,3-dibromo-4,5-dihydroxybenzyl units and are highly brominated, inhibit Tyrosine-protein phosphatase non-receptor type 1 also known as protein-tyrosine phosphatase 1B (PTP1B) activity (IC_{50} values were 2.4, 1.7, 1.5, and 0.84 μM, respectively) and the *R. confervoides* extracts could decrease the blood glucose level in diabetic rats, and bis(2,3,6-tribromo-4,5-dihydroxybenzyl) ether (with an IC_{50} of 0.03 μM) inhibited α-glucosidase *in vitro* (Liu et al. 2011b) and protein tyrosine phosphatase 1B ($IC_{50} = 0.84\,\mu mol\,l^{-1}$ *in vitro* assay) (PTP1B is a negative signaling modulator mediated by tyrosine kinase receptors in insulin resistance in type II diabetes), which could be of interest for the development of antidiabetic pharmaceutical products (Shi et al. 2013).

19.2.3 Sterols

Sterols are not only found in terrestrial plants but also in marine algae. *Phaeophyceae* such as *H. elongata*, *U. pinnatifida*, and *Laminaria ochroleuca* mainly contain fucosterol (83–97% of total sterol content; 662–2320 $\mu g\, g^{-1}$ dry weight [DW]); *Rhodophyceae* such as *Palmaria* sp. and *Porphyra* sp. primarily contain cholesterol and its derivatives (desmosterol, 87–93% of total sterol content; 187–337 $\mu g\, g^{-1}$ DW); and *Chlorophyceae* contain ergosterol and 24-ethylcholesterol (Sánchez-Machado et al. 2004). Fucosterol (3β-hydroxy-5,24(28)-stigmastadiene, 5,24(28)-stigmastadien-3β-ol) is the most researched derivative due to its different biological activities (Yoon et al. 2008; Wong et al. 2018). *In vitro* studies performed with fucosterol extracted from *Ecklonia stolonifera* Okamura showed that it has anticholinesterase activities, which is a selective inhibitor of Butyrylcholinesterase (BChE) in neurotransmitter breakdown with relevance in the treatment of Alzheimer's disease (Yoon et al. 2008; Wong et al. 2018). *In vivo* studies in rats with hepatic damage induced by CCl4, carried out to investigate the antioxidant properties of fucosterol (Lee et al. 2003; Kim and Ta, 2011), showed that it caused a significant increase in hepatic free radical scavenging enzyme activities such as SOD, catalase, and glutathione peroxidase (GSH-Px). Moreover, an increase in hepatic catalase activity indicated that fucosterol can play an important role in quenching hydrogen peroxide radicals, while an increase in SOD indicated that it can help in cellular defense mechanisms by preventing oxidation of membranes (Lee et al. 2003). Moreover, an increase in glutathione peroxidase activity indicates that fucosterol may also assist in the restoration of endogenous antioxidant molecules such as glutathione. Algal sterols may also play a role in actions related to metabolic disorders (Lee et al. 2003; Kim and Ta, 2011). *In vivo* studies have shown that fucosterol from *P. siliquosa* may be beneficial in diabetes management by inducing a fall in blood glucose levels and glycogen breakdown (administered orally at 30 $mg\, kg^{-1}$ in streptozotocin-induced diabetic rats) (Lee et al. 2004). Plaza et al. (2008), in a review related to "new functional food ingredients from algae," indicated that sterols from *H. elongata*, *U. pinnatifida*, *Porphyra* spp., *Chondrus crispus*, *Cystoseira* spp., and *Ulva* spp. reduced plasma total cholesterol and LDL-C (Plaza et al. 2008). Other studies carried out with fucosterol extracted from *E. stolonifera* suggested that it can inhibit the expression of peroxisome proliferator-activated receptor γ (PPARγ) and CCAAT/enhancer binding protein α (C/EBPα), in a concentration-dependent manner (12.5–50 $\mu g\, ml^{-1}$) with a consequent decrease in lipid accumulation in cell lines 3T3-L1 pre-adipocytes, and thus the potential to use fucosterol as an antiobesity agent (Jung et al. 2014a). Recent studies conducted by Paul and Raja (2018) also reported hepatoprotective effects of methanolic extracts from *Gracilaria corticata*. An acute oral toxicity study was performed as per OECD-423 guidelines on Wistar albino rats ($n = 6$) of either sex selected through random sampling technique. The animals were kept fasting overnight providing only water, after which the extract (50% methanolic extract) was administered orally at the dose level of 5 $mg\, kg^{-1}$ body weight by gastric intubation and observed for 14 days. Methanolic extracts reduced activities of the liver enzymes serum glutamic oxaloacetic transaminase (SGOT), serum glutamic pyruvic transaminase (SGPT), and alkaline phosphatase (ALP), as well as bilirubin levels (Paul and Raja 2018).

Although the anti-inflammatory effects of algal compounds have been associated mainly with SPs and phlorotannins, algal sterols may also have anti-inflammatory activities *in vitro* (Yoo et al. 2012; Jung et al. 2013). Several studies have shown that fucosterol derived from *U. pinnatifida* and *E. bicyclis* had effects associated with the suppression of nuclear factor kappa B (NF-κB) and p38 MAPK pathways in lipopolysaccharide (LPS)-induced RAW 264.7 macrophages (doses between 5 and 10 μM) (Table 19.1; Yoo et al. 2012; Jung et al. 2013).

Another biological activity of sterols of interest is their antibacterial properties (Lee et al. 2011; Begun et al. 2018). Sterol derivatives (e.g. saringosterol; 24-vinyl-cholest-5-ene-3beta,24-diol) isolated from *Sargassum ringgoldianum*, *Lessonia nigrescens*, and *Isochrysis galbana* have been reported to inhibit the growth of *Mycobacterium tuberculosis in vitro*, which shows its potential for development as a natural low-toxicity drug for tuberculosis treatment (Lee et al. 2011). Another recent study has shown that, in addition to the antibacterial activities of fucosterol (and also a sesquiterpenoid, debromolaurinterol) from *Cystoseira myrica* and *Padina boryana*, these compounds have exhibited antiparasitic activities against *Plasmodium falciparum in vitro* as potential antimalarial agents (Begun et al. 2018).

One field of interest in drug development is the antiproliferative and antitumoral activities of sterols such as fucosterol from *Turbinaria ornata*, and oxysterol from red coral alga *Jania rubens* (Kim and Ta 2011). Kim and Ta (2011) described the cytotoxic effects on human cancer cell lines (such as mouse lymphocytic leukemia cells, human colon carcinoma, and KB cells, among others) of sterols obtained from *Turbinaria conoides*, *T. ornata*, *Sargassum carpophyllum*, *J. rubens*, and *Peyssonnelia* sp. For example, the authors cited two sterol glycosides isolated from red alga *Peyssonnelia* sp. that displayed significant cytotoxicity toward human breast cancer MDA-MB-468 cells and human lung cancer cell line A549 with IC_{50} 0.71 and 0.86 mM, respectively, which were often more resistant to cytotoxins than those of other common cancer cells that inhibited with values of IC_{50} 0.93 and 0.97 mM, and concluded that sterols from algae may have potential for use as chemo-preventive agents in cancer therapy (Kim and Ta, 2011).

There is growing interest in the study and possible applications of microalgal phytosterols due to the possibility of cultivating large amounts of their biomass (Luo et al. 2015). Luo et al. (2015) described the main types of phytosterols (crinosterol, stigmasterol, sitosterol, fucosterol, and ergosterol among others) obtained from diverse microalgae such as *I. galbana*, *Nannochloropis gaditana*, *Nannochloropsis* sp., *Phaeodactylum tricornutum*, *Pavlova lutheri*, and *Tetraselmis* sp., and their biological activities such as the reduction of total and LDL-C levels in patients with hypercholesterolemia, and their anti-inflammatory activities on 12-*O*-tetradecanoylphorbol-13-acetate (TPA)-induced mice with 0.2–0.7 mg ear^{-1} as 50% inhibitory dose. In addition, stigmasterol (stigmasta-5,22-dien-3beta-ol; $C_{29}H_{48}O$) extracted from the microalga *Navicula incerta* was reported to induce apoptosis in human hepatoma HepG2 cells in a dose-dependent manner (5, 10, 20 μM) (Kim et al. 2014a). It is worth highlighting the antiproliferative potential of sterols obtained from the microalga *Nannochloropsis oculata* against lipopolysaccharide-stimulated RAW 264.7 macrophages cells with IC_{50} values less than 6.25 μg ml^{-1} (Sanjeewa et al. 2016), another source for research and development of these types of pharmacological compounds.

19.2.4 PUFAs and Other Lipidic Compounds

It is well known that fatty acids are abundant in oil seeds (sunflower, maize, and soy), nuts, fatty fish, and seafood such as oysters and shrimp, but it is the marine macroalgae that by far have the greatest proportion of long-chain PUFAs as compared with terrestrial plants, and thus, have potential as a source of essential fatty acids and the long-chain PUFAs (Sánchez-Machado et al. 2002, 2004; Hamed et al.

2015; Yuan 2008). Microalgae also have abundant PUFAs in the lipid fraction and have also become a source of these fatty acids for nutrition due to their ease of cultivation (Hamed 2016). PUFAs (mostly represented by eicosapentaenoic acid [EPA] and docosahexaenoic acid [DHA]) are involved in mediating the inflammatory response through the production of inflammatory mediators from arachidonic acid, namely the eicosanoids, including prostaglandins, thromboxanes, and leukotrienes (Abdolmaleki et al. 2019). The ratio of omega-3 to omega-6 of macroalgae is close to ideal, therefore they are used as dietary complement as part of a balanced diet (Hamed et al. 2015). Rhodophyta and Phaeophyta have a high percentage of omega-3 fatty acids (linolenic acid, DHA, and EPA) and omega-6 fatty acids (linoleic acid, γ-linolenic acid [GLA], arachidonic acid) (Hamed et al. 2015). Red and brown algae have high levels of omega-3 fatty acids (EPA) and the omega-6 fatty acids (arachidonic acid [AA] and linoleic acid). In fact, Sánchez-Machado et al. (2004) showed that the omega-3 fatty acid octadecatetraenoic acid is rich in two brown algae, *L. ochroleuca* and *U. pinnatifida* (Sánchez-Machado et al. 2004). However, green seaweeds, for instance *U. pertusa*, are characterized by hexadecatetraenoic (omega-3), oleic (omega-9), and palmitic acids (saturated fatty acids [SFAs]) (Hamed et al. 2015). These are directly and indirectly responsible for the biosynthesis of powerful anti-inflammatory mediators such as thromboxane A_3 and leukotriene B_5, and therefore may play a role in modulating inflammation through different immune cell-mediated processes (Robertson et al. 2013, 2015). Some examples (*in vitro* and *in vivo*) of anti-inflammatory PUFAs derived from algae are EPA and stearidonic acid (SDA: C18:4, ω3) (Khan et al. 2007). They have been extracted from *U. pinnatifida* and were able to reduce inflammation, with IC_{50} values of 160, 314, and 235 μg per ear for edema, erythema, and blood flow, respectively, in mice when phorbol myristate acetate (PMA) was applied topically (Khan et al. 2007). The anti-inflammatory effects of DHA and docosapentaenoic acid (DPA; C22:5, n-6) have also been observed both in human peripheral mononuclear cells *in vitro* and paw edema *in vivo* (Nauroth et al. 2010). Likewise, PUFAs extracted from *Ishige okamurae* (EPA, eicosatrienoic acid, linolenic acid, and GLA) were able to relieve allergic inflammation by reducing the release of histamine and regulating cytokine production in human basophilic cells *in vitro* (Vo et al. 2011).

Barbosa et al. (2014) reported that EPA and DHA may have neuroprotective actions in the brain via moderation of Acetylcholinesterase (AChE) activity (Barbosa et al. 2014), which in turn opens up prospects for use in degenerative diseases such as Alzheimer's disease. Several mechanisms have been proposed to explain the protective role of PUFAs in neurological disorders such as promotion of neuronal survival by the maintenance of basal Akt activity (Akbar et al. 2005) or increasing cortical brain derived neurotrophic factor (BDNTF) (Rao et al. 2007).

PUFAs such as EPA, GLA, and DHA extracted from microalgae have been the focus of study in recent years (Raposo et al. 2013). In this review, microalgae are said to have several antimicrobial and anti-inflammatory properties, among others, and are obtained from *Phaeodactylum tricornutum*, *Porphyridium cruentum*, *Crypthecodinium* sp., *Odontella* sp., *Nannochloropsis* sp., *Pavlova lutheri*, and *I. galbana* (Raposo et al. 2013). Other work showed that EPA extracted from the marine diatom *Cocconeis scutellum* induced apoptosis in BT20-human breast cancer cells (up to 26.1% of apoptotic cells at 2.5 ng ml^{-1} of diatoms) (Nappo et al. 2012). However, the authors were not certain whether this effect was solely due to the EPA or its synergy with other compounds in the same extract. Other authors highlighted the use of PUFAs as nutraceuticals in cancer prevention (Ulmann et al.

2017). Other lipid compounds of algae such as sulfoglycolipids (sulfoquinovosyl diacylglycerols; 1,2-di-O-acyl-3-O-(6-deoxy-6-sulfo-α-D-glucopyranosyl)-*sn*-glycerol; sulfoquinovosyldiacylglycerols [SQDGs]) obtained from *Porphyra crispata* have also exhibited growth inhibition of human hepatocellular carcinoma cell lines (HepG2) (the IC_{50} was 126 μg ml^{-1}) (Tsai and Pan 2012). Monogalactosyldiacylglycerols (MGDGs) obtained from *Solieria chordalis* and digalactosyldiacylglycerols (DGDGs), extracted from *Ulva armoricana* exhibited antiproliferative properties in *in vitro* studies carried out in bronchopulmonary carcinoma cell lines (NSCLC-N6) with an IC_{50} of 23 μg ml^{-1} for MGDGs isolated from *S. chordalis* and 24 μg ml^{-1} for DGDGs from *U. armoricana* (Kendel et al. 2015). In other work, a galactoglycerolipid ((2R)-1-O-(palmitoyl)-2-O-(5,8,11, 14,17-eicosapentanoyl)-3-O-b-D-galactopyranosyl-sn-glycerol) extracted from the alga *Chondria armata* (Kützing) Okamura showed antibacterial activity against *Klebsiella* sp. (between 65 μg disk^{-1} and 130 μg disk^{-1}) (Al-Fadhli et al. 2006). Terme et al. (2018) studied the antioxidant activities of glycolipids and phospholipids obtained from *Solieria chordalis* and *Sargassum muticum*, by extraction with supercritical CO_2, and discovered that they have a higher anti-free radical activity (using DPPH radical scavenging assays) than fractions extracted with chloroform/methanol (Terme et al. 2018).

19.2.5 Carotenoids and Other Pigments

Carotenoids are a group of more than 600 natural photosynthetic pigments that have been reported to exhibit numerous biological activities and include two main subclasses: the non-polar hydrocarbon, carotenes (e.g. α- and β-carotene, lycopene) and the polar compounds named xanthophylls (e.g. lutein, zeaxanthin, neoxanthin, violaxanthin, flavoxanthin, and α- and β-cryptoxanthin, etc.) (Déléris et al. 2016). Fucoxanthin (acetic acid [(1S,3R)-3-hydroxy-4-[(3E,5E,7E,9E,11E,13E,15E)-18-[(1S,4S,6R)-4-hydroxy-2,2,6-trimethyl-7-oxabicyclo[4.1.0]heptan-1-yl]-3,7,12,16-tetramethyl-17-oxooctadeca-1,3,5,7,9,11,13,15-octaenylidene]-3,5,5-trimethylcyclohexyl] ester; $C_{42}H_{58}O_6$) is the most studied of the xanthophylls present in brown algae and diatoms, and *U. pinnatifida* is a rich source of this carotenoid among other algae such as *Fucus* sp., *Dictyota* sp., *Laminaria* sp., and *H. elongata* (Mori et al. 2004; Rajauria et al. 2017). Several studies have shown that the antioxidant capacity (by DPPH radical scavenging and FRAP assays) of fucoxanthin is mainly as a radical scavenger (Zhang et al. 2015; Rajauria et al. 2017). In a review, Peng et al. (2011) discussed several potential biological activities of fucoxanthin: antioxidant (effective radical scavenger, inhibits formation of intracellular ROS, DNA damage, and H_2O_2-induced apoptosis, possibly because it increases catalase); anti-inflammatory (by inhibiting the effects of cytokines and other inflammatory mediators); anticancer (inducing apoptosis of tumor cells); antidiabetic (improving insulin resistance and lowering blood glucose levels); and protection of the liver (by reducing lipid levels in the liver). Several studies showed that fucoxanthin exerted antiproliferative effects and may reduce the risk of diet-related cancers (Satomi 2017). This author reviewed the fucoxanthin antitumor and cancer-preventive functions and reported that it does so via different molecules and cell signaling pathways, including modulating proteins Ccl-2, MAPK, NF-kB, caspases, and GADD45, and fucoxanthin has been mainly observed to induce G_1 cell cycle arrest in many tumor cell lines, thereby showing cytotoxicity in cancer cells (such as colon carcinoma WiDr cells, $HepG_2$ human hepatocarcinoma cells, and human gastric adenocarcinoma MGC-803 cells) (Satomi 2017). Fucoxanthin has been observed to have low toxicity in healthy liver cells. The study was carried out in mice; animals were orally administered with fucoxanthin suspension at a volume of $10\,ml\,kg^{-1}$ (dose were 1000 and $2000\,mg\,kg^{-1}$ in a single dose study, and 500 and $1000\,mg\,kg^{-1}$ in a repeated dose study), and, after sacrificing, microscopy was conducted on abdominal tissues, and liver, spleen, kidney, and gonadal tissues (Beppu et al. 2009). Foo et al. (2017), using 2,2′-azino-bis(3-ethylbenzothiazoline-6-sulphonic acid) (ABTS) radical cation scavenging assay, showed that fucoxanthin extracted from *Chaetoceros calcitrans* (16.92 ± 0.87 mg Trolox equivalent [TE] g^{-1} DW) and *I. galbana* (21.55 ± 1.58 mg TE g^{-1} DW) exhibited high antioxidant activity, while that obtained from *Odontella sinensis* and *Skeletonema costatum* displayed moderate bioactivity. The authors also studied gallic acid and indicated that the antioxidant activities were increased when both fucoxanthin and gallic acid were present (Pearson correlation and multiple regression analysis). Castro-Puyana et al. (2017) analyzed extracts from the microalga *Neochloris oleoabundans* (abundant in lutein and monoester carotenoids such as astaxanthin and violaxanthin) and observed *in vitro* that violaxanthin exhibited antiproliferative effects at concentrations of $250\,\mu g\,ml^{-1}$, and that low concentrations of lutein ($\sim 15\,\mu g\,ml^{-1}$) were able to significantly inhibit the proliferation of the HT-29 colon cancer cells. Moreover, to confirm the actions of extracts containing violaxanthin, concentrations of ~ 1.8 and $\sim 2.8\,\mu g\,ml^{-1}$ were investigated and also found to inhibit proliferation of colon cancer cells, thus confirming earlier research performed by Pasquet et al. (2011) with violaxanthin from *Dunaliella tertiolecta* (Pasquet et al. 2011), and Cha et al. 2008, with violaxanthin from *Chlorella ellipsoidea* (Cha et al. 2008). It has also been observed that fucoxanthin and its derivative, fucoxanthinol (8-oxo-trans-neoxanthin; $C_{40}H_{56}O_5$), obtained from *U. pinnatifida* ($15\,\mu g\,ml^{-1}$) exhibited neuroprotective effects on rat hippocampal neurons in both hypoxia-induced oxidative stress and normoxic conditions through antiexcitatory and antioxidative actions (Mohibbullah et al. 2018), which could be of interest in the prevention of neurodegenerative diseases.

The food industry is increasingly interested in other photosynthetic pigments: chlorophylls *a* and *b*, which are also present in micro- and macroalgae (Grimi et al. 2014; Barba et al. 2015). Fernandes et al. (2017) studied the production of chlorophyll from the microalga *Phormidium autumnale* due to its antioxidant properties, using a peroxyl radical (ROO)·scavenging assay, and noted that both chlorophyll a and chlorophyll b (40, 80, 160, 250, and 310 µMol) have a high peroxyl radical scavenging capacity: 200 times higher than the α-tocopherol standard (25, 50, 150, 250, and 350 µMol). The antioxidant activity of the chlorophylls has been associated with the conjugated double bonds of the pyrrole rings as well as oxidation of the cyclopentanone rings (Fernandes et al. 2017).

19.2.6 Peptides and Proteins

The bioactivities of peptides and proteins derived from algae have mainly been studied for their nutritional value, as well as their capacities as antioxidants, antihypertensives, immunomodulators, anticarcinogens, hepatoprotectors, and also for pharmaceutical or cosmetic uses as reviewed by Samarakoon and Jeon (2012). These authors reviewed studies on more than 40 different peptides (mainly pepsins) extracted from macroalgae and microalgae such as *Porphyra yezoensis*, *U. pinnatifida*, *Chlorella vulgaris*, and *N. incerta* and a cyanobacterium (*Spirulina platensis*) with antioxidant, antiproliferative, antihypertensive, and ACE-1 inhibitory properties.

Pangestuti and Kim (2017) reviewed a variety of peptides such as a tri-decapeptide (papain hydrolysates) obtained from *P. palmata*, which exhibited antihypertensive activity on spontaneously hypertensive rats (SHR) (dose $50\,mg\,kg^{-1}$ body weight); dipeptide obtained by enzymatic hydrolysis (protease S) from *U. pinnatifida*, with anti-ACE-1 activity in SHR (dose 1.5 μM); tri, tetra, and pentapeptides obtained from *C. ellipsoidea* (dose of $10\,mg\,kg^{-1}$ significantly decreased systolic blood pressure in SHR); and *S. platensis* with similar antihypertensive activities (dose 11.4 μM), as well as cyanobacterial lipopeptides with cytotoxic activities and antitumoral activity such us malyngamides A and B from *Moorea producens* (formerly *Lyngbya majuscula*) with concentrations ranging from 10 to $0.0026\,mg\,ml^{-1}$ on lung carcinoma (A549, ATCC CCL-185), colorectal carcinoma (HT29, ATCC HTB-38), and breast adenocarcinoma cells (MDA-MB-231, ATCC HTB-26) (Pangestuti and Kim 2017).

In a review Singh et al. (2015) highlighted the role of macro- and microalgal lectins in human health, and described several of these antinutrient proteins from macroalgae such as *Ulva rigida*, *Gracilaria* sp., *Bryothamnion* sp., *Bryopsis* sp., and microalgae such as *Chlorella* sp., *Microcystis aeruginosa*, and *Oscillatoria agardhii* among others, and their biomedical applications as antiviral, anticancer, anti-inflammatory, or analgesic (antinociceptive) agents. The authors discussed that the specificity of lectins in their bonding with sugars on host cell membranes to form glycoconjugates is important since this property makes them useful for developing tools for therapeutic applications including diagnosis and prognosis of cancer (as pathological markers of different diseases), cellular communication, bioadhesion, and for controlling different types of infections (Singh et al. 2015).

19.2.7 Other Bioactive Compounds

Other macro- and microalgal compounds have come to light in recent years because of their potential pharmacological applications (Gallé et al. 2013; Lim et al. 2018). Gallé et al. (2013) studied the antiparasitic activity of 20 species of macroalgae from the French coast, and found that organic extracts of *Bifurcaria bifurcata* exhibited a strong antiparasitic effect that inhibited the growth of *Trypanosoma brucei* and *P. falciparum*, mainly due to the activity of a diterpene, eleganolone ((E,E,E)-16-hydroxy-2,6,10,14-tetramethyl-2,6,10,14-hexadecatetraen-4-one; $C_{20}H_{32}O_2$). Other molecules of interest are the meroterpenoids (MES): *in vitro* studies have shown the potential hepatoprotective effects of the MES present in ethanolic extracts of *Sargassum serratifolium* (Lim et al. 2018). Research carried out with *tert*-butyl hydroperoxide (*t*-BHP)-treated HepG2 cells showed that the ethanolic extracts rich in MES obtained from *S. serratofolium* have strong antioxidant activity (dose $0.25 \sim 1.0\,\mu g\,ml^{-1}$). The authors concluded that it will be critical to further investigate molecular and biochemical targets in order to better understand the pharmacological and toxicological profiles of the active components (Lim et al. 2018).

Other studies have shown the anti-inflammatory activities of ethanolic extracts of *S. serratifolium* (in mouse peritoneal macrophages stimulated with lipopolysaccharides), where they were found to inhibit the production of inflammatory mediators and proinflammatory cytokines (nitric oxide (NO), prostaglandin E2 [PGE_2], TNF-α, IL-1β, and

IL-6) at low concentrations 0, 1.0, 2.5, and 5.0 mg l^{-1} of ethanolic extract of *S. serratifolium* (Joung et al. 2017). The active compounds have been identified as sargahydroquinoic acid ((2*Z*,6*E*,10*E*)-12-(2,5-dihydroxy-3-methylphenyl)-6,10-dimethyl-2-(4-methylpent-3-enyl)dodeca-2,6,10-trienoic acid; $C_{27}H_{38}O_4$), sargachromenol ((2*Z*,6*E*)-9-[(2*R*)-6-hydroxy-2,8-dimethylchromen-2-yl]-6-methyl-2-(4-methylpent-3-enyl)nona-2,6-dienoic acid; $C_{27}H_{36}O_4$), and sargaquinoic acid ((2Z,6E,10E)-6,10-dimethyl-12-(5-methyl-3,6-dioxo-1,4-cyclohexadien-1-yl)-2-(4-methyl-3-penten-1-yl)-2,6,10-dodecatrienoic acid; $C_{27}H_{36}O_4$) (Jung et al. 2017). Other *in vivo* studies in high-fat-fed C57BL/6J mice fed a high-fat diet (fed with MES 60 and 120 mg kg^{-1} body weightday^{-1}) showed that MES (sargahydroquinoic acid, sargachromenol, and sargaquinoic acid) obtained from ethanolic extracts of *S. serratifolium* operated by activating AMPK-related fatty acid oxidation signaling and inhibiting sterol regulatory element-binding protein 1 (SREBP1c)-related lipogenesis signaling in liver and adipose tissues (60–120 mg kg^{-1}), and that these compounds could thereby potentially be used as preventive drugs against obesity and metabolic syndrome (Kwon et al. 2018).

Another molecule of interest is caulerpin (dimethyl (2*E*,13*E*)-11,22-diazapentacyclo [13.7.0.0^{4,12}.0^{5,10}.0^{16,21}]docosa-1(15),2,4(12),5,7,9,13,16,18,20-decaene-2,13-dicarboxylate; $C_{24}H_{18}N_2O_4$; an alkaloid characteristic to the genus *Caulerpa*), which has, ever since its isolation in 1968 (Ayyad and Badria 1994), shown biological properties such as antitumoral (Vairappan 2004), antiviral (Macedo et al. 2012), analgesic (antinociceptive), and anti-inflammatory activities (Souza et al. 2009). Subsequent studies (writhing test) suggested that caulerpin exerts the analgesic (antinociceptive) effect through pathways that involve α2-adrenoceptors and 5-HT3 on the cortex of Wistar rats (Cavalcante-Silva et al. 2013, 2014). A recent study analyzed the effect of caulerpin in murine models of zymosan-induced peritonitis and ulcerative colitis through chemical induction, and noted that a dose of 4 mg kg^{-1} body wt improved the disease activity index (DAI) as an indicator of ulcerative colitis disease, and attenuated colonic epithelial damage (Lucena et al. 2018). This dose decreased levels of TNF-α, IFN-γ, IL-6, IL-17, and NFκB p65, and increased levels of IL-10 in colonic tissue, which are promising results for the possible development of an ulcerative colitis treatment (Lucena et al. 2018).

19.3 Potential Pharmaceutical Formulations from Algae

As evident in the works cited above, micro- and macroalgae can be a rich source of a wide variety of bioactive compounds with possible pharmacological activities. Table 19.1 shows a summary of: (i) the most studied bioactive compounds, (ii) examples of specific compounds, and (iii) potential pharmaceutical applications.

19.3.1 Potential Anticancer, Cytotoxic, and Antiproliferative Pharmaceutical Formulations

Antitumoral activity is perhaps the most researched of all pharmaceutical activities due to the prevalence of this type of disease. *In vitro* and *in vivo* studies with fucoidans show that they inhibit tumor growth by: (i) activating intrinsic and extrinsic pathways for apoptosis, (ii) by suppressing angiogenesis, (iii) reducing the adhesion of tumor cells to platelets, and (iv) by increasing the immune response (Koyanagi et al. 2003; Li et al. 2008; Wijesekara et al. 2011; Vo and Kim 2013; Moghadamtousi et al. 2014; Bae et al. 2015; Kalimuthu and Kim 2015; Alves et al. 2018; Pereira 2018a). A recent study has also shown that fucoidan isolated from two species of the genus *Fucus* is a potent stimulator of sirtuin 6 (SIRT6), involved in numerous molecular processes associated with aging, including DNA repair, maintenance of telomeres, glycolysis, and inflammation (Rahnasto-Rilla et al. 2017), and can thus be another avenue in the search for cancer treatment molecules.

One of the most interesting aspects of the possible use of fucoidan as an anticarcinogenic agent is its low toxicity on healthy cells, thus avoiding the important side effects of most chemotherapy treatments (Déléris et al. 2016).

Other studies show that an oligosaccharide obtained from alginates derived from seaweed has been able to reduce the progression of osteosarcoma in operated patients, and has improved its status as an antioxidant and anti-inflammatory drug (Chen et al. 2017). MS80, another oligosaccharide derived from algae, has been shown to be effective as an antitumoral agent. It does so by inhibiting the activation signals of transforming growth factor (TGF)-β/Smad in lung and breast cancer cells, and in the 4T1 Orthotopic Xenograft Model, by reversing the migration and invasion of tumors (Zhou et al. 2016).

Microalgal compounds are also of interest in the manufacture of pharmaceutical products. A recent study on an exopolysaccharide extracted from *Thraustochytriidae* sp. has shown antiproliferative capacity in BG-1 ovarian cancer cells, MCF-7 breast cancer cells, and SW-620 colon cancer cells. It also showed immunomodulatory activity and induces proliferation of B cells even at low dilutions, besides producing alterations in the production of cytokines by T cells (Park et al. 2017a).

Although less studied, it has also been reported that porphyran is able to induce apoptosis through activation of caspase-and/or caspase-6, while simultaneously reducing phosphorylation of insulin-like growth factor receptor (IGF-IR) and exerts a negative regulation of serine/threonine kinase (Akt) phosphorylation (Kwon and Nam 2006).

Fucoxanthin has also been widely studied due to its ability to inhibit growth in tumor cells and induce apoptosis (Hosokawa et al. 2004; Peng et al. 2011; Mori 2004; Moghadamtousi et al. 2014; Yousefi et al. 2018). Satomi (2017) recently reviewed the mechanisms of action, which can be summed up as G1 cell cycle arrest and induction of apoptosis in diverse types of cancers (duodenal, skin, colon, liver, melanoma, etc., in carcinogenesis and xenograft models). Another recent review by Rocha et al. (2018) confirms the above action mechanisms and also cites the inhibition of angiogenesis. Jin et al. (2018) demonstrated that fucoxanthin-induced apoptosis in cervical cancer cell lines is via its action on the PI3K/Akt/NF-κB pathways (Jin et al. 2018). A recent study highlights that fucoxanthinol induces anoikis (apoptosis induced by loss of cell anchorage to the extracellular matrix or because the cell-matrix interactions are insufficient or inappropriate) in human colorectal cancer cells, apparently by inhibiting the signals of integrins (Terasaki et al. 2017). This is an interesting aspect, since anoikis is a potential survival mechanism of cancer cells during metastasis.

Laminarin shows antitumoral activity by inducing apoptosis and inhibiting growth of tumors (Park et al. 2013; Déléris et al. 2016). Carrageenan acts as an antiangiogenic agent but with gastrointestinal side effects (Zhou et al. 2005; Tobacman, 2001).

The antitumoral activity of phlorotannins has also been widely demonstrated in numerous publications that indicate antiproliferative activity against breast cancer and liver cell lines through the induction of apoptosis (Kong et al. 2009; Wijesekara et al., 2010; Li et al. 2011a; Namvar et al. 2013; Narasimham et al. 2013). Moreover, *in vivo* studies show that phloroglucinol suppresses tumorigenicity. It also sensitizes tumor cells to chemotherapy and also acts on stem cells, thereby preventing relapses (Kim et al. 2015b). Worth mentioning among the *in vivo* studies is the study of Sadeeshkumar et al. (2017) on the effects of dieckol obtained from *E. cava* that causes suppression of N-nitrosodiethylamine (NDEA)-induced hepatocarcinogenesis in mice by modulating xenobiotic-metabolizing enzymes, thus producing cell proliferation and induction of apoptosis via mitochondrial pathways (Sadeeshkumar et al. 2017).

There is abundant scientific literature on the cytotoxic capacity of bromophenols. Rocha et al. (2018) listed 10 different compounds with cytotoxic activity against lung, gastric, breast, melanoma, ovarian, and colon cancer cell lines via different action mechanisms (mainly by inducing apoptosis) and that the activity is influenced by the location and the number of bromine atoms – aspects that may be of interest in the future development of cancer treatment drugs (Rocha et al. 2018). Another major field of research is that of obtaining cytotoxic terpenes, mainly monoterpenes, diterpenes, and MES, among which we can cite halomon (halogenated monoterpene), one of the first terpenes from algae studied as a possible anticarcinogenic agent, because it has been shown to possess a potent inhibitory activity of DNA methyltransferase-1 (DNMT-1); laurinterol, a sesquiterpene that has been postulated as a potential anticancer metabolite against melanoma cells (B16F1); and dactylon, a halogenated sesquiterpenoide that inhibits epidermal growth factor-induced transformation in JB6P+Cl41 cells, and induces G1-S cell progression arrest and apoptosis of tumor cells (Rocha et al. 2018). Firdaus et al. (2018) identified benzene propanoic acid as the agent responsible for reducing cervical cancer cell viability (HeLa cells) (Firdaus et al. 2018).

Other molecules derived from algae can have indirect benefits in cancer treatment; thus, ulvan has been cited as a cytotoxic agent (Alves et al. 2013), laminarin as an inducer of apoptosis (Pereira 2018a), ascophyllan as a promoter of the immune response (Zhang et al. 2016), and caulerpin, which acts by activating the AMPKα1 pathway (Yu et al. 2017).

In a recent review on the development of cancer therapy drugs based on bioactive compounds derived from microalgae and cyanobacteria, Bajpai et al. (2018) cite eight compounds: brentuximab vedotin 63 (Adcetris™), glembatumumab vedotin, desmethoxymajusculamide C (DMMC (cyclic depsipeptide)), largazole, apratoxin A, cryptophycin 1, tasipeptins A–B, and coibamide A, two of which are already on the market (brentuximab vedotin 63 and cryptophycin 1), while the others are in various stages of preclinical and clinical studies. This increases the expectations for research, since they are marine organisms that are easy togrow.

19.3.2 Potential Antithrombotic, Anticoagulant, and Antihypertensive Pharmaceutical Formulations

Preclinical studies with rats fed on a modified diet with algal supplementation showed that some bioactive algal compounds could act as effective antihypertensive agents (Cha et al. 2006). Thus, Sato et al. (2002), using extracts from *U. pinnatifida*, identified four types of peptides that inhibit ACE, causing antihypertensive effects in hypertensive rats after a single oral administration.

Phlorotannins obtained from various brown algae also show antihypertensive activity (as referred to in Section 19.2.2), and furthermore inhibit the activity of ACE (Jung et al. 2006; Li et al. 2011a).

On the other hand, the anticoagulant activity of SPs has been known since the 1990s, and two main types with high anticoagulant activity were identified: sulfated galactan, commonly known as carrageenan, and sulfated fucoidan (Wijesekara et al. 2011). Different studies have described that the anticoagulant property of SPs is similar to or greater than that of heparin (Costa et al. 2010; Sun et al. 2018), so they are ideal candidates for the production of drugs. Other galactans from green algae and microalgae also have anticoagulant properties, but not as pronounced as fucoidan and carrageenan (Ngo and Kim 2013).

Insofar as the antithrombotic activity is concerned, fucoidan appears to be the most active compound. A randomized, 5-week double-blind study performed by Ren et al. (2013) showed that the intake of fucoidan reduces thrombolysis time by elevating the secretion of prostacyclin (PDI2) as a result of an increased production of H_2O_2 in the blood (Ren et al. 2013).

19.3.3 Potential Antilipidemic and Anticholesterolemic Pharmaceutical Formulations

A diet rich in fiber reduces cholesterol levels and some studies show that dietary fiber with ion exchange capacity has a very potent cholesterol-reducing effect (Guillon and Champ 2000). SPs are excellent agents for this function; thus, Yu et al. (2003a,b) demonstrated that ulvans can be potential antilipidemic agents and that they can reduce levels of serum triglycerides, total cholesterol, and LDL-C, and moreover, raise HDL-C levels in mice. Later *in vivo* studies showed that ulvans can improve the lipid profile through mRNA expression of farnesoid X receptor (FXR) and PPARγ and downregulate the expression of liver X receptor (LXR) (Qi and Sheng 2015). Other *in vivo* research carried out using the SP porphyran shows that it is able to lower levels of triglycerides, total cholesterol, and the ratio of LDL-C/HDL-C after 28 days of oral treatment in mice fed on a high-fat diet, thereby improving the rates of liver damage (Cao et al. 2016). Recent studies in hyperlipidemic mice confirm these data and suggest that porphyran could be a good candidate for the development of drugs for prevention of hyperlipidemia (Wang et al. 2017).

Lastly, algal phytosterols have been suggested as potential agents to reduce cholesterol levels (Lopes et al. 2013), but the possible action mechanism is yet to be deciphered.

19.3.4 Potential Antiobesity and Antidiabetic Pharmaceuticals Formulations

There is epidemiological evidence for the protective effect of algae in metabolic syndrome and that their consumption can reduce the progression of diabetes (Lee et al. 2010a). The most studied antiobesity bioactive compounds are fucoidan, fucoxanthin, and alginates, the more recent ones being phlorotannins and fucosterol. Different *in vivo* studies have shown that the consumption of fucoidan can prevent hyperglycemia by improving glucose utilization, and lowering blood glucose levels and concentrations of serum insulin in mice (Kim et al. 2012), improving glucose tolerance and insulin sensitivity by increasing serum concentrations of adiponectin (Jeong et al. 2013), or by stimulating the release of insulin from the pancreas (Wang et al. 2014). With regard to obesity, a study on obese mice also demonstrated that fucoidan lowered body weight and significantly reduced plasma levels of total cholesterol, low-density lipoproteins, and triglycerides (Kim et al. 2014a,b).

Other *in vitro* and *in vivo* studies show that fucoidan can act as a potent inhibitor of α-glucosidase and that this compound can be used in the treatment of type II diabetes mellitus (Shan et al. 2016). Although clinical trials in humans are scarce, Hernández-Corona et al. (2014) conducted a random, double-blind study by administering fucoidan to a group of obese or overweight patients, and noted that over a period of 3 months, it lowered blood pressure and levels of LDL-C, and increased insulin secretion (Hernández-Corona et al. 2014).

Other research has shown that fucoxanthin has antidiabetic properties. It has been shown *in vivo* that fucoxanthin improves insulin resistance and lipid metabolism (Maeda et al. 2009; Fumiaki et al. 2012), stimulates β-oxidation, and reduces lipogenesis in obese mouse models, by activating key lipid metabolism enzymes such as AMPK and acetyl-CoA carboxylase (ACC) in epididymal adipose tissue (Kang et al. 2012). Also worth highlighting is the study by Hu et al. (2012) in which a combination of fucoxanthin and conjugated linoleic acid managed to reduce serum levels of triacylglycerols, glucose, and leptin in obese rats (Hu et al. 2012). Moreover, a double-blind study with placebo control has shown that ingestion (between 1 and 3 mg day^{-1}) of fucoxanthin for 4 weeks reduces body mass index, abdominal fat, and other parameters related to obesity in obese patients (Hitoe and Shimoda 2017).

Alginates have also been studied for diabetes control, where *in vitro* studies have shown that they inhibit the activity of pancreatic lipase, especially alginates with a high guluronic acid content (Wilcox et al. 2014). A review by Georg Jensen et al. (2013) concluded that the consumption of alginates has beneficial effects on postprandial glucose absorption and response to insulin.

Lee et al. (2017) showed that fucosterol inhibited adipogenesis of 3T3-L1 preadipocytes through modulation of the FoxO signaling pathway (linked to insulin growth factor) (Lee et al. 2017).

Phlorotannins can also be candidates for the control of obesity and diabetes. A comprehensive review of literature on the role of phlorotannins in type II diabetes mellitus shows up to 15 compounds (including 6,6′-bieckol, 8,8′-bieckol, dieckol, dioxinodehydroeckol, diphlorethohydroxycarmalol, eckol, fucodiphloroethol-G, phlorofucofuroeckol-A, 2-phloroeckol, and 7-phloroeckol), whose action mechanisms are mainly the inhibition of α-glucosidase and α-amylase (Lopes et al. 2016).

Other bioactive algal compounds can also be of interest in the prevention of obesity and related diseases. Kang et al. (2017) isolated diverse indole derivatives, noting that they have inhibitory effects on adipogenesis via activation of the AMPK signal pathway. Lee et al. (2007) showed that methanolic extracts from the algae *Derbesia marina* and *Symphycladia latiscula* inhibit activity of the protein tyrosine phosphatase 1B (a negative regulator of insulin receptors associated with signal transduction) (Lee et al. 2007). A recent *in vivo* study on mice with induced type II diabetes showed that an extract rich in flavonoids obtained from the green alga *Enteromorpha prolifera* regulates glucose metabolism and attenuates hyperglycemia via activation of insulin receptor substrate 1 (IRS1) and PI3K/AKT, and inhibition of the c-Jun N-terminal kinases (JNK1/2) insulin pathway in the liver (Yan et al. 2019). Moreover, it modifies the intestinal microbiota, yet another aspect of interest related to the release of intestinal hormones that can regulate the release of insulin.

19.3.5 Potential Antibacterial, Antiviral, and Antifungal Pharmaceutical Formulations

The antibacterial activity of both macroalgae and microalgae is well known (Malini et al. 2014; El Shafay et al. 2016; Amri et al. 2017; Razarinah et al. 2018; Li et al. 2012b). Studies of macroalgae show that extracts obtained with organic solvents (ethanol, chloroform) have higher antibacterial activity than those extracted with aqueous solvents (Al-Saif et al. 2014) and that phenolic compounds may act against both Gram-negative and Gram-positive human pathogens (Vijayabaskar and Shiyamala 2011). One of the most studied algae for its antimicrobial capacity is *E. cava*, whose extracts have been shown to be active against different microorganisms (Kim et al. 2015d; Lee et al. 2016). It has recently been determined that the lipophilic fractions of *B. bifurcata* are active against Gram-positive and Gram-negative bacteria, and that extracts from this alga boost the action of other conventional antibiotics (Santos et al. 2017). It is therefore of great interest to identify the molecules responsible for these activities. The antiviral activity of SPs has been widely studied, as mentioned earlier (Girond et al. 1991; Boisson-Vidal et al. 1995; Santoyo et al. 2011; Peng et al. 2013). Of great interest is the study of anti-HIV agents, where fucoidan is the most active algal compound (Wijesekara et al. 2011; Dinesh et al. 2016) in addition to sulfated galactans (Yasuhara and Lu, 2010). *In vitro* studies of galactofucans obtained from *Adenocystis utricularis* have been shown to inhibit replication of the virus (Trinchero et al. 2009). Ahmadi et al. (2015) cites several SPs with anti-HIV properties, both in macroalgae such as carrageenan, galactan, alginate, fucan, and laminarin, and in microalgae such as naviculan, calcium spirulan, and nostaflan (Ahmadi et al. 2015). An example of interest is iota-carrageenan (Carragelose®), the first product developed from algae in the pharmaceutical market (Marinomed Biotech AG). It is a type of carrageenan isolated from a red edible alga (strains such us *Chondrus*, *Gigartina*, *Eucheuma*, *Furcellaria*, *Phyllophora*) belonging to a family of linear SPs. Carragelose has the ability to block viral attachment to host cells and is effective against a broad spectrum of respiratory viruses (https://www.carragelose.com/en/mode-of-action) (Ludwig et al. 2013; Calado et al. 2018).

Phlorotannins can likewise be potential antiviral agents, in particular 8.4″-dieckol, which selectively inhibits the activity of HIV-1 reverse transcriptase (Karadeniz et al. 2014). Moreover, a lectin, cyanovirin-N, extracted from cyanobacteria can inhibit the penetration of the virus into target cells (Zappe et al. 2008) and it has also been shown to be effective against the Ebola virus (Matei et al. 2016). Cyanobacterial lectins are also being researched for their potential anti-HIV action (Akkouh et al. 2015). Other microalgal and cyanobacterial compounds have been the subject of study to obtain antibacterial and antiviral substances. A recent review by Bule et al. (2018) cites several compounds, including SPs and bromophenols. Worth mentioning in this group of potential drugs is the antiprotozoal activity of some algal compounds such as diterpenes, sesquiterpenes (e.g. elatol), or fucoidan, but more studies are needed to verify their effectiveness (Torres et al. 2014).

19.3.6 Potential Immunomodulatory Anti-Inflammatory Pharmaceutical Formulations

Polysaccharides are the most studied algal bioactive compounds due to their anti-inflammatory action. Recent *in vitro* and *in vitro* studies have shown that lectins and polysaccharides obtained from *U. lactuca* show anti-inflammatory and immunomodulatory activity associated with the inhibition of TNF-α cytokine release and downregulation of NO production (Mezdour et al. 2017). Xu et al. (2017) reviewed the immunomodulatory activities of algal polysaccharides and indicated the different possible action mechanisms, which include stimulation of macrophages and enhanced production of cytokines (such as TNF-α, IL-1β, IL-6, and IL-10), where once again, fucoidan, which promotes the activation of NK cells, stands out. Also studied were the algal polysaccharides that enhance the immune response as a coadjuvant during vaccination (Li et al. 2012b), and therefore the need to isolate and identify the molecules that can perform these actions and be possible candidates for the development of immunomodulatory drugs.

Several studies have likewise shown the anti-inflammatory capacity of astaxanthin and that this activity is dose-dependent (Ohgami et al. 2003; Shiratori et al. 2005; Lee et al. 2003). It works by inhibiting the secretion of IL-1β, IL-6, and TNF-α, or the production of NO and PGE_2.

Other possible anti-inflammatory molecules such as sargaquinone or aryl polyketide lactones inhibit the biosynthesis of leukotrienes (Tziveleka et al. 2005) and both are extracted from species belonging to the genus *Sargassum* (Maneesh and Chakraborty 2017). The isoprenoid (3-hydroxy-4,7-megastigmadien-9-one) obtained from *U. pertusa* is postulated as a powerful anti-inflammatory agent since it has inhibitory effects on the production of inflammatory cytokines by downregulating TLR9-dependent AP-1 and NF-κB activation (Ali et al. 2017).

Another aspect of pharmacological interest is the treatment of osteoarthritis with aqueous extracts obtained from *Codium fragile*. They have showed ability to inhibit disease progression, decrease loss of proteoglycans, and reduce the osteoarthritis cartilage histopathology assessment system indexes (Moon et al. 2018). This warrants the need to study the active compounds involved for their potential pharmacologicaluse.

Microalgae and cyanobacteria can also be potential sources of anti-inflammatory substances and worth highlighting are the malyngamides, which inhibit production of NO in murine macrophages (Villa et al. 2010).

19.3.7 Potential Neuroprotective Pharmaceutical Formulations for a Healthy Nervous System

There are estimates that neurodegenerative diseases will surpass cancer cases in the future (Pangestuti and Kim 2011). Mechanisms and strategies for safe and effective neuroprotection against several types of damage, apoptosis, dysfunction, and degeneration of the central nervous system should therefore be developed (Pangestuti and

Kim 2011). The neuroprotective action of certain algal compounds has been studied in recent years and examples of these are: pigments such as fucoxanthin, probably due to its antioxidant capacity (Pangestuti and Kim 2011; Mohibbullah et al. 2018), and pheophytin, which promotes neuronal development in embryogenesis. Pheophytin did not itself promote neurite outgrowth of PC12 cells. However, when PC12 cells were treated with a low concentration of pheophytin a ($3.9\ \mu\ ml^{-1}$) in the presence of a low level of nerve growth factor ($10\ ng\ ml^{-1}$), the compound produced neurite outgrowth similar to that produced by a high level of nerve growth factor ($50\ ng\ ml^{-1}$) (Ina et al. 2007).

Fucosterol could likewise be a compound of interest, since *in vitro* studies have shown that it presents a dose-dependent inhibitory activity against acetylcholinesterase and butyrylcholinesterase, and it can significantly inhibit the production of cytokines, such as interleukins (IL-6, IL-1β), TNF-α, NO, and PGE_2 in lipopolysaccharide- and β-amyloid (Aβ)-induced microglial cells (Wong et al. 2018). The role of two alkaloids, racemosins A and B, extracted from *Caulerpa racemosa* have likewise been studied. *In vitro* studies have shown a certain neuroprotective activity vis-à-vis Aβ-induced SH-SY5Y cell damage (Liu et al. 2013).

On the other hand, the role of 3-amino-1-propanesulfonic acid (also called homotaurine and tramiprosate) present in different red algae species has been studied both *in vivo* and *in vitro* and found to have neuroprotective effects by preventing neurotoxicity of the Aβ peptide through reduction of amyloid aggregation. This may be of interest in the prevention of Alzheimer's disease (Kocis et al. 2017). Homotaurine is an aminosulfonate compound naturally found in red algae (Bossù et al. 2018). Homotaurine has been shown to have effects on the memory of Parkinson's patients and on cognitive deficits in double-blind studies (Ricciardi et al. 2015; Bossù et al. 2018). Bossù et al. (2018), in an *in vivo* study in patients at the earliest stages of Alzheimer's disease, i.e. suffering from amnestic mild cognitive impairment (aMCI), suggested that homotaurine supplementation in aMCI individuals carrying apo lipoprotein E (APOE) $\varepsilon4$ has a positive consequence on episodic memory loss due, at least in part, to homotaurine anti-inflammatory effects targeting IL-18, and this has aroused interest in this molecule for the prevention of degenerative diseases.

Two phlorotannins, eckol and dieckol, have also been studied for their ability to inhibit peroxisome proliferator-activated receptor c (Jung et al., 2014b), which protects against neurodegeneration in Parkinson's disease (Carta 2013). Subsequent *in vitro* studies suggest that eckol and dieckol inhibit monoamine oxidases (MAOs) (Jung et al. 2017).

Barbosa et al. (2014) reviewed literature on neuroprotective algal bioactive compounds for their action mechanisms and suggest that the use of molecules extracted from algae can reduce the risk of toxicity in the body and prevent certain undesirable effects (Barbosa et al. 2014).

19.3.8 Other Potential Pharmacological Formulations from Algae

Algae are known to promote intestinal health and one of the reasons for this is their high fiber content, which confers a protective effect (Hamed et al. 2015). However, the action mechanism of fibers appears to be related to the prebiotic properties of algal polysaccharides (Brown et al. 2014; Hamed et al. 2015; Gómez-Guzmán et al. 2018;

Yang and Lee 2016), an aspect of great interest because we now know that intestinal microbiota play a fundamental role in human health. The role of porphyran-rich algal extracts has been related to changes in intestinal microbiota (Kearney et al. 2018) and more clinical studies are needed to confirm this hypothesis and progress toward these new pharmacological uses of algal bioactive compounds.

Another interesting study on inflammatory bowel disease shows that fucoidan improves the intestinal epithelial barrier function by regulating the expression of claudín-1 (Iraha et al. 2013). A study, conducted on H_2O_2-induced tight junction destruction in human intestinal epithelial cells, showed that fucoidan protected the epithelial barrier function from oxidative injury of the tight junction as well as barrier disruption by upregulating the expression of claudin-1 (Iraha et al. 2013).

In relation to gastrointestinal health, other studies have shown that fucoidan (in patients, dose 1.5–4.5 mg $kg^{-1}\cdot day^{-1}$, 10 days) can relieve symptoms of non-ulcer dyspepsia (two-way crossover test) and furthermore has preventive and curative actions on gastric ulcers by preventing the adhesion of *Helicobacter pylori* to the gastric cells (Nagaoka et al. 2000).

Another aspect of pharmacological interest is the influence of certain algal compounds in bone metabolism and in the prevention of osteoporosis. Although there are *in vivo* and *in vitro* studies on the role of some algal compounds such as (i) fucoidan in inducing differentiation of osteoblasts and inhibition of the differentiation of osteoclasts (Kim et al. 2015c), and (ii) fucoxanthin, which induces apoptosis of osteoclasts (Das et al. 2010), there is nevertheless a lack of clinical studies to confirm these effects in humans in order to develop pharmaceutical formulae to improve bone health.

Other applications of algal compounds are the development of products for wound healing (Zhang et al. 2018), development of biocomposites (Gómez d'Ayala et al. 2008), and microencapsulation and other drug delivery systems (Gomez d'Ayala et al., 2008; Laurienzo 2010; Wang et al. 2012b; Barbosa et al. 2019). With regard to the drug delivery systems, progress has been made in recent years in the development of biosilicate materials from diatoms that have already been used in cancer therapy (Uthappa et al. 2018).

19.4 Algae as a Source of Active Ingredients for Cosmeceuticals

The cosmetics industry is continually seeking new agents for cosmetics, not only for marketing reasons but also because certain ingredients (or raw materials) are prohibited by cosmetovigilance committees from time to time (as has been the case of raw materials sourced from bovine brain, spinal cord, and eyes) (https://publications.europa.eu), or because consumers reject them (https://knowledge.ulprospector.com). Therefore, the marine environment is of interest to the cosmetics industry as a source of active substances with numerous bioactive compounds in animals, algae, bacteria and even sea water (Pereira 2018b; Mourelle et al. 2017).

Polysaccharides such as agar-agar, alginates, and carrageenans from red algae have been used since time immemorial, as thickeners in cosmetic formulations such as creams, shampoos, etc. (Pereira 2018b). However, the current interest is focused on bioactive compounds for hydration, sun protection, skin detoxification, weight loss treatments, and prevention of aging, etc., and this is supported by the trend toward using natural products (organic cosmetics; www.marketwatch.com).

Cosmetics are products aimed at improving the structure, morphology, and appearance of skin, with the assistance of excipients (defined as a constituent of a medicine or a cosmetic other than the active substance, added in the formulation for a specific purpose, such as long-term stabilization, bulking up solid formulations, etc.) and active ingredients adapted to different skin types (normal, oily, combination, sensitive) (Mourelle et al. 2017).

Cosmeceuticals (also called cosmeceutics), although the term is not legally recognized, for example, in the Food, Drugs and Cosmetics Act of the USA, are defined as "cosmetic products with biologically active ingredients purporting to have medical or drug-like benefits" (Mourelle et al. 2017). In dermatology, cosmeceuticals encompass the topical application of biologically active ingredients, which affect the skin barrier and overall skin health (Vermeer and Gilcherst, 1996; Draelos 2014).

Marine algae, microalgae, and cyanobacteria provide numerous agents and other ingredients for the food and nutritional supplements industry. Macroalgae are a source of minerals, vitamins, polysaccharides, PUFAs, and polyphenols, while microalgae provide pigments, mainly carotenoids and vitamins, and cyanobacteria are rich in protein and pigments that can be used as active ingredients in cosmetics and cosmeceuticals. There is abundant literature on the use of algal bioactive compounds in cosmetics (Azam et al. 2017; Kim et al. 2017; Pereira 2018b), but less on compounds from microalgae and cyanobacteria. Table 19.2 provides a summary of the most interesting ones for cosmeceuticals.

19.4.1 Polysaccharides

As stated above, these are the most widely used algal thickening compounds and are currently also associated with other properties such as moisturizing, antioxidant, anti-inflammatory, antiaging, and skin whitening (Kim et al. 2018; Wang et al. 2013). Some of the most promising active compounds are fucoidans, which inhibited the expression of MMPs (MMP-I; collagenase, involved in skin aging) induced by UVB at the protein level and mRNA in human fibroblasts (HS68) and could help prevent skin aging (Moon et al. 2009). Fucoidans also stimulated the production of fibroblasts by promoting skin regeneration and increasing expression of α6-integrin in CCD-25Sk human fibroblasts seeded with various concentrations of fucoidan (0~50 $\mu g\,ml^{-1}$) (Song et al. 2014). Fucoidans also stimulated the proliferation of fibroblasts by increasing the expression of cyclin D1, a protein involved in cell cycle regulation (Song et al. 2014).The above reports support the potential use of fucoidans in antiaging applications and creams, and especially against photoageing. Fucoidans may also be useful in the preparation of regeneration and healing cosmeceuticals, since fucoidans from brown algae such as *A. nodosum* have been shown to stimulate fibroblasts and extracellular matrix deposition (on human dermal fibroblast from prepuce of healthy subjects aged 3–4 years and from one cell strain after breast plastic surgery on a mid-aged patient, dose at 10 and 100 $\mu g\,ml^{-1}$) (Senni et al. 2006), and low molecular fucoidan inhibited protease leucocyte elastase which protects the elastic fiber network of the dermis against enzymatic proteolysis from *in vitro* studies (0.01–0.03% concentrations, residue weight %, *F. vesiculosus* extract) (Table 19.2; Fujimura et al. 2000; Fitton et al. 2007). Other studies show the capacity of fucoidans

Table 19.2 Bioactive compounds from macroalgae and microalgae and their potential uses as active ingredients in cosmeceuticals.

General class of bioactive compounds	Examples of bioactive compounds	Potential uses in cosmeceuticals	References
Polysaccharides	Fucoidans (from *Undaria pinnatifida*, *Ascophyllum nodosum*, *Fucus vesiculosus*)	Antiaging: stimulation of fibroblast and extracellular matrix deposition (increased type I procollagen mRNA and protein expression in a dose-dependent manner) Antiaging: increased fibroblast proliferation; wound healing	Moon et al. (2009); Song et al. (2014); Senni et al. (2006); Park et al. (2017a)
	Agaro-oligosaccharides	Moisturizing agents	Kim et al. (2017);
	Carrageenan-oligosaccharides (obtained by enzymatic hydrolysis)	Skin whitening (inhibit melanin synthesis and cellular tyrosinase activity in B16F10 cells)	Yun et al. (2013); Kim et al. (2017)
	3,6-Anhydro-L-galactose	Reduction of melanin production in B16F10 cells (reduce melanin secretion)	Kim et al. (2017)
	Alginates	Thickening agent in cosmetics	Pereira et al. (2018a)
	Carrageenans	Wound healing Thickening agent in cosmetics	Pereira et al. (2013)
	Ulvans	Moisturizing agent Antioxidant (scavenging activity on hydroxyl radical) Promotes hyaluronan (hyaluronic acid) synthesis (in cultured dermal fibroblasts)	Fabrowska et al. (2015); Qi et al. (2005) Adrien et al. (2017)

(*continued*)

Table 19.2 (*continued*)

General class of bioactive compounds	Examples of bioactive compounds	Potential uses in cosmeceuticals	References
	Laminarans	Prevents photoaging (by downregulating MMP-1 and upregulating TIMP-1 and hydroxyproline content) in dermis of Kunming SPF mice Promotes dermis matrix production; Wound healing (in wounded Wistar female rats)	Li et al. (2013) Ayoub et al. (2015) Sellimi et al. (2018)
	Porphyrans	Antioxidant (scavenging activity toward superoxide anion and hydroxyl radical); Anti-inflammatory (in RAW264.7 macrophages)	Zhang et al. (2009); Isaka et al. (2015); Jiang et al. (2012)
	ß-1,3-Glucan	Free radical quencher; immune system booster Anti-inflammatory	Spolaore et al. (2006) Koller et al. (2014)
Phenols and polyphenols	Phlorotannins (e. g. phloroglucinol, eckol, and dieckol)	Antioxidant; anti-photoageing: prevents expression of matrix metalloproteinases in human dermal fibroblasts Reduces hyaluronidase activity (HAase assay)	Liu et al. (2017) Pallela et al. (2010) Shibata et al. (2002)
	Bromophenols	Antioxidant (DPPH radical scavenging method)	Liu et al. (2011a)
Terpenes	Sargaquinoic acid	Attenuates melanin synthesis (by inhibiting the expression of the melanogenic enzymes): TYR, TRP1, and TRP2; also inhibited cellular TYR activity in α-MSH-stimulated B16F10 cells	Azam et al. (2017, 2018)

(*continued*)

Table 19.2 (*continued*)

General class of bioactive compounds	Examples of bioactive compounds	Potential uses in cosmeceuticals	References
Pigments	Chlorophyll a, b; astaxanthin, phycocyanobilins, and phycoerythrobilins from microalgae (*Arthrospira*, *Dunaliella*, *Haematococcus*, and *Chlorella*)	Colorants; to mask odors in dentifrices and deodorants	Hosikian et al. (2010) Borowitzka (2013)
	Astaxanthin	Antioxidant Sunscreen protection Skin whitening (melanin synthesis inhibition) in open-labeled non-controlled clinical study by combining both oral supplementation and topical treatment of astaxanthin	Koller et al. (2014) Tominaga et al. (2012)
	Fucoxanthin	Protection against UVB-induced photoaging *in vitro* and *in vivo* (mice) and in human dermal fibroblasts ROS scavenging activity (DCFH-DA assay)	Urikura et al. (2011); Liu et al. (2016); Chen et al. (2016); Matsui et al. (2016)
		Stimulates restoration of the skin barrier protein filaggrin in human dermal fibroblasts (filament aggregating protein) Protective and therapeutic effects against sunburn in human dermal fibroblasts	Matsui et al. (2016)
	β-Cryptoxanthin	Anti-inflammatory Promotes hyaluronan (hyaluronic acid) synthesis in human foreskin keratinocytes	Tang and Suter (2011)
	ß-carotene	Free radical scavenging	Gammone et al. (2015)

(*continued*)

Table 19.2 (*continued*)

General class of bioactive compounds	Examples of bioactive compounds	Potential uses in cosmeceuticals	References
PUFAs and other lipids	PUFAs	Emollient, epidermal lipid repair protection against TEWL	Bedoux et al. (2014)
	Stearic acid, arachidonic acid, and eicosapentaenoic acid	Calming and restoring the skin Anti-inflammatory; antiallergic Immune system booster Antiaging	Łęska et al. (2018)
	Sterols (e.g. fucosterol)	ROS scavenging activity; Prevents aging on human dermal fibroblasts of skin (inhibition of IL-6 and MMP-1 production)	Hwang et al. (2014) Kim et al. (2005)
Proteins and amino acids	Amino acids: alanine, serine, proline, histidine tyrosine, tryptophan	Moisturizing agents	Pereira et al. (2018a)
	Taurine (2-aminoethanesulfonic acid)	Free radical quencher Protecting in oxidative stress on skin	Widiastuti and Khairani (2018)
	Mycosporine-like amino acids	Sunscreens and photoaging prevention in UV-induced apoptosis in HaCaT cells Prevented extrinsic skin aging: inhibitory properties against MMPs, increased procollagen secretion levels, and enhancing the expression of type I collagen and elastin in human skin fibroblasts	Suh et al. (2017) Chrapusta et al. (2017)
Other compounds	Ectoine (1,4,5,6-tetrahydro-2-methyl-4-pyrimidinecar-boxylic acid) (from halophilic bacteria as *Halomonas elongata*, *alpha*- and *gamma-proteobacteria*, and *Actinobacteridae*)	Osmoprotectant (skin moisturizing) by topical applications in humans Immune protection, UV protection Stress protection of skin Decreased skin inflammation (clinical trial)	Guillerme et al. (2017) Kim et al. (2008) Marini et al. (2014)

(*continued*)

Table 19.2 (*continued*)

General class of bioactive compounds	Examples of bioactive compounds	Potential uses in cosmeceuticals	References
	Scytonemin	Photoprotective effect (*in vitro*)	Rastogi et al. (2013)
	Vitamin C (ascorbic acid), vitamin D, and vitamin E (α-tocopherol)	Antioxidant activities	Pereira et al. (2018a)
	Pantothenic acid (Vitamin B_5)	Wound healing (in HaCaT keratinocytes)	Kobayashi et al. (2011)
	Microelements: Zn, Mg, Cu, I, Fe, Mn	Skin conditioning (moisturizing, protection)	Pereira et al. (2018a)
	Macroelements: Ca, Na, K,Cl		Mourelle and Gómez (2015)
Algae extracts	*Chondrus crispus*, *Codium tomentosum*, *Undaria pinnatifida*, *Durvillaea antarctica*, *Ascophyllum nodosum*, and *Polysiphonia lanosa*	Moisturizing Skin protection from UV irradiation	Kim et al. (2008)
	Laminaria saccharina	Anti-inflammatory Regulates sebaceous gland activity	Kim et al. (2008)
	Ascophyllum nodosum and *Asparagopsis armata*	Anti-irritant (for sensitive skin)	Kim et al. (2008)
	Enteromorpha compressa	Increases blood circulation in skin	Kim et al. (2008)
	Arthrospira and *Chlorella*	Skin protection against UV irradiation Antioxidant (DPPH assay; chelating and SOD activity) ROS scavenging activity (chelating activity and SOD, catalase, and peroxidase activities)	Ismaiel et al. (2014)
	Corallina pilulifera	Prevents photoaging: protective effect on dermal fibroblast against UVA matrix metalloproteinases 2 and 9 inhibition in human fibroblasts	Pallela et al. (2010)
	Ecklonia cava and *Sargassum siliquastrum*	Skin whitening: tyrosinase inhibition *in vivo* assay with adult zebrafish	Cha et al. (2011)

α-MSH, α-melanocyte stimulating hormone; DCFH-DA, dichlorofluorescin diacetate; DPPH, 2,2-diphenyl-1-picrylhydrazyl; IL, interleukin; MMP-1, matrix metalloproteinase 1; PUFA, polyunsaturated fatty acid; ROS, reactive oxygen species; SOD, superoxide dismutase; SPF, specific pathogen free; TEWL, transepidermal water loss; TIMP-1, metallopeptidase inhibitor 1; TRP1, tyrosinase-related protein 1; TYR, tyrosinase; UV, ultraviolet.

for wound healing is possibly a result of a complex coordination mechanism between an antioxidant, anti-inflammatory, and antigrowth factor-dependent activities. The study was conducted in in a full-thickness dermal excision rat model treated with low molecular weight fucoidan (dose 50–200 mg ml^{-1}) from *U. pinnatifida* with three-way ANOVA for the kinetics of wound contraction in comparison with Madecassol Care™ containing 1% *Centella asiatica* as a commercial natural source (Park et al. 2017b).

As we mentioned before, agar and carrageenan are widely used in the cosmetics industry as thickeners and stabilizers in emulsions (Kim et al. 2017), but present attention is inclined toward oligosaccharides, agaro-oligosaccharides, and carrageenan-oligosaccharides derived from agar and carrageenan, respectively, through enzymatic hydrolysis, for use as active ingredients, because it has been shown that they can act as moisturizers and skin whiteners by reducing the production of melanin. Yun et al. (2013) carried out a study where they obtained oligosaccharides from a commercial agarose (Intron Biotechnology, Seongnam, Korea) pre-hydrolysis of agarose into agaro-oligosaccharides by using acetic acid, hydrolysis of the agaro-oligosaccharides into neoagarobiose by an exo-agarase, and hydrolysis of neoagarobiose into 3,6-anhydro-L-galactose and galactose by a neoagarobiose hydrolase. They treated a murine melanoma cell line B16F10 with 1, 10, and 100 μg ml^{-1}, and after 4 days of cultivation with α-melanocyte-stimulating hormone (α-MSH), melanine was determined by measuring the absorbance at 475 nm with an enzyme-linked immunosorbent assay (ELISA) reader (Yun et al. 2013) (Table 19.2; Yun et al. 2013). It has been observed in *in vitro* studies that the 3,6-anhydro-L-galactose monosaccharide obtained by enzymatic hydrolysis from commercial agarose (Intron Biotechnology, Seongnam, Korea) also reduced the production of melanin in B16F10 melanoma cells exposed to 100 nM α-MSH (the levels of melanin were determined by measuring the absorbance at 495 nm using an ELISA reader) (Kim et al. 2017).

Alginates are also used as gelling agents in multiple cosmetic products (creams, shampoos, face masks, etc.) (Pereira 2018b) to form a flexible film that promotes adhesion to the skin (Pereira 2018b), with the advantage that emulsions form a surface film that prevents transepidermal water loss (TEWL) through clinical testing. They have also been used to develop formulae that boost wound healing composed by alginate and *Aloe vera* gel in different proportions (95:5, 85:15, and 75:25, v/v) and testing mechanical properties (such as tensile strength and elongation at break), and also swelling behavior (Pereira et al. 2013). Similarly, the different types of carrageenan, kappa (κ), iota (ι), and lambda (λ), have been used to increase viscosity in cosmetic formulations and produce a protective film on the skin to prevent TEWL (Pereira 2018b).

Ulvans are polysaccharides of interest in cosmeceuticals, since they have been observed to have moisturizing, protective, and antioxidant properties (Fabrowska et al. 2015). Ulvans extracted from *Ulva* sp. have not only been studied for their antioxidant activity by DPPH and ABTS assays (Qi et al. 2005), but also their antiaging capacity due to their ability to stimulate the production of hyaluronic acid in commercial normal human dermal fibroblasts and quantification by an ELISA-like hyaluronan test plate (R&D Systems, USA) (Adrien et al. 2017).

Laminarins from brown algae are one of the little studied algal polysaccharides for potential cosmetic uses. Laminarin from *Saccharina longicruris* has been shown to reduce damage caused by UVA/UVB radiation in *in vivo* models, by downregulating MMP-1 and tissue inhibitor of metalloproteinases (TIMP-1) and upregulating hydroxyproline content. In this study, Kunming SPF mouse skin was abdominally injected with 1 mg kg^{-1} and 5 mg kg^{-1} of laminarin polysaccharide twice on a daily basis and exposed to ultraviolet rays; hydroxyproline content was measured by chemical colorimetry after collecting the exposed skin (Li et al. 2013). Laminarins, isolated from the brown seaweed *S. longicruris*, have also been reported to promote the formation of the dermal matrix in monolayer-cultured human skin fibroblasts (Ayoub et al. 2015), which makes it an equally interesting active compound in cosmeceuticals. Sellimi et al. (2018), in an *in vivo* study, demonstrated the healing ability of laminarins from *Cystoseira barbata* seaweed in healthy Wistar female rats treated with laminaran based-cream at 50 mg ml^{-1} (in a full-thickness circular area of approximately 150 mm^2 wound) for 13 days; results were expressed in percentage of healed wound area (Sellimi et al. 2018).

The antioxidant activities of porphyrans from *Porphyra yezoensis* have been widely studied (Zhang et al. 2009; Isaka et al. 2015); porphyrans from *P. yezoensis* inhibited NO production in LPS-stimulated RAW264.7 cells (Isaka et al. 2015) and porphyrans from *Porphyra haitanensis* also showed antioxidant activities (scavenging effect of superoxide, hydroxyl, and 1,1-diphenyl-2-picrylhydrazyl radicals) (Zhang et al. 2009). They have also been reported to be anti-inflammatory agents as porphyran from *P. yezoensis* showed anti-inflammation activity in LPS-stimulated macrophages (suppressed LPS-induced NO production and iNOS level by blocking NF-κB activation in RAW264.7 cells) (Jiang et al. 2012), with potential use in cosmeceuticals for dermatitis. An ß-1,3-glucan, a natural soluble fiber from microalgae such as *Chlorella* sp. that acts as immune-stimulator and antioxidant, has to be mentioned for antiaging cosmeceuticals formulations (Koller et al. 2014; Spolaore et al. 2006).

19.4.2 Phenols and Polyphenols

Algal phenolic compounds can have numerous uses such as antioxidant, anti-free radical, anti-inflammatory, antibacterial, antiviral, and for protection against UV radiation as discussed above (Table 19.1; Thomas and Kim 2013). The most widely used in antiageing cosmetics are phlorotannins, whose antioxidant activity has been amply demonstrated as discussed above (Table 19.1; Liu et al. 2017). Several studies have also shown their anti-photoageing ability via preventing the expression of MMPs (Pallela et al. 2010). In this review, the authors mention the photoprotective effect of phlorotannins from *E. cava* against the photo-oxidative stress induced by UVB radiation via dichlorodihydrofluorescein diacetate (DCFH-DA), MTT, comet assay, and microscopic analysis (Heo and Jeon 2009), and methanol extracts of alga *Corallina pilulifera* possess high phenolic content, which reduces the expression of UV-induced MMP-2 and -9 in human dermal fibroblast (HDF) cells in a dose-dependent manner, thereby attaining the capability of inhibiting free radicals (Ryu et al. 2009). They also have the ability to decrease hyaluronidase activity *in vitro* with an IC_{50} value of 40 μM (hyaluronidase, an enzyme that depolymerizes the polysaccharide hyaluronic acid in the extracellular matrix of connective tissue, is known to be involved in allergic effects) (Kim et al. 2008). Their action as a potential inhibitor of tyrosinase and thereby as a potential skin whitening/lightening agent has also been studied by Kang et al. (2004), who found five phloroglucinol derivatives from *E. stolonifera* (phloroglucinol, eckstolonol, eckol, phlorofucofuroeckol, and dieckol) that inhibited the oxidation of L-tyrosinase catalized by mushroom tyrosinase with IC_{50} values of 92.8, 126, 33.3, 177, and 2.16 μg ml^{-1} (Kang et al. 2004).

Algal bromophenols have been found to have different biological activities, including antioxidant, and evidence indicates that this activity is directly related to the number of hydroxyl groups in the molecule as discussed above (Tables 19.1 and 19.2; Liu et al. 2011a). This makes them part of the potential group of compounds that are of interest in cosmetics.

19.4.3 Terpenes

Algal terpenes are a very heterogeneous group of secondary metabolites and there are few studies on their use in cosmetics or cosmeceuticals (Azam et al. 2017, 2018). It has recently been determined that sargaquinoic acid obtained from *S. serratifolium* reduced the synthesis of melanin by inhibiting the expression of enzymes involved in melanogenesis, including tyrosinase-related protein 1 and 2, and, furthermore inhibits tyrosinase activity in a dose-dependent manner in α-MSH-stimulated B16F10 cells to reduce hyperpigmentation (Azam et al. 2017).

19.4.4 Pigments

Pigments are abundant in algae and microalgae and many of them have antioxidant properties, as discussed in Section 19.2.5 and Tables 19.1 and 19.2. Chlorophyll a and b are used as colorants in cosmetics, and also in deodorants due to their bactericidal and odor-masking properties (Table 19.2; Hosikian et al. 2010). Carotenoids are the commercially most exploited pigments and are obtained mainly from microalgae such as *Haematococcus pluvialis* (Shah et al. 2016). They are known for their antioxidant potential as discussed above (Borowitzka 2013) and are also used as colorants in the cosmetic industry (Arad and Yaron 1992); the most used are β-carotenes, astaxanthin, phycocyanobilins, and phycoerythrobilins for orange, pink, blue, and red colors (Arad and Yaron 1992). Astaxanthin can protect the skin against UV-induced photo-oxidation (Koller et al. 2014) and can hence be used in cosmetic sunscreens. In another report, astaxanthin acted by inhibiting melanin synthesis and therefore prevented hyperpigmentation under UV irradiation, both in topical application when combining 6 mg per day oral supplementation and 2 ml (78.9 μM solution) per day topical application of astaxanthin (from *H. pluvialis*) (Tominaga et al. 2012). Similarly, fucoxanthin, one of the carotenoids with several biological activities as discussed above (Table 19.1), has been reported to protect against UVB-induced photoageing. Matsui et al. (2016) studied the protective effect of fucoxathin in UVB-induced skin photoaging in hairless mice; the skin was analyzed by immunohistochemistry and immunoblot assay and they found that fucoxanthin protected from filaggrin downregulation (filaggrin is a protein with an important role in the terminal differentiation of skin and formation of the cornified envelope that protects the skin) (Matsui et al. 2016). This protection against photoageing has also been observed by other authors (Urikura et al. 2011; Liu et al. 2016; Chen et al. 2016) and it seems that the main mechanism involved is the ROS scavenging activity. Matsui et al. (2016) also have shown that fucoxanthin promotes repair of the protein filaggrin likely by enhancement of metabolism in the dermis, involved in the epidermal barrier (Table 19.2;

Matsui et al. 2016). ß-cryptoxanthin, a carotenoid extracted from *Dunaliella salina*, among other microalga (Tang and Suter 2011), induced the synthesis of hyaluronic acid ($(C_{14}H_{21}NO_{11})_n$) in human foreskin keratinocytes and bovine pituitary extracts (quantification made by spectrophotometric techniques) (Sayo et al. 2013), a glycosaminoglycan involved in skin hydration. And ß-carotene, abundant in microalgae, especially in *D. salina*, is known to quench ROS as discussed above (Tables 19.1 and 19.2; Gammone et al. 2015), hence they are potential candidates for the formulation of preventive antiaging cosmeceuticals.

19.4.5 PUFAs and Other Lipid Compounds

Lipids present in macro- and microalgae include triacylglycerols, glyco- and phospholipids, and sterols (Stengel et al. 2011). The most well-known are the PUFAs due to their skin care properties (Kim et al. 2006). Even though algal PUFAs are known for their anti-inflammatory properties as discussed above (Hamed et al. 2015; Robertson et al. 2013, 2015) and in Table 19.2, there are few studies on their topical activities. They are considered as good emollients and repairers of intercorneocitary lipids, and thus protect against water loss from the epidermis after topical application and forming a lipid occlusive film (Bedoux et al. 2014). Other studies showed that stearic acid, arachidonic acid, and EPA are soothing and regenerative to the skin, and have anti-inflammatory and antiallergy functions, besides improving the immune barrier of the skin and slowing aging (Łęska et al. 2018).

With respect to sterols, a study in UVB-irradiated normal human dermal fibroblasts (HDFs) by using ELISA, Western blot analysis, and reverse transcription-polymerase chain reaction showed that fucosterol has free radical DPPH scavenging activity and inhibited the secretion of IL-6 and the production of MMP-1, and therefore may protect against photoageing as in habitually UV-irradiated skin, MMPs are stimulated, and type I procollagen synthesis is suppressed (Hwang et al. 2014) owing to effects on collagen synthesis and inflammation (Table 19.2).

19.4.6 Proteins and Amino Acids

Algae may contain endogenous amino acids such as alanine, serine, proline, and exogenous amino acids, such as histidine, tyrosine, and tryptophan (Pereira 2018a). Amino acids are used in moisturizing cosmetics because many of them are constituents of the natural moisturizing factor (NMF) in the outer layers of the epidermis that helps to maintain skin moisturizing (Fabrowska et al. 2015). Taurine (2-aminoethanesulfonic acid) isolated from *Sargassum* sp. and *Gracilliaria* sp., may play a role in controlling biochemical changes due to aging and cell damage caused by free radicals as well as protecting against oxidative stress in *in vivo* studies in male mice by measuring the number of blood cells (red blood cells and leucocytes) and blood protein profile of mice induced by benzo(α)pyrene (the amount given of *Sargassum* sp. and *Gracillaria* sp. extraction each was 8 mg body weight^{-1} and the amount given of taurine was 15.6 mg body weight^{-1}) (Widiastuti and Khairani 2018).

Researchers have also focused their attention on extracting MAAs from cyanobacteria such as *Nostoc commune*, *Glenodinium foliaceum*, *Oxyrrhis marina*, *N. oculata*, and *Rhodomonas baltica* (Llewellyn and Airs 2010; Guillerme et al. 2017), and red macroalgae such as *P. palmata*, *C. crispus*, *Mastocarpus stellatus*, and *Devaleraea ramentacea* (Athukorala et al. 2016; Bedoux et al. 2014), for their potential use in sunscreens and photoaging prevention (Chrapusta et al. 2017). Recent research has demonstrated that protective effects of porphyra-334 against UVA (home solarium sun lamp) stimulated apoptosis in human keratinocytes (HaCaT cells) involving the suppression of the caspase pathway by lowering the level of caspase-3 protein expression when cells were incubated with porphyra-334 at 0.1 mg ml^{-1} for 30 minutes prior to UV irradiation (Suh et al. 2017). The abilities of MAAs such as shinorine, porphyra, and palythine isolated from the marine red algae *Porphyra* sp. and *P. palmata* to prevent extrinsic skin aging was also confirmed *in vitro* evaluating for their inhibitory properties against *Clostridium histolyticum* collagenase (IC_{50} values of 104.0 μM for shinorine, 105.9 μM for porphyra, and 158.9 μM for palythine) (Hartmann et al. 2015). Porphyra-334 in *in vivo* studies (in UV-damaged human skin fibroblasts) showed inhibitory properties against MMPs, increasing procollagen secretion levels, and enhancing the expression of type I collagen and elastin (Ryu et al. 2014).

19.4.7 Other Compounds

There are other less studied algal compounds that may be of great interest in skincare: the ectoins, vitamins, and macro- and micronutrients such as copper, iron, and zinc (Guillerme et al. 2017). Ectoin (1,4,5,6-tetrahydro-2-methyl-4-pyrimidinecarboxylic acid) is an osmoprotectant present in halophilic bacteria such as *alpha*-and *gamma-proteobacteria* and *Actinobacteridae* whose water-binding capacity is similar to other wetting agents used in cosmetics such as glycerol (Guillerme et al. 2017), and therefore has potential use in moisturizing cosmeceuticals. Ectoin provides multiple cosmetic benefits such as immune protection, cell protection, UV protection, and membrane protection (Kim et al. 2008; Guillerme et al. 2017), as well as being a stress protective agent (Buommino et al. 2005). Ectoin has been reported to protect against the effects of UVA-induced and accelerated skin aging (Bownik and Stępniewska 2016). Buommino et al. (2005) reported that heat-stressed keratinocytes incubated with ectoin had higher levels of heat shock protein 70 (hsp70) and inhibited the production of proinflammatory signals (Buommino et al. 2005), and is therefore being used as a dermatological cosmetic additive in moisturizers for the care of aged, dry, or irritated skin (e.g. https://www.bitop.de/en/products). Ectoin also decreases skin inflammation in atopic dermatitis and is currently being investigated for the treatment of moderate atopic dermatitis (Marini et al. 2014).

Other photoprotective compounds such as scytonemin (a dimer of indolic and phenolic subunits) have been reported to reduce the risk of skin cell damage caused by UVA or B light (Singh et al. 2017; Mourelle et al. 2017). The reported research by Rastogi et al. (2013) studied cultures of cyanobacterium, *Rivularia* sp., irradiated with artificial UVA and UVB and analyzed the photoprotective role of scytonemin by exposing the cultures continuously for 24 hours with or without partially purified scytonemin; ROS and thymine dimers were analyzed showing the radical scavenging activity. The dose-dependent antioxidant activity of scytonemin was 12, 33, and 57% at concentrations of 0.5, 1.0, and 2.0 mg ml^{-1}, respectively (Rastogi et al. 2013).

Algae are an important source of vitamins including vitamin A (β-carotene as a provitamin A) and other carotenoids such as lutein, and zeaxanthin with vitamin A activity, B complex vitamins (B_1-thiamine, B_2-riboflavin, B_3-niacin, B_5-pantothenic acid, B_6-pyridoxine, B_7-biotin, and B_{12}-cobalamin), vitamin C (ascorbic acid), vitamin D, and vitamin E (α-tocopherol) (Pereira 2018b; Sonani et al. 2018; Agatonovic-Kustrin and Morton 2013). These may be of interest in the formulation of cosmeceuticals, especially the vitamins with antioxidant activities (A, E, and C), used either as active agents or as preservatives in cosmetics (e.g. tocopherol; https://ec.europa.eu/growth/tools-databases/cosing/index.cfm?fuseaction=search.details_v2&id=80273) by companies such as GreenTech (http://www.greentech.fr/en) or Pentapharm (https://www.pentapharm.com). Pantothenic acid (B_5) is essential for the healing of wounds and maintaining an intact skin barrier. Kobayashi et al. (2011) investigated the effect of pantothenic acid deficiency on the proliferation of HaCaT keratinocytes using the MTT assay and cell counting. These assays revealed that the proliferation of HaCaT keratinocytes cultured in pantothenic acid-deficient medium was suppressed compared with HaCaT keratinocytes cultured in the control medium (Kobayashi et al. 2011).

Depending on their natural habitat and thereby growth conditions, algae may contain differing amounts of microelements including zinc (Zn), magnesium (Mg), copper (Cu), iodine (I), iron (Fe), and manganese (Mn), and macroelements, such as calcium (Ca), sodium (Na), potassium (K), and chlorine (Cl), essential for healthy skin and general good health (Pereira 2018b). Many of these minerals (Cu, Zn, etc.) are cofactors for endogenous antioxidant enzymes including Mn or Cu/Zn SOD, glutathione peroxidase. Other minerals are involved in the regulation of the proliferation of keratinocytes (i.e. Ca) by increasing caspase-14 expression (Huang et al. 2006) and also regulate water and ion balance in cells and tissues (i.e. Na, Cl) (Mourelle and Gómez 2015).

19.4.8 Algal Extracts

Algal extracts from different species (macro- and microalgae) such as *P. cruentum*, *U. lactuca*, *Laminaria saccharina*, *C. crispus*, etc, are currently widely used in cosmetics such as moisturizers, sun protection, or antiaging products; some examples are GreenSea (http://greensea.fr) and Pentapharm (https://www.pentapharm.com). Macro- and microalgal hydroalcoholic aqueous extracts have been reported to contain various water-soluble substances such as proteins, amino acids, polysaccharides, water-soluble vitamins, macro- and microelements, MAAs, etc. (Athukorala et al. 2016), while organic extracts contain phospholipids, glycolipids, fatty acids, and fat-soluble vitamins (Pereira 2018b). These crude algal extracts have been used in moisturizing, nutritional, regenerating, and protective cosmeceuticals (Kim et al. 2008) (https://www.seppic.com/bioplasma-fa).

There is abundant scientific literature on the use of extracts from algae and microalgae in cosmetics, but not all of their bioactive compounds have been identified (Kim et al. 2008). In a review article about cosmeceuticals, Kim et al. (2008) discussed aqueous alcoholic extracts from *C. crispus* (rich in polysaccharides and minerals), *Codium tomentosum* (source of glucuronic acid), *U. pinnatifida*, *Durvillaea antarctica*, *A. nodosum*, and *Polysiphonia lanosa*, among others for their potential to act as moisturizer, skin conditioning, or antiageing agents. The article went on to summarize that these extracts were rich in polysaccharides, vitamins, and minerals, and exhibited moisturizing and protective actions on the skin. For example,

Undaria-derived fucoidan inhibited the enzyme hyaluronidase, and a fucoidan extract from *F. vesiculosus* increased skin elasticity; this activity is in part modulated by growth factor potentiation (Fitton et al. 2007). Extracts from *L. saccharina* exhibited anti-inflammatory activities associated with the biological activities of phlorogine and regulated secretion of sebaceous glands, inhibiting PAR2 activation of keratinocytes (US Patent number: 20110097286) in clinical trials; those from *A. nodosum* and *Asparagopsis armata* exhibited anti-itching activities by reducing the level of vascular endothelial growth factor (VEGF) in clinical studies (healthy women and men with some degree of skin redness with telangiectasia (spider veins), and the evaluation was made through colorimetric and visual analysis) (Dupont et al. 2012), which influenced expression of intermediates *in vitro* with epithelial cells; while extracts from *Enteromorpha compressa* improved circulation and acted as antiallergenics by alleviating IgE levels in murine models (Raman et al. 2004) and because of that it is used for sensitive skin (Dermasooth™). Extracts from microalgae (e.g. *Chlorella* sp.) and cyanobacteria (e.g. *Arthrospira* sp.) have also been reported to have cosmeceutical applications; for example, extracts from *Arthrospira* sp. and *Chlorella* sp. are used in skin protection and in antiaging products owing to their antioxidant and free radical scavenging properties (Kim et al. 2008; Ismaiel et al. 2014). Some examples are Dermochlorella (www.codif-tn.com) or Bioplasma FA™ (https://www.seppic.com/bioplasma-fa).

Other algae have been studied for their sun protection and antiaging properties; for example, the methanolic extracts from *C. pilulifera* have been reported to protect human fibroblasts *in vitro* from UVA damage and cell DNA against MMP-2 and -9, reducing the expression of UV-induced MMP-2 and -9 in HDF cells in a dose-dependent manner, there by attaining the capability of inhibiting free radicals (Ryu et al. 2009). On the other hand, aqueous extracts from *E. cava* and *Sargassum siliquastrum* have been reported to exhibit inhibition of tyrosinase, similar to that of kojic acid, in an *in vivo* assay with adult zebrafish of skin whitening with clinical testing (Cha et al. 2011).

There are companies in the cosmetic and cosmeceutical markets that commercialize algal extracts, either as raw materials for manufacturers, or include them in their own formulations: some examples are Seppic (lipophilic extracts obtained from *Alaria esculenta* to reduce hyperpigmentation) (https://www.seppic.com), Codif (www.codif-tn.com) (extract obtained from *Dictyopteris membranacea*, also reduces hyperpigmentation), and Biosil Technologies, Inc. (www.biosiltech.com) (extracts obtained from *A. nodosum* and *Halopteris scoparia*, which are rich in phytohormones).

19.5 Potential Cosmeceutical Formulations from Algae

Cosmeceutical formulations can be divided into four large groups: moisturizers, anti-aging and anti-photoageing, antipigmentary, and formulations for certain types of dermatosis, such as dermatitis, skin allergies, or psoriasis.

The use of algal extracts (and micronized particles or preparations) in cosmetics and cosmeceuticals depends on the type and concentration of the active substances they contain. Thus, the presence of amino acids, proteins, and fatty acids indicates their potential use as moisturizing and water loss prevention agents (e.g. Algil® from Biosil

Technologies). The presence of antioxidants such as carotenoids, tocopherol, ascorbic acid, and polyphenols indicates a potential antiaging effect that promotes the synthesis of collagen and elastin, thereby enhancing skin elasticity, firmness, and regeneration, while delaying aging and protecting against free radicals (e.g. products by GreenTech (www.greentech.fr/en) or Pentapharm (https://www.pentapharm.com)). The presence of terpenes and zinc regulates the activity of sebaceous glands, detoxifies the skin, reduces inflammation, and exerts a bacteriostatic effect (Schroeder et al. 2016) that may be of interest in cosmeceuticals for the treatment of acne.

19.5.1 Moisturizing Cosmeceutical Formulations

Skin hydration is linked to the water content of the dermis, but at the epidermis level it depends on the natural moisturizing factor (NMF), ceramides and aquaporins (Draelos 2014). The amino acids that are included in cosmetic formulations are biomimetic agents that mimic the action of NMF (acting as hydro-captors), while the PUFAs facilitate the reconstruction of the epidermal barrier and thus prevent excessive TEWL. Given that many species of algae are rich in both components, their inclusion in this type of cosmetics is justified, and either use individual bioactive compounds or extracts obtained from algae rich in them. Moreover, DNA extracted from seaweed such as *U. pinnatifida*, *D. antarctica*, and *A. nodosum* is used in cosmetics for skin hydration (Couteau and Coiffard 2016) and, as mentioned earlier, algal polysaccharides are of great interest because of their moisturizing and skin protection properties. And lastly, worth mentioning is the use of ectoin to regulate hydration and to protect the skin from external aggressions (Guillerme et al. 2017).

There are companies that presently commercialize different active agents derived from algae and cyanobacteria for use in cosmeceuticals. An example is ectoin obtained from *Halomonas elongata*, marketed by Bitop (Germany), which claims that ectoin (ectoin®) protects the epithelium against allergens, UV light, air pollution, and temperature changes.

19.5.2 Antiaging and Photoageing Cosmeceutical Formulations

The skin aging process takes place in parallel to the rest of the body, although there are differences between chronological aging and that from sun exposure or photoageing. Premature aging appears whenever skin is exposed to excessive solar radiation or tanning booth lamps. There are some clear differences such as greater thickness, dryness and roughness in the epidermis, presence of hyper pigmentation, elastosis, actinic keratoses and vascular disorders such as telangiectasia, and purpura, among others (Durai et al. 2012). As indicated in the previous sections, algae contain bioactive compounds that are of great interest in the prevention of aging (especially photoageing), these being phlorotannins (eckol and dieckol) that inhibit matrix metalloproteinases; astaxanthin and fucoxanthin, with potent antioxidant action; as well as the ulvan polysaccharides, laminarin and fucoidan, with preventive antiaging actions related to the inhibition of MMPs and protection against UVA/UVB light, or porphyran with antioxidant and anti-inflammatory action. Antiaging cosmeceuticals can also include PUFAs since they possess anti-inflammatory and antiallergy properties, and it is worth highlighting fucosterol, due to its radical scavenging capacity. Mention should also be made of MAAs, characterized by their protective action against UVA radiation, where the most well-known ones are obtained from *Porphyra umbilicalis*. MAAs are of great interest in the development of sun and antiaging creams. As an example, one can cite the product Helioguard 365®, marketed by Mibelle Biochemistry (Switzerland), which contains porphyra-334, an MAA obtained from *P. umbilicalis*, and claims to be "a natural UVA protection factor for everyday use." Another example is the extract obtained from *C. vulgaris* (marketed under the trade name Dermochlorella D), which is said to "reactivate collagen synthesis and also protect it."

19.5.3 Skin Whitening Cosmeceutical Formulations

Hyperpigmentation of melanic origin is a common concern in women from the Eastern and Western worlds, although it is more frequent in phototypes III and IV. The development of depigmenting cosmeceuticals has passed through several phases, beginning with the synthesis of depigmenting agents such as hydroquinone, recently replaced by substances of natural origin like kojic acid, produced by a type of fungus, and arbutin, extracted from *Arctostaphylos* sp.; both act as tyrosinase inhibitors. Recent research has been focused on obtaining depigmenting compounds from algae and microalgae. Therefore, nowadays included in cosmetics are extracts from *E. cava*, whose depigmenting activity is attributed to phorotannins: phloroglucinol, dioxinodehydroeckol, and 7-phloroeckol, where the antityrosinase activity of the latter is greater than that of arbutin and kojic acid (Yoon et al. 2009). The dioxinodehydroeckol extracted from *E. stolonifera* is also postulated as a promising active inhibitor of melanogenesis (Lee et al. 2012). Azam et al. (2017) recently identified different depigmenting compounds from algae that operate through two main mechanisms: inhibition of tyrosinase and downregulation of melanocyte inducing transcription factor (MITF); among which are phlorotaninns, fucoidan, fucoxanthin, and meroterpenoids.

There are few studies on the use of microalgal compounds as depigmenting agents and worth mentioning is zeaxanthin obtained from *N. oculata* known for its antityrosinase activity (Shen et al. 2011). Examples of depigmenting agents marketed are: 3M3.WHITERIS G®, a concentrate obtained from *D. membranacea* (Codif, France; www.codif-tn.com), where the company claims that it "reduces melanin synthesis and transfers to the surface of the skin," and WHITONYL® (Silab, France; www.silab.fr), obtained from *P. palmata*, which claims that it "inhibits melano-genesis by acting at the heart of the melanocyte while limiting the impact of its environment (epigenetics, intercellular communication via exosomes)."

19.5.4 Other Potential Cosmeceutical Formulations

There are other interesting cosmeceutical formulations for skin affected by certain types of dermatosis such as allergies or dermatitis, psoriasis, and even acne, which can be improved through the application of moisturizing cosmetics, emollients, soothing, and anti-inflammatory drugs. As explained earlier, SPs can act as moisturizers and anti-inflammatory agents, and, in particular, fucoidan inhibits IgE production by preventing the NFκB p52-mediated pathways activated by CD40 (Kim and Thomas 2011; Iwamoto et al. 2011; Kim et al. 2018). Other studies show that the SPs obtained from

Porphyra tenera display anti-inflammatory action (Senevirathne et al. 2010), just like the SPs of *Sargassum cristaefolium* (Wu et al. 2016) and hence could be possible active ingredients in formulations aimed at care of atopic dermatitis.

Extracts of 342 species of marine algae were collected from Japanese coastlines for antibacterial activity against *Propionibacterium acnes*, and exhibited a novel antibacterial compound, named Sargafuran, from the MeOH extract of the marine brown alga, *Sargassum macrocarpum*. Sargafuran has low cytotoxicity, showing a broad antibacterial activity against Gram-positive bacteria. These results suggest that Sargafuran might be useful as a lead compound to develop new types of anti-*P. acnes* substances and new skin care cosmetics to prevent or improve acne (Kamei et al. 2009).

Phlorotannins from different algae (*E. arborea*, *E. bicyclis*, *E. kurome*, and *Ecklonia cava*) have also been researched for their anti-inflammatory and antihyaluronidase activity as potential agents in the treatment of atopic dermatitis (Kim and Thomas 2011). Hence, it would be of interest to study them in-depth for use in cosmeceuticals.

On the other hand, studies with an extract obtained from *I. okamurae* have shown antiallergenic properties, which the authors attribute to its content of EPA, eicosatrienoic acid, linolenic acid, and GLA (Vo et al. 2011), agents that can be included in cosmeceutical formulations since they also have emollient and restorative effects on the epidermal barrier.

19.6 Conclusion and Future Trends

The previous discussion outlined numerous review articles and studies that showed the potential of algal compounds, especially of the secondary metabolites, as possible bioactive molecules in pharmacology. However, even though there are a large number of *in vitro* and *in vivo* studies, there is a paucity of well-designed, randomized, clinical trials, to ascertain whether these molecules are promising candidates for the development of pharmaceuticals and nutraceuticals. Toxicity studies are also needed to determine the safety of these compounds.

The reality is that most of these compounds fail in the clinical study phases and some such cases can be reformulated. One example is a new peptide produced by the cyanobacteria *Symploca hydnoides* and *Lyngbya majuscule,* called dolostatin 10, which exhibits high antineoplastic activity, with ED_{50} values in the picomole range. It failed as it progressed into Phase III clinical studies due to its low *in vivo* activity. Researchers rectified its action by conjugating an analogue of dolostatin 10 to a monoclonal antibody that targets CD30, an antigen present on the surface of Hodgkin's lymphoma cells. The antibody–drug conjugate called brentuximab vendotin was approved by the US Food and Drug Administration in 2011, and a year later, by the European Medicines Agency under the trade name Adcetris for the treatment of Hodgkin's and systemic anaplastic large cell lymphoma (Soldatou 2017). Another similar case is that of the molecule kahalalide F obtained from the green alga *Bryopsis pennata*, which showed potent cytotoxic activity. However, it failed in phase II clinical studies due its limited spectrum of activity and poor response in patients. But its high potential as a cytotoxic agent inspired the development of synthetic analogues that have addressed the above limitations and increased potency and half-life (Alves et al. 2018).

This shows that the path toward the development of pharmaceutical formulations is long and arduous; hence research in this field should be promoted through investment in R&D and the use of new technologies and procedures. Studies should also be carried out using metabolomics, genomics, and proteomics for the identification and isolation of new molecules. Improvements in the cultivation of algae and microalgae can facilitate access to these compounds and maintain constancy in their composition, and thus avoid the impact of climatic changes or seasonal variations.

With regard to the development of cosmeceutical formulations from algal compounds, the cosmetics industry has currently been deeply involved in the cultivation of algae, obtaining of extracts and isolation of biologically active compounds of interest. The advantage here is that, despite legislation and regulation being quite demanding, there are actually fewer impediments to launching a product on the market. Algal compounds presently have many specific applications in sun protection and prevention of aging, but more research into others for treating dermatological disorders (dermatitis, rosacea, psoriasis, etc.) is needed. Another interesting subject is the development of biovectors (liposomes, microspheres, etc.) as carriers, to ensure that a particular active ingredient is delivered to its site of action and/or produces sustained release, and this is where algal compounds have a promising future. Therefore, in order to achieve these objectives, research in this area also needs to be intensified.

References

Abdolmaleki, F., Kovanen, P.T., Mardani, R. et al. (2019). Resolvins: emerging players in autoimmune and inflammatory diseases. *Clinical Reviews in Allergy and Immunology* **2**: 1–10.

Adrien, A., Bonnet, A., Dufour, D. et al. (2017). Pilot production of ulvans from *Ulva* sp. and their effects on hyaluronan and collagen production in cultured dermal fibroblasts. *Carbohydrate Polymers* **157**: 1306–1314.

Adrien, A., Bonnet, A., Dufour, D. et al. (2019). Anticoagulant activity of sulfated ulvan isolated from the green macroalga *Ulva rigida*. *Marine Drugs* **17**: 291. https://doi.org/10.3390/md17050291.

Agatonovic-Kustrin, S. and Morton, D.W. (2013). Cosmeceuticals derived from bioactive substances found in marine algae. *Oceanography* **1**: 106. https://doi.org/10.4172/2332-2632.1000106.

Agregán, R., Lorenzo, J.M., Munekata, P.E.S. et al. (2017). Assessment of the antioxidant activity of *Bifurcaria bifurcata* aqueous extract on canola oil. Effect of extract concentration on the oxidation stability and volatile compound generation during oil storage. *Food Research International* **99** (3): 1095–1102.

Ahmadi, A., Zorofchian Moghadamtousi, S., Abubakar, S., and Zandi, K. (2015). Antiviral potential of algae polysaccharides isolated from marine sources: a review. *BioMed Research International* **2015**: 825203. http://dx.doi.org/10.1155/2015/825203.

Ahn, M.J., Yoon, K.D., Min, S.Y. et al. (2004). Inhibition of HIV-1 reverse transcriptase and protease by phlorotannins from the brown alga *Ecklonia cava*. *Biological and Pharmaceutical Bulletin* **27** (4): 544–547. https://doi.org/10.1248/bpb.27.544.

Akbar, M., Calderon, F., Wen, Z., and Kim, H.-Y. (2005). Docosahexaenoic acid: a positive modulator of Akt signaling in neuronal survival. *Proceedings of the National Academy of Sciences USA* **102**: 10858–10863.

Akkouh, O., Ng, T.B., Singh, S.S. et al. (2015). Lectins with anti-HIV activity: a review. *Molecules* **20**: 648–668.

Al-Fadhli, A., Wahidulla, S., and D'Souza, L. (2006). Glycolipids from the red alga *Chondria armata* (Kütz.) Okamura. *Glycobiology* **16** (10): 902–915.

Ali, I., Manzoora, Z., Kooa, J.E. et al. (2017). 3-Hydroxy-4,7-megastigmadien-9-one, isolated from *Ulva pertusa*, attenuates TLR9-mediated inflammatory response by down-regulating mitogen-activated protein kinase and NF-jB pathways. *Pharmaceutical Biology* **55** (1): 435–440.

Al-Saif, S.S.A., Abdel-Raouf, N., El-Wazanani, H.A., and Aref, I.A. (2014). Antibacterial substances from marine algae isolated from Jeddah coast of Red Sea, Saudi Arabia. *Saudi Journal of Biological Sciences* **21** (1): 57–64.

Alves, A., Sousa, R.A., and Reis, R.L. (2013). In vitro cytotoxicity assessment of ulvan, a polysaccharide extracted from green algae. *Phytotherapy Research* **27** (8): 1143–1148.

Alves, C., Silva, J., Pinteus, S. et al. (2018). From marine origin to therapeutics: the anti-tumor potential of marine algae-derived compounds. *Frontiers in Pharmacology* **9**: 777. https://doi.org/10.3389/fphar.2018.00777.

Amri, E., Armaini, D.A., and Tjong, D.H. (2017). Screening anti-acne potency of microalgae: antibacterial and antioxidant activities. *Der Pharma Chemica* **9** (4): 28–31.

Arad, S. and Yaron, A. (1992). Natural pigments from red microalgae for use in foods and cosmetics. *Trends in Food Science & Technology* **3**: 92–97.

Artan, M., Li, Y., Karadeniz, F. et al. (2008). Anti-HIV-1 activity of phloroglucinol derivative, 6,6′-bieckol, from *Ecklonia cava*. *Bioorganic and Medicinal Chemistry* **16**: 7921–7926.

Athukorala, Y., Trang, S., Kwok, C., and Yuan, Y.V. (2016). Antiproliferative and antioxidant activities and mycosporine-like amino acid profiles of wild-harvested and cultivated edible Canadian marine red macroalgae. *Molecules* **21** (1): 119. https://doi.org/10.3390/molecules21010119.

Ayoub, A., Pereira, J.M., Rioux, L.E. et al. (2015). Role of seaweed laminaran from *Saccharina longicruris* on matrix deposition during dermal tissue-engineered production. *International Journal of Biological Macromolecules* **75**: 13–20.

Ayyad, S.E.N. and Badria, F.A. (1994). Caulerpin: an antitumor indole alkaloid from *Caulerpa racemosa*. *Alexandria Journal of Pharmaceutical Sciences* **8**: 217–219.

Azam, M.S., Choi, J., Lee, M.S., and Kim, H.R. (2017). Hypopigmenting effects of brown algae-derived phytochemicals: a review on molecular mechanisms. *Marine Drugs* **15** (10): 297. https://doi.org/10.3390/md15100297.

Azam, M.S., Kwon, M., Choi, J., and Kim, H.R. (2018). Sargaquinoic acid ameliorates hyperpigmentation through cAMP and ERK-mediated downregulation of MITF in α-MSH-stimulated B16F10 cells. *Biomedicine & Pharmacotherapy* **104**: 582–589.

Bae, M.J., Karadeniz, F., Ahn, B.-N., and Kong, C.-S. (2015). Evaluation of effective MMP inhibitors from eight different brown algae in human fibrosarcoma HT1080 cells. *Preventive Nutrition and Food Science* **20** (3): 153–161.

Bajpai, V.K., Shukla, S., Kang, S.-M. et al. (2018). Developments of cyanobacteria for nano-marine drugs: relevance of nanoformulations in cancer therapies. *Marine Drugs* **16** (6): 179. https://doi.org/10.3390/md16060179.

Barba, F., Grimi, N., and Vorobiev, E. (2015). New approaches for the use of non-conventional cell disruption technologies to extract potential food additives and nutraceuticals from microalgae. *Food Engineering Reviews* **7**: 45–62.

Barbosa, M., Valentão, P., and Andrade, P.B. (2014). Bioactive compounds from macroalgae in the new millennium: implications for neurodegenerative diseases. *Marine Drugs* **12**: 4934–4972.

Barbosa, A.I., Costa Lima, S.A., and Reis, S. (2019). Development of methotrexate loaded fucoidan/chitosan nanoparticles with anti-inflammatory potential and enhanced skin permeation. *International Journal of Biological Macromolecules* **124**: 1115–1122.

Bedoux, A., Hardouin, K., Burlot, A.S., and Bourgougnon, N. (2014). Bioactive components from seaweeds: cosmetic applications and future development. *Advances in Botanical Research* **71**: 345–378.

Beetul, K., Gopeechund, A., Kaullysing, D. et al. (2016). Challenges and opportunities in the present era of marine algal applications. In: *Algae – Organisms for Imminent Biotechnology* (eds. N. Thajuddin and Dhanasekaran). InTech (Open Access) https://doi.org/10.5772/63272.

Begun, S., Nyandoro, S., Buriyo, A. et al. (2018). Bioactivities of extracts, debromolaurinterol and fucosterol from macroalgae species. *Tanzania Journal of Science* **44** (2): 104–116.

Beppu, F., Niwano, Y., Tsukui, T. et al. (2009). Single and repeated oral dose toxicity study of fucoxanthin (FX), a marine carotenoid, in mice. *The Journal of Toxicological Science* **34**: 501–510.

Blunt, J.W., Copp, B.R., Keyzers, R.A. et al. (2017). Marine natural products. *Natural Product Reports* **34**: 235–294.

Boisson-Vidal, C., Haroun, F., Ellouali, M. et al. (1995). Biological activities of polysaccharides from marine algae. *Drugs of the Future* **20** (12): 1237–1249.

Borowitzka, M.A. (2013). High-value products from microalgae-their development and commercialisation. *Journal of Applied Phycology* **25**: 743–756.

Bossù, P., Salani, F., Ciaramella, A. et al. (2018). Anti-inflammatory effects of homotaurine in patients with amnestic mild cognitive impairment. *Frontiers in Aging Neuroscience* **10**: 285. https://doi.org/10.3389/fnagi.2018.00285. . eCollection 2018.

Bownik, A. and Stępniewska, Z. (2016). Ectoine as a promising protective agent in humans and animals. *Archives of Industrial Hygiene and Toxicology* **67** (4): 260–265. https://doi.org/10.1515/aiht-2016-67-2837.

Brown, E.S., Allsopp, P.J., Magee, P.J. et al. (2014). Seaweed and human health. *Nutrition Reviews* **72**: 205–216.

Bule, M.H., Ahmed, I., Maqbool, F. et al. (2018). Microalgae as a source of high-value bioactive compounds. *Frontiers in Bioscience* **10**: 197–216.

Buommino, E., Schiraldi, C., Baroni, A. et al. (2005). Ectoine from halophilic microorganisms induces the expression of hsp70 and hsp70B′ in human keratinocytes modulating the proinflammatory response. *Cell Stress & Chaperones* **10**: 197–203. https://doi.org/10.1379/CSC-101R.1.

Byun, J.-H., Kim, J., and Choung, S.-Y. (2018). Hepaprotective effect of standardized *Ecklonia stolonifera* formulation on CCl4-induced liver injury in Sprague-Dawley rats. *Biomolecules & Therapeutics* **26** (2): 218–223.

Calado, R., Costa Leal, M., Gaspar, H. et al. (2018). How to succeed in marketing marine natural products for pharmaceutical, cosmetics & nutraceutical markets. In: *Grand Challenges in Marine Biotechnology* (eds. P.H. Rampelotto and A. Trincone), 317–403. Basel: Springer.

Cao, J., Wang, S., Yao, C. et al. (2016). Hypolipidemic effect of porphyran extracted from *Pyropia yezoensis* in ICR mice with high fatty diet. *Journal of Applied Phycology* **28**: 1315–1322.

Cardozo, K., Guaratini, T., Barros, M. et al. (2007). Metabolites from algae with economical impact. *Comparative Biochemical Physiology. Part C: Toxicology & Pharmacology* **146** (1–2): 60–78.

Carta, A.R. (2013). PPAR-c: therapeutic prospects in Parkinson's disease. *Current Drug Targets* **14** (7): 743–751.

Castro-Puyana, M., Pérez-Sánchez, A., Valdés, A. et al. (2017). Pressurized liquid extraction of *Neochloris oleoabundans* for the recovery of bioactive carotenoids with anti-proliferative activity against human colon cancer cells. *Food Research International* **99**: 1048–1055.

Cavalcante-Silva, L.H.A., de Carvalho Correia, A.C., Barbosa-Filho, J.M. et al. (2013). Spasmolytic effect of caulerpine involves blockade of Ca^{2+} influx on guinea pig ileum. *Marine Drugs* **11** (5): 1553–1564.

Cavalcante-Silva, L.H.A., Falcão, M.A.P., Vieira, A.C.S. et al. (2014). Assessment of mechanisms involved in antinociception produced by the alkaloid caulerpine. *Molecules* **19**: 14699–14709.

Cha, S.-H., Lee, K.-W., and Jeon, Y.-J. (2006). Screening of extracts from red algae in Jeju for potentials marine angiotensin-I converting enzyme (ACE) inhibitory activity. *Algae* **21**: 343–348.

Cha, K.H., Koo, S.Y., and Lee, D.U. (2008). Antiproliferative effects of carotenoids extracted from *Chlorella ellipsoidea* and *Chlorella vulgaris* on human colon cancer cells. *Journal of Agricultural and Food Chemistry* **56**: 10521–10526.

Cha, S.-H., Ko, S.-C., Kim, D., and Jeon, Y.-J. (2011). Screening of marine algae for potential tyrosinase inhibitor: those inhibitors reduced tyrosinase activity and melanin synthesis in zebrafish. *Journal of Dermatology* **38**: 354–363.

Chandini, S.K., Ganesan, P., and Bhaskar, N. (2008). In vitro antioxidant activities of three selected brown seaweeds of India. *Food Chemistry* **107** (2): 707–713.

Chen, D., Wu, X.Z., and Wen, Z.Y. (2008). Sulfated polysaccharides and immune response: promoter or inhibitor? *Panminerva Medica* **50**: 177–183.

Chen, S.-J., Lee, C.-J., Lin, T.-B. et al. (2016). Inhibition of ultraviolet B-induced expression of the proinflammatory cytokines TNF-α and VEGF in the cornea by fucoxanthin treatment in a rat model. *Marine Drugs* **14** (1): 13. https://doi.org/10.3390/md14010013.

Chen, J., Hu, Y., Zhang, L. et al. (2017). Alginate oligosaccharide DP5 exhibits antitumor effects in osteosarcoma patients following surgery. *Frontiers in Pharmacology* **8**: 623.

Chrapusta, E., Kaminski, A., Duchnik, K. et al. (2017). Mycosporine-like amino acids: potential health and beauty ingredients. *Marine Drugs* **15** (10): 326. https://doi.org/10.3390/md15100326.

Collins, K.G., Fitzgerald, G.F., Stanton, C., and Ross, R.P. (2016). Looking beyond the terrestrial: the potential of seaweed derived bioactives to treat non-communicable diseases. *Marine Drugs* **14** (3): 60.

Costa, L.S., Fidelis, G.P., Cordeiro, S.L. et al. (2010). Biological activities of sulfated polysaccharides from tropical seaweeds. *Biomedicine & Pharmacotherapy* **64**: 21–28.

Couteau, C. and Coiffard, L. (2016). Seaweed application in cosmetics. In: *Seaweed in Health and Disease Prevention* (eds. J. Fleurence and I. Levine), 423–441. Nantes: Academic Press.

Damonte, E.B., Matulewicz, M.C., and Cerezo, A.S. (2004). Sulfated seaweed polysaccharides as antiviral agents. *Current Medicinal Chemistry* **11** (18): 2399–2419.

Das, S.K., Ren, R., Hashimoto, T., and Kanazawa, K. (2010). Fucoxanthin induces apoptosis in osteoclast-like cells differentiated from RAW264.7 cells. *Journal of Agricultural and Food Chemistry* **58**: 6090–6095.

Déléris, P., Nazih, H., and Bard, J.-M. (2016). Seaweeds in human health. In: *Seaweed in Health and Disease Prevention* (eds. J. Fleurence and I. Levine), 319–367. Nantes: Academic Press.

Dinesh, S., Menon, T., Hanna, L.E. et al. (2016). In vitro anti-HIV-1 activity of fucoidan from *Sargassum swartzii*. *International Journal of Biological Macromolecules* **82**: 83–88.

Draelos, Z.D. (2014). Cosmeceuticals. Efficacy and influence on skin tone. *Dermatologic Clinics* **32**: 137–143.

Dupont, E., Léveillé, C., Gomez, J. et al. (2012). Clinical efficacy of a serum integrating multiple cosmetic ingredients in the management of erythema of the face in aging skin. *Journal of Cosmetic Dermatology* **11** (3): 207–212. https://doi.org/10.1111/j.1473-2165.2012.00623.x.

Durai, P.C., Thappa, D.M., Kumari, R., and Malathi, M. (2012). Aging in elderly: chronological versus photoaging. *Indian Journal of Dermatology* **57** (5): 343–352.

El Shafay, S.M., Ali, S.S., and El-Sheekh, M.M. (2016). Antimicrobial activity of some seaweeds species from Red Sea, against multidrug resistant bacteria. *Egyptian Journal of Aquatic Research* **42**: 65–74.

Fabrowska, J., Łeska, B., Schroeder, G. et al. (2015). Biomass and extracts o algae as material for cosmetics. In: *Marine Algae Extracts: Processes, Products, and Applications* (eds. S.-K. Kim and K. Chojnacka), 681–706. Hoboken, NJ: Wiley.

Farias, W.R.L., Valente, A.P., Pereira, M.S., and Mourao, P.A.S. (2000). Structure and anticoagulant activity of sulfated galactans. Isolation of a unique sulfated galactan from the red algae *Botryocladia occidentalis* and comparison of its anticoagulant action with that of sulfated galactans from invertebrates. *The Journal of Biological Chemistry* **275**: 29299–29307.

Fernandes, A.S., Mercadante, A.Z., Cichoski, A.J. et al. (2017). Identification of chlorophyll molecules with peroxyl radical scavenger capacity in microalgae *Phormidium autumnale* using ultrasound-assisted extraction. *Food Research International* **99**: 1036–1041.

Firdaus, M., Setijawati, D., Islam, I. et al. (2018). The reducibility of heLa cell viability by *Sargassum polycystum* extracts. *IOP Conference Series Earth and Environmental Science* **137**: 012064.

Fitton, J., Irhimeh, M., and Falk, N. (2007). Macroalgal fucoidan extracts: a new opportunity for marine cosmetics. *Cosmetics and Toiletries* **122**: 55–64.

Fitzgerald, C., Gallagher, E., Tasdemir, D., and Hayes, M. (2011). Heart health peptides from macroalgae and their potential use in functional foods. *Journal of Agricultural and Food Chemistry* **59** (13): 6829–6836.

Foo, S.C., Yusoff, F.M., Ismail, M. et al. (2017). Antioxidant capacities of fucoxanthin-producing algae as influenced by their carotenoid and phenolic contents. *Journal of Biotechnology* **241**: 175–183.

Fujimura, T., Tsukahara, K., Moriwaki, S. et al. (2000). Effects of natural product extracts on contraction and mechanical properties of fibroblast populated collagen gel. *Biological and Pharmaceutical Bulletin* **23** (3): 291–297. https://doi.org/10.1248/bpb.23.291.

Fumiaki, B., Masashi, H., Yoshimi, N., and Kazuo, M. (2012). Effects of dietary fucoxanthin on cholesterol metabolism in diabetic/obese KK-Ay mice. *Lipids in Health and Disease* **11**: 112. https://doi.org/10.1186/1476-511X-11-112.

Gallé, J.-B., Attioua, B., Kaiser, M. et al. (2013). Eleganolone a diterpene from the French marine alga *Bifurcaria bifurcata* inhibits growth of the human pathogens *Trypanosoma brucei* and *Plasmodium falciparum*. *Marine Drugs* **11**: 599–610.

Gammone, M.A., Riccioni, G., and D'Orazio, N. (2015). Marine carotenoids against oxidative stress: effects on human health. *Marine Drugs* **13**: 6226–6246.

Garcia-Vaquero, M., Rajauria, G., O'Doherty, J., and Torres, S. (2017). Polysaccharides from macroalgae: recent advances, innovative technologies and challenges in extraction and purification. *Food Research International* **99**: 1011–1020.

Georg Jensen, M., Pedersen, C., Kristensen, M. et al. (2013). Review: efficacy of alginate supplementation in relation to appetite regulation and metabolic risk factors: evidence from animal and human studies. *Obesity Reviews* **14** (2): 129–144.

Girond, S., Crance, J.M., Van Cuyck-Gandre, H. et al. (1991). Antiviral activity of carrageenan on hepatitis A virus replication in cell culture. *Research in Virology* **142** (4): 261–270.

Gomez d'Ayala, G., Malinconico, M., and Laurienzo, P. (2008). Marine derived polysaccharides for biomedical applications: chemical modification approaches. *Molecules* **13**: 2069–2106.

Gómez-Guzman, M., Rodríguez-Nogales, A., Algieri, F., and Gálvez, J. (2018). Potential role of seaweed polyphenols in cardiovascular-associated disorders. *Marine Drugs* **16** (8): 250.

Gómez-Ordoñez, E., Jiménez-Escrig, A., and Rupérez, P. (2010). Dietary fibre and physicochemical properties of several edible seaweeds from the northwestern Spanish coast. *Food Research International* **43** (9): 2289–2294.

Granert, C., Raud, J., Xie, X. et al. (1994). Inhibition of leukocyte rolling with polysaccharide fucoidin prevents pleocytosis in experimental meningitis in the rabbit. *Journal of Clinical Investigation* **93**: 929–936.

Grimi, N., Dubois, A., Marchal, L. et al. (2014). Selective extraction from microalgae *Nannochloropsis* sp. using different methods of cell disruption. *Bioresource Technology* **153**: 254–259.

Guillerme, J.-B., Couteau, C., and Coiffard, L. (2017). Applications for marine resources in cosmetics. *Cosmetics* **4** (3): 35.

Guillon, F. and Champ, M. (2000). Structural and physical properties of dietary fibres, and consequences of processing on human physiology. *Food Research International* **33**: 233–245.

Hamed, I. (2016). The evolution and versatility of microalgal biotechnology: a review. *Comprehensive Reviews in Food Science and Food Safety* **15**: 1104–1123.

Hamed, I., Özogul, F., Özogul, Y., and Regenstein, J.M. (2015). Marine bioactive compounds and their health benefits: a review. *Comprehensive Reviews in Food Science and Food Safety* **14** (4): 446–465.

Hartmann, A., Gostner, J., Fuchs, J.E. et al. (2015). Inhibition of collagenase by mycosporine-like amino acids from marine sources. *Planta Medica* **81** (10): 813–820. https://doi.org/10.1055/s-0035-1546105.

Hassan, S., El-Twab, S.A., Hetta, M., and Mahmoud, B. (2011). Improvement of lipid profile and antioxidant of hypercholesterolemic albino rats by polysaccharides extracted from the green alga *Ulva lactuca* Linnaeus. *Saudi Journal of Biological Sciences* **18** (4): 333–340.

Heo, S.J. and Jeon, Y.J. (2009). Protective effect of fucoxanthin isolated from *Sargassum siliquastrum* on UV-B induced cell damage. *Journal of Photochemistry and Photobiology B: Biology* **95** (2): 101–107.

Hernández-Corona, D.M., Martínez-Abundis, E., and González-Ortiz, M. (2014). Effect of fucoidan administration on insulin secretion and insulin resistance in overweight or obese adults. *Journal of Medicinal Food* **17**: 830–832.

Hitoe, S. and Shimoda, H. (2017). Seaweed fucoxanthin supplementation improves obesity parameters in mildly obese Japanese subjects. *Functional Foods in Health and Disease* **7** (4): 246–262.

Hosikian, A., Lim, S., Halim, R., and Danquah, M.K. (2010). Chlorophyll extraction from microalgae: a review on the process engineering aspects. *International Journal of Chemical Engineering* **2010**: 391632.

Hosokawa, M., Kudo, M., Maeda, H. et al. (2004). Fucoxanthin induces apoptosis and enhances the antiproliferative effect of the PPARγ ligand, troglitazone, on colon cancer cells. *Biochimica et Biophysica Acta (BBA) General Subjects General Subjects* **1675** (1–3): 113–119. https://doi.org/10.1016/j.bbagen.2004.08.012.

Hu, X., Li, Y., Li, C. et al. (2012). Combination of fucoxanthin and conjugated linoleic acid attenuates body weight gain and improves lipid metabolism in high-fat diet-induced obese rats. *Archives of Biochemistry and Biophysics* **519**: 59–65.

Huang, Y.-C., Wang, T.-W., Sun, J.-S., and Lin, F.-H. (2006). Effect of calcium ion concentration on keratinocyte behaviors in the defined media. *Biomedical Engineering: Applications, Basis and Communications* **18**: 37–41.

Hwang, E., Park, S.Y., Sun, Z.W. et al. (2014). The protective effects of fucosterol against skin damage in UVB-irradiated human dermal fibroblasts. *Marine Biotechnology* **16** (3): 361–370.

Ina, A., Hayashi, K., Nozaki, H., and Kamei, Y. (2007). Pheophytin a, a low molecular weight compound found in the marine brown alga *Sargassum fulvellum*, promotes the differentiation of PC12 cells. *International Journal of Developmental Neuroscience* **25** (1): 63–68.

Iraha, A., Chinen, H., Hokama, A. et al. (2013). Fucoidan enhances intestinal barrier function by upregulating the expression of claudin-1. *World Journal of Gastroenterology* **19** (33): 5500–5507.

Isaka, S., Cho, K., Nakazono, S. et al. (2015). Antioxidant and anti-inflammatory activities of porphyran isolated from discolored nori (*Porphyra yezoensis*). *International Journal of Biological Macromolecules* **74**: 68–75.

Ismaiel, M.M.S., El-Ayouty, Y.M., and Piercey-Normore, M.D. (2014). Antioxidants characterization in selected cyanobacteria. *Annals of Microbiology* **64** (3): 1223–1230.

Iwamoto, K., Hiragun, T., Takahagi, S. et al. (2011). Fucoidan suppresses IgE production in peripheral blood mononuclear cells from patients with atopic dermatitis. *Archives of Dermatological Research* **303**: 425–431.

Jeong, Y.-T., Kim, Y.D., Jung, Y.-M. et al. (2013). Low molecular weight fucoidan improves endoplasmic reticulum stress-reduced insulin sensitivity through AMP-activated protein kinase activation in L6 myotubes and restores lipid homeostasis in a mouse model of type 2 diabetes. *Molecular Pharmacology* **84**: 147–157.

Jiang, Z., Hama, Y., Yamaguchi, K., and Oda, T. (2012). Inhibitory effect of sulphated polysaccharide porphyran on nitric oxide production in lipopolysaccharide-stimulated RAW264.7 macrophages. *Journal of Biochemistry* **151**: 65–74.

Jiao, G., Yu, G., Zhang, J., and Ewart, H.S. (2011). Chemical structures and bioactivities of sulfated polysaccharides from marine algae. *Marine Drugs* **9** (2): 196–223.

Jin, W., Ren, L., Liu, B. et al. (2018). Structural features of sulfated glucuronomannan oligosaccharides and their antioxidant activity. *Marine Drugs* **16** (9): 291.

Joung, E., Gwon, W., Shin, T. et al. (2017). Anti-inflammatory action of the ethanolic extract from *Sargassum serratifolium* on lipopolysaccharide-stimulated mouse peritoneal macrophages and identification of active components. *Journal of Applied Phycology* **29**: 563–573. https://doi.org/10.1007/s10811-016-0954-9.

Jung, H.A., Hyun, S.K., Kim, H.R., and Choi, J.S. (2006). Angiotensin-converting enzyme I inhibitory activity of phlorotannins from *Ecklonia stolonifera*. *Fisheries Science* **72**: 1292–1299.

Jung, H.A., Jin, S.E., Ahn, B.R. et al. (2013). Anti-inflammatory activity of edible brown alga *Eisenia bicyclis* and its constituents fucosterol and phlorotannins in LPS-stimulated RAW264.7 macrophages. *Food and Chemical Toxicology* **59**: 199–206.

Jung, H.A., Jung, H.J., Jeong, H.Y. et al. (2014a). Phlorotannins isolated from the edible brown alga *Ecklonia stolonifera* exert anti-adipogenic activity on 3T3-L1 adipocytes by downregulating C/EBPa and PPARc. *Fitoterapia* **92**: 260–269.

Jung, H.A., Jung, H.J., Jeong, H.Y. et al. (2014b). Anti-adipogenic activity of the edible brown alga *Ecklonia stolonifera* and its constituent fucosterol in 3T3-L1 adipocytes. *Archives of Pharmacal Research* **37** (6): 713–720.

Jung, H.A., Roy, A., Jung, J.H., and Choi, J.S. (2017). Evaluation of the inhibitory effects of eckol and dieckol isolated from edible brown alga *Eisenia bicyclis* on human monoamine oxidases A and B. *Archives of Pharmacal Research* **40** (4): 480–491.

Kalimuthu, S. and Kim, S.-K. (2015). Fucoidan, a sulfated polysaccharides from brown algae as therapeutic target for cancer. In: *Handbook of Anticancer Drugs from Marine Origin* (ed. S.-K. Kim), 145–164. Cham: Springer https://doi.org/10.1007/7978-3-319-07145-9.

Kamei, Y., Sueyoshi, M., Hayashi, K. et al. (2009). The novel anti-*Propionibacterium acnes* compound, Sargafuran, found in the marine brown alga *Sargassum macrocarpum*. *The Journal of Antibiotics* **62** (5): 259–263.

Kang, H.S., Kim, H.R., Byun, D.S. et al. (2004). Tyrosinase inhibitors isolated from the edible brown alga *Ecklonia stolonifera*. *Archives of Pharmacal Research* **27**: 1226–1232.

Kang, K.A., Lee, K.H., Chae, S. et al. (2006). Cytoprotective effect of phloroglucinol on oxidative stress induced cell damage via catalase activation. *Journal of Cellular Biochemistry* **97** (3): 609–620.

Kang, S.I., Shin, H.S., Kim, H.M. et al. (2012). *Petalonia binghamiae* extract and its constituent fucoxanthin ameliorate high-fat diet-induced obesity by activating AMP-activated protein kinase. *Journal of Agricultural and Food Chemistry* **60**: 3389–3395.

Kang, M.-C., Wijesinghe, W.A.J.P., Lee, S.-H. et al. (2013). Dieckol isolated from brown seaweed *Ecklonia cava* attenuates type II diabetes in db/db mouse model. *Food and Chemical Toxicology* **53**: 294–298.

Kang, M.C., Ding, Y., Kim, E.A. et al. (2017). Indole derivatives isolated from brown alga *Sargassum thunbergii* inhibit adipogenesis through AMPK activation in 3T3-L1 preadipocytes. *Marine Drugs* **15**: 119. https://doi.org/10.3390/md15040119.

Karadeniz, F., Kang, K.H., Park, J.W. et al. (2014). Anti-HIV-1 activity of phlorotannin derivative 8,4′′'-dieckol from Korean brown alga *Ecklonia cava*. *Bioscience, Biotechnology, and Biochemistry* **78**: 1151–1158.

Kearney, S.M., Gibbons, S.M., Erdman, S.E., and Alm, E.J. (2018). Orthogonal dietary niche enables reversible engraftment of a gut bacterial commensal. *Cell Reports* **24**: 1842–1851.

Kendel, M., Wielgosz-Collin, G., Bertrand, S. et al. (2015). Lipid composition, fatty acids and sterols in the seaweeds *Ulva armoricana*, and *Solieria chordalis* from Brittany (France): an analysis from nutritional, chemotaxonomic, and antiproliferative activity perspectives. *Marine Drugs* **13** (9): 5606–5628.

Khan, M.N., Cho, J.Y., Lee, M.C. et al. (2007). Isolation of two anti-inflammatory and one pro-inflammatory polyunsaturated fatty acids from the brown seaweed *Undaria pinnatifida*. *Journal of Agricultural and Food Chemistry* **55** (17): 6984–6988.

Kim, S.-K. and Ta, Q.V. (2011). Potential beneficial effects of marine algal sterols on human health. *Advances in Food and Nutrition Research* **64**: 191–198.

Kim, S.-K. and Thomas, N.V. (2011). Potential cosmeceutical applications of phlorotannins and fucoidans from marine algae in the treatment of atopic dermatitis. In: *Marine Cosmeceuticals: Trends and Prospects* (ed. S.-K. Kim). Boca Raton, FL: CRC Press.

Kim, H.H., Shin, C.M., Park, C.H. et al. (2005). Eicosapentaenoic acid inhibits UV-induced MMP-1 expression in human dermal fibroblasts. *Journal of Lipid Research* **46**: 1712–1720.

Kim, M.M., Ta, Q.V., Mendis, E. et al. (2006). Phlorotannins in *Ecklonia cava* extract inhibit matrix metalloproteinase activity. *Life Sciences* **79** (15): 1436–1443.

Kim, S.-K., Ravichandran, Y.D., Khan, S.B., and Kim, Y.T. (2008). Prospective of the cosmeceuticals derived from marine organisms. *Biotechnology and Bioprocess Engineering* **13** (5): 511–523.

Kim, K.J., Yoon, K.Y., and Lee, B.Y. (2012). Fucoidan regulate blood glucose homeostasis in C57BL/KSJ m+/+db and C57BL/KSJ db/db mice. *Fitoterapia* **83** (6): 1105–1109.

Kim, Y.-S., Li, X.-F., Kang, K.-H. et al. (2014a). Stigmasterol isolated from marine microalgae *Navicula incerta* induces apoptosis in human hepatoma HepG2 cells. *BMB Reports* **47**: 433–438.

Kim, M.-J., Jeon, J., and Lee, J.-S. (2014b). Fucoidan prevents high-fat diet-induced obesity in animals by suppression of fat accumulation. *Phytotherapy Research* **28**: 137–143.

Kim, B.S., Kang, H.-J., Park, J.-Y., and Lee, J. (2015a). Fucoidan promotes osteoblast differentiation via JNK- and ERK-dependent BMP2-Smad 1/5/8 signaling in human mesenchymal stem cells. *Experimental and Molecular Medicine* **47**: e128. https://doi.org/10.1038/emm.2014.95.

Kim, R.-K., Uddin, N., Hyun, J.-W. et al. (2015b). Novel anticancer activity of phloroglucinol against breast cancer stem-like cells. *Toxicology and Applied Pharmacology* **286** (3): 143–150. https://doi.org/10.1016/j.taap.2015.03.026.

Kim, R.-K., Suh, Y., Yoo, K.-C. et al. (2015c). Phloroglucinol suppresses metastatic ability of breast cancer cells by inhibition of epithelial-mesenchymal cell transition. *Cancer Science* **106**: 94–101.

Kim, S.-Y., Kim, Y.M., Kim, E., and Lee, M.S. (2015d). Synergistic antibacterial activity of *Ecklonia cava* extract against anti-biotic resistant *Enterococcus faecalis*. *Korean Journal of Fisheries and Aquatic Science* **48**: 51–57.

Kim, J.H., Yun, E.J., Yu, S. et al. (2017). Different levels of skin whitening activity among 3,6-anhydro-L-galactose, agarooligosaccharides, and neoagarooligosaccharides. *Marine Drugs* **15** (10): 321. https://doi.org/10.3390/md15100321.

Kim, J.H., Lee, J.-E., Kim, K.H., and Kang, N.J. (2018). Beneficial effects of marine algae-derived carbohydrates for skin health. *Marine Drugs* **16** (11): 459.

Kobayashi, D., Kusama, M., Onda, M., and Nakahata, N. (2011). The effect of pantothenic acid deficiency on keratinocyte proliferation and the synthesis of keratinocyte growth factor and collagen in fibroblast. *Journal of Pharmacological Sciences* **115** (2): 230–234.

Kocis, P., Tolar, Y.J., Sinko, W. et al. (2017). Elucidating the Aβ42 anti-aggregation mechanism of action of tramiprosate in Alzheimer's disease: integrating molecular analytical methods, pharmacokinetic and clinical data. *CNS Drugs* **31** (6): 495–509.

Koller, M., Muhr, A., and Braunegg, G. (2014). Microalgae as versatile cellular factories for valued products. *Algal Research* **6**: 52–63.

Kong, C.-S., Kim, J.-A., Yoon, N.-Y., and Kim, S.-K. (2009). Induction of apoptosis by phloroglucinol derivative from *Ecklonia cava* in MCF-7 human breast cancer cells. *Food and Chemical Toxicology* **47** (7): 1653–1658.

Korukanti, V.P., Ponnam, H., and Akondi, B.R. (2013). Evaluation of antiobesity activity of *Fucus vesiculosus*. *Indian Journal of Research in Homoeopathy* **7**: 126–132.

Koyanagi, S., Tanigawa, N., Nakagawa, H. et al. (2003). Oversulfation of fucoidan enhances its anti-angiogenic and antitumor activities. *Biochemical Pharmacology* **65** (2): 173–179.

Kwon, M.-J. and Nam, T.-J. (2006). Porphyran induces apoptosis related signal pathway in AGS gastric cancer cell lines. *Life Sciences* **79** (20): 1956–1962.

Kwon, M., Lim, S.J., Joung, E.J. et al. (2018). Meroterpenoid-rich fraction of an ethanolic extract from *Sargassum serratifolium* alleviates obesity and non-alcoholic fatty liver disease in high fat-fed C57BL/6J mice. *Journal of Functional Foods* **47**: 288–298.

Laurienzo, P. (2010). Marine polysaccharides in pharmaceutical applications: an overview. *Marine Drugs* **8** (9): 2435–2465.

Le, Q.T., Li, Y., Qian, Z.J. et al. (2009). Inhibitory effects of polyphenols isolated from marine alga *Ecklonia cava* on histamine release. *Process Biochemistry* **44**: 168–176.

Leal, M.C., Munro, M.H.G., Blunt, J.W. et al. (2013). Biogeography and biodiscovery hotspots of macroalgal marine natural products. *Natural Product Reports* **30**: 1380–1390.

Lee, S.-H. and Jeon, Y.-J. (2013). Anti-diabetic effects of brown algae derived phlorotannins, marine polyphenols through diverse mechanisms. *Fitoterapia* **86**: 129–136.

Lee, S.J., Bai, S.K., Lee, K.S. et al. (2003). Astaxanthin inhibits nitric oxide production and inflammatory gene expression by suppressing I(kappa)B kinase-dependent NF-kappaB activation. *Molecules and Cells* **16**: 97–105.

Lee, Y.S., Shin, K.H., Kim, B.K., and Lee, S. (2004). Anti-diabetic activities of fucosterol from *Pelvetia siliquosa*. *Archives of Pharmacal Research* **27** (11): 1120–1122.

Lee, H.J., Kim, Y.A., Lee, J.I. et al. (2007). Screening of Korean marine plants extracts for inhibitory activity on protein tyrosine phosphatase 1B. *Journal of Applied Biological Chemistry* **50** (2): 74–77.

Lee, H.J., Kim, H.C., Vitek, L., and Nam, C.M. (2010a). Algae consumption and risk of type 2 diabetes: Korean National Health and nutrition examination survey in 2005. *Journal of Nutritional Science and Vitaminology* **56** (1): 13–18.

Lee, S.-H., Park, M.-H., Heo, S.-J. et al. (2010b). Dieckol isolated from *Ecklonia cava* inhibits α-glucosidase and α-amylase in vitro and alleviates postprandial hyperglycemia in streptozotocin-induced diabetic mice. *Food and Chemical Toxicology* **48** (10): 2633–2637. https://doi.org/10.1016/j.fct.2010.06.032.

Lee, O.H., Yoon, K.Y., Kim, K.J. et al. (2011). Seaweed extracts as a potential tool for the attenuation of oxidative damage in obesity-related pathologies. *Journal of Phycology* **47**: 548–556.

Lee, M.-S., Yoon, H.-D., Kim, J.-L. et al. (2012). Dioxinodehydroeckol inhibits melanin synthesis through PI3K/Akt signalling pathway in a-melanocyte-stimulating hormone-treated B16F10 cells. *Experimental Dermatology* **21** (6): 471–473.

Lee, W., Ahn, G., Oh, J.Y. et al. (2016). A prebiotic effect of *Ecklonia cava* on the growth and mortality of olive flounder infected with pathogenic bacteria. *Fish & Shellfish Immunology* **51**: 313–320.

Lee, J.H., Jung, H.A., Kang, M.J. et al. (2017). Fucosterol, isolated from *Ecklonia stolonifera*, inhibits adipogenesis through modulation of FoxO1 pathway in 3T3-L1 adipocytes. *Journal of Pharmacy and Pharmacology* **69**: 325–333.

Lee, A.-R., Roh, S.-S., and Kim, H.-K. (2018). Anti-microbial activity and anti-inflammatory effects of fucoidan extracts. *Asian Journal of Beauty and Cosmetology* **16** (2): 191–200.

Łęska, B., Messyasz, B., and Schroeder, G. (2018). Application of algae biomass and algae extracts in cosmetic formulations. In: *Algae Biomass: Characteristics and Applications*, Developments in Applied Phycology, vol. **8** (eds. K. Chojnacka, P. Wieczorek, G. Schroeder and I. Michalak), 89–101. Cham: Springer https://doi.org/10.1007/978-3-39-74703-3.

Li, B., Lu, F., Wei, X.J., and Zhao, R.X. (2008). Fucoidan: structure and bioactivity. *Molecules* **13** (8): 1671–1695.

Li, Y., Qian, Z.J., Kim, M.M., and Kim, S.K. (2011a). Cytotoxic activities of phlorethol and fucophlorethol derivatives isolated from Laminariaceae *Ecklonia cava*. *Journal of Food Biochemistry* **35**: 357–369.

Li, Y.-X., Wijesekara, I., Li, Y., and Kim, S.-K. (2011b). Phlorotannins as bioactive agents from brown algae. *Process Biochemistry* **46**: 2219–2224.

Li, K., Li, X.M., Gloer, J.B., and Wang, B.G. (2012a). New nitrogen-containing bromophenols from the marine red alga *Rhodomela confervoides* and their radical scavenging activity. *Food Chemistry* **135**: 868–872.

Li, L.J., Li, M.-Y., Li, Y.-T. et al. (2012b). Adjuvant activity of *Sargassum pallidum* polysaccharides against combined Newcastle disease, infectious bronchitis and avian influenza inactivated vaccines. *Marine Drugs* **10**: 2648–2660.

Li, J., Xie, L., Qin, Y. et al. (2013). Effect of laminarin polysaccharide on activity of matrix metalloproteinase in photoaging skin. *China Journal of Chinese Materia Medica* **38**: 2370–2373.

Lim, S., Kwon, M., Joung, E.-J. et al. (2018). Meroterpenoid-rich fraction of the ethanolic extract from *Sargassum serratifolium* suppressed oxidative stress induced by tert-butyl hydroperoxide in HepG2 Cells. *Marine Drugs* **16** (10): 374. https://doi.org/10.3390/md16100374.

Liu, M., Hansen, P.E., and Lin, X. (2011a). Bromophenols in marine algae and their bioactivities. *Marine Drugs* **9**: 1273–1292.

Liu, M., Zhang, W., Wei, J., and Lin, X. (2011b). Synthesis and α-glucosidase inhibitory mechanisms of bis(2,3-dibromo-4,5-dihydroxybenzyl) ether, a potential marine bromophenol α-glucosidase inhibitor. *Marine Drugs* **9**: 1554–1565.

Liu, D.-Q., Mao, S.-C., Zhang, H.-Y. et al. (2013). Racemosins A and B, two novel bisindole alkaloids from the green alga *Caulerpa racemosa*. *Fitoterapia* **91**: 15–20.

Liu, M., Wang, G., Xiao, L. et al. (2014). Bis(2,3-dibromo-4,5-dihydroxybenzyl) ether, a marine algae derived bromophenol, inhibits the growth of *Botrytis cinerea* and interacts with DNA molecules. *Marine Drugs* **12**: 3838–3851.

Liu, Y., Liu, M., Zhang, X. et al. (2016). Protective effect of fucoxanthin isolated from *Laminaria japonica* against visible light-induced retinal damage both in vitro and in vivo. *Journal of Agricultural and Food Chemistry* **64**: 416–424.

Liu, X., Yuan, W., Sharma-Shivappa, R., and Van Zanten, J. (2017). Antioxidant activity of phlorotannins from brown algae. *International Journal of Agricultural and Biological Engineering* **10** (6): 184–191.

Llewellyn, C.A. and Airs, R.L. (2010). Distribution and abundance of MAAs in 33 species of microalgae across 13 classes. *Marine Drugs* **8**: 1273–1291.

Lopes, G., Sousa, C., Valentão, P., and Andrade, P.B. (2013). Sterols in algae and health. In: *Bioactive Compounds from Marine Foods* (eds. B. Hernández-Ledesma and M. Herrero). Hoboken, NJ: Wiley https://doi.org/10.1002/9781118412893.ch9.

Lopes, G., Andrade, P.B., and Valentao, P. (2016). Phlorotannins: towards new pharmacological interventions for diabetes mellitus type 2. *Molecules* **22** (1): 56.

Lucena, A.M.M., Souza, C.R.M., Jales, J.T. et al. (2018). The bisindole alkaloid caulerpin, from seaweeds of the genus *Caulerpa*, attenuated colon damage in murine colitis model. *Marine Drugs* **16**: 318. https://doi.org/10.3390/md16090318.

Ludwig, M., Enzenhofer, E., Schneider, S. et al. (2013). Efficacy of a carrageenan nasal spray in patients with common cold: a randomized controlled trial. *Respiratory Research* **14**: 124. https://doi.org/10.1186/1465-9921-14-124.

Luo, X., Su, P., and Zhang, W. (2015). Advances in microalgae-derived phytosterols for functional food and pharmaceutical applications. *Marine Drugs* **13**: 4231–4254.

Macedo, N.R.P.V., Ribeiro, M.S., and Villaça, R.C., Ferreira, W., Pinto, A.M., Teixeira, V.L., Cirne-Santos, C., Paixão, I.C.N.P., & Giongo, V. (2012). Caulerpine as a potential antiviral drug against herpes simplex virus type 1. *Brazilian Journal of Pharmacognosy* **22**: 861–867.

Maeda, H., Hosokawa, M., Sashima, T. et al. (2009). Anti-obesity and anti-diabetic effects of fucoxanthin on diet-induced obesity conditions in a murine model. *Molecular Medicine Reports* **2** (6): 897–902.

Malini, M., Ponnanikajamideen, M., Chelladurai, M., and Shanmugam, R. (2014). Explore the antimicrobial potential from organic solvents extract of brown seaweed (*Sargassum longifolium*) alleviating to pharmaceuticals. *International Journal of Pharmaceutical Research* **6** (1): 28–35.

Maneesh, A. and Chakraborty, K. (2017). Unprecedented antioxidative and anti-inflammatory aryl polyketides from the brown seaweed *Sargassum wightii*. *Food Research International* **100** (1): 640–649.

Marini, A., Reinelt, K., Krutmann, J., and Bilstein, A. (2014). Ectoine-containing cream in the treatment of mild to moderate atopic dermatitis: a randomised, comparator-controlled, intra-individual double-blind, multi-center trial. *Skin Pharmacology and Physiology* **27**: 57–65.

Matei, E., Basu, R., Furey, W. et al. (2016). Structure and glycan binding of a new cyanovirin-N homolog. *Journal of Biological Chemistry* **291** (36): 18967–18976.

Matsui, M., Tanaka, K., Higashiguchi, N. et al. (2016). Protective and therapeutic effects of fucoxanthin against sunburn caused by UV irradiation. *Journal of Pharmacological Sciences* **132**: 55–64.

Mezdour, H., Menad, A., Abdelfettah, G. et al. (2017). Immunomodulatory and anti-inflammatory activities of algerian *Ulva lactuca*. *World Journal of Pharmaceutical Research* **6** (11): 72–95.

Mikalak, I. and Chojnacka, K. (2015). Algae as production systems of bioactive compounds. *Engineering in Life Sciences* **15**: 160–176.

Moghadamtousi, S.Z., Karimian, H., Khanabdali, R. et al. (2014). Anticancer and antitumor potential of fucoidan and fucoxanthin, two main metabolites isolated from brown algae. *The Scientific World Journal* **2014**: 768323.

Mohamed, S., Hashim, S.N., and Rahman, H.A. (2012). Seaweeds: a sustainable functional food for complementary and alternative therapy. *Trends in Food Science & Technology* **23** (2): 83–96. https://doi.org/10.1016/j.tifs.2011.09.001.

Mohibbullah, M., Haque, M.N., Khan, M.N.A. et al. (2018). Neuroprotective effects of fucoxanthin and its derivative fucoxanthinol from the phaeophyte *Undaria pinnatifida* attenuate oxidative stress in hippocampal neurons. *Journal of Applied Phycology* **30** (6): 3243–3252.

Mohsen, M.S.A., Mohamed, S.F., Ali, F.M., and El-Sayed, O.H. (2007). Chemical structure and antiviral activity of water-soluble sulfated polysaccharides from *Sargassum latifolium*. *Journal of Applied Sciences Research* **3**: 1178–1185.

Moon, H.J., Lee, S.H., Ku, M.J. et al. (2009). Fucoidan inhibits UVB-induced MMP-1 promoter expression and down regulation of type I procollagen synthesis in human skin fibroblasts. *European Journal of Dermatology* **19**: 129–134.

Moon, S.-M., Lee, S.A., Han, S.H. et al. (2018). Aqueous extract of *Codium fragile* alleviates osteoarthritis through the MAPK/NF-κB pathways in IL-1β-induced rat primary chondrocytes and a rat osteoarthritis model. *Biomedicine & Pharmacotherapy* **97**: 264–270.

Mori, K., Ooi, T., Hiraoka, M. et al. (2004). Fucoxanthin and its metabolites in edible brown algae cultivated in deep seawater. *Marine Drugs* **2**: 63–72.

Mourelle, M.L. and Gómez, C.P. (2015). Cosmética termal. Aplicaciones en el ámbito de la salud y la belleza. In: *Proceedings of 1st International Symposium on Healing SPA and Life Quality* (eds. J.M. Failde, A. Fornella, J.A. Fraiz, et al.), 389–398. Ourense: Campus da Agua.

Mourelle, M.L., Gómez, C.P., and Legido, J.L. (2017). The potential use of marine microalgae and cyanobacteria in cosmetics and thalassotherapy. *Cosmetics* **4**: 46. https://doi.org/10.3390/cosmetics4040046.

Nagaoka, M., Shibata, H., Kimura-Takagi, I. et al. (2000). Anti-ulcer effects and biological activities of polysaccharides from marine algae. *BioFactors* **12**: 267–274.

Nagayama, K., Iwamura, Y., Shibata, T. et al. (2002). Bactericidal activity of phlorotannins from the brown alga *Ecklonia kurome*. *Journal of Antimicrobial Chemotherapy* **50** (6): 889–893.

Namvar, F., Mohamad, R., Baharara, J. et al. (2013). Antioxidant, antiproliferative, and antiangiogenesis effects of polyphenol-rich seaweed (*Sargassum muticum*). *BioMed Research International* **2013**: 604787.

Nappo, M., Berkov, S., Massucco, C. et al. (2012). Apoptotic activity of the marine diatom *Cocconeis scutellum* and eicosapentaenoic acid in BT20 cells. *Pharmaceutical Biology* **50**: 529–535.

Narasimham, M.K., Pavithra, S.K., Krishnan, V., and Chandrasekaran, M. (2013). In vitro analysis of antioxidant, antimicrobial and antiproliferative activity of *Enteromorpha antenna*, *Enteromorpha linza* and *Gracilaria corticata* extracts. *Jundishapur Journal of Natural Pharmaceutical Products* **8** (4): 151–159.

Nauroth, J.M., Liu, Y.C., Van Elswyk, M. et al. (2010). Docosahexaenoic acid (DHA) and docosapentaenoic acid (DPAn-6) algal oils reduce inflammatory mediators in human peripheral mononuclear cells in vitro and paw edema in vivo. *Lipids* **45** (5): 375–384.

Ngo, D.-H. and Kim, S.-K. (2013). Sulfated polysaccharides as bioactive agents from marine algae. *International Journal of Biological Macromolecules* **62**: 70–75.

Nwosu, F., Morris, J., Lund, V.A. et al. (2011). Anti-proliferative and potential anti-diabetic effects of phenolic-rich extracts from edible marine algae. *Food Chemistry* **126**: 1006–1012.

Ohgami, K., Shiratori, K., Kotake, S. et al. (2003). Effects of astaxanthin on lipopolysaccharide induced inflammation in vitro and in vivo. *Journal of Investigative Ophthalmology & Visual Science* **44**: 2694–2701.

Pallela, R., Na-Young, Y., and Kim, S.K. (2010). Anti-photoaging and photoprotective compounds derived from marine organisms. *Marine Drugs* **8**: 1189–1202.

Pangestuti, R. and Kim, S.-K. (2011). Biological activities and health benefit effects of natural pigments derived from marine algae. *Journal of Functional Foods* **3**: 255–266.

Pangestuti, R. and Kim, S.-K. (2017). Bioactive peptide of marine origin for the prevention and treatment of non-communicable diseases. *Marine Drugs* **15** (3): 67. https://doi.org/10.3390/md15030067.

Park, H.-K., Kim, I.-H., Kim, J., and Nam, T.-J. (2013). Induction of apoptosis and the regulation of ErbB signaling by laminarin in HT-29 human colon cancer cells. *International Journal of Molecular Medicine* **32**: 291–295.

Park, G.T., Go, R.-E., Lee, H.-M. et al. (2017a). Potential anti-proliferative and immunomodulatory effects of marine microalgal exopolysaccharide on various human cancer cells and lymphocytes in vitro. *Marine Biotechnology* **19**: 136–146.

Park, J.-H., Choi, S.-H., Park, S.-J. et al. (2017b). Promoting wound healing using low molecular weight fucoidan in a full-thickness dermal excision rat model. *Marine Drugs* **15**: 112. https://doi.org/10.3390/md15040112.

Pasquet, V., Morisset, P., Ihammouine, S. et al. (2011). Antiproliferative activity of violaxanthin isolated from bioguided fractionation of *Dunaliella tertiolecta* extracts. *Marine Drugs* **9**: 819–831.

Paul, J.P. and Raja, P. (2018). Hepatoprotective activity of methanolic extract of *Gracilaria corticata* J.AG. in Hare Island, Thoothukudi, Tamil Nadu, India. *World Journal of Pharmaceutical Research* **7** (7): 1517–1522.

Peng, J., Yuan, J.P., Wu, C.F., and Wang, J.H. (2011). Fucoxanthin, a marine carotenoid present in brown seaweeds and diatoms: metabolism and bioactivities relevant to human health. *Marine Drugs* **9**: 1806–1828.

Peng, Y., Xie, E., Zheng, K. et al. (2013). Nutritional and chemical composition and antiviral activity of cultivated seaweed *Sargassum naozhouense* Tseng et Lu. *Marine Drugs* **11**: 20–32.

Pengzhan, Y., Ning, L., Xiguang, L. et al. (2003a). Antihyperlipidemic effects of different molecular weight sulfated polysaccharides from *Ulva pertusa* (Chlorophyta). *Pharmacological Research* **48**: 543–549.

Pengzhan, Y., Quanbin, Z., Ning, L. et al. (2003b). Polysaccharides from *Ulva pertusa* (Chlorophyta) and preliminary studies on their antihyperlipidemia activity. *Journal of Applied Phycology* **15**: 21–27.

Pereira, L. (2018a). Biological and therapeutic properties of the seaweed polysaccharides. *International Biology Review* **2** (2): 1–50.

Pereira, L. (2018b). Seaweeds as source of bioactive substances and skin care therapy – cosmeceuticals, algotheraphy, and thalassotherapy. *Cosmetics* **5** (4): 68.

Pereira, R., Carvalho, A., Vaz, D. et al. (2013). Development of novel alginate based hydrogel films for wound healing applications. *International Journal of Biological Macromolecules* **52**: 221–230.

Plaza, M., Cifuentes, A., and Ibáñez, E. (2008). In the search of new functional food ingredients from algae. *Trends in Food Science and Technology* **19**: 31–39.

Qi, H. and Sheng, J. (2015). The Antihyperlipidemic mechanism of high sulfate content ulvan in rats. *Marine Drugs* **13**: 3407–3421.

Qi, H., Zhang, Q., Zhao, T. et al. (2005). Antioxidant activity of different sulfate content derivatives of polysaccharide extracted from *Ulva pertusa* (Chlorophyta) in vitro. *International Journal of Biological Macromolecules* **37**: 195–199.

Raguraman, V., Abraham, S., Jyotsna, J. et al. (2019). Sulfated polysaccharide from *Sargassum tenerrimum* attenuates oxidative T stress induced reactive oxygen species production in in vitro and in zebrafish model. *Carbohydrate Polymers* **203**: 441–449.

Rahnasto-Rilla, M.K., McLoughlin, P., Kulikowicz, T. et al. (2017). The identification of a SIRT6 activator from brown algae *Fucus distichus*. *Marine Drugs* **2017** (15): 190. https://doi.org/10.3390/md15060190.

Rajauria, G. (2018). Optimization and validation of reverse phase HPLC method for qualitative and quantitative assessment of polyphenols in seaweed. *Journal of Pharmaceutical and Biomedical Analysis* **148**: 230–237. https://doi.org/10.1016/j.jpba.2017.10.002.

Rajauria, G., Foley, B., and Abu-Ghannam, N. (2017). Characterization of dietary fucoxanthin from *Himanthalia elongata* brown seaweed. *Food Research International* **99**: 995–1001.

Raman, B.V., Rao, D.N., and Radhakrishnan, T.M. (2004). *Enteromorpha compressa* (L.) Greville an edible green alga as a source of antiallergic principle (S). *Indian Journal of Clinical Biochemistry* **19** (1): 105–109. https://doi.org/10.1007/BF02872402.

Rao, J.S., Ertley, R.N., Lee, H.J. et al. (2007). n-3 polyunsaturated fatty acid deprivation in rats decreases frontal cortex BDNF via a p38 MAPK-dependent mechanism. *Molecular Psychiatry* **12**: 36–46.

Raposo, M.F.J., Morais, R.M., and Morais, A.M.M.B. (2013). Bioactivity and applications of sulphated polysaccharides from marine microalgae. *Marine Drugs* **11**: 233–252.

Rastogi, R.P., Sinha, R.P., and Incharoensakdi, A. (2013). Partial characterization, UV-induction and photoprotective function of sunscreen pigment, scytonemin from *Rivularia sp*. HKAR-4. *Chemosphere* **93** (9): 1874–1878. https://doi.org/10.1016/j.chemosphere.2013.06.057.

Razarinah, W., Rizlan Ross, E.E., Nor Farinna, A.R. et al. (2018). Antimicrobial activity of marine green algae extract against microbial pathogens. *Malaysian Journal of Bichemistry and Molecular Biology* **2**: 42–46.

Ren, R., Azuma, Y., Ojima, T. et al. (2013). Modulation of platelet aggregation-related eicosanoid production by dietary F-fucoidan from brown alga *Laminaria japonica* in human subjects. *British Journal of Nutrition* **110**: 880–890.

Ricciardi, L., De Nigris, F., Specchia, A., and Fasano, A. (2015). Homotaurine in Parkinson's disease. *Neurological Science* **36** (9): 1581–1587.

Robertson, R., Guihéneuf, F., Schmid, M. et al. (2013). Algae-derived polyunsaturated fatty acids: implications for human health. In: *Polyunsaturated Fatty Acids: Sources, Antioxidant Properties and Health Benefits* (ed. A. Catalá), 45–99. Hauppauge, NY: Nova Sciences Publishers, Inc.

Robertson, R.C., Guihèneuf, F., Bahar, B. et al. (2015). Anti-inflammatory effect of algae-derived lipid extracts on lipopolysaccharide (LPS)-stimulated human THP-1 macrophages. *Marine Drugs* **13** (8): 5402–5424.

Rocha de Souza, M., Marques, C., Guerra Dore, C. et al. (2007). Antioxidant activities of sulfated polysaccharides from brown and red seaweeds. *Journal of Applied Phycology* **19**: 153–160.

Rocha, D.H.A., Seca, A.M.L., and Pinto, D.C.A. (2018). Seaweed secondary metabolites in vitro and in vivo anticancer activity. *Marine Drugs* **16** (11): 410. https://doi.org/10.3390/md16110410.

Ryu, B.M., Qian, Z.J., Kim, M.M. et al. (2009). Anti-photoaging activity and inhibition of matrix metalloproteinase (MMP) by marine red alga, *Corallina pilulifera* methanol extract. *Radiation Physics and Chemistry* **78** (2): 98–105. https://doi.org/10.1016/j.radphyschem.2008.09.001.

Ryu, J., Park, S.J., Kim, I.H. et al. (2014). Protective effect of porphyra-334 on UVA-induced photoaging in human skin fibroblasts. *International Journal of Molecular Medicine* **34** (3): 796–803. https://doi.org/10.3892/ijmm.2014.1815.

Sadeeshkumar, V., Duraikannu, A., Ravichandran, S. et al. (2017). Modulatory efficacy of dieckol on xenobiotic-metabolizing enzymes, cell proliferation, apoptosis, invasion, and angiogenesis during NDEA-induced rat hepatocarcinogenesis. *Molecular and Cellular Biochemistry* **433**: 195–204.

Samarakoon, K. and Jeon, Y.-J. (2012). Bio-functionalities of proteins derived from marine algae – a review. *Food Research International* **48**: 948–960.

Sánchez-Machado, D.I., López-Cervantes, J., López-Hernández, J., and Paseiro-Losada, P. (2002). Fatty acids, total lipid, protein and ash contents of processed edible seaweeds. *Food Chemistry* **85**: 439–444.

Sánchez-Machado, D.I., López-Hernández, J., Paseiro-Losada, P., and López-Cervantes, J. (2004). An HPLC method for the quantification of sterols in edible seaweeds. *Biomedical Chromatography* **18** (3): 183–190.

Sanjeewa, K.K.A., Fernando, I.P.S., Samarakoon, K.W. et al. (2016). Anti-inflammatory and anti-cancer activities of sterol rich fraction of cultured marine microalga *Nannochloropsis oculata*. *Algae* **31** (3): 277–287.

Santos, S.A.O., Trindade, S.S., Oliveira, C.S.D. et al. (2017). Lipophilic fraction of cultivated *Bifurcaria bifurcata* R. Ross: detailed composition and in vitro prospection of current challenging bioactive properties. *Marine Drugs* **15** (11): 340. https://doi.org/10.3390/md15110340.

Santoyo, S., Plaza, M., Jaime, L. et al. (2011). Pressurized liquids as an alternative green process to extract antiviral agents from the edible seaweed *Himanthalia elongata*. *Journal of Applied Phycology* **23**: 909–917.

Sato, M., Hosokawa, T., Yamaguchi, T. et al. (2002). Angiotensin-I converting enzyme inhibitory peptides derived from wakame (*Undaria pinnatifida*) and their antihypertensive effect in spontaneously hypertensive rats. *Journal of Agricultural and Food Chemistry* **50**: 6245–6252.

Satomi, Y. (2017). Antitumor and cancer-preventative function of fucoxanthin: a marine carotenoid. *Anticancer Research* **37**: 1557–1562.

Sayo, T., Sugiyama, Y., and Inoue, S. (2013). Lutein, a nonprovitamin A, activates the retinoic acid receptor to induce HAS3-dependent hyaluronan synthesis in keratinocytes. *Bioscience, Biotechnology, and Biochemistry* **6**: 1282–1286.

Schieber, M. and Chandel, N.S. (2014). ROS function in redox signaling and oxidative stress. *Current Biology* **24** (10): 453–462.

Schroeder, G., Messyasz, B., and Łęska, B. (2016). Identification of biologically active compounds and commercial properties assessment of algal extracts as cosmetic ingredients. In: *Algal Extracts in Products for Human, Animal and Plants* (ed. K. Chojnacka), 1–14. New York: Nova Science Publishers, Inc.

Sellimi, S., Maalej, H., Rekik, D.M. et al. (2018). Antioxidant, antibacterial and in vivo wound healing properties of laminaran purified from *Cystoseira barbata* seaweed. *International Journal of Biological Macromolecules* **119**: 633–644.

Senevirathne, M., Ahn, C.-B., and Je, J.-Y. (2010). Enzymatic extracts from edible red algae, *Porphyra tenera*, and their antioxidant, anti-acetylcholinesterase, and anti-inflammatory activities. *Food Science and Biotechnology* **19** (6): 1551–1557.

Senni, K., Gueniche, F., Foucault-Bertaud, A. et al. (2006). Fucoidan a sulfated polysaccharide from brown algae is a potent modulator of connective tissue proteolysis. *Archives of Biochemistry and Biophysics* **445**: 56–64.

Shah, M.R., Liang, Y., Cheng, J.J., and Daroch, M. (2016). Astaxanthin-producing green microalga *Haematococcus pluvialis*: from single cell to high value commercial products. *Frontiers in Plant Science* **7**: 531. https://doi.org/10.3389/fpls.2016.00531.

Shan, X., Liu, X., Hao, J. et al. (2016). In vitro and in vivo hypoglycemic effects of brown algal fucoidans. *International Journal of Biological Macromolecules* **82**: 249–255.

Shen, C.T., Chen, P.Y., Wu, J.J. et al. (2011). Purification of algal anti-tyrosinase zeaxanthin from *Nannochloropsis oculata* using supercritical anti-solvent precipitation. *Journal of Supercritical Fluids* **55**: 955–962.

Shi, D., Guo, S., Jiang, B. et al. (2013). HPN, a synthetic analogue of bromophenol from red alga *Rhodomela confervoides*: synthesis and anti-diabetic effects in C57BL/KsJ-db/db mice. *Marine Drugs* **11**: 350–362.

Shibata, T., Fujimoto, K., Nagayama, K. et al. (2002). Inhibitory activity of brown algal phlorotannins against hyaluronidase. *International Journal of Food Science & Technology* **37**: 703–770.

Shibata, T., Ishimaru, K., Kawaguchi, S. et al. (2008). Antioxidant activities of phlorotannins isolated from Japanese Laminariaceae. *Journal of Applied Phycology* **20**: 705. https://doi.org/10.1007/s10811-007-9254-8.

Shiratori, K., Ohgami, K., Ilieva, I. et al. (2005). Effects of fucoxanthin on lipopolysaccharide-induced inflammation in vitro and in vivo. *Experimental Eye Research* **81**: 422–428.

Shoeib, N.A., Bibby, M.C., Blunden, G. et al. (2004). In-vitro cytotoxic activities of the major bromophenols of the red alga *Polysiphonia lanosa* and some novel synthetic isomers. *Journal of Natural Products* **67**: 1445–1449.

Singh, R.S., Thakur, S.R., and Bansal, P. (2015). Algal lectins as promising biomolecules for biomedical research. *Critical Reviews in Microbiology* **41** (1): 77–88.

Singh, V., Pathak, J., Richa, R. et al. (2017). Do cyanobacteria have enough mechanisms to counteract UV stress? In: *New Approaches in Biological Research* (eds. R.P. Sinha and Richa). New York: Nova Science Publishers.

Siriwardhana, N., Lee, K.W., and Jeon, Y.J. (2005). Radical scavenging potential of hydrophilic phlorotannins of *Hizikia fusiformis*. *Algae* **20** (1): 69–75.

Smit, A.J. (2004). Medicinal and pharmaceutical uses of seaweed natural products: a review. *Journal of Applied Phycology* **16**: 245–262.

Soldatou, S. (2017). Marine biodiscovery from Floridian mangrove forests and Irish waters. PhD Thesis. NUI Galway. http://hdl.handle.net/10379/6935 (accessed September 18, 2020).

Sonami, R.R., Rastogi, R.P., and Madamwar, D. (2018). The phycobiliproteins: the source, biosynthesis, spectral properties and possible applications in nutraceuticals and cosmetic industries. In: *Sunscreens: Source, Formulations, Efficacy and Recommendations* (ed. R.P. Rastogi), 79–98. New Delhi: Nova Science Publishers, Inc.

Song, Y.-S., Li, H., Balcos, M.C. et al. (2014). Fucoidan promotes the reconstruction of skin equivalents. *Korean Journal of Physiology and Pharmacology* **18**: 327–331.

Souza, E.T., Lira, D.P., Queiroz, A.C. et al. (2009). The antinociceptive and anti-inflammatory activities of caulerpine, a bisindole alkaloid isolated from seaweeds of the genus Caulerpa. *Marine Drugs* **7**: 689–704.

Spolaore, P., Joannis-Cassan, C., Duran, E., and Isambert, A. (2006). Commercial applications of microalgae. *Journal of Bioscience and Bioengineering* **101**: 87–96.

Stengel, D.B., Connan, S., and Popper, Z.A. (2011). Algal chemodiversity and bioactivity: sources of natural variability and implications for commercial application. *Biotechnology Advances* **29**: 483–501.

Suh, S.S., Oh, S.K., Lee, S.G. et al. (2017). Porphyra-334, a mycosporine-like amino acid, attenuates UV-induced apoptosis in HaCaT cells. *Acta Pharmaceutica* **67**: 257–264.

Sun, Y., Chen, X., Liu, S. et al. (2018). Preparation of low molecular weight *Sargassum fusiforme* polysaccharide and its anticoagulant activity. *Journal of Oceanology and Limnology* **36** (3): 882–891.

Tang, G. and Suter, P.M. (2011). Vitamin A, nutrition, and health values of algae: *Spirulina, Chlorella*, and *Dunaliella. Journal of Pharmacy and Nutrition Sciences* **1**: 111–118.

Terasaki, M., Maeda, H., Miyashita, K., and Mutoh, M. (2017). Induction of anoikis in human colorectal cancer cells by fucoxanthinol. *Nutrition and Cancer* **69** (7): 1043–1052. https://doi.org/10.1080/01635581.2017.1339814.

Terme, N., Boulho, R., Kucma, J.-P. et al. (2018). Radical scavenging activity of lipids from seaweeds isolated by solid-liquid extraction and supercritical fluids. *Oil Seeds and Facts, Crops and Lipids* **25** (5): D505.

Thomas, N. and Kim, S.-H. (2011). Potential pharmacological applications of polyphenolic derivatives from marine brown algae. *Environmental Toxicology and Pharmacology* **32**: 325–335.

Thomas, N.V. and Kim, S.K. (2013). Beneficial effects of marine algal compounds in cosmeceuticals. *Marine Drugs* **14**: 146–164. https://doi.org/10.3390/md11010146.

Tobacman, J.K. (2001). Review of harmful gastrointestinal effects of carrageenan in animal experiments. *Environmental Health Perspectives* **109**: 983–994.

Tominaga, K., Hongo, N., Karato, M., and Yamashita, E. (2012). Cosmetic benefits of astaxanthin on humans subjects. *Acta Biochimica Polonica* **59** (1): 43–47.

Torres, F.A.E., Passalacqua, T.G., Velásquez, A.M.A. et al. (2014). New drugs with antiprotozoal activity from marine algae: a review. *Revista Brasileira de Farmacognosia* **24** (3): 24265–24276.

Trinchero, J., Ponce, N.M., Cordoba, O.L. et al. (2009). Antiretroviral activity of fucoidans extracted from the brown seaweed *Adenocystis utricularis*. *Phytotherapy Research* **23**: 707–712.

Tsai, C.-J. and Pan, B.S. (2012). Identification of sulfoglycolipid bioactivities and characteristic fatty acids of marine macroalgae. *Journal of Agricultural and Food Chemistry* **60** (34): 8404–8410.

Tziveleka, L.-A., Abatis, D., Paulus, K. et al. (2005). Marine polyprenylated hydroquinones, quinones, and chromenols with inhibitory effects on leukotriene formation. *Chemistry & Biology* **2**: 901–909.

Ulmann, L., Blanckaert, V., Mimouni, V. et al. (2017). Microalgal fatty acids and their implication in health and disease. *Mini-Reviews in Medicinal Chemistry* **17**: 1112–1123.

Urikura, I., Sugawara, T., and Hirata, T. (2011). Protective effect of fucoxanthin against UVB-induced skin photoaging in hairless mice. *Bioscience, Biotechnology, and Biochemistry* **75**: 757–760.

Uthappa, U.T., Brahmkhatri, V., Sriram, G. et al. (2018). Nature engineered diatom biosilica as drug delivery systems. *Journal of Controlled Release* **281**: 70–83.

Vairappan, C.S. (2004). Antibacterial activity of major secondary metabolities: found in four species of edible green macroalgae genus *Caulerpa*. *Asian Journal of Microbiology, Biotechnology and Environmental Sciences* **6**: 197–201.

Vermeer, B.J. and Gilchrest, B.A. (1996). Cosmeceuticals. A proposal for rational definition, evaluation and regulation. *Archives of Dermatology* **132** (3): 337340.

Vijayabaskar, P. and Shiyamala, V. (2011). Antibacterial activities of brown marine algae (*Sargassum wrightii* and *Turbinaria ornata*) from the Gulf of Mannar. *Advances in Biological Research* **5**: 99–102.

Villa, F.A., Lieske, K., and Gerwick, L. (2010). Selective MyD88-dependent pathway inhibition by the cyanobacterial natural product malyngamide F acetate. *European Journal of Pharmacology* **629** (1–3): 140–146.

Vo, T.-S. and Kim, S.-K. (2013). Fucoidans as a natural bioactive ingredient for functional foods. *Journal of Functional Foods* **5** (1): 16–27.

Vo, T.-S., Kim, J.-A., Wijesekara, I. et al. (2011). Potent effect of brown algae (*Ishige okamurae*) on suppression of allergic inflammation in human basophilic KU812F cells. *Food Science and Biotechnology* **20** (5): 1227–1234.

Vo, T.-S., Ngo, D.-H., and Kim, S.-K. (2012). Marine algae as a potential pharmaceutical source for anti-allergic therapeutics. *Process Biochemistry* **47**: 386–394.

Wang, Y., Xu, Z., Bach, S., and MacAllister, T. (2009). Sensitivity of *Escherichia coli* to seaweed (*Ascophyllum nodosum*) phlorotannins and terrestrial tannins. *Asian-Australian Journal of Animal Science* **22**: 238–245.

Wang, J., Luo, T., Li, S., and Zhao, J. (2012a). The powerful applications of polyunsaturated fatty acids in improving the therapeutic efficacy of anticancer drugs. *Expert Opinion on Drug Delivery* **9**: 1–7.

Wang, T., Jónsdóttir, R., Liu, H. et al. (2012b). Antioxidant capacities of phlorotannins extracted from the brown algae *Fucus vesiculosus*. *Journal of Agricultural and Food Chemistry* **60** (23): 5874–5883.

Wang, J., Jin, W., Hou, Y. et al. (2013). Chemical composition and moisture-absorption/retention ability of polysaccharides extracted from five algae. *International Journal of Biological Macromolecules* **57**: 26–29.

Wang, S.K., Li, Y., White, W.L., and Lu, J. (2014). Extracts from New Zealand *Undaria pinnatifida* containing fucoxanthin as potential functional biomaterials against cancer in vitro. *Journal of Functional Biomaterials* **5**: 29–42.

Wang, X., Li, W., Xiao, L. et al. (2017). In vivo antihyperlipidemic and antioxidant activity of porphyran in hyperlipidemic mice. *Carbohydrate Polymers* **15** (174): 417–420.

Weelden, G.V., Bobinski, M., Okla, K. et al. (2019). Fucoidan structure and activity in relation to anti-cancer mechanisms. *Marine Drugs* **17** (1): 32. https://doi.org/10.3390/md17010032.

Widiastuti, E.L. and Khairani, I.A. (2018). Antioxidant effect of taurine and macroalgae (*Sargassum* sp. and *Gracilaria* sp.) extraction on numbers of blood cells and protein profile of mice induced by benzo(α)piren. *Journal of Physics: Conference Series* **1116**: 052073.

Wijesekara, I., Yoon, N.Y., Li, Y., and Kim, S.-K. (2010). Phlorotannins from *Ecklonia cava* (Phaeophyceae): biological activities and potential health benefits. *BioFactors* **36**: 408–414.

Wijesekara, I., Pangestuti, R., and Kim, S.-K. (2011). Biological activities and potential health benefits of sulfated polysaccharides derived from marine algae. *Carbohydrate Polymers* **84**: 14–21.

Wijesinghe, W.A.J.P. and Jeon, Y. (2012). Biological activities and potential industrial applications of fucose rich sulfated polysaccharides and fucoidans isolated from brown seaweeds: a review. *Carbohydrate Polymers* **88** (1): 13–20.

Wilcox, M.D., Brownlee, I.A., Richardson, J.C. et al. (2014). The modulation of pancreatic lipase activity by alginates. *Food Chemistry* **146**: 479–484.

Wong, C.H., Gan, S.Y., Tan, S.C. et al. (2018). Fucosterol inhibits the cholinesterase activities and reduces the release of pro-inflammatory mediators in lipopolysaccharide. *Journal of Applied Phycology* **30** (6): 3261–3270.

Wu, G.-J., Shiu, S.-M., Hsieh, M.-C., and Tsai, G.-J. (2016). Anti-inflammatory activity of a sulfated polysaccharide from the brown alga *Sargassum cristaefolium*. *Food Hydrocolloids* **53**: 16–23.

Xu, N., Fan, X., Yan, X. et al. (2003). Antibacterial bromophenols from the marine red alga *Rhodomela confervoides*. *Phytochemistry* **62**: 1221–1224.

Xu, X., Yin, L., Gao, L. et al. (2013). Two new bromophenols with radical scavenging activity from marine red alga *Symphyocladia latiuscula*. *Marine Drugs* **11** (3): 842–847. https://doi.org/10.3390/md11030842.

Xu, S.-Y., Huang, X., and Cheong, K.-L. (2017). Recent advances in marine algae polysaccharides: isolation, structure, and activities. *Marine Drugs* **15**: 388. https://doi.org/10.3390/md15120388.

Yan, X., Yang, C., Lin, G. et al. (2019). Antidiabetic potential of green seaweed *Enteromorpha prolifera* flavonoids regulating insulin signaling pathway and gut microbiota in type 2 diabetic mice. *Journal of Food Science* **84** (1): 165–173.

Yang, H. and Lee, Y. (2016). Seaweed derived oligosaccharides and its health beneficial effects on gut health. *The Journal of the Korea Contents Association* **16** (7): 465–475.

Yasuhara-Bell, J. and Lu, Y. (2010). Marine compounds and their antiviral activities. *Antiviral Research* **86**: 231–240.

Yoo, M.S., Shin, J.S., Choi, H.E. et al. (2012). Fucosterol isolated from *Undaria pinnatifida* inhibits lipopolysaccharide-induced production of nitric oxide and pro-inflammatory cytokines via the inactivation of nuclear factor-κB and p38 mitogen-activated protein kinase in RAW264.7 macrophages. *Food Chemistry* **135** (3): 967–975.

Yoon, N.Y., Chung, H.Y., Kim, H.R., and Choi, J.S. (2008). Acetyl- and butyrylcholinesterase inhibitory activities of sterols and phlorotannins from *Ecklonia stolonifera*. *Fisheries Science* **74**: 200–207.

Yoon, W.-J., Ham, Y.M., Kim, S.-S. et al. (2009). Suppression of pro-inflammatory cytokines, iNOS, and COX-2 expression by brown algae *Sargassum micracanthum* in RAW 264.7 macrophages. *EurAsian Journal of BioScience* **3**: 130–143.

Yotsu-Yamasita, M., Kondo, S., Segawa, S. et al. (2013). Isolation and structural determination of two novel phlorotannins from the brown alga *Ecklonia kurome* Okamura, and their radical scavenging activities. *Marine Drugs* **11**: 165–183.

Yousefi, M.K., Hashtroudi, M.S., Moradi, A.M., and Ghasempour, A.R. (2018). In vitro investigating of anticancer activity of fucoxanthin from marine brown seaweed species. *Global Journal of Environmental Science Management* **4** (1): 81–90.

Yu, P., Ning, L., Xiguang, L. et al. (2003a). Antihyperlipidemic effects of different molecular weight sulfated polysaccharides from *Ulva pertusa* (Chlorophyta). *Pharmacological Research* **48**: 543–549.

Yu, P., Quanbin, Z., Ning, L. et al. (2003b). Polysaccharides from *Ulva pertusa* (Chlorophyta) and preliminary studies on their antihyperlipidemia activity. *Journal of Applied Phycology* **15**: 21–27.

Yu, H., Zhang, H., Dong, M. et al. (2017). Metabolic reprogramming and AMPKα1 pathway activation by caulerpin in colorectal cancer cells. *International Journal of Oncology* **50** (1): 161–172.

Yuan, Y.V. (2008). Marine algal constituents. In: *Marine Nutraceuticals and Functional Foods* (eds. C. Barrow and F. Shahidi), 197–227. Boca Raton, FL: CRC Taylor & Francis Press Inc.

Yuan, Y.V. and Walsh, N.A. (2006). Antioxidant and antiproliferative activities of extracts from a variety of edible seaweeds. *Food and Chemical Toxicology* **44**: 1144–1150.

Yuan, Y.V., Bone, D.E., and Carrington, M.F. (2005). Antioxidant activity of dulse (*Palmaria palmata*) extract evaluated in vitro. *Food Chemistry* **91**: 485–494.

Yun, E.J., Lee, S., Kim, J.H. et al. (2013). Enzymatic production of 3,6-anhydro-L-galactose from agarose and its purification and in vitro skin whitening and anti-inflammatory activities. *Applied Microbiology and Biotechnology* **97**: 2961–2970.

Zappe, H., Snell, M.E., and Bossard, M.J. (2008). PEGylation of cyanovirin-N, an entry inhibitor of HIV. *Advanced Drug Delivery Reviews* **60** (1): 79–87.

Zhang, Z.S., Zhang, Q.B., Wang, J. et al. (2009). Preparation of the different derivatives of the low-molecular-weight porphyran from *Porphyra haitanensis* and their antioxidant activities in vitro. *International Journal of Biological Macromolecules* **45**: 22–26.

Zhang, H., Tang, Y., Zhang, Y. et al. (2015). Fucoxanthin: a promising medicinal and nutritional ingredient. *Evidence-based Complementary and Alternative Medicine*: 1–723515, 10.

Zhang, W., Okimura, T., Xu, L. et al. (2016). Ascophyllan functions as an adjuvant to promote anti-cancer effect by dendritic cell activation. *Oncotarget* **7**: 19284–19298.

Zhang, X., Kang, X., Jin, L. et al. (2018). Stimulation of wound healing using bioinspired hydrogels with basic fibroblast growth factor (bFGF). *International Journal of Nanomedicine* **13**: 3897–3906.

Zhou, G., Xin, H., Sheng, W. et al. (2005). In vivo growth-inhibition of S180 tumor by mixture of 5-Fu and low molecular lambda-carrageenan from *Chondrus ocellatus*. *Pharmacological Research* **51**: 153–157.

Zhou, J., You, W., Sun, G. et al. (2016). The marine-derived oligosaccharide sulfate MS80, a novel transforming growth factor b1 inhibitor, reverses epithelial mesenchymal transition induced by transforming growth factor-b1 and suppresses tumor metastasis. *Journal of Pharmacology and Experimental Therapeutics* **359**: 54–61.

20
Economic Status of Seaweed: Production, Consumption, Commercial Applications, Hazards, and Legislations

Anushree Priyadarshini[1], Akanksha Priyadarshini[2], and Gaurav Rajauria[3]
[1]*College of Business, Technological University Dublin, Dublin, Ireland*
[2]*UCD Michael Smurfit Graduate Business School, University College Dublin, Dublin, Ireland*
[3]*School of Agriculture and Food Science, University College Dublin, Dublin, Ireland*

20.1 Introduction

Seaweed or marine algae is a very versatile organism. It comes in various shades of red, brown, and green that can be collected from the wild or cultivated. It is widely used as food for human consumption because of to its rich composition of macronutrients and was considered the only source of food for coastal communities in the earliest times. Seaweed as food has a very prominent presence in Asian countries such as China, Japan, and the Republic of Korea, but the demand for seaweed as food is increasingly spreading across the globe, especially, in North America, South America, and Europe. China is currently the largest seaweed producer followed by the Republic of Korea and Japan (Ferdouse et al. 2018).

Apart from consumption as food, seaweeds, particularly the red and brown seaweeds, are also used to produce the hydrocolloids alginate, agar, and carrageenan that are commonly used as thickening and gelling agents. They are used in the cosmetics industries as ingredients and as fertilizers and animal feed additives (McHugh 2003).

Approximately 221 species of seaweeds are commercially exploited, of which 145 species are for food and about 101 species for phycocolloid production. These comprise approx. 32 chlorophytes, 125 rhodophytes, and 64 phaeophytes (Zemke-White and Ohno 1999). Seaweed species that are extensively cultivated,

Recent Advances in Micro- and Macroalgal Processing: Food and Health Perspectives, First Edition.
Edited by Gaurav Rajauria and Yvonne V. Yuan.

include the brown algae *Laminaria japonica* and *Undaria pinnatifida*, and the red algae *Porphyra* spp., *Porphyra tenera*, *Eucheuma* spp., *Kappaphycus alvarezii*, *Gracilaria* spp., and *Gracilaria verrucosa* (Nayar and Bott 2014; Wikfors and Ohno 2001).

The Food and Agriculture Organization of the United Nations (FAO)'s annual publications, such as *The State of World's Fisheries and Aquaculture*, are primarily the only source of statistics on seaweed. The purpose of this chapter is to review the recent published literature on commercial aspects of seaweed including its production statistics and usage details and present a comprehensive business overview of this unique resource.

20.2 World Seaweed Utilization

20.2.1 World Seaweed Production

Globally about 30 million t of seaweeds are utilized annually, either harvested as wild or cultivated in farms (Ferdouse et al. 2018). In 2005, of the total seaweed production of 14.7 million t, 13.5 million t was cultivated while the harvest from the wild was about 1.2 million t. Environmental concerns for natural resources and industrial pollution have led to the focus on cultivation more and FAO (2012), highlights that the bulk of seaweed produced worldwide is from aquaculture, identified as cultivated production. Seaweed biomass production, which was 6.4 million t in the year 2000, grew to 20.8 million t in 2012, and 30.4 million t in 2015, with seaweed farming being particularly profitable in Asian countries where it provides income, employment, and foreign trade, and is hence economically important (Ferdouse et al. 2018). The Asian countries leading production include Indonesia, China, and the Philippines. In 2014, the aggregated production by China and Indonesia was 23 million t. Indonesia produces the carrageenophytes *Kappaphycus* and *Eucheuma*, which accounted for 27% of total world seaweed production in 2012 (FAO 2016). China mainly produces kelp for food and red algae, including *Laminaria* (4.8 million t; 23% of total), *Gracilaria* (1.9 million t; 9% of total), *Undaria* (1.7 million t; 8% of total), and *Porphyra* (1.1 million t; 5% of total), while the Philippines produced 1.7 million t *Eucheuma* accounting for 8% of the total global seaweed production (White and Wilson 2015). Furthermore, Chile, China, and Norway are the leading producers of the wild species of seaweeds and Chilean kelp (Buschmann et al. 2017). The world seaweed output (wild and cultured), by species and by country, 2006– 015 is outlined in Tables 20.1 and 20.2, respectively.

20.2.2 Trends in Seaweed Production and Consumption

Seaweed production and utilization have grown rapidly over the past decade but, despite the massive growth of seaweed aquaculture, demand for seaweed-based products has surpassed supply (Nayar and Bott 2014). The seaweed industry involves a large and diverse array of applications and a wide variety of macroalgal products that have an estimated total annual value of US$6 billion, of which food products for human consumption contribute about US$5 billion. Seaweed derived extracts – hydrocolloids – account for the majority of the remaining billion dollars, and miscellaneous uses, such as fertilizers and animal feed additives, contribute to the remaining. While seaweed is harvested either from naturally growing (wild)

Table 20.1 World seaweed output (wild and cultured), by species, 2015.

Species	**2006**	**2007**	**2008**	**2009**	**2010**	**2011**	**2012**	**2013**	**2014**	**2015**
	World wild seaweed output, by species, weight in t, 2006–2015									
Aquatic plants nei	288 062	364 437	403 642	303 031	274 445	306 643	287 570	314 189	274 093	285 056
Brown seaweeds	198 239	163 726	184 611	186 505	185 127	179 994	171 587	185 946	186 704	175 642
Red seaweeds	78 177	59 645	55 956	74 530	63 471	43 948	42 876	70 487	120 402	119 986
Chilean kelp	161 834	136 766	202 262	222 628	190 746	241 633	268 722	313 341	219 998	115 311
Lessonia trabeculata	27 552	31 010	33 754	54 120	62 734	46 239	48 040	38 724	60 531	72 071
Japanese kelp	84 677	72 795	73 246	80 469	74 232	61 429	73 107	56 948	66 766	71 610
Gracilaria seaweeds	44 153	69 739	63 967	1169	45 089	42 224	24 340	46 053	32 352	45 344
North Atlantic rockweed	61 390	51 736	52 508	53 763	56 332	47 374	50 588	51 371	48 991	44 203
Leister	17 135	12 297	14 941	34 289	30 194	29 559	36 758	34 153	34 693	41 077
Giant kelps nei	12 377	10 960	20 814	18 340	15 370	22 387	28 285	33 914	29 169	31 959
Skottsberg's gigartina	33 331	41 879	41 896	29 159	19 725	14 616	26 336	40 756	27 068	27 327
Tangle	15 991	28 949	28 191	20 714	23 774	42 299	15 998	53 590	28 052	12 509
Green seaweeds	20 650	19 700	18 750	17 850	16 875	15 935	15 035	14 135	12 289	12 171
North European kelp	2 891	8 114	8 114	2 806	2 677	9 481	5 309	21 384	37 314	10 489
Bull kelp	2 292	4 274	4 872	5 872	6 048	6 468	2 649	8 304	8 509	9 441
Wakame	7 144	6 384	3 114	3 882	4 783	2 742	2 184	2 848	3 547	4 188
Mazzaella laminarioides	3 731	5 108	4 372	4 225	1 172	2 096	1 574	3 181	4 607	3 013
Gelidium seaweeds	1 618	1 337	1 290	1 395	1 148	1 241	1 267	1 367	2 892	2 707
Seaweeds nei	176	8 855	8 885	18	—	3 236	27 368	1 366	701	2 533
Chondracanthus chamissoi	1 590	980	1 031	2 001	914	998	1 400	2 475	2 715	2 199
Others	4 544	6 212	3 808	3 175	1 052	2 456	2 275	1 904	2 111	2 986
Total	**1 063 010**	**1 098 691**	**1 226 216**	**1 116 766**	**1 074 856**	**1 120 542**	**1 130 993**	**1 294 532**	**1 201 393**	**1 088 836**

Table 20.1 *(continued)*

Species	2006	2007	2008	2009	2010	2011	2012	2013	2014	2015
	World cultured seaweed production, by species, weight in t, 2006–2015									
Eucheuma seaweeds nei	1 159 422	1 582 286	2 016 230	2 870 448	3 481 401	4 615 764	5 852 837	8 430 343	9 033 651	**10 189 939**
Japanese kelp	4 497 518	4 613 060	4 765 213	4 930 705	5 146 883	5 257 201	5 682 078	5 941 658	7 699 383	**8 026 782**
Gracilaria seaweeds	1 054 024	1 272 509	1 386 547	1 526 393	1 691 028	2 171 031	2 762 556	3 460 203	3 751 396	**3 880 748**
Wakame	2 027 763	1 765 619	1 756 197	1 694 540	1 537 339	1 754 504	2 139 477	2 079 099	2 359 413	**2 296 468**
Elkhorn sea moss	1 452 632	1 495 118	1 674 739	1 772 669	1 888 392	1 956 576	1 962 952	1 726 016	1 710 631	**1 753 686**
Nori nei	822 100	904 170	814 660	1 074 750	1 072 350	1 027 450	1 123 290	1 139 000	1 141 710	**1 158 750**
Seaweeds nei	2 334 424	2 290 534	2 452 424	2 489 230	3 121 938	2 886 482	2 812 530	2 859 389	443 568	**769 781**
Laver (nori)	585 242	606 741	562 783	554 064	564 234	608 791	691 425	721 778	673 992	**686 784**
Spiny eucheuma	154 622	187 587	216 424	220 555	258 652	266 122	287 975	233 048	240 817	**273 600**
Fusiform sargassum	114 230	136 260	87 480	79 490	78 210	111 310	112 260	151 520	175 430	**189 050**
Spirulina nei	55 870	66 920	62 320	70 890	96 942	73 048	80 266	82 025	85 705	**89 441**
Brown seaweeds	21 943	21 209	18 961	21 272	22 747	27 701	16 962	15 819	19 149	**30 450**
Green laver	682	684	8003	5903	4531	6085	6002	5034	6055	**6748**
Fragile codium	165	158	1186	1796	1394	1005	855	2045	5550	**3895**
Aquatic plants nei	1776	1102	3597	4647	4144	2183	2741	4729	5023	**3823**
Caulerpa seaweeds	5444	5177	4288	3881	4309	5145	3928	3029	1199	**1219**
Bright green nori	10 160	10 550	12 540	10 600	11 150	9100	8900	4390	1000	**1000**
Warty gracilaria	5944	9382	6861	4383	4888	4865	3478	3210	936	**634**
Haematococcus pluvialis	1544	107	116	188	162	205	215	241	226	**200**
Spirulina platensis	50	50	70	70	70	100	100	121	100	**84**
Others nei	6221	3771	7563	1512	1520	523	4575	55	9	**77**
Total, including other countries	**14 311 776**	**14 972 993**	**15 858 203**	**17 337 986**	**18 992 284**	**20 785 191**	**23 555 401**	**26 862 752**	**27 354 942**	**29 363 158**

nei: "Not elsewhere identified."
Source: Ferdouse et al., 2018.

Table 20.2 World seaweed output (wild and cultured), by country, 2015.

Country	2006	2007	2008	2009	2010	2011	2012	2013	2014	2015
					World wild seaweed output, by country, weight in t, 2006–2015					
Chile	301 115	313 551	384 563	368 032	368 580	403 496	436 035	517 929	417 331	345 704
China	270 410	328 600	366 100	276 170	246 620	274 060	257 640	283 010	245 550	261 770
Norway	145 429	134 671	154 215	160 361	158 516	152 382	140 998	154 150	154 230	147 391
Japan	113 665	103 602	104 668	104 103	97 231	87 779	98 514	84 498	91 601	93 300
Indonesia	4 996	4 643	2 917	3 030	2 697	5 479	7 641	17 136	70 514	78 230
Ireland	29 500	29 500	29 500	29 500	29 500	29 500	29 500	29 500	29 500	29 500
France	19 160	39 757	29 757	18 907	22 597	47 307	41 229	69 126	58 512	19 110
India	32 500	31 000	29 500	28 000	26 500	25 000	23 500	22 000	18 890	18 650
Iceland	20 964	21 867	22 559	22 563	21 014	15 737	18 079	17 168	18 427	16 830
Peru	3 434	10 786	13 779	5 677	4 368	5 801	3 585	22 089	25 827	14 824
Canada	43 191	19 382	17 715	43 300	43 431	14 824	13 833	14 842	14 360	11 573
Mexico	4 532	5 093	4 900	5 152	1 128	5 072	5 725	10 122	8 484	11 331
Korea, Republic of	13 754	18 189	13 866	10 843	13 043	14 787	10 123	8 566	9 687	7 826
South Africa	9 776	11 507	10 788	10 748	11 821	10 901	16 234	12 583	13 211	7 131
Russian Federation	11 614	8 342	10 242	5 828	5 917	6 639	6 597	5 341	7 070	6 662
United States of America	6 362	2 272	6 951	8 207	9 027	9 614	9 382	11 388	8 373	6 469
Morocco	14 870	12 373	9 037	10 368	7 405	5 797	5 150	6 138	2 688	5 284
Spain	485	109	97	64	124	261	525	1 215	2 151	2 386
Australia	15 504	2 223	1 923	1 923	1 923	1 923	1 923	1 923	1 923	1 923
Portugal	765	495	198	351	498	461	801	839	782	1 574
Others	5 528	6 941	6 749	6 814	3 968	6 178	6 254	6 873	4 393	4 354
Total	**1 062 026**	**1 097 962**	**1 223 275**	**1 113 127**	**1 071 940**	**1 116 820**	**1 127 014**	**1 289 563**	**1 199 111**	**1 087 468**

Table 20.2 (*continued*)

Country	2006	2007	2008	2009	2010	2011	2012	2013	2014	2015
World cultured seaweed production, by country, weight in t, 2006–2015										
China	9 744 210	9 745 025	9 933 885	10 495 905	11 092 270	11 549 555	12 832 060	13 561 445	13 326 315	13 924 535
Indonesia	1 170 000	1 728 475	2 145 061	2 963 556	3 915 017	5 170 201	6 514 854	9 298 474	10 076 992	11 269 341
Philippines	1 468 905	1 505 070	1 666 556	1 739 995	1 801 272	1 840 833	1 751 071	1 558 378	1 549 576	1 566 361
Korea, Republic of	765 595	792 953	921 024	858 659	901 672	992 283	1022 326	1 131 305	1 087 048	1 197 129
Korea, Dem. People's Rep	444 300	444 300	444 300	444 300	444 300	444 300	444 300	444 300	48 900	48 900
Japan	490 062	513 964	456 337	456 426	432 796	349 737	440 754	418 365	373 908	399 300
Malaysia	60 000	90 269	111 298	138 857	207 892	239 450	331 490	269 431	245 332	260 760
Zanzibar	76 760	84 850	107 925	102 682	125 157	130 400	150 876	110 438	133 020	172 490
Madagascar	5 300	3 650	3 650	3 600	4 000	1 699	1 400	3 575	6 970	15 377
Solomon Islands	1 354	866	1 159	4 029	7 104	7 218	6 990	11 812	12 162	12 200
Chile	38 219	26 387	27 703	88 193	12 179	14 694	4126	12 512	12 836	11 952
Viet Nam	15 000	15 000	15 000	15 000	18 221	14 019	18 544	13 561	14 327	11 822
Tanzania, United Rep. of	3 200	4 000	5 000	5 520	6 885	6 601	6 510	6 689	6 705	6 750
Sri Lanka	—	—	—	—	—	1	23	25	9	4 760
Papua New Guinea	—	—	—	—	100	250	1 400	2 500	3 000	4 000
Kiribati	8 837	1 112	1 083	1 788	4 745	4 290	8 280	2 250	3 580	3 600
India	1 954	2 522	4 706	6 922	4 242	4 502	4 502	4 502	3 002	3 002
Myanmar	—	—	288	1 200	2 094	2 336	3 200	1 600	2 100	2 324
Russian Federation	818	300	260	739	614	821	1 584	642	2 386	2 036
South Africa	3 000	3 000	1 834	1 900	2 015	2 000	2 000	2 000	2 000	2 000
Others	142 612	11 250	11 134	8 716	9 709	10 001	9 111	8 947	4 674	44 189
Total	**14 311 776**	**14 972 993**	**15 858 203**	**17 337 986**	**18 992 284**	**20 785 191**	**23 555 401**	**26 862 752**	**27 354 942**	**293 631 583**

Source: FAO 2018.

seaweed or from cultivated (farmed) crops, seaweed production from the wild harvest is declining globally and now contributes to less than 5% of the global seaweed production (FAO 2010, 2012). Commercial harvesting spans the northern and southern hemispheres, in waters extending from cold, temperate, to tropical, but global concern has been increasing with regard to the impact climate change can have on the quality, availability, and distribution of seaweed (Buschmann et al. 2017; Straub et al. 2016).

Industrially, the trend in the usage of seaweed biomass has shifted from exploiting seaweeds as fertilizers and a source of potash, to hydrocolloid extraction (Synytsya et al. 2015). Researchers outline that seaweeds are being grown for more valuable purposes such as raw materials for speciality polysaccharides (e.g. agar, carrageenan, and alginates) rather than as mere commodity food and feeds (Neori 2016; Bixler and Porse 2011). Conversion of the biomass into functional ingredients (Fleurence 2016), cosmeceuticals (Balboa et al. 2015), nutraceuticals (Himaya and Kim 2015), pharmaceuticals (Vo et al. 2012; Anis et al. 2017), speciality agronomic applications (Craigie 2011), and bioenergy application (Korzen et al. 2015) are other current trends in seaweed consumption.

An important trend in terms of the sustainability of the seaweed industry within the context of the current boom in the production and processing has been the "increasing need to address new challenges imposed by trade and market demand" as outlined by the United Nations University policy brief 2016 (Cottier-Cook et al. 2016). The brief highlights the need for efficient resource management in coastal areas, safeguarding against pathogens and pests, and preventing displacement of wild stocks.

20.2.3 Economic Relevance of Seaweed

In 2016, about 1 million t (product weight) of seaweed, as dried or processed, with an approximate value of US$4 billion was exported to almost 100 markets globally. Asia, Europe, and North America were the main trading locations with the top 35 countries importing about 650 000 t (product weight) of seaweed of an estimated value of US$2 billion (Table 20.3). This accounted for nearly 80% of the worldwide seaweed trade and 70% of the global production of farmed seaweed that year, highlighting the exponential increase in the production of seaweed owing to its expanding usage and worldwide trade (Ferdouse et al. 2018). China, the European Union (EU), Japan, and the United States are the primary import markets. Table 20.4 lists the imports by weight and value.

Developing countries are the primary suppliers of dried seaweed that is further processed for the production of agar-agar, alginate, and carrageenan. While hydrocolloid products are very widely traded in many countries for their numerous applications, the trade for edible seaweed is almost exclusively concentrated in countries like China, Japan, Korea, and Taiwan. In the case of nonedible seaweed, while China, the United States, and EU continue to be the major markets, but the global trade for nonedible seaweed is declining as the producing countries are themselves using it for further processing into industrial usage products (Ferdouse et al. 2018).

Table 20.3 Seaweed imports into the top 35 countries, 2013–2016.

	Weight in t; value in US$ thousands					
	2014		**2015**		**2016**	
	Weight	**Value**	**Weight**	**Value**	**Weight**	**Value**
Edible seaweed	247 527	692 978	251 709	633 915	250 735	648 719
Nonedible seaweed	244 514	348 059	244 777	271 209	245 381	269 473
Carrageenan	115 467	913 486	111 852	891 776	110 555	759 844
Agar-agar	11 738	243 316	11 771	231 958	12 052	225 624
Total	**619 246**	**2 197 839**	**620 109**	**2 028 858**	**618 723**	**1 903 660**

Source: FAO 2018.

Table 20.4 Top four importers of dried seaweed and hydrocolloid products, 2014–2016.

	Weight in t; value in US$					
	2014		**2015**		**2016**	
	Weight	**Value**	**Weight**	**Value**	**Weight**	**Value**
China	257 959	377 389	234 424	250 727	252 683	255 775
European Union	154 924	725 090	167 170	688 326	178 467	613 162
Japan	51 880	296 750	48 705	272 589	49 718	312 749
United States	38 102	256 442	38 278	253 227	40 861	209 143
Total	**502 865**	**1 655 671**	**488 577**	**1 464 869**	**521 729**	**1 390 829**

Source: FAO 2018.

20.3 Commercial Usage of Seaweed and Seaweed Functional Components

Seaweeds are well recognized for their richness in polysaccharides, minerals, and vitamins (Arasaki and Arasaki 1983), but the seaweed biomass has diverse and multiple applications not just as a source of food, but for various industrial applications and for fertilizer. Used in a broad variety of formats like fresh, dried, powder or flakes, salted, canned, liquid extracts, or as prepared foods, seaweeds are consumed directly by humans or processed into products such as food additives and nutraceuticals, feeds, fertilizers, biofuels, cosmetics, and medicines (McHugh 2003; Bixler and Porse 2011; Anis et al. 2017).

20.3.1 Food Applications of Seaweed

Seaweeds have enormous potential as a supplement in functional food or for the extraction of compounds as these contain bioactive substances like polysaccharides, proteins, lipids, and polyphenols, with antibacterial, antiviral, and antifungal properties (Kumar et al. 2008). This gives seaweed great potential as a food source – one that is extensively utilized in many maritime countries, particularly in Asia, e.g. Japan, Korea, and China.

Red macroalgae (*Gracilaria* spp.) are popularly marketed as fresh food in Hawaii. Species like *Gracilaria coronopifolia*, *Gracilaria parvispora*, *Gracilaria salicornia*, and *Gracilaria tikvahiae*, though they have a short postharvest life, are commonly used (Paull and Chen 2008). Carrageenan from red seaweed and alginates from brown seaweed have various uses ranging from being used as thickening agents in confectionaries, bakery products, salad dressings, ice creams, puddings, chewing gum, jams, jellies, to being used in clarifying beers and wines, to processing of meats, sausages, and fish.

They also have a usage in the pharmaceutical industry as binders, stabilizers, emulsifiers, and for creating molds in dentistry. Oral medications such as cough medicine also use alginates.

20.3.2 Nonfood Applications of Seaweed

The use of seaweeds as fertilizers dates back to the nineteenth century. Owing to its high fiber content seaweed acts as a soil conditioner and aids in moisture retention, together with its mineral content and trace elements, this means that seaweed acts as a useful fertilizer. With the growing popularity of organic farming, the market for seaweed as a fertilizer has grown exponentially (McHugh 2003).

Seaweeds have commonly been used an additive to animal feed as they build resistance to disease by ensuring a complete balance of micronutrients. Seaweed is also known to improve fertility and birth rate of animals and yolk color in eggs (Chapman and Chapman 1980). Commonly called seaweed meal, feed additives are made from brown seaweeds that are collected, dried, and milled. Species such as *Gracilaria*, *Gelidiella*, *Hypnea*, and *Sargassum* containing minerals, amino acids, and carbohydrates are used as feed for fish and prawn culture as these maintain water quality in aquaculture (Kaladharan et al. 1998; Pati et al. 2016)

Seaweed is increasingly being used in cosmetic products, such as creams and lotions. Hydrocolloids extracted from seaweed, alginate or carrageenan, are added to cosmetic products as these can improve the skin's moisture retention properties. Seaweed baths as a treatment for arthritis, rheumatism, and other aches and pains are also gaining in popularity. Thalassotherapy, wherein pastes of seaweed are applied to the person's body and then warmed under infrared radiation in conjunction with seawater hydrotherapy, is said to provide relief and improvement for rheumatism and osteoporosis patients (McHugh 2003; Pati et al. 2016).

Seaweed is also finding potential usage in wastewater treatment as it can absorb heavy metal ions such as zinc and cadmium from polluted water. The effluent water from fish farms usually contains high levels of waste and much of this waste material can be used by seaweeds as a nutrient, so trials are underway to exploit seaweed for wastewater treatments.

20.4 Hazards Associated with Seaweed Applications

Hazards associated with seaweed applications are primarily because of heavy metal accumulation in seaweed depending on the growing time in the sea and the levels of heavy metals in the water. Also, depending upon the species, collection time, growth phase, and collection site, the type of metals accumulated in seaweed vary (Murphy et al. 2007; Smith et al. 2010). The heavy metals reported to be accumulated by seaweeds include arsenic, copper, cadmium, chromium, nickel, vanadium, mercury, lead, cesium-137, and radium-226 (Riosmena-Rodríguez et al. 2010; Akköz et al. 2011). Owing to the spatially and temporally variable concentration of ammonium in the seawater and driven by the size of the plant, seaweed also accumulates ammonium (Rees 2003).

Pesticides and dioxins of industrial origin are some of the other contaminants found in seaweeds. For example, seaweeds are contaminated by polychlorinated dibenzo-p-dioxins (PCDDs) and polychlorinated dibenzofurans (PCDFs) (Hashimoto and Morita 1995). Pesticides such as azametiphos, diflubenzuron, teflubenzuron, propoxur (Lorenzo et al. 2012), and organic micropollutants (polychlorinated biphenyls [PCBs], chlorinated pesticides, and polycyclic aromatic hydrocarbons [PAHs]) are commonly found contaminants (Pavoni et al. 2003; Van der Spiegel et al. 2013).

20.5 Legislation

The General Food Law (Regulation [EC] 178/2002,1 GFL) provides the framework for EU legislation on food and feed and applies to all stages of food and feed production. However, for novel food and novel food ingredients that were not consumed in the EU prior to May 15, 1997 to be introduced into the market they must be authorized according to Regulation (EC) 258/97, the Novel Food Regulation (NFR). The four categories of novel food and food ingredients to which the NFR applies are identified in art. 1 (2) c–f (a and b pertaining to genetically modified organisms were later included in separate regulations) (see *italics below*):

(a) *Foods and food ingredients with a new or intentionally modified primary molecular structure.*
(b) *Foods and food ingredients consisting of or isolated from microorganisms, fungi, or algae.*
(c) *Foods and food ingredients consisting of or isolated from plants and food ingredients isolated from animals, except for foods and food ingredients obtained by traditional propagating or breeding practices and having a history of safe food use.*
(d) *Foods and food ingredients to which has been applied a production process not currently used, where the process gives rise to significant changes in the composition or structure of the foods or food ingredients which affect their nutritional value, metabolism, or level of undesirable substances.*

Seaweed as a novel food comes under the NFR depending upon if the variety is considered novel. The Novel Food Catalogue is used to verify the same. For instance, the brown seaweed *Fucus vesiculosus* is not regarded as a novel food according to the catalogue, while the red seaweed *Rhodymenia palmata* L. (*Palmaria palmata*) is, as this seaweed has only been used before in food supplements.

For use in feed, authorization is not required. Seaweeds are mentioned in Annex I of Regulation (EC) 396/2005. When seaweeds are used for human consumption, a maximum residue limit applies but not if they are used as feed for animals. Seaweed used as feed must comply with the maximum levels included in Directive 2002/32/EC. For seaweed meal and feed materials maximum levels for arsenic are set out in Directive 2002/32/EC (Van der Spiegel et al. 2013).

20.6 Conclusion

Commercial exploitation of seaweeds is primarily focused on farming edible species or production of hydrocolloids. Currently, seaweeds are used as food for direct consumption, as food ingredients, in cosmetics, fertilizers, and in the production of gelling agents, such as agar and alginate. Further opportunities for commercial exploitation of seaweed may include processing for bioactives, of which some 15 000 have been chemically isolated to date (Cardozo et al. 2007; Holdt and Kraan 2011), processing of meats, sausages, and fish, nutraceuticals, pharmaceuticals and dentistry, clarifying alcohol, the health and beauty industries, animal stock feeds, soil conditioners, fertilizers, biofuels, water filtration, and livestock and fishery diets (Winberg et al. 2009). Global seaweed production is experiencing steady growth in recent years, as have the by-products and co-products derived from them.

References

Akköz, C., Arslan, D., Ünver, A. et al. (2011). Chemical composition, total phenolic and mineral contents of enteromorpha intestinalis (l.) kütz. And cladophora glomerata (l.) kütz. Seaweeds. *Journal of Food Biochemistry* **35** (2): 513–523.

Anis, M., Ahmed, S., and Hasan, M.M. (2017). Algae as nutrition, medicine and cosmetic: the forgotten history, present status and future trends. *World Journal of Pharmacy and Pharmaceutical Sciences* **6** (6): 1934–1959.

Arasaki, S. and Arasaki, T. (1983). *Vegetables from the Sea*. Tokyo: Japan Pub. Inc.

Balboa, E.M., Conde, E., Soto, M.L. et al. (2015). Cosmetics from marine sources. In: *Springer Handbook of Marine Biotechnology* (ed. S.-K. Kim), 1015–1042. Berlin, Heidelberg: Springer.

Bixler, H.J. and Porse, H. (2011). A decade of change in the seaweed hydrocolloids industry. *Journal of Applied Phycology* **23** (3): 321–335.

Buschmann, A.H., Camus, C., Infante, J. et al. (2017). Seaweed production: overview of the global state of exploitation, farming and emerging research activity. *European Journal of Phycology* **52** (4): 391–406.

Cardozo, K.H., Guaratini, T., Barros, M.P. et al. (2007). Metabolites from algae with economical impact. *Comparative Biochemistry and Physiology Part C: Toxicology & Pharmacology* **146** (1-2): 60–78.

Chapman, V.J. and Chapman, D.J. (1980). *Seaweed and their Uses*, 3e, 63–65. New York: Chapman and Hall.

Cottier-Cook, E.J., Nagabhatla, N., Badis, Y. et al. (2016). Safeguarding the future of the global seaweed aquaculture industry. United Nations University and Scottish Association for Marine Science Policy Brief. https://inweh.unu.edu/wp-content/uploads/2016/09/unu-seaweed-aquaculture-policy.pdf (accessed September 22, 2020).

Craigie, J.S. (2011). Seaweed extract stimuli in plant science and agriculture. *Journal of Applied Phycology* **23** (3): 371–393.

FAO (2010). *The State of World Fisheries and Aquaculture*. Rome: Food and Agriculture Organization of the United Nations.

FAO (2012). *The State of World Fisheries and Aquaculture. Opportunities and Challenges.* Rome: Food and Agriculture Organization of the United Nations.

FAO (2016). *The State of Fisheries and Aquaculture 2016. Contributing to Food Security and Nutrition for all.* Rome: Food and Agriculture Organization of the United Nations.

Ferdouse, F., Holdt, S., Smith, R. et al. (2018). *The Global Status of Seaweed Production, Trade and Utilization.* Rome: Food and Agriculture Organization of the United Nations.

Fleurence, J. (2016). Seaweeds as food. In: *Seaweed in Health and Disease Prevention* (eds. J. Fleurence and I. Levine), 149–167. London: Academic Press.

Hashimoto, S. and Morita, M. (1995). Analysis of PCDDs, PCDFs, planar and other PCBs in seaweed from Japanese coast. *Chemosphere* **31** (8): 3887–3897.

Himaya, S.W.A. and Kim, S.K. (2015). Marine nutraceuticals. In: *Springer Handbook of Marine Biotechnology* (ed. S.-K. Kim), 995–1014. Berlin, Heidelberg: Springer.

Holdt, S.L. and Kraan, S. (2011). Bioactive compounds in seaweed: functional food applications and legislation. *Journal of Applied Phycology* **23** (3): 543–597.

Kaladharan, P., Kaliaperumal, N., and Ramalingam, J.R. (1998). Marine fishery information series. *Marine Fishery Information Series* **157**: 1–10.

Korzen, L., Pulidindi, I.N., Israel, A. et al. (2015). Single step production of bioethanol from the seaweed *Ulva rigida* using sonication. *RSC Advances* **5** (21): 16223–16229.

Kumar, C.S., Ganesan, P., Suresh, P.V., and Bhaskar, N. (2008). Seaweeds as a source of nutritionally beneficial compounds – a review. *Journal of Food Science and Technology* **45** (1): 1.

Lorenzo, R.A., Pais, S., Racamonde, I. et al. (2012). Pesticides in seaweed: optimization of pressurized liquid extraction and in-cell clean-up and analysis by liquid chromatography–mass spectrometry. *Analytical and Bioanalytical Chemistry* **404** (1): 173–181.

McHugh, D.J. (2003). *A Guide to the Seaweed Industry FAO Fisheries Technical Paper 441.* Rome, Rome: Food and Agriculture Organization of the United Nations.

Murphy, V., Hughes, H., and McLoughlin, P. (2007). Cu (II) binding by dried biomass of red, green and brown macroalgae. *Water Research* **41** (4): 731–740.

Nayar, S. and Bott, K. (2014). Current status of global cultivated seaweed production and markets. *World Aquaculture* **45** (2): 32–37.

Neori, A. (2016). Can sustainable mariculture match agriculture's output. *Global Aquaculture Advocate.* https://www.aquaculturealliance.org/advocate/can-sustainable-mariculture-match-agricultures-output/ (accessed September 22, 2020).

Pati, M.P., Sharma, S.D., Nayak, L., and PANDA, C.R. (2016). Uses of seaweed and its application to human welfare: a review. *International Journal of Pharmacy and Pharmaceutical Sciences* **8** (10): 12–20.

Paull, R.E. and Chen, N.J. (2008). Postharvest handling and storage of the edible red seaweed Gracilaria. *Postharvest Biology and Technology* **48** (2): 302–308.

Pavoni, B., Caliceti, M., Sperni, L., and Sfriso, A. (2003). Organic micropollutants (PAHs, PCBs, pesticides) in seaweeds of the lagoon of Venice. *Oceanologica Acta* **26** (5–6): 585–596.

Rees, T.A.V. (2003). Safety factors and nutrient uptake by seaweeds. *Marine Ecology Progress Series* **263**: 29–42.

Riosmena-Rodríguez, R., Talavera-Sáenz, A., Acosta-Vargas, B., and Gardner, S.C. (2010). Heavy metals dynamics in seaweeds and seagrasses in Bahía Magdalena, BCS, México. *Journal of Applied Phycology* **22** (3): 283–291.

Smith, J.L., Summers, G., and Wong, R. (2010). Nutrient and heavy metal content of edible seaweeds in New Zealand. *New Zealand Journal of Crop and Horticultural Science* **38** (1): 19–28.

Straub, S.C., Thomsen, M.S., and Wernberg, T. (2016). The dynamic biogeography of the Anthropocene: the speed of recent range shifts in seaweeds. In: *Seaweed Phylogeography* (eds. Z.-M. Hu and C. Fraser), 63–93. Dordrecht: Springer.

Synytsya, A., Čopíková, J., Kim, W.J., and Park, Y.I. (2015). Cell wall polysaccharides of marine algae. In: *Springer Handbook of Marine Biotechnology* (ed. S.-K. Kim), 543–590. Berlin, Heidelberg: Springer.

Van der Spiegel, M., Noordam, M.Y., and Van der Fels-Klerx, H.J. (2013). Safety of novel protein sources (insects, microalgae, seaweed, duckweed, and rapeseed) and legislative aspects for their application in food and feed production. *Comprehensive Reviews in Food Science and Food Safety* **12** (6): 662–678.

Vo, T.S., Ngo, D.H., and Kim, S.K. (2012). Marine algae as a potential pharmaceutical source for anti-allergic therapeutics. *Process Biochemistry* **47** (3): 386–394.

White, W.L. and Wilson, P. (2015). World seaweed utilization. In: *Seaweed Sustainability: Food and Non-Food Applications* (ed. B.K. Tiwari), 7–25. London: Academic Press.

Wikfors, G.H. and Ohno, M. (2001). Impact of algal research in aquaculture. *Journal of Phycology* **37** (6): 968–974.

Winberg, P.C., Ghosh, D., and Tapsell, L. (2009). Seaweed culture in integrated multi-trophic aquaculture-nutritional benefits and systems for Australia. RIRDC Publication 09/005. Canberra: Australian Government. https://ro.uow.edu.au/cgi/viewcontent.cgi?referer=http://scholar.google.co.uk/&httpsredir=1&article=1004&context=smfc (accessed September 22, 2020).

Zemke-White, W.L. and Ohno, M. (1999). World seaweed utilisation: an end-of-century summary. *Journal of Applied Phycology* **11** (4): 369–376.

Index

Recent Advances in Micro- and Macroalgal Processing: Food and Health Perspectives, First Edition.
Edited by Gaurav Rajauria and Yvonne V. Yuan.